Essentials of Pediatric Nursing

Essentials of Pediatric Nursing

(As per Revised INC Syllabus)

A Sudhakar
MSc (N), MBA (Hospital Mgmt), PGDC (NICU and ICU)
Associate Professor and HOD
Pediatric Nursing Department
Heritage Institute of Medical Science
Heritage College of Nursing
Varanasi, Uttar Pradesh, India

Foreword
Prof Dr M Kandasamy

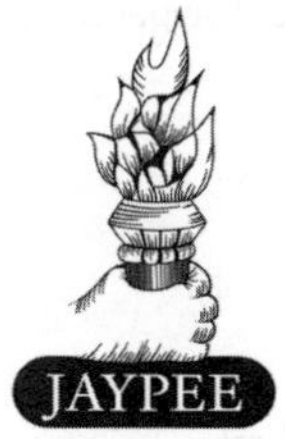

JAYPEE BROTHERS MEDICAL PUBLISHERS
The Health Sciences Publisher
New Delhi | London

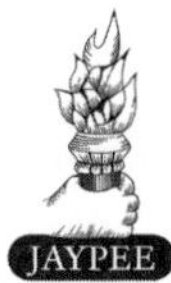

Jaypee Brothers Medical Publishers (P) Ltd

Headquarters
EMCA House, 23/23-B
Ansari Road, Daryaganj
New Delhi 110 002, India
Landline: +91-11-23272143, +91-11-23272703
+91-11-23282021, +91-11-23245672
e-mail: jaypee@jaypeebrothers.com

Corporate Office
4838/24, Ansari Road, Daryaganj
New Delhi 110 002, India
Phone: +91-11-43574357
Fax: +91-11-43574314
e-mail: jaypee@jaypeebrothers.com

Overseas Office
JP Medical Ltd.
83, Victoria Street, London
SW1H 0HW (UK)
Phone: +44-20 3170 8910
e-mail: info@jpmedpub.com

EU GPSR Authorised Representative
Logos Europe, 9 rue Nicolas Poussin
17000, La Rochelle, France
Phone: +33 (0) 6 67 93 73 78
e-mail: contact@logoseurope.eu

Website: www.jaypeebrothers.com
Website: www.jaypeedigital.com

Inquiries for bulk sales may be solicited at: jaypee@jaypeebrothers.com

Essentials of Pediatric Nursing

First Edition: 2017

Reprint: 2024, 2025, **2026**

ISBN: 978-93-85999-21-5

Printed in India at Sterling Graphics Pvt. Ltd.

Florence Nightingale

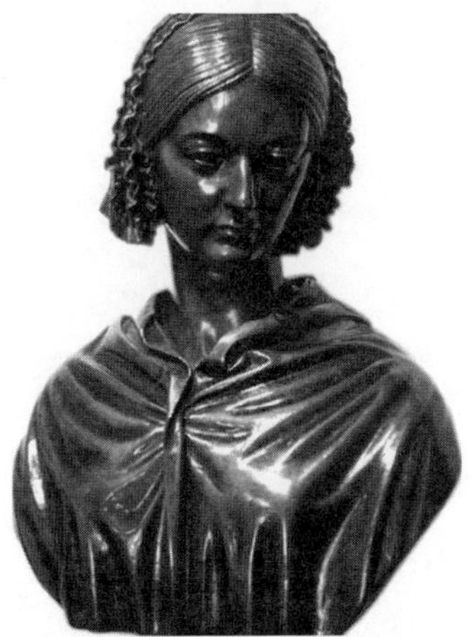

May 12, 1820–August 13, 1910

'Pioneer of Modern Nursing'

The 'Nightingale Pledge'

I solemnly pledge in the presence of this assembly
To render nursing services with due respect
For the dignity and rights of the people I serve
I will, at all times, respect the values and beliefs
Of the people entrusted to my care
And will make no distinction of caste, creed or race
In the Performance of my duties
I will strive in the practice of my profession
To promote health, prevent illness, alleviate sufferings,
And restore health of the people I serve
I will hold in trust personal information
Of a confidential nature
And use my best judgement in sharing this
With responsible persons
I will strive to maintain co-operative relationship
With fellow-workers in nursing and other fields
I will try to maintain standard of personal conduct
That will reflect credit upon my profession.
I will strive to observe the code of nursing Ethics
As laid down by my profession.

Ref: Nightingale Pledge and code for nurses 1973

Dedicated to

My parents and dear wife

Ms Syama Sudhakar

Foreword

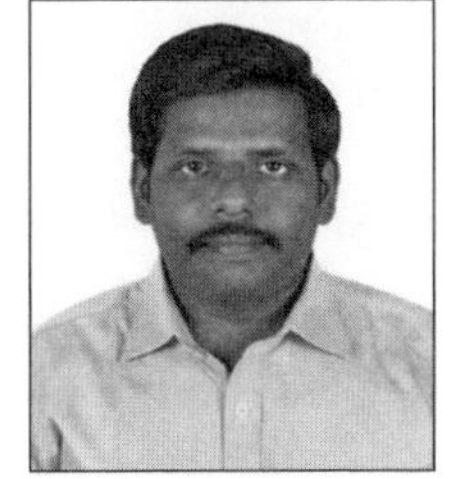

Child health nursing is an unique and complex discipline, which demands highly specialized knowledge and skill from the nurses. But, the sources of literature related to care of children in Indian context are limited in comparison with abroad. The pediatric nurses should be prepared to deliver quality care incorporating the local culture that depends on the material which suits the local conditions.

Essentials of Pediatric Nursing authored by Prof A Sudhakar, Associate Professor, is focused on care of newborn, healthy and sick child with emphasising on detailed nursing assessment, latest version of *NANDA (North American Nursing Diagnosis Association) diagnosis and interventions*. Further, the book has incorporated recent trends in care of children's health and illness with appropriate illustrations.

Being written in simple language it will be widely used by diploma, graduate and postgraduate nursing students. The author is to be congratulated on his success in bringing out this textbook.

Prof Dr M Kandasamy
Vice Principal
College of Nursing
Andaman Nicobar Islands Institute of
Medical Sciences (ANIIMS)
Port Blair, Andaman Nicobar, India

Preface

Pediatric nursing is very essential profession in care of the child health. In the medical field, the pediatric nurses have more responsibility to take care of the child and parents. It must be expected that all child health nurses have competence and independent practices, good judgement, skill-based subspecialized up-to-date knowledge and positive attitude towards care of the child health.

A pediatric nursing student should be talented to understand the problems of the children and ready to help them whenever health care is needed. The entire pediatric nursing students must have special preparation and training to contribute the effective health care towards children.

Being in a nursing profession for the last 15 years, I feel that a pediatric nursing textbook is required for everyone as per revised INC (Indian Nursing Council) syllabus. The main concept of this textbook is to make the students comfortable in their studies. I decided to take this project from my hardworking schedule to help pediatric nursing students.

This textbook covers complete **BSc Nursing** and **GNM Nursing** revised INC syllabus. The **Post Basic BSc and MSc nursing students** also can refer this textbook. I hope this textbook will help the pediatric nurses student to review their knowledge and practice in different aspects of child health care.

In this textbook, most of the reference journals are written by eminent Indian and International authors, foreign books, WHO news, IAP and NNF Bulletins.

I have invested my best effort to prepare and enrich this textbook considering the level of the students and placement of the course according to INC syllabus. In this book, unintentional mistakes are regretted and will be rectified.

Constructive criticism and comments are always heartily welcome for further enrichment of this book and will be gladly accepted. I hope my hard work will be useful to all the pediatric nursing students and clinical nurses.

A Sudhakar

Acknowledgments

This is my duty to pay sincere gratitude to Almighty Lord for His love and kind grace in the completion of this textbook. Hereby, I credit my lovable thanks to my parents, **Mr P Anumanthan** and **Ms Dhanalakshmi** who made me to achieve all success in my life.

I honor to convey my special thanks and gratitude to our respected Vice Chairman of Heritage foundation **Dr Siddarth Rai** for his great support and blessing to publish my project a grand success.

This is my great job to say thanks to respected **Prof Tamil Selvi**, Principal, Heritage School and College of Nursing, Varanasi, UP, India, who has supported me to publish this project successfully.

It is my duty to convey my special thanks to my respected teacher, **Prof Dr M Kandasamy** PhD, Vice Principal, College of Nursing, Andaman Nicobar Island Institute of Medical Sciences, Port Blair, India, an inspiring personality and who has given me positive thoughts to complete this project without delay.

This is my great job to say thanks to my respected principal, **Prof Dr A Jayasudha**, former Principal of Sri Gokulam College of Nursing, Salem, Tamil Nadu, India, and Associate Professor of Female College of Applied Medical Sciences, King Khalid University, Bisha, Kingdom of Saudi Arabia who makes me to do grand success of this project.

I would like to show my gratitude to my dear brother and senior **Prof Dr J Sathis Kumar,** PhD, independent Researcher cum Professor in Pediatric Nursing Department, Sridevi College of Nursing, Ponnari, Tamil Nadu, India, who has positively motivated me to complete this project in grand success.

I would like to take the opportunity to thank honorable **Prof Dr I Clement** and **Prof Ms Nisha Clement** who have helped and inspired me to make this project.

I wish to express my special thanks to my dear friend Vice Principal, **Prof Ravi Kumar BR,** MSc (N), PhD (Scholar), Vivekananda College of Nursing, Lucknow, UP, India, for his truthful prayer and efforts to complete this project success. I extend my warm gratitude to my beloved Gokulam College of Nursing Family Members, who have supported me directly and indirectly to complete this project without trouble.

I wish to express my special thanks to my dear close friends **Mr Nagaraj,** MSc (N), **Mr Prabu,** MSc (N), **Ms Rathika,** MSc (N), **Ms Anitha,** MSc (N) and **Ms T Chandra,** MSc (N), Associate Professor and Vice Principal in various reputed institutes in Tamil Nadu, for their truthful support to make this project success.

It is my special thanks to my dear younger brother and juniors **Mr Dhanasekar** and **Mr Boobalan**, staff nurse in AIIMS, New Delhi and Staff Nurse in Tamil Nadu Government, for their wishes and special contribution to success of this project.

My sincere thanks are due to all my seniors, colleagues, friends and my beloved students who encouraged me to write and publish this textbook.

I convey my special thanks to my dear Father and Mother-in-law, **Mr Sankaran and Ms Umadevi** for their special prayer to complete my project a grand success.

I convey my lovable thanks to my dear wife, **Ms Syama Sudhakar**, my sister-in-law **Ms Hema Anil NS** and my brother-in-law **Mr Anil** and their kids Aishwarya and Kashinathan, who always encouraged to complete this textbook.

I convey my heartiest thank to my dear sweet daughters, **SS Jayani Sree** and **SS Navanya Sree** for showing enough patience and sacrifices at the time of my project work and also for the contribution of their photographs in this project.

I express my deep sense of gratitude and thanks to the backbone of my family lovable Grandmother, **Ms Parvathi (Kanniyammal),** my dear brother and sister-in-law, **Mr A Gajendra Prasad** and **G Sathya** and their kids, **Ms Pooja** and **Master Bhavan** for rendering emotional support during the hardworking period for preparation of this project.

I would like to convey my gratitude and special thanks to **Mr Venugopal V,** (Associate Director) Jaypee Brothers Medical Publishers (P) Ltd., Bengaluru, who has helped me to publish my project.

Also, I convey my sincere thanks to Jaypee Brothers Medical Publishers (P) Ltd, New Delhi, India for their efforts and suggestions, especially Shri Jitendar P Vij (Group Chairman), Mr Ankit Vij (Group President), Ms Chetna Malhotra Vohra (Associate Director–Content Strategy) and Ms Ruby Sharma (Project Manager) for helping me through my idea.

भारतीय नर्सिंग परिषद्
संयुक्त परिषद् भवन, कोटला रोड,
टेम्पल लेन, नई दिल्ली - 110002

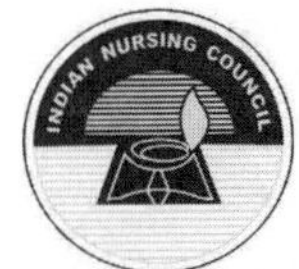

INDIAN NURSING COUNCIL
COMBINED COUNCIL BUILDING, KOTLA ROAD,
TEMPLE LANE, NEW DELHI – 110002

नर्सिंग शिक्षा के समान स्तर को प्राप्त करने का प्रयास
Striving to achieve uniform standards of Nursing Education

F. No. 1-16/2015-INC Dated: 12 JUN 2015

To

All Secretary (Health)

All DME

All DHS

Subject: - Revision of General Nursing and Midwifery (GNM) syllabus 2015 implementation – regarding.

Sir/Madam,

Indian Nursing Council (INC) revised the syllabus in the year 2001. There are a lot of changes that have taken place in the health policy and different national Health & Family Welfare programmes. The duration of B.Sc. (N) programme is 4 years whereas the duration of diploma in General Nursing and Midwifery (GNM) is 3½ years. Many requests from different nursing associations and students that there should be a distinct difference between the diploma and degree programme in the format of duration. The six months internship prescribed for GNMs was also not properly implemented by the nursing educational institutions. A committee was constituted by the Indian Nursing Council to review the syllabus of the GNM. The stakeholders were consulted by the said committee accordingly the General Body of INC has approved the revision of the syllabus by keeping in mind health trends, existing health care delivery system, needs of the students and career prospects. **Accordingly the duration of the diploma of GNM has been reduced from 3½ years to 3 years. The internship is integrated into the revised syllabus. This will be effective from the academic year 2015-16.**

The revision of the syllabus made by INC as per the section 16 (g)(h)(i) and the resolution passed by the General Body with regard to revision of the syllabus was included in the Annual Report 2013-14 and the same was laid in the Parliament.

The orientation programme was organized at national level for the registrars of State Nursing Council and examination boards who are responsible for implementation of syllabus.

Website : www.indiannursingcouncil.org **E-mail** secy2010@indiannursingcouncil.org
Phone : 011-23235619, 23235570, 23233762, 23233763, 23233764 **Fax:** 011-23236140

भारतीय नर्सिंग परिषद्
संयुक्त परिषद् भवन, कोटला रोड,
टेम्पल लेन, नई दिल्ली - 110002

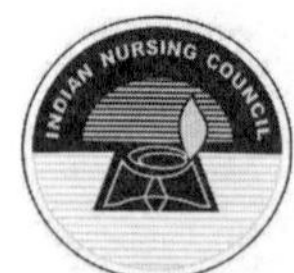

INDIAN NURSING COUNCIL
COMBINED COUNCIL BUILDING, KOTLA ROAD,
TEMPLE LANE, NEW DELHI – 110002

नर्सिंग शिक्षा के समान स्तर को प्राप्त करने का प्रयास
Striving to achieve uniform standards of Nursing Education

All State Nursing Councils have been instructed that they should organize orientation workshop for the teachers of the diploma of the GNM programme to make them get to know the revised syllabus 2015. The INC has sent the resource material to the Registrars of the state Councils and examination boards in the fom1 of powerpoint presentation to organize the orientation workshop for the teachers of the Schools of Nursing of their State. The expenditure to organize the orientation programme will be met by the INC. The revised syllabus and regulation of the GNM programme has been posted in the INC website.

In order to have a uniformity of the nursing education in the country and also to allow hassle free migration of candidates from one state to another state, that is taking place rapidly it is mandatory that all the states should implement the revised syllabus with effect from 2015-16 academic year. Otherwise candidates may face difficulty in getting reciprocal registration from the State Nursing Council due to change in duration. It is requested that necessary action may be taken to implement the revised syllabus.

An early reply in this regard will be appreciated.

Yours faithfully,

(Surekha Sama)
SECRETARY

Copy for the information to: -

1. All State Nursing Councils
2. All Examination Boards

Website : www.indiannursingcouncil.org **E-mail** secy2010@indiannursingcouncil.org
Phone : 011-23235619, 23235570, 23233762, 23233763, 23233764 **Fax:** 011-23236140

Revised INC Syllabus

Child Health Nursing

Placement: GNM Second Year

Course Description

This course is designed to help the students to develop and understand the concept of child health, the trends in child care and the health problems of children. This shall enable the students to meet the needs of the children, in health and sickness.

General Objective

Upon completion of this course, the students shall able to:

1. Explain the concept of child health, the principles underlying child care trends in pediatric nursing.
2. Describe normal growth and development of children, so as to recognize the deviations for normal health and care of healthy children
3. Demonstration skill in meeting the needs of the sick infants and children based on the IMNCI (Integrated Management of Neonatal and Childhood Illness) guidelines of Government of India (GoI).

Total hours: 70

Unit	Learning objective	Content	Hours	Teaching learning activities	Assess-ment methods	Chapter
I	Understand the concept of the child health care, trends and emerging challenges for pediatric nurses Describe the role of pedi-atric nurses in clinics, hospitals and com-munity	**Introduction** a. Modern concept in child health care b. Trends in pediatric nursing c. Role of pediatric nurses in child care d. Emerging challenges, nursing process related to pediatric nursing e. Concept of preventive pediatric f. Vital statistics related to pediatrics as per the NRHS (National Rural Health Mission) and GoI	5	• Lecture • Discussion • Project on collection of vital statistics related to child health	• Short answers • Essay type • Objective type	1

Unit	Learning objective	Content	Hours	Teaching learning activities	Assessment methods	Chapter
II	Describe normal growth and development of children	**Growth and Development** a. Definition, principles, factors affecting growth and development, techniques of assessment, plotting of growth chart **b. Infant:** Growth and development, health promotion, breastfeeding and weaning, immunization, infant and young child feeding **c. Toddler:** Growth and development, nutrition counseling, toilet training, safety, prevention of accidents, play **d. Preschoolers:** Growth and development, daycare centers, role of parents in sex education **e. School agers:** Growth and development, rest, sleep, physical exercises and activity, dental health, sex education **f. Adolescent:** - Growth and development, adaptation to puberty, menstrual hygiene, nutritional guidance, sex education, - Role of parents in health promotion of adolescents - Control of iron deficiency anemia (WIFS guidelines)	15	• Lecture • Discussion • Role play • Videos • Plotting of growth chart	• Short answers • Essay type • Objective type	3
III	Describe the role of nurse in caring for a sick child Develop skill in carrying out nursing intervention while caring for pediatric age group	**The Sick Child** a. Child's reaction to hospital b. Effect of hospitalization on the family of the child c. Role of nurse in helping child and family in coping with stress of hospitalization and illness **Pediatric Procedures** a. Preparation of child for diagnostic tests, collection of specimens b. Calculation and administration of oral and parenteral medication c. Procedures related to feeding - Katori and spoon - Ryle's tube and gastrostomy - Pediatric resuscitation d. Procedures relating to elimination - Enema - Colostomy irrigation e. Administration and analysis of oxygen concentration, steam inhalation, nebulization,	8	• Lecture • Discussion • Demonstration • Simulation role play	• Short answers • Essay type • Objective type • Return demonstration	4

Unit	Learning objective	Content	Hours	Teaching learning activities	Assess-ment methods	Chapter
		f. Other procedures: – Pediatric resuscitation – Surgical dressing				
IV	Describe the man-agement of behavioral disorders and com-mon health problems of children Demon-strate skills in the prevention and imple-mentation of medical and nursing manage-ment of behavioral	**Disorders and health problems of a child** **a. Infancy:** – Failure to thrive – Diarrhea and vomiting **b. Childhood:** – Communicable diseases – Tonsillitis – Otitis media – Child abuse – Breath holding spasms – Enuresis, nail biting, thumb sucking, thumb sucking, somnambulism – Protein energy malnutrition – Helminthic infections – Bites and stings – Pica – Tics **c. Adolescent:** – Precocious puberty – Gynecomastia – Accident, sport injuries – Obesity and anorexia nervosa – Juvenile delinquency	6	• Seminars • Lecture • Discussion	• Short answers • Essay type • Objective type	5
V	Demon-strate skills in providing comprehen-sive nursing care to the children having congenital defects/ malforma-tion	**Child with Congenital Disorders:** Etiology, signs, symptoms, diagnosis, complications and medical, surgical and nursing management of children with: • Malformations of CNS (Central Nervous System), cranial deformities, spina bifida, hydrocephalus, cerebral palsy, meningocele • Skeletal defects, cleft lip and cleft palate • Gastrointestinal tract (GIT) defects, fistula, anorectal malformations, hernia, congenital hypertrophic pyloric stenosis • **Defects of Genitourinary tract:** Hypospadias and epispadias, exstrophy of bladder, phimosis and paraphimosis, cryptorchidism, polycystic kidney • Sexual abnormalities, ambiguous genitalia	15	• Lecture • Discussion • Presentation of picture of congenital anomalies supervised by clinical practices	• Short answers • Essay type • Objective type	6

Unit	Learning objective	Content	Hours	Teaching learning activities	Assess-ment methods	Chapter
		Defects of Cardiovascular System (CVS) **Cyanotic and Acyanotic:** • Tetralogy of Fallots (TOF) • Transposition of Great Vessels (TGV) • Total Anomalous Pulmonary Venous Connection (TAPVC) • Atrial Septal Defect (ASD) • Ventricular Septal Defect (VSD) • Coarctation of aorta • Patent Ductus Arteriosus (PDA)				
VI	Demon-strate skills in providing comprehen-sive nurs-ing care to children with various dis-orders and diseases	**Children with Various Disorders and Diseases:** Etiology, signs and symptoms, complications, prevention, medical, surgical and nursing management of: **a. Renal system:** – Nephrotic syndrome – Acute glomerulonephritis – Acute renal failure (ARF) and Chronic renal failure (CRF) **b. Respiratory system:** – Upper respiratory infections (URI) and lower respiratory infections (LRI) – Asthma, pneumonia **c. GI (Gastrointestinal) system:** – Intestinal obstruction (Mechanical) – Hirschsprung's disease – Malabsorption syndrome – Inflammatory conditions—appendicitis, Meckel's diverticulum, ulcerative colitis – Worm infestation **d. CVS System:** – Rheumatic fever – Congestive cardiac failure (CCF) – Infective endocarditis **e. Hematological system:** – Anemia – Leukemia, thalassemia – Hemophilia – Sickle cell anemia – Thrombocytopenic purpura	15	• Lecture • Discussion -Presentation • Clinical teaching, simulation, videos • Visit to Blind, deaf and dumb school and rehabilitation center	• Short answers • Essay type • Objective type	7

Unit	Learning objective	Content	Hours	Teaching learning activities	Assess-ment methods	Chapter
		f. Neurological system: - Meningitis - Encephalitis - Convulsive disorders - Craniocerebral trauma **g. Endocrine:** - Pituitary disorders - Hypo and hyperthyroidism - Juvenile diabetes - Adrenal disorders **h. Developmental problems:** - Handicapped children - Mental retardation - Dyslexia - Hearing and vision impairment **i. Others:** - Fluid and electrolyte imbalance - Burns **j. Problems with locomotion:** - Poliomyelitis - Osteomyelitis - Kyphosis, lordosis, scoliosis - Fractures **k. Pre-and postoperative care of children undergoing surgery.**				
VII	Describe the various child welfare services provided by Governmental and non-governmental agencies. Explain the ethical and legal implication in pediatric nursing.	**Child Welfare Services** **a. Child welfare services and agencies:** - Integrated Child Development Services (ICDS) - Mid-day meal program - Balwadi, anganwadi - Daycare centers - National Polio Surveillance Project (NPSP) **b. Law pertaining to pediatrics:** - National child labour policy - Child act - Juvenile justice act - Internationally accepted rights of the child - Rehabilitation of delinquent and destitute children - Adoption laws and services - Adolescent health programs—menstrual hygiene, Weekly Iron Folic Acid Supplementation program, adolescent safety program	6	• Lecture • Discussion -Visit to anganwadi schools, remand homes and adoption centers	• Short answers • Essay type • Objective type	8

Child Health Nursing–Practical Placement: GNM Second Year

Time: 320 hours (8 weeks)

Internship: 96 hours (2 weeks)

Areas	Duration	Objectives	Skill	Assignments	Assessment methods	Chapter
Pediatric medicine ward	3 weeks	• Perform physical assessment • Assist in diagnostic procedure and provide pre and post care related to diagnostic procedure • Administer the drugs • Provide health education • Perform basic resuscitation	• Taking pediatric history • Perform physical examination and assessment of children • Administration of oral, intramuscular (IM), and intravenous (IV), medicine/ fluid • Calculation of fluid requirements • Prepare different strengths of IV fluids • Apply restraints • Administer O_2 inhalation by different methods • Feed children by katori (bowl) and spoon, pallada, etc. • Collect specimens for common investigations • Assist with common diagnostic procedure • Teach mothers/ parents on balance diet for child of different age group • Oral rehydration therapy • Feeding and weaning • Play therapy • Check vital signs • Give enema • Insert suppositories	• Give care to assigned pediatric patients • Nursing care plan-1 -Case study or presentation 1 • Health talk-1	• Assess performance with rating scale • Assess each skill with checklist • Evaluation of nursing care plan, case study, health talk, case presentation • Completion of activity record	2 and 4
Pediatric surgery ward	3 weeks	• Recognize different pediatric surgical condition • Provide pre and postoperative care to children with common pediatric surgical conditions/ malformation	• Do bowel wash • Care for ostomies: – Colostomy irrigation – Ureterostomy – Gastrostomy – Enterostomy • Urinary catheterization and drainage	• Give care to three assigned pediatric surgical patients • Nursing care plan 1 Case study or presentation 1	• Assess performance with rating scale • Assess each skill with checklist • Evaluation of nursing care plan, case study, case presentation	4

Areas	Duration	Objectives	Skill	Assignments	Assessment methods	Chapter
		• Counsel and educate parents	• Feeding: – Nasogastric – Gastrostomy – Jejunostomy • Care of surgical wound: – dressing – suture removal		• Completion of activity record	
Pediatric OPD/ Immunization room/ well baby clinic / adolescent clinic	2 weeks	• Perform assessment of children, health development and anthropometric • Perform immunization • Give health education/ nutritional education	• Assessment of children: – Health assessment – Developmental assessment – Anthropometric assessment • Immunization • Health/ nutritional education	Health assessment of the child Health talk 1	• Assess performance with rating scale • Completion of activity record • Assessment of the health talk	2 and 3

Child Health Nursing
Placement: BSc Nursing Third Year

Time: Theory: 90 hours
Practical: 300 hours
Internship: 145 hours

Course description: This course is designed for developing an understanding of the modern approach to child-care, identification, prevention and nursing management of common health problems of neonates and children.

Unit	Time (Hrs)	Learning objectives	Content	Teaching learning activities	Assessment methods	Chapter
I	15	• Explain the modern concept of child care and principles of child health nursing • Describe national policy programs and legislation in relation to child health and welfare • List major causes of death during infancy, early and late childhood • Describe the major functions and role of the paediatric nurse in caring for a hospitalized child • Describe the principles of child health nursing	**Introduction** **Modern concepts of childcare** • Internationally accepted rights of the child • National policy and legislation in relation to child health and welfare • National programmes related to child health and welfare • Agencies related to welfare services to the children • Changing trends in hospital care, preventive, promotive and curative aspects of child health • Child morbidity and mortality rates • Differences between an adult and child • Hospital environment for a sick child • Impact of hospitalisation on the child and family • Grief and bereavement • The role of a Child health nurse in caring for a hospitalised child • Principles of pre and post operative care of infants and children • Child health nursing procedures	• Lecture Discussion • Demonstration of common paediatric procedures	• Short answers • Objective type • Assessment of skills with checklist	1, 2, 4 and 8

Unit	Time (Hrs)	Learning objectives	Content	Teaching learning activities	Assessment methods	Chapter
II	25	• Describe the normal growth and development of children at different ages • Identify the needs of children at different ages and provide parental guidance • Identify the nutritional needs of children at different ages and ways of meeting the needs • Appreciate the role of play for normal and sick children • Appreciate the preventive measures and strategies for children	**The healthy child** • Principles of growth and development • Factors affecting growth and development • Growth and development from birth to adolescence • The needs of normal children through the stages of developmental and parental guidance • Nutritional needs of children and infants: breastfeeding, exclusive breastfeeding supplementary! artificial feeding and weaning, • Baby friendly hospital concept • Accidents: causes and prevention • Value of play and selection of play material • Preventive immunization, immunization programme and cold chain • Preventive paediatrics • Care of under five and under five clinics/ well baby clinics	• Lecture Discussion • Develop-mental study of infant and children • Observation study of normal and sick child • Field visit to Anganwadi, child guidance clinic • Film show on breast-feeding • Clinical practice/ field	• Short answers • Objective type • Assess-ment of field visits and develop-mental study reports	1, 2 and 3
III	15	• Provide care to normal and high risk neonates • Perform neonatal resuscitation • Recognize and manage common neonatal problems	**Nursing care of a neonate** • Nursing care of a normal newborn/Essential newborn care • Neonatal resuscitation • Nursing management of a low birth weight baby • Kangaroo mother care • Nursing management of common neonatal disorders • Organization of neonatal unit • Identification and nursing management of common congenital malformations	• Lecture Discussion • Workshop on neonatal resuscita-tion • Demonstra-tion • Practice session • Clinical practice	• Short answers • Objective type • Assess-ment of skills with checklist	2 and 4

Unit	Time (Hrs)	Learning objectives	Content	Teaching learning activities	Assessment methods	Chapter
IV	10		**Integrated management of neonatal and childhood illnesses (IMNCI)**			2
V	23	• Identify measures to prevent common childhood diseases including immunization • Provide nursing care in common childhood diseases	**Nursing management in common childhood diseases** • Nutritional deficiency disorders • Respiratory disorders and infections • Gastrointestinal infections, infestations and congenital disorders • **Cardiovascular problem:** Congenital defects and rheumatic fever, rheumatic heart disease • **Genitourinary disorders:** acute glomerulonephritis, Nephrotic syndrome, Wilms' tumor, infection and congenital disorders. • Neurological infections and disorders: convulsions, epilepsy, meningitis, hydrocephalus, spinabifida • **Hematological disorders:** Anemia, thalassemia, ITP, Leukemia, hemophilia • **Endocrine disorders:** Juvenile Diabetes Mellitus • **Orthopedic disorders:** club feet, hip dislocation and fracture. • Disorders of skin, eye, and ears • Common communicable diseases in children, their identification, nursing management in hospital and home and prevention • **Child health emergencies:** poisoning, foreign bodies, hemorrhage, burns and drowning. Nursing care of infant and children with HIV/AIDS	• Lecture discussion • Demonstration • Practice session • Clinical practice	• Objective type • Assessment of skills with checklist • Short answers	5 and 6

Unit	Time (Hrs)	Learning objectives	Content	Teaching learning activities	Assessment methods	Chapter
VI	12	• Manage the child with behavioural social problems • Identify the social and welfare services for challenged children	**Management of behavioural and social problems in children** • Management of common behavioural disorders • Management of common psychiatric problems • Management of challenged children: Mentally, physically, and socially challenged • Welfare services for challenged children in India • Child guidance clinics	• Lecture discussion • Field visits to child guidance clinics, school for mentally and physically, socially challenged	• Short answers • Objective type • Assess-ment of field • Reports	7 and 8

Child Health Nursing–Practical
Placement: BSc Nursing Third Year, Fourth Year

Time: 300 hours (9 weeks)
Internship: 145 hours (3 weeks)

Areas	Duration in week	Objectives	Skills	Assignments	Assessment methods	Chapter
Paediatric Medicine Ward	3	• Provide nursing care to children with various medical disorders • Counsel and educate parents	• Taking paediatric history' physical examination and assessment of children • Administer of oral, J/M and IV medicine/fluids • Calculation of fluid requirements • Prepare different strengths of IV fluids • Apply restraints • Administer 02 inhalation by different methods • Give baby bath • Feed children by Katori spoon, etc • Collect specimens for common investigations • Assist with common diagnostic procedures • Teach mothers/parents malnutrition • Oral rehydration therapy • Feeding and Weaning • Immunization schedule • Play therapy • Specific disease conditions	• Give care to three assigned paediatric patients • Nursing Care Plan I • Case study/ presentation I Health Talk I	• Assess clinical performance with rating scale • Assess each skill with checklist OSCE/ OSPE • Evaluation of case study! presentation and health education session • Completion of activity record	2 and 4

Areas	Duration in weeks	Objectives	Skills	Assignments	Assessment methods	Chapter
Pediatric Surgery Ward	4	• Recognize different pediatric surgical conditions/ Malformations • Provide pre and post operative care to children with common paediatric surgical conditions/ Malformation • Counsel and educate parents	Calculate, prepare and administer IV fluids • Bowel wash • Care for ostomies • Colostomy irrigation • Ureterostomy • Gastrostomy • Enterostomy • Urinary catheterization and drainage • Feeding • Nasogastric • Gastrostomy • Jejunostomy • Care of surgical wounds • Dressing • Suture removal	• Give care to three assigned paediatric surgical patients • Nursing Care Plan-1 • Case study/ Presentation-1	• Assess clinical performance with rating scale • Assess each skill with checklist • OSCE/ OSPE • Evaluation of case study • presentation Completion of activity record	2 and 4

Areas	Duration in weeks	Objectives	Skills	Assign-ments	Assessment methods	Chapter
Pediatric OPD/ Immuni-zation room	1	• Perform assessment of children: health, developmental and anthropo-metric perform immunization • Give health education/ nutritional education	• Assessment of children - Health assessment - Developmental assessment • Anthropometric assessment • Immunization • Health/Nutritional education	Develop-mental study - I	• Assess clinical performance with rating scale • Completion ofactivity record	2, 3 and 4
Paediatric medicine and surgery ICU	1+1	Provide nursing care to critically ill children	• Care of a baby in incubator/warmer • Care of a child on ventilator • Endotracheal suction • Chest physiotherapy • Administer fluids with infusion pump • Total parenteral nutrition • Phototherapy • Monitoring of babies • Cardiopulmonary resuscitation	• Nursing care plan I • Obser-vation report 1	• Assess clinical performance with rating scale • Completion of activity record • Evaluation of observation report	2 and 4

Internship

Areas	Duration in week	Objectives	Skills	Assignments	Assessment methods
Pediatric medicine ward/ICU	1	Provide comprehensive care to children with medical conditions	Integrated practice		Assess clinical performance with rating scale
Pediatric surgery ward/ICU	1	Provide comprehensive care to children with surgical conditions	Integrated practice		Assess clinical performance with rating scale
NICU	1	Provide intensive care to neonates	Integrated practice		Assess clinical performance with rating scale

Contents

Chapter 1

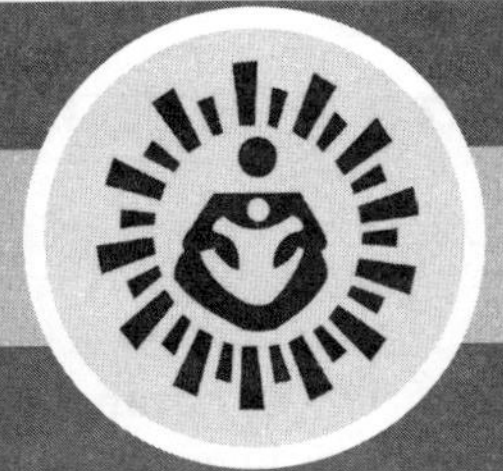

Introduction to Pediatrics and Pediatric Nursing

- **Factors Affecting Child Health**
- **International Rights of Child**
- **The National Rights of the Child**
- **United Nations Declaration of the Rights of the Child**
- **Modern Concept in Child Health Care**
  - Historical Development of Pediatric Nursing
- **Trends in Pediatric Nursing and Nursing Practice**
  - Ethics in Pediatric Nursing
- **Role of Pediatric Nurses in Child Care**
- **Emerging Challenges in Pediatric Nursing**
- **Concept of Preventive Pediatrics**
  - Differences between Children and Adult
  - Purpose of Differentiating Adult and Child
  - Anatomical/Physiological Difference
  - Psychosocial Differences
  - Social Differences
  - Emotional Differences
  - Cognitive Differences
  - Adolescence
  - Role of Nurse
- **Vital Statistics Related to Pediatrics as per the NRHS and GOI**

Introduction

Pediatric nursing involves taking the responsibility of care for children and families throughout the lifespan. This task includes health promotion, illness care, health restoration, and rehabilitation of the child health.

Pediatric nursing requires understanding the developmental aspects of children and the physical differences between children and adults. Pediatric nurses must also recognize the role that families play in the child's health and reflect family-centered care in practice (Taylor, 2006).

Dr Abraham Jacobi (1830–1919), is referred to as the **'Father of Pediatrics'** because of his achievements during this time period.

The word 'Pediatrics' comes from the Greek words.

- **'Pedia'** which means child.
- **'Iatrike'** which means treatment.
- **'Ics'** which means branch of science.

Pedia + iatrike + ics = Pediatrics

This means **'Pediatric nursing'** is the science of child care and scientific treatment of childhood. This branch of medical science deals with the care of children from conception to adolescence in health care.

Definition of Nursing

The unique function of the nurse is to assist the individual, sick or well, in the performance of those activities contributing to health or its recovery (or to peaceful death) that he would perform unaided, if he had the necessary strength will, or knowledge and to do this in such a way as to strength, will or knowledge, and to do this is such a way as to help him gain independence as rapidly as possible' **—Virginia Henderson, 1966**

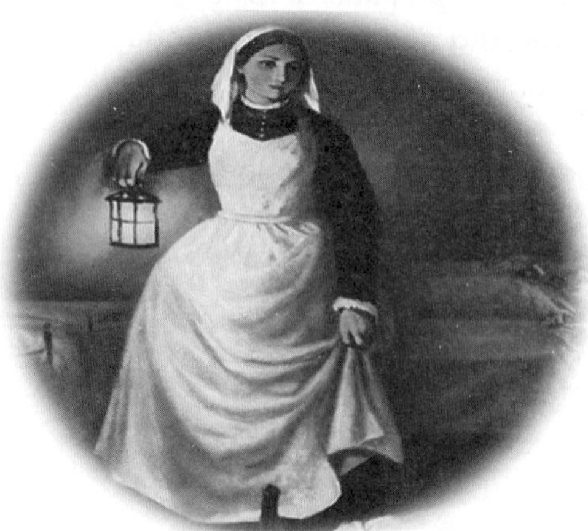

The American Nurses Association (ANA) states nursing is the protection, promotion, and optimization of health and abilities, prevention of illness and injury, alleviation of suffering through the diagnosis and treatment of human response, and advocacy in the care of individuals, families, communities, and populations.

—American Nurses Association (ANA)

Definition of Pediatrics

Pediatrics can be defined as the branch of medical science that deals with the care of the children, from conception to adolescence, in health and illness. It is concerned with preventive, curative, and rehabilitative care of children.

Definition of Pediatric Nursing

Pediatric nursing is defined as the specialized area of the nursing practice concerning the care of children during wellness and illness, which includes preventive, promotive, curative and rehabilitative care of children.

Importance of Pediatric Nursing

The children are the major consumers of health care. 35 to 40% of total population are children below the age of 15 years.

- More vulnerable to various health problems
- Majority of children morbidity and mortality preventable
- Needs special care to survive and thrive
- Wealth of tomorrow's society and Nation
- The branch of nursing concerned with the care of infants and children. Pediatric nursing requires knowledge of normal psychomotor, psychosocial, and cognitive growth and development, as well as of the health problems and needs of people in this age group. Preventive care and anticipatory guidance are integral to the practice of pediatric nursing **(Mosby medical dictionary).**

Goals of Pediatric Nursing

- To provide skillful, intelligent, need based comprehensive care to the children in health and sickness.
- To interpreted the basic needs of the children to their parents and family members and to guide them in child care.
- To prevent disease and alleviate suffering in children.
- To promote growth and development of children towards optimum state of health for functioning at the peak of their capacity in future.
- Build a working relationship with the parents and their children from the time of first contact.
- Should be aware that all behaviors should be meaningful.
- Should accept parents and their children exactly as they are.
- Allow them to know that their problems are important, and the nurse is there to aid in their solutions.

Common Themes in Pediatric Nursing

- Nursing is caring
- Nursing is an art
- Nursing is science
- Nursing is client centered
- Nursing is holistic
- Nursing is adaptive.

Nursing is concerned with health promotion, health maintenance, and health restoration. Nursing is a basically helping profession.

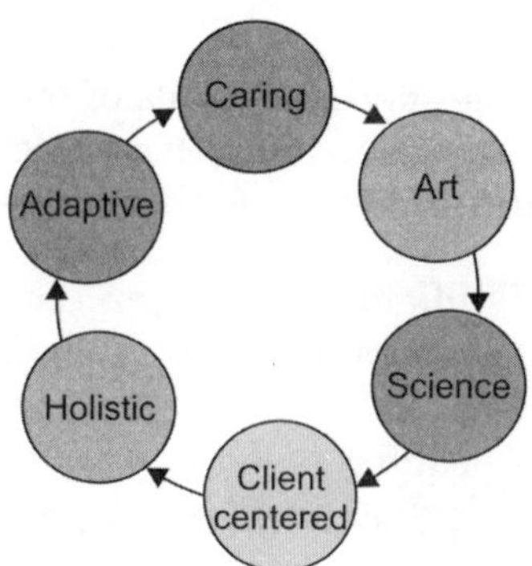

Fig. 1.1: Common themes in pediatric nursing

Scope of Pediatric Nursing and Nurse

Nurses have the responsibility in providing nursing interventions either in ambulatory or institutional settings. Ambulatory setting: such as home, schools and or physician's clinic, where children and their parents have health or counseling needs. While institutional settings are mainly hospitals (general or specialized hospitals) where the care is provided to sick children and their parents.

Qualities of Good Pediatric Nurse

- Good observer
- Honest and truthful
- Sympathetic, kind, patient and cheerful
- Love to work with children
- Interested in family care
- Able to provide teaching to children and their families.

FACTORS AFFECTING CHILD HEALTH

The Child well-being is determines the health of the next generation and can help predict future public health challenges for families, communities, and the health care system. The objectives of the Maternal, Infant, and Child Health topic area address a wide range of conditions, health behaviors, and health systems indicators that affect the health, wellness, and quality of life of women, children, and families.

Concept of Child Health

- Social Development
- Environments
- Genetics
- Nurturing
- Emotional Security.

Common Maternal and Child Health Problems

- Hypertension and heart disease
- Juvenile diabetes mellitus

- Maternal depression
- Genetic conditions [Sickle cell anemia]
- Sexually transmitted diseases (STDs)
- Malnutrition or PEM
- Low birth weight [LBW]
- Childhood infection
- Accident and poisoning
- Behavioral problems.

Maternal Factors

The maternal and infant mortality rates and pregnancy-related complications can be reduced by increasing access to quality preconception (before pregnancy) and interconception (between pregnancies) care.

- Multiple pregnancies
- Poverty in during pregnancy
- Lack of spacing between two child
- Improper antenatal care
- Maternal age [below 16 and above 35 years]
- Preeclampsia
- Maternal infection
- Imbalanced maternal diet
- Illegal drugs exposure during pregnancy
- Smoking and alcoholism.

Socioeconomic Factors

These include prepregnancy health behaviors and health status, which are influenced by a variety of environmental and social factors such as access to health care and chronic stress.

The social determinants that influence maternal health also affect pregnancy outcomes and infant health. Racial and ethnic disparities in infant mortality exist. Child health status varies by both race and ethnicity, as well as by family income and related factors, including educational attainment among household members and health insurance coverage.

- Modified life style
- Culture and customs
- Gender bias
- Poor child rearing practice
- Large family size
- Poor economic status of the family
- Parents illiteracy ratio
- Poverty.

Environmental Factors

In India environmental factors are most common reason for childhood mortality and morbidity.

- Poor environmental sanitation
- Homemade accidents
- Open airway defecation
- Improper disposal of wastes
- Unhygienic practice in home
- Insect threat
- Unsafe drinking water supply.

Promotion of Child Health

The maintenance and promotion of child and mother health following child health services, maternal and child health programme.

- To create the health awareness
- School health programme
- RCH and MCH Programme
- Community health Programme
- National child health policy
- Immunisation programme.

INTERNATIONAL RIGHTS OF CHILD

'Declaration of the Rights of the Child 1959'

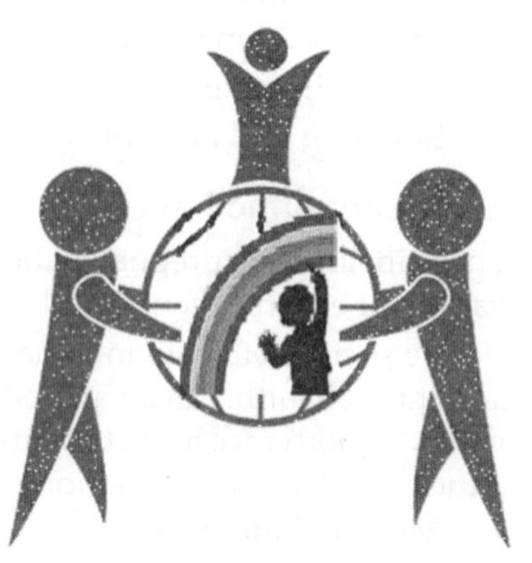

First it was documented on prior to World War II, the League of Nations had adopted the Geneva Declaration of the Rights of the Child in 1924. The United Nations (UN) took its first step towards declaring the importance of child rights by establishing the United Nations International Children's Emergency Fund in 1946 (The name was shortened to United Nations Children's Fund in 1953, but kept the popular acronym UNICEF). Two years later the UN General Assembly adopted the Universal Declaration of Human Rights, making it the first UN document to recognize children's need for protection.

The Preamble notes that children need 'special safeguards and care, including appropriate legal protection, before as well as after birth,' reiterates the 1924 Declaration's pledge that 'mankind owes to the child the best it has to give,' and specifically calls upon voluntary organizations and local authorities to strive for the observance of children's rights.

Principles of Child Rights

There are four general principles for children's rights:

1. Nondiscrimination means that all children have the same right to develop their potential in all situations and at all times. For example, every child should have equal access to education regardless of the child's gender, race, ethnicity, nationality, religion, disability, parentage, sexual orientation or other status.

2. The best interests of the child must be 'a primary consideration' in all actions and decisions concerning a child, and must be used to resolve conflicts between different rights. For example, when making national budgetary decisions affecting children, Government must consider how cuts will impact on the best interests of the child.
3. The right to survival and development underscores the vital importance of ensuring access to basic services and to equality of opportunity for children to achieve their full development. For example, a child with a disability should have effective access to education and health care to achieve their full potential.
4. The views of the child mean that the voice of the child must be heard and respected in all matters concerning his or her rights. For example, those in power should consult with children before making decisions that will affect them.

THE NATIONAL RIGHTS OF THE CHILD

Basic 10 rights

1. Right to develop in an atmosphere of affection and security and wherever possible in the cars and under the responsibility of his / her parents.
2. Right to enjoy the benefits of social security including nutrition housing and medical care.
3. Right to free education
4. Right to full opportunity for play and recreation
5. Right to a name and nationality
6. Right to special care if handicapped
7. Right to be among the first to receive protection and relief in times of disaster
8. Right to learn to be useful member of society and to develop in a healthy and normal manner and in conditions of freedom and dignity
9. Right to be brought up in a spirit of understanding tolerance friendship among people, peace is universal brotherhood.
10. Right to enjoy these rights, regardless of race, color, sex, religion National or Social origin.

UNITED NATIONS DECLARATION OF THE RIGHTS OF THE CHILD

- To be free from discrimination
- To develop physically and mentally in freedom and dignity to have a name and nationality
- To have adequate nutrition, housing recreation and medical services
- To receive special care if handicapped
- To receive love, understanding and material security
- To receive on education and develop lies or her abilities
- To be the first to receive protection in dictates
- To be protected from neglect, cruelty exploitation
- To be brought up in spirit of friendship among people.

MODERN CONCEPT IN CHILD HEALTH CARE

Concept of Pediatric Nursing

Nurses who specialize in pediatrics devote their knowledge and skills to caring for children from infancy through the adolescents and their families. These specialized nurses usually complete advanced training in pediatrics and collaborate closely with physicians and other health care providers who share their dedication to children's health.

Pediatric nurses can perform:

- Physical examinations
- Measure vital statistics
- Take blood and urine samples
- Order diagnostic tests.

Nurses with advanced training can interpret test results to form diagnoses and develop treatment plans.

Parents often prefer to have their children treated by nurses and other health providers who are pediatric specialists, because children have special health care needs. Their bodies are growing and changing, and they often react differently to injury, illness and even common medications.

In addition, children get scared and can not always clearly communicate 'what hurts.' Pediatric nurses know how to talk to children and how to dispel their fears. They also know how to ask children questions about their health, so they can gather complete and accurate information to aid in diagnosis and treatment.

In addition to caring for child with injuries and illnesses, pediatric nurses spend a significant amount of time educating parents and other caregivers about how to care for their children and protect children's health. For families of children with chronic conditions, such as juvenile diabetes or paralysis, they design home care plans to help the families meet their child's special needs.

Prevention and health education is a big part of pediatric nursing. Pediatric nurses often staff community health fairs and visit schools to perform:

- Physical examination
- Growth and Development monitoring
- Immunize children
- Provide routine developmental health screenings
- Pediatric nursing is a very special vocation, because it provides the opportunity to play a key role in a child's life when that child needs you most.

HISTORICAL DEVELOPMENT OF PEDIATRIC NURSING

The continuance of any successful society depends on the succeeding new generation. Once upon a time there was no specialty of pediatrics and pediatric nursing as we understand today. Since primitive times, the welfare of the child has been sensitive index of the general welfare of the people. Whenever general health conditions have been good, the death rate among children has fallen.

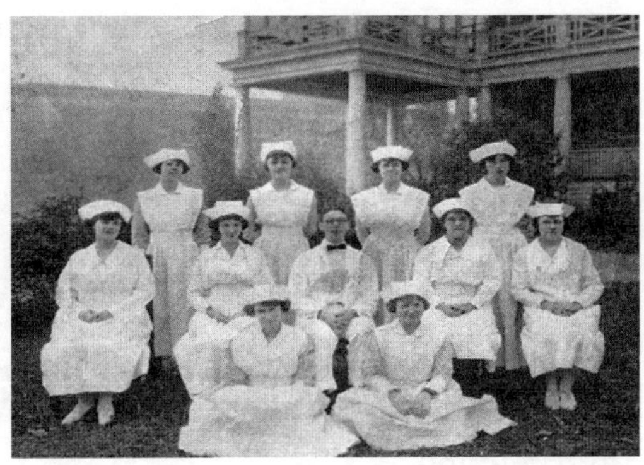

It raises with deterioration in the health conditions. Children, however, are so helpless that their health depends not only on the general factors influencing all society but also on what adults do for them–feeding, clothing and training them. Thus the history of the pediatric nursing is linked with that of sanitation, hygiene discoveries in the medical science and general culture of the group.

Many specific recommendations for the care of the child are found in the records of ancient civilizations:

- As early as 225 BC in the Indian **Susruta Samhita**, there is a description of qualities of breast milk and child hygiene.
- In ancient Egypt mothers were advised to dress the infants loosely and feed at breast.
- Christian charity greatly influenced pediatric nursing. In the Christian hospitals, at an early date, there was provision for the fondling homes.
- Pediatrics as a specialty came into being in 1860. Dr Abraham Jacob established the first children's clinic in New York and gave special lectures in diseases of children.
- In 1888 the first department of pediatrics was established the first children's clinic in New York and gave special lectures on disease of children.
- In 1888 the first department of pediatrics was established in Harvard Medical School. It was realized that diseases of children differed somewhat from the diseases of adults.
- Antenatal health care and pediatrics are essentially developments of the 20th century in so far as the modern system of medicine is concerned.
- It is difficult to say when pediatric nursing began to be considered a speciality, for it developed gradually as nursing became a profession and as nurses recognized children's needs for nursing care.
- A century ago the knowledge of child development was limited. It was not known what is needed for the sound personality development nor was it known how hospitalization affected to the child.
- The increased knowledge of developmental needs has influenced nursing and made pediatric nursing a speciality.
- The Lady Chelmsford All India League for Maternity and Child Welfare was established in 1920. Efforts were made to create public awareness about health problems of children by exhibition, publishing a journal and celebrating baby weeks.
- The first crèche in the country was opened in 1923.
- Presently, pediatric nursing is being taught in all nursing courses at undergraduate level. Postgraduate education is necessary for those who expect to specialize in the care of the children.

The present concept of health care is prevention of illness and promotion of health rather than medical care alone.

These changes which are as a result of various factors are:

- Concepts of wellness and illness
- Changing needs of the society
- Medical and technological advances in the field of health and medical care
- Trends within the nursing profession
- Increased understanding of the psychological aspects of illness and hospitalization
- Increased consumer demands due to awareness of health needs.

TRENDS IN PEDIATRIC NURSING AND NURSING PRACTICE

Introduction

Changes in the standard of care for pediatric patients are not something the medical community takes lightly. In the world of medicine, clinical care guidelines are typically developed around sound clinical research; however, there is an exception to this rule when developing clinical care guidelines for use with the pediatric patient.

Child health nursing is undergoing tremendous advancements just like pediatric medicine and surgery. The current trends in the practice are based on researches that have taken place in the field of pediatric nursing. The common trends are as following:

Family Centered Care (FCC)

It is based on the philosophy that quality care can be provided in an environment that support family integrity and promote psychological and physiological health of the family. It assumes that if the family gains adequate information and support, it is capable of making health care decisions (McKay and Philips, 1984).

Features of FCC

- It provides a holistic approach than simply providing medical and nursing care.
- Parents know best about their child's needs, more aware of their child's behavior and habits.
- The parent's right to know about the condition of their child, need to be considered while caring children.
- Attention must be given to parents must be taken into confidence as partners in the provision of care that aid in better stability to the child psychologically.

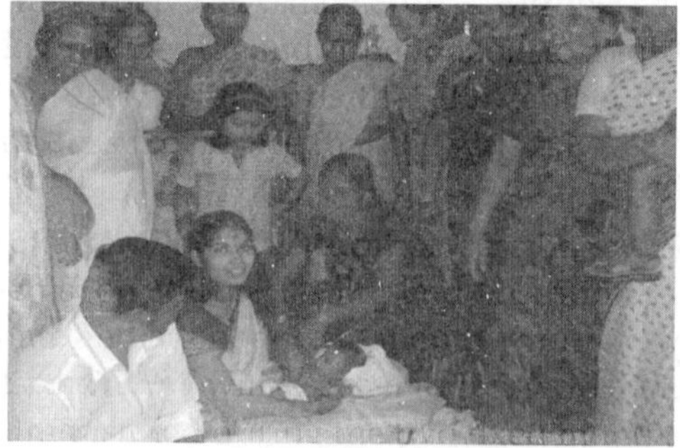

Fig. 1.2: Family centered care

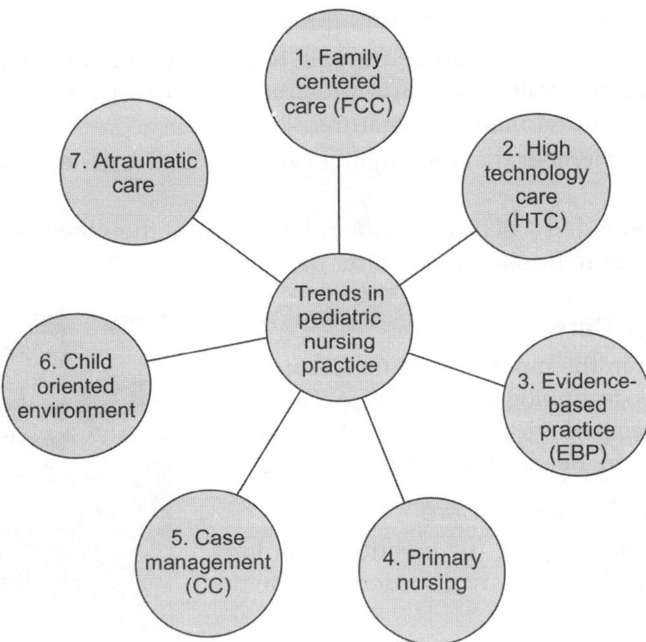

Fig. 1.3: Trends in nursing practices

- The nurse should not take over the care without due importance to the parents.
- Make an involvement of the parents in the care of their children facilitates better coping in parents and reduce separation trauma to children that help quick recovery.

Concept of FCC

There are two basic concepts of family centered care are enabling and empowering.

1. **Enabling:** In the process of enabling, all the family members are helped by the professional to create opportunities and means to utilize their present abilities, competence and acquire new skills that are necessary to provide care to their sick children.
2. **Empowering:** It helps to foster the strengths of family members to cope up and withstand stress related to sickness of their children.

   Interact such that families maintain or acquire a sense of control over their lives and acknowledge positive changes.

Role of Nurse in FCC

- Nurses should help families to make responsible decision through education.
- Nurses need to act as interpreter and develop mutually respectful and trusting relationship with parents.
- She should be Recognizing parents as unique autonomous individuals by creating humanistic empowered environment is the responsibility of the nurse in FCC. This promotes parental support and makes parents capable for providing vital elements of care to their children.

- This form of empowering parents is of supreme personnel and forms foundation for FCC.
- FCC expects the nurse should be capable to provide humane care that incorporates hopes, dreams and values, cultural preferences and concerns of children and their parents that are individualistic in nature.
- Nurses must remember that the nursing care provided will be same but the customer changes.
- The care we provided will be remembered throughout their lifetime and to nurses their work can appear to be similar day after day.

High Technology Care

The advancement in the medical field has created the care of children too technologically versatile. The nurse also needs to be technologically competent enough to meet the nursing care needs of children.

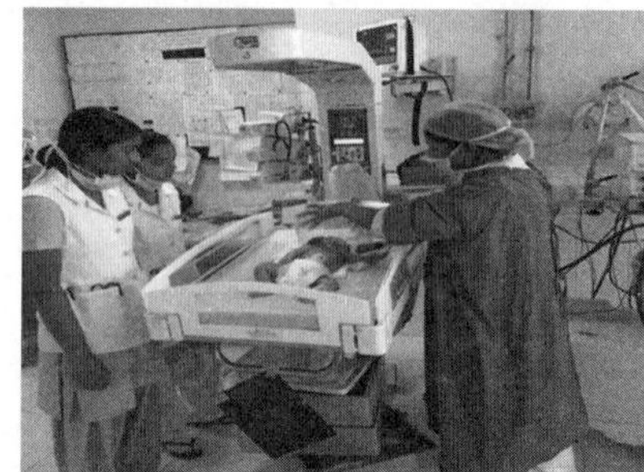

Fig. 1.4: Staff nurses are providing high technology care to newborn baby

Features of High Technology Care

- The advancement in the diagnostic technology has made detection of many disorders even in the fetal period.
- Laboratory methods to assess fetal maturity and health of the fetus in the womb.
- USG (ultra sound in diagnosis and aggressive technology to the care of premature and sick basics have created many ethical dilemma even in nursing practice.

Role of Nurse in High Technology Care

- Nurse need to be alert to these advances.
- Advanced technology and computer skills in working place challenge nurses for continuing nursing education.
- High technology induced ethical dilemmas include controversial fetal surgeries like:
  - Fetal blood transfusions
  - Medical termination of pregnancy
  - Cloning
  - Invitro fertilization
  - Female feticide, etc.

Here the nurse need to be technically competent and must possess soft skills to cope with technological advancements.

Evidence-based Practice

In evidence-based practice (EBP), nurses need to make decisions on the best available sources of evidences.

Features of EBP

- An evidence-based practice in nursing profession, it will provides a systematic approach to enable nurses to effectively perform in nursing practice.

- Nurse need to search the literature to analyze evidences using biostatistics rules to identify generalizabilty of findings. Here comes the significance of EBP as it involves the ability to access.
- It summarize and apply information from literature to day-to-day clinical problems.
- It warrants reliance on the research literature to substantiate nursing decisions.
- This ensures that our accomplishments make sense to patients.
- Nursing focus is on the illness aspect of care the human response during disease and therapy.
- Nurses should find data necessary to identify and support their contribution to patient outcomes.
- EBP can be applied to any problem that seeks solutions.
- The problem seeking solution needs to be framed as question. A problem may have many subproblems, all need to be framed as questions. After framing questions the nurse need to search for evidences in literature.
- EBP is relatively less practiced in child health nursing as small number of children is nursed for long-term basis and due to ethical limitations.

Evidence-based Medicine

Evidence-based medicine (EBM) is defined as judicious use of the best current evidence in making decisions about the care of an individual patient. The intent of EBM is to integrate clinical expertise with the best available research evidence while observing the psychosocial needs of the child.

Evidence-based medicine follows four steps:

1. Formulate a clear clinical question from a patient's problem
2. Conduct a literature search of peer-reviewed journals for relevant clinical articles
3. Evaluate the literature for its value to EMS practice and collaborate with your medical director
4. Implement changes to the patient care protocols.

Primary Nursing

The system of primary nursing provides extreme commitment to client accountability. 24 hour responsibility and accountability by one nurse for the care of a small group of patients is possible with primary nursing.

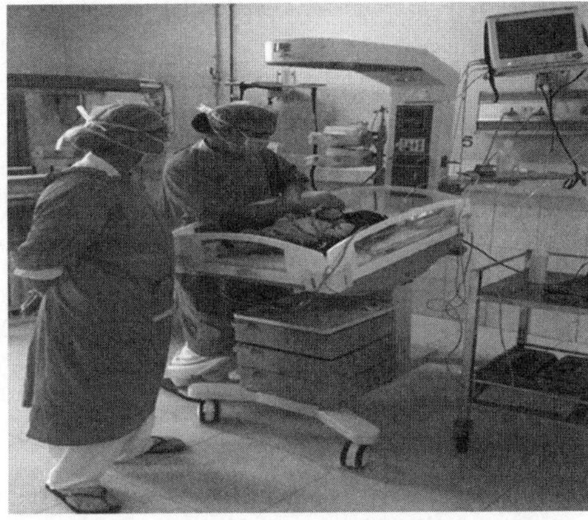

Fig. 1.5: Staff nurse providing primary nursing care

Primary nurse is the bedside nurse with few duties delegated to other nurses. When primary is not working, an associate primary nurse will maintain continuity of care. This system provides better client satisfaction and they have the privilege to get all necessary information from one person. At this juncture, maintenance of primary care is essential. To maintain the consistency of care is to designate one primary nurse and as many associates to provide the pediatric care to provide consistent caregivers to care for the child. It also focuses family unit as an integral component in planning and implementing care.

Case Management

It is considered as an extension of primary nursing. It is usually used in outpatient setting by assigning child or group of children.

It utilizes time line or critical path or based on practice guidelines. Vitiations in timelines are noted to identify delay in provision of care that helps to resolve the problems related to patient system or community.

Case management system is widely used in countries where health insurance paying is prevalent. In this system, care delivery need to be balanced as per cost and quality, i.e. delivery of health care in a cost effective manner.

Advantages

- Improved patient family satisfaction
- Decreased fragmentation of care
- Ability to describe and measure outcomes for a homogenous group of patients.

Case management system utilizes set guidelines that are prepared. Many forms or models of guidelines are used such as critical path, care maps and standardized care plan.

Child-oriented Environment

A child Eco-friendly environment should be provided to a child who is admitted to hospital. Child should be admitted to a Pediatric ward.

The outlay of the ward should be one of child friendly with adequate safety precautions. Education and facilities for play should be provided. Removing young children from their familiar environment to strange ward is frightening to the child.

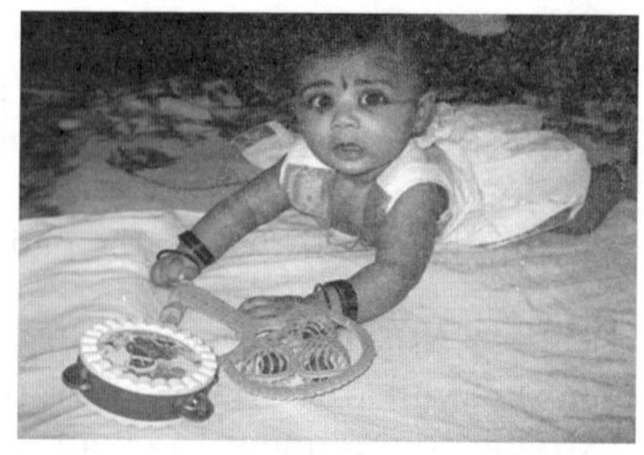

It also disrupts family routines not only for the child but also for the siblings and others at home. Staff should be sensitive to the family's individual needs according to the social educational, cultural and religious background.

Pediatric ward should be equipped with skilled staff Nurse. There should be a 'named nurse' responsible for planning and coordinating the care by other nurses.

Ensure that families receive all information they need and the nurse need to provide a link between the team members as child health care is essentially a multidisciplinary care.

She should maintain the liberal visiting hours and permitting the parents be with their hospitalized children, this also promotes child-oriented environment in a hospital.

Atraumatic Care

It is the provision of therapeutic care in settings by personnel and with interventions that eliminates or minimizes the psychological and physical distress experienced by children and their families in the health care system.

Therapeutic care includes the prevention, diagnosis, treatment or palliation of chronic or acute condition and settings refers to whatever places that care is provided.

Concept of Atraumatic Care

The concept of therapeutic care is intended to reduce mental and physical harm and to provide an environment with minimum physical and mental trauma. There are three principles to be followed in the provision of a atraumatic care:

1. Prevent or minimize the child's separation from family members
2. Promote sense of comfort
3. Prevent or minimize bodily injury and pain.

Though there is tremendous technological advancement in the provision of therapeutic care, the injury and pain produced with this is not reduced.

A child who receives therapeutic intervention needs to be treated with tender loving care. By inculcating the above-mentioned principles, atraumatic care encompasses many aspects such as:

- Reducing separation anxiety
- Providing adequate information to care givers and equip them to minimize trauma of hospitalization
- Preparing parents to utilize positive coping and performing procedures with utmost skill and right attitude
- Even the provision of child-oriented environment and skilled staff are essential component of atraumatic care.

Suggested nursing interventions are as following:

- Promote foster parent-child relationship during hospitalization
- Prepare the child before any procedure
- Control pain
- Provide child privacy
- Provide play for expression fear and aggression
- Minimize loss of control
- Respect cultural religious differences especially in Indian set up.

Trends in Nursing Managements

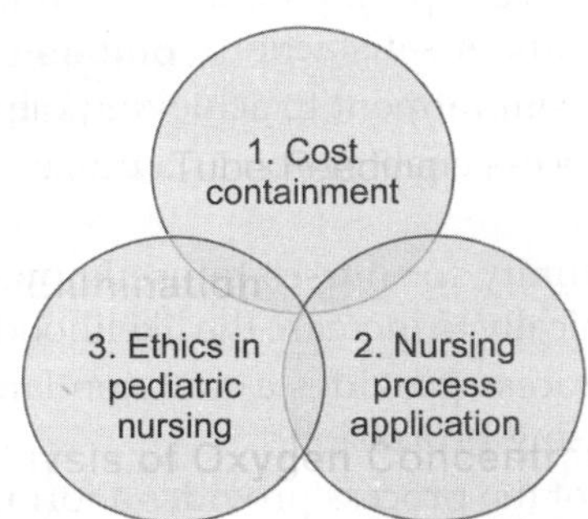

Fig. 1.6: Trends in nursing managements

Cost Containment

Cost containment is maximum utilization of advanced technique to reduce the cost of hospitalization. It is achieved in many ways in hospitals either by cutting nursing positions or by improving the process of care and tightening nonlabor resources.

- This is reducing mortality rates and length of hospital stay.
- Cost containment reduced complications and by increasing family satisfaction and readiness and ability of function upon discharge.
- Nurses make significant contribution to both the quality of hospital services and the containment of hospital costs. The case management model outlines and activates strategic management of quality patient outcomes and costs.
  - Cost containment strategy transforms primary nurse approach to care managers and changes the focus of nursing process to multidisciplinary outcomes.
  - Cost effective care will exist only in situations in which the patient is known where there is continuity of care provided by expert caregivers.
  - Excellent results obtained when nurses provide intuitive, scientific care to patients and families.
  - Enabling and empowerment are yet another concept followed in cost containment strategy too where nurses are on the position of expect caregiver helping parents to learn and provide care to their children; by obtaining the necessary knowledge and skill from nurses as mentioned along with FCC.

Nursing Process Application

Definition: The nursing process is a series of organized steps designed for nurses to provide excellent client and family care. Learn the five phases, including assessing, diagnosing, planning, implementing, and evaluating.

Purpose of nursing process in child care:

The nursing process provides an organizing framework for meeting the individual needs of the child and family.

- The nursing process provides an organized, systematic method of problem-solving (while still allowing for creative solutions) that may minimize dangerous errors or omissions in care giving and avoid time-consuming repetition in care and documentation.
- The use of the nursing process promotes the active involvement of clients in their healthcare, enhancing consumer satisfaction.
- It strengthens the client's commitment to achieving the identified goals.
- The use of the nursing process enables you as a nurse to have more control over your practice during child care.
- This enhances the opportunity for nurses to use knowledge, expertise, and intuition constructively and dynamically to increase the likelihood of a successful client outcome.
- The use of the nursing process provides a common language (nursing diagnosis) for practice, unifying the nursing profession.
- In addition, the structure of the process provides a format for documenting the client's response to all aspects of the planned care.

- The use of the nursing process provides a means of assessing nursing's economic contribution to client care.
- The nursing process supplies a vehicle for the quantitative and qualitative measurement of nursing care that meets the goal of cost-effectiveness and still promotes holistic care towards child health.

Steps in nursing process

In nursing practices, this process is one of the foundations of practice. It offers a framework for thinking through problems and provides some organization to a nurse's critical thinking skills. It is important to point out that this process is flexible and not rigid. It is a tool to use in nursing care, but one that should allow for creativity and thinking outside of the nursing process table.

Nursing process which stand for 'ADPIE'

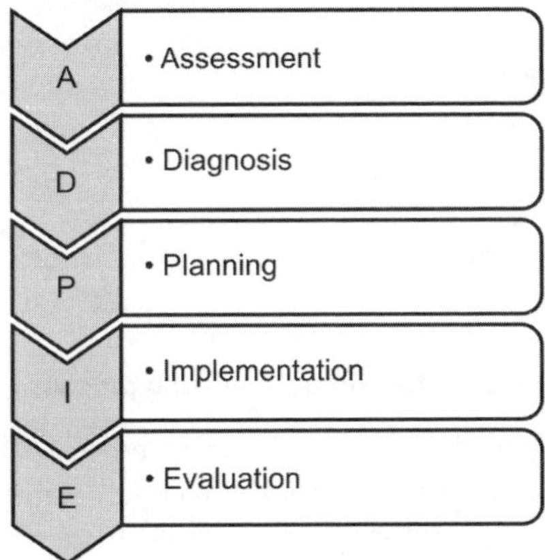

Fig. 1.7: ADPIE–nursing process

Assessment phase: The first step of the nursing process is assessment. During this phase, the nurse gathers information about a patient's psychological, physiological, sociological, and spiritual status. This data can be collected in a variety of ways. Generally, nurses will conduct a patient interview. Physical examinations, referencing a patient's health history, obtaining a patient's family history, and general observation can also be used to gather assessment data. Patient interaction is generally the heaviest during this evaluative phase.

Diagnosing phase: The diagnosing phase involves a nurse making an educated judgment about a potential or actual health problem with a patient. Multiple diagnoses are sometimes made for a single patient. These assessments not only include an actual description of the problem (e.g. sleep deprivation) but also whether or not a patient is at risk of developing further problems. These diagnoses are also used to determine a patient's readiness for health improvement and whether or not they may have developed a syndrome. The diagnoses phase is a critical step as it is used to determine the course of treatment.

Planning phase: In this phase once a client and nurse agree on the diagnoses, a plan of action can be developed. If multiple diagnoses need to be addressed, the head nurse will prioritize each assessment and devote attention to severe symptoms and high risk factors. Each problem is assigned a clear, measurable goal for the expected beneficial outcome. For this phase, nurses generally refer to the evidence-based Nursing Outcome Classification, which is a set of standardized terms and measurements for tracking patient wellness. The Nursing Interventions Classification may also be used as a resource for planning.

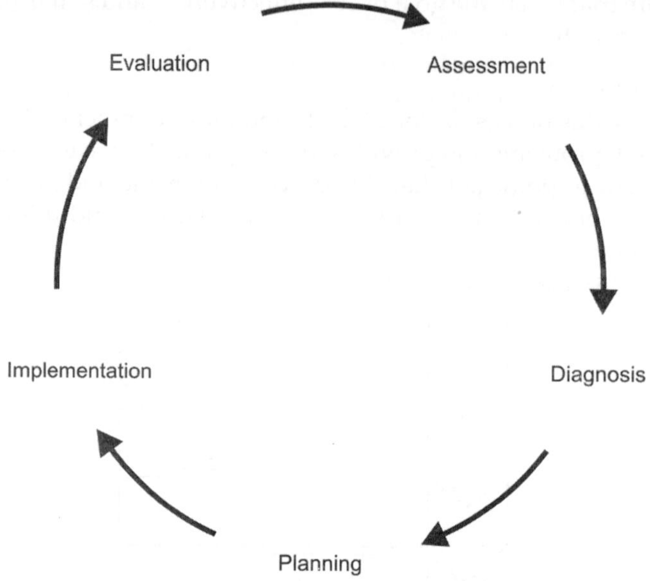

Fig. 1.8: Steps in nursing process

Implementing phase: The implementing phase is where the nurse follows through on the decided plan of action. This plan is specific to each patient and focuses on achievable outcomes. Actions involved in a nursing care plan include monitoring the patient for signs of change or improvement, directly caring for the patient or performing necessary medical tasks, educating and instructing the patient about further health management, and referring or contacting the patient for follow-up. Implementation can take place over the course of hours, days, weeks, or even months.

Evaluation phase: In this once all nursing intervention actions have taken place, the nurse completes an evaluation to determine of the goals for patient wellnesses have been met. The possible patient outcomes are generally described under three terms: patient's condition improved, patient's condition stabilized, and patient's condition deteriorated, died, or discharged. In the event the condition of the patient has shown no improvement, or if the wellness goals were not met, the nursing process begins again from the first step.

ETHICS IN PEDIATRIC NURSING

Introduction

Ethical issues permeate all interaction between physicians and patients. Nurses are most often the primary care providers whatever the setting and are therefore the first health come to become are of an ethical issue. In addition to understand the legal parameters of safe practice. The performance of nurse must ground her or his daily activities in a solid ethical foundation.

Ethics is the study of the nature and justification of principles that guide human behavior and that are applied when minor problems area.

Ethical principles

- Autonomy
- Justice
- Beneficence
- Nonmaleficence
- Veracity
- Fidelity
- Accountability
- Rights
- Right of self determination
- Right of privacy and confidentiality.

Ethical issues in child care:

- Refusal of treatments
- Informed consent
- Scare resources
- Ethical decision-making
- Ethical issues/dilemma
  - Autonomy
  - Competence
  - Beneficiary
  - Paternalism
  - Genetic testing
  - Autopsies of children
  - Organ donation and transplantation
  - Using children as subjects research
  - Children assent to treatments.

Ethical theories: Ways of thinking about ethical problems and issues all represented in a variety of theoretical positions of framework.

Normative ethics: It provides the standards to justify our moral actions and choices. Ethical issues is health care generally involve normative ethics.

Descriptive ethics: It differs from normative (or) that it seeks to identify actual preferences on dispositions in ethical situations as they occur. Descriptive ethics looks at what is actually done in any given ethical situation whereas normative ethics looks at what 'ought' to be done.

Four main groups of theory ball under the normative ethics.

1. ***Deontological theory:*** It uses principles or rules to guide the decision making process. The rightness or wrongness of acts is clear cut regardless of consequences. Duty to atheism is emphasized. This theory is regarded by some as the key theory to be used for ethical decision making.

2. ***Teleological theory:*** It uses the consequentiality approach to set criteria for justifying any moral action. The desired outcome serve as the basic norm the moral action rather than examining what should be done for example rationing of health cone may deprive some vulnerable groups such as develop mentally disabled children of the full array of health cone services, but it would serve the greater good by providing health care to longer, broader segment of the general populations.
3. ***Virtue theory:*** It looks at the content of the moral agent development of traits of character such as excellence truthfulness, gentleman, politician, and trust worth lead to appreciation of a situation and the resulting appropriate decision. An example the general public's response to nurse belonging unions asking fox contracts on going on strike.
4. ***Care theory:*** It incorporates advocacy or acting on the client's behalf based on empathy and caring. It kinds to use the individual needs ore concerns as the framework for ethical decision making.

Table 1.1: Ethical principles in pediatric nursing

Ethical principle	Definition	Example
Autonomy	The eight of client to freedom and self determination. As health care provides, nurses may not always agree with clients eight to make these choices.	Allowing a teen to refuse a home visit
Justice	Treating individuals equally or with fairness regardless of gender, ethnicity, and culture on socioeconomic states.	Provide care to children reg and less of the family is ability to pay for services.
Beneficence	Doing good for and to others in health care, competent care is the primary goal of health care providers and is thus viewed as the 'good'	Teaching a school-aged child about sports safety.
Nonmaleficence	Doing no harm to the client, it also evolves preventing harm to clients who are underage incompetent, non response we or unable in any way to protect themselves.	No leaving a pediatric client an all distress
Veracity	Telling the truth particularly in health care regarding diagnosis treatment or prognosis client cannot be misled or internationally delivered under this principle	Answering terminally all child is questions about his or her contents.
Fidelity	Keeping one's promise on word	Taking a pediatric client is the play room on a preschool day

Ethical decision-making: Ethical decision-making is a rational way on resoling ethical dilemmas in nursing practice. It is used in situations in which there are conflicts of rights and duties. It includes five step processes.

Step 1	Collect information about the situation
Step 2	Start the dilemma
Step 3	List all possible courier of action for resolution
Step 4	Analyze the advantages and disadvantages of each action
Step 5	Make the decision

- **Step 1:** It involves connecting information about the situation including client and family wishes and biopsychological problems and circumstances.

- **Step 2:** It entails stating the dilemma which should be done as quaintly as possible and a brief stalemate of the main ethical issues.
- **Step 3:** It consists of listing all possible courses of action to resolve this dilemma though results of these options are not considered at this point input from colleagues and experts is helpful at this brain staining stage.
- **Step 4:** It involves analysis of the advantages and disadvantages of each course of action.
- **Step 5:** Making the decision consequences of the decisions must be accepted and framed within the client's wishes and collaborators health team perfectives.

Role of nurse

- To educate the hospital staff on utilization of the ethics committee and basic issues involved in ethical decision-making
- To lead multidisciplinary discussion involving the team versus specific disciplines in ways to resolve conflict and classify values.
- To allocate resources quality outcomes are cost effective
- To document and disseminate the hospital's mission philosophy image and community identity
- To formulate policies related to ethical issues
- To consult and assured medical and other health care providers in difficult decisions.

ROLE OF PEDIATRIC NURSES IN CHILD CARE

Introduction

The pediatric nurse's role is unique because of developmental immaturity and vulnerability of children. The goals of nursing care of children, based on primary health care are:

- Promote the healthy maturation of the child as a physical, intellectual and emotional being within the context of his family and communities (primary level).
- Provide health care for the child who requires treatment from disease(s) (secondary level).
- Dealing with the child's disabilities (tertiary level). Therefore, the role of the pediatric nurse includes:

Different Role of Nurse in Child Health Care

- Primary caregiver
- Health teacher
- Nurse counselor
- Social worker
- Co-ordinator and collaborator
- Child care advocate
- Nurse manager
- Nurse recreationist
- Nurse consultant
- Nurse researcher.

Primary Caregiver

Pediatric nurses are providing basic care to children. Like hospitalized child Physical, Growth and developmental assessment, immunization, feeding. It should be focused on four concept of child health.

1. Preventive aspect of care
2. Promotive aspect of care
3. Curative aspect of care
4. Rehabilitative aspect of care

Health Teacher

A child health teaching is very basic duty for nurses since they are the ones responsible for monitoring the child as well as carry out the physician's discharge orders. She must be anticipating parent's doubts regarding improvement of their children's health status such as parenting and disease process so as to prevent future hospital admission as much as possible.

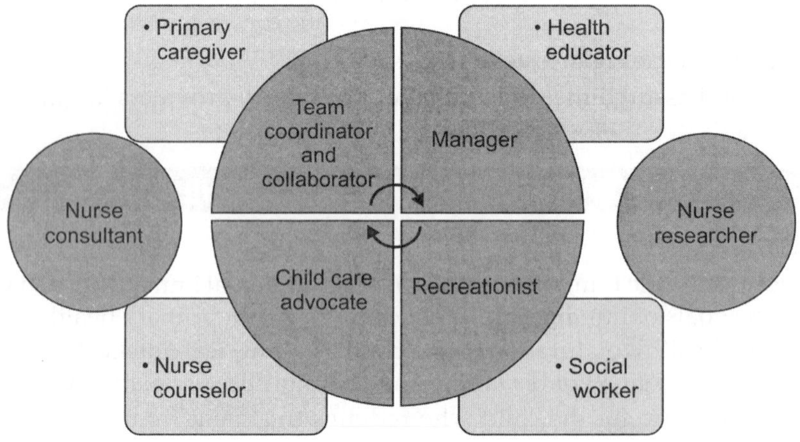

Fig. 1.9: Different role of nurse in child health care

Nurse Counselor

Providing guidance to parents in health hazards of children and health them for own decision making in different situations. Nurse counselor must be active listeners in order to establish a therapeutic relationship between parents and child, making health care plans easier.

Nurse counselor will be solving the parent's problem towards their child care. She helps the parents to take the independent decision for betterment of their child health care.

Social Worker

Pediatric nurse can participate in social services or refer child family to child welfare agencies for necessary support. In child health care, sometimes, pediatric nurse act as a social worker, try to reduce the social problems which is going to affect the child health. She should guide the parents related to child welfare agencies for improvement of child health.

Coordinator and Collaborator

Pediatric nurses are sometimes or most of the time works with other health care team members, where he or she is the avenue of important information that other health team members need in delivering competent care. So it is a must that pediatric nurses need to be a good information giver and communicator among health team members to promote a harmonious working environment.

There are many roles that a pediatric nurse could perform as health care settings evolved from one stage to another. The challenge lies behind the application of evidenced-based practice to provide competent care to children. Last but not the least, having a heart for children matters a lot when the work load at the area seems to be heavy – children could make you smile no matter how harsh the world could be.

Child Care Advocate

Pediatric nurses are expected to be sensible enough in voicing out the needs of their child and folks in behalf of them when it is impossible for them to readily address their needs. She can help the child and parents to receive the best quality of care from the hospital.

Nurse Manager

A pediatric nurse managers should help the child and parents by managing the nurses who care for them. While these nurses are mainly responsible for recruitment and retention of the nursing staff and overseeing them, they should be collaborate with doctors on child care, and help to assist child and their families when needed.

Nurse Recreationist

The pediatric nurse plays supportive role for the child to provide play facilities for recreation and diversion. It helps to decrease crisis imposed by illness or hospitalization.

Nurse Consultant

The pediatric nurse can act as consultant to guide parents and family members for maintenance and promotion of health. For example, Guiding parents about feeding practices, accident prevention, drowning and childhood poisoning.

Nurse Researcher

Pediatric nurse researchers are more important in pediatric nursing field for improvement of child health status. A change is constant in the health care setting, so it is must to practice evidenced-based practice. This means that pediatric nurses should have the ability to improve themselves in order to give updated care to children.

Level of Nursing Care in Child Health

Primary Level

Through heath education to child and his parents and providing child's basic needs and immunization, she can:

- Maintain child's health status
- Help the child achieves his optimal growth and development
- Prevent diseases condition and their complications.

Secondary Level

The nurse has to provide care to sick children and their families by:
- Assessing their needs
- Planning for their care
- Implementing the plan
- Evaluating children's condition
- Providing heath teaching to children and their parents.

Tertiary Level

The nurse should assist children to return to their maximal level of functioning following illness and/or disabilities.

Family Centered Care Approach

Family and child centered care is family oriented, yet individualized and co-ordinated, recognizing the worth of each person as a member of the family constellation. Health team should be flexible and creative in caring for the child within his family as their intervention are based on the needs of parent and child and on their coping resources.

Although the family is the ultimate coordinator of its own care, the nurse can help establish a positive environment for family members and help them accept and utilize the care provided. She can guide family members through the unknown of new experiences in seeking holistic health.

Parent Education

One of the major roles of the nurse is teaching both the child (according to his age) and his family members especially his parent. The nurse has many opportunities in providing health education to parents' daily either for child's parent alone or in-group (group teaching of parents and children).

Her education may be specific to information on:
- Growth and development needs
- Child's health promotion and maintenance as nutritional need and hygienic care
- Preventive aspects, such as, accident prevention, immunization, periodic examination
- Child's illness (nature of illness and care needs)
- Plan for child's discharge, such as, child's medication; follow-up, nutrition..., etc.

Job Description of Pediatric Nurse

- Assessing, observing and reporting on the condition of patients
- Preparing patients for operations and procedures
- Recording pulse, temperature and respiration and keeping accurate records of these observations
- Setting up drips and blood transfusions
- Maintaining and checking intravenous infusions
- Administering drugs and injections
- Assisting with tests and evaluations
- Responding quickly to emergencies

- Explaining treatment and procedures to enable parents/guardians to consent to treatment
- Supporting, advising and educating patients and close relatives
- Engaging in and promoting multidisciplinary teamwork, including working alongside specialist doctors and nurses, health visitors, social workers, radiographers and physiotherapists
- Observing strict hygiene and safety rules and ensuring that visitors also observe any rules on the ward or unit
- Writing reports and updating records before completing a shift.

EMERGING CHALLENGES IN PEDIATRIC NURSING

Introduction

The pediatric nurse practitioner role in the tertiary setting is one of several emerging roles gaining recognition in the various groups of advanced practice nursing programs today.

The advanced practice nurse (APN) who is a pediatric nurse practitioner (PNP) in an acute care setting helps to provide cost-effective, quality patient care for critically and chronically ill children.

Emerging Challenges in Pediatric Nursing

- Child welfare systems present particular challenges to the process of assessing health needs and the development and implementation of plans of care.
- A lack of coordination between the health care system and the child welfare system also interferes with the development of comprehensive health services for the children.
- The foundation of advanced practice nursing in this role incorporates the general role expectations of advanced nursing preparation, including case management, clinical pathway development, consultation and education, research, and collaboration, with the specific knowledge and skills of the pediatric nurse practitioner to function effectively with sick children in the acute care areas.
- The acute care nurse practitioner (ACNP) specializing in pediatrics is one of several new and emerging advanced clinicians being developed in nursing.
- Health promotion, disease prevention and anticipatory guidance are the hallmarks of nursing practice, particularly in pediatrics.
- Adolescence is a unique time of development incorporating a transition from child centered to adult centered health care.
- Constantly changing, expanding medical and nursing practice, emerging challenges in different aspects of child care, consumer demands, technology advancements, variation of roles/responsibilities remain the same.
- Interpersonal communication coordinates nursing care with disciplines, e.g. social workers.
- Promotion and maintenance of optimal family health to ensure cycles of optimal childbearing and childrearing.
- Affordability, high tech care, liability, and high cost of care for LBW babies, Access to care, inability to pay, lack of transportation , and dependent child care are barriers, health disparities.

- Rooming in family centered care.
- Legal issues related to consumer protection act malpractice and negligence are great challenges in all areas of nursing practices.
- Poverty and illiteracy are two big problems must overcome to improve the child health.
- Psychological problems among the children due to unhealthy competition, comparison, and single parents family.
- Disrupted communication among various care providers during the removal and placement process can easily lead to a health need for any child being unattended. Establishing protocols and development of collegial rapport with care providers is essential for successful management of the health needs of these children.
- Being able to meet children's health needs immediately after placement becomes complicated by multiple actors and modes of communication. Failure to meet a child's health needs stems from the failure to develop necessary rapport and effective communication among care providers.
- Childhood problems lead to frustrating and stressful situation. Nurse also must adjust and scope with those problems and develop tolerance of own feelings.

CONCEPT OF PREVENTIVE PEDIATRICS

Introduction

Pediatrics which is synonymous with child health is that branch of medical science that deals with the care of children from conception to adolescents, in health is scores pediatric and one of the first clinical subjects to link itself to preventive medicine recent years have witnessed further specialization within the bread field of pediatrics *viz* preventive pediatrics, social pediatrics, developmental pediatrics so on.

It has been defined as the prevention of desease and prostration of physical, mental and social well series of children with the aim of attaining a positive health. Preventive pediatrics aims at the prevention of disease in children rather than focusing on cure of disease. The child health care depends upon preventive care. Majority of the child health problems are preventable. Preventive pediatrics is a specialized area of child health comprises efforts to prevent rather than cure disease and disabilities.

There are three aspects of preventive pediatrics:

1. Social Preventive Pediatrics

It has been defined as the application of the principles of social medicine to pediatrics to obtain a more complete understanding of the problems of children in order to percent and treat disease and promote their adequate growth and development through organizes health structure.

To ensure adequate physical, mental and social growth of the child, total health needs should be provided as:

- Health and happy parents
- Balanced and nutritious diet
- Clean, healthful house is loving environment

- Developmental needs like play, relocation love and affection, safety and security recognition and companionship as emotional food
- Educational provisions is opportunities.

Prevention of disease can be best achieved through primary healthcare activities such as

- Growth monitoring
- Promotion of breastfeeding
- Oral rehydration
- Community feeding
- Immunization
- Nutritional surveillance
- Regular health checkups.

2. Antenatal Preventive Pediatrics

Care of the pregnant mothers with adequate nutrition, prevention of communicable disease, preparation of the mother for delivery, breastfeeding and mother craft trainings, etc. Pregnant health status of the mother also influences the child health promotion of health of girl child and nonpregnant state should be emphasized as the future mother who is soil and sold of future generations.

- Care of antenatal mothers
- Prevention of communicable diseases
- Preparation for delivery and breastfeeding
- Adequate nutrition
- Mother craft training.

Care of Antenatal Mothers

Antenatal care is the clinical assessment of mother and fetus during pregnancy, for the purpose of obtaining the best possible outcome for the mother and child.

To achieve this objective compulsory:

- Antenatal history collection
- Physical examination
- Screening text and assessment, including
- Biochemical investigation
- Hematological investigation
- Ultrasound scan (USG)
- Efforts are made to maintain maternal physical and mental well-being
- Prevent preterm delivery
- To anticipate difficulties and complications at delivery, ensure the birth of a live health infant.

Maternity care remains a mixture of both art and science, with advantages in medical technology now allowing us to focus more on the specific requirements of the mother and fetus, with an increasing drive towards the reappraisal of current practices.

The Essential Elements of Antenatal Care

- Identification and surveillance of the pregnant woman and her expected child
- Recognition and management of pregnancy-related complications, particularly pre-eclampsia
- Recognition and treatment of underlying or concurrent illness
- Screening for conditions and diseases such as anemia, STIs (particularly syphilis), HIV infection, mental health problems, and/or symptoms of stress or domestic violence
- Preventive measures, including tetanus toxoid immunization, de-worming, iron and folic acid, intermittent preventive treatment of malaria in pregnancy (IPTp), insecticide treated bed nets (ITN)
- Advice and support to the woman and her family for developing healthy home behaviors and a birth and emergency preparedness plan to:
  - Increase awareness of maternal and newborn health needs and self care during pregnancy and the postnatal period, including the need for social support during and after pregnancy.
  - Promote healthy behaviors in the home, including healthy lifestyles and diet, safety and injury prevention, and support and care in the home, such as advice and adherence support for preventive interventions like iron supplementation, condom use, and use of ITN.
  - Support care seeking behavior, including recognition of danger signs for the woman and the newborn as well as transport and funding plans in case of emergencies.
  - Help the pregnant woman and her partner prepare emotionally and physically for birth and care of their baby, particularly preparing for early and exclusive breastfeeding and essential newborn care and considering the role of a supportive companion at birth.
  - Promote postnatal family planning/birth spacing.

The Preconception Visit

The ideal first 'antenatal' visit is at a preconception clinic where health education and risk assessment can be directed towards the planned pregnancy. At that time the patient's general health and wellbeing can be fully assessed, rubella, hepatitis and HIV status can be established, and appropriate action taken where indicated. General advice regarding nutrition and lifestyle can be given at this time. Even a single antenatal nutritional education session during pregnancy has a significant effect on birth weight.

Advice can be given regarding the avoidance of teratogens, including those linked with excesses such as vitamin A, cigarette smoking, while ensuring an optimal dietary intake of folic acid. Following the demonstration that folate supplementation reduces the risk of a subsequent **Neural Tube Defect** by 72%, in those at high risk by virtue of a previous affected pregnancy, it is recommended that at least 0.4 mg folic acid is taken daily during the periconceptional period. Abnormal blood glucose control during the periconceptional period is associated with increased fetal complications and this is also an ideal time to ensure that such factors have been taken care of by sound dietary education and adjustment, and where necessary, medication.

Schedule of Visits During Pregnancy

The pregnant woman is seen by her general practitioner as soon as possible following the first missed menstrual period and after an initial assessment is referred on to the hospital for her first (booking) hospital visit between 8–14 weeks. Hospital referrals are increasingly instituted earlier nowadays, especially among the more health conscious older educated women, who may request screening tests for the early detection of fetal abnormality.

Previously the antenatal visits were: monthly until 32 weeks gestation, then fortnightly until 36 weeks, and weekly thereafter until delivery, resulting in up to 14 hospital visits during pregnancy. Although 'antenatal care' improves the outcome in terms of maternal and perinatal morbidity and mortality, there appears to be little difference in outcome between a four-visit schedule and a twelve-visit schedule. Currently the trend is towards reducing the number of attendance's, while at the same time establishing clearly defined objectives to be achieved at each visit.

The Mid-Trimester Risk Assessment Visit (20–24 Weeks)

The results of the tests performed at the first trimester visit and at 16 weeks are reviewed with the woman. The results of the ultrasound scan for fetal abnormality are also reviewed. In some centres, Doppler ultrasound screening of the uterine arteries is used to identify women at high risk of subsequent pre-eclampsia and intrauterine growth restriction is offered at this stage. Further care is then planned in line with risk assessment based on the ultrasound scan and other findings.

Antenatal Visits in the Second Half of Pregnancy

Assessment of maternal health and fetal growth and well-being are pursued through these visits, which can take place in the community setting. Any incidental maternal symptoms are dealt with. This period is also important in ensuring the education of the woman regarding the rest of pregnancy and her delivery. Contraception and plans for the birth should also be discussed from an early stage especially with regards to sterilization or other permanent contraception. This is in order to avoid unnecessary duress under emergency conditions if a cesarean operative delivery is decided upon during labor.

Antenatal Classes and the Familiarization Hospital Visit

During the antenatal visits informal education is provided for the pregnant woman and those supporting her through pregnancy. There are formal parenting (or parentcraft) classes organized in most units where the prospective parents are encouraged to discuss the pregnancy and delivery, and any apprehensions they may have. There are also usually sessions with others involved in their care to discuss topics like breastfeeding, pain management during the delivery etc. The common objectives of these formal educational sessions include the promotion of good health habits, allaying anxiety, increasing the feelings of control and satisfaction with the pregnancy and delivery by the mother, preparation for the postnatal period, infant feeding, and subsequent contraception.

Antenatal Visit with Hospital Team (Usually Around 36–38 Weeks)

The primary objective of this visit is to anticipate any problems regarding the prospective delivery. Several factors are considered, including the past obstetric history, e.g. a previous cesarean delivery for lack of progress in labor. Fetal malpresentation or malposition is sought because these may also indicate a high likelihood of operative delivery. With the increasing number of planned home births, the final place of choice for the delivery is also decided. This is also a good time to finalize the discussions on planned contraception after delivery, especially sterilization.

The Postdates Visits–Induction of Labor (41–42 Weeks)

At this visit a joint decision is taken as to whether an induction of labor is appropriate. This is current practice because of the reported association between postdates pregnancies and poor pregnancy outcome, particularly in order to prevent stillbirths due to the lack of an accurate, reliable test of fetoplacental reserve during those final few weeks of pregnancy. Induction of labor is usually performed by the 42nd week.

There are still two main methods of induction; amniotomy or surgical induction, and the medical methods using prostaglandin or oxytocin. When appropriately selected, there is a high probability of a safe uneventful vaginal delivery. If spontaneous labor does not occur by the 43rd week the likelihood of a Cesarean delivery is high, irrespective of the mode of onset labor. As the perinatal morbidity and mortality continue to rise at this stage, intervention is recommended.

Counseling

- Type and timing of antenatal information for all pregnant women
- Appropriate form of and setting for giving of information
- Antenatal classes
- Cultural and individual sensitivity
- Lifestyle considerations (working, nutritional supplements, infection prevention, use of medications, exercise, sexual intercourse, alcohol, tobacco or cannabis smoking, travel).

Evaluation/Screening

- Clinical examination of the pregnant woman
  - Measurement of weight and body mass index
  - Assessment of female genital mutilation
  - Assessment for domestic violence
- Prediction, detection and initial management of mental disorders
- Assessment of fetal growth and well-being
- Screening for hematologic conditions
- Screening for structural fetal anomalies or Down's syndrome
- Screening for infections
  - *Recommended:* Asymptomatic bacteruria, hepatitis B virus, HIV, rubella, syphilis
  - *Not recommended routinely:* Bacterial vaginosis, cytomegalovirus, group B streptococcus, hepatitis C virus, toxoplasmosis
  - *Referral for testing recommended as appropriate:* Chlamydia trachomatis.
- Screening for clinical conditions
  - Gestational diabetes in the presence of risk factors (screening using fasting plasma glucose, random blood glucose, glucose challenge test, and urinalysis not recommended)

 - Pre-eclampsia
 - Preterm birth (not recommended).
- Assessment of placenta previa, if appropriate.

Management

- Provision and organization of care
- Gestational age assessment
- Management of common symptoms (nausea and vomiting, heartburn, constipation, hemorrhoids, varicose veins, vaginal discharge, backache)
- Management of pregnancy after 41 weeks
- Management of breech presentation at birth.

Prevention of Communicable Diseases

Pregnant women are at risk for developing viral and bacterial infections. Infections are a particular concern during pregnancy since some infections are more severe in pregnant women or may harm the fetus or newborn. However, you can take steps to decrease the chance of developing a potentially harmful illness during pregnancy.

Types of common infection in pregnancy

- Cytomegalovirus infection (CMV)
- Toxoplasmosis
- Listeria
- Chickenpox and rubella
- Group B streptococcus
- Genital herpes
- HIV.

Immunization

Mother should be up-to-date on her immunizations before pregnancy. Some of the immunizations, such as

- TT
- Influenza
- Pertussis
- Hepatitis B, can and should be given during pregnancy.

Children and other family household members should also be up-to-date with their immunizations; this decreases a pregnant woman's risk of exposure to infections during pregnancy. Vaccine safety during pregnancy is discussed separately.

Hygiene

Pregnant women can get infections by person-to-person contact, such as:

- Kissing
- Sexual contact
- Handling another person's body fluids (e.g. saliva or urine)
- Touching their eyes, nose, or mouth.

Good hygiene practices, such as frequent handwashing and avoiding contact with another person's saliva through shared foods, drinks, or utensils, can lessen your chances of becoming infected with potentially harmful illnesses. Good hygiene is particularly important for pregnant women who have young children or work with them, as in day care centers or schools. Some potentially harmful infections, such as cytomegalovirus, are more prevalent in young children.

Handwashing

Handwashing is an essential and very effective way to prevent the spread of infection. Hands should be washed before and after preparing food and eating, after going to the bathroom, after changing a diaper or assisting a child with toileting, after wiping a young child's nose or drool, after handling garbage or dirty laundry, after touching animals or pets, after handling children's toys, after contact with another person's saliva, and after gardening or touching dirt/soil.

Hands should be wet with water and a plain or antimicrobial soap and then rubbed together for 15 to 30 seconds. Pay special attention to the fingernails, between the fingers, and the wrists. Rinse the hands thoroughly and, ideally, dry with a single use towel.

Alcohol-based hand rubs are a good alternative for disinfecting hands if a sink is not available. Spread hand rubs over the entire surface of hands, fingers, and wrists until dry. Hand rubs are available as a liquid or wipe in small, portable sizes that are easy to carry in a pocket or handbag. When a sink is available, visibly soiled hands should be washed with soap and water.

Food Precautions

Expert groups like the Food Safety and Inspection Services and the Centers for Disease Control and Prevention have guidelines for food safety for everyone, not just pregnant women.

Preparation for Delivery and Breastfeeding

The birth of baby is usually a happy occasion for expectant parents and their families. Since pregnancy and childbirth are a normal physiological process, the woman usually goes through the 9 month pregnancy expecting everything to be perfect at the end.

Preparation for Delivery

Admission to the birth center

The Decision to go to the Hospital or Birth Center during the last trimester, the woman needs to know when she should go to the hospital or birth center.

Factors to consider include:

- Number and duration of any previous labors, distance from the hospital, available transportation, child care needs, nurses instruct women to distinguish between false and true labor.
- Nurses teach guidelines for going to the birth center and reinforce those given by the physician or nurse midwife.

Nursing responsibilities during admission

- Establish a therapeutic relationship
- Assess the condition of the mother and fetus.

Establishing a therapeutic relationship

The nurse must quickly establish a therapeutic relationship with the woman and her significant other. The woman's first impression influences her perception of the quality of her entire birth experience.

A warm greeting makes the woman and her significant other feel valued. Even if the unit is busy, the nurse should communicate interest, friendliness, caring, and competence. People understand if the nurse is busy, but they do not understand rudeness and insensitivity to their needs. Nurses often encounter women who speak a language other than English. Arranging for a culturally acceptable interpreter who is fluent in the woman's language makes the woman and her family feels welcome and promotes safety because it enhances understanding among the woman, her family, and the nurse.

Role of Nurse in preparation of mother for delivery

- Making the family feel welcome
- Determining family expectations about birth
- Conveying confidence
- Assigning a primary nurse
- Respecting cultural values
- Prepare legal documentation.

Preparation for Breastfeeding

The nurse can provide information about, and support of, breastfeeding. The prenatal nurse can inform the mother of the advantages of breastfeeding to herself and her baby. The labor and delivery nurse can aid the mother in her first contact with the baby and reassure the mother who has a cesarean birth, or a premature or sick infant, that she too can nurse. The postpartum nurse can help breastfeeding to continue by providing frequent maternal-infant contact during the mother's hospital stay.

The nursery nurse supports breastfeeding by refraining from giving the baby other fluids. The pediatric nurse continues the helping pattern by reinforcing the statements and actions of others which will further impress the mother with the appropriateness of her infant feeding method.

Weight before pregnancy	1st trimester	2nd trimester	3rd trimester
110 lbs. (49.9 kg)	6 oz (ounce)	8 oz	8 oz
140 lbs. (63.5 kg)	7 oz	9 oz	9 oz
128 lbs. (58.1 kg)	7 oz	9 oz	9 oz
162 lbs. (73.5 kg)	8 oz	10 oz	10 oz

Mothers need to be informed about infant feeding options in order to make a knowledgeable choice based on awareness of alternatives. The nurse's role in support of breastfeeding varies with the time and place where patient care is provided. In each setting, however, the nurse plays a significant role in helping the mother to begin breastfeeding and to enjoy it, at the same time providing her infant with optimum nutrition for his early growth and development.

Adequate Nutrition in Pregnancy

Eating a healthy diet during pregnancy is one of the best food for mothers and baby. After all, the food pregnant women eating are her baby's main source of nutrition. Smart choices about pregnancy nutrition can help mothers to promote her baby's growth and development.

Grains

Grains provide essential carbohydrates, your body's main source of energy. Many whole-grain and enriched products also contain fiber, iron, B vitamins and various minerals. Fortified bread and cereal can help you get enough folic acid.

Make sure at least half of your grains each day are whole grains. If that sounds like a lot, do not worry. It might not be as much as you think. You can get most of your day's grains with a bowl of fortified cereal for breakfast, a lunchtime sandwich made with two slices of whole-wheat bread and whole-wheat pasta for dinner.

To optimize pregnancy nutrition, trade sugary cereals and white bread for whole-grain cereals, brown rice, whole-wheat pasta and whole-grain bread. Try wild rice or barley in soups, stews, casseroles and salads. Look for products that list whole grains, such as whole-wheat flour, first in the ingredients list.

Table 1.2: Suggested daily servings of grains for a woman age 25, 5'4"

Weight before pregnancy	1st trimester	2nd trimester	3rd trimester
110 lbs. (49.9 kg)	4 1/2 cups	5 cups	5 cups
140 lbs. (63.5 kg)	5 cups	5 1/2 cups	5 1/2 cups

Source: USDA Daily Food Plan for Moms, 2013

Fruits and Vegetables

Fruits and vegetables contain many important nutrients for pregnancy especially, Vitamin C and Folic Acid. Pregnant women need at least 70 mg of Vitamin C daily, which is contained in fruits such as oranges, grapefruits and honeydew, and vegetables such as broccoli, tomatoes, and brussel sprouts.

Fruits and vegetables are critical components of pregnancy nutrition, since they provide various vitamins and minerals, as well as fiber to aid digestion. Vitamin C, found in many fruits and vegetables, helps you absorb iron. Dark green vegetables have vitamin A, iron and folate other important nutrients during pregnancy.

Dairy Products

The calcium in dairy products and calcium-fortified soy milk helps build your baby's bones and teeth. Dairy products also have vitamin D and protein. Eat yogurt for your afternoon snack. Drink the milk in your cereal bowl. Have a glass of skim milk with dinner. Add low-fat cheese to a salad.

Meat, Poultry, Fish, Eggs and Beans

Foods in this group have plenty of protein, as well as B vitamins and iron. Protein is crucial for your baby's growth, especially during the second and third trimesters. Try whole-wheat toast with peanut butter for breakfast. Eat a scrambled egg or an omelet for lunch. Serve a salmon fillet for dinner. Add chickpeas or black beans to your salad. Snack on a handful of soy nuts.

Good Sources

Table 1.3: Suggested daily servings of fruits and vegetables for a woman age 25, 5'4"

Nutrition	Sources
Protein	Chicken, fish, beef, pork, turkey, tofu, nuts, legumes (beans), milk, eggs, cottage cheese, whole grains, wheat gluten, soy cheese
Whole grains	Brown rice, kasha (buckwheat groats), whole oats, whole wheat bread, whole grain cereals, quinoa, wild rice, wheat gluten, wheat germ, whole wheat pastas
Fruits	Strawberries, kiwi fruit, apples, oranges, bananas, mangos, cantaloupe, pears, grapefruit, plums, nectarines, and peaches
Green vegetables	Spinach, broccoli, zucchini, dark green lettuces, kale, Swiss chard, green beans, asparagus, arugula, lambs lettuce
Dairy	Milk, yogurt, hard cheese, cottage cheese, egg
Other good whole foods	Baked potatoes, sweet potatoes, carrots, squash, green peas, soy products, corn
Iron	Red meats, organ meats, eggs, fish poultry, blackstrap molasses, cherry juice, green leafy vegetables, dried fruits (raisins, apricots, etc.)
Zinc	Pumpkin seeds, squash seeds, sunflower seeds, seafood, organ meats, mushrooms, brewer's yeast, soybeans, eggs, wheat germ, meats, turkey
Folic acid	Spinach, asparagus, turnip greens, Brussels sprouts, lima beans, soybeans, organ meats, brewer's yeast, root vegetables, whole grains, wheat germ, bulger wheat, kidney beans, white beans, salmon, orange juice, avocado, milk

Sample Daily Menu

The following sample menu will give you some idea of what a pregnant woman should typically consume in a day for a healthy diet during pregnancy. Three small, but balanced, meals and three light snacks throughout the day are a good rule of thumb to ensure you and your baby's nutritional needs are met.

- *Breakfast:* Oatmeal cereal, banana, 1 slice whole wheat toast, 2 tsp jam, 1 cup skim milk
- *Snack:* 1 cup yogurt, grapes
- *Lunch:* Turkey and cheese sandwich on whole wheat bread, small bag potato chips, pear, and 1 cup skim milk
- *Snack:* Raw veggies and low calorie dip
- *Dinner:* 4 oz chicken, 1 cup wild rice, 1 cup veggies, 1 cup skim milk
- *Snack:* Fresh fruit or low-fat frozen yogurt

Mother Craft Training

This program is designed to provide basic information to individuals interested in providing child care in their own homes and in no way guarantees that the participant has achieved any level of child development knowledge usually determined through course examination. There is no admission requirement or assessment of participants, therefore Mothercraft cannot guarantee the level of understanding and knowledge acquired through attendance in the program.

3. Postnatal Preventive Pediatrics

Family Health Services

Child health depends upon the family's members, physical condition, social, economical and environmental conditions, which include family size, family income, standard of living, parent's educational status, culture, family custom, traditional habits, child bearing and child rearing practices, family relationship, family stability, etc.

Family health means the overall health of the individual family members; it is influenced by the interrelationship and interdependence of the physical and mental health status of the individual member of the family.

- Promotion of breastfeeding
- Introduction of complementary feeding is appropriate age
- Immunization
- Prevention of accidents
- Tender loving care with emotional security
- Growth monitoring
- Periodic medical supervision
- Health check-up
- Psychological assessment, etc.

Aims of family health service

- Reduction of material, infant and child mortality and morbidity rates
- Improvement of family planning practices and to ensure planned parenthood
- Improvement of nutritional status of all family members
- Increasing health accursedness through health education in all protective, premature curative and rehabilitative aspects of health care.

Subareas of family health

- Maternal and child health service
- Immunization
- Family welfare services
- Nutritional services
- Health education.

Factors influencing family health

Environmental factors

- Housing, sanitation
- Drinking center supply
- Pollution.

Economical factors
- Family income
- Family medical expenditure.

Educational factors
- Parent educational status
- Mother's education
- Level of education of other family members.

Social factors
- Culture
- Family customs
- Health status
- Food pattern
- Size of family
- Fertility rate, etc.

Maternal and Child Health Programme (MCH)

The Maternal and Child Health Care refers to broad and currently accepted approach of promotive, preventive, curative and rehabilitative health care for mother and child.

Maternal and child health (MCH) is an integral part of our efforts. We have worked to strongly advocate and place on the national agenda the issue that children have a basic right to live, and live well, and that this right should be recognized by both, the family and the state.

Objectives
- To reduce maternal, infant and childhood mortality, mobility
- To promote reproductive health
- To promote physical and psychological development of children and adolescents.

Components
- Surveillance of health of women from 15 to 45 years and of children during first year of life.
- Antenatal care of the first and subsequent pregnancy
- Intranatal, postnatal care of women
- Provision of family planning
- Care of child including the newborn
- Supplementary nutrition to child at risk and nutrition rehabilitation of the malnourished children.
- Educating men and women about small family norms, nutrition, and child care.

Target Population
- Services of all pregnant and lactating women and that reproductive age group
- All children below 5 years
- Population of about 30,000 the services are expected to be delivered to about 6000
- Children 4200 under five years.

The important elements of the programme

- Provision of antenatal care, including at least three antenatal care visits, iron prophylaxis for pregnant and lactating mothers, two doses of tetanus toxoid
- Vaccine, detection and treatment of anemia in mothers, and management and referral of high-risk pregnancies
- Encouragement of institutional deliveries or home deliveries assisted by trained health personnel
- Provision of postnatal care, including at least three postnatal visits
- Identification and management of reproductive tract infections, including sexually transmitted infections.

Implementation of MCH Programme

For away 5000 population in rural area and 3000 population in table area there is a sub-centre what fixed by day MCH clinics/immunization clinics conducted. Integrated child Development services ICDS. It was initiated by the govt. of India in the ministry of social and women's welfare in 1975.

Deliver Services

Supplementary nutrition: The Supplementary nutrition is given to children below 6 years.

Age	Calorie	Protein
Below 1 year	200 cal	8–10 gm
1–6 years	300 cal	15 gm
Pregnant	500 cal	25 gm

The supplementary nutrition given to children sufficing from 2nd and 3rd degree malnutrition, children suffering from 4th degree malnutrition are recommended hospitalization.

- Nutrition and health education
- Immunization
- Health check-up.

This include as antenatal care:

- Postnatal care and care of newborn
- Care of children under 5 years
- The health care of children under 6 years
- Record weight and height of children at periodical interval
- Watch over milk storage.

Reproductive and Child Health (RCH)

Introduction

The rapidly growing population had been a major concern for health planners and administrators in India since independence. The result was the launching of National Family Planning Programme by the Government of India. India was the first country to have taken up the family planning programme at the national level.

The Reproductive and Child Health (RCH) Programme was launched in October 1997. The main aim of the programme is to reduce infant, child and maternal mortality rates.

Objectives of the Programme

To improve the implementation and management of policy by using a participatory planning approach and strengthening.

- Institutions to maximum utilization of the project resources
- To improve quality, coverage and effectiveness of existing Family Welfare services
- To gradually expand the scope and coverage of the Family Welfare services to eventually come to a defined package of essential RCH services
- Progressively expand the scope and content of existing FW services to include more elements of a defined package of essential
- Give importance to disadvantaged areas of districts or cities by increasing the quality and infrastructure of Family Welfare services.

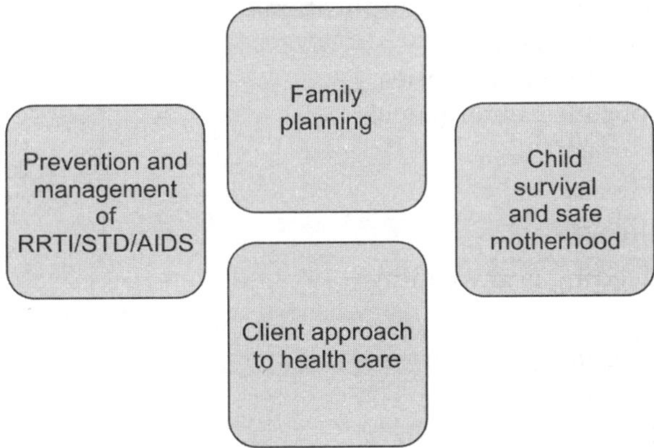

Fig. 1.10: Package of RCH programme

Aims of the Programme

- Expand services to the entire sector of Family Welfare beyond RCH scope
- Holding states accountable by involving them in the development of the programme
- Decentralization for better services
- Allowing states to adjust and improve programmes features according to their direct needs.
- Improving monitoring and evaluation processes at the district, state and the central level to ensure improved program implementation.
- Give performance-based funding, by rewarding good performers and supporting weak performers.
- Pool together financial support from external sources
- Encourage coordination and convergence, within and outside the sector to maximize use resources as well as infrastructural facilities.

Components of RCH Programme

- Integrated delivery of services for fertility regulation
- Maternal health
- Child health
- Safe abortions
- Nutrition
- Communication for behavior changes
- RTIs / STIs
- Adolescent health.

RCH Services

For the mothers:

- Tetanus Toxoid Immunization
- Prevention and treatment of anemia
- Antenatal care
- Early identification of maternal complications
- Deliveries by trained personnel
- Promotion of institutional deliveries
- Management of obstetric emergencies
- Birth spacing.

For the children:

- Essential newborn care
- Exclusive breastfeeding and weaning
- Immunization
- Appropriate management of diarrhea
- Appropriate management of ARI
- Vitamin A prophylaxis
- Treatment of anemia

For eligible couple:

- Prevention of pregnancy
- Safe abortion (MTP).

Other services:

- Services for Recognition and Referral of RTI/STIs.
  - Adolescent health
  - Involvement of male.
- Prevention and treatment of reproductive tract infection (RTI) and sexually transmitted diseases (STD).

Integrated Child Development Services (ICDS)

Introduction

The Integrated Child Development Services was launched on 2nd October 1975. Presently ICDS Scheme represents one of the world's largest and most unique programme for early childhood development. ICDS is the foremost symbol of India's commitment to children, India's response to the challenge of providing pre-school education on one hand and breaking the vicious cycle of malnutrition, morbidity, reduced learning capacity and mortality, on the other.

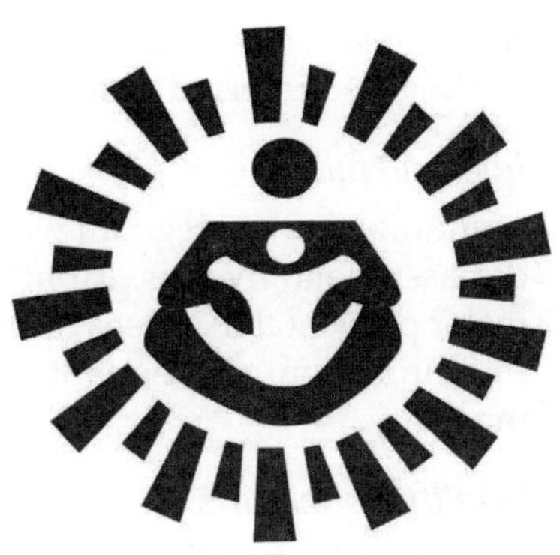

Concept of ICDS

The concept of providing a package of services is based primarily on the consideration that the overall impact will be much larger if the different services develop in an integrated manner as the efficacy of a particular service depends upon the support it receives from related services.

Objectives

The Integrated Child Development Services (ICDS) Scheme was launched in 1975 with the following objectives:

- To improve the nutritional and health status of children in the age group 0–6 years
- To lay the foundation for proper psychological, physical and social development of the child
- To reduce the incidence of mortality, morbidity, malnutrition and school dropout
- To achieve effective coordination of policy and implementation amongst the various departments to promote child development
- To enhance the capability of the mother to look after the normal health and nutritional needs of the child through proper nutrition and health education.

Services of ICDS

The above objectives are sought to be achieved through a package of services comprising:

- Supplementary nutrition
- Immunization
- Health check-up
- Referral services
- Preschool nonformal education
- Nutrition and health education.

Nutrition Including Supplementary Nutrition

This includes supplementary feeding and growth monitoring; and prophylaxis against vitamin A deficiency and control of nutritional anemia. All families in the community are surveyed, to identify children below the age of six and pregnant and nursing mothers. They avail of supplementary feeding support for 300 days in a year. By providing supplementary feeding, the Anganwadi attempts to bridge the caloric gap between the national recommended and average intake of children and women in low income and disadvantaged communities.

Growth Monitoring and nutrition surveillance are two important activities that are undertaken. Children below the age of three years of age are weighed once a month and children 3–6 years of age are weighed quarterly. Weight-for-age growth cards are maintained for all children below six years. This helps to detect growth faltering and helps in assessing nutritional status. Besides, severely malnourished children are given special supplementary feeding and referred to medical services.

Immunization

Immunization of pregnant women and infants protects children from six vaccine preventable diseases-poliomyelitis, diphtheria, pertussis, tetanus, tuberculosis and measles. These are major preventable causes of child mortality, disability, morbidity and related malnutrition. Immunization of pregnant women against tetanus also reduces maternal and neonatal mortality.

Health Check-ups

This includes health care of children less than six years of age, antenatal care of expectant mothers and postnatal care of nursing mothers. The various health services provided for children by anganwadi workers and Primary Health Centre (PHC) staff includes regular health check-ups, recording of weight, immunization, management of malnutrition, treatment of diarrhea, de-worming and distribution of simple medicines, etc.

Referral Services

During health check-ups and growth monitoring, sick or malnourished children, in need of prompt medical attention, are referred to the primary.

The anganwadi worker has also been oriented to detect disabilities in young children. She enlists all such cases in a special register and refers them to the medical officer of the Primary Health Centre/Subcentre.

Preschool Nonformal Education (PSE)

The Nonformal Preschool Education (PSE) component of the ICDS may well be considered the backbone of the ICDS programme, since all its services essentially converge at the anganwadi a village courtyard. Anganwadi Centre (AWC), a village courtyard is the main platform for delivering of these services.

These AWCs have been set-up in every village in the country. In pursuance of its commitment to the cause of India's Children, present government has decided to set-up an AWC in every human habitation/ settlement. As a result, total number of AWC would go up to almost 1.4 million.

This is also the most joyful play-way daily activity, visibly sustained for three hours a day. It brings and keeps young children at the anganwadi centre—an activity that motivates parents and communities. PSE, as envisaged in the ICDS, focuses on total development of the child, in the age up to six years, mainly from the underprivileged groups. Its programme for the three-to six years old children in the anganwadi is directed towards providing and ensuring a natural, joyful and stimulating environment, with emphasis on necessary inputs for optimal growth and development.

The early learning component of the ICDS is a significant input for providing a sound foundation for cumulative lifelong learning and development. It also contributes to the universalization of primary education, by providing to the child the necessary preparation for primary schooling and offering substitute care to younger siblings, thus freeing the older ones—especially girls—to attend school.

Nutrition and Health Education

Nutrition, Health and Education (NHED) is a key element of the work of the Anganwadi worker. This forms part of BCC (Behavior Change Communication) strategy. This has the long-term-goal of capacity-building of women—especially in the age group of 15–45 years—so that they can look after their own health, nutrition and development needs as well as that of their children and families.

The ICDS team members:

- Anganwadi Workers
- Anganwadi Helpers
- Supervisors
- Child Development Project Officers (CDPOs)
- District Programme Officers (DPOs)

Anganwadi worker, a lady selected from the local community, is a community based frontline honorary worker of the ICDS Programme. She is also an agent of social change, mobilizing community support for better care of young children, girls and women. Besides, the medical officers, Auxiliary Nurse Midwife (ANM) and Accredited Social Health Activist (ASHA) form a team with the ICDS functionaries to achieve convergence of different services.

International Partners of ICDS

Government of India partners with the following international agencies to supplement interventions under the ICDS:

- United Nations International Children' Emergency Fund (UNICEF)
- Cooperative for Assistance and Relief Everywhere (CARE)
- World Food Programme (WFP).

Recent Initiatives

The Ministry has recently initiated a process of consultations with the States and other stakeholders to review and identify gaps in the existing training system and make suggestions to strengthen the ICDS Training programme including its contents/syllabi, training methodology and the existing monitoring mechanism under ICDS training programme.

School Health Programme

Introduction

School Health programme is a program for school health service under National Rural Health Mission, which has been necessitated and launched in fulfilling the vision of NRHM to provide effective health care to population throughout the country It also focuses on effective integration of health concerns through decentralized management at district with determinant of health like sanitation, hygiene, nutrition, safe drinking water, gender and social concern. The School Health Programme intends to cover 12,88,750 Government and private aided schools covering around 22 Crore students all over India.

Rationale for School Health Programme

The school health programme is the only public sector programme specifically focused on school age children. Its main focus is to address the health needs of children, both physical and mental, and in addition, it provides for nutrition interventions, yoga facilities and counseling. It responds to an increased need, increases the efficacy of other investments in child development, ensures good current and future health, better educational outcomes and improves social equity and all the services are provided for in a cost effective manner.

The programme at the national level has been developed to provide uniformity/guidance to States who are already implementing or plan to implement their own versions of programme and to give guidance in proposing a coherent strategy for school health programme in next year's NRHM PIP to those States who have not yet started their programme.

Process Adopted for Developing the Programme

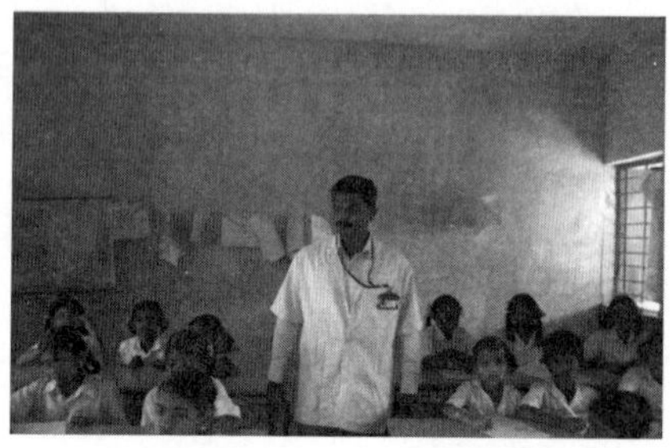

The decentralized framework of implementation under NRHM has enabled various states to devise and implement their own version of School Health Programme. A detailed study was undertaken through which the programmes being implemented in various States was documented. Through the analysis of the strengths and weaknesses of these programmes being implemented in various 2 States a broad strategy for the school health programme was developed. This strategy was shared in meeting chaired by HFM and attended by Secretary (HFW) apart from various other senior officers. The contours of the programme were shaped after this consultation.

Components of School Health Programme

Screening, health care and referral: The Screening of general health, assessment of Anemia/Nutritional status, visual acuity, hearing problems, dental check-up, common skin conditions, heart defects, physical disabilities, learning disorders, behavior problems, etc.

- Basic medicine kit will be provided to take care of common ailments prevalent among young school going children.
- Referral Cards for priority services at District/Sub-District hospitals.

Immunization

- As per national schedule
- Fixed day activity
- Coupled with education about the issue.

Micronutrient (Vitamin A and IFA) Management

- Weekly supervised distribution of Iron-Folate tablets coupled with Education about the issue
- Administration of Vitamin A in needy cases.

Deworming

- As per national guidelines
- Biannually supervised schedule
- Prior IEC
- Siblings of students also to be covered.

Health Promoting Schools

- Counseling services
- Regular practice of Yoga, physical education, health education
- Peer leaders as health educators
- Adolescent health education-existing in few places
- Linkages with the out of school children
- Health clubs, health cabinets
- First Aid room/corners or clinics.
  - Capacity building
  - Monitoring and Evaluation
  - Mid-Day Meal (see the national nutritional programme).

Management Structure for Effective Management

The management structure has been provided for in the guidelines at national, State and District levels. The NRHM convergence mechanism will apply to this programme as well. The involvement of MSG, State Health Mission and District Health Mission has been ensured by placing the school health programme management committees under the overall supervision/guidance of these overarching structures.

In addition, emphasis has been placed at making these management committees multi-departmental involving the functionaries of various related departments/organizations, such as Education, Rural Development, WCD, NACO, etc. Various School Health Promotion Committees recommended at State, District, Block and School levels is detailed in the enclosed write-up of the programme. School Health Coordinator on contract basis at the State and District levels has been provided to support the programme in the areas of coordination and monitoring and evaluation of programme.

Mid-day Meal Programme (Scheme)

Introduction

National Programme of Nutritional Support to Primary Education, popularly known as the Mid-day Meal Scheme (MDM) was started in 1995 in an attempt to enhance enrollment, retention and attendance while simultaneously improving nutritional levels among children in school. It currently covers nearly 12 crore children.

Objectives of the Scheme

- Improve the nutritional status of children in classes one through five in government schools and government aided schools

- To encourage children from disadvantaged backgrounds to attend school regularly and help them concentrate in school activities
- As well as provide nutritional support to students in drought- ridden areas throughout summer vacation.

Concept of Programme

The concept and the purpose of initiating anything is always good but when it comes to the management then we are miserable. The same thing has happened to Mid-Day Meal Scheme in India. It has been found by the Human Resource Development (HRD) ministry that most of the states are receiving complaints regarding the schemes but no one is acting on these complaints that are filed against the programme.

The programme is being carried out by local authorities with assistance from village panchayat, village education committees, school management committees, parent teacher associations, etc. In rural areas the cooking is being done by women self-help groups.

In urban areas, some NGOs have taken responsibility for cooking the food and bringing it to the primary schools. Free mid-Day meals can achieve a great deal with regard to child education and health.

They promote the participation of the child in school, reduce classroom hunger, facilitate the healthy growth of a child, promotes good eating habits like washing ones hands, finishing ones food, etc. and fosters social and gender equality as all children get the same food and must eat together.

Special Nutrition Programme (SNP)

The programme was launched in the country in 1970–71. It provides supplementary feeding of about 300 calories and 10 grams of protein to preschool children and about 500 calories and 25 grams of protein to expect at and nursing mothers for six days a week. This programme was operated under Minimum Need Programme. The programme was taken up in rural areas inhibited predominantly by lower socioeconomic groups in tribal and urban slums. Fund for nutrition component of ICD programme is taken from the SNP budget.

The target groups are:

- Children under 6 years
- Pregnant and lactating mothers.

The program is operated in the following locations:

- Urban slums
- Tribal areas
- Backward rural areas.

Supplementary nutrition is provided for 300 days every year

- Children under 6 years—300 kcal, 10–12 g protein
- Pregnant and lactating women—500 kcal, 25 g protein

Initially the programme was under the Central Government. The responsibility was later shifted to the state government under the Minimum Needs Programme. Now the special nutrition programme is integrated with the ICDS (Integrated Child Development Services).

Baby Friendly Hospital Initiative (BFHI)

Baby Friendly hospital initiative was launched in 1992 in India, as part of innocent declaration on breastfeeding the baby friendly hospital campaign was launched by the WHO/UNICEF in mid 1991 in Ankara to boost the breastfeeding practices and to counter the trend of bottle feeding and to counter the trends of bottle feeding 10 steps of successful breastfeeding as recommended by code of practice of WHO/UNICEF.

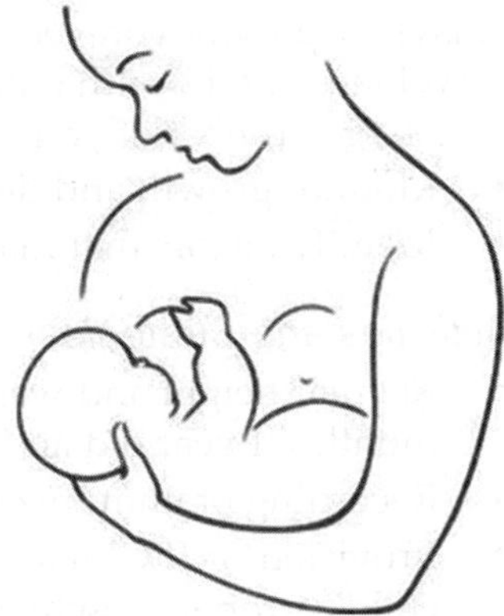

Fig. 1.11: Theme image of BFHI

- Have a written breastfeeding policy, that Is untimely communicated to all health care staff.
- Train all health care staff in skills necessary be implement this policy.
- Inform all pregnant women about the benefits and management of breastfeeding.
- Help mothers to ciliate breastfeeding in half an hour of birth.
- Show mother how to breastfeed and how to maintain lactabon even if they should be separated from their infants.
- Give newborn infants no food or drink other than breast milk, unless medically in indicated.
- Practice rooming in Allow mothers and infants to remain together 24 hours a day.
- Encourage breastfeeding on demand.
- Give an artificial treats of pacifiers to breastfeeding infants.
- Foster the establishment of breastfeeding support groups and refer mothers to them on discharge from the hospital or clinch.

Besides promotion of breastfeeding, baby friendly hospital initiative in India also proposes to provide:

- Improved antenatal care
- Mother friendly delivery services
- Standardized institutional support of immunization
- Diarrhea management
- Promotion of health growth and good nutrition
- Widespread availability and adoption of family planners.

Under-five Clinics

Introduction

The first five years of life form the foundations of the child's physical and mental growth and development. Studies have shown the mortality and morbidity are high among this age group. The Department of Health established the Under-Five Clinic Programme to address this problem.

Concept of Under-five Clinic

The concept of under-five clinic is derived from the well Baby clinic of the west for comprehensive health case of children below five years of the age.

Objective and Goals

This clinic provides preventive services along with health supervision, treatment, nutritional surveillance and health education. The services are economical within available resources for a large number of young children:

- Monitor growth and development of the child until 5 years of age.
- Identify factors that may hinder the growth and development of the child.

Activities and Strategies

- Regular height and weight determination/monitoring until 5 years old. 0–1 year old = monthly 1 year old and above = quarterly
- Recording of immunization, vitamins supplementation, deforming and feeding.
- Provision of IEC materials (ex. Posters, charts, and toys) that promote and enhance child's proper growth and development.
- Provision of a safe and learning – oriented environment for the child.
- Monitoring and Evaluation.

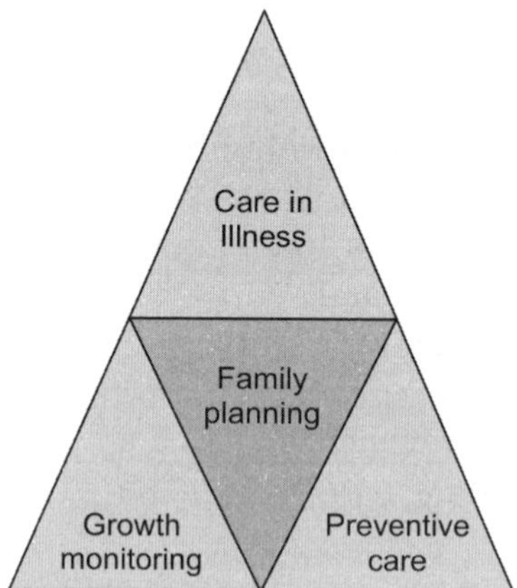

Fig. 1.12: Symbol of under-five clinic

Symbol of Under-five Clinic

The services provided by the clinic are set out is the symbol, which has been proposed for under five clinics in India. The apex of the large triangle represents care is illness, the left triangle represents adequate nutrition, the right triangle represents immunization and the central red triad represents family planning. The line bordering the big triangle represents health teaching to the mother.

Function

Care is illness: This is the felt need of the mother and child for which any child is brought to the clinic. The usual illnesses encountered in children under-five are fever, diarrhea, ARI, infections of the skin and helminthiasis. The facility should provide for essential laboratory investigations, X-ray facilities and referral services.

Preventive care: This involves primarily the immunization services during the 1st five years of life, vitamin A supplementation and administration of Iron supplementation and antihelminthic treatment to prevent anemia. The preventive care also provides for regular health check-up and use of ORS during diarrhea to prevent dehydration from developing.

Growth monitoring: This is one of the most important functions of the clinic. The child is weighed periodically – every month during the first year, every 2 monthly from 1 to 3 years of age and every 3 monthly in 4th and 5th years. Besides weighing, measuring height, mid arm circumference can also be carried out depending upon the availability of trained manpower and equipments. The growth is plotted on the growth chart and any faltering in the growth is detected and suitable action initiated.

Family planning: Family planning is central to any program directed towards women and children. The mothers are more receptive to family planning during early Puerperium and lactation. Mother is counselled on the various options available, their merits and de-merits so that she can make a choice. The months attending the clinic receives counseling with different aspects of family planning practices, which is a significant concern for the health and well-being of the child.

Health education: Health education to the other is an essential and compulsory activity of the under five–clinic. The mother should receive the information on various aspect of child care and child rearing practices prevent measures against malnutrition, ARI, diarrhea, tuberculoses worm infestations, etc. should be informed to the mother to improve averseness about the disease and its prevention.

Child Labor

The term **'child labor'** is often defined as work that deprives children of their childhood, their potential and their dignity, and that is harmful to physical and mental development. The child labor refers to the employment of children in any work that deprives children of their childhood, interferes with their ability to attend regular school, and that is mentally, physically, socially or morally dangerous and harmful. This practice is considered exploitative by many international organizations. Legislations across the world prohibit child labor.

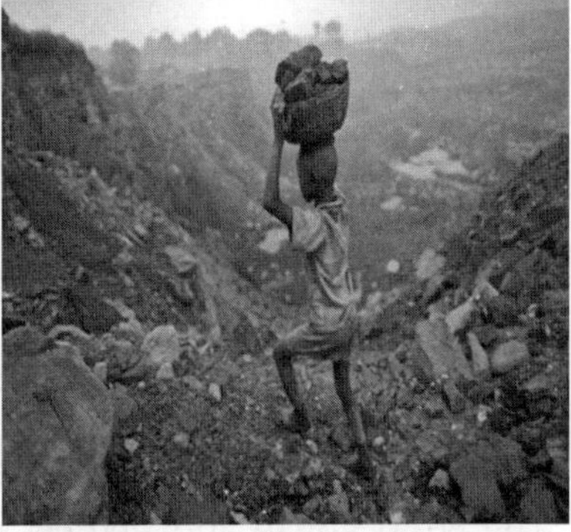

Fig. 1.13: Child labor below 14 years of children

Causes of Child Labor

- Primary causes
- Cultural causes
- Macroeconomic causes.

The factors affecting child labor

- Poverty
- Lack of education
- Unemployment
- Exploitation by selfish is lazy parents
- Bad company
- Beggar

- School dropout
- Maladjustment in the family
- Broken family
- Death of parents
- Child of unmarried pregnancy, etc.

Child labor is a social problem and needs special attention from all levels to eliminate the basic causes behind it. It is now difficult to abolish child labor in the present situation of our country but these children can be improved and regulated. Regular health cheek up and early detection of health problems with necessary treatment should be arranged for them.

While the Bonded Labour Liberation Front placed 10 million bonded children in India alone. In 1998 the government of India labelled bonded child labour as a marginal problem with only 3000 or so cases. A survey in Tamil Nadu in 1995 found 125,000 bonded child laboures in the state alone.

Child bonded labour in India is mostly in the agricultural sector but has in recent times been moving into other sectors as well, such as beedi-rolling, brick kilns, carpet weaving, commercial sexual exploitation, construction, fireworks and matches factories, hotels, hybrid cottonseed production, leather, mines, quarries, silk, synthetic gems, etc.

The Child Labour (Prohibition and Regulation) Act, 1986 is one the most debated acts regarding children in India. It outlines where and how children can work and where they cannot. The provisions of the act are meant to be acted upon immediately after the publication of the act, except for part III that discusses the conditions in which a child may work. Part III can only come into effect as per a date appointed by the Central Government (which was decided as 26th of May, 1993).

Child Abuse and Neglect

Definition

Child abuse is the physical, sexual or emotional maltreatment or neglect of a child or children.

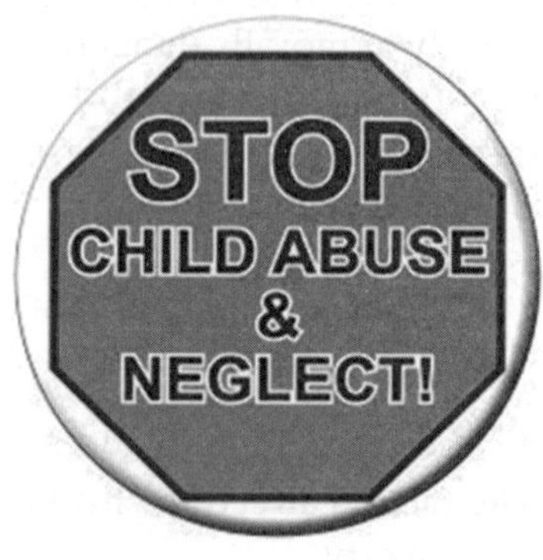

Risk Factors for Child Abuse and Neglect

The child abuse and neglect occurs in all types of families even in those that look happy from the outside children are at a much greater risk in certain situations.

- Domestic violence
- Alcohol and drug abuse
- Untreated mental illness
- Lack of parenting skills
- Stress and lack of support.

Types

- Physical abuse
- Psychological abuse

- Sexual abuse
- Maltreatment with negligence
- Maternal deprivation

Physical Abuse

Physical abuse involves physical harm or injury to the child. It may be the result of a deliberate attempt to hurt the child, but not always. It can also result from severe discipline, such as using a belt on a child, or physical punishment that is inappropriate to the child's age or physical condition.

The physically abusive parents and caregivers insist that their actions are simply forms of discipline ways to make children learn to behave. But there is a big difference between using physical punishment to discipline and physical abuse. The point of disciplining children is to teach them right from wrong, not to make them live in fear.

Psychological Abuse

The emotional abuse can severely damage a child's mental health or social development, leaving lifelong psychological scars. Examples of emotional child abuse include:

- Constant belittling, shaming, and humiliating a child
- Calling names and making negative comparisons to others
- Telling a child he or she is 'no good,' 'worthless,' 'bad,' or 'a mistake'
- Frequent yelling, threatening, or bullying
- Ignoring or rejecting a child as punishment, giving him or her the silent treatment
- Limited physical contact with the child—no hugs, kisses, or other signs of affection
- Exposing the child to violence or the abuse of others, whether it be the abuse of a parent, a sibling, or even a pet.

Warning signs of child abuse and neglect

The earlier child abuse is caught, the better the chance of recovery and appropriate treatment for the child. Child abuse is not always obvious. By learning some of the common warning signs of child abuse and neglect, pediatric nurse can catch the problem as early as possible and get both the child and the abuser the help that they need.

Warning signs of emotional abuse in children

- Excessively withdrawn, fearful, or anxious about doing something wrong
- Shows extremes in behavior (extremely compliant or extremely demanding; extremely passive or extremely aggressive)
- Does not seem to be attached to the parent or caregiver
- Acts either inappropriately adult (taking care of other children) or inappropriately infantile (rocking, thumbsucking, throwing tantrums).

Warning signs of physical abuse in children

- Frequent injuries or unexplained bruises, welts, or cuts
- It is always watchful and 'on alert,' as if waiting for something bad to happen

- Injuries appear to have a pattern, such as marks from a hand or belt
- Shies away from touch, flinches at sudden movements, or seems afraid to go home
- Wears inappropriate clothing to cover up injuries, such as long-sleeved shirts on hot days.

Warning signs of neglect in children

- Clothes are ill-fitting, filthy, or inappropriate for the weather
- Hygiene is consistently bad (unbathed, matted and unwashed hair, noticeable body odor)
- Untreated illnesses and physical injuries
- It is frequently unsupervised or left alone or allowed to play in unsafe situations and environments
- It is frequently late or missing from school.

Warning signs of sexual abuse in children

- Trouble walking or sitting
- Displays knowledge or interest in sexual acts inappropriate to his or her age, or even seductive behavior
- Makes strong efforts to avoid a specific person, without an obvious reason
- Does not want to change clothes in front of others or participate in physical activities
- An STD or pregnancy, especially under the age of 14
- Runs away from home.

Management

The first step is to provide a safe environment to prevent further harm. The sooner this happens, the better the child's chance for physical and emotional recovery. This includes separating the child, as well as any other children in the household, from the person suspected of abuse.

Any physical injuries will be treated, either in a hospital or at a doctor's office, depending on how serious they are.

Counseling is always recommended for abused or neglected children. It usually focuses on:

- How they feel about themselves
- Their past experiences
- Fears and concerns they may have about the present and future
- For very young children, counseling may involve play therapy.

Treatment for parents or caregivers

Parents or caregivers who have abused or neglected a child also need treatment. The type of treatment depends on the specific abuse that occurred. Some people need to learn more about how to raise and care for children. Others may need treatment for other serious problems, such as:

- Drug or alcohol abuse
- Depression or other mental health problems
- Low self-esteem
- Violent behavior.

Gender Bias

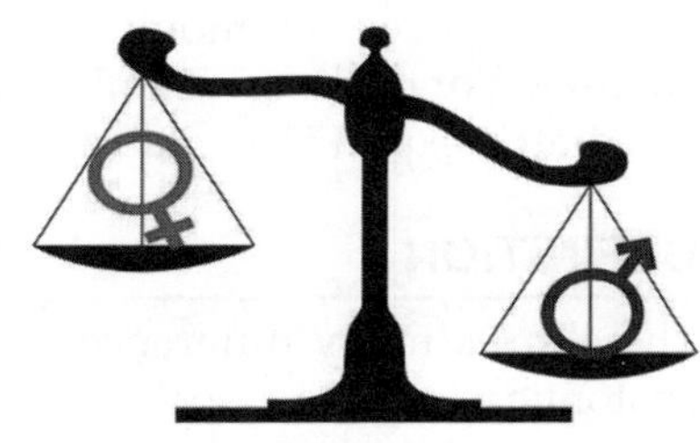

Gender equity refers to the equal valuing of males and females and equal opportunities for life and work regardless of gender. Since the Universal Declaration of Human Rights by the United Nations in 1948, gender equity has been accepted as a fundamental principal of human rights. Promoting gender equity is about working for fairness in relationships between males and females and being alert to the ways that gender may create inequality.

The purpose of promoting gender equity in child care services is to create equitable and enriching lives for all children. To achieve this child care professionals can work to identify inequities for boys and girls, and plan to overcome these through an ongoing process of self-reflection, observation, planning and evaluation.

National Health Programmes for Children in India

Various national health programmes are currently in operation for the improvement of child health and prevention of child hood diseases.

- Reproductive and Child Health Programme (RCH)
- Universal Immunisation Programme (UIP)
- Intensified Pulse Polio Immunization (PPI)
- Integrated Child Development Services Scheme (ICDS)
- School Health Programme (SHP)
- Nutritional Programme (AIP)
  - Mid-Day Meal Programme
  - Special Nutrition Programme
  - Nutritional Blindness Prevention Programme.

Nursing Responsibilities in Preventive Pediatrics

- Creating awareness
- Provide appropriate antenatal mothers care
- Adequate intranatal care
- Promoting breastfeeding
- Nutrition education
- Promoting community hygiene
- Promoting self-care attitude
- Participating and contributing in the planning of child health programmes.

DIFFERENCES BETWEEN CHILDREN AND ADULT

INTRODUCTION

The anatomical, physiological, developmental, and psychological differences between children and adults require that special resources (e.g. medications, equipment, and protocols) be available to ensure appropriate pediatric care in a disaster or an emergency. Many resources commonly used for treating adults will not be appropriate for treating children. For this reason, unless absolutely necessary, do not begin specific treatment until a pediatric expert is available to provide guidance.

DEFINITION

There are a many differences between children, adolescents and adults—physiological, anatomical, cognitive, social and emotional—which all impact on the way illness and disease present in children and young people, as well as the way healthcare is provided.

PURPOSE OF DIFFERENTIATING ADULT AND CHILD

- Pediatric treatment for biologic agents: Antibiotic contraindications and immunization difficulties
- Pediatric treatment for chemical events
- Pediatric treatment for radiologic events
- Triage protocols
- Caring for children separated from their families/guardians
- Pediatric decontamination

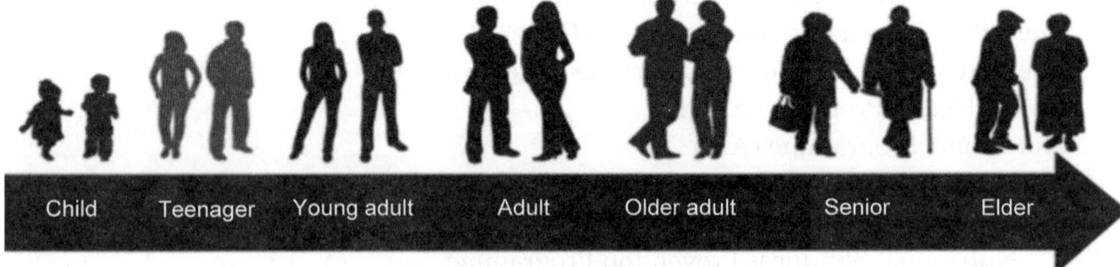

Fig. 1.14: Developmental stages

ANATOMICAL/PHYSIOLOGICAL DIFFERENCE

- **Larger BSA:** Children have a proportionately larger body surface area (BSA) than adults do. The smaller the patient, the greater the ratio of surface area (skin) to size. As a result, children are at greater risk of excessive loss of heat and fluids; children are affected by more quickly and easily toxins that are absorbed through the skin.
- **Thinner skin:** Children have thinner skin than adults. Their epidermis is thinner and under-keratinized, compared with adults. As a result, children are at risk for increased absorption of agents that can be absorbed through the skin.
- **Rapidly dividing cells:** Children's cells divide more rapidly than adults to assist in their rapid rate of growth. As a result, children are more susceptible to the effects of radiation than adults.
- **Higher heart rate (HR) and respiratory rate (RR)**: Children have higher respiratory rates than adults. Higher respirator rates lead to proportionately higher minute volumes. As a result, children may be more susceptible to agents absorbed through the pulmonary

route than adults with the same exposure. Children may also respond more rapidly to such agents. Signs and symptoms in children may be an 'early warning' of a chemical, biological, or radiological incident.

- **Immature blood brain barrier**: Children have immature blood-brain barriers and enhanced central nervous system (CNS) receptivity. As a result, children may exhibit a prevalence of neurological symptoms. Nerve agents may produce more symptoms in pediatric patients, requiring levels of treatment for children that are not indicated for adults with the same level of exposure.

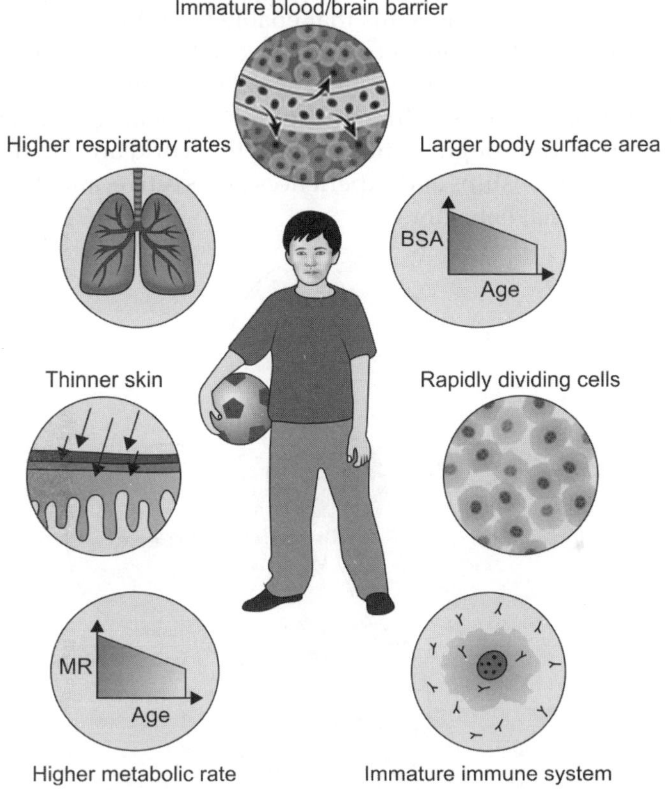

Fig. 1.15: Adult and pediatric systems difference

- **Higher metabolic rate (MR)**: More susceptible to contaminants in food or water; greater risk for increased loss of water and when ill or stressed. Medication doses must be carefully calculated based on the child's weight and body size.
- **Immature immune systems:** Greater risk of infection; less hard immunity from some infections.

PSYCHOSOCIAL DIFFERENCES

Although adults continue to develop psychosocially, their values/behavior/social circles are generally far more defined and stable, whereas children and adolescents are rapidly developing and using the world around them and picking up cues from their environment to aid in that development. It is essential to be mindful of the way clinicians interact and communicate with children, adolescents and their families as they play a role in this development, and to be well aware of the broader context of a child or adolescent's life, as this has a much more significant impact on the way they experience and recover from illness or injury.

SOCIAL DIFFERENCES

The adult, children and adolescents are still in a period of social development which involves learning the values, knowledge and skills that enable them to relate to others. The goal is for children and adolescents to build a positive sense of their own identity and their role in relationships with people around them. These social skills and lessons can be learnt from those who care for them, as well as indirectly through negotiating social relationships with family or with friends, and through participation in the world around them, e.g. coming to hospital. Not of these relationships and experiences are positive, and the impact of negative influences also shapes social behaviors.

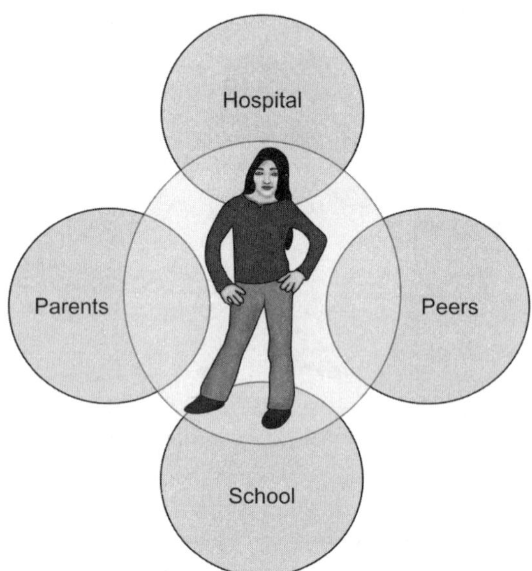

Fig. 1.16: Social difference

Hospitals and their staff can be part of a child/families social environment and therefore it is important for clinicians to be mindful of how they conduct themselves in their social or professional relationships with a child's family and toward the child and adolescent themselves, as this has an impact on learning and development of their own social identity. It is also important to be mindful of different circumstances which shape social skills during the developmental process and influence behaviors and interactions with other people. Children and to a lesser extent adolescents, typically present more explicitly with their immediate social circle shown to the clinician with the presentation of parents, grandparents, aunts and uncles, etc. at appointments.

EMOTIONAL DIFFERENCES

Children and adolescents are still developing their ability to recognize and manage their emotions or feelings, and this can be influenced by many social and environmental factors. For infants and young children, their emotional bond of affection or 'attachment' to their caregivers is crucial to their emotional development.

Effects of Secure Attachment

- More resilient, competent toddlers with high self-esteem
- In preschool display more persistence, curiosity, self-reliance, leadership and have better peer relations
- After age 11—better social skills, > close friends.

Clinicians in a pediatric setting should be mindful of the disruption to this bond that may result in separation anxiety which is emotional distress seen in many infants when they are separated from people with whom they have formed an attachment. They should also be mindful that not all children and adolescents will come from an environment where they will have the consistency and stability in their everyday lives to allow them to form secure attachments, and this may be reflected in their coping and behavior.

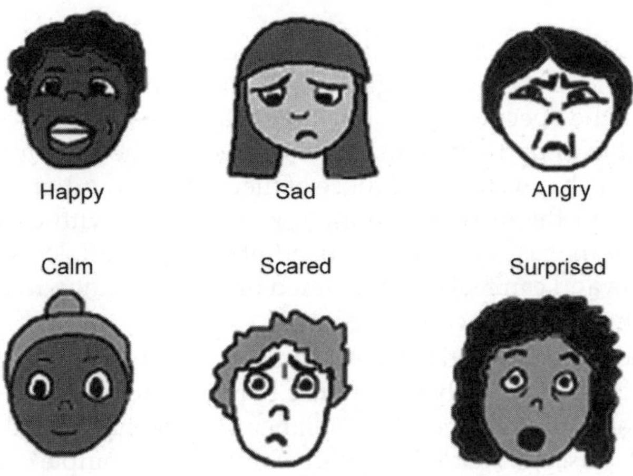

COGNITIVE DIFFERENCES

The growth of thought in children more so that in an adult environment, a clinician must be mindful of how they communicate with a patient, taking into account a child or adolescent's level of cognitive development.

Examples:

- **Example for a younger child:** Four year old Susan was asked where she got her name.
  - She answered, 'My mummy named me',
  - 'What if your mother called you Jack?'
  - 'Then I'd be a boy'
- Example for an older child:

Concrete: 'You said I'd get it if I missed my asthma inhalers, but I forgot them twice and I stayed fine so I don't need them anymore'

Abstract: 'I missed my inhalers a couple of times but I think I got away with it because I wasn't doing much exercise. I think I'll still need them in the future if I'm doing lots of exercise or in cold weather'.

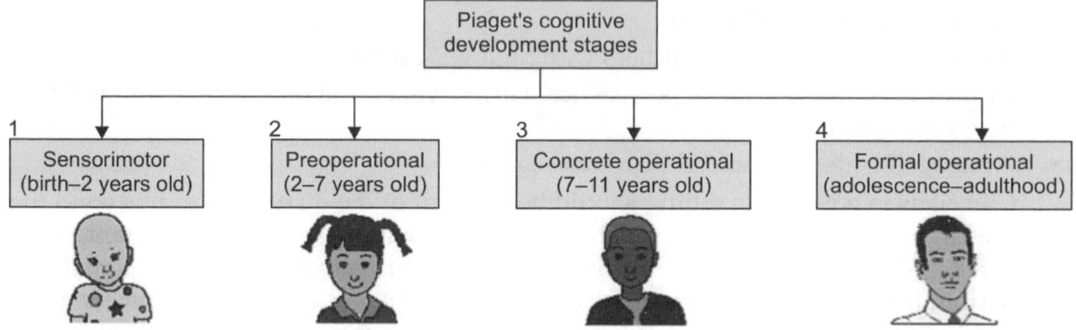

Fig. 1.17: Cognitive development

ADOLESCENCE

This is important to not only acknowledge the differences in a child *vs* adult population but also adolescence and the specific developmental challenges that it presents. Adolescents are generally more able to participate in decision-making about their own care, and have opinions and views which can challenge those of their families and/or health care providers so it is necessary to find the most appropriate way to work with each adolescent on an individual basis. This is the case in a pediatric or adult setting, as adolescents can often be seen in adult environments and can feel overwhelmed or insignificant without the opportunity to participate in their own health care decisions.

Adolescents can be more inclined to be experimental and take part in high-risk behaviors which impact on their health and their response to intervention. Adolescents and children are also more vulnerable as a result of their reliance on others to meet their different needs, and they can be more susceptible to the negative impacts of complex social situations and exploitation as they are not yet fully developed or independent. These factors can have a major impact on their presentation and behaviors, and are also a major factor in planning for discharge/future health care and wellness.

Adolescents will eventually transition to adult health care environments, which can be a vastly different environment with new challenges and staff. It is important to help adolescents prepare for this transition by taking more responsibility for their own health care and enable them to negotiate their way through this new environment.

ROLE OF NURSE

Present with illness differently, so people working with children need the skills and knowledge to identify and diagnose illness in a child or adolescent, and be aware of illnesses specific to different age groups.

- Often require different treatment or approaches to treatment, so require specific age-appropriate treatment approaches and environments (where possible).

Children and Adults Health Programs

- Children and adolescents come with families, who generally have a greater role in their well-being, so health professionals need to work with family as well as the patient.
- Activities are different for different ages—play becomes less important with age, but the need for stimulation and employment in other activities remains important. School in older children and adolescents moving towards work for older adolescents and adults.

Children and adolescents are still developing, so their responses to similar situations will be different and experiences they have will impact on their future development.

As well as the more obvious physiological and cognitive differences between children and adults, working with children and adolescents requires the consideration of future development—physical, social, emotional cognitive—as of primary importance. The needs to be aware of the context in which a child or adolescent lives and functions are crucial for both the provision of appropriate management as well as planning for meet the future health care demands.

VITAL STATISTICS RELATED TO PEDIATRICS AS PER THE NRHS AND GOI

Introduction

Vital statistics are statistics on live births, deaths rate, fetal deaths rate, marriages and divorces. The most common way of collecting information on these events is through civil registration, an administrative system used by governments to record vital events which occur in their populations.

The number of births and deaths can be obtained by enumeration at certain points in time (e.g. censuses and surveys), civil registration collects this information on a continuous basis and is the only source that provides individuals with a legal document.

United Nations Children's Fund (UNICEF) and a number of non-governmental organizations (Plan International, Save the Children Fund, World Vision, etc.) have particularly promoted the human rights aspects of registration, while the United Nations Statistics Division (UNSD), United Nations Population Fund (UNPF) and World Health Organization (WHO) have focused more on the statistical aspects of civil registration.

Vital registration systems that include medical certification of the cause of death captured about 18.8 million deaths of an estimated annual total of 51.7 million deaths in 2005, which is the latest year for which the largest number of countries reported deaths from a vital registration system.

Even for these deaths, the comparability of findings on the leading causes of death is affected by variation in certification skills among physicians, the diagnostic and pathological data available at the time of completing a death certificate, variations in medical culture in choosing the underlying cause, and legal and institutional frameworks for governing mortality reporting.

India has been at the forefront of the global effort to reduce child mortality and morbidity. Its continuous commitment and ongoing efforts have resulted in a 59% reduction in under-5

(U5) child mortality since 1990. India has proven, that it can reach even the most hard-to-reach and vulnerable Children with affordable life-saving interventions, as also is evident from its polio eradication strategies.

The Government of India (GOI)

The GOI recognizes child survival and development as essential for the overall development of the society. This is reflected in its policies committed to providing adequate services for children before and after birth and throughout childhood to facilitate their full physical, mental, and social development. India contributes more than any other country to global under-5 and newborn deaths.

Despite considerable strides, progress within India has not been uniform, i.e. reduction in neonatal mortality lags behind reduction in postneonatal deaths.

- The demographic and cultural diversity, India does face numerous challenges with significant such as:
- Rural-urban
- Poor-rich
- Gender
- Socioeconomic
- Regional differences.

In India more girls than boys are dying, and newborns delivered in rural setting are twice as likely to die as those born in urban areas. Furthermore, neonatal mortality varies considerably between states and regions.

The four large states of Uttar Pradesh, Bihar, Madhya Pradesh, and Rajasthan together account for more than half of the country's neonatal mortality, which accounts for about 14% of global newborn deaths. Newborn health has captured the attention of policymakers at the highest level in India.

This has resulted in strong political commitment to end preventable newborn deaths and stillbirths, and recognize newborn health as a national development necessity.

In this regard, the **GOI** is building on a series of efforts, policy Introduction INAP: India Newborn Action Plan 19 decisions and programmes introduced over the past two decades to address maternal and newborn health. Major milestones so far include: launch of the Child Survival and Safe Motherhood Programme (CSSM) in 1992.

Reproductive and Child Health Programme Phase I (RCH I) in 1997, followed by RCH II in 2005; the National Rural Health Mission (NRHM) in 2005 which, along with the National Urban Health Mission, became part of the National Health Mission in 2013; the Call to Action for Child Survival and Development, and the subsequent Reproductive, Maternal, Newborn, Child and Adolescent Health (RMNCH+A) strategic framework in 2013.

National Rural Health Mission (NRHM)

Progress since the Launch of the National Rural Health Mission (NRHM) – 2005

- Janani Suraksha Yojana (JSY) has increased the number of women delivering in public health facilities to 107 lakhs each year.
- 470 new maternal and child health wings (30/50/100 bedded) have been sanctioned in the public health system, adding more than 28,000 beds.

- A nationwide network of facility-based newborn care has been established at various levels: 14,135 Newborn Care Corners at the point of child birth; 1,810 Newborn Stabilization Units; 548 Special Newborn Care Units (SNCUs) for sick and small newborns, with care to more than 6 lakhs newborns being provided in SNCUs each year.
- Janani Shishu Suraksha Karyakram (JSSK) has entitled all pregnant women and infants to free delivery, drugs, diagnostics, treatment, food, and transportation to and from facilities.
- 38,300 public health facilities constructed/ upgraded and more than 20,000 ambulances have been sanctioned.
- The total number of technical HR supported under NRHM increased to 3.45 lakhs which includes 30,429 doctors/specialists including AYUSH doctors, 38,421 staff nurses, 21,965 para-medics and 2.39 lakhs ANMs.
- Incentivized Home-Based Newborn Care programme has been launched in 2011: 8.95 lakhs ASHAs selected and more than 6 lakhs ASHAs trained to improve newborn practices at the community level; early detection and referral of sick newborn babies by making home visits as per schedule during the first 42 days after birth.

India Newborn Action Plan (INAP)

The India Newborn Action Plan (INAP) is India's committed response to the Global Every Newborn Action Plan (ENAP), launched in June 2014 at the 67th World Health Assembly, to advance the Global Strategy for Women's and Children's Health.

INAP lays out a vision and a plan for India to end preventable newborn deaths, accelerate progress, and scale up high-impact yet cost-effective interventions. INAP has a clear vision supported by goals, strategic intervention packages, priority actions, and a monitoring framework. For the first time, INAP also articulates the Government of India's specific attention on preventing stillbirths. INAP is guided by the principles such as:

- Integration
- Equity
- Gender
- Quality of care
- Convergence
- Accountability
- Partnerships.

It includes six pillars of intervention packages across various stages with specific actions to impact stillbirths and newborn health.

The six pillars are:

1. Preconception and antenatal care
2. Care during labour and child birth
3. Immediate newborn care
4. Care of healthy newborn
5. Care of small and sick newborn
6. Care beyond newborn survival.

The India Newborn Action Plan is a concerted effort towards translating commitments into meaningful change for newborns. It will serve as a framework for the States to develop their area-specific action plans.

Morbidity and Mortality

Morbidity

The word morbid is related to sickness and disease. As a concept, morbidity can be applied to an individual (e.g. someone with diabetes) or to a population in the form of a morbidity rate (e.g. the incidence of seasonal flu). There is also comorbidity, which refers to two or more illnesses affecting an individual at the same time. For example, gout is often comorbid with diabetes.

Mortality

All humans are mortal, subject to death. A 'crude death rate' the total number of deaths in a year, per 1,000 individuals can be used to see how many people are dying in the world. This rate is often paired with those used to calculate the number of people being born (e.g. crude birth rate), so as to estimate the total living human population on the planet.

Mortality rates	Death rates
Infant Mortality Rate	Crude Death Rate
Neonatal Mortality Rate	Age-Specific Death Rate
Postneonatal Mortality rate	Cause-Specific Death Rate
Perinatal Mortality Rate	Age-Adjusted Death Rate
Fetal Mortality Rate	
Maternal Mortality Rate	

Neonatal Mortality Rate (NMR)

India has witnessed a significant reduction in the number of neonatal deaths from 1.35 million in 1990, to around 0.76 million in 2012. Over that period, from 1990–2012, while neonatal deaths reduced by 44%, child deaths (under 5 years) reduced by 59%. As a result, the contribution of neonatal deaths to under-5 deaths increased from 41% in 1990 to 56% in 2012, which is higher when compared to the contribution observed globally (44%). During the same period, the global under-5 death rate reduced by 50%, and the global neonatal mortality rate by only 37%.

Stillbirth Rates

The estimated Stillbirth Rate (SBR) in the country is 22 per 1000 live births (Lancet, 2011). The SBR estimates from the Sample Registration System (SRS) however require careful interpretation because of underestimation due to unavailable pregnancy history for women and misclassification of deaths.

Trends of Mortality Rates

During the last 12 year period, i.e. 2000–2012, the Average Annual Rate of Reduction (AARR) for Neonatal Mortality Rate (NMR) has been 3.4% per year. After a period of stagnation (2003–2007), the decline in neonatal mortality gained pace with more than 6% annual decline recorded in the last 2 consecutive years.

Geographical Differences

The neonatal mortality rate is not uniform across India. While the state of Kerala has already attained Single Digit NMR (7/1000 live births); Odisha, Madhya Pradesh, Uttar Pradesh, Rajasthan, and Chhattisgarh have a higher neonatal mortality rate at 30 or more per 1000 live births.

In terms of absolute numbers, four states alone Uttar Pradesh, Madhya Pradesh, Bihar, and Rajasthan contribute to 56% of total neonatal deaths in India and about 14% of the global neonatal deaths that occur every year.

Causes of NMR

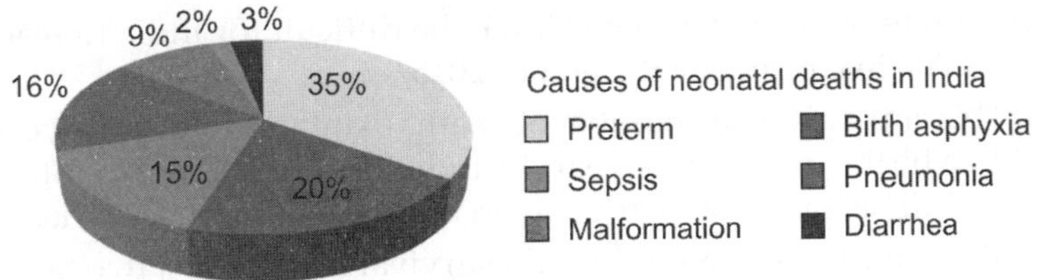

NMR calculation formula:

Neonatal mortality rate is the number of neonates dying before reaching 28 days of age, per 1,000 live births in a given year.

$$\text{NMR} = \frac{\text{Number of children died under the 28 days of age in year}}{\text{Total live birth in the same year}} \times 1000$$

Perinatal Mortality Rate (PMR)

Definition

The perinatal mortality rate is the sum of the number of resident fetal deaths of 28 or more weeks gestation plus the number of resident newborns dying under 7 days of age in a specified geographic area (country, state, county, etc.) divided by the sum of the number of resident live births plus the number of resident fetal deaths of 28 or more weeks gestation for the same geographic area (for a specified time period, usually a calendar year) and multiplied by 1,000. 2.

Calculation formula: Number of resident fetal deaths 28 or more weeks gestation + Number of resident newborns dying under 7 days of age)/(Number of resident live births + Number of resident fetal deaths of 28 or more weeks gestation)] × 1,000

$$\text{PMR} = \frac{\text{(Number of resident fetal deaths of 28 or more weeks gestation + number of resident newborns dying under 7 days of age)}}{\text{(Number of resident live births + resident fetal deaths of 28 or more weeks gestation)}} \times 1000$$

Examples

700 fetal deaths of 28 or more weeks gestation in 2008 among state residents 300 newborns dying under 7 days of age in 2008 among state residents 150,000 live births in 2005 among

state residents [(700 + 300)/(150,000 + 700)] × 1,000 = 6.6 perinatal deaths per 1,000 live births and fetal deaths of 28 or more weeks gestation in 2008 among state residents.

Infant Mortality Rate (IMR)

Introduction

The current pace of decline, India is unlikely to achieve its target of reducing the infant mortality rate to less than 39 per 1,000 live births by 2015-end, said a senior UNICEF official.

'The current Infant Mortality Rate (IMR) of India, as per the Sample Registration System (SRS) 2013, is 40 per 1,000 live births while the Under-5 Mortality Rate (U5MR) as per SRS 2012 is 52 per 1,000 live births.

'At this current rate of decline it seems it will be difficult for India to reach the target of less than 39 per 1,000 live births by the end of 2015,'

Definition: This entry gives the number of deaths of infants under one year old in a given year per 1,000 live births in the same year; included is the total death rate, and deaths by sex, *male* and *female*. This rate is often used as an indicator of the level of health in a country.

India has realized impressive gains in child survival over the last two decades. However, at the current pace, the country is unlikely to achieve the Millennium Development Goal (MDG).

Aims

- To reduce the Under-Five Mortality (U5MR) by two thirds between 1990 and 2015.
- Unless the related socioeconomic; maternal and demographic; and environmental determinants are urgently addressed.

This is one of the conclusions of The Infant and Child Mortality India Report released by UNICEF and the National Institute of Medical Sciences (NIMS), Indian Council of Medical Research.

Types

- Perinatal mortality rate is late fetal death (22 weeks gestation to birth), or death of a newborn up to one week postpartum.
- Neonatal mortality rate is newborn death occurring within 28 days postpartum. Neonatal death is often attributed to inadequate access to basic medical care, during pregnancy and after delivery. This accounts for 40–60% of infant mortality in developing countries.

Causes

- Malformations
- Sudden infant death syndrome
- Maternal complications
- Accidents in during pregnancy
- Infections
- Premature births
- Complications during delivery
- Perinatal asphyxia
- Birth injuries.

Preventive Measures

- Ensure pregnant women have access to and receive adequate prenatal care.
- Reduce the number of teen pregnancies.
- Reduce the number of preterm babies (Ensure pregnant women have access to and receive adequate prenatal care.
- Reduce the number of teen pregnancies.
- Reduce the number of pre-term babies (< 37 weeks gestation) by:
  - Reducing the number of women using drugs and alcohol during pregnancy
  - Reducing the number of women who smoke during pregnancy
  - Increase the amount of folic acid a woman gets before and during pregnancy
  - Increase the number of women that maintain a healthy weight during pregnancy, since obesity has been linked to preterm labor.
  - Increase the number of women that choose natural child birth, by reducing planned c-sections or medically induced labors.
- Increase the number of mothers that breastfeed their infants.
- Decrease infant exposure to secondhand smoke and other risk factors for Sudden Infant Death Syndrome (SIDS).
- Encourage 'back to sleep' programs that highlight the importance of putting babies to sleep on their backs.
- Teach parents the dangers of 'shaken baby syndrome' and offer skills to cope with stressful situations.
- Teach parents how to correctly install and use infant car seats and reduce other safety hazards.
- Increase the number of women that graduate high school. Higher levels of education are linked to better infant care.

Under-five Mortality Rate

Definition

The child mortality, also known as under-5 mortality, refers to the death of infants and children under the age of five or between the age of one month to four years depending on the definition.

Under-five mortality rate is the probability per 1,000 that a newborn baby will die before reaching age five, if subject to age-specific mortality rates of the specified year.

The risk of a child dying before completing five years of age is still highest in the WHO African Region (90 per 1000 live births), about 7 times higher than that in the WHO European Region (12 per 1000 live births).

Many countries still have very high under-five mortality particularly those in WHO Africa Region, home to 11 of the 12 countries with an under-five mortality rate above 100 deaths per 1000 live births.

In addition, inequities in child mortality between high-income and low-income countries remain large.

In 2013, the under-five mortality rate in low-income countries was 76 deaths per 1000 live birth almost 13 times the average rate in high-income countries (6 deaths per 1000 live births). Reducing these inequities across countries and saving more children's lives by ending preventable child deaths are important priorities.

Causes

The leading causes of death of children under five include:

- Diarrhea
- Malaria
- Malnutrition
- Pneumonia
- Preterm birth conditions.

Preventive Measures

- Poverty reduction.
- Women's empowerment and improving their status in society.
- Resource mobilization to ensure adequate resources for health care.
- Sustained political commitment to implement enabling policies and translate knowledge into action.
- Strengthening national health systems and capacity building at all levels of health care in order to improve quality of care.
- Ensuring equitable provision of health services.
- Support for scaling up and increasing coverage of cost-effective interventions to all children.
- Documenting and disseminating lessons learnt to ensure national coverage.
- Regular monitoring and evaluation to assess coverage and collect data for re-planning.

Vital Statistics Calculation Formulas

$$\text{(Crude) live birth rate} = \frac{\text{Total number of live births}}{\text{Total population}} \times 1{,}000$$

$$\text{(Crude) death rate} = \frac{\text{Total number of deaths}}{\text{Total population}} \times 1{,}000$$

$$\text{(Crude) marriage rate} = \frac{\text{Total number of marriages}}{\text{Total population}} \times 1{,}000$$

$$\text{(Crude) divorce rate} = \frac{\text{Total number of divorces and annulments}}{\text{Total population}} \times 1{,}000$$

$$\text{Cause-specific mortality rate} = \frac{\text{Number of deaths from a specific cause}}{\text{Total population}} \times 1{,}000$$

$$\text{Maternal mortality rate} = \frac{\text{Number of maternal deaths}}{\text{Total number of live births}} \times 100{,}000$$

Contd...

Contd...

$$\text{Neonatal mortality rate} = \frac{\text{Number of neonatal deaths}}{\text{Total number of live births}} \times 1{,}000$$

$$\text{Postneonatal mortality rate} = \frac{\text{Number of postneonatal deaths}}{\text{Total number of live births}} \times 1{,}000$$

$$\text{Infant mortality rate} = \frac{\text{Number of infant deaths}}{\text{Total number of live births}} \times 1{,}000$$

$$\text{Fetal mortality rate} = \frac{\text{Number of fetal deaths}}{\text{Total number of fetal deaths (stillbirths) plus live births}} \times 1{,}000$$

$$\text{Induced abortion ratio} = \frac{\text{Number of induced abortions}}{\text{Total number of live births}} \times 100$$

$$\text{Percentage of live births to unmarried women} = \frac{\text{Number of children born alive to unmarried women}}{\text{Total number of live births}} \times 100$$

$$\text{Percentage of low birth weight births} = \frac{\text{Number of low birth weight infants born alive}}{\text{Total number of live births}} \times 1{,}000$$

MODEL QUESTIONS

Multiple Choice Questions

1. **Who is the father of pediatrics?**
   (a) Abraham Jacob
   (b) Karl Menninger
   (c) Kashyapa and Jeevaka
   (d) Hippocrates
2. **International child rights started at_____year**
   (a) 1959
   (b) 1969
   (c) 1972
   (d) 1982
3. **How many international child rights_____**
   (a) 8
   (b) 10
   (c) 12
   (d) 1
4. **Which year pediatric specialty started in the field of medicine?**
   (a) 1860
   (b) 1852
   (c) 1868
   (d) 1870
5. **The first children clinic started at_________**
   (a) New York
   (b) Italy
   (c) Japan
   (d) China

6. **First pediatric hospital was opened in________**
   (a) Japan (c) Paris
   (b) Bangladesh (d) India
7. **Which age group belongs to pediatric up to __________**
   (a) 8 years (c) 4 years
   (b) 16 years (d) 12 years
8. **Who is the first pediatrician_______________**
   (a) Hippocrates (b) Abraham Jacob
   (b) Kashyapa and Jeevaka (d) Charaka
9. **In 1923 the first creche was opened in________**
   (a) India (c) London
   (b) Nepal (d) Sri Lanka

Fill in the Blanks

(a) …………………is known as 'Father of Pediatrics'.
(b) …………………..was the first author to write known manuscript devoted to pediatrics.
(c) The first English book on children's disease was written by………
(d) The world's first pediatrician were ……………..and………………..
(e) ……....is the branch of medical science which deals with treatment and care of a child.
(f) The word pediatrics is derived from Greek words……………………..
(g) Recent trend in pediatric nursing are…………………..……………..…

Full Forms

(a) MCH
(b) BFHI
(c) UNICEF
(d) RCH
(e) CAN

True or False

(a) The world's first pediatricians Kashyapa and Jeevaka were Indians.
(b) Aristotic is the father of modern medicine.
(c) Thomas Phare wrote the first book in English on children disease.
(d) Abram Jacob is known as 'Father of pediatrics'.

Short Answer Questions

(a) Trends in pediatric nursing.
(b) Role of pediatric nurse in child care.
(c) Child care in India
(d) Goals of pediatric nursing.
(e) Concept of preventive pediatrics.
(f) Nursing responsibilities in preventive pediatrics.
(g) List down the national health programmes for children in India.
(h) Female feticide.

Long Answer Questions

(a) Define the term pediatrics and describe in detail about concepts of child care.
(b) What do you understand by the term health and illness.
(c) Discuss the modern concept of pediatric nursing.
(d) Describe in brief about historical development of pediatrics in India.
(e) What is RCH? Explain its components.

ANSWER KEY

Multiple Choice Questions

1. (a)	2. (a)	3. (b)	4. (a)	5. (a)	6. (c)	7. (c)
8. (b)	9. (a)					

Fill in the Blanks

(a) Abraham Jacob
(b) Kashyapa and Samhita
(c) Thomas Phare
(d) Kashyapa and Jeevaka
(e) Pediatric
(f) Pedia + iatrike + ics
(g) Ethical decision, legal safeguards and quality assurance

True and False

(a) True	(b) False	(c) True	(d) True

Chapter 2

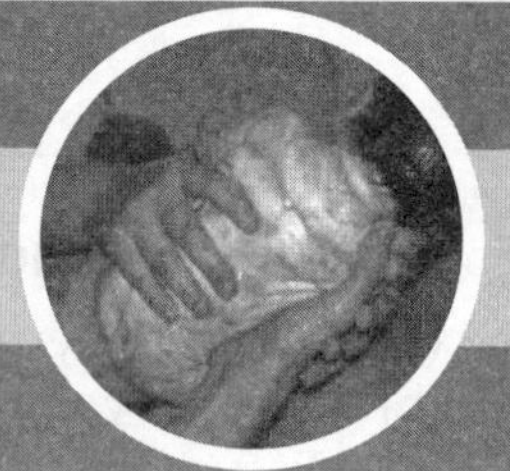

Nursing Care of a Neonate

- **Characteristics of the Normal Newborn Baby**
  - Assessment of the Newborn Baby
  - Nursing Care of the Normal Newborn Baby and Home Care
  - Breastfeeding
  - Baby-Friendly Hospital Initiative (BFHI)
- **Nursing Management of Low Birth Weight Baby/Preterm Baby**
  - Risk Factors and Causes of LBW
  - Clinical Features of LBW Baby
  - Complications of LBW
  - Prevention of LBW
  - Management of LBW Babies
  - Nursing Care of LBW Baby
  - Complication of LBW
- **Intrauterine Growth Retardation (IUGR)**
- **Care of Preterm Babies**
- **Nursing Management of Common Neonatal Disorders**
  - Hyperbilirubinemia of the Newborn
  - Hemolytic Disorders
  - Neonatal Hypoglycemia
  - Neonatal Sepsis
  - Oral Thrush
  - Impetigo
  - Erythema Toxicum
  - Hypothermia
  - Neonatal Convulsion
  - Birth Injury

- **Organization of Neonatal Care Unit (NICU and PICU)**
  - Pediatric Intensive Care Unit (PICU)
  - Importance of PICU
  - Practice and Standards of PICU
  - Emergency Procedures
  - Physical Set-up of Pediatric Intensive Care Unit
  - PICU Personnel
  - Equipment Required for a PICU
- **Neonatal Intensive Care Unit (NICU)**
  - Types of Procedures in the Neonatal Intensive Care Unit
- **Level of Neonatal Care in NICU and PICU**
- **An Integrated Evidence-based Syndromic Approach to Case Management**
  - Components of the Integrated Approach
  - The Principles of Integrated Care
  - The IMNCI Case Management Process

CHARACTERISTICS OF THE NORMAL NEWBORN BABY

Introduction

The nurse is a unique position to care the newborn baby in the stressful transition from a warm, dark, fluid-filled environment to an outside world filled with light, sound, and novel tactile stimuli. During this period of the newborn adjusting from intrauterine to extrauterine life, the nurse must be knowledgeable about a newborn's normal biopsychosocial adaptations to recognize any deviations.

To begin life as an independent being, the baby must immediately establish pulmonary ventilation in conjunction with marked circulatory changes. These radical and rapid changes are crucial to the maintenance of life. All other neonatal body systems change their functions or establish themselves over a longer period of time. The nurse performs an initial assessment to evaluate the neonate, its immediate post birth adaptations, and the need for further support.

Physical Characteristics of Newborn

Temperature Regulation

The newborn baby body temperature drops immediately after birth in response to the extrauterine environment. His internal organs are poorly insulated and his skin is very thin and does not contain much subcutaneous fat. The newborn baby heat regulating mechanism has not fully developed. His temperature rapidly reflects that of his environment. The flexed position that the newborn baby assumes is a safeguard against heat loss because it substantially diminishes the amount of body surface exposed.

Pediatric Nursing implications are centered on regulating an environment to provide constant body temperature of a neutral thermal environment. The newborn baby is placed in blankets, hat, and a controlled temperature environment after birth to counteract the drop in body temperature that occurs immediately after birth. After admission to the nursery, the infant is placed in isolation (isolate) and a temperature probe may be used for continuous monitoring. The newborn baby axillary temperature is maintained at 36.4 to 37.2 °C.

- **Pulse:** The normal pulse range for a newborn baby is 120 to 140 beats per minute (bpm). The rate may rise to 160 bpm when the newborn baby is crying or drop to 100 bpm when the infant is sleeping. The apical pulse is considered the most accurate.
- **Blood Pressure:** The average blood pressure (BP) of an infant at birth is 72/42. A drop in systolic BP of about 15 mm Hg the first hour after birth is common. The newborn's BP may be taken with a Doppler blood pressure device. This greatly improves accuracy.
- **Respirations:** The respirations of a newborn baby are irregular in depth, rate, and rhythm and vary from 30 to 60 beats per minute. Respirations are affected by the infant's activity (that is, crying). Normally, respirations are gentle, quiet, rapid, and shallow. They are most easily observed by watching abdominal movement because the infant's respirations are accomplished mainly by the diaphragm and abdominal muscles No sound should be audible on inspiration or expiration.

Characteristics of the Newborn Baby Head

The newborn baby head represents one-fourth of his total body length. Its circumference is equal to that of his abdomen or chest. The average size is 13" to 14" (33–35 cm).

The head is shaped or molded as it is forced through the birth canal in vertex presentations.

Molding

During delivery, for the large head to pass through the small birth canal, the skull bones may actually overlap in a process referred to as molding. Such molding reduces the diameter of the skull temporarily. This elongated look usually disappears a few hours after birth as the bones assume their normal relationships.

Fontanels

The newborn baby skull is separated into six bones one from another along the suture lines. Where more than two bones come together, the space is called a fontanel. This is the

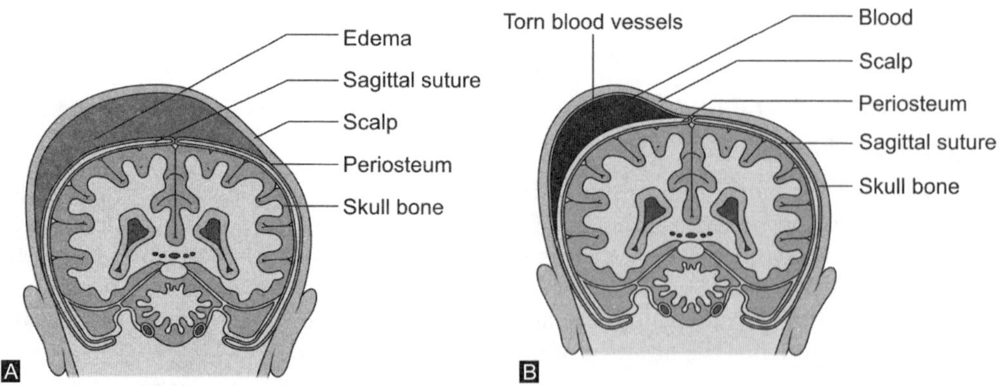

Figs. 2.1 (A and B): A. Cephalophematoma, B. Caput succedaneum

unossified space or soft spot between the cranial bones of the skull in a newborn baby. The newborn baby pulse is sometimes visible there.

The anterior fontanel is located at the intersection of the sutures of the two parietal bones and the frontal bones. It is diamond-shaped and strongly pulsatile. It normally closes at 9 to 18 months of age.

The posterior fontanel is located at the junction of the sutures of the two parietal bones and one occipital bone. It is small, triangular shaped, and less pulsatile. It normally closes at 1 1/2 to 3 months of age. The anterior fontanel is the large size of the two bones.

Cephalohematoma

This is a collection of blood between a cranial bone and its overlying periosteum. Bleeding is limited to the surface of the particular bone. It is caused by pressure of the fetal head against the maternal pelvis during a prolonged or difficult labor.

This pressure loosens the periosteum from the underlying bone, therefore rupturing capillaries and causing bleeding. It may be apparent at birth but sometimes are not seen until 24 to 48 hours of life because subperiosteal bleeding is slow. It varies in size, rather firm to the touch and tends to increase in size from 1 to 3 days and then become softer and more fluctuant. Most Cephalohematoma are absorbed within several weeks. No treatment is required in the absence of unexplained neurologic abnormalities.

Caput Succedaneum

This is an abnormal collection of fluid under the scalp on top of the skull that may or may not cross the suture lines, depending on the size. Pressure on the presenting part of the fetal head against the cervix during labor may cause edema of the scalp. This diffuse swelling is temporary and will be absorbed within 2 or 3 days.

Characteristics of the Newborn Baby Eyes and Ears

Eyes

The newborn baby eyes may be folded and creased and may seem out of shape because they contain little hardened cartilage. The newborn baby eyes may not track properly and may cross (strabismus) or twitch (nystagmus). This will cause concern if it extends beyond six months.

Color

At birth, the iris color is usually grayish-blue in Caucasians and grayish brown or brown in dark-complexioned races. A gradual deposition of pigment produces the final eye color of the baby at the age of three to six months and sometimes it may take a year.

Pupils

The pupils do react to light and the infant can focus on objects about eight inches away. The newborn baby blinking is a natural protection reflex.

Lacrimal apparatus

The lacrimal apparatus is small and nonfunctioning at birth and tears are not usually produced with crying until one to three months of age.

Ears

The newborn baby ears tend to be folded and creased. A line drawn through the inner and outer canthus of the eye should come to the top notch of the ear where it joins the scalp. The newborn baby usually responds to sound at birth.

Characteristics of the Newborn Baby Skin

The newborn baby has delicate skin at birth that appears dark red because it is thin and layers of subcutaneous fat have not yet covered the capillary beds. This redness can be seen through heavily pigmented skin and becomes even more flushed when the baby cries.

Vernix Caseosa

This is a soft, white, cheesy, yellowish cream on the newborn baby skin at birth. It is caused by the secretions of the sebaceous glands of the skin. It offers protection from the watery environment of the uterus, is absorbed in the skin after birth, and serves as a natural moisturizer. If there is a large amount of vernix caseosa present, it should be meticulously removed as it is thought to be a good culture medium for bacteria.

Lanugo

This is a long, soft growth of fine hair on the newborn baby shoulders, back, and forehead. It disappears early in postnatal life.

Mongolian Spots

These are blue-black colorations on the infant's lower back, buttocks, and anterior trunk. They are often seen in infants of Black, Indian, Mongolian, or Mediterranean ancestry. These spots occur less frequently in Caucasian babies. The spots are not bruises nor are they associated with mental retardation. They disappear in early childhood.

Jaundice

This is a yellow discoloration that may be seen in the newborn baby skin or in the sclera of the eye. Jaundice is caused by excessive amounts of free bilirubin in the blood and tissue.

Petechiae

These are small, blue-red dots on the newborn baby body caused by breakage of tiny capillaries. They may be seen on the face as a result of pressure exerted on the head during birth. True petechiae do not blanch on pressure.

Milia

These are tiny sebaceous retention cysts. They appear as small white or yellow dots and are common on the nose, forehead, and cheeks of the newborn baby. They are of pin head size and opalescent. Milia are due to blocked sweat and oil glands that have not begun to function properly. They disappear spontaneously within a few weeks.

Birthmarks

- These are small, reddened areas sometimes present on the newborn baby eyelids, mid-forehead, and nape of the neck. They may be the result of local dilatation of skin capillaries and abnormal thinness of the skin. They are sometimes called stork bites or telangiectasia. These marks usually fade and disappear altogether. They may be noticeable when the infant blushes, is extremely warm, or becomes excited.

- A hemangioma or strawberry mark is a type of birthmark that is characterized by a dark or bright red raised, rough surface. They do not develop for several days. They may regress spontaneously or may even increase in size. Surgical removal is not recommended. There is a 'wait-and-see' attitude advocated before surgical removal.

Characteristics of the Newborn Gastrointestinal System

Mouth

The newborn baby lips should be pink and the tongue smooth and symmetrical. The tongue should not extend or protrude between the lips. The connective tissue attached to the underside of the tongue should not restrict the mobility of the tip of the tongue.

The gums may have tooth ridges along them, and rarely a tooth or two may have erupted before birth. The roof of the mouth should be closed, and the uvula should be present. Sometimes there are glistening spots (firm white or grayish-white nodules, usually multiple) on the palate that are referred to as Epstein's pearls. A common site for them is at the junction of the hard and soft palates.

Stomach

The capacity of the newborn baby stomach is about one to two ounces (30 to 60 ml) at birth, but increases rapidly. Milk passes through the infant's stomach almost immediately. The infant is capable of digesting simple carbohydrates and proteins, but has a limited ability to digests fats.

Intestines

Irregularity in peristaltic motility slows stomach emptying. Peristaltic increases in the lower ileum, which results in one to six stools a day. The first stools after birth and for three to four days afterwards are called meconium. Meconium is stringy, tenacious, and black and has a tarry texture. With the ingestion of colostrum or formula, a gradual transition occurs. There may be few greenish stools and the stools will gradually become more yellow. Formula stools are lemon yellow and curdy. Breast milk stools are yellow-orange, soft, and more frequent.

Characteristics of the Newborn Circulatory System

Blood Flow

The umbilical blood stops flowing at birth, sudden pressure differences occur within the circulatory system. These differences cause the blood flowing to the lungs and liver to increase and the blood flowing through the bypass channels to decrease. Peripheral circulation refers to residual cyanosis in hands and feet. This may be apparent for one to two hours after birth and is due to sluggish circulation. Blood is shunted to vital organs immediately after birth.

Blood Coagulation

During the first few days of life, the prothrombin level decreases and clotting time in all infants is prolonged. This process is most acute between the second and fifth postnatal days. It can be prevented to a large extent by giving vitamin K to the newborn baby after birth.

With the ingestion of food, establishment of digestion, and maturation of the liver, vitamin K is manufactured by the baby and clotting time stabilizes within a week to ten days.

Characteristics of the Newborn Respiratory System

Until the newborn baby first breath of air is taken, the alveoli (air sacs) in the lungs are in an almost complete state of collapsed. The lungs should be in this state because the lung must not fill with amniotic fluid or other liquids. However, the fluid/liquid that flows in the lungs during normal delivery is squeezed or drained from the infant lungs. The major portion of the fluid is absorbed after delivery by the vacuolar membranes into the blood capillaries.

The most frequent cause of respiratory difficulty in the first few hours of birth has been due to the too liberal use of sedatives, tranquilizers, analgesics, and anesthetics that affect not only the mother, but pass over the placenta to the infant. These drugs make the baby sleepy and disinclined to take the first breath.

Characteristics of the Newborn Endocrine System

The endocrine glands are considered better organized than other systems. Disturbances are most often related to maternally provided hormones (estrogen, luteal, and prolactin) that may cause the following conditions:

- Vaginal discharge and/or bleeding may occur in female infants. This discharge is white fucoids in color. Bleeding may occur as a result of withdrawal from maternal hormones at the time of birth. There are usually only a few blood spots seen on the diapers. The entire process terminates in one to two days.
- Enlargement of the mammary glands may occur in both sexes. This is particularly noticeable about the third day of life. Breast secretion may also occur. Swelling usually subsides in two to three weeks. The breast should not be squeezed; it only increases the chances of infection and injuries to the tender tissue.

Characteristics of the Newborn Neuromuscular System

The newborn baby exhibits remarkable sensory development and an amazing ability for self-organization in social interactions. The newborn baby muscles are firm and resilient. He has the ability to contract when stimulated, but lacks the ability to control them. He wiggles and stretches, but movements are uncoordinated.

Cephalocaudal (Head to Toe) in Development

The gross motor development occurs first, followed by finer motor development. Reflex actions present at birth serve the newborn baby until neuromuscular development is improved. Absence of reflex activity often indicates some form of brain damage.

Common Infant Reflexes

- *Rooting:* The newborn baby turns his head to the side when the side of his face is touched.
- *Moro reflex:* The newborn baby total body responds to a startling event. His arms extend out and up, legs flex toward abdomen. This reflex is usually lost by three months of age.
- *Tonic neck reflex:* The newborn baby assumes a fencer's position. His arm and leg on one side is extended, the opposite side is flexed. His head is turned toward extended side. This is not evident after four months of age.

Table 2.1: Normal newborn baby appearance

Features	Description	Image
Color	A baby's skin coloring can vary greatly, depending on the baby's age, race or ethnic group, temperature, and whether or not the baby is crying. Skin color in babies often changes with both the environment and health. When a baby is first born, the skin is a dark red to purple color. As the baby begins to breathe air, the color changes to red. This redness normally begins to fade in the first day. A baby's hands and feet may stay bluish in color for several days. This is a normal response to a baby's immature blood circulation. Jaundice can often be seen by gently pressing on the baby's forehead or chest and watching the color return. Laboratory tests may be needed to assess jaundice.	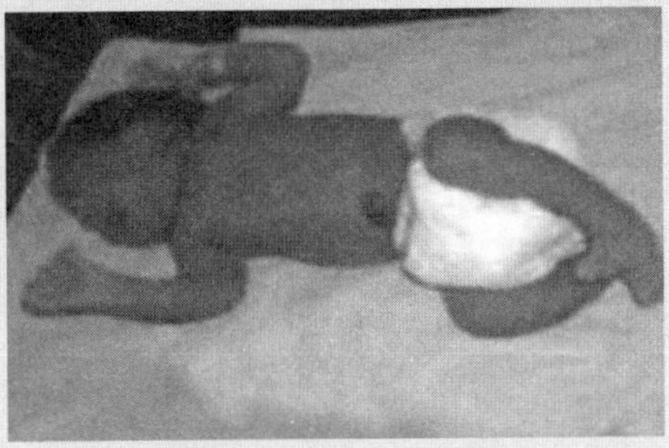
Molding	Molding is the elongation of the shape of a baby's head. It occurs when the movable bones of the baby's head overlap to help the baby pass through the mother's birth canal. Normal shape usually returns by the end of the first week.	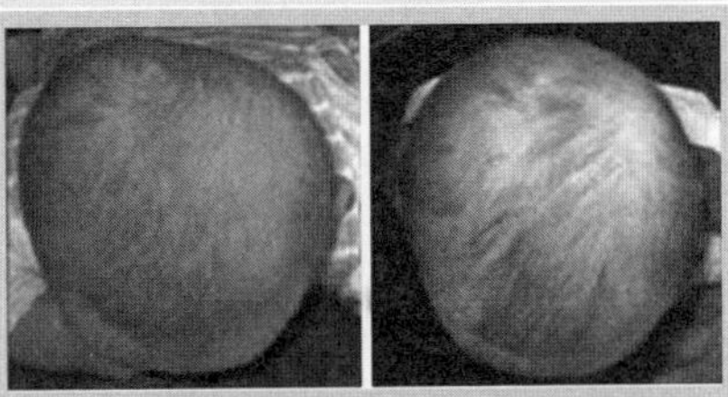 Before After
Vernix	This is a white, greasy, cheese-like substance that covers the skin of many babies at birth. It is formed by secretions from the baby's oil glands and protects the baby's skin in the amniotic fluid during pregnancy. Vernix may not be present in babies who are born post-term (after 41 weeks of pregnancy). It does not need to be removed and usually absorbs into the skin.	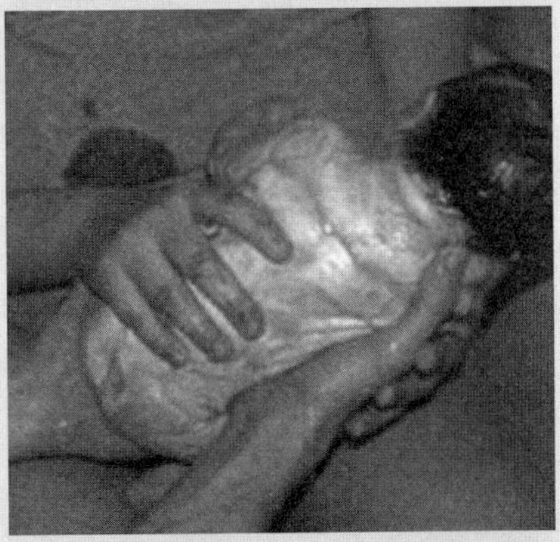
Lanugo	This is soft, downy hair on a baby's body, especially on the shoulders, back, forehead, and cheeks. It is more noticeable in premature babies, but is not usually seen in babies born very late in pregnancy.	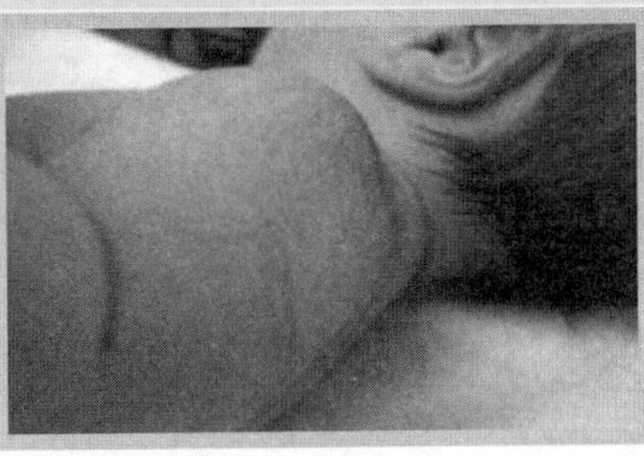

Contd...

Contd...

Features	Description	Image
Milia	Milia are tiny, white, hard spots that look like pimples on a newborn's nose. They may also appear on the chin and forehead. Milia form from oil glands and disappear on their own. When these occur in a baby's mouth and gums, they are called Epstein pearls.	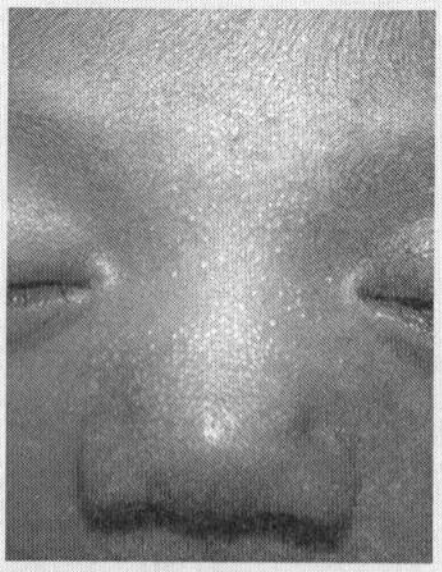
Stork bites or salmon patches	These are small pink or red patches often found on a baby's eyelids, between the eyes, upper lip, and back of the neck. The name comes from the marks on the back of the neck where, as the myth goes, a stork may have picked up the baby. They are caused by a concentration of immature blood vessels and may be the most visible when the baby is crying. Most of these fade and disappear completely.	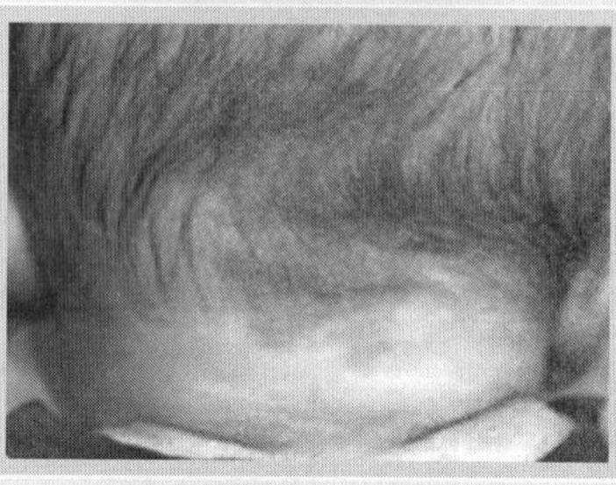
Mongolian spots	Mongolian spots are blue or purple-colored splotches on the baby's lower back and buttocks. Over 80 percent of African-American, Asian, and Indian babies have Mongolian spots, but they occur in dark-skinned babies of all races. The spots are caused by a concentration of pigmented cells. They usually disappear in the first four years of life.	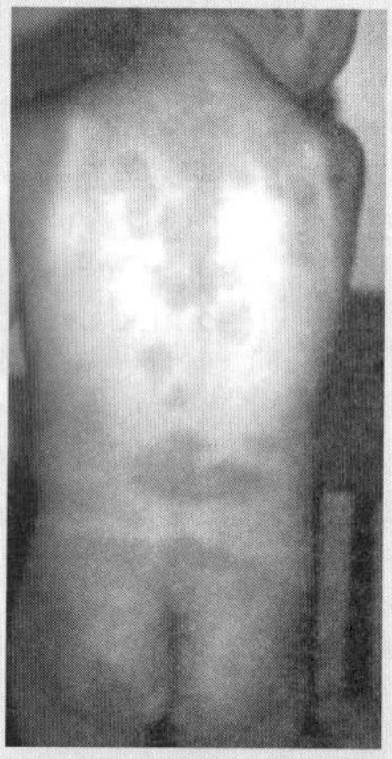
Erythema toxicum	Erythema toxicum is a red rash on newborns that is often described as 'flea bites.' The rash is common on the chest and back, but may be found all over. About half of all babies develop this condition in the first few days of life. It is less common in premature babies. The cause is unknown but it is not dangerous. Erythema toxicum does not require any treatment and disappears by itself in a few days.	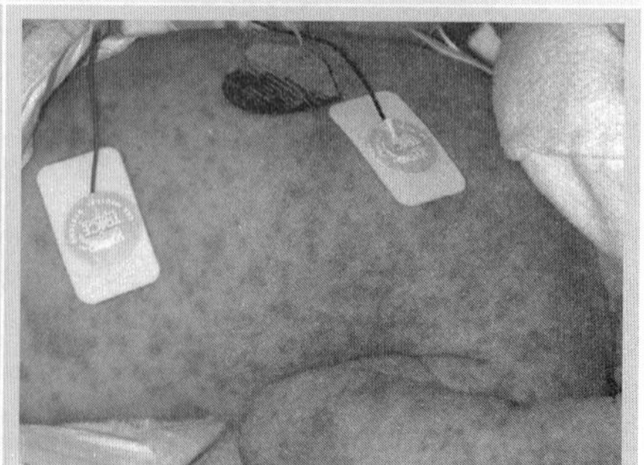

Contd...

Contd...

Features	Description	Image
Acne neonatorum (baby acne)	About one-fifth of newborns develop pimples in the first month. These usually appear on the cheeks and forehead. It is thought that maternal hormones cause these, and they usually disappear within a few months. Do not try to break open or squeeze the pimples, as this can lead to infection.	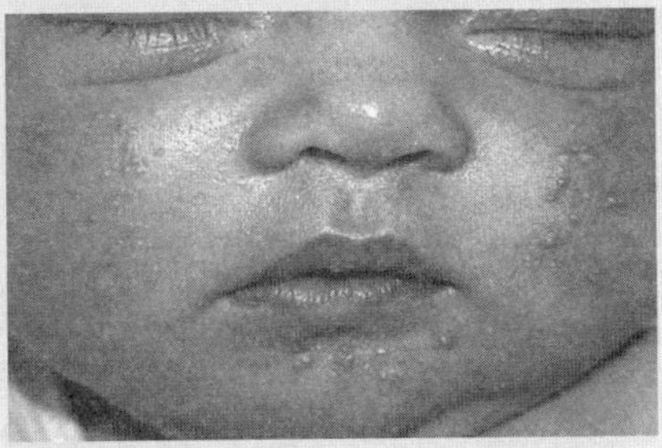
Strawberry hemangioma	This is a bright or dark red, raised or swollen, bumpy area that looks like a strawberry. Hemangiomas are formed by a concentration of tiny, immature blood vessels. Most of these occur on the head. They may not appear at birth, but often develop in the first two months. Strawberry hemangiomas are more common in premature babies and in girls. These birthmarks often grow in size for several months, and then gradually begin to fade. Nearly all strawberry hemangiomas completely disappear by nine years of age.	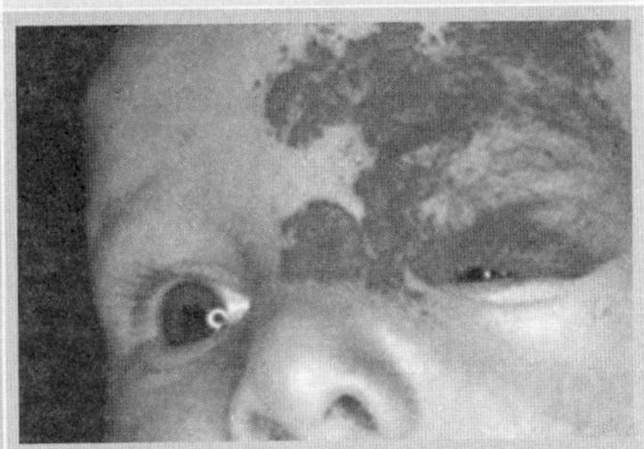
Port-wine stain	A port-wine stain is a flat, pink, red, or purple colored birthmark. These are caused by a concentration of dilated tiny blood vessels called capillaries. They usually occur on the head or neck. Port-wine stains on the face may be associated with more serious problems. Skin-colored cosmetics may be used to cover small port wine stains. The most effective way of treating port wine stains is with a special type of laser. This is done when the baby is older by a plastic surgery specialist.	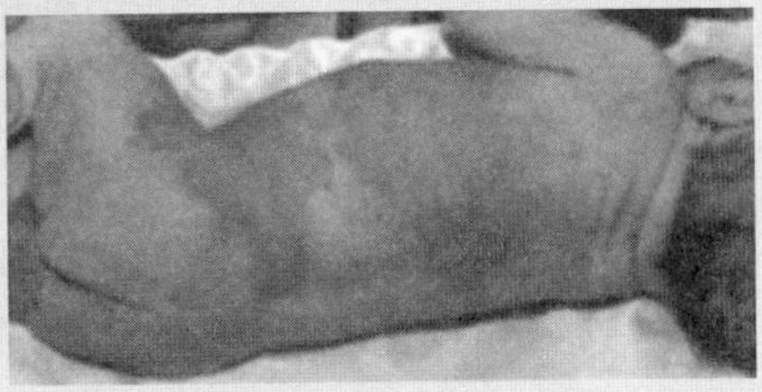
Newborn breast swelling	Breast enlargement may occur in newborn boys and girls around the third day of life. In the first week, a milky substance, sometimes called 'witch's milk,' may leak from the nipples. This is related to the mother's hormones and goes away within a few days to weeks. Do not massage or squeeze the breasts or nipples, as this may cause an infection in the breast.	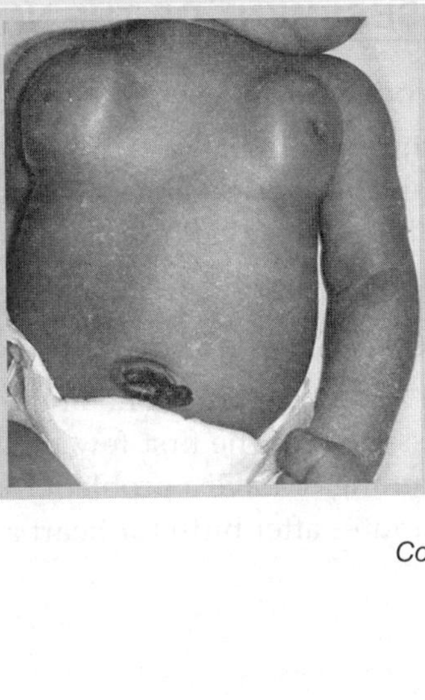

Contd...

Contd...

Features	Description	Image
Swollen genitals/ discharge	A newborn's genitals may appear different depending on the gestational age (the number of weeks of pregnancy). Premature baby girls may have a very prominent clitoris and inner labia. A baby born closer to full-term has larger outer labia. Girls may have a small amount of whitish discharge or blood-tinged mucus from the vagina in the first few weeks. This is a normal occurrence related to the mother's hormones. Premature boys may have a smooth, flat scrotum with undescended testicles. Boys born later in pregnancy have ridges in the scrotum with descended testicles.	Penis Vagina

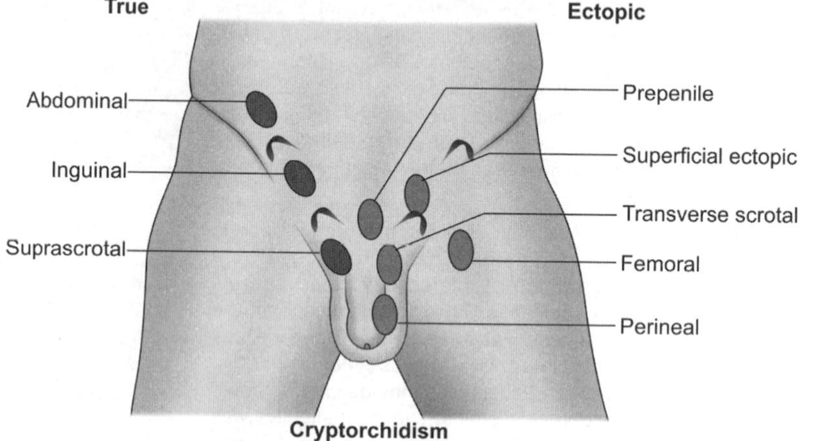

Cryptorchidism

ASSESSMENT OF THE NEWBORN BABY

Introduction

Each newborn baby is carefully checked at birth for signs of problems or complications. A complete physical assessment will be done that includes every body system. Throughout the hospital stay, doctors, nurses, and other health care providers continually assess the health of the baby, observing for signs of problems or illness. Assessment may include:

APGAR Scoring

The APGAR score is one of the first checks of your new baby's health. The APGAR score is assigned in the first few minutes after birth to help identify babies that have difficulty breathing or have a problem that needs further care. The baby is checked at 1 minute and 5 minutes after birth for heart and respiratory rates, muscle tone, reflexes, and color.

Each area can have a score of 0, 1, or 2, with 10 points as the maximum. A total score of 10 means a baby is in the best possible condition. Nearly all babies score between 8 and 10, with 1 or 2 points taken off for blue hands and feet because of immature circulation. If a baby has a difficult time during delivery, this can lower the oxygen levels in the blood, which can lower the APGAR score. APGAR scores of 3 or less often mean a baby needs immediate attention and care.

	0 Points	1 Points	2 Points	Points totaled
Activity (muscle tone)	Absent	Arms and legs flexed	Active movement	
Pulse	Absent	Below 100 bpm	Over 100 bpm	
Grimace (reflex irritability)	Flaccid	Some flexion of Extremities	Active motion (sneeze, cough pull away)	
Appearance (skin color)	Blue, pale	Body pink, Extremities blue	Completely pink	
Respiration	Absent	Slow, irregular	Vigorous cry	

Severely depressed	0–3
Moderately depressed	4–6
Excellent condition	7–10

Fig. 2.2: Assessment of newborn baby with APGAR scoring scale

Birth Weight

A baby's birth weight is an important indicator of health. The average weight for term babies (born between 37 and 41 weeks gestation) is about 7 lbs. (3.2 kg). In general, small babies and very large babies are at greater risk for problems. Babies are weighed daily in the nursery to assess growth, fluid, and nutrition needs. Newborn babies may often lose 5 to 7% of their birth weight. This means that a baby weighing 7 pounds 3 ounces at birth might lose as much as 8 ounces in the first few days. Babies will usually gain this weight back by 2 weeks of age. Premature and sick babies may not begin to gain weight right away.

Anthropometric Measurements

The measurement of the human individual. An early tool of physical anthropology, it has been used for identification, for the purposes of understanding human physical variation, in paleoanthropology and in various attempts to correlate physical with racial and psychological traits. Anthropometry involves the systematic measurement of the physical properties of the human body, primarily dimensional descriptors of body size and shape.

History Collection

History taking in children is likely to be compromised by a variety of factors, not least that the child may be distressed and ill and the parents extremely anxious. This is particularly true where most pediatric histories are taken—that is, in general practice and in accident and emergency departments. In general practice such histories will usually be gathered within consultations which are of necessity brief and focused.

Physical Examination (Head to Toe)

The purpose of the newborn physical examination is to assess the baby's transition from intrauterine line to extrauterine existence and to detect congenital malformations and actual or potential disease. The baby should be examined briefly immediately after birth. This should be confined to quick assessment of respiration, circulation, temperature, neurological status, and screening for anomalies or disease that might mandate emergency treatment. The initial examination should be done with minimal disturbance to the baby, taking particular care to prevent excessive cooling from exposure.

A complete examination should be performed within the first 24 hours and again at discharge from the nursery. The full examination should be performed when the baby is quiet. The baby should be observed from a distance before being touched since a great deal can be learned by observing the infant's spontaneous activity. See, and then touch.

Auscultate the heart and chest and feel the pulses before the baby begins to cry, and then proceed systematically to the rest of the examination.

Head

- Shape, presence of fontanels and whether normal, sunken or bulging
- Measure and record head circumference on the growth chart
  - Assess facial appearance and eye position
  - Look for any asymmetry or abnormality of facial form.

Eyes

- Establish that they are of normal shape and appearance
- Check for presence of red reflex
- Look for obvious cataracts or signs of ophthalmic infection.

Ears

- Note shape and size
- Establish whether they are set at the normal level or 'low-set'
- Check patency of external auditory meatus.

Mouth

- Check the color of the mucous membrane; observe the palate
- Check suckling reflex by inserting a clean little finger gently inside the baby's mouth.

Arms and hands

- Establish whether they are of normal shape and moving normally
- Look for evidence of traction birth injury (e.g. Erb's palsy) by checking the neck, shoulders and clavicles
- Count the fingers and observe their shape; check for any evidence of clinodactyly (incurving of fingers)
- Check palmar creases—whether they are multiple or single. A single palmar crease may be normal, but can be a sign of Down's syndrome (trisomy 21).

Peripheral pulses

- Check brachial, radial and femoral pulses for rate, rhythm and volume
- A hyperdynamic pulse may suggest patent ductus arteriosus
- A weak pulse may occur with a congenital cardiac anomaly (impairing cardiac output and in conjunction with other signs from the examination)
- Check for radiofemoral delay (aortic coarctation).

Heart

- Check the cardiac position by palpation and feel for any thrill or heave
- Listen to the heart sounds carefully and for any added sounds or murmurs
- Suspected abnormalities require further examination (and often more expert opinion and investigation).

Lungs

- Watch the respiratory pattern, rate and depth for a few seconds
- Look for any evidence of intercostals recession
- Listen for stridor
- Auscultate lung fields for added sounds.

Abdomen

- Look at abdominal girth and shape
- Carefully check the umbilical stump for infection or surrounding hernia
- Palpate gently for organs, masses or hernia
- It is common to be able to feel the liver and/or spleen in healthy newborns
- Check the external genitalia carefully (see the separate article on ambiguous genitalia)
- Palpate for testes in boys
- Inspect the anus (establish whether meconium been passed).

Back

- Look carefully at the skin over the back and at the spinal curvature/symmetry
- Observe whether there is any evidence of spina bifida occulta or pilonidal sinus hidden by flesh creases or dimples
- Palpate the spine gently.

Hips

Specifically test for congenital dislocation of the hip (congenital hip dysplasia) using a combination of Barlow and Ortolani manoeuvres (follow the link for more detail).

Legs

- Watch movements at each joint
- Check for any evidence of talipes equinovarus
- Count toes and check their shape.

Central nervous system (CNS)

- Observe tone, behavior, movements and posture.
- Elicit newborn reflexes only if there is cause for concern.

- Further examination should be conducted as necessary according to any abnormalities that are detected, or suspicions of undetected illness in the baby.

Record the findings

Always document the findings of the examination in the postnatal care plan and personal child health record. A proforma for the examination, kept within the notes, can save time and act as a prompt to ensure that no element of the examination is missed.

Gestational Assessment

Assessing a baby's physical maturity is an important part of care. Maturity assessment is helpful in meeting a baby's needs if the dates of a pregnancy are uncertain. For example, a very small baby may actually be more mature than it appears by size, and may need different care than a premature baby.

An examination called The Dubowitz/Ballard Examination for gestational age is often used. A baby's gestational age often can be closely estimated using this examination. The Dubowitz/Ballard Examination evaluates a baby's appearance, skin texture, motor function, and reflexes. The physical maturity part of the examination is done in the first two hours of birth. The neuromuscular maturity examination is completed within 24 hours after delivery.

Physical Maturity

The physical assessment part of the Dubowitz/Ballard Examination looks at physical characteristics that look different at different stages of a baby's gestational maturity. Babies who are physically mature usually have higher scores than premature babies. Points are given for each area of assessment, with a low of -1 or -2 for extreme immaturity to as much as 4 or 5 for post maturity. Areas of assessment include the following:

- *Skin textures* (for example, sticky, smooth, or peeling)
- *Lanugo* (the soft downy hair on a baby's body). Absent in immature babies, then appears with maturity, and then disappears again with postmaturity
- *Plantar creases:* These creases on the soles of the feet range from absent to covering the entire foot, depending on the maturity
- *Breast:* The thickness and size of breast tissue and areola (the darkened ring around each nipple) are assessed
- *Eyes and ears:* Eyes fused or open and amount of cartilage and stiffness of the ear tissue.
- *Genitals, male:* Presence of testes and appearance of scrotum, from smooth to wrinkled.
- *Genitals, female:* Appearance and size of the clitoris and the labia.

Neuromuscular Maturity

At the time of assessment six evaluations of the baby's neuromuscular system are done. A score is assigned to each assessment area. Typically, the more neurologically mature the baby, the higher the score. The areas of assessment include:

- *Posture:* How does the baby hold his or her arms and legs.
- *Square window:* How far the baby's hands can be flexed toward the wrist.
- *Arm recoil:* How much the baby's arms 'spring back' to a flexed position.
- *Popliteal angle:* How far the baby's knees extend.

- *Scarf sign:* How far the elbows can be moved across the baby's chest.
- *Heel to ear:* How close the baby's feet can be moved to the ears.

When the physical assessment score and the neuromuscular score are added together, the gestational age can be estimated. Scores range from very low for immature babies (less than 26 to 28 weeks) to very high scores for mature and post mature babies. All of these exams are important ways to learn about your baby's well-being at birth. By identifying any problems, your baby's doctor can plan the best possible care.

Assessment of High-risk Newborn

The New Ballard Score

Score sheet: Use this score sheet to assess the gestational maturity of baby. At the end of the examination the total score determines the gestational maturity in weeks.

Make sure that the following things are available for the newborn

- The room where the delivery takes place should be clean, warm, well-lighted and ventilated, but draught-free.
- Two clean and warm towels/cloths for keeping the baby warm; one for drying and wrapping the baby initially, the other one for covering the newborn to prevent heat loss.
- Ensure the 'five cleans during' delivery have soap, water, new razor blade, a clean plastic sheet and a clean piece of thread.
- A clean delivery kit for cord care.
- An oral mucus extractor.
- A blanket.
- A watch to note the time delivery.

Routine care at birth: Over 90% of newborns do not require any active resuscitation at birth. Efforts are directed to maintain asepsis and prevent infection of the newborn, prevent hypothermia and keep the airways patent.

Asepsis: Wash your hands with soap and water when preparing for the birth. Use gloves; Deliver the newborn under aseptic conditions. Note the time (hour and minute).

Airways and breathing: If the baby is crying and the breathing is normal, then there is no need for resuscitation. Provide normal care and clear the upper airway by wiping the nose and mouth of the baby and removing the secretions present therein. If the baby is not crying, assess the breathing; if the chest is rising symmetrically and the respiratory rate is >30/minute, no immediate action is needed. Remember, occasional gasps are not considered breathing.

Feeding: Initiate breastfeeding within half an hour of a normal delivery. Ensure that the baby is sucking well. If suckling is poor, ensure correct positioning and attachment of the baby to the breast.

Clamping of the cord: The umbilical cord should be clamped 2–3 minutes after the neonate is delivered completely. Wait till the cord has stopped pulsating before clamping and cutting it. This will result in an extra amount of blood being transfused in the neonate and prevent neonatal anemia. However, early and immediate clamping of the cord is recommended in newborns with severe birth asphyxia, cord around the neck and rhesus isoimmunization.

Maintenance of body temperature in the newborn: Newborns may be hypothermic at birth. Hypothermia is a body temperature of < 36 °C. The simplest way to measure body temperature in a newborn is by placing a thermometer in the axilla of the child. The thermometer should be kept for at least five minutes before taking the reading off the thermometer. The normal temperature of the body is between 36.50 °C and 37.0 °C.

Physical maturity								
	Score							Sign score
Sign	–1	0	1	2	3	4	5	
Skin	Sticky, friable, transpaent	Gelatinous, red, trans-lucent	Smooth, pink, visible veins	Superficial peeling and/ or rash, few veins	Crack-ing, pale, areas, rare, veins	Parchment, deep, cracking, no vessels	Leath-ery, cracked, wrinkled	
Lanugo	None	Sparse	Abundant	Thinning	Bald Areas	Mostly Bald		
Plantar surface	Heel-toe 40–50 mm: –1 < 40 mm: –2	> 50 mm no crease	Faint red marks	Anterior transverse crease only	Creases ant. 2/3	Creases over entire sole		
Breast	Impercep-tible	Barely perceptible	Flat areola no bud	Stippled areola 1–2 mm bud	Raised areola 3–4 mm bud	Full areola 5–10 mm bud		
Eye/Ear	Lids fused loosely: –1 tightly : –2	Lids open pinna flat stays folded	Sl.curved pinna; soft; slow recoil	Well-curved pinna; soft but ready recoil	Formed and firm instant recoil	Thick cartilage ear stiff		
Genitals (Male)	Scrotum flat, smooth	Scrotum empty faint rugae	Testes in upper canal, rare rugae	Testes descending few rugae	Testes down, good rugae	Testes pendulous. deep rugae		
Genitals (Female)	Clitoris prominent and labia flat	Prominent clitoris and small labia minora	Prominent clitoris and enlarging minora	Majora and minora equally prominent	Labia majora large, labia minora small	Majora cover clitoris and minora		
Total physical maturity score								

Table 2.2: Neuromuscular maturity assessments

Neuromuscular maturity								
	Score							
Sign	–1	0	1	2	3	4	5	**Sign score**
Posture								
Square window								

Contd...

Contd...

Neuromuscular maturity								
	Score							
Sign	–1	0	1	2	3	4	5	**Sign score**
Arm recoil								
Popliteal angle								
Scarf sign								
Total neuromuscular score								

Table 2.3: Maturity rating assessments table

Maturity rating	
Total score (Neuromuscular + Physical Maturity)	**Weeks**
–10	20
–5	22
0	24
5	26
10	28
15	30
20	32
25	34
30	36
35	38
40	40
45	42

Role of Nurse

The pediatric nurse should counsel them when to come and meet the health facility immediately. It is particularly important to watch out for the signs mentioned below. Teach the mother these sings. Ask her check questions to be sure that she knows when to come to a healthy facility immediately.

Pediatric nurse plays a critical role in providing newborn care at district and subdistrict facilities. They, and not the physicians, conduct newborn deliveries at these facilities.

They also provide care to sick neonates brought from the community. Nurses are the interface with the community and the family in regard to the promotion of healthy newborn care practices. Nurses perform critical newborn care procedures and look after the neonatal equipment. It is not an overstatement to mention that nurses from the backbone of newborn care at DHs, FRUs, CHCs and PHCs and play a more important role than the physicians.

Advise the mother to come to a health facility immediately if the baby has any of these signs.

- Poor breastfeeding or drinking
- Looks ill
- Develops a fever or is cold to the touch
- Fast breathing
- Difficult breathing
- Blood in the stool
- Nurse in thermal comfort (the baby) should be warm to the touch at the abdomen and the soles of the feet should be pink
- Check the umbilicus, skin and eyes
- Ensure good sucking at the breast
- Screen for danger signs
- Advise the family, especially the mother, on immunization.

Care for umbilical stump:

- Inspect the cord for bleeding two hours after typing
- Do not apply anything on the stump; keep the cord clean and dry
- Inspect for discharge or infection till healing occurs.

The purpose of umbilical cord care:

The umbilical cord must be cut with a pair of sterile scissors/blade 3.5 cm from the abdominal skin surface. Not the following

- Nothing needs to be applied to the cord. The cord is frequently infected because many mothers apply substance which may not be clean. The cord will dry and fall off on its own.
- Advices the mother to prevent the cord from getting soiled with the newborn's urine or feces.
- The mother should wash her hands with soap and water after cleaning the baby every time it passes stools.

Babies receive nourishment and oxygen in the womb through the placenta, which is connected to the inner wall of the mother's uterus.

The placenta is connected to the baby by the umbilical cord through an opening in the baby's stomach. After your baby is born, the umbilical cord is clamped and cut in a painless procedure, leaving a 2–3 cm umbilical stump.

The cord may be clamped and cut immediately after birth or when the cord has stopped pulsating; as part of a natural or physiological third stage of labor, this allows time for blood in the placenta to transfuse to the baby. Sometime between five and 15 days after birth, the stump will dry up, turn black and drop off; leaving a small wound that may take a few days to heal.

It must be kept clean and dry to prevent infection. Harmful bacteria that live naturally on out skin can track up the cord stump causing infection. Avoid the traditional practice of taping a coin to retract the belly button as it may encourage infection and delay the healing process.

Always wash your hands before handling your baby's cord stump, before and after nappy changes and other care. Avoid the cord stump getting urine on it by folding the nappy down away from it, leaving the stump exposed to the air.

If the stump gets urine on it, wash it off using clean water and soap, or just water alone. It is better to use a mild soap to wash-off, as the higher percentage of fatty deposits found in baby feces can make it difficult to remove with just water.

A major concern with bathing newborns is preventing body heat loss. Experts recommend waiting until your baby's body temperature has stabilised after birth before bathing; wait at least six hours after birth, or longer if possible. Make sure the room is warm, dry your baby immediately and wrap him up well afterwards to minimize heat loss.

After the stump falls off, it usually takes about seven to 10 days for the area to heal over completely. When the stump falls off, you may see a little blood on your baby's nappy, which is normal. Sometimes, when the umbilical stump takes a long time to heal, bits of lumpy flesh (a type of connective tissue) appear in the wound and which soon disappear.

In the past, cord stumps have been cleaned with antiseptic tissues or sprinkled with an antiseptic powder. Studies of the healing process have found to advantage to using antiseptics over simply keeping the cord clean, unless the baby is premature or in intensive care. Antiseptics also cause the cord to take longer to fall off, which causes anxiety to parents.

- The newborn baby develops a fever, becomes lethargic, starts to feed poorly, or appears unwell generally.
- The naval and the surrounding area become swollen or red.
- The cord stump becomes swollen or smelly. It is normal for the cord stump to look a bit 'mucky', or appear to have pus at the base, as it dries up and heals, but this does not mean that it is infected.

NURSING CARE OF THE NORMAL NEWBORN BABY AND HOME CARE

Introduction

Neonatal morbidity and mortality is directly related to the birth weight and gestational maturity of the newborn, high-risk and gestational maturity of the newborn.

High-risk pregnancies (which are associated with the birth of high-risk infants) must be identified during antenatal period and referred to an appropriate center for skilled management. Simplified scoring system should be evolved to detect at-risk pregnancy in a community set up. Based upon birth weight and gestational age, a three tier system of neonatal care is proposed for developing countries.

Care of Newborn Baby in Level-I

In care of newborn baby overall 80 percent of newborn babies require minimal care which can be provided by their mothers under the supervision of basic health professionals.

Neonates weighing above 2000 gm or having gestational maturity of 37 weeks or more belong to this category.

The care can be provided at home, subcenter and primary health center level. Basic care at birth, provision of warmth, maintenance of asepsis and promotion of breastfeeding form the mainstay of level I care.

Traditional birth attendants and community health workers must be trained in the art of essential perinatal care.

Care of Newborn Baby in Level-II

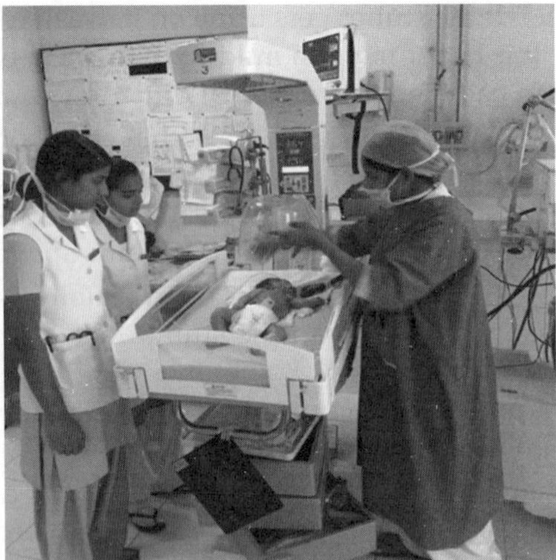

Fig. 2.3: Care of newborn baby in level II

An infants weighing between 1500–2000 gm or having gestational maturity of 32–36 weeks need specialized neonatal care supervised by trained nurses and pediatricians.

District hospitals, teaching institutions and nursing homes should be equipped to provide intermediate neonatal care. Equipment for resuscitation, maintenance of thermoneutral environment, intravenous infusion and gavages feeding, phototherapy and exchange blood transfusion should be provided.

There should be no compromise on the basis needs of adequate space, nursing staff and maintenance of asepsis including provision for disposable gamma-irradiated suction catheters, feeding tubes, endotracheal tubes, small vein infusion sets, etc.

Intermediate neonatal care is needed for about 10 to 15 percent of newborn population and should be available at all hospitals catering to 1000 to 1500 deliveries per year.

Care of Newborn Baby in Level-III

Intensive neonatal care is required for babies weighing less than 1500 gm or those born before 32 weeks of gestation.

Apex institutions or regional perinatal centers equipped with centralized oxygen and suction facilities, servo-controlled incubators, vital sign and transcutaneous monitors, ventilators and infusion pumps, etc. are best suited to provide intensive neonatal care. Skilled nurses and neonatologists are required to organize this service. About 3 to 5 percent of newborn populations qualify for intensive care.

Establishment of intensive care neonatal center demands a sound infrastructure and should be envisaged only when optimal intermediate neonatal care facilities have already been in existence for sometime.

The capital and recurring expenditure for level III care is exorbitant and it is not cost effective unless service is regionalized.

Basic Care of Normal Newborn Babies

It is desirable to keep the normal term babies with their mothers rather than in a separate nursery. Rooming-in promotes better emotional rapport between the mother and the baby. The mother can participate in the nursing care of her baby. This infuses self-confidence in her and reduces demands on nursing personnel. Cross infection is prevented and breast feeding is established easily.

The baby should be open-back and covered adequately depending upon the environmental temperature. The baby's color, respiration, temperature and umbilical stump should be checked on arrival in the lying-in ward. Skin temperature should be recorded twice a day.

Mother's Role in the Care of the Baby at Home

The health and survival of the newborn baby depends upon the health status of the mother and her awareness, education and skills in mothercraft.

A mother is the best primary health worker. She has the advantages of instinct, concern and interest to look after her baby.

A mother looks after her baby with love, affection and sense of sacrifice. Early involvement of the mother in the care of her baby is the best way to promote and encourage breast-feeding. The healthy babies should never by house in the nursery. Mother is the best person to identify minor developmental deviations and early evidences of disease process because she is constantly and closely watching her baby.

The basic knowledge and skills pertaining to mothercraft, child nutrition, immunizations, environmental sanitation and personal hygiene, and common problems in children, etc. should be manuals and Anganwadis should organize regular teaching and training programs in mothercraft.

The simple messages for basic care of pregnant women and healthy babies should be widely disseminated through available media including radio and television.

Care of Breastfeeding

All mothers must be emotionally and physically prepared and motivated during pregnancy so that they do not encounter any difficulties to establish successful breastfeeding. The inverted and cracked nipples must be managed during pregnancy so that baby is not faced with any mechanical difficulties during breastfeeding.

- The baby should be put straight to the breast as soon as the mother has recovered from the fatigue of labor. The first feed is usually offered within 1 to 2 hours after birth.
- There is no need to administer any prelacteal feeds in the form of honey, glucose water, tea, etc. The colostrums (milk secretions during the first three days of lactation) must never by discarded and all babies should invariably receive it because it is rich in energy, proteins, protective antibodies and cellular elements.
- The physiological inadequacy of lactation during first three days of nursing should never be considered as an excuse for supplementing the feeding because it does not impose and hazards to a healthy newborn baby because he has a large pool of extracellular fluid volume and enough quota of glycogen in the liver.
- The introduction of supplemental feeds during this period will lead to refusal on the part of the baby to suck on the breast resulting in delayed establishment of lactation.
- The mother must be explained and reassured that the act of sucking is the best stimulus for milk production and the small amount of concentrated milk produced during first two to three days of lactation is adequate to meet the nutritional needs of healthy normal babies.
- During first six months of life the baby should receive exclusive breast feeds and there is no need to give any water even during summer months because all the fluid requirements of the baby are met through milk.
- The exclusively breast fed babies are likely to have better weight gain because they will drink more milk when thirsty.

- The child should be on demand feeding and most babies are satisfied with feeds taken every two to three hours. The mother should sit up comfortably and keep the baby's head slightly raised and supported on her elbow.
- The baby should not allowed to merely suck on the nipple but he must grasp the areola and part of the breast tissue into his mouth.
- The baby should be allowed to suck at the breast till he is satisfied which usually takes 15–20 minutes. Some babies are satisfied with one breast while others may need to suck at both the breasts during each feeding session.
- During each feed one breast must be completely emptied before the baby is put to the other breast. Alternate breast should be offered first at the next feed. The mother should actively interact with the baby while breastfeeding. She should intently look at the baby and fondle with him so that he does not fall asleep half way through the feed.
- The baby is receiving adequate feeds if he sleeps well after a feed for at least 2 hours, gains weight regularly on an average of 30 g per day (after the first week of life) and voids urine six or more times a day.
- During first four to six weeks many babies need to be fed round-the-clock and after that gradually the night feeds can be reduced to one late night feed and one early morning feed. The regurgitation of feeds is often due to faulty technique of feeding and swallowing of air during sucking.
- The mother must be advised to burp the child after each feed to safeguard against the risk of regurgitation. Many babies feel uncomfortable till they eructate out the swallowed air.
- During lactation the mother should be advised to take extra liquids and additional 450 calories per day and supplements of micronutrients in order to maintain her own health and nutrition, and improve the nutritional quality of milk.

Care of Newborn Baby Temperature

The body temperature in newborn babies is usually unstable and they are particularly vulnerable to develop hypothermia in winter. The environmental temperature that may feel uncomfortable to an adult may impose serious cold stress to a newborn baby. The baby bath should not be given at birth and delayed till next day when his temperature has stabilized.

The child should be nursed in close proximity to the mother so that the baby gains heat from maternal warmth. In winter, the linen and clothes of the baby should be prewarmed.

He should be provided with a cap, socks and mittens. The rooms should be kept warm. The mother and health workers should be trained to assess the temperature of the baby by touch alone.

The trunk should feel warmer than the perceiving hand. The hands and feet of the baby should be warm and pink. The presence of warm and pink extremities are reassuring that baby is not having any cold stress.

The cultural practice of keeping the mother-baby dyad isolated from 40 days is useful and needs to be promoted. It prevents exposure of the baby to cold and safeguards against occurrence of infections. The oil massage is also both culturally and scientifically acceptable as it provides insulation against heat and insensible water loss.

Baby Body Massage

Body Message is culturally accepted and has scientifically proven benefits. Oil massage of the baby should be postponed till he is 3 to 4 weeks old and his body weight is more than 3 kg. Most babies enjoy an oil massage; they cry less and sleep better.

It improves the circulation and tone of the muscles, gives comfort to the baby, strengthens maternal bonding and provides additional energy to the baby because oil can get absorbed from the thin skin of the baby. Oil massage is credited to improve weight gain, reduce stress and enhance immunological functions of the baby.

It prevents dryness and chaffing of skin. Use a nonirritating oil like olive oil or coconut oil but avoid mustard oil in young infants. There are no additional virtues of doing a message with butter oil or almond oil.

The baby should be massaged before giving the bath in a room which is comfortably kept warm and free from draughts. In winter massage is best done by placing the baby in front of a closed window through which sunrays are peeping in the room.

The exposure of the skin to sunrays is an important source of endogenous production of vitamin D in the skin.

Care of Baby Skin and Baby Bath

The baby must be cleaned off blood, mucus and meconium before he is presented to the mother. Effective cleaning and drying of skin at birth minimizes the risk of potential infection by microorganisms such as hepatitis B virus, HIV and herpes simplex virus.

She should be bathed or sponged next morning using unmediated soap and clean lukewarm water. The barrier nursing with separate articles for each baby in their individual lockers is desirable.

There should be no centralized bathing of babies as this often results in cross infection. The nursing toilet of each baby should be carried out by the cot-side as this has the advantage of providing education and ensuring active participation of the mother.

Routine use of hexachlorophene is not recommended because of its neurologic toxicity to the newborn babies. In the event of an epidemic of staphylococcal infection, use of chlorhexidine gluconate lotion or medicated soap is recommended, taking care that skin is rinsed thoroughly, after its application. It has been shown, that 'no bath' regimen during hospital stay of the baby reduces incidence of superficial infections.

During summer months, the baby can be given a bath. The rooms should be reasonably warm and free of any draught. Take clean, warm water in a plastic basin.

Avoid dip baths till the cord has fallen. Use any mild unmediated soap. The baby should be held over the forearms or over the thighs. Bath by wetting and applying soap to small areas beginning from head and proceeding downwards to prevent exposure. Eyes should be cleaned by using one sterile water soaked swab for each eye.

The bottom should be washed in the end to avoid contamination of healthy areas of skin. The infant should be promptly dried with a soft towel to prevent damage to the delicate skin of the baby. No vigorous attempts should be made to rub off the vernix caseosa which provides protection to the delicate skin.

During winter months the baby should preferably be sponged rather than bathed to avoid the risk of exposure.

The use of talcum powder is unnecessary except for aesthetic purpose. Talcum powder should be taken on the fingers or cotton ball and applied over the axilla and groins taking care that it is not sprinkled over the eyes and nostrils. After the baby should be given a breastfeed. Most babies go to sleep after the ritual of a bath and breastfeed. They wake up after 2 to 3 hours fully refreshed and ready for the next feed. Bathing provides a good opportunity to the nurse to identify any developmental peculiarities and superficial skin infections which should be brought to the notice of the physician.

Care of the Umbilical Stump

The umbilical cord is an important site for entry of spores of tetanus. The health personnel must use sterile instruments to cut and clamp the cord to prevent occurrence of tetanus neonatorum. The cord must be inspected after 2 to 4 hours of birth. Bleeding commonly occurs at this time due to shrinkage of cord and loosening of ligatures. Ligation of cord with rubber band or disposable clip safeguards against this hazard.

Triple dye, ethyl alcohol or betadine should be applied at the tip and around the base of the umbilical stump daily to prevent colonization. The dressing should not be applied. The stump need not be kept moistened in babies with future need for exchange transfusion but precautions should be taken to keep the stump bacteria free by using polybactericidal powder containing neomycin, bacitracin and polymyxin. The cord normally falls after 5 to 10 days but may 6 take longer, if it is dry and shriveled or when infected. The delayed falling of the cord is also a useful marker of immunodeficiency state.

Care of the Eyes

Eyes should be cleaned daily with sterile cotton swabs soaked in normal saline using one swab for each eye. If the eyes are sticky, 10 percent solution of sulfacetamide should be instilled in the eyes every two to four hours. Prophylactic instillation of human colostrums into the eyes has been shown to reduce the incidence of sticky eyes. The practice of applying kajal in the eyes is not recommended because it may transmit infection like trachoma and may even cause lead poisoning.

Dresses for the Baby

The clothes should be loose, soft and preferably made of cotton. They should be open on the front or back for ease of wearing. Avoid the use of large buttons which may hurt the tender skin of the baby. The nappies in order to readily soak the urine and stools. The use of plastic napkin should be avoided at home due to increased risk of nappy rash.

The woolen clothes should not be stored and preserved with moth balls because there is a potential risk of development of severe jaundice in a baby who is deficient in glucose-6-phosphate dehydrogenate enzyme in his red blood cells. When woolens had been protected with moth balls, they should be exposed to bright sunlight for one to two days before being worn.

Early Detection of Serious Disease

The pediatricians can justify their presence in the maternity wards only if they exercise due vigilance to diagnose neonatal abnormalities at the earliest. Most healthy term babies do not pose any serious health problems except appearance of certain developmental peculiarities and minor problems which need identification, reassurance and advice to the mother. However, when a newborn baby is genuinely sick and refuses to take adequate feeds or manifest any other danger signs he should be considered as seriously ill. The following danger signs should be closely watched and brought to the notice of the consultant.

Bleeding from any site; appearance of jaundice within 24 hours of age or deep jaundice; failure to pass meconium within 24 hours and urine within 48 hours; vomiting or diarrheal poor feeding; undue lethargy or excessive crying; excessive frothiness or drooling; chocking at feeds; respiratory difficulty, apneic attacks and/or cyanosis; seizures; sudden rise or fall in the body temperature and any evidences of superficial infection (conjunctivitis, pustules, umbilical sepsis and oral thrush, etc.)

Weight Record

Most babies lose weight during first 2 to 3 days of life. The weight loss varies between 5–8 percent of birth weight. The weight remains stationary during next 1 to 2 days and birth weight is regained by the end of first week. The factors contributing to initial weight loss include removal of vernix, mucus and blood from skin, passage of meconium and reduction of extracellular fluid volume. The transition from in utero parenteral nutrition to postnatal oral feeding is growth of babies. Deliberate starvation and delayed feeding is associated with excessive weight loss. Exclusively breastfed babies tend to lose relatively more weight due to inadequacy of lactation during initial 2 to 3 days. Malnourished small-for-dates babies, if fed early and adequately, do not lose weight and start gaining weight within 2 to 3 day after birth.

During first year of life average daily weight gain is around 30 g, 20 g and 10 g during first, second and third 4 months periods respectively. Most infants double their birth weight by 4–5 month of age and triple it by their first birth day. It is mandatory that periodic weight record should be taken and charted on Road-To-Health cards during preschool years.

Immunizations

BCG and first dose of OPV and hepatitis B vaccine (HBV) are given at birth or before the baby is discharged from the hospital. The OPV may preferably be given after 3 days because colostrums may interfere with its uptake.

The BCG site should be checked for 'take' response after 4 weeks. Persistent and recurrent ulceration at the site of vaccination or regional adenitis responds to oral administration of erythromycin in a dose of 30 mg/kg/day for 14 days or INH 10 mg/kg/day for 3 months. The modified national vaccination schedule along with optional vaccines is depicted in:

- The suggested schedule may be modified by the consultant pediatrician as per the local needs
- Breastfeeding can be given after oral polio vaccine and it does not interfere with development of satisfactory immunity.
- Most immunization can be given in the presence of a minor illness. Paracetamol should be routinely given following a vaccination for relief of local pain and fever.
- There is no need to give HIB vaccine (Hemophilus influenza type B vaccine) if it has not been taken by the age of 1 ½ years.

- Chicken pox is a mild disease among healthy children and natural infection provides a lifelong protection. If the natural infection does not occur by the age of 10 years chicken-pox vaccine may then be given as a single dose.
- HAV (Hepatitis A vaccine) is not usually required after the age of 5 years because most children become seropositive by contracting natural subclinical infection.
- The need and cost-effectiveness of optional vaccines must be explained to the parents before they are recommended.
- Live vaccines should be avoided in immune compromised children and symptomatic HIV-positive infants.
- A number of vaccines can be administered together simultaneously without interfering with development of protection against different antigens. But, after having given a vaccine, the minimum interval for administration of next vaccine should be at least 4 weeks.
- When a dose of a vaccine is missed, the remaining dose should be administered at the earliest opportunity while keeping in mind that the vaccine dose already given is valid.

Supplements and Follow-up

Human milk of healthy mothers receiving adequate nutrition and supplements of micronutrients is a complete food to look after all the nutritional needs of their healthy normal weight babies. Vitamin-K 1.0 mg 1M is given to all babies at birth to prevent occurrence of hemorrhagic disease of the newborn.

There are recent reports to suggest that some healthy breast fed babies may develop rickets at 3–4 months of age and should be provided supplements of vitamin-D.

The infants should be followed-up in the Well Baby Clinic for evaluation of their growth and development, immunizations, nutritional advice, early diagnosis of abnormalities and guidance to the parents for the management of day-to-day problems of their children. When complementary feeds are started after 6 months of age, supplements of vitamins and minerals should be provided.

BREASTFEEDING

Introduction

The practice of breastfeeding is widely prevalent in India except among the urban elites. In urban areas bottle is replacing the breast (with disastrous result) because of several reasons.

Definition

Breastfeeding is the normal way of providing young infants with the nutrients they need for healthy growth and development. Virtually all mothers can breastfeed, provided they have accurate information, and the support of their family, the health care system and society at large.

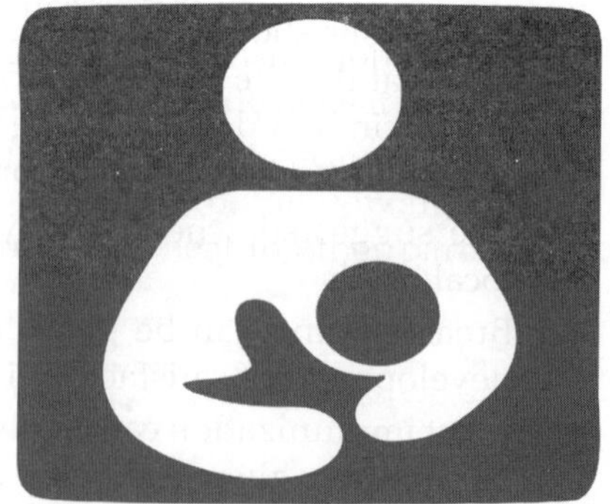

Fig. 2.4: Breastfeeding

Colostrums, the yellowish, sticky breast milk produced at the end of pregnancy, is recommended by WHO as the perfect food for the newborn, and feeding should be initiated within the first hour after birth.

Exclusive breastfeeding is recommended up to 6 months of age, with continued breastfeeding along with appropriate complementary foods up to two years of age or beyond.

Physiology of Lactation

Lactation involves three physiological processes

1. Development of mammary glands
2. Milk synthesis and its maintenance
3. Ejection or propulsion of milk from the alveoli to the nipple.

By the end of pregnancy the breasts are fully developed but do not secrete. Milk starts coming in on the third or fourth day after delivery. Nevertheless to promote the let down reflex baby has to be put to breast within a couple of hours after his birth. The let down reflex heavily depends upon the act of sucking and positive psychological confidence of the mother. Anxiety and stress depress the reflex.

Prolactin is stimulated by the act of suckling and is responsible for milk secretion. The let down reflex is psychosomatic, being stimulated by confidence and inhibited by anxiety and stressful by confidence and inhibited by anxiety and stressful conditions. This reflex can be significantly enhanced by judicious antenatal preparation of the mother. Anxiety, uncertainty and lock of interest can lead to lactation failure. Pain, sore nipple, cracked nipple, bacterial invasion and breast abscess can lead to poor let-down reflex causing breast engorgement and subsequent lactation failure. No particular food is definitely known to increase the milk quantity. At the beginning of a feed the milk contains less fat and more proteins and may look watery.

Towards the end, the fat content rises and milk is more opaque, whiter and appears thicker. After the first month of lactation volume of milk increases a little. As the baby's weight increases greatly, the fat and energy content of milk rises. As the feed proceeds there are changes in taste and texture. After a fairly long period, milk yield tends to diminish.

Lactation can continue from 6 months to 1 year. Sucking stimulation is the best galactogouge. In maternal malnutrition, fat and other constituents may be lowered and total volume is decreased and the milk quantity is reduced by about 3–4 months. Breastfeeding at night, should be encouraged in early months as prolactin levels are high at night giving a good milk yield during night. Prelacteal feeds, e.g. water, honey, herbs are not necessary and may actually depress lactation if the baby does not suck at the breast during this period.

The Advantages of Breastfeeding are as Follows

Nutritive Value

- Breast milk contains all the nutrients in the right proportion which are needed for optimum growth and development of the baby up to 4 to 6 months.
- It is essential for brain growth of the infant because it has high percentage of lactose and galactose which are important components of galactocerebroside.
- It facilitates absorption of calcium which helps in bony growth.

- It contains amino acids like taurine (2-aminoethanesulfonic acid) and cysteine which are necessary for the myelination of the nervous system.
- It has vitamins, minerals, electrolytes and water in the right proportion for the infant which are necessary for the maturation of the intestinal tract.
- It provides 66 calories per 100 ml and contains 1.2 g protein, 3.8 g fat, 7 g lactose and vitamin 'A' 170 to 670 IU, vitamin C' to 6 mg. The total amount of milk secretion per day is about 600 to 700 ml, which is sufficient for the baby. Its composition is ideal for an infant.
- It provides specific nutrition for preterm baby in preterm delivery.

Digestibility

Breast milk is easily digestible. The protein of breast milk is mostly lacto albumin and loctoglobulin which form soft curds that is easy to digest. The enzyme lipase in the breast milk helps in the digestion of fats and provides free fatty acids.

Protective Value

Breast milk contains 1gA, 1gM, macrophages, lymphocytes, bifida factors, unsaturated lactoferrin, lysozyme, complement and interferon. Thus breastfed body less likely to develop infections especially gastrointestinal and respiratory tract infections, e.g. diarrhea and ARI.

It also provides protection against malaria and various viral and bacterial infections like skin infections, septicemia, etc.

Breastfeeding protects in infant from allergy and bronchial asthma. It also products against neonatal hypocalcemia, tenancy, necrotizing enterocolitis, deficiencies of vitamin-E and zinc, neonatal convulsions and sudden infant death syndrome.

Exclusive breastfeeding baby has less chance of developing malnutrition, hypertension, diabetes mellitus, coronary artery disease, arteriosclerosis, uncreative mellitus, coronary artery disease, arteriosclerosis, ulcerative colitis, appendicitis, childhood lymphoma, liver disease, celiac disease and dental caries.

Psychological Benefits

- Breastfeeding promotes close physical and emotional bondage with the mother by frequent skin to skin contact, attention and interaction.
- It stimulates psychomotor and social development. It leads to better parent child adjustment, fewer behavioral disorders in children and less risk of child abuse and neglect.
- Breastfeeding promotes development of higher intelligence and feeling of security in infant.

Maternal Benefits

- Breastfeeding reduces the chance of postpartum hemorrhage and helps in better uterine involution, lactational amenorrhea promotes in recovery or iron stores. It can protect from pregnancy for first 6 months if exclusive breastfeeding is carried out.
- Breastfeeding improves metabolic efficiency and dissatisfaction with sense of fulfillment of the mother.

- It reduces the risk of breast and ovarian cancer of the mother.
- It improves slimming of the mother by consuming extra fat which accumulated during pregnancy.
- It is more convenient and time saving for the mother. Mother can provide fresh, pure, ready-made, clean uncontaminated milk to her baby at right temperature without any preparations. Mother feels comfortable to feed the baby especially at night.

Family and Community Benefits

- Breastfeeding is economical in terms of saving of many, time and energy.
- Family has to spend less on milk, health care and illness.
- Community expenditure of health care and contraception are reduced. It is economic for the families, hospitals, communities and for countries.

Preparation for Breastfeeding

Preparation for breastfeeding must begin in the antenatal period. The idea of breastfeeding can be introduced in childhood period and during school education about its importance. Mothercraft training should be provided and includes benefits of breastfeeding which should be given in the prepregnant state.

In the antenatal period, examination of breast and identification of problems, like retracted nipple, should be done with necessary advice for interventions. Adequate diet in prenatal period should be consumed in terms of energy and nutrients. Prevention of micronutrient deficiencies, rest, regular exercise, hygienic measures, etc. should be advices for better health in antenatal period.

Antenatal counseling, family support, mother-support group also should be emphasized as the preparation of mothers for breastfeeding. Mother should be psychologically prepare to feed her baby immediate after birth.

Initiation of Breastfeeding

Breastfeeding should be initiated within first half-an-hour to one hour of birth or as soon a possible. It should be to one hour of birth after cesarean section delivery.

Early suckling provides warmth, security and colostrums, the baby's first immunization. Although little in amount, the first milk, colostrums, is most suitable and contains a high concentration of protein and other nutrients, the baby needs. It is in anti-infective factors and protects the baby from respiratory infections and diarrheal diseases.

Mothers should be demonstrated about the techniques of breastfeedings. Rooming—in or bedding—in should be done with infant and mother as soon as possible to prevent separation. Mother should be advised for exclusive breastfeeding up to 4 to 6 months and as demand feeding.

No food or drink other than breast milk should be given to neonates. No water, glucose water, animal milk, gripe water, indigenous medicines, vitamins and minerals drops or syrup should be given. No bottle and pacifier are followed.

In case of preterm babies or sick babies, being in special care unit, they should be fed with expressed breast milk (EBM).

Nursing staff is responsible to ensure that nothing except breast milk is given. Mother should be instructed to assess the indicators of adequacy of breastfeeding and importance of increasing her own dietary intake with extra 550 cal and to drink fluids in response to her thirst. Rest and relaxation of mother are important for recovery from delivery and successful lactation in postnatal period.

Indicators of Adequacy of Breastfeeding

Adequacy of breastfeeding in indicated and established by the followings:

- Audible swallowing sound during the feed.
- Let down sensation in mother's breast.
- Breast is full before feed and softer afterward.
- Wet nappies 6 or more in 24 hours.
- Frequent soft bowel movements, 3 top 8 times in 24 hours.
- Average weight gain of 18 to 30 gm per day.
- Baby sleeps well and does not cry frequently.
- Baby has good muscle tone and healthy skin.

Different Composition of Breast Milk

The composition of breast milk varies at different stages in the postnatal period to fulfill the needs of the baby.

Colostrum: It is secreted during first three days after delivery. It is thick, yellow and small in quantities. It contains more antibodies and cells with higher amount of proteins and fat soluble vitamin (A, D, E, K). It is sufficient and protective for the baby and should not be discarded.

Transitional milk: It follows the colostrums and secretes during first two weeks of postnatal period. It has increased fat and sugar content and decreased protein and immunoglobulin content.

Mature milk: It is secreted usually from 10 to 12 days after delivery. It is watery but contains all nutrients for optimal growth of the baby.

Preterm milk: The breast milk secreted by a mother who has delivered a preterm baby is different from milk of a mother who has delivered a full term baby. This milk contains more proteins, sodium, iron, immunoglobulin and calories appropriate for the requirements of the preterm neonates.

Fore milk: It is secreted at the starting of the regular breastfeeding. It is more watery to satisfy the baby's thirst and contains more proteins, sugar, vitamins and minerals.

Hind milk: It is secreted towards the end of regular breastfeeding and contains more fat and energy. The mother should feed the baby allowing one breast to empty of provides both fore milk and hind milk, before offering other breast. For optimum growth and to fulfill adequate fluid and nutritional requirements, both fore milk and hind milk are needed for the baby.

Technique of Breastfeeding

Majority of mothers can feed their babies successfully. Some mothers need help in the technique of breastfeeding, specially the prime mother, mothers having breastfeeding problems in previous pregnancy, nonmotivated mothers about breastfeeding and the mother having retracted nipples. Nursing personnel should help the mother to follow the technique of breastfeeding.

- Mother should be comfortable and relaxed physically and mentally before giving breast feed. She should wash her hands and can have a glass of water or milk.
- Mother should have no due work in her hands. Baby should be cleaned and dried before feeding, otherwise baby may feel discomfort or may noncooperate during feeding.
- Correct positioning of mother and baby is an important aspect of successful breastfeeding. Mother can be in flat with infant on top of the mother, especially following LUCS delivery. Baby should be supported by the mother's forearm in slight head elevated position and with head, neck and back in a straight line. Baby should be hold close to mother with trunk to trunk in touch and facing towards breast.
- Latching after proper positioning, when baby's chin touches the breast, cheek touches the nipple, baby will open the mouth in rooting reflex. Then the baby will be quickly moved on to the breast with the lower lip below the nipple; so that the nipple and most of the areola go into the baby's mouth.
- The suckling of breast stimulates the milk secretion or prolactin reflex, which promotes the milk production and secretion. Then by the milk ejection or oxytocin reflex, milk flows out from the glands into the lactiferous sinuses and ducts and then to the baby's mouth. When baby suckles again and again in regular slow deep sucks with good sucking reflex, the adequate milk flows out and there baby's cheeks become full with milk.

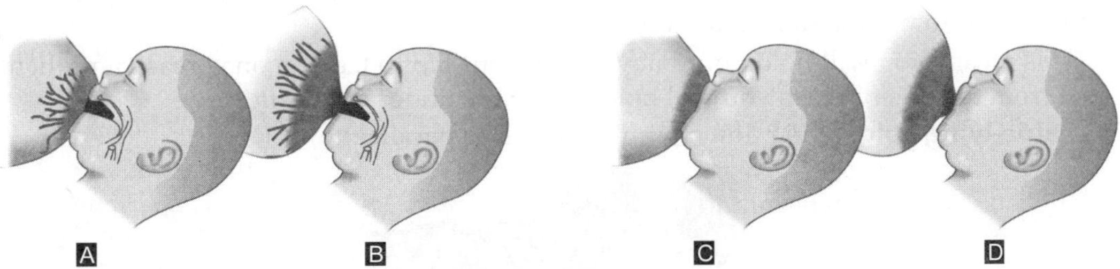

Figs. 2.5 (A to D): A. Good attachment; B. Poor attachment; C and D. Outside appearance: C. Good attachment, D. Poor attachment

- The mother may hear the swallowing sound and does not feel pain in the nipple. All these indicate favorable signs of good attachment or latching and breastfeeding.
- The baby should have good swallowing reflex to take adequate feed with sufficient flow of milk. If the baby fall asleep after few sucks, mother should arouse the baby by gently tap behind the ear or no the sole of the foot.
- Initially breastfeeding can be given at 1–2 hours interval and then on self-demand by the baby. A baby usually cries when feel hungry and then must be put into the breast.
- Duration of feeding should be continued till the baby is satisfied. The duration of sucking depends upon the vigor of the baby and on the let-down reflex. One breast should be emptied completely before starting with another breast. Next feeding should be started with opposite breast, i.e. which was fed last in the previous feeding.
- Burping is usually not necessary, if the baby is having good latching and attachment during feeding which prevent air entry into the baby's mouth.
- Baby should be placed on right side after feeding. Usually the baby falls asleep. Mother should make the baby dry and comfortable.

- Breastfeeding should be continued exclusively up to 4 months of age or preferably may be up to 6 months if adequate breast milk is available the baby should be given only breast milk and nothing else, not even water for first 4 months of life, even in summer months. Frequent sucking helps to have adequate amount of milk for the baby.
- Complementary foods can be started between 4 to 6 months, exact age may vary, but breastfeeding should be continued up to 2 years of age or beyond and especially at night.
- Mother should maintain hygienic measures, take daily bath and wash her breast during bath and wear clean blouse during this period to prevent contamination of breast milk.

Breastfeeding Positions

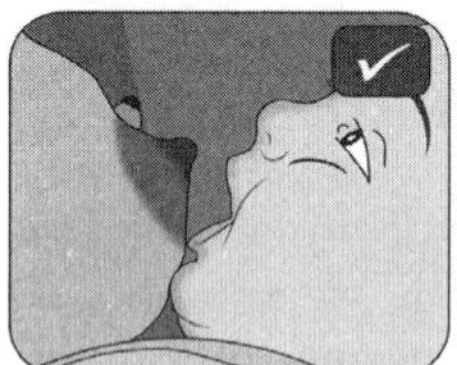
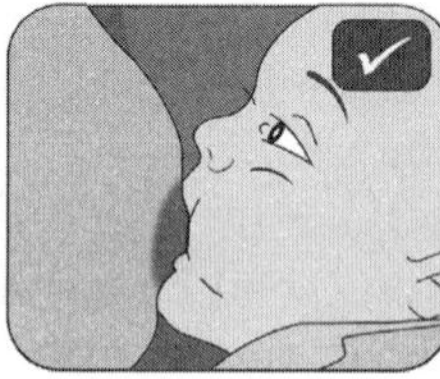
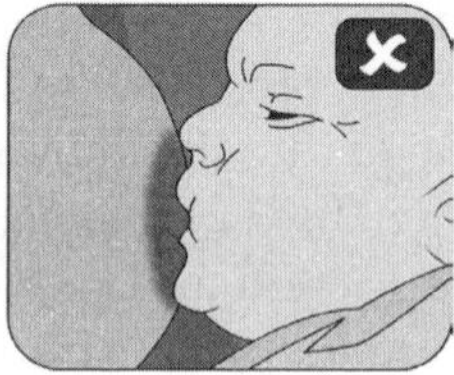

Fig. 2.6: Breastfeeding positions

There is no one correct position for breastfeeding. Any of these styles may work well for you and your baby. In the early days of breastfeeding, while you are still learning, you may find it easier to use the same hand for both breasts.

This means you will hold your baby across your lap to feed on one breast, and then to feed from the other breast, you will hold your baby under your arm.

- **Side-lying hold:** Lying down with your bodies parallel.

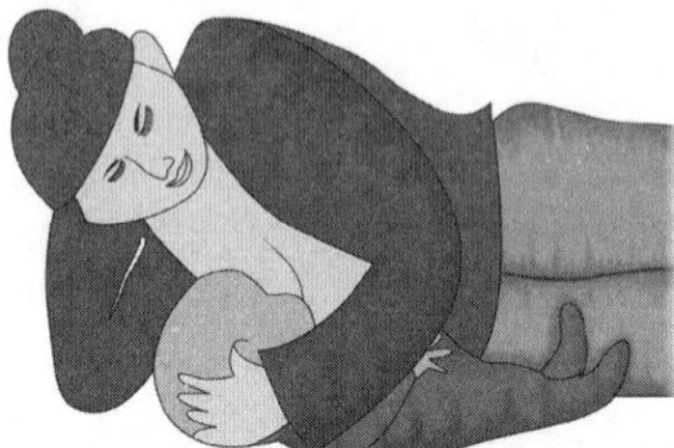

Fig. 2.7: Side-lying hold

- **Cradle hold (same arm):** Holding your baby across your lap, supporting her with the same arm as your breast.

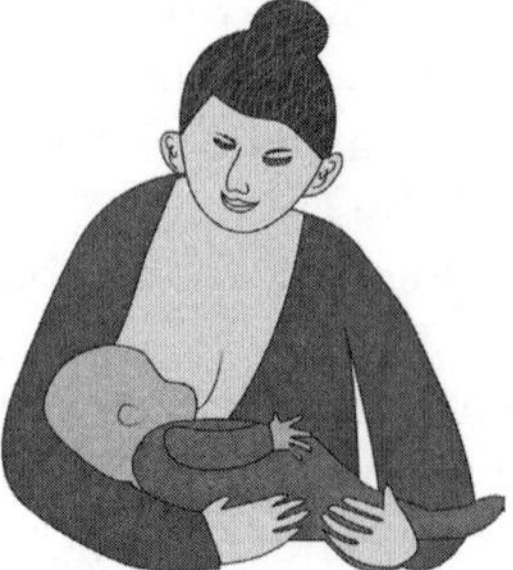

Fig. 2.8: Cradle hold

- **Cross-cradle hold (opposite arm):** Holding your baby across your lap, using the opposite arm to the breast she is feeding from to support her.

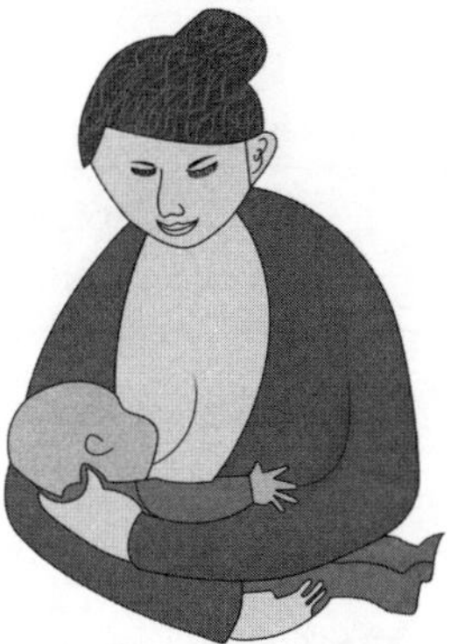

Fig. 2.9: Cross-cradle hold (opposite arm)

- **Food (rugby) ball hold:** Holding your baby underarm.

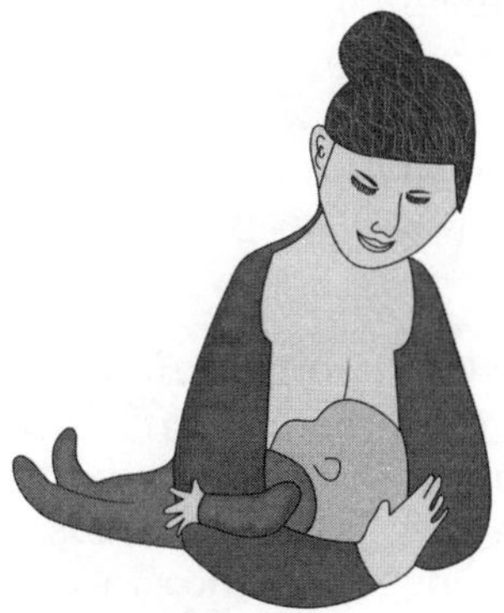

Fig. 2.10: Food (rugby) ball hold

- **Twins hold:** Using a cushion (pillow) under your babies as you gently support them with your hands on their upper backs.

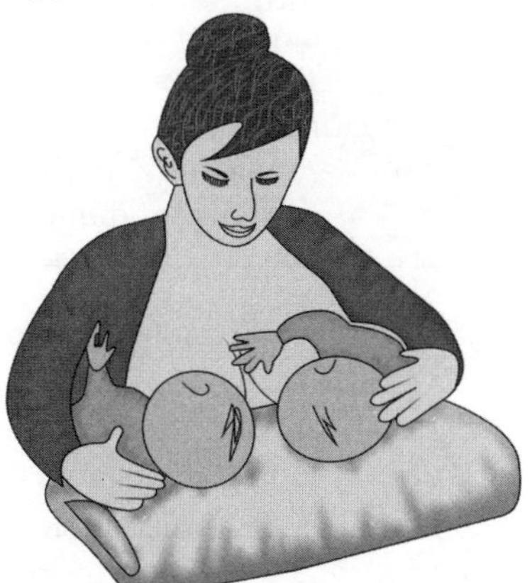

Fig. 2.11: Twins hold

- **Koala hold:** Supporting your baby while she has straddled across your knees in an upright position.

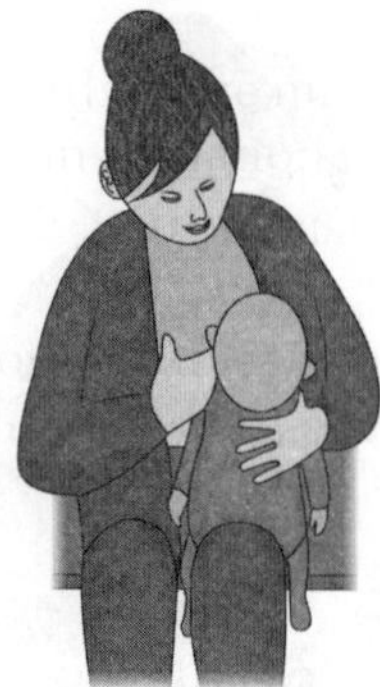

Fig. 2.12: Koala hold

- **Laid-back breastfeeding (Biological nurturing):** Semireclined, with your baby lying across your stomach or shoulder.

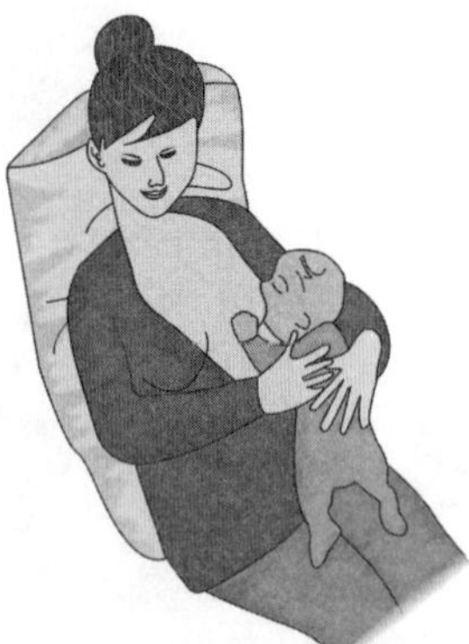

Fig. 2.13: Laid-back breastfeeding (biological nurturing)

- **Laid-back breastfeeding after a cesarean:** Semireclined, with your baby lying vertically on you, to protect your cesarean wound.

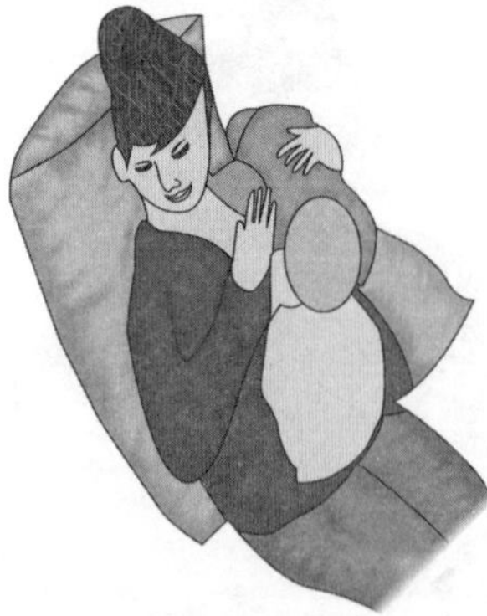

Fig. 2.14: Laid-back breastfeeding after a cesarean

Breastfeeding after a Cesarean

Semireclined, with your baby lying vertically on you, to protect your cesarean wound.

Contraindication of Breastfeeding

The true contraindications of breastfeeding are galactosemia and phenylketonuria. Maternal conditions which can be considered as REAL contraindications are Radiotherapy, Ergometrine therapy, Antimetabolites therapy and Lithium therapy.

Maternal illness should not result in interruption of breastfeeding. Expressed breast milk (EBM) can be given to the baby, whenever needed, from the mother or mother's substitute.

Problems of Breastfeeding

The measures to be taken to overcome the problems are as follows:

The baby who does not suckle

- No unneeded drugs to be given to breastfeeding mothers.
- No artificial food or water to be given to the baby.
- Breastfeeding to be given when the baby is alert and ready.
- Milk to be expressed into the nipple just prior to feed the baby.
- Nipple should be placed slightly upward towards the roof of the baby's mouth.
- Keeping the baby's nose free during breastfeeding.

The baby who refused on breast

- Baby should be hold in comfortable position with good attachment to the breast and should be kept dry and warm.
- Avoiding pressure on potentially painful areas during feeding.
- Express breast milk to maintain lactation in both breasts.
- Allowing the baby to geed only one breast.

Inverted Nipples

- Treatment should be started after birth of the baby.
- The nipple is manually stretched and rolled out several times a day.
- A pump or a plastic syringe is use to draw out the nipple and the baby is then put of the breast.

Sore Nipple

- Correct positioning and latching of the baby to the breast.
- Frequent washing with soap and water should be avoided.
- Baby should not be pull off the breast while still sucking.
- Hind milk to be applied to the nipple after a feeding.
- Nipples should be aired and allowed to heal in between feeds.

Breast Engorgement

- Frequent feeding and correct attachment of the baby to the breast during feeding to be done to prevent engorgement.

- Treatment of this condition to be done with local warm packs and analgesics to the mother to relieve the pain.
- Milk should be expressed gently to soften the breast and then baby to be put of the breast with good latching.

Breast Abscess

- Treatment to be done with analgesics and antibiotics.
- Abscess any need incision and drainage.
- Breastfeeding must be continued.

Expressed Breast Milk

Expressing is a way of taking breast milk from your breast without your baby needing to suckle. You can do this by using:

- Manual hand methods
- A manual pump methods
- An electric pump methods.

Techniques

Consciously try to relax, using whatever method suits you. Try to express in a quiet, warm, relaxing area, away from distractions. While expressing, breathe slowly and deeply. You could express in the place you usually sit to feed. Some mothers have a warm drink first or listen to soft music. Warmth (expressing after a warm shower, warm face washers on the breast for a few minutes before starting) may also help.

Manual Hand Methods

- Gently massaging your breasts by stroking down towards the nipple, and gently rolling the nipple between your fingers. While you cannot actually push the milk out of your breasts by massage, you can help trigger the let-down by touching your breasts.
- Thinking about your baby and how much your breastmilk is helping her will encourage your let-down reflex. If she is premature or sick in hospital, you might find it easier to express near her crib or just after you leave her. If you are away from her, looking at her photo can help.
- Having someone support you. Many mothers find they manage much better when they have an encouraging partner or friend. Your ABA breastfeeding counselor can also give you ideas and encouragement as you learn to express.

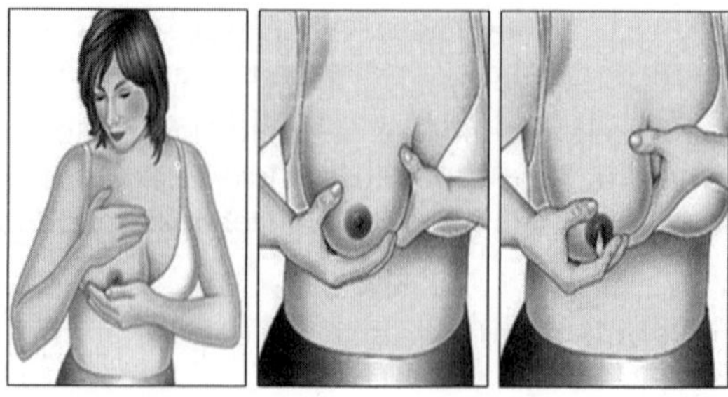

Fig. 2.15: Manual hand methods

A Manual Pump Methods

Hand expressing a little breast milk can help soothe engorgement and plugged ducts. And if you have sore, cracked nipples, you might want to express a bit of breast milk by hand after each nursing session to rub over them and soothe them.

Many women find that expressing milk by hand is time-consuming, though, so it is not usually feasible if you need to express a larger amount of milk regularly.

- Wash your hands before you start.
- You may find it helpful to massage your breasts a bit or apply a warm towel before expressing.
- Sit up and lean forward—gravity helps!
- Place your thumb and index finger on each side of the breast, about an inch or so behind the areola, forming a C with your hand.
- Press your fingers back toward your chest wall and then gently together. (You want to compress the area under the areola, not the nipple itself.) Use a rolling motion rather than pulling or yanking. You may need to experiment a bit to find the right spot—when you do, you will squirt milk.
- Rotate your fingers around the areola (starting on top and bottom and moving to the sides, for example) as you continue to milk each breast. At first you may only get a few drops. That is okay—you will get more with practice.

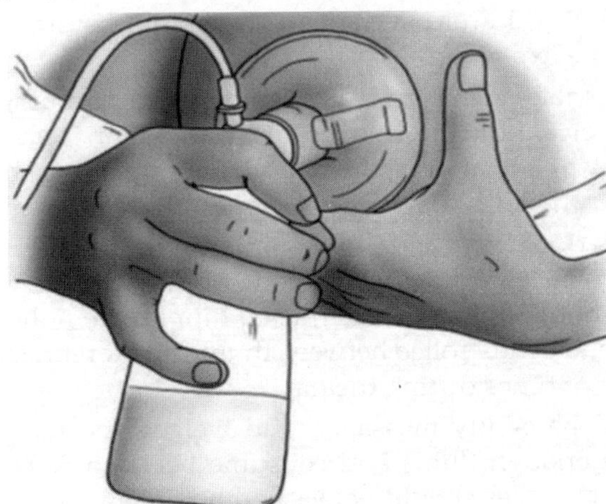

Fig. 2.16: Manual pump method

There are different opinions on how long breast milk stays fresh once it is left your body. The Centers for Disease Control and Prevention (CDC) says milk can be kept at room temperature for six to eight hours, though it is best to refrigerate it immediately. Use fresh, refrigerated milk within five days. (Store it in the back of the main part of the refrigerator.)

In the freezer compartment of a refrigerator (5 degrees F), milk can be frozen for two weeks. If there is a freezer compartment with separate doors (0 degree F), it can be stored for three to six months. And in a chest or upright deep freezer (–4 degrees F), it will be good for six to 12 months. (Use the lower numbers—three months and six months—for best quality. At the higher end, the milk is still safe, but the quality will be a bit lower.)

Once you have thawed frozen milk, you can keep it in the refrigerator for up to 24 hours. If it is at room temperature, use it within one hour. (If you have not used it in that time, you will have to throw it away, since you cannot refreeze it.) If you need to transport milk, keep it cold until just before using.

Reasons for avoiding breastfeeding by women

- Effect of high pressure promotional activities of manufactures of powdered milk.
- Doctor's or health worker's ignorance or apathy especially those working in hospitals where women deliver.
- Mother's fear that baby may not get enough milk.
- Feeling of revulsion at the idea of breastfeeding.
- Embarrassment about baring the breast.
- Fear of failure, sore nipples, breast abscess, exhaustion, spoiling the shape of the breasts.
- Feeling that bottle feeding is easier.
- A working mother
- Lack of confidence.
- Illness in the mother or baby.

Breastfeeding hence has to be positively promoted by pediatricians, general practitioners, obstetricians, nurses, midwives and other paramedical workers in child welfare centers. Preparations for breastfeeding should start during the antenatal period. Beneficial effects, nutritional, physical and psychological—should be emphasized. Advantages of breastfeeding should be explained.

Artificial feeding of babies in maternity homes should be discouraged except in exceptional circumstances. Mother should be relaxed and confident. Traditional beliefs prohibit breastfeeding for a day or two after birth. Actually breastfeeding should be initiated within a couple of hours after the birth of the baby, once mother has recovered.

During antenatal period breast and nipples must be cleaned. Skin over the nipple should not be dry. Retracted nipples are pulled out gently by holding the nipple must be cleaned. Skin over the nipple should not be dry. Retracted nipples are pulled out gently by holding the nipple at the base and gently rolled between thumb and forefinger. The procedure should be repeated a number of times during the day.

The breasts should be gently massaged and well supported. Nursing and pregnant mothers should have enough fluids and consume between 2500–3000 calories from the daily diet. Breasts and nipples should be washed before and after each feed with a gauze pad wetted in water. Lanoline cream can be applied to keep nipple moist. Erroneous beliefs concerning the disadvantages of breastfeeding be dispelled so that more mothers return to the tradition of breastfeeding.

Advantages of Breastfeeding

For the Infant

- Significant lower death rate due to avoidance of infection.
- Significant lower morbidity rate as number of infections are prevented. Various antibodies, lactoferrin, lysozyme, leucocytes and preponderance of lactobacilli giving acid pH are the factors preventing infections like E-coli, poliomyelitis, salmonella, gastroenteritis and necrotizing enterocolitis.

- Babies are less likely to become fat.
- Asthma, eczema, hypernatremia, dehydration, cot deaths, metabolic acidosis in the first three weeks, pyridoxine deficiency, calcium deficiency, tetany, dental caries and hypomagnesemia do not occur in breastfed babies.
- Breastfeeding in convenient, easy and cheap.
- Phychological bonding occurs between mother and baby.
- Breast milk has less solute load.
- Bioavailability of iron in breast milk is better.
- Breast milk is easily digestible because of higher level of lactalbumin and less of casein.
- Unsaturated fatty acids aid calcium absorption.
- Human milk is rich in cysteine which is essential for brain development.
- The anti-infective factors are present in significant amount even at 1 year of age of infant.
- Breast milk is postulated to be protective against future arteriosclerosis.

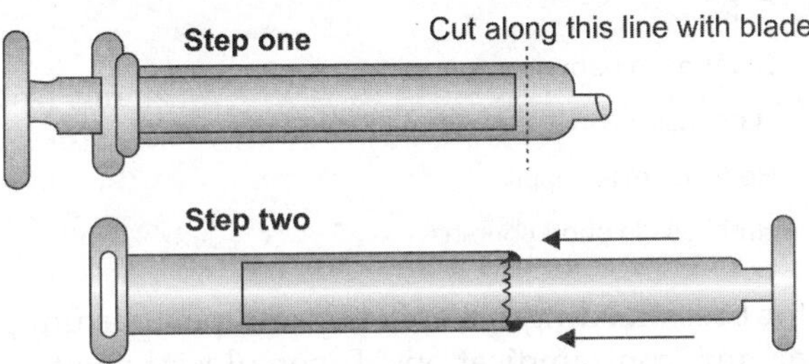

Fig. 2.17: Insert piston from cut end

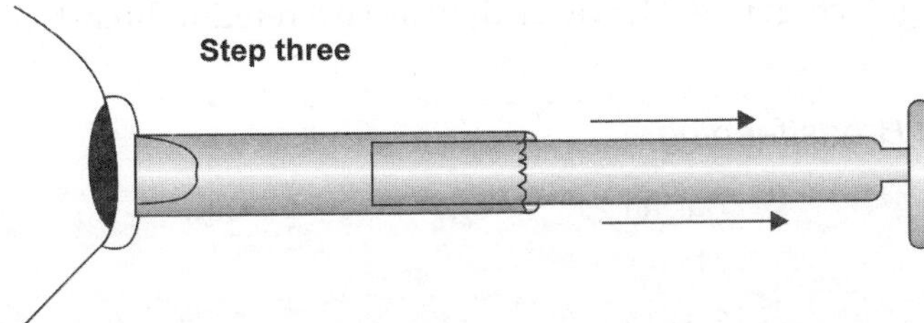

Fig. 2.18: Mother applies the smooth end to her breast and gently pulls the piston

For the Mother

- Mothers in whom lactation is suppressed by estrogens are liable to get thrombo-embolism. Continued breastfeeding prevents this.
- Breastfeeding facilitates normal evolution of uterus.
- Placental expulsion is facilitated by early initiation of breastfeeding.
- Lactation suppresses ovulation. This can be adopted as a family planning measure.
- No expense in involved for the milk itself, bottles or fuel. It is therefore a great national resource.
- Breast cancer is less common in women who feeding their babies.

Drugs Excreted in Breast Milk

Alcohol	Affects the baby
Nicotine	Reduces milk output. No effect on baby
Caffeine	Harmless
Antithyroid drugs	Harmful
Aspirin	Bleeding tendency in baby.
Antibiotics	Penicillin sensitivity can occur. Sulfonamides, Cotrimoxazole, Nitrofurantoin can cause hemolysis
Anticoagulants	Harmful
Sedatives	Sedation of baby
Morphine	Fairly safe
Bronchodilators	Harmless
Digoxin, Propranolol	Safe
Senna	Diarrhea in baby
Iron	Harmless
Oral Contraceptive	Reduces milk supply
Corticosteroids	Harmless in short courses

The contraindications for breastfeeding are epilepsy and postpartum psychosis. Breast milk jaundice and allergy are rare contraindications. Tuberculosis in mother is also a relative contraindication as breastfeeding involves close contact. Drugs taken by the mother are often excreted in breast milk. Onset of menstruation is not a contraindication for breastfeeding.

Psychotropic drugs (phenothiazine and tricyclic antidepressants) may increase prolactin level and can act as galactogouge. However they are excreted in breast milk and can over sedate a baby.

First Two Weeks of Breastfeeding

Items	**Human**	**Cow**
Calories	71	69
Proteins	1 g.	3.3 g.
Caseinogens	0.4 g.	2.7 g.
Lactose	7 g.	4.8 g.
Fat	3.8 g.	3.8 g.
Ash	0.21 mg.	0.71 mg.
Calcium/Phosphate	34/16 mg.	126/99 mg.
Iron	21 mg.	1.5 mg.
Folate	0.18 microgm.	0.23 microgm.
Vit B_{12}	0.04 microgm.	0.41 microgm.
Vit C	4.3 mg.	1.8 mg.

Artificial Feeding

Feeding an infant with artificial milk is a practice of great antiquity, but only in the last 50 years artificial feeding has become safe enough to be widely used. In developing countries where property is more of rule than exception amongst the masses, breastfeeding has to be positively encouraged.

Replacement of breast by bottle in developing countries, often leads to an increased incidence of diarrhea, malnutrition and death. In poor environment with shortage of fuel, clean water, clean utensils and proper storage facilities it is extremely difficult to prepare storage facilities it is extremely difficult of prepare a hygienic bottle feed. Feeds are often very dilute. Mother does not follow written instructions. Over concentrated feeds also pose a danger to the babies.

A wide range of tinned milk powders present a confusing picture to semiliterate mothers. In India bottle is thus a dangerous killer. Artificial feeding should be employed only and only if breastfeeding is not feasible. The decision to resort to artificial feeding must be taken after all the efforts to breastfeed the baby have proved futile.

Indications for Artificial Feeding

Death of mother, working mother, chronic illnesses in mother, another pregnancy, lactation failure, intolerance to breast milk.

Usually cow and buffalo milk are used. Rarely goat or camel or ass milks are used for infant feeding. Dry powered milk is also available commercially. Several preparations are available. These are modified to resemble human milk. A hygienically prepared feed as per instructions of the manufacturer can be fairly safe for infant feeding. These preparations are generally expensive. High pressure advertising has resulted in widespread, injudicious resort to artificial feeding by mothers who psychologically are too willing to give up nursing their babies on flimsiest of grounds. Mothers from the weaker section are too eager to follow women from higher strata, powdered milk feed being turned into a status symbol.

Condensed milk powders are unsuitable for infant feeding as on reconstitution of formula is unbalanced and contains excessive sugar. Dried skimmed milk on reconstitution provides fewer calories than the natural milk. Low fat dry milk powders are suitable for premature and infants with diarrhea.

They are not advisable for routine infant feeding. Advantages of dried milk are that it can be easily stored and carried during travelling; the composition remains constant at all times. It is sterile and fortified with vitamins and iron. Whole dried milk, humanized milk, half-cream milk, skimmed milk, low fat high protein milk, hypoallergenic milk powders are available. Dried milk should be reconstituted at the time of feeding. In most formulae one level measure of milk powder is to be added to 30 ml of boiled cooled water. Whole dried milk can be given to babies above 3 months. Half cream, low fat, high protein milk powders are used in premature and low weight babies.

Vegetable milks prepared from groundnuts, soybean, coconut and Bengal gram are also used in South East Asia. One teaspoon of Bengal gram powder is added to 3 ml of water with 1 to 2 teaspoon of sugar. These milk are still not very popular in India. Soybean milk (fresh, powdered) is used in lactose intolerance.

Animal milk is hence modified by:

- Dilution with water to reduce fat and protein content
- Addition of sugar to given adequate energy as well as sweet taste.

Cow milk needs less dilution. Full strength cow milk can be given from the second month. Buffalo milk has to be diluted in equal proportion with water in the first two months, 2 parts milk and 1 part water in 3rd and 4th months and given undiluted from the 5th month 1 Teaspoon (5 gms) of sugar is added to 120 ml. of milk mixture.

Methods of Feeding

Bottle is the commonest mode of feeding. Spoon and pipette feeding is done in some circumstances. A baby with recurrent diarrhea is fed with a spoon. Pipette feeding is done in premature. In some cases tube feeding is resorted to. A wide mouth vertical bottle over which a cap is screwed, holding in place the wide based rubber teat is preferred, it can be easily cleaned. Teat can be turned inside the bottle after sterilization. Disposable plastic bottles are also in use. Boat shaped bottles are not used.

Weaning: Most mothers do not have enough milk to satisfy the baby's nutritional needs after 4 months. Breast milk will hence have to be supplemented by semisolid foods and other liquids. By 4 to 5 months baby's sucking reflex starts waning and he is able to do initial masticators movements with his gums.

Hence by the time baby is 5 months old some food other than milk should be introduced, which has a thicker consistency. The process of weaning has to be a gradual one. The process should start by 4 months and completed by 9 months. Actually in developing countries, especially amongst low socioeconomic classes, breastfeeding can be continued in the early months of second year so as to make good quality of proteins available to the baby for a longer time. However this may have inherent danger of breast addiction and refusal of the baby of chew of eat solids.

The new foods have to be given initially in small quantities and with a spoon. Any one type of food should be given for three or four days continuously before another type of food is introduced. Solids if introduced earlier than 4 months of age can cause hypernatremia. Baby's tastes will have to respect. One should be familiar with seasonal foods available their prices and methods of cooking them. Certain fears and prejudices must be allayed.

All the food should be freshly and hygienically cooked. Utensils should be clean and hands should be washed before cooking or feeding. Food should be kept covered to protect from dust and files. Simplest recipes made by modifying family food should be advised. Solids should be given before breastfeed. Baby should not be hurried. Initially baby spits out. Learning to swallow semisolids can take a little time. Initially everything must be thoroughly mashed. Food should not contain chilies and spices. By the time he is nine months old he should be made to hold a cup or a tumbler. Parents must allow the child to learn by him.

Human Milk Bank

The first human milk bank in India was established in Bombay in 1989. In developing countries at present establishment and maintenance of milk bank has low priority because of the financial commitments. A neonatal unit runs a milk bank where the milk (either drip or expressed at the end of a feed) is delivered within 24 hours of collection to the bank and then frozen. Milk is then batched, pasteurized and refrozen.

Sterilization

- Heating the bottle after cleaning and washing with cold water and a brush so as to remove the milk film which may form over the hole of the teat. Bottle along with the cap is boiled for 10 minutes. Teat is boiled for 5 minutes. They are then kept covered till used next time. Bottle filled with sterile milk or water can be kept in a refrigerator. Spoon also should be boiled for 10 minutes. Boiling of bottles and teats should be done preceding every feed.
- Chlorine sterilization is done by 1% electrolytic sodium hypochlorite. Solution is prepared (15 ml solution to 1 liter water) daily and is effective for 24 hours. Plastic or glass bottles can be sterilized this way.
- Pasteurization involves heating to temperature of 145 °F for 30 minutes and then cooled to 55 °F.
- *Terminal heating:* This method does not require presterilization of bottles or utensils. Formula is poured in clean bottles and teats are applied.
- Teats are then loosely covered with glasses and bottles are kept in a rack in a container tall enough to prevent bottles from touching the lid.
- Container is filled with water to about midpoints of bottles, covered and placed and placed over a moderate flame. Water allowed boiling gently for 25 minutes. Bottles are the removed with tongs and placed in a container for minutes. Caps are then tightened and bottles store a refrigerator.

Breast Milk Storage Duration

Storage location	Duration	Recommendation notes
Countertop (room temperature less than 78 °F/26 °C)	6–8 hours	Store in a covered container and attempt to keep the milk as cool as possible.
Insulated cooler bag (less than 40 °F/4 °C)	24 hours	Keep ice packs in contact with milk containers at all times, limit opening cooler bag.
Refrigerator (39 °F/4 °C)	5 days	Write the date on each container. Store milk in the back of the fridge where temperature are cooler.
Freezer section inside the fridge (5 °F/–15 °C)	2 weeks	Temperatures vary more in a style of refrigerator with one door, and which provides a section inside the refrigerator for freezing. As a result, breast milk lasts less time. DO NOT REFREEZE.
Freezer with it's own door (0 °F/–20 °C)	3–6 months	Store milk towards back of freezer where temperature is most constant. Milk stored for longer periods in the range, up to 6 months, are still safe but some of the lipids in milk undergo degradation resulting in lower quality. DO NOT REFREEZE.
Deep freezer (–4 °F/–20 °C)	6–12 months	Milk stored for longer in the range, up to 12 months, are still safe but some of the lipids in milk undergo degradation resulting in lower quality. DO NOT REFREEZE.

General Considerations in Bottle-fed Infants

These infants need more water than the breast babies for elimination of waste products. Risk of infect is very high.

Cleanliness is essence which often is possible in many households. These babies need vitamin and iron supplements. (Breastfed babies also need vitamin and iron supplements).

Bottle should be held inclined that the teat is full with milk and not air. Baby must burped after the feed. Most babies prefer warm milk flabby teats should be discarded.

A rapid sucker require a larger volume of feed. An average term infant require 150 ml/kg/day of milk to satisfy its need for proteins and calories, through the first year.

The estimated quantity milk is offered in divided feeds at intervals of about 4 hours. Night feeds are given in the first months, after which they are replaced by water. However a consider able flexibility is needed in the schedule. A little more quantity than the estimate need should be offered to the baby. As he grows his need also increases. His milk intents should keep pace with his growth.

Working Mother

- Mother should express her milk in a clean, wide mouthed container and this milk should be fed to her baby by the caretaker, in the absence of the mother.
- Express breast milk (EBM) can be stored at room temperature for 8 hours and in the refrigerator for 24 hours.
- EBM feeding should be given with cup and spoon.
- Express of milk should be done by hands which is more easier then other methods.

Table 2.4: Suggested plan of weaning food

6 months	Fruit juice/soup	
7 months	Mashed banana, soft cooked rice, porridge, precooked cereal. Give 1 to 2 teaspoonful and increase slowly	
8 months	One banana, ½ cup porridge, other seasonal fruits	
9 months	Rice khichadi, soft bread, chappati, yellow of egg, dal, biscuits, thickened soup	
10 to 12 months	All the above + egg (10 months), fish and meat (12 months)	
1 to 1.5 year	All household diet. Food has to be softened. More frequent feeds may be necessary. Baby should use a cup. Milk 250 ml. 4 times.	
2 years	Idlis, bread, rice with dhal, custards, puddings, fruits, fish, minced meat, 1 egg, 600 ml milk and other items in the family diet.	
3 to 6 years	• Calories: 1300 • Proteins: 35 g. • Fat: 40 g. • Iron: 12 mg. • Vit A: 2500 IU • Vit D: 100 IU • Vit C: 40 mg.	• **Breakfast** – fruit juice, 250 ml milk, Porridge, Cereal, bread slice, Full egg • **Lunch** – 2 wati rice, 1 wati vegetables, 1 wati Dhal, 2 chappatis, 2 teasp, butter, meat of fish. • **Tea** – 250 ml. milk biscuits/shira/upama, flaked rice. • **Dinner** – As lunch • **Bed time** – 250 ml. milk.
7 to 12 years	• Calories: 2000 • Proteins: 30 g. • Iron: 15 mg. • Vit A: 4000 IU • Vit D: 400 IU	• Cereals: 350 g. • Pulse: 60 g. • Nuts: 30 g. • Milk: 150 ml. • Meat or fish: 60 g.

Contd...

Contd...

	• Vit C: 40 mg. • Diet has to be arranged taking into consideration the time spent in school and the school timings.	• Egg: 1 • Fruits: 100 g. • Fat: 30 g. • Sugar: 60 g.
Adolescence	• Calories: 2500–5000 • Proteins: 50 g. • Vitamin requirements • Same as above • Diet has to be arranged taking into consideration the time spent outside home	• Cereals: 450 g. • Pulse: 100 g. • Nuts: 60 g. • Milk: 300 ml. • Meat or fish: 60 g. • Vegetables: 100 g. • Fruits: 100 g. • Oil/fats: 60 g. • Sugar: 60 g.

BABY-FRIENDLY HOSPITAL INITIATIVE (BFHI)

Introduction

The Baby-friendly Hospital Initiative (BFHI) was launched by WHO and UNICEF in 1991, following the Innocent Declaration of 1990. The initiative is a global effort to implement practices that protect, promote and support breastfeeding. To help in the implementation of the initiative, different tools and materials were developed, field-tested and provided, including a course for maternity staff, a self-appraisal tool and an external assessment tool.

Since 1991, the Global Strategy for IYCF was launched with nine operational targets, including BFHI. New evidence became available in the area of infant and young child feeding. Additionally the HIV pandemic raised concerns and queries in relation to feeding recommendations for children of HIV-infected mothers slowing down the process of implementation of BFHI.

In response to the HIV pandemic and other new evidence, WHO and UNICEF collaborated on an effort to update the Baby-friendly hospital initiative materials and promote the initiative in the context of the IYCF strategy. The updated material integrates Code implementation, mother-friendliness, care of pregnant women and mothers in the context of HIV, emergencies as well as expansion towards other type of health facilities and the community. The updated process was also used for strengthening the BFHI-related training courses.

The revised BFHI package includes:

- Section 1 background and implementation, summarizes the background of the initiative and describes the process of implementation
- Section 2 includes all material for training/raising the awareness of policy and decision-makers in relation of BFHI and IYCF in general
- Section 3 corresponds to a 20 hours course for training facility staff (clinical and non-clinical)
- Section 4 includes self-appraisal and monitoring tools
- Section 5 includes the assessment and reassessment tools

Baby-friendly Hospital Initiative (2009)

Revised, Updated and Expanded for Integrated Care

The Baby-friendly Hospital Initiative (BFHI) is a worldwide programme of the World Health Organization and UNICEF, launched in 1991 following Declaration of 1990. The initiative is a global effort for improving the role of maternity services to enable mothers to breastfeed babies for the best start in life. It aims at improving the care of pregnant women, mothers and newborns at health facilities that provide maternity services for protecting, promoting and supporting breastfeeding, in accordance with the international code of marketing of breast milk substitutes.

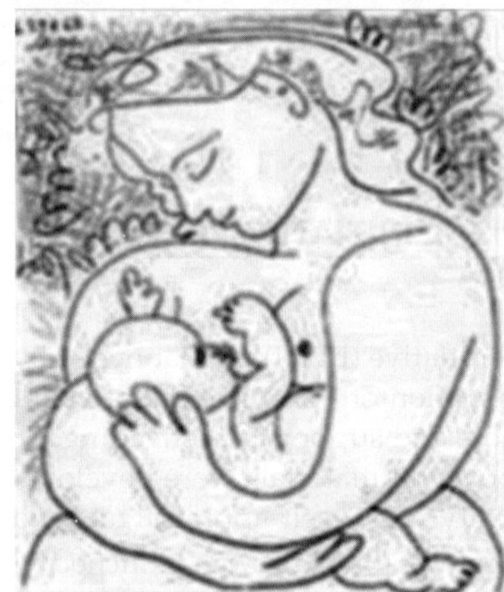

Fig. 2.19: 2003 Estate of Pablo Picasso/Artists Rights Society (ARS), New York

Criteria

The criteria for a hospital's baby friendly accreditation include:

- Have a written breastfeeding policy that is routinely communicated to all health care staff.
- Train all health care staff in skills necessary to implement this policy.
- Inform all pregnant women about the benefits and management of breastfeeding.
- Help mothers initiate breastfeeding within one and half hour of birth.
- Show mothers how to breastfeed and maintain lactation, even if they should be separated from their infants.
- Give newborn infants no food or drink other than breast milk, not even sips of water, unless medically indicated.
- Practice rooming in—that is, allow mothers and infants to remain together 24 hours a day.
- Encourage breastfeeding on demand.
- Give no artificial teats or pacifiers (also called dummies or soothers) to breastfeeding infants.
- Foster the establishment of breastfeeding support groups and refer mothers to them on discharge from the hospital or clinic

The program also restricts use by the hospital of free formula or other infant care aids provided by formula companies. Between 1991 and 2005, approximately 15,000 facilities worldwide have been inspected and accredited as 'Baby-Friendly.'

National Schemes

United Kingdom (UK): The UNICEF UK baby-friendly initiative was launched in 1994 and, in 1998, its principles were extended to cover the work of community health care services with the Seven Point Plan for Supporting Breastfeeding in the Community. In 2005, it introduced an accreditation programme for university departments responsible for midwifery, health visitor and public health nurse education. Its emphasis on applying the standards in post-natal and education settings makes it unique amongst the various baby-friendly programmes in other countries.

In the UK, the baby-friendly initiative works with the National Health Service to ensure a high standard of care for pregnant women and breastfeeding mothers and babies in hospitals and community health settings.

The baby-friendly initiative accredits health care facilities that adopt internationally recognized best practice standards for breastfeeding. During each stage of accreditation, the baby-friendly Initiative provides support as facilities implement standards relating to policies and procedures, staff education, effective auditing, educating pregnant women and mothers, and other relevant areas.

There is also a baby-friendly university standards programme aimed at university departments responsible for midwifery and health visitor/public health nurse education.

This ensures that newly qualified midwives and health visitors are equipped with the basic knowledge and skills they need to support breastfeeding effectively. There are now 52 Baby Friendly-accredited maternity hospitals in the UK and ten accredited community health-care providers.

In 2009, the Department of Health awarded a total of £4 million to 40 Primary Care Trusts in areas with low rates of breastfeeding to support them in seeking baby-friendly accreditation.

Australia

- Baby-friendly Health Initiative.
- Baby-friendly USA.

Health Benefits

Breastfeeding offers benefits for both mother and baby: UNICEF, and World Health Organization and the UK Government all recommend that babies are breastfed exclusively for their first six months of life. Studies have shown that breastfed babies are less likely to suffer from serious illnesses, including gastroenteritis, asthma, eczema, and respiratory and ear infections.

Adults who were breastfed as babies are less likely to develop risk factors for heart disease such as obesity and high blood pressure. There are benefits for mothers too: Women who breastfeed have a lower risk of developing breast cancer, ovarian cancer and hip fractures in later life.

NURSING MANAGEMENT OF LOW BIRTH WEIGHT BABY/PRETERM BABY

Introduction

A baby's weight at birth is a strong indicator of maternal and newborn health and nutrition. Being undernourished in the womb increases the risk of death in the early months and years of a child's life. Those who survive tend to have impaired immune function and increased risk of disease; they are likely to remain undernourished, with reduced muscle strength, cognitive abilities and IQ throughout their lives. As adults, they suffer a higher incidence of diabetes and heart disease.

Incidence

The incidence of low birth weight (LBW), defined as the proportion of newborns weighing less than 2,500 grams, is monitored through both health system surveillance and household surveys. In 2013, nearly 22 million newborns an estimated 16% of all babies born globally that year had low birth weight. Accurate monitoring is challenging, however, since nearly half of the world's infants are not weighed at birth. — *UNICEF*

RISK FACTORS AND CAUSES OF LBW

- Poor socioeconomic condition
- Illiteracy
- Maternal malnutrition and anemia
- Maternal illness like DM, hypertension
- Low maternal weight
- Teenage pregnancy
- Too frequent child birth
- Maternal smoking and drug addition
- Multiple pregnancy
- Placental dysfunction
- Antepartum hemorrhage
- Pregnancy-induced hypertension
- Acute emotional stress
- Premature onset of labor
- Intrauterine infection
- Congenital malformations, etc.

CLASSIFICATION

Preterm babies: They are born before 37 wks completed weeks of gestation. They weight between 10th–90th percentile of man weight for their gestational age.

Small for date (SFD) babies: They are born at term but their growth rate was retarded. They are also called intrauterine growth restriction (IUGR) baby. They weigh < 10th percentile below mean weight for their gestational age. SFD baby may be have delivered prematurely, they are both preterm.

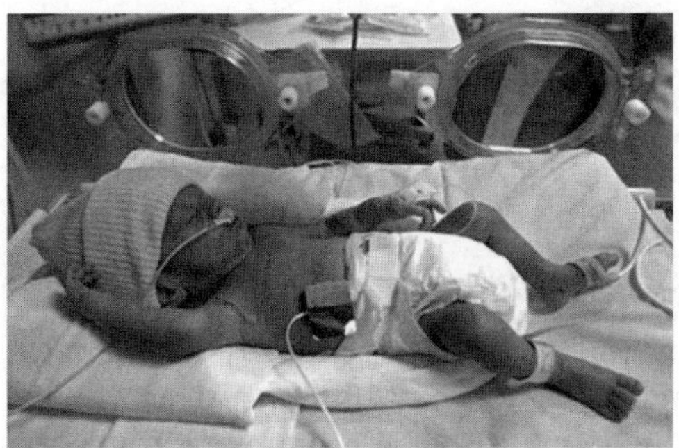

CLINICAL FEATURES OF LBW BABY

Physical Characteristics

- Weight less than 2500 gm
- Length < 47cm
- Head circumference < 33 cm
- Chest circumference < head circumference by more than 3 cm
- General activity poor and weak cry
- Attitude relaxed and limbs extended with poor tone
- Sucking, swallowing, cough and Moro reflexes are sluggish or incomplete
- Skin shiny, loose thin, delicate, pink with scanty vernix and plenty lanugo
- Less subcutaneous fat and edema
- Head large than body skill bones are soft sutures and fontanelles are wide
- Ears are soft and flat, cartilage not fully developed
- Eyes remain closed and protruding
- Hairs are scanty, wooly and fuzzy
- Face is small with small chin and less buccal fat
- Breast nodules are absent or < 4 mm, nipples and areola are flat
- Abdomen full, soft and round with prominent veins
- Nails are short and not grown up to fingertips
- Deep creases over palms and soles due absent
- Genitalia—in male testes are undescended and scrotum poorly developed
- In female, labia majora is exposed due to poorly developed labia majora clitoris is hypertrophied.

Physiological Handicaps

Alteration of Respiratory Function

Respiration is rapid, shallow, and irregular with periods of apnea and cyanosis, cough and gag reflex are weak or absent. Primary atelectasis is common and hyaline membrane disease may develop. These are due to weak respiratory muscles. Poor expansion of lungs, inefficient respiratory center and deficiency of surfactant in the alveoli.

Impaired Thermoregulation

The LBW baby has poor control over thermoregulation. There may be variations of body temperature and hypothermia may develop. These are due to poor developed heat regulating center, large body surface area in relation to body weight, poor insulating subcutaneous fat, poor muscular activity and less brown fat.

Disturbance in Food and Nutrition

Sucking and swallowing reflex are poor, capacity of stomach is less; cardioesophageal sphincter is incompetent leading to regurgitation and aspiration. There is lack of digestive enzymes which leads to inadequate digestion and absorption of essential nutrients resulting malnutrition. They are prone to develop iron deficiency anemia and deficiency of vitamin A, D, E, and K.

Lack of Immunity

Inefficient immunological system of LBW babies makes them susceptible to infections cellular immunity and antibody level are low. Incubator care, resuscitation and invasive procedures are the source of infections for LBW baby.

Metabolic Disturbances

Hypoglycemia, hypocalcemia, hypoxia, acidosis, may develop in LBW babies due to poor metabolic function, poor glycogen store, delayed feeding and birth asphyxia.

Inefficient Hepatic Function

Results in hyperbilirubinemia and kernicterus as unconjugated bilirubin is not effectively converted to conjugated bilirubin by enzymatic action. Physiological jaundice is severe in LBW baby as immature liver is not able to cope with the bilirubin produced by hemolysis, poor vitamin-K synthesis in liver and poor prothrombin production leads to hemorrhagic disease.

Impaired Renal Functions

Due to deficiency of nephro and low glomerular filtrating rate, acidosis develops as acid base balance is not well-maintained in LBW baby. They may be dehydrated due to inability to conserve water and urination may be delayed.

Inadequate renal clearance along with poor hepatic function makes the LBW baby more vulnerable to drug toxicity due to poor detoxification of drugs.

Inefficient Neurological Function

There is absent or incomplete Moro reflex or traction reflex in LBW baby. They have poor, cough reflex, sucking and swallowing reflex. Immaturity of nervous systems leads to poor reflex, lethargy and inactivity.

Other Handicap Conditions

These are hypofunciton of bone marrow weak and fragile blood vessels leading to hemorrhagic problems. LBW baby is more prone to develop retinopathy due to higher concentration of O_2 which constrict retinal arteries and result anoxic damage and retinal detachment. This condition is termed as retrolental fibroplasia which can cause blindness.

COMPLICATIONS OF LBW

- Birth asphyxia
- Hyaline membrane disease (RDS)
- Intra-alveolar hemorrhage
- Intra-ventricular hemorrhage
- Anemia
- Kernicterus
- Cardiac failure
- Renal failure
- Retinopathy of prematurity
- Infections.

PREVENTION OF LBW

The preventive measures are

- Detection of high-risk antenatal mother and management of risk mother according.
- Emphasis on recommended dietary intake in pregnancy for the expected fetal weight gain.
- Necessary measure to be taken to avoid preterm labor.
- Efficient management of premature labor and prevention of complications.
- Delivery of LBW baby must be attended by expert neonatologist for prompt management.

MANAGEMENT OF LBW BABIES

Due to high incidence of LBW babies and limited resources to care for them, the segregation of high-risk LBW neonates is required for special care. They are with birth weight 2000 gm or less, inability to such the breast and swallow unable to regulate baby temperature and to control cardiorespiratory function.

Immediate Care of LBW Baby at Birth

- Air passage to be cleared promptly and gently
- Adequate of warmth by drying and wrapping the baby and rooming in with mother
- Administration of 'vitamin K' to prevent hemorrhagic problems
- Initiating of breastfeeding as early as possible
- Body can be caused in prone position
- Gentle handing and care in special neonatal care unit (NICU).

NURSING CARE OF LBW BABY

Maintenance of Respiratory Function

- Position the baby with neck slightly extended'
- Clear the air passage by gentle sucking
- Monitor and record respiratory rate, rhythm, signs of distress, retraction, nasal cleaning apnea cyanosis, etc.
- Providing tactile stimulation by sole flicking to stimulate respiratory effort.

- Administer O_2 therapy with bag and mask initially in 100% concentration then reduced to 40% to prevent retrolental fibroplasia.
- Provide chest physiotherapy by percussion, vibration, postural drainage to loosen and remove respiratory secretions.

Maintenance of Thermoregulation

- Environmental temperature to be maintained at 30 ± 2 °C by air conditioner, radiant warmer. Hot blowers, room heater, etc. to provide thermoneutral surroundings.
- Skin temperature of the baby to be maintained at 36.5–37.5 °C.
- Baby need to be kept in incubator with desired level of humidity (60– 65%), and O_2.
- Constant monitoring of the baby's temperature is essential, low reading thermometer is useful measures to be taken to prevent heat loss during care.

Maintenance of Nutrition and Fluid

LBW baby required 120–150 Kcal/kg body wt/day. Water 150–200 ml/kg/day, protein 4-6 gm/kg/day for first few days to meet the requirement for optimum growth.

- Early feeding should be to prevent hypoglycemia, hyperbilirubinemia and kernicterus
- Frequent feeding should be given
- In poor sucking reflex, IV fluid and nasogastric tube feeding may be needed. Flopper, spoon and pipette can be use to feed the LBW baby.
- Weight to be recorded daily to assess wt gain preferably before feeding, in same machine and same amount of clothing.

Prevention of Infections

- Poor immunity power makes of LBW baby more prone to infection measures to be taken to prevent infections.
- Through handwashing with antiseptics must be done before touching and caring each baby. Each neonates should have separate clothing's, feeding articles, thermometer, stethoscope, etc.
- All personnel working in special care unit must change their shoes and wear nursery slippers and sterile gown and mask.
- Any person having any infections should not enter the neonatal care unit.
- Visitors should be restricted in the unit.
- Nursery floors and surfaces to be mopped detergents or carbolic solution in every shift.
- Incubators and baby cots should be cleaned with soap water and antiseptics.
- Clothing and linen must be autoclaved.
- Infected baby should be kept in separate unit.
- Baby bath to be withheld in the unit but general cleanliness to be maintained.
- Any complications found to be treated promptly.

Provide Stimulation

Nurse should provide sensory stimulation to the LBW baby by talking, singing, cuddling, and gentle touching during care. Visual stimulation can be provided by colorful hanging object. Baby's position to be changed at interval—Baby should be placed on right side after feeding to prevent regurgitation and aspiration. Mother should be allowed to care the body with necessary precautions or to visit nursery to sea, to touch and to handle the baby.

Informing the Parent about Infant's Progress

Baby's condition and progress to be explained to the parent plan to be discussed. Parent should allow seeing the baby care after discharge to be discussed with the parent. Parent should learn about warmth, feeding, follow up and hygienic practices at home.

The LBW baby's usually discharged from special care unit when the baby gained sufficient weight approximately 2000 gm or more, having good vigor and able to suck successfully. Ultimate survival of the baby depends upon continued care.

COMPLICATION OF LBW

Respiratory Distress Syndrome (RDS)

- This breathing problem is common in babies born before 34 weeks of pregnancy. Babies with RDS do not have a protein called surfactant that keeps small air sacs in the lungs from collapsing.
- Treatment with surfactant helps these babies breathe more easily. Babies with RDS also may need oxygen and other breathing help to make their lungs work.

Bleeding in the Brain (Intraventricular Hemorrhage or IVH)

- Bleeding in the brain can affect low-birth weight premature babies, usually in the first 3 days of life. Brain bleeds usually are diagnosed with an ultrasound.
- Most brain bleeds are mild and fix themselves with no or few lasting problems. More severe bleeds can cause pressure on the brain that can cause fluid to build up in the brain. This can cause brain damage. To reduce the fluid, your baby may be treated with medicine. In some cases, a surgeon may insert a tube into the baby's brain to drain the fluid.

Patent Ductus Arteriosus (PDA)

- PDA is a common heart problem for premature babies. Before birth, a large artery called the ductus arteriosus lets the baby's blood bypass his lungs.
- This artery usually closes after birth so that blood can travel to the baby's lungs and pick up oxygen. When the artery does not close properly, it can lead to heart failure.
- Providers use tests like ultrasound to check for PDA. Babies with PDA are treated with a drug that helps close the artery. If the drug does not work, a baby may need surgery.

Necrotizing Enterocolitis (NEC)

- This is a problem in a baby's intestines. The intestines are long tubes below the stomach that help digest food. NEC usually develops 2 to 3 weeks or later after birth.
- It can be dangerous for a baby. It can lead to feeding problems, swelling in the belly and other complications. Babies with NEC are treated with antibiotics (medicines that kill infections) and fed intravenously (through a vein) instead of by mouth while the intestine heals.
- In some cases, a baby may need surgery to remove damaged parts of intestine.

Retinopathy of Prematurity (ROP)

- ROP affects blood vessels in the eye. It mostly affects babies born before 32 weeks of pregnancy. Most cases heal themselves with little or no vision loss. Some babies need treatment, though, to prevent vision loss.

INTRAUTERINE GROWTH RETARDATION (IUGR)

Introduction

Intrauterine growth restriction (IUGR) is a term used to describe a condition in which the fetus is smaller than expected for the number of weeks of pregnancy. Another term for IUGR is fetal growth restriction. Newborn babies with IUGR are often described as small for gestational age (SGA).

Intrauterine growth restriction (IUGR) refers to poor growth of a baby while in the mother's womb during pregnancy. The causes can be many, but most often involve poor maternal nutrition or lack of adequate oxygen supply to the fetus. Intrauterine growth retardation, dysmaturity, small for date, chronic placental insufficiency.

Definition

Intrauterine growth restriction is said to be presented in those babies whose birth weight is below the tenth percentile of the average for the gestational age. Growth restriction can occur in preterm or post-term babies.

Incidence

Dysmaturity comprises about one third of low birth weight babies. In developed countries, its overall incidence is about 2–8%. The incidence amount the term babies is about 5% and that amount the post-term babies is about 15%.

Classification

Where growth is restricted by pathological process (true IUGR). Depending upon the relative size of their hear, abdomen and femur, the fetuses are subdivided into:

- Symmetrical or type I
- Asymmetrical or type II

Classification of IUGR

Type	Symmetric/Type 1 (20%)	Asymmetric/Type 2 (80%)
Onset	• Early in utero	• Later onset
Etiology	• Congenital infections, genetic disorders	• Utero-placental insufficiency, maternal malnutrition, hypertension
Pathophysiology	• Impaired cell division • Decreased cell number • Irreversible	• Impaired cellular hypertrophy • Decreased cell size • Reversible
Clinical features	• Inadequate growth of head and body • Head:abdomen ratio may be normal	• Brain is spared, therefore head:abdomen ratio increased
Prognosis	• Poor prognosis	• More favorable prognosis

Causes

The causes of fetal growth restriction can be divided into four groups.

Maternal Condition

- **Constitutional:** Small women, maternal genetic and racial background are associated with small babies. These babies are not at increased risk.
- **Maternal nutrition before and during pregnancy:** Critical substrate requirement for fetal growth such as glucose, amino acids and oxygen are deficient during pregnancy. This is an important cause of IUGR in women with undernutrition.

Maternal Diseases

Anemia, hypertension, thrombophilia, heart disease, chronic renal disease, collagen vascular diseases are the important causes. Toxins—Alcohol, smoking, cocaine, heroin, drugs.

Fetal

There is enough substrate in the maternal blood and also crosses the placenta but is not utilized by the fetus. The failure of nonutilization may be due to:

- Structural anomalies either cardiovascular, renal or others
- Chromosomal abnormality is associated with 8–12% of growth retarded infants. The common abnormalities are triploidy and aneuploidy. Trisomy (13, 18 and 21) and Turner's syndrome are commonly observed
- Infection TORCH agents (toxoplasmosis, rubella, cytomegalovirus and herpes simples) and malaria
- **Multiple pregnancies:** There is mechanical hindrance to growth and excessive fetal demand.

Placental

The causes include cases of poor uterine blood flow to the placental site for a long time. This leads to chronic placental insufficiency with inadequate substrate transfer. The placental pathology includes: Placenta previa, circumvallates placenta, infarction and mosaicism.

Unknown causes: The cause remains unknown in about 40%.

Factors

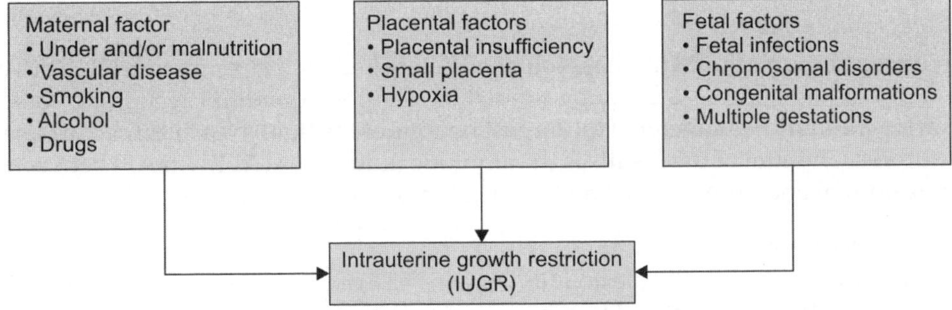

Pathophysiology

Basic pathology in small for gestational age is due to reduce availability of nutrients in the mother or its reduced transfer by the placenta to the fetus. It may also be due to reduced ultilization by the fetus. Brain cell size (asymmetric– SGA) as well as cell number (symmetric–SGA) are reduced. Liver glycogen content is reduced.

There is oligohydramnios as the renal and pulmonary contributions to amniotic fluid are diminished due to reduction in blood flow to these organs. The SGA fetus is at risk of intrauterine hypoxia and acidosis, which if severe may lead to intrauterine fetal death.

Diagnostic Evaluation

Significant improvements have been made by clinical and biophysical methods in detecting a growth restricted fetus. Clinical palpation of the uterus for the fundal height, liquor volume and fetal mass may be used for screening. But it is less sensitive. Symphysis fundal height (SFH) measurement in centimeters closely correlate with gestational age after 24 weeks.

It is a fairly sensitive parameter (30–80%). Serial measurement is important. Maternal weight gain remains stationary or at times falling during the second half of pregnancy. Measurement of the abdominal girth showing stationary or falling values.

Biophysical Examination

The first examination should confirm the clinical estimation of gestational age. USG is extremely useful not only to diagnose the growth retardation but also to identify a fetus of symmetrical or asymmetrical one.

Sonographic Predictive Values

Hear circumference (HC) and abdominal circumference (AC) ration: In a normally growing fetus the HC/AC ration exceeds 1.0 before 32 weeks. It is approximately 1.0 at 32 to 34 weeks. After 34 weeks it falls below 1.0. If the fetus is affected by asymmetric IUGR, the HC remains larger.

The HC/AC is than elevated. In symmetric IUGR, both the HC and AC are reduced. The HC/AC ratio remains normal. Using HC/AC ratio, 85% of IUGR fetuses are detected. AC is the single most sensitive parameter to detect IUGR. Serial measurements of AC and estimation of fetal weight are more diagnostic to fetal growth restriction. Femur length (FL) is not affected in asymmetric IUGR. The FL/AC ratio is 22 at all gestational ages from 21 weeks term. FL/AC ratio greater than 23.5 suggests IUGR.

Amniotic Fluid Volume

The reduced amniotic fluid volume is too often associated with asymmetrical IUGR. Vertical pocket of amniotic fluid < 2 cm suggests IUGR. The four quadrant technique consists of measuring the vertical diameter of the largest pockets of the fluid in each of the four quadrant of the uterus. The sum of the results is the amniotic fluid index (AFI). An AFI between 5 and 25 cm is normal and an AFI less than 5 indication of oligohydramnios.

Doppler Velocimetry

Elevated uterine artery systolic/diastolic (S/D) ratio (> 2.6) and or presence of diastolic notch are associated with IUGR and intrauterine fetal death. The presence of diastolic notch in uterine artery suggests incomplete invasion of placental trophoblasts to the uterine spiral arteries.

Physical Features at Birth

Weight deficit at birth is about 600 gm below the minimum in percentile standard. Every hospital should have their own birth weight—gestational age chart. Length is unaffected.

Head circumference is relatively larger than the body in asymmetric variety. Physical features show dry and wrinkled skin because of less subcutaneous fat, scaphoid abdomen, thin meconium stained vernix caseosa and thin umbilical cord. All these give the baby an 'old man look'. Pinna of ear has cartilaginous ridges. Plantar creases are well defined. The baby is alert, active and having normal cry. Eyes are open. Reflexes are normal including moro-reflex.

Signs and Symptoms

The main symptom of IUGR is a small for gestational age baby. Specifically, the baby's estimated weight is below the 10th percentile—or less than that of 90% of babies of the same gestational age.

Depending on the cause of IUGR, the baby may be small all over or look malnourished. They may be thin and pale and have loose, dry skin. The umbilical cord is often thin and dull instead of thick and shiny.

Management

Whenever, a small for gestation age fetus is suspected, careful search is made to determine the presence of growth restriction with the help of sonographic images. If it is present, the type of IUGR and the possible cause are sought for. If a fetus is symmetrically growth retarded, a meticulous search should be made to detect fetal anomalies including fetal blood sampling and karyotyping to prevent unnecessary CS in a malformed baby screening for TORCH organisms is usually not rewarding. Majority of fetal deaths occur after the 36th week of gestation. So current diagnosis and timed intervention is essential.

General

At present, there is no proven therapy for reversing growth restriction once it is established. However, the following may be tried with some success.

- Adequate bed rest specially in left lateral position
- **To correct malnutrition by balanced diet:** 300 extra calories per day are to be taken.
- To institute appropriate therapy for the associated complicating factors likely to produce growth restriction.
- Avoidance of smoking and alcohol.
- Maternal hyper oxygenation (55%) for short-term prolongation of pregnancy.
- Low dose aspirin (50 mg daily) may be helpful in much selected cases with history of recurrence.

Termination of Pregnancy

The factors to be considered are:

- Presence of fetal abnormality
- Duration of pregnancy
- Degree of growth restriction

- Associated complicating factor
- Degree of fetal compromise
- Previous obstetric history
- Facilities available at the place of delivery.

The condition may we reversed and in such cases, the pregnancy is allowed to continue but the tendency to overrun the expected date is to be curtailed by termination.

Severe Degree of IUGR

If the lung maturation is achieved as evidenced by presence of phosphatidylglycerol and L:S ratio of a least 2 form the amniotic fluid study (amniocentesis), termination is done.

Methods of Termination

Low rapture of the membranes followed by oxytocin is employed in cases such as pregnancy beyond 34 weeks favorable cervix and the head is deep in the perils. Prostaglandin (PGE) gel could used when the cervix in unfavorable. The color of the liquor could be a guide for further management.

Complications

Fetal

- **Antenatal:** Chronic fetal distress, fetal death
- **Intranatal:** Hypoxia and acidosis
- After birth

Immediate

- 1) Asphyxia (intrauterine and neonatal) and RDS. 2) Hypoglycemic due to shortage of glycogen reserve in the liver as a result of chronic hypoxia. 3) Meconium aspiration syndrome
- Micro coagulation leading to DIC during first day of life
- Hypothermia
- Pulmonary hemorrhage
- Polycythemia
- Hyperviscosity syndrome
- Necrotizing enterocolitis due to reduced intestinal blood flow
- Intraventricular hemorrhage (IVH).

CARE OF PRETERM BABIES

Introduction

A premature birth is a birth that takes place more than three weeks before the baby is due. In other words, a premature birth is one that occurs before the start of the 37th week of pregnancy. Normally, a pregnancy usually lasts about 40 weeks.

The World Health Organization (WHO) defines prematurity as babies born before 37 weeks from the first day of the last menstrual period. Recent data indicate that > 1 in 10 babies born around the world in 2010 were premature and this translates to an estimated 15 million preterm births.

All babies born before 37 weeks as premature fails to illustrate the marked gradation in terms of severity of the problem with increasing prematurity:

- A baby born at 36 weeks will probably be a little slow to feed.
- A baby born before 33 weeks will have more serious problems including, possibly, immature lungs.
- Birth before 28 weeks causes very significant problems but the survival rate is quite remarkable.

It is not uncommon for babies to be both early and to have intrauterine growth restriction (IUGR), which adversely affects their prognosis. IUGR is a condition where the baby's growth slows down or becomes static while still in the uterus. It is part of a wider group referred to as small for gestational age (SGA) fetuses where the fetus is smaller than expected for the gestational age. The SGA includes fetuses which are constitutionally small and those whose growth has been restricted.

Definition

Preterm Birth

The preterm baby is birth of a baby less than 37 weeks gestational age; such a baby is sometimes referred to as a 'preemie' or 'premmie', depending on local pronunciation. The cause of preterm birth is in many situations elusive and unknown; many factors appear to be associated with the development of preterm birth, making the reduction of preterm birth a challenging proposition.

Premature birth is defined either as the same as preterm birth or the birth of a baby before the developing organs are mature enough to allow normal postnatal survival. Premature infants are at greater risk for short- and long-term complications, including disabilities and impediments in growth and mental development. Significant progress has been made in the care of premature infants, but not in reducing the prevalence of preterm birth. Preterm birth is among the top causes of death in infants worldwide.

Types of Preterm Baby

- **Late preterm:** Born between 34 and 36 weeks of pregnancy
- **Moderately preterm:** Born between 32 and 34 weeks of pregnancy
- **Very preterm:** Born at less than 32 weeks of pregnancy
- **Extremely preterm:** Born at or before 25 weeks of pregnancy.

Risk Factors

- Having a previous premature birth
- Pregnancy with twins, triplets or other multiples
- An interval of less than six months between pregnancies
- Conceiving through *in vitro* fertilization
- Problems with the uterus, cervix or placenta
- Smoking cigarettes or using illicit drugs
- Poor nutrition

- Not gaining enough weight during pregnancy
- Some infections, particularly of the amniotic fluid and lower genital tract
- Some chronic conditions, such as high blood pressure and diabetes
- Being underweight or overweight before pregnancy
- Stressful life events, such as the death of a loved one or domestic violence
- Multiple miscarriages or abortions
- Physical injury or trauma.

Causes of 'Prematurity'

The mechanisms initiating normal labor are not clearly understood and much less is known about the triggers that imitate labor before term. There may be spontaneous onset of premature labor or it may be induced by the obstetrician to safe guard the interests of the mother or baby.

Spontaneous

The cause of premature onset of labor is uncertain in most instances. The known causes include poor socioeconomic status, low maternal weight, chronic and acute systemic maternal disease, antepartum hemorrhage, cervical incompetence, maternal genital colonization and infections, cigarette smoking during pregnancy, threatened abortion, acute emotional stress, physical exertion, sexual activity, trauma, bicornuate uterus, multiple pregnancy and congenital malformations.

Premature births are relatively common among very young and unmarried mothers. Past history of preterm birth(s) is associated with 3 to 4 times increased risk of prematurity in the subsequent pregnancies.

Induced

The labor is often induced before term when there is impending danger to mother or fetal life *inutero,* e.g. maternal diabetes mellitus, placental dysfunction as indicated by unsatisfactory fetal growth, eclampsia, fetal hypoxia, antepartum hemorrhage and severe rhesus isoimmunization.

Clinical Features

Measurements

Their size is small with relatively large head. Crown-heel length is less than 47cm; head circumference is less than 33 cm but exceeds the chest circumference by more than 3 cm.

Activity and Posture

The general activity is poor and their automatic reflex responses, such as Moro response, sucking and swallowing are sluggish or incomplete. The baby assumes an extended posture due to poor tone.

Face and Head

Face appears small for the disproportionately large head size, sutures are widely separated and the fontanels are large. Other characteristic features include small chin, protruding eyes due to shallow orbits and absent buccal pad of fat.

Optic nerve is often unmyelinated but presence of pupillary membrane makes its visualization difficult. Ear cartilage is deficient or absent with poor recoil. Hair appears woolly and fuzzy and individual hair fibers can be seen separately.

Skin and Subcutaneous Tissues

Skin is thin, gelatinous, shiny and excessively pink with abundant lanugo and very little vernix caseosa. Edema may be present. Subcutaneous fat is deficient and breast nodule is small or absent. Deep sole creases are often not present.

Genitals

In males, testes are undescended and scrotum is poorly developed. In female infants, labia majora are widely separated exposing labia minora and hypertrophied clitoris.

Physiological Handicaps

The functional immaturity of various system results in different clinical problems and their knowledge is essential for the satisfactory management of these babies.

Central Nervous System

The immaturity of central nervous system is expressed as inactivity and lethargy, poor cough reflex and in coordinated sucking and swallowing in babies weighing less than 1,800 g or born before 35 weeks of gestation. Resuscitation difficulties at birth and requirement apneic attacks are common. Retrolental fibroplasia due to oxygen to toxicity are limited to babies with a gestation of less than 35 weeks. On the other hand, they are more resistant to toxic effects of hypoxia as compared to the term babies.

They are extremely vulnerable to develop intraventricular and periventricular hemorrhage due to relative deficiency of vitamin-K dependent coagulation factors and increased capillary fragility. The blood-brain barrier, which is possibly a function of available serum proteins, is inefficient in preterm babies; the brain damage may occur at lower serum bilirubin levels.

Respiratory System

The cuboidal alveolar lining in babies with a gestational age of less than 26 weeks results in poor alveolar diffusion of gases and therefore the infant may not be viable. They pose resuscitation difficulties at birth, often followed by hyaline membrane disease, if associated with deficiency of pulmonary surfactant.

The breathing is mostly diaphragmatic, periodic and associated with intercostals recession due to soft ribs. Pulmonary aspiration and atelectasis are common. They are vulnerable to develop chronic pulmonary insufficiency due to bronchopulmonary dysplasia.

Cardiovascular System

The closure of ductus arteriosus is delayed among the preterm infants. About one-third infants with gestational age of 34 weeks or less manifest clinical evidences of patent ductus arteriosus with or without congestive heart failure. Its incidence is much higher among preterm infants with hyaline membrane disease or protracted hypoxia due to any cause. In grossly immature infants (less than 32 weeks) ECG shows left ventricular preponderance. They are at risk to develop thromboembolic complications and hypertension due to indwelling venous and arterial catheters.

Gastrointestinal System

Due to poor or incardinated sucking and swallowing there are difficulties in self-feeding, although their digestive ability is generally good. Animal fat is not tolerated as well as the vegetable fat. Regurgitation and aspiration are common because of in coordinated sucking, small capacity of stomach, incompetence of cardioesophageal junction and poor cough reflex.

Gastroesophageal reflux and is consequences are common. Abdominal distension and functional intestinal obstruction are due to hypotonic. Enterocolitis occurs when other predisposing factors are present. Immaturity of glucuronyl transferase system in the liver leads to hyperbilirubinemia.

Which may be aggravated by dehydration, delayed feeding and hypoglycemia? Relatively low serum albumin, acidosis and hypoxia in these babies predispose to the development of kernicterus at lower serum bilirubin levels. The poor hepatic glycogen stores, delayed feeding, birth and respiratory distress syndrome contribute to the development of hypoglycemia.

Thermoregulation

Hypothermia is invariable and life-threatening unless environmental temperature is monitored. Excessive heat loss is due to relatively large surface area and poor generation of heat due to paucity of brown fat in a baby who is equipped with an inefficient thermostat.

Infections

Infections are an important cause of neonatal mortality in low birth weight babies. The low levels of IgG antibodies and inefficient cellular immunity predispose them to infection. Excessive handling, humid and warm atmosphere, contaminated incubators and resuscitators expose them to infecting organisms, thus contributing to high incidence of infections.

Renal Immaturity

The blood nitrogen is high due to low glomerular filtration rate. The renal tubular ammonia mechanism is poorly developed thus acidosis occurs early. They are vulnerable to develop late metabolic acidosis especially when fed with a high protein milk formula.

The maximum tubular diluting ability in the newborn is satisfactory but ability to concentrate urine is very poor, preterm baby has to pass 4 to 5 ml of urine to excrete one milliosmole of solute as compared to 0.7 ml by an adult for the same purpose. Therefore, the baby cannot conserve water and gets dehydrated readily. The solute retention and low serum proteins explain occurrence of edema in some preterm infants.

Toxicity of Drugs

Poor hepatic detoxification and reduced renal clearance make a preterm baby vulnerable to toxic effects of drugs unless caution is exercised during their administration.

Nutritional Handicaps

Low birth weight babies are prone to develop anemia around 6 to 8 weeks of age. This is due to diminished total stores of iron due to short gestation. They may also manifest deficiencies of folic acid and vitamin E. Vitamin E deficiency occurs among infants is prone to develop hemolytic anemia, thrombocytopenia, and edema at 6 to 10 weeks of age.

Vitamin E being an antioxidant, its deficiency state may be associated with oxygen toxicity to the vulnerable tissues in the form of retrolental fibroplasia and bronchopulmonary dysplasia. Rapid growth following adequate feeding may result in osteropenia and rickets unless calcium phosphorus and vitamin D are administered.

Biochemical Disturbances

These babies are prone to develop hypoglycemia, hypocalcemia, hypoproteinemia, acidosis and hypoxia.

Symptoms

A premature birth means that your baby has not had the usual amount of time to develop in the womb before needing to adapt to life outside the womb.

The signs that a baby's gestation has been cut short include:

- Small size, with a disproportionately large head
- Sharper looking, less rounded features than a full-term baby's features, due to a lack of fat stores
- Fine hair (lanugo) covering much of the body
- Low body temperature, especially immediately after birth in the delivery room, due to a lack of stored body fat
- Labored breathing or respiratory distress
- Lack of reflexes for sucking and swallowing, leading to feeding difficulties.

Management

High-risk mother should be identified early during the course of pregnancy and referred for confinement to an appropriate health care facility which is equipped with good quality obstetrical and neonatal care facilities. Mother is indeed an ideal transport incubator.

Arrest of Premature Labor

Advantages in perinatal care including fabrication of a variety of electronic gadgets cannot compare with unique security and optimal care provided to the fetus by the uteroplacental unit. Efforts should always be made to arrest the progress of premature labor.

The onset of 'true' labor is suspected by occurrence of two or more uterine contractions lasting at least 30 seconds during a 15-minute period in association with dilatation and effacement of cervix. Apart from bed rest and sedation, a variety of tocolytic agents are recommended, but none is entirely safe or effective. Ethanol though popular at one stage is rarely used now due to its dangers of inebriation, vomiting, headache, flushing, restlessness, disorientation and dieresis.

Magnesium sulfate is more effective and is being increasingly used though there is a potential risk of respiratory depression in the newborn, The treatment with magnesium sulfate is associated with reduced risk of IVH, cerebral palsy and mental retardation in their preterm babies.

Sympathomimetic agents specially mediating via beta 2-adrenergic receptors are powerful tocolytic agents and currently used. Isoxsurprine (duvadilan) is useful but its effect is mediated both through beta-1 and beta-2 receptors. Its use is associated with untoward beta-1 receptor side effects such as apprehension, palpitation, hypotension, fetal tachycardia and neonatal hypoglycemia,

Therapy is initiated by intravenous infusion of 20 mg isoxsuprine diluted in 200 ml of 5% dextrose at a rate of 40-50 drops/minute. This is followed by intramuscular administrating of 10 mg isoxsuprine every 4 hours for 24 and 48 hours. Oral therapy is continued for at least 2 weeks with maintenance doses of 10 mg every 6 hours. Ritodrine has been approved by US Food and Drug Administration for treatment of premature labor and is more effective than ethanol.

The common side effects are maternal and fetal tachycardia. The usual dose is 100–400 µg/minute intravenously through an infusion pump for a period of 12 hours followed by oral ritodrine 10 mg every 2 hours. Salbutamol and terbutaline are selective beta 2-receptor stimulators and are very effective tocolytic agents. They are generally safe but an occasional patient may develop tachycardia and pulmonary edema. Terbutaline is administered as an intravenous bolus of 0.25 mg followed by constant infusion of 10-80 µg/minute for 1–2 hours.

After control of uterine contractions, maintenance therapy is continued by administration of 0.25 mg of terbutaline subcutaneously (or 0.25 mg orally) every 4 hours. Indomethacin, an inhibitor of prostaglandin-synthesize has also offered some hope in arresting premature uterine contractions. It must be used with caution because it may also block production of prostaglandin E, thus markedly decreasing uteroplacental perfusion and may cause closure of ductus arteriosus.

Induction of Premature Labor

When induction of labor is contemplated before term, either in the interest of mother or the fetus, maturity of fetus should is ascertained by examination of amniotic fluid for phosphatidyl glycerol or lecithin/sphingomyelin (L/S) ratio. As far as possible, delivery should be postponed till fetal pulmonary maturity is assured. When delivery can be safely delayed for 36 to 48 hours, corticosteroids should be administered to the mother to enhance fetal lung maturity.

Antenatal Corticosteroids

Antenatal administration of corticosteroids is one of the most cost-effective perinatal strategies which must be universally exploited. It is associated with 50 percent reduction in the incidence of RDS due to surfactant deficiency. It provides additional benefits by reducing the incidence of intraventricular hemorrhage and necrotizing enterocolitis.

The overall neonatal mortality is reduced by 40 percent by this simple and cheap intervention. Injection betamethasone 12 mg IM every 24 hours for 2 doses or dexamethasone 6 mg IM every 12 hours for 4 doses should be administered to the mother if labor starts or is induced before 34 weeks of gestation. Betamethasone is more potent and is associated with reduced risk of side effects.

The optimal effect is seen if delivery occurs after 24 hours of the initiation of therapy and its therapeutic effect lasts for 7 days. The beneficial effects are better in female babies compared to the male. The need and safety of repeat course of antenatal steroids is controversial and is under investigation by multicenteric clinical trials. Tocolytic therapy should be continued concomitantly.

Corticosteroids can be given even in the presence of maternal hypertension or diabetes mellitus but should preferably be avoided if preterm premature rupture of membranes (PPROM) is associated with definitive clinical evidence of chorioamnionitis.

Prevention

Interventions to reduce the morbidity and mortality of preterm birth can be primary (directed to all women), secondary (aimed at eliminating or reducing existing risk), or tertiary (intended to improve outcomes for preterm infants). Most efforts so far have been tertiary interventions.

Primary Prevention

The problems of social deprivation, poor maternal nutrition and substance abuse must all be addressed. Smoking should cease and, as explained in the article on fetal alcohol syndrome, alcohol consumption should be avoided, as there may be no safe lower limit.

Secondary Prevention

Antenatal care is important and should be easily accessible to all women.

Tertiary Prevention

The interventions when complications arise, e.g. regionalized care, treatment with antenatal corticosteroids, tocolytic agents and antibiotics. More recently the role of progesterone treatment of women at risk of preterm labor, to prevent preterm birth, has been recognized.

NURSING MANAGEMENT OF COMMON NEONATAL DISORDERS

HYPERBILIRUBINEMIA OF THE NEWBORN

Introduction

Newborn jaundice is when a baby has a high level of bilirubin in the blood. Bilirubin is a yellow substance that the body creates when it replaces old red blood cells. The liver helps break down the substance so it can be removed from the body in the stool.

Jaundice usually appears in the first 5 days of life. Many babies have left the hospital by the time jaundice starts. So your doctor may want to do a follow-up exam when your baby is 3 to 5 days old.

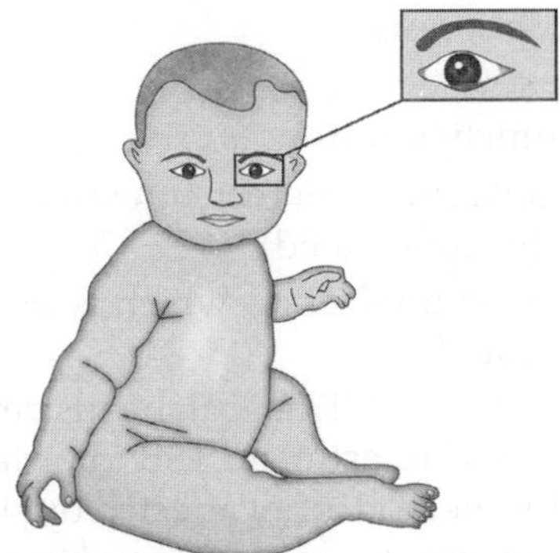

Fig. 2.20: Hyperbilirubinemia baby

Definition

The bilirubin (unconjugated) level raises more than the arbitrary cut-off point of 10 mg% the condition is called hyperbilirubinemia of the newborn.

An excessive accumulation of bilirubin in the blood and is characterized by jaundice or icterus neonatorum yellowish discoloration of the skin and other organs.

Causes

- **Unconjugated:** Hemolytic disease due to Rh (Common) or ABO (rare) incompatibility. Increased red cell fragility prematurity, glucose-6-phosphate dehydrogenises deficiency, sepsis, iatrogenic (drugs) breast milk jaundice, cephalohematoma, infant of diabetic mother, cretinism, idiopathic.
- **Conjugated:** Neonatal hepatitis, bacterial infection intrauterine TORCH infection, trisomy 21, 18, galactosemia, biliary atresia, etc.

Diagnostic Evaluation

- *Clinical study:* Evaluation of jaundice is done by blanching the skin with digital pressure. Clinical jaundice in a neonate indicates serum bilirubin of more than 5 mg/dl Cephalo-caudal progression of dermal icterus is a useful clinical tool.

  Dermal icterus zone and serum bilirubin (indirect) level in a term infant.
- *Laboratory studies:* A serum bilirubin level > 12 mg/dl.
  - Total conjugated bilirubin and unconjugated bilirubin
  - CBC
    - *Hemolytic anemia:* ↑ Hb%
    - Increased reticulocyte count, presence of nucleated red cells
    - Polycythemia: Hematocrit (> 65%)
    - *Sepsis:* WBC count (total and differential) increased
  - Hereditary spherocytosis
  - Serum albumin to detect total bilirubin binding sites and to assess the need of albumin infusion
  - Other laboratory tests:
    - Urine for reducing substance (Galactosemia)
    - Culture for infection
    - Hemoglobin electrophoresis
    - Osmotic fragility test
    - Thyroid and liver function test.
- *Radiology and ultrasonography:* It to detect intestinal obstruction, intraventricular hemorrhage complication (unconjugated)

  Kernicterus is the important complication which is more often fatal, if not promptly detected and adequately treated.
- *Transcutaneous Bilirubin Measurement:* Transcutaneous devices that use multiwavelength spectral reflectance can be used to estimate TSB in order to avoid blood sampling. In contrast to older devices, this method is not affected by skin pigmentation. In one report of a racially and ethnically diverse group of 490 newborns, a close correlation was found between transcutaneous and TSB measurements.

Management

To prevent rise of serum bilirubin to toxic level, this may cause kernicterus.

- **Phototherapy**
- *Tin Metalloporphyrins:* Since this inhibits mono-oxygenases decreasing their breakdown to bilirubin. This needs further confirmation.
- *Exchange transfusion:* Effectively reduces the bilirubin level and removes the sensitized red cells from circulation in erythroblastosis fetalis.

Indications

- Elevation of unconjugated bilirubin (above 25–28 mg/dl in nonhemolytic cases and > 18–20 mg/dl in children with hemolysis
- Serum bilirubin protein ralio of more than 3.5
- In erythroblastosis fetalis exchange transfusion should be seriously considered if the maternal antibody titer is above 1:64 red blood cells of the newborn show positive direct comb's test, etc.

Administration of 25% solution of salt-free albumin is a dose of 1g of albumin /kg, ½ to 1 hour before the exchange transfusion may be useful as it binds the bilirubin that has diffused into the interstitial tissues.

It should be avoided if there is evidence of congestive cardiac failure or severe anemia.

HEMOLYTIC DISORDERS

Hemolytic Disease of the Newborn (HDN)

Introduction

Hemolytic disease of the newborn (HDN) otherwise known as erythroblastosis fetalis, it is a blood disorder of newborn that occurs when the blood types of a mother and baby are incompatible. It is more likely to happen during a mother's second or subsequent pregnancy. There are two causes, Rh incompatibility and ABO incompatibility. HDN due to Rh incompatibility occurs more frequently and is often called Rh disease.

Definition

Hemolytic disease of the newborn, also known erythroblastosis fetalis, is an autoimmune condition that develops in a fetus, when the IgG molecules (one of the five main types of antibodies) produced by the mother pass through the placenta.

Causes

Hemolytic disease of the newborn (HDN) occurs when the blood types of a mother and baby are incompatible. If the baby's incompatible red blood cells crossover to his mother, through the placenta during pregnancy or at delivery, her immune system sees them as foreign and responds by developing proteins called antibodies to attack and break them down. This can lead to several complications that range from mild to very severe.

The mother's immune system also keeps these antibodies in case the incompatible red blood cells appear again, making her 'sensitized.' Because of this, HDN is more likely to occur during a mother's second or subsequent pregnancy, or following a miscarriage or abortion.

Types

- *Rh incompatibility:* Hemolytic disease of the newborn most frequently occurs when a mother with Rh-negative blood becomes pregnant by an Rh-positive father, resulting in an Rh-positive baby. This type of hemolytic disease of the newborn is often called Rh disease.
- *ABO incompatibility:* Although it is not as common, hemolytic disease of the newborn can also occur when a mother and baby have incompatible blood types.

Table 2.5: ABO incompatibility

Mother's blood type	O	A	B
Baby's blood type	A or B	B	A

Signs and Symptoms of Hemolytic Disease

- Pale skin
- Yellow color of the amniotic fluid, umbilical cord, skin and eyes
- Enlarged liver or spleen
- Severe swelling of the body.

Pathophysiology

Complications of the Newborn During Pregnancy

Mild anemia: In this condition the baby's red blood cell count is deficient; his blood cannot carry enough oxygen from the lungs to all parts of his body, causing his organs and tissues to oxygen insufficiency.

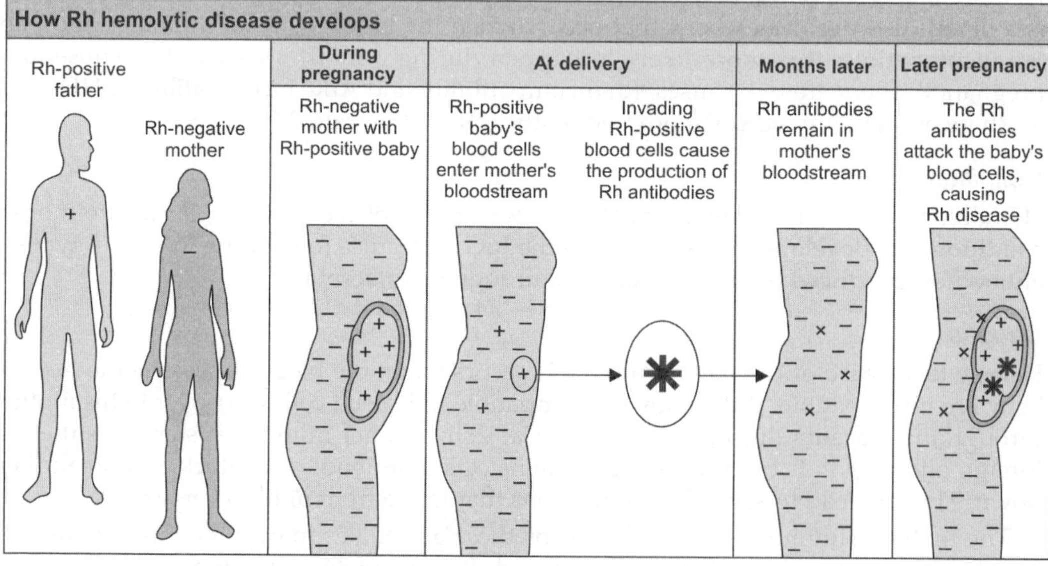

Fig. 2.21: Rh hemolytic disease

Hyperbilirubinemia and jaundice: The breakdown of red blood cells produces bilirubin, a brownish yellow substance that is difficult for a baby to discharge and can build up in his blood (hyperbilirubinemia) and make his skin appear yellow.

Severe anemia with enlargement of liver and spleen: The baby's body tries to compensate for the breakdown of red blood cells by making more of them very quickly in the liver and spleen, which causes the organs to get bigger. These new red blood cells are often immature and unable to function completely, leading to severe anemia.

Hydrops fetalis: In this condition newborn baby's body cannot cope with the anemia, his heart begins to fail and large amounts of fluid buildup in his tissues and organs.

Complications of HDN for Newborn after Birth

- *Severe hyperbilirubinemia and jaundice:* Excessive build-up of bilirubin in the baby's blood causes his liver to become enlarged.
- *Kernicterus:* Build-up of bilirubin in the blood is so high that it spills over into the brain, which can lead to permanent brain damage.

Management

Treatment during pregnancy:

- Blood transfusion
- Early delivery of the baby if severe complications arise and baby's lungs are mature.

Treatment after the birth:

- Blood transfusion
- Intravenous fluids
- Oxygen or mechanical breathing machine
- Exchange transfusion to replace the baby's damaged blood with fresh blood.

Preventive Measures

The hemolytic disease of the newborn is very preventable. Today, nearly all women with Rh-negative blood are identified in early pregnancy through blood tests. If a mother is Rh-negative and has not been sensitized, she is usually given a drug called **Rh immunoglobulin, or RhoGAM**.

This specially developed blood product prevents an Rh-negative mother's antibodies from reacting to her baby's Rh-positive red blood cells. Mothers are typically given RhoGAM around the 28th week of pregnancy and again within 72 hours of giving birth.

Hemolytic Anemia

Definition

Hemolytic anemia is a blood disorder that occurs when red blood cells are destroyed faster than the bone marrow can make them. There are two types of hemolytic anemia: intrinsic, which is inherited, and extrinsic which can be caused by certain infections, medications or autoimmune disorders.

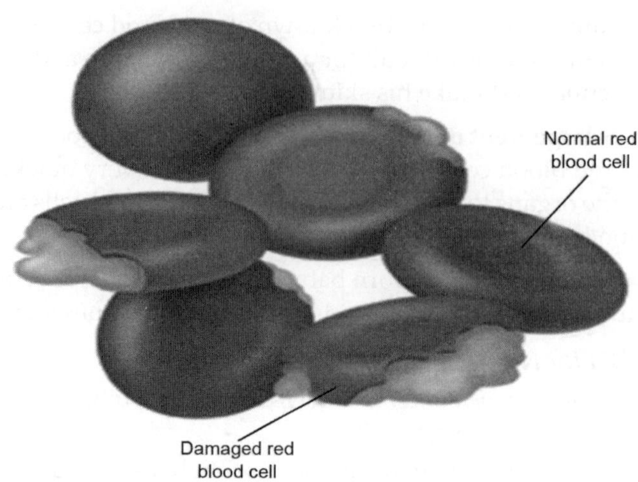

Fig. 2.22: Hemolytic anemia

Classification of Hemolytic Anemia

	Intracorpuscular defects	Extracorpuscular factors
Hereditary	• Hemoglobinopathies • Enzymopathies • Membrane cytoskeletal defects	• Familial hemolytic uremic syndrome
Acquired	• Paroxysmal hemoglobinuria	• Mechanical destruction (microangiopathic) • Toxic agents • Drugs • Infectious • Autoimmune

Types

- *Intrinsic hemolytic anemia:* The destruction of the red blood cells is due to a defect within the red blood cells themselves. Intrinsic hemolytic anemia are often inherited, such as sickle cell anemia, thalassemia, or erythrocytosis.

  These conditions produce red blood cells that do not live as long as normal red blood cells.
- *Extrinsic hemolytic anemia:* Red blood cells are produced healthy, but are later destroyed by getting trapped in the spleen, destroyed by infection, or destroyed from drugs that can affect red blood cells. In severe cases the destruction takes place in the circulation.

Causes

- Infections such as:
  - Hepatitis virus
  - Cytomegalovirus (CMV)
  - Epstein-Barr virus (EBV)

  - Typhoid fever
  - E. Coli, or streptococcus.
- Medications such as:
  - Penicillin
  - Antimalarial medications
  - Sulfa medications, or acetaminophen.
- Leukemia or lymphoma
- Autoimmune disorders such as:
  - Systemic lupus erythematous (SLE, or lupus), rheumatoid arthritis
  - Wiskott-Aldrich syndrome
  - Ulcerative colitis.
- Various tumors
- Hypersplenism.

Some types of extrinsic hemolytic anemia are temporary and resolve over several months. Other types can become chronic with periods of remissions and recurrence.

Signs and Symptoms

The following are the most common symptoms of hemolytic anemia. However, each child may experience symptoms differently. Symptoms may include:

- Paleness or lack of color of the skin
- Jaundice, or yellowing of the skin and eyes
- Dark-colored urine
- Fever
- Weakness
- Dizziness
- Confusion
- Intolerance to physical activity
- Enlargement of the spleen and live
- Increased heart rate (Tachycardia)
- Heart murmur sound.

Diagnostic Evaluation

Hemolytic anemia may be suspected from general findings on a complete medical history and physical examination of child, such as complaints of tiring easily, pale skin and lips, or a fast heartbeat (tachycardia). In addition to a complete physical examination.

Following diagnostic tests:

- *Blood tests:* These tests measure hemoglobin and Reticulocyte count and will reveal how many new red blood cells are being produced.
- *Other blood tests:* These tests will check lactate dehydrogenase, bilirubin, and hepatoglobin, as well as the presence of certain antibodies. Blood smear or look at the red blood cells under a microscope to aid in the diagnosis.
- *Urine tests for hemoglobin*

- *Bone marrow aspiration and/or biopsy:* A procedure that involves taking a small amount of bone marrow fluid (aspiration) and/or solid bone marrow tissue (called a core biopsy), usually from the hip bones, to be examined for the number, size, and maturity of blood cells and/or abnormal cells.

Management

Treatment for hemolytic anemia

- Blood transfusions
- Corticosteroid medications
- Treatment with intravenous immunoglobulin (to strengthen the immune system)
- Rituximab or other immune suppressing drugs
- Antibiotics if the cause is an infection.

In more severe cases, the following treatments may be necessary and usually require hospitalization:

- Exchange transfusion (similar to a blood transfusion, but with more blood being given and an equal amount of the child's hemolyzed blood being removed)
- Surgical removal of the spleen (usually reserved for children who do not respond to other therapies)
- Immunosuppressive therapy.

Nursing Management

Nursing Diagnosis

a. Ineffective tissue perfusion

Goal: Adequate tissue perfusion

Nursing Intervention for anemia:

- Monitor vital signs, capillary refill, skin color, mucous membranes.
- Exalt the position of head of in bed
- Examine and document the presence of pain.
- Observation of a delay in verbal response, confusion, or restlessness
- Observe and document the presence of the cold.
- Maintain the ambient temperature to keep warm the body needs.
- Provide oxygen as needed.

b. Activity Intolerance

Goal: Tolerant of activity

Nursing Intervention

- Assess the capability of doing the activity
- Monitor vital signs during and after activity, and noted a physiological response to activity (increased heart rate increased blood pressure, or rapid breathing).
- Provide information to the patient or family to stop doing activities if teladi symptoms of increased heart rate, increased blood pressure, rapid breathing, dizziness or fatigue).
- Provide support to perform their daily activities according to the ability of the child.
- Creating a schedule of activities involving other health team.

NEONATAL HYPOGLYCEMIA

Introduction

Blood glucose concentrations in the newborn baby, irrespective of its birth weight and gestational age, are generally lower than those found in older children and adults. The infant is born with a blood glucose concentration of 60 to 70 percent of the maternal level and it falls during first 24 hours, the lowest value is seen at the age of three hours. This is followed by a transient rise in blood glucose level during next 24 hours and again dangerously low levels may be encountered at the age of 3 to 4 days before stability is achieved.

There is a controversy and confusion regarding the universally accepted definition of hypoglycemia in the newborn baby. The operational threshold for hypoglycemia is defined as 'that concentration of plasma or whole blood glucose at which the clinician should consider intervention, based on the evidence currently available in the literature.' Most workers now agree that a true blood glucose level of less than 40 mg per 100 ml (irrespective of period of gestation), if associated with symptoms of hypoglycemia or if confirmed on repeat analysis in asymptomatic babies, is indicative of hypoglycemia (1.0 mMol/l of glucose is equivalent to 18.02 mg/dl).

Predisposing Factors

Intrauterine Growth Retardation

In malnourished babies and smaller of the discordant twins, the liver weight is much reduced whereas the brain weight remains within normal limits so that the ratio of brain weight to liver weight is greater than five. This discrepancy in the size of the utilizer (brain) and provider (liver glycogen) of glucose leads to hypoglycemia. The other predisposing factors in these babies include higher incidence of fetal and neonatal asphyxia, raised basal metabolic rate and higher oxygen uptake, excessive responsiveness to insulin, inability to increase adrenaline output in response to hypoglycemia and possibly disturbed hypothalamic mechanism in the brain. Hypoglycemia occurs in about 15 percent of small-for-dates babies and is often symptomatic especially in male babies. It generally manifests between 24 and 72 hours and is preventable by early feeding.

Maternal Diabetes Mellitus

The fetus by virtue of being exposed to high concentrations of glucose *in utero* respond by hyperplasia of islet-cells. The high insulin concentrations may lead to hypoglycemia in about 50 percent of such babies which is observed mostly during first 12 hours after birth and is asymptomatic in majority of infants.

About one-fifth of babies born to mothers with gestational diabetes mellitus may show hypoglycemia. The administration of chlorpropamide during the latter parts of pregnancy my lead to intractable hypoglycemia in the baby which may need exchange blood transfusion.

Immaturity

There is a direct correlation between blood glucose levels and gestational maturity and birth weight of the baby. The low hepatic glycogen stores and relatively high incidence of hypoxia, hypothermia and respiratory distress syndrome in these babies contribute to hypoglycemia. Maternal tocolytic therapy with beta-sympathomimetic agents (ritodrine, isoxsuprine, salbutamol, terbutaline) can predispose to hypoglycemia. These agents decrease peripheral utilization of glucose leading to hyperglycemia in the mother and hyperinsulinemia in the fetus. The incidence of hypoglycemia in preterm babies varies between 5 to 10 percent and is higher in babies with a birth weight of less than 50th percentile for their gestational age. About three-fourth of hypoglycemic low birth babies are symptomatic.

Erythroblastosis fetal is due to rhesus incompatibility: The hyperplasia of islet cells may lead to asymptomatic hypoglycemia during the first 24 hours of life in about 5 percent of babies with erythroblastosis. The incidence of hypoglycemia is directly related to the severity of rhesus hemolytic disease. There is some evidence to suggest that breakdown products of hemolyzed red blood cells (glutathione) inactivates circulating insulin leading to hyperplasia of islet-cells to maintain adequate insulin levels. Exchange transfusion with heparinised blood is associated with hypoglycemia while following exchange transfusion with CPD-blood, rebound hypoglycemia occurs.

Miscellaneous Disorders

Hypoglycemia is common following severe birth asphyxia, hypothermia, septicemia and polycythemia. Rarely, recurrent and often intractable hypoglycemia may occur due to a number of metabolic and developmental disorders. They include glycogen storage disease, organic acidemias, adrenal insufficiency, leucine sensitivity, and insulinoma.

Large-for-dates infants due to any cause (maternal diabetes, erythroblastosis fetalis, Wiedemann-Beckwith syndrome, transposition of great vessels) are associated with islet-cells hyperplasia and are predisposed to develop hypoglycemia. Their overgrowth appears to be due to consumption of large quantities of glucose in utero. Therefore, their organs arereplete with glycogen. Neonatal hypoglycemia can be classified on the basis of underlying patho-physiological mechanism. The hypoglycemia would be provoked by milk feeding in leucine sensitivity, galactosemia, fructosemia (sucrose added to the milk) and in some cases of islet cell hyperplasia and tumor. Maternal therapy with beta blockers especially propranolol is also associated with neonatal hypoglycemia.

Indication

To prevent brain damage, blood glucose should be routinely estimated in the following high-risk situations.

- Small-for-dates babies and smaller of the discordant twins
- Infants of diabetic mothers or those with a birth weight of above 90th percentile for their period of gestation
- Preterm infants < 35 weeks gestation
- Rhesus hemolytic disease of the newborn
- Babies with symptoms suggestive of hypoglycemia
- Babies with prolonged hypoxia, hypothermia, polycythemia, septicemia, cardiac failure and suspected metabolic disorders
- Infants born to mothers receiving therapy with terbutaline, propranolol and oral hypoglycemic agent
- Infants on IV fluid or total parenteral nutrition.

The routine monitoring of blood glucose in above high-risk situations is recommended at the ages of 3, 12, 24, 48 and 72 hours prior to feeding. Following exchange transfusion with

CPD blood, glucose level should be checked 2 hours after the procedure to detect rebound hypoglycemia. In an asymptomatic infant with hypoglycemia on a feed trial, blood glucose should be checked after one hour of feed.

Methods for Estimation of Blood Glucose

It is imperative to measure the level of true glucose rather than the reducing ability of the blood either by glucose oxidase, glucose electrode and Nelson and Somogyi methods. The blood glucose level is the sum total of glucose in the plasma and red blood cells, although the latter is unavailable to the brain.

The rapid glycolysis of red cell glucose demands that whenever there is a delay in doing the estimation, sample should be stored in the refrigerator or should be immediately precipitated with sodium fluoride to inhibit glycolysis otherwise falsely low values may be obtained. If these precautions are not taken, the glucose level of sample may drop at a rate of 15 to 20 mg per 100 ml per hour. Glucose strips (dextrostix) are very useful and essential for screening glucose on capillary samples with the help of a dextrometer. They are not accurate for monitoring low glucose levels. Reagent strips measure whole blood glucose which is 15 percent lower than plasma level. If dextrotix reveals blood glucose concentration of less than 40 mg/dl, treatment should not be delayed while one is awaiting confirmation of hypoglycemia by laboratory analysis.

Classification of neonatal hypoglycemia on the basis of underlying physiologic mechanisms

Fetal/Neonatal Hyperinsulinism

- Maternal diabetes mellitus
- Erythroblastosis fetalis
- Weidemann-Beckwith syndrome
- Transposition of great vessels
- Maternal therapy with beta-sympathomimetic tocolytic agents (ritodrine, isoxsuprine, salbutamol, terbutaline) and propranolol.
- Insulin producing tumors (nesidioblastosis, islet cell adenoma, islet cell dysmaturity).

Decreased glycogen stores and/or increased utilization of glucose

- Intrauterine growth retardation
- Prematurity
- Birth asphyxia
- Hypothermia
- Polycythemia
- Septicemia
- Starvation.

Miscellaneous

- Inborn errors of metabolism (glycogen storage disease, galactosemia, fructose intolerance, congenital adrenal hyperplasia, cretinism).
- Maternal therapy with chlopropamide and beta-blockers (propranonol and labetalol)
- Exchange transfusion with heparinized or ACD/CPD blood
- Congenital hypopituitrism.

Signs and Symptoms

There are no pathognomonic symtoms of hypoglycemia in the newborn and there is poor correlation between the level of blood glucose and symptomatology. The various factors which result in poor correlation between blood glucose concentration and development of symptoms include probable utilization of lactate and glycerol as an alternative substrate by the brain, reduced peripheral utilization of glucose level rather than the total or red cell glucose content and susceptibility or threshold of brain to hypoglycemic insult which may be altered by anoxia and intracranial injury.

Irritability of the central nervous system is manifested by jitteriness, course tremors, twitching and convulsions. Jitteriness alone is not a reliable sign of hypoglycemia. The babies may manifest with refusal of feeds, apathy, limpness and come.

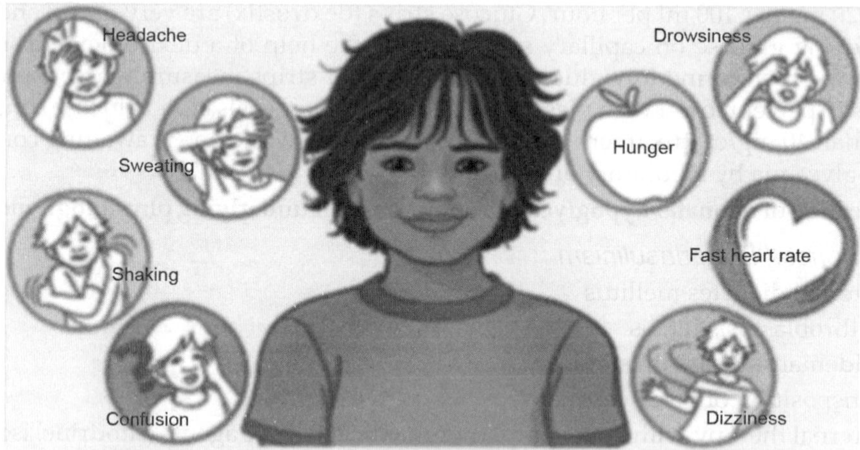

Fig. 2.23: These symptoms and others can be signs of hypoglycemia

Episodes of apnea with cyanosis and tachypnea with irregular breathing may occur due to hypoglycemia in preterm babies. There may be episodes of sudden pallor, limpness and hypothermia. Tachycardia and sweating may reflect excess of catecholamine secretion. Cardiomegaly and occasionally cardiac failure may occur in hypoglycemic babies. Septicemic babies may also have associated hypoglycemia.

In view of the fact that there are no diagnostic symptoms or signs of hypoglycemia and above clinical manifestations can occur from a variety of causes, the proof of hypoglycemic etiology of symptoms rests solely upon prompt disappearance of symptoms on administration of intravenous glucose.

Diagnostic Evaluation

- *Asymptomatic hypoglycemia:* The true blood glucose level is below 40 mg/dl on two occasions in a baby without any clinical symptoms of hypoglycemia.
- *Symptomatic hypoglycemia:* The diagnosis is made on the basis of Whipple's triad:
  - Presence of symptoms attributable to hypoglycemia
  - Low true blood glucose documented by an accurate and sensitive laboratory method

- Disappearance of clinical symptoms when blood glucose level is normalized. If the clinical symptoms or signs attributed to hypoglycemia are not resolved on administration of glucose, other diagnostic possibilities should be considered.

Management

Prevention: Infants at increased risk to develop hypoglycemia (SFD's, LFD's. IGDM's, IDM's, smaller of twin) should be nursed in thermoneutral environment so that glucose is not wasted for metabolic thermogenesis. First feed should be given within first hour of birth. Breastfeeding should be continued and formula feeds fortified with 5 g sucrose/dl should be offered every 2-hourly during first 3 days of life.

Instead of adding sucrose, formula feeds can be prepared in 5 percent dextrose water. The mother should not be asked to buy the feeding bottle or the formula which should be provided from the nursery. The supplementary feeds should be given with a cup and spoon. Blood glucose should be checked after one hour of complementary feed. After 3 days of age, the infant should receive exclusive breastfeeding. If hypoglycemia develops despite administration of fortified feeds, the protocol for management of hypoglycemia should be followed.

Treatment

In symptomatic cases therapy should be administered immediately after withdrawing a blood sample for glucose estimation. The baby should be kept warm by nursing in a thermoneutral environment. In a symptomatic infant with seizures, give 5 – 10 ml/kg of 10% dextrose intravenously as a bolus. In the absence of seizures, symptomatic infant is given a mini-bolus of 2 ml/kg of 10% dextrose.

This is followed by continuous infusion of 10% dextrose at a rate of 8 mg/kg/minute preferably with the help of an infusion pump. Calculate separately glucose intake (mg/kg/min) and water requirements everyday. For example, if fluid ml/kg/min. in this case 10% dextrose (100 mg dextrose/ml) would provide the glucose infusion rate of 5.5 mg/kg/min while 15% dextrose (150 mg/ml) solution would provide 8.25 mg glucose/kg/min. depending upon the daily fluid requirements, the concentration of dextrose solution to be infused can be worked out to provide the desired amount of constant delivery of glucose.

The maximal glucose concentration is usually limited to 15% to safeguard against the risk of thrombophlebitis. To prepare 14.5 percent solution of dextrose, add 30 ml of 10% dextrose (7.5 g dextrose) to 70 ml of 10% dextrose (7.0 g dextrose). Blood glucose is monitored every 2 hours. The glucose infusion rate is gradually increased by 2 mg/kg/minute every 2 hours till a maximum infusion rate of 12 mg/kg/minute is reached or the blood glucose has crossed the level of 40 mg/dl.

The glucose level should be checked after 30 min of each change in infusion rate. When blood glucose level crosses 502 mg/dl, glucose infusion rate is gradually tapered with decrements of 2 mg/kg/minute every 6 hourly till glucose infusion rate comes down to 4 mg/kg/minute with satisfactory blood glucose values (> 50 mg/dl). Oral feeds are introduced gradually when glucose infusion is being tapered. The infant is completely weaned off intravenous infusion when his blood glucose values are stable at an infusion rate of 4 mg/kg/minute. Refer to Algorithm for stepwise management of hypoglycemia.

Note

- Check blood glucose after 30 min of every hypoglycemia
- Change in infusion rate
- Reduce glucose infusion rate if last 2 blood
- Glucose values are > 50 mg/dl. In case of resistant hypoglycemia, exclude polycythemia
- There is no role of drugs in infants with IUGR. Stop hydrocortisone in 3 to 5 days
- BG: Blood glucose.

Investigate for resistant hypoglycemia. Serum cortisol and Insulin levels. CT scan of pancreas and screening for inborn error of metabolism.

Flowchart 2.1: Algorithm for stepwise management of hypoglycemia

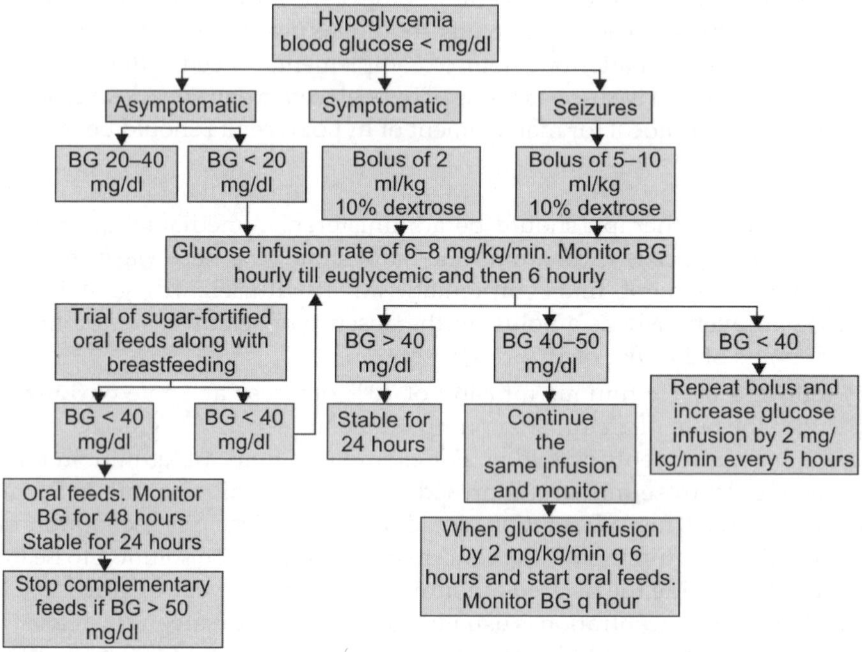

Hypoglycemia blood glucose < mg/dl

Asymptomatic

Symptomatic

Seizures

BG 20–40 mg/dl

BG < 20 mg/dl

Bolus of 2 ml/kg 10% dextrose

Bolus of 5–10 ml/kg 10% dextrose

Glucose infusion rate of 6–8 mg/kg/min. Monitor BG hourly till euglycemic and then 6 hourly

Trial of sugar-fortified oral feeds along with breastfeeding

BG < 40 mg/dl

BG < 40 mg/dl

Oral feeds. Monitor BG for 48 hours Stable for 24 hours

Stop complementary feeds if BG > 50 mg/dl

BG > 40 mg/dl

Stable for 24 hours

BG 40–50 mg/dl

Continue the same infusion and monitor

When glucose infusion by 2 mg/kg/min q 6 hours and start oral feeds. Monitor BG q hour

BG < 40

Repeat bolus and increase glucose infusion by 2 mg/kg/min every 5 hours

NEONATAL SEPSIS

Introduction

Neonatal sepsis is any type of infection involving an infant during the first 28 days of life. Neonatal sepsis is also known as **sepsis neonatorum.** The infection may involve the infant globally or may be limited to just one organ (such as the lungs with pneumonia).

Definition

Neonatal sepsis is defined as the presence bacterial or virus in the newborn baby blood stream called newborn infection or sepsis, such as meningitis, pneumonia, Pyelonephritis, or gastroenteritis) in the setting of high fever.

Types

Sepsis may be acquired prior to birth (intrauterine sepsis) or after birth (extrauterine sepsis). Viral (such as herpes, rubella [German measles), bacterial (such as group B strep) and more rarely fungal (such as Candida) causes may be implicated.

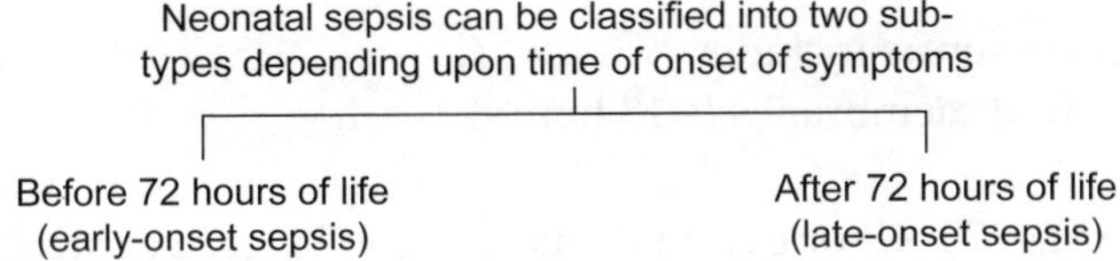

Causes

Neonatal sepsis can be caused by bacteria, such as *Escherichia coli* (*E. coli*), *Listeria*, and some strains of streptococcus. The herpes virus can also cause a severe infection in a newborn baby.

Causes of Early-onset Neonatal Sepsis

This type of sepsis most often appears within 24 hours of birth. The baby gets the infection from the mother before or during delivery. The following increases an infant's risk of early-onset sepsis:

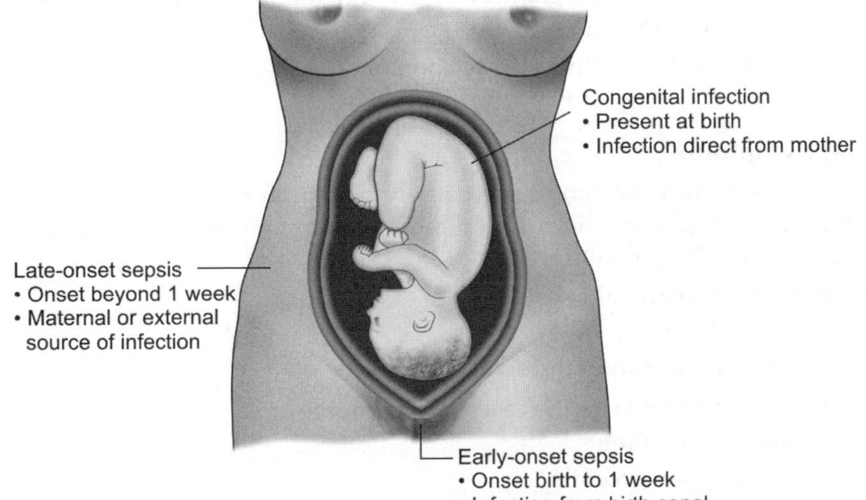

Fig. 2.24: Causes of neonatal sepsis

- Group B streptococcus infection during pregnancy
- Preterm delivery
- Water breaking (rupture of membranes) longer than 24 hours before birth
- Infection of the placenta tissues and amniotic fluid (chorioamnionitis).

Causes of Late-onset Neonatal Sepsis

This type of sepsis Babies with late-onset neonatal sepsis get infected after delivery. The following increase an infant's risk of sepsis after delivery:

- Having a catheter in a blood vessel for a long time
- Staying in the hospital for an extended period of time.

Risk Factors for Sepsis

Early-onset Sepsis

Features of early-onset sepsis include:

- Prolonged ruptured membranes (> 18 hours)
- Fetal distress
- Maternal pyrexia (> 38 °C) or overt infection, e.g. UTI, gastroenteritis/diarrheal illness
- Multiple obstetric procedures, including cervical sutures
- Preterm delivery
- History of GBS infection in previous infant
- GBS bacteriuria in this pregnancy.

Late-onset Sepsis

Features of late-onset sepsis include:

- Prolonged hospitalization, e.g. preterm infant in a NICU
- Presence of foreign bodies, e.g. intravenous catheters, endotracheal tubes, etc.
- Cross infection by staff and parents
- Malformations, such as urinary tract anomalies (e.g. vesicoureteric reflux) or neural tube defects.

Signs and Symptoms

Most common signs and symptoms are usually nonspecific since other conditions cause similar clinical states (e.g. cardiac or respiratory failure, metabolic disorders). Often gut feeling of baby being 'not quite right'.

Common features of neonatal sepsis

- Pallor, lethargy, jaundice
- Fever, hypothermia, temperature instability.

Note: One third of confirmed sepsis cases are normothermia

- Poor tolerance to handling
- Hypoglycemia/hyperglycemia
- Blood gas derangements (including acidosis and lactate accumulation).

Respiratory Symptoms

- Increased respiratory rate
- Apnea
- Grunting
- Cyanosis.

Cardiovascular System Symptoms

- Tachycardia
- Bradycardia episodes

- Poor perfusion
- Hypotension.

Cutaneous Symptoms
- Petechiae
- Bruising
- Bleeding from puncture sites.

Gastrointestinal Tract (GIT) Symptoms
- Poor feeding
- Vomiting
- Abdominal distension
- Feed intolerance
- Bilious aspirates/vomits
- Loose stools.

Central Nervous System (CNS) Symptoms
- Lethargy
- Irritability
- Seizures.

Diagnostic Evaluation
- Blood culture
- C-reactive protein
- Complete blood count (CBC)
- A lumbar puncture (spinal tap) will be done to look at the spinal fluid for bacteria. Skin, stool, and urine cultures may be done for herpes virus if the mother has a history of infection.
- The initial blood culture is positive. LP must be performed to exclude meningitis since the presence of meningitis alters the length of antibiotic treatment as well as prognosis. A lumbar puncture may still be useful within four hours of commencing antibiotics as growth may still occur.
- A chest X-ray will be done if the baby has a cough or problems breathing.
- Urine culture tests are done in babies older than a few days.

Management
Antibiotic Choice
- Antibiotics therapy usual given on causative organisms following regimes are recommended initially.
- Antibiotic choice can then be rationalized on the basis of culture results and clinical course.

Early Onset Sepsis
- *Benzylpenicillin:* 60 mg/kg IV 12 hourly. 120 mg/kg/dose 12 hourly if meningitis suspected
- *Gentamicin:* 5 mg/kg IV 36 hourly if > = 1200 g, 48 hrly if < 1200 g

- Antiviral medication called acyclovir will be used for infections that may be caused by the herpesvirus.

Complications

- Disability
- Death.

Preventive Measures

Antibiotics therapy [during Pregnancy]:

- Infection in the placenta
- Group B strep infection
- Given birth in the past to a baby with sepsis caused by bacteria.

Other measures to prevent the sepsis include:

- Preventing and treating infections in mothers, including herpes infection
- Providing a clean place for birth
- Delivering the baby within 24 hours of when the membranes break.

Nursing Management

General Nursing Care

- Provide thermal care by radiant warmer
- Incubator nursing care
- Phototherapy if needed
- Monitoring of oxygen saturation, heart rate and blood pressure.

Specific Nursing Care

Oxygen therapy to Support the apnoea

  - Hypoxia
  - Hypercapnea
  - Respiratory distress.

ORAL THRUSH

Introduction

Oral thrush is a very common infection in infants that causes irritation in and around a baby's mouth. It is caused by the overgrowth of a yeast (a type of fungus) called Candida albicans.

Definition

Oral thrush is defined as an infection caused by a yeast germ called Candida. The newborn mouth is a common site where Candida causes infection. Candidal infection otherwise known as oral thrush. Characterized by it looks like spots or patches of cottage cheese or milk curds in and around newborn baby mouth. These patches may appear:

- Inside the cheeks
- On the roof of the mouth
- On the gums
- On the tongue.

Causes

Thrush is caused by forms of a fungus called Candida. A small amount of this fungus lives in the mouth. It is usually kept in check by the immune system and other types of germs that also normally live in the mouth.

When the child immune system is weaker, the fungus can grow, leading to sores and lesions in the mouth and on the tongue. Oral thrush may occur in babies because their immune systems take time to mature, making them less able to resist infection.

- Premature infants are especially predisposed to thrush due to their immature immune system.
- In older child who are immunocompetent, predisposing factors are often present, such as a recent course of antibiotic therapy that disrupts the normal flora, or steroid use.
- Immunosuppressed child are more susceptible to oral candidiasis, as well as cutaneous and systemic infections.

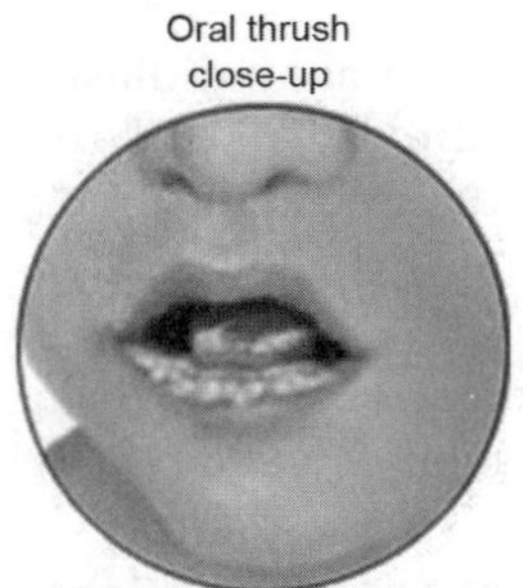

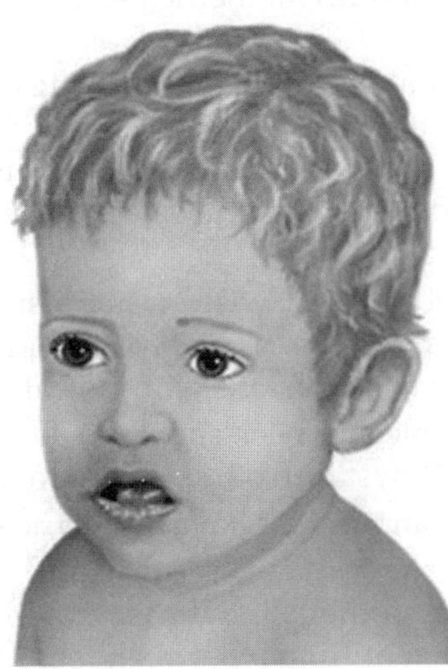

Fig. 2.25: Oral thrush

Signs and Symptoms

- White spots usually develop in newborn mouth and on their tongue. The spots may join together to form larger spots called plaques. They may become yellow or gray.
- Infants with thrush may present with pain, poor feeding, or fussiness, but patients are more often asymptomatic and thrush presents no interference with eating.
- Esophagitis due to Candida infection may present with chest pain and poor feeding.

Pathophysiology

- Based on causes oral thrush represents an overgrowth of yeast when either normal host immunity or normal host flora has been disrupted.
- Yeast overgrowth on the oral mucosa causes the epithelial cells to desquamate.
- Bacteria, keratin, and necrotic tissue accumulate and form a pseudomembrane.

- Oral candidiasis is common in infants. Neonates with thrush have usually been colonized when they passed through the birth canal, but other sources of transmission may include colonized breasts, hands, or bottle nipples.
- Thrush can also develop as an adverse effect from inhaled corticosteroids for asthma.
- Immunosuppressed patients may also develop candidal esophagitis.

Diagnostic Evaluation

- History collection
- Physical Examination of oral Cavity
- Blood test to check the child level of iron, and vitamin B_{12} or folate.
- *Oral mucous swab*: The swab is then sent to the laboratory to be examined under a microscope. It help to identify the grow the *Candida* in the laboratory.

Management

The two main antifungal medicines used to treat oral thrush in babies are miconazole and nystatin:

- Nystatin oral suspension is the drug of choice for oral candidiasis. Various reports have reported cure rates between 50 and 80% on standard 100,000 units per dose 4 times a day. May have to double the dose or apply it directly to the lesions with a cotton swab. Nystatin does not adhere well to the lesions and is swallowed rapidly and this interferes with its efficacy.
- Older children can swish nystatin suspension around in their mouth and swallow it. For infants, parents can apply 1 to 2 ml of the solution inside each cheek between meals, or directly to the lesions with a swab.
- Gentian violet has been shown to be effective as a second-line agent for oral candidiasis resistant to nystatin, but is messy to use and should not be swallowed.
- These oral antifungals have little to no systemic absorption, so there are minimal adverse effects.
- In nursing mothers, the breast may be a reservoir for the yeast so that the application of a topical antifungal between feeds to the breast may help eradicate the infection.
- Always continue to check for diaper dermatitis because often associated with oral monilia infection.

Nursing Management

- Advise the mothers should avoid damp or wet nursing pads and consider air-drying their nipples.
- Advise the parents before feeding the child feeding bottle should be clean with soap and hot water.
- Ask parents to maintain the hygiene for bottle nipples and pacifiers for reduce the oral candida infections.
- If child had a asthma provide the daily-inhaled corticosteroids for effective control.
- She should be use the spacer when using a Metered Dose Inhaler (MDI) and rinsing and spitting out with water following MDI or nebulizer administered corticosteroids is imperative.

IMPETIGO

Introduction

Childhood impetigo is the most common pyoderma diseases, manifests as thin superficial vesiculopustules which soon rupture to form honey-colored crusts with a 'stuck-on' appearance. Bullous lesions can occur in neonates and infants (bullous impetigo) which on rupture spread peripherally causing annular lesions. Lesions develop most commonly on the face and heal without scarring.

Definition

Impetigo is defined as superficial infection of the skin caused by bacteria. The lesions are often grouped and have a red base. The lesions open and become crusty and have a honey color, which is typical of impetigo. Impetigo is contagious and can be spread throughout a household, with children reinfection themselves or other family members.

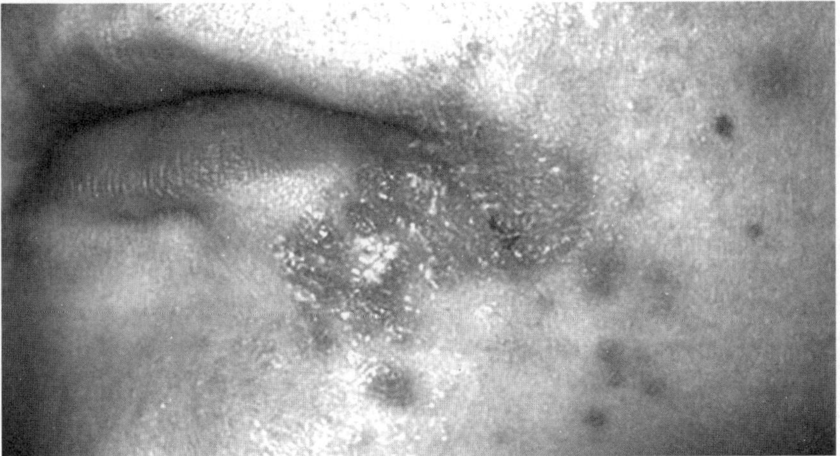

Fig. 2.26: Impetigo

Causes

Common bacteria, some of which are found normally on the skin, cause impetigo. When the bacteria enter an open area in the skin, the infection can occur. The most common bacteria that cause impetigo include the following:

- Group A β-hemolytic streptococcus
- Staphylococcus aureus.

Signs and Symptoms

Impetigo usually occurs on the face, neck, arms, and limbs, but the lesions may appear on any part of the body. Impetigo starts as a small vesicle or fluid-filled lesion. The lesion then ruptures and the fluid drains, leaving areas that are covered with honey-colored crusts.

The lesions may all look different, with different sizes and shapes. In more advanced cases, your child may also have swollen lymph nodes (small lumps that are located mostly in the neck, arm, under the arm, and in the groin area). The lymph nodes become enlarged when child's body is fighting an infection.

Diagnostic Evaluation

- Impetigo is usually diagnosed based on a complete medical history
- Physical examination of the child. The lesions of impetigo are unique and usually allow for a diagnosis based simply on physical examination
- In additional investigation like culture of child's lesion to confirm the diagnosis and the type of bacteria that are present.

Management

Treatment of impetigo typically involves local wound care in conjunction with either a topical antibiotic or a combination of systemic and topical agents. In general, the antibiotic selection has coverage against both S aureus and S pyogenes.

In areas with a high prevalence of community-acquired MRSA [Methicillin-resistant *S. aureus*] with susceptible isolates, children older than 8 years may take clindamycin or doxycycline in cases.

Specific treatment for impetigo will be determined by:

- The child's age, overall health, and medical history
- Extent of the condition
- Child's tolerance for specific medications, procedures, or therapies
- Expectations for the course of the condition
- Parents opinion or preference.

Treatment may include

- If child with many lesions, oral antibiotics may be prescribed.
- Child has only a few lesions, she may prescribe a topical antibiotic applied directly to the lesions.

Preventive Management

- Discourage the child to touching the lesions
- Advice the parents about early and proper care of predisposing factors (e.g. insect bites, minor trauma)
- She should be advised the mother regarding proper cleanse and apply a topical antibiotic to minor skin traumas
- Because of the contagious nature, children should not return to day care or school until 24 hours after the initiation of appropriate antimicrobial therapy
- Caretakers should be instructed about hygienic issues and prevention
- A history of poor hygiene and crowded living situations are common. This infection is transmitted by direct contact and by fomites, including hygiene items, clothing, and toys.

Nursing Management

- Child should wash daily with an antibacterial soap
- Everyone in the household should practice proper handwashing
- Advice the mother should short the child's fingernails it will help to decrease the chance of scratching and spreading the infection
- Avoid sharing clothing, towels and other household items.

ERYTHEMA TOXICUM

Introduction

Erythema toxicum neonatorum condition is very common and completely benign condition usually arises in the first 2 days of life. The eruption is characterized by small, erythematous papules, vesicles, and, occasionally, pustules. The lesions are usually surrounded by a distinctive diffuse, blotchy, erythematous halo. Individual lesions are transitory, often disappearing within hours and then appearing elsewhere on the body.

Definition

Erythema toxicum is defined as common harmless rash that appears in at least half of all infants who are carried to term baby. The condition is also sometimes called erythema toxicum neonatorum (ETN) or toxic erythema of the newborn.

Other terminology:

- Erythema toxicum neonatorum
- Erythema toxicum
- Urticaria neonatorum and toxic erythema.

It appears in up to half of newborns carried to term, usually between day 2 and 5 after birth.

Erythema toxicum is defined as rash that consists of tiny bumps that are firm, yellowish or white, and surrounded by a ring of redness. Characterized by bumps are filled with a fluid that looks like pus filled sac. Sometimes there are no bumps at all only a splotchy redness.

Causes

The cause is unknown; various ideas have been suggested, including the possibility that it is a normal inflammatory or immune system response in babies. It has not been proven to be an allergic problem. It is also not related to whether the baby is breastfed or formula-fed.

Risk Factors

It includes higher birth weight [above 3 kg], greater gestational age [40-weeks], and vaginal delivery. A positive correlation has been recognized between the length of labor and both the incidence of erythema toxicum neonatorum and the duration of the cutaneous manifestations.

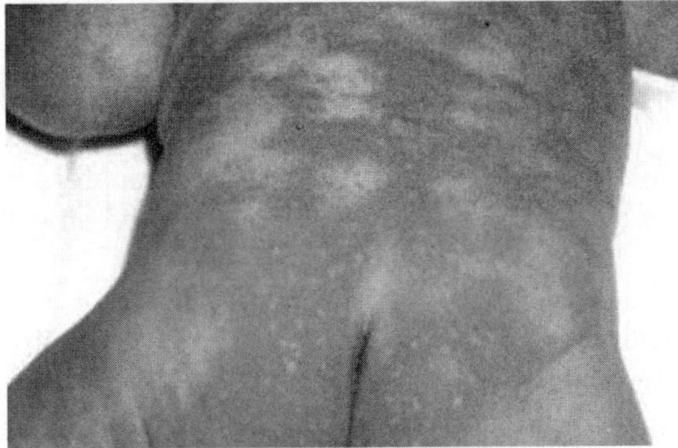

Fig. 2.27: Erythema toxicum

Signs and Symptoms

It occurs in healthy babies born at full term, between 3 and 14 days of age. The rash can occur in the first 48 hours of life but 9 out of 10 cases are in babies more than 2 days old.

Overall, it seems to be more common in male babies (about half of male babies get it) compared with female babies (about a third of female babies get it). It is more common in babies who are heavier at birth and in babies who are fed milk powder substitute or a mixed diet.

The rash usually appears on the baby's face, chest, arms, and legs. It may be concentrated on only one area of the body or it may cover much of the child's skin, although it usually does not affect the palms or soles of the feet.

Erythema toxicum neonatorum most commonly presents with a blotchy, evanescent, macular erythema, often on the face or trunk.

Diagnostic Evaluation

Erythema toxicum is usually diagnosed on the History collection and physical examination. It is sometimes confused with other benign conditions, such as **milia**, **miliaria**, or **baby acne**. It is sometimes also confused with serious infections, such as **herpes**. If the diagnosis is not clear, lab tests are sometimes required.

Management

The eruption is transient and self-limiting, no treatment is indicated.

HYPOTHERMIA

Introduction

Newborn baby, infants, and young children are more common to develop hypothermia because they have a larger surface area compared to body weight so they can lose body heat faster than older children and adults. Newborn baby is a homoeothermic, but his ability to stay warm may easily be overwhelmed by extremes of environmental temperatures. Neonatal hypothermia often due to lack of attention by health care providers continues to be a very important cause of neonatal deaths.

Definition

A newborn is more prone to develop hypothermia because of large surface area per unit of body weight. A low birth weight baby has decreased thermal insulation due to less subcutaneous fat and reduced amount of brown fat. Brown fat is the site of heat production.

It is localized around the adrenal glands, kidneys, nape of neck, inter scapular area and axillary region. Metabolism of brown fat results in heat production. Blood flowing through the brown fat becomes warm and through circulation transfers heat to other parts of the body. This mechanism of heat production is called nonshivering thermogenesis.

Types of Hypothermia

According to WHO temperature values for hypothermia levels in infants:

- Cold stress or mild hypothermia: 36 to 36.4 °C (96.8–97.5 °F)
- Moderate hypothermia: 32 to 35.9 °C (89.6 to 96.6 °F)
- Severe hypothermia: < 32 °C (89.6 °F)

Causes

Hypothermia may be caused by environmental factors, disorders that impair thermoregulation
- Sepsis [Neonatal Sepsis]
- Intracranial hemorrhage
- Drug withdrawal [Prenatal Drug Exposure].

Risk factors for hypothermia include:
- Maternal hypertension
- Cesarean delivery (Cesarean Delivery)
- Low Apgar scores (Neonatal Assessment).

Mechanism of Thermoregulation

Newborn baby loses body heat by such as:
- *Evaporation* particularly soon after birth (due to evaporation of amniotic fluid from skin surface), conduction (by coming in contact with cold objects-cloth, tray, etc.)
- *Convection* (by air currents in which cold air replaces warm air around baby-open windows, fans)
- *Radiation* (to colder solid objects in vicinity-walls)
- *Conduction:* The process of heat gain is by conduction
- *Convection and radiation* in addition to nonshivering thermogenesis.

Signs and Symptoms

- An accurate axillary (armpit) or rectal temperature below 36.4 °C (97.5 °F)
- A weak cry
- Low energy level
- Lethargic
- Reddish and cold skin
- Cool feeling of extremities and abdomen
- Poor feeding
- Hypoglycemia (low blood sugar)
- Hypoxia (low levels of blood oxygen) or apneic (absence of breathing) episodes
- Heart arrhythmias.

Chronic hypothermia symptoms of:
- Weight loss
- No weight gains
- Failure to thrive.

Temperature Monitoring Technique

Advice the nurses to use the low reading thermometer which can record temperature as low as 30 °C should be used in the newborn.

Axillary Temperature

It is as good as rectal and probably safer (less risk of injury or infection). It is recorded by placing the bulb of thermometer against the roof of dry axilla, free from moisture. Baby's arm is held close to the body to keep thermometer in place. The temperature is read after three minutes.

Rectal Temperature

Advice the nurse does not use this method for routine monitoring. However, it is the best guide for core temperature in cold (hypothermic) sick neonates. It is recorded by inserting the greased bulb of the thermometer backwards and downwards to a depth of 3 cm in a term baby (2 cm in a preterm baby). Keep thermometer in place at least for 2 minutes.

Rectal temperature is not recorded as a standard procedure in neonate. Record rectal temperature only for sick hypothermic neonates.

Skin Temperature

Skin temperature is recorded by a thermister. The probe of the thermister is attached to the skin over upper right abdomen. The thermister senses the skin temperature and displays it on the panel.

The Concept of 'Warm Chain'

Hypothermic newborn baby must be kept under the warm place at the time of birth (home or hospital) and during transportation for special care either from home to hospital or within the hospital. Satisfactory control demands both prevention of heat loss and promotion of heat gain. The 'warm chain' is a set of ten interlinked procedures carried out at birth and later, which will minimize the likelihood of hypothermia in all newborns.

- Warm delivery room (> 25 °C)
- Warm resuscitation
- Immediate drying
- Skin-to-skin contact between baby and mother
- Breastfeeding
- Bathing and weighing postponed
- Appropriate clothing and bedding
- Mother and baby together
- Warm transportation
- Training/awareness of health care providers.

Management

Hypothermia baby is treated by rewarming in an incubator or under a radiant warmer. The neonate should be monitored and treated as needed for hypoglycemia, hypoxemia, and apnea. Underlying conditions, such as sepsis, drug withdrawal, or intracranial hemorrhage require specific treatment.

- Rewarming in an incubator or under a radiant warmer
- Kangaroo mother care.

A hypothermic baby has to be rewarmed as quickly as possible. The method selected will depend on the severity of hypothermia and availability of staff and equipment.

The methods of controlling the hypothermia include:

- Skin-to-skin contact
- Warm room or bed

- Use the 200 watt bulb
- Radiant heater or an incubator
- Infection should be suspected if hypothermia persists despite above measures
- Monitor axillary temperature every half an hour till it reaches 36.5 °C, then hourly for next 4 hours, 2 hourly for 12 hours thereafter and 3 hourly as a routine.
- Moderate hypothermia (> 32 to < 36 °C) Skin-to-skin contact should be in a warm room and warm bed. Warmer/incubator may be used, if available. Continue rewarming till temperature reaches normal range. Monitor every 15–30 minutes.

Temperature maintenance during transport:

- Always stabilize the baby's temperature before transport.
- Record temperature before transport and take remedial measures. If temperature cannot be documented, use touch to judge temperature. Hands and feet should be as warm as abdomen.
- Carry the baby close to the chest of mother.
- Cover head, legs and hands. Avoid undressing the infant for cleaning, weighing or examination. Postpone these until baby is warm.
- Thermocol box with pre warmed linen or plastic bubble sheet or silver swaddler may be used during transport.
- Water filled mattress with thermostat to control temperature may be used for transport, if available.

Preventive Measures

- Hypothermia can be prevented by immediately drying and then swaddling the neonate (including the head) in a warm blanket to prevent evaporative, conductive, and convective losses.
- Preterm very-low-birth-weight infants also benefit from a polyethylene occlusive wrapping at the time of delivery.
- A neonate exposed for resuscitation or observation should be placed under a radiant warmer to prevent radiant losses.
- Sick neonates should be maintained in a neutral thermal environment to minimize the metabolic rate.
- The proper incubator temperature varies depending on the neonate's birth weight and postnatal age, and humidity in the incubator.
- Alternatively, heating can be adjusted with a servomechanism set to maintain skin temperature at 36.5° C.

NEONATAL CONVULSION

Introduction

Neonatal seizures otherwise known as neonatal convulsions, Epileptic, fits. It is occurring from birth to the end of the neonatal period. The neonatal period is the most vulnerable of all periods of life for developing seizures, particularly in the first 1–2 days to the first week from birth.

They may be short-lived events lasting for a few days only. However, they often signify serious malfunction of or damage to the immature brain and constitute a neurological emergency demanding urgent diagnosis and management.

Definition

A seizure is a paroxysmal behavior caused by hypersynchronous discharge of a group of neurons. Neonatal seizures are the most common overt manifestation of neurological dysfunction in the newborn.

Neonatal seizures defined as an abnormal electrical discharge in the CNS of neonates and usually manifest as stereotyped muscular activity or autonomic changes.

Causes

- Hypoxic ischemic encephalopathy
- Brain damage due to prenatal distress
- Malformations of cortical development
- Intracranial hemorrhage and infarction
- Stroke and prenatal
- Neonatal infections are common
- Acute metabolic disturbances, such as electrolyte and glucose abnormalities have been minimized because of improved neonatal intensive care and awareness of nutritional hazards
- Inborn errors of metabolism such as urea cycle disorders are rare
- In most cases, the neonate may present with a combination of different neurological disturbances, each of which can cause seizures.

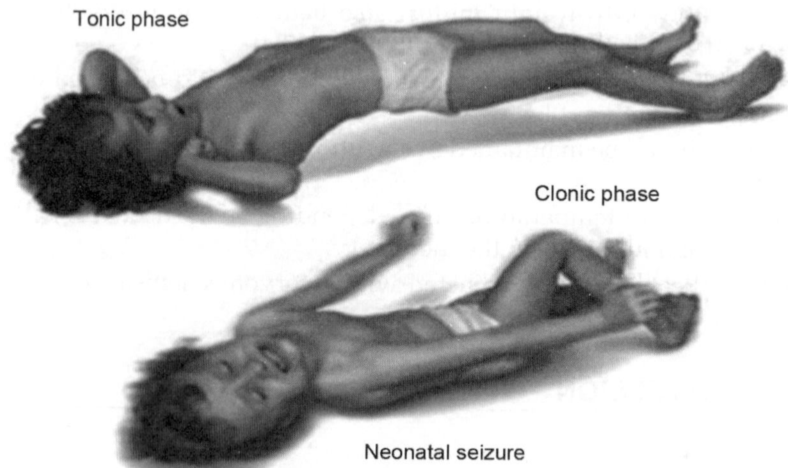

Fig. 2.28: Types of neonatal seizure or convulsion

Neonatal Seizure Classification

Subtle Seizures

Subtle seizures are far more common than other types of neonatal seizures. They are described as *subtle* **because the clinical manifestations are frequently overlooked.**

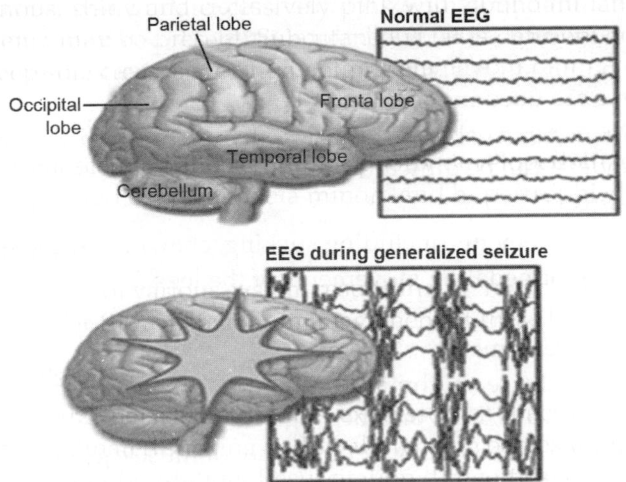

Fig. 2.29: Anatomical view of normal and seizure brain

These include the following:

- *Ocular movements,* which range from random and roving eye movements to sustained conjugate tonic deviation with or without jerking. Eyelid blinking or fluttering, eyes rolling up, eye opening, fixation of a gaze or nystagmus may occur alone or with other ictal manifestations.
- *Oral–buccal–lingual movements* (sucking, smocking, chewing and tongue protrusions).
- *Progression movements* (rowing, swimming, pedalling, bicycling, thrashing or struggling movements).
- *Complex purposeless movements* (sudden arousal with episodic limb hyperactivity and crying.

Motor Seizures

- *Clonic seizures:* These movements most commonly are associated with electrographic seizures. They often involve one extremity or one side of the body. The rhythm of the clonic movements is usually slow, at 1 to 3 movements per second.
- *Tonic seizures:* These may involve one extremity or the whole body. Focal tonic seizures involving 1 extremity often are associated with electrographic seizures.
- *Generalized tonic seizures:* It is often manifesting with tonic extension of the upper and lower limbs and also may involve the axial musculature in an opisthotonic fashion. Generalized tonic seizures mimic decorticate posturing; the majority are not associated with electrographic seizures.
- *Myoclonic seizures:* These may occur focally in one extremity or in several body parts (in which case they are described as multifocal myoclonic seizures). Focal and multifocal

myoclonic seizures typically are not associated with electrographic correlates. Generalized Myoclonic jerks are possibly the clinical equivalent of infantile spasms.

Signs and Symptoms

Neonatal seizures are usually focal and may be difficult to recognize. Common manifestations include migratory clonic jerks of extremities, alternating hemiseizures, and primitive subcortical seizures (which cause respiratory arrest, chewing movements, persistent eye deviations or nystagmoid movements, and episodic changes in muscle tone). Generalized tonic-clonic seizures are uncommon.

Neonatal seizures occur in babies who are less than 28 days old. Seizures in a newborn are often short and subtle; it can be difficult to tell whether a baby is actually having a seizure.

Seizures in newborns

- Repetitive facial movements, including sucking, chewing, or eye movements
- Unusual bicycling or pedaling movements of the legs
- Staring
- Apnea (stopping breathing)
- *Clonic seizures:* Which are rhythmic jerking movements that may involve the muscles of the face, tongue, arms, legs, or other regions
- *Tonic seizures:* Which are stiffening or tightening or muscle groups; the head or eyes may turn to one side, or the baby may bend or stretch one or more arms or legs
- *Myoclonic seizures:* Which are quick, single jerks involving one arm or leg or the whole body.

Duration of neonatal seizures

The duration of neonatal seizures is usually brief (10 s to 1–2 min) and repetitive with a median of 8 min in between each seizure. Longer seizures and status epilepticus develop more readily at this age, but convulsive neonatal status epilepticus is not as severe as that of older infants and children.

Diagnostic Procedures

- EEG
- Laboratory testing [e.g. serum glucose, electrolytes]
- CSF analysis
- Urine and blood cultures
- Usually cranial imaging.

MRI or CT is done when infants are stable: Cranial CT can detect intracranial bleeding and some brain malformations. MRI shows malformations more clearly and can detect ischemic tissue within a few hours of onset. Magnetic resonance spectroscopy may help determine the extent of an ischemic injury or identify build-up of certain neurotransmitters associated with an underlying metabolic disorder.

Pathology tests

Initial investigations recommended to determine cause include:

- Blood glucose level (BGL)
- Serum electrolytes including calcium magnesium

- Serum ammonia
- Full blood count
- Blood cultures
- Arterial blood gas
- Serum amino acids
- Urine amino acids and organic acids
- Thrombophilia screen (after stroke)
- Lumbar puncture.

Management

Neonatal seizures require urgent treatment to prevent brain injury. Give anticonvulsant medication only after adequate ventilation and perfusion have been established and the blood glucose concentration has been measured.

- **Ensure adequate ventilation and perfusion.**
- **Correct metabolic disturbances.**

Hypoglycemia (10% glucose in water) 2 ml/kg IV (0.2 g/kg) as bolus. Follow with continuous infusion at up to 8 mg/kg/min.

Hypocalcemia (calcium gluconate 10%) 100 mg/kg IV over 1 to 3 minutes (Note: Monitor cardiac rhythm for bradycardia) Follow with maintenance of 500 mg/kg/24 hrs IV or PO.

Hypomagnesemia (magnesium sulfate) 25–250 mg/kg/dose IV/IM.

Begin Anticonvulsant Therapy

- *Phenobarbital:* 20 mg/kg IV. If necessary, additional 10–20 mg/kg IV in 10 mg/kg aliquots (Note: monitor blood pressure and respiration) Maintenance: 4–6 mg/kg/24 hrs IV/PO If 40 mg/kg of Phenobarbital is not effective, proceed to Lorazepam and obtain consult with the Neurology Service for advice regarding seizure treatment. (While the literature supports the use of Phenytoin as a second line agent, our experience is that Lorazepam is more effective in the acute setting.)
- *Lorazepam:* 0.05 mg/kg to 0.10 mg/kg IV in 0.05 mg/kg increments over several minutes. (Note: Monitor closely for respiratory depression.) The half-life in asphyxiated newborns is ~40 hours; duration of action 6–24 hours.
- *Phenytoin:* 20 mg/kg IV (diluted in 0.9% NaCl) (Maximal rate: 1 mg/kg/min monitor cardiac rate and rhythm). Maintenance 5–10 mg/kg/24h IV (Phenytoin is VERY poorly absorbed PO in the newborn). Fourth line anticonvulsants include Paraldehyde. If you must proceed to this stage, then Neurology should have been consulted for guidance with dosage and other management issues.

Nursing Management

A family centered model of care with early Social Worker involvement provides support:

- Early and ongoing communication is established with parent(s) to convey:
  - Information regarding baby's condition as soon as possible (information may have to be repeated as stress levels may affect information reception and retention).
  - Anticipated management plan and prognosis. This information should be delivered with honesty and sensitivity by the treating team. If the baby is not expected to survive, the parents should have an understanding of this process.

- Early communication with the Obstetric team to convey information regarding the baby's assessment, management plan and prognosis is necessary to facilitate consistent counseling for parents.
- Document all communication regarding the management plan, prognosis and parental decisions to enable consistency of information transfer.
- Specialist (Neonatologist/Pediatric Neurologist) follow-up for babies discharged on anticonvulsant drugs
- General Pediatrician follow-up for all babies, in their local area
- Multidisciplinary follow-up to identify physical or cognitive deficit and provide timely neurorehabilitation intervention.

Prognosis

Prognosis depends on the etiology. About 50% of neonates with seizures due to hypoxia-ischemia develop normally. Most neonates with seizures due to subarachnoid hemorrhage, hypocalcemia, or hyponatremia do well. Those with severe intraventricular hemorrhage have a high morbidity rate. For idiopathic seizures or seizures due to malformations, earlier onset is associated with worse neurodevelopmental outcomes.

BIRTH INJURY

Introduction

Injuries to the infant that result from mechanical forces (i.e. compression, traction) during the birth process are categorized as birth trauma. Factors responsible for mechanical injury may coexist with hypoxic-ischemic insult; one may predispose the infant to the other.

Lesions that are predominantly hypoxic in origin are not discussed in this article. Significant birth injury accounts for fewer than 2% of neonatal deaths and stillbirths in the United States; it still occurs occasionally and unavoidably, with an average of 6–8 injuries per 1000 live births. In general, larger infants are more susceptible to birth trauma. Higher rates are reported for infants who weigh more than 4500 g.

Most birth traumas are self-limiting and have a favorable outcome. Nearly one half are potentially avoidable with recognition and anticipation of obstetric risk factors. Infant outcome is the product of multiple factors. Separating the effects of a hypoxic-ischemic insult from those of traumatic birth injury is difficult.

Risk factors include large-for-date infants, especially infants who weigh more than 4500 g; instrumental deliveries, especially forceps (midcavity) or vacuum; vaginal breech delivery; and abnormal or excessive traction during delivery.

Mortality/Morbidity

Birth injuries account for fewer than 2% of neonatal deaths. From 1970–1985, rates of infant mortality due to birth trauma fell from 64.2 to 7.5 deaths per 100,000 live births, a remarkable decline of 88%. This decrease reflects, in part, the technologic advancements that allow today's obstetrician to recognize birth trauma risk factors using ultrasonography and fetal monitoring prior to attempting vaginal delivery. The use of potentially injurious instrumentation, such as midforceps rotation and vacuum delivery, has also declined. The accepted alternative is a cesarean delivery.

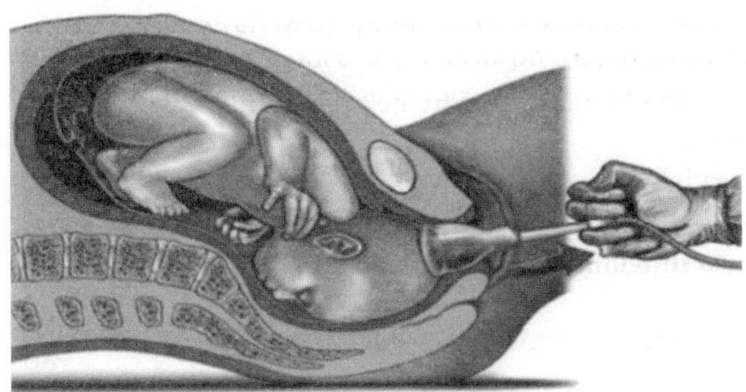
Fig. 2.30: Vacuum delivery

Causes

The birth process is a blend of compression, contractions, torques, and traction. When fetal size, presentation, or neurologic immaturity complicates this event, such intrapartum forces may lead to tissue damage, edemas, hemorrhages, or fracture in the neonate. The use of obstetric instrumentation may further amplify the effects of such forces or may induce injury alone. Under certain conditions, cesarean delivery can be an acceptable alternative but does not guarantee an injury-free birth.

Factors predisposing to injury include the following:

- Primigravida
- Cephalopelvic disproportion, small maternal stature, maternal pelvic anomalies
- Prolonged or rapid labor
- Deep transverse arrest of descent of presenting part of the fetus
- Oligohydramnios
- Abnormal presentation (breech)

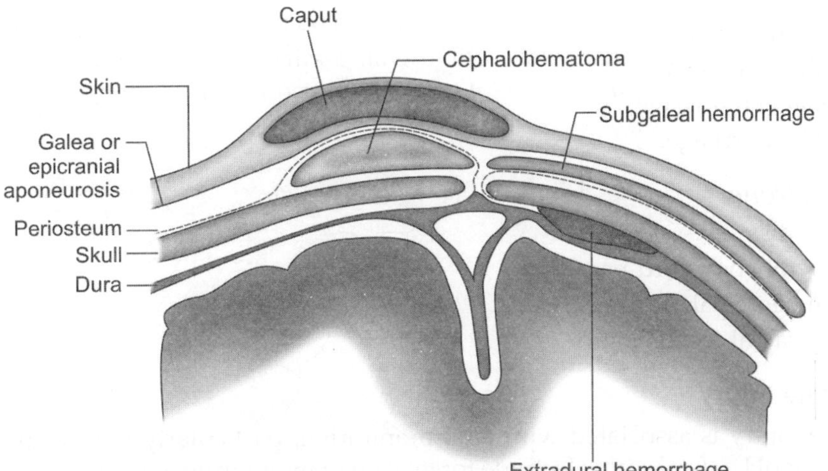

Fig. 2.31: Location of injury in soft tissue planes on the scalp and head

- Use of midcavity forceps or vacuum extraction
- Versions and extractions
- Very low birth weight infant or extreme prematurity
- Fetal macrosomia
- Large fetal head
- Fetal anomalies.

Injuries with favorable long-term prognosis

- Abrasions
- Erythema petechiae
- Ecchymosis
- Lacerations
- Subcutaneous fat necrosis.

Skull

- Caput succedaneum
- Cephalohematoma
- Linear fractures.

Face

- Subconjunctival hemorrhage
- Retinal hemorrhage.

Musculoskeletal Injuries

- Clavicular fractures
- Fractures of long bones
- Sternocleidomastoid injury.

Intra-abdominal Injuries

- Liver hematoma
- Splenic hematoma
- Adrenal hemorrhage
- Renal hemorrhage.

Peripheral Nerve

- Facial palsy
- Unilateral vocal cord paralysis
- Radial nerve palsy
- Lumbosacral plexus injury.

Soft Tissue Injury

Soft tissue injury is associated with fetal monitoring, particularly with fetal scalp blood sampling for pH or fetal scalp electrode for fetal heart monitoring, which has a low incidence of hemorrhage, infection, or abscess at the site of sampling.

Cephalohematoma

Cephalohematoma is a subperiosteal collection of blood secondary to rupture of blood vessels between the skull and the periosteum; suture lines delineate its extent. Most commonly parietal, cephalohematoma may occasionally be observed over the occipital bone.

The extent of hemorrhage may be severe enough to cause anemia and hypotension, although this is uncommon. The resolving hematoma predisposes to hyperbilirubinemia. Rarely, cephalohematoma may be a focus of infection that leads to meningitis or osteomyelitis. Linear skull fractures may underlie a cephalohematoma (5–20% of cephalohematomas). Resolution occurs over weeks, occasionally with residual calcification.

No laboratory studies are usually necessary. Skull radiography or CT scanning is performed if neurologic symptoms are present. Usually, management solely consists of observation. Transfusion for anemia, hypovolemia, or both is necessary if blood accumulation is significant. Aspiration is not required for resolution and is likely to increase the risk of infection. Hyperbilirubinemia occurs following the breakdown of the RBCs within the hematoma. This type of hyperbilirubinemia occurs later than classic physiologic hyperbilirubinemia. The presence of a bleeding disorder should be considered. Skull radiography or CT scanning is also performed if concomitant depressed skull fracture is a possibility.

Subgaleal Hematoma

Subgaleal hematoma is bleeding in the potential space between the skull periosteum and the scalp galea aponeurosis. Ninety percent of cases result from vacuum applied to the head at delivery. Subgaleal hematoma has a high frequency of occurrence of associated head trauma (40%), such as intracranial hemorrhage or skull fracture. The occurrence of these features does not significantly correlate with the severity of Subgaleal hemorrhage.

The diagnosis is generally a clinical one, with a fluctuant boggy mass developing over the scalp (especially over the occiput). The swelling develops gradually 12 to 72 hours after delivery, although it may be noted immediately after delivery in severe cases. The hematoma spreads across the whole calvaria; its growth is insidious, and subgaleal hematoma may not be recognized for hours. Patients with subgaleal hematoma may present with hemorrhagic shock. The swelling may obscure the fontanelle and cross suture lines (distinguishing it from Cephalohematoma). Watch for significant hyperbilirubinemia. In the absence of shock or intracranial injury, the long-term prognosis is generally good.

Laboratory studies consist of a hematocrit evaluation. Management consists of vigilant observation over days to detect progression and provide therapy for such problems as shock and anemia. Transfusion and phototherapy may be necessary. Investigation for coagulopathy may be indicated.

Caput Succedaneum

Caput succedaneum is a serosanguineous, subcutaneous, extraperiosteal fluid collection with poorly defined margins; it is caused by the pressure of the presenting part against the dilating cervix. Caput succedaneum extends across the midline and over suture lines and is associated with head moulding. Caput succedaneum does not usually cause complications and usually resolves over the first few days. Management consists of observation only.

Abrasions and Lacerations

Abrasions and lacerations sometimes may occur as scalpel cuts during cesarean delivery or during instrumental delivery (i.e. vacuum, forceps). Infection remains a risk, but most uneventfully heal. Management consists of careful cleaning, application of antibiotic ointment, and observation. Bring edges together using Steri-Strips. Lacerations occasionally require suturing.

Subcutaneous Fat Necrosis

Subcutaneous fat necrosis is not usually detected at birth. Irregular, hard, nonpitting, subcutaneous plaques with overlying dusky red-purple discoloration on the extremities, face, trunk, or buttocks may be caused by pressure during delivery. No treatment is necessary. Subcutaneous fat necrosis sometimes calcifies.

Peripheral Nerve Injury

Brachial Plexus Injury

Brachial plexus injury occurs most commonly in large babies, frequently with shoulder dystocia or breech delivery. Incidence for brachial plexus injury is 0.5–2 per 1000 live births. Most cases are Erb palsy; entire brachial plexus involvement occurs in 10% of cases.

Traumatic lesions associated with brachial plexus injury include fractured clavicle (10%), fractured humerus (10%), subluxation of cervical spine (5%), cervical cord injury (5–10%), and facial palsy (10–20%). Erb palsy (C5-C6) is most common and is associated with lack of shoulder motion. The involved extremity lies adducted, prone, and internally rotated. Moro, biceps, and radial reflexes are absent on the affected side. Grasp reflex is usually present. Five percent of patients have an accompanying (ipsilateral) phrenic nerve paresis.

The chest should be examined to rule out associated phrenic nerve injury. Electromyography (EMG) and nerve conduction studies are occasionally useful. Fast spin-echo MRI can be used to evaluate plexus injuries noninvasively in a relatively short time, minimizing the need for general anesthesia. MRI can define meningoceles and may distinguish between intact nerve roots and pseudomeningoceles (indicative of complete avulsion). Carefully performed, intrathecally enhanced CT myelography may show preganglionic disruption, pseudomeningoceles, and partial nerve root avulsion. CT myelography is more invasive and offers few advantages over MRI.

Management consists of prevention of contractures. Immobilize the limb gently across the abdomen for the first week and then start passive range of motion exercises at all joints of the limb. Use supportive wrist splints. Best results for surgical repair appear to be obtained in the first year of life. Several investigators recommend surgical exploration and grafting if no function is present in the upper roots at age 3 months, although the recommendation for early explorations is far from universal. Complications of brachial plexus exploration include infection, poor outcome, and burns from the operating microscope. Patients with root avulsion do not do well. Palliative procedures involving tendon transfers have been of some use. Latissimus dorsi and teres major transfers to the rotator cuff have been advocated for improved shoulder function in Erb palsy. One permanent and 3 transitory axillary nerve palsies have been reported from the procedure.

Cranial Nerve and Spinal Cord Injury

Cranial nerve and spinal cord injuries result from hyperextension, traction, and overstretching with simultaneous rotation; they may range from localized neurapraxia to complete nerve or cord transaction.

Cranial Nerve Injury

Unilateral branches of the facial nerve and vagus nerve, in the form of recurrent laryngeal nerve, are most commonly involved in cranial nerve injuries and result in temporary or permanent paralysis.

Compression by the forceps blade has been implicated in some facial nerve injury, but most facial nerve palsy is unrelated to trauma from obstetrical instrumentation (e.g. forceps). The compression appears to occur as the head passes by the sacrum.

Physical findings for central nerve injuries are asymmetric faces with crying. The mouth is drawn towards the normal side, wrinkles are deeper on the normal side and movement of the forehead and eyelid is unaffected. The paralyzed side is smooth with a swollen appearance, the nasolabial fold is absent, and the corner of the mouth droops. No evidence of trauma is present on the face.

Physical findings for peripheral nerve injuries are asymmetric faces with crying. Sometimes evidence of forceps marks is present. With peripheral nerve branch injury, the paralysis is limited to the forehead, eye, or mouth. The differential diagnosis includes nuclear genesis (Möbius syndrome), congenital absence of the facial muscles, unilateral absence of the orbicularis oris muscle, and intracranial hemorrhage.

Most infants begin to recover in the first week, but full resolution may take several months. Palsy that is due to trauma usually resolves or improves, whereas palsy that persists is often due to absence of the nerve. Management consists of protecting the open eye with patches and synthetic tears (methylcellulose drops) every 4 hours. Consultation with a neurologist and a surgeon should be sought if no improvement is observed in 7–10 days.

Diaphragmatic paralysis secondary to traumatic injury to the cervical nerve roots that supply the phrenic nerve can occur as an isolated finding or in association with brachial plexus injury. The clinical syndrome is variable. The course is biphasic; initially the infant experiences respiratory distress with Tachypnea and blood gases suggestive of hypoventilation (i.e. hypoxemia, hypercapnia, acidosis). Over the next several days, the infant may improve with oxygen and varying degrees of ventilator support. Elevated hemidiaphragm may not be observed in the early stages. Approximately 80% of lesions involve the right side and about 10% are bilateral.

The diagnosis is established by ultrasonography or fluoroscopy of the chest, which reveals the elevated hemidiaphragm with paradoxic movement of the affected side with breathing. The mortality rate for unilateral lesions is approximately 10–15%. Most patients recover in the first 6–12 months. An outcome for bilateral lesions is poorer. The mortality rate approaches 50%, and prolonged ventilatory support may be necessary. Management consists of careful surveillance of respiratory status, and intervention, when appropriate, is critical.

Laryngeal Nerve Injury

Disturbance of laryngeal nerve function may affect swallowing and breathing. Laryngeal nerve injury appears to result from an intrauterine posture in which the head is rotated and flexed laterally. During delivery, similar head movement (when marked) may injure the laryngeal nerve, accounting for approximately 10% of cases of vocal cord paralysis attributed to birth trauma. The infant presents with a hoarse cry or respiratory stridor, caused most often by unilateral laryngeal nerve paralysis. Swallowing may be affected if the superior branch is involved. Bilateral paralysis may be caused by trauma to both laryngeal nerves or, more commonly, by a CNS injury, such as hypoxia or hemorrhage that involves the brainstem. Patients with bilateral paralysis often present with severe respiratory distress or asphyxia.

Direct laryngoscopic examination is necessary to make the diagnosis and to distinguish vocal cord paralysis from other causes of respiratory distress and stridor in the newborn. Differentiate from other rare etiologies, such as cardiovascular or CNS malformations or a meditational tumor.

Paralysis often resolves in 4 to 6 weeks, although recovery may take as long as 6 to 12 months in severe cases. Treatment is symptomatic. Once the neonate is stable, small frequent feeds minimize the risk of aspiration. Infants with bilateral involvement may require gavage feeding and tracheotomy.

Spinal Cord Injury

Spinal cord injury incurred during delivery results from excessive traction or rotation. Traction is more important in breech deliveries (minority of cases), and torsion is more significant in vertex deliveries. True incidence is difficult to determine. The lower cervical and upper thoracic region for breech delivery and the upper and midcervical region for vertex delivery are the major sites of injury.

Major neuropathologic changes consist of acute lesions, which are hemorrhages, especially epidural, intraspinal, and edema. Hemorrhagic lesions are associated with varying degrees of stretching, laceration, and disruption or total transaction. Occasionally, the dura may be torn, and rarely, the vertebral fractures or dislocations may be observed.

The clinical presentation is stillbirth or rapid neonatal death with failure to establish adequate respiratory function, especially in cases involving the upper cervical cord or lower brainstem. Severe respiratory failure may be obscured by mechanical ventilation and may cause ethical issues later. The infant may survive with weakness and hypotonia, and the true etiology may not be recognized. A neuromuscular disorder or transient hypoxic ischemic encephalopathy may be considered. Most infants later develop spasticity that may be mistaken for cerebral palsy.

Prevention is the most important aspect of medical care. Obstetric management of breech deliveries, instrumental deliveries, and pharmacologic augmentation of labor must be appropriate. Occasionally, injury may be sustained *in utero*.

The diagnosis is made using MRI or CT myelography. Little evidence indicates that laminectomy or decompression has anything to offer. A potential role for methylprednisolone is recognized. Supportive therapy is important.

Bone Injury

Fractures are most often observed following breech delivery, shoulder dystopia, or both in infants with excessive birth weights.

Clavicular Fracture

The clavicle is the most frequently fractured bone in the neonate during birth; this is most often an unpredictable, unavoidable complication of normal birth. Some correlation with birth weight, midforceps delivery, and shoulder dystocia is recognized. The infant may present with pseudoparalysis. Examination may reveal crepitus, palpable bony irregularity, and sternocleidomastoid muscle spasm. Radiographic studies confirm the fracture. Healing usually occurs in 7 to 10 days. In order to decrease pain, arm motion may be limited by pinning the infant's sleeve to the shirt. Assess other associated injury to the spine, brachial plexus, or humerus.

Long Bone Fracture

Loss of spontaneous arm or leg movement is an early sign of long bone fracture, followed by swelling and pain on passive movement. The obstetrician may feel or hear a snap at the time of delivery. Radiographic studies of the limb confirm the diagnosis.

Femoral and humeral shaft fractures are treated with splinting. Closed reduction and casting is necessary only when displaced. Watch for evidence of radial nerve injury with humeral fracture. Callus formation occurs, and complete recovery is expected in 2 to 4 weeks. In 8 to 10 days, the callus formation is sufficient to discontinue immobilization. Orthopedic consultation is recommended. Radiographic studies distinguish this condition from septic arthritis.

Epiphysial Displacement

Separation of humeral or femoral epiphysis occurs through the hypertrophied layer of cartilage cells in the epiphysis. The diagnosis is clinically based on swelling around the shoulder, crepitus, and pain when the shoulder is moved. Motion is painful, and the arm lies limp by the side. Because the proximal humeral epiphysis is not ossified at birth, it is not visible on radiography. Callus appears in 8 to 10 days and is visible on radiography. Management consists of immobilizing the arm for 8 to 10 days. Fracture of the distal epiphysis is more likely to have a significant residual deformity than is fracture of the proximal humeral epiphysis.

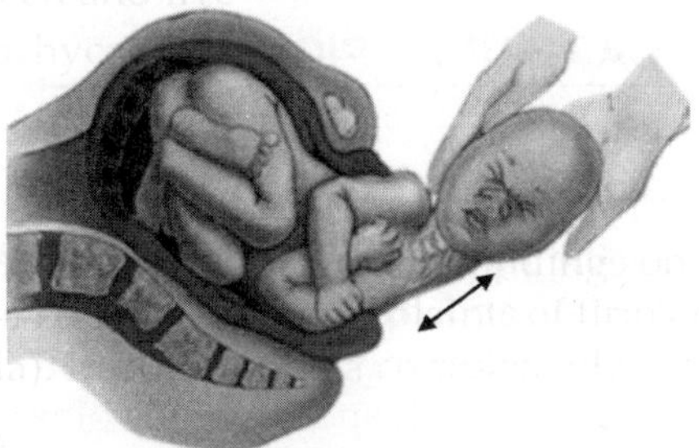

Fig. 2.32: Shoulder dystocia

Intra-abdominal Injury

Intra-abdominal injury is relatively uncommon and can sometimes be overlooked as a cause of death in the newborn. Hemorrhage is the most serious acute complication, and the liver is the most commonly damaged internal organ.

Signs and Symptoms of Intraperitoneal Bleed

Bleeding may be fulminate or insidious, but patients ultimately present with circulatory collapse. Intra-abdominal bleeding should be considered for every infant who presents with shock, pallor, unexplained anemia, and abdominal distension. Overlying abdominal skin may have bluish discoloration. Radiographic findings are not diagnostic but may suggest free peritoneal fluid. Paracentesis is the procedure of choice.

Hepatic Rupture

The most common lesion is subcapsular hematoma, which increases to 4–5 cm before rupturing. Symptoms of shock may be delayed. Lacerations are less common, often caused by abnormal pull on peritoneal support ligaments or effect of excessive pressure by the costal margin. Infants with hepatomegaly may be at higher risk. Other predisposing factors include prematurity, postmaturity, coagulation disorders, and asphyxia. In cases associated with asphyxia, vigorous resuscitative effort (often by unusual methods) is the culprit. Splenic rupture is at least a fifth as common as liver laceration. Predisposing factors and mechanisms of injury are similar.

Rapid identification and stabilization of the infant are the keys to management, along with assessment of coagulation defect. Blood transfusion is the most urgent initial step. Persistent coagulopathy may be treated with fresh frozen plasma, transfusion of platelets, and other measures. Hepatic rupture has no specific racial predilection and has equal sex distribution. Patients usually present immediately following birth, or rupture becomes obvious within the first few hours or days.

Conclusion

Recognition of trauma necessitates a careful physical and neurologic evaluation of the infant to establish whether additional injuries are present. Occasionally, injury may result from resuscitation. Symmetry of structure and function should be assessed as well as specifics, such as cranial nerve examination, individual joint range of motion, and scalp/skull integrity.

ORGANIZATION OF NEONATAL CARE UNIT (NICU AND PICU)

PEDIATRIC INTENSIVE CARE UNIT (PICU)

Introduction

The practice of pediatric critical care has matured dramatically throughout the past three decades. Knowledge of the pathophysiology of life-threatening processes and the technological capacity to monitor and treat pediatric patients suffering from them has advanced rapidly during this period. Along with the scientific and technical advances has come the evolution of the PICU, in which special needs of critically ill or injured children and their families can be met by pediatric specialists. All critically ill infants and children cared for in hospitals, regardless of the physical setting, are entitled to receive the same quality of care.

History of PICU

In 1985, the American Board of Pediatrics recognized the subspecialty of pediatric critical care medicine and set criteria for subspecialty certification. The American Boards of Medicine,

Surgery, and Anesthesiology gave similar recognition to the subspecialty. In 1990, the Residency Review Committee of the Accreditation Council for Graduate Medical Education completed its first accreditation of pediatric critical care medicine training programs. In 1986, the American Association of Critical Care Nurses developed a certification program for pediatric critical care, and in 1999, a certification program for clinical nurse specialists in pediatric critical care was initiated.

In view of recent developments, the Pediatric Section of the Society of Critical Care Medicine and the Section on Critical Care Medicine and Committee on Hospital Care of the American Academy of Pediatrics believe that the original guidelines for levels of PICU care from 1993 should be updated.

This report represents the consensus of the three aforementioned groups and presents those elements of hospital care that are necessary to provide high-quality pediatric critical care. The concept of level I and level II PICUs as established in the guidelines set forth in 1993 will be continued in this report. Individual states may have PICU guidelines, and it is not the intent of this report to supersede already established state rules, regulations, or guidelines; however, these guidelines represent the consensus report of critical care experts.

Pediatric critical care is ideally provided by a PICU that meets level I specifications. The level I PICU must provide multidisciplinary definitive care for a wide range of complex, progressive, and rapidly changing medical, surgical, and traumatic disorders occurring in pediatric patients of all ages, excluding premature newborns. Most, although not all, level I PICUs should be located in major medical centers or within children's hospitals. It is also recognized that in the appropriate clinical setting and as a result of many forces, including but not limited to the presence of managed care, the insufficient supply of trained pediatric intensivists, and geographic and transport limitations, level II PICUs may be an appropriate alternative to the transfer of all critically ill children to a level I PICU.

Definition

The PICU is the section of the hospital that provides sick children with the highest level of medical care. It differs from other parts of the hospital, like the general medical floors, in that the PICU allows intensive nursing care and monitoring things like heart rate, breathing, and blood pressure.

Purposes

- The provision of specialized care for children with critical illness which may best be provided by concentrating these patients in areas under the supervision of skilled and specially trained team of physicians and nurses.
- The continuing education of health care team members.
- Any child who is seriously ill and needs intensive care and whose medical needs can not be met on the hospital's main medical floors goes to the PICU.
- Kids in the PICU might include those with severe breathing problems from asthma, serious infections, certain heart defects, some complications of diabetes, or those involved in a serious automobile accident or near-drowning.
- Some kids may have been stable enough to initially be cared for on the hospitals main medical floor, but may be transferred to the PICU if they become more acutely ill. Following major surgery, many children are cared for in the PICU for several days.

- How long kids will be in the PICU depends on their condition—some might stay a single day; others might need to stay for weeks or even months. As always, ask the doctor or nurse caring for your child if you have questions.

IMPORTANCE OF PICU

Introduction

The progress in medical science, it is now possible to offer to children with complex life-threatening illness and unstable vital system function, therapeutic measures to support and stabilize vital functions, and sustains life till the underlying primary illness is treated.

PICU is an integral part of the health care services being offered in a particular set-up, an assessment of its need should primarily be based on the existing patient load and type of illness cared. Development of separate PICU is only a logical corollary in this process, as physiological and psychological needs and disease pattern of young infants and children are distinct from adults.

Pediatric Intensive Care Unit

- To provide the advanced care in an organized manner.
- To monitor the seriously ill patients for early detection of life-threatening events and for assessment of response to therapeutic measures.
- To provide life sustaining therapeutic measures and intensive continuous monitoring to defect and correct life-threatening events.
- To reduce pediatric mortality and morbidity.

Pediatric Patients Need Intensive Care

Common Conditions

- Respiratory conditions
  - Upper airway obstruction
  - Abnormal respiratory rate (or) pattern
  - Patient unable to protect on airway (post-trauma, unconsciousness)
  - Severe pulmonary disease (pneumonia, acute asthma, bronchiolitis)
  - Respiratory paralysis.
- Cardiovascular conditions
  - Myocarditis/myocardial failure
  - Unstable arrhythmias.
- Shock
  - Hypovolemic shock
    - Septic shock
    - Severe burns.
- Central nerves system
  - Increased intracranial pressure
  - Seizures
  - Infections (meningitis, encephalitis)

- Hypoxic-ischemic encephalopathy
- Head injury
- Coma

- Major trauma/major surgery
- Serious poisoning
  - Organophosphates
  - Barbiturates
  - Iron poisoning
  - Aluminum phosphate.
- Bites and envenomations
  - Snakebites
  - Scorpion bites.
- Acute hepatic failure
  - Acute fulminate hepatitis
  - Reye's syndrome.
- Acute renal failure
  - Hemolytic–uremic syndrome
  - Acute tubular necrosis.

PRACTICE AND STANDARDS OF PICU

Intensive Care for Children

The PICU addresses a diverse range of serious medical and surgical concerns. Some of the most common conditions seen in the PICU are:

- Heart disease
- Postsurgical complications
- Respiratory failure
- Serious infection
- Severe head injury
- Trauma

The PICU Team

The pediatric intensive care team members are skilled in the care of critically ill children. They promote healing and recovery using the most-advanced treatments possible. PICU team members include:

- Children's Memorial specialists, board certified in critical care and pediatrics
- Additional Children's Memorial specialists including pediatric cardiologists, pediatric surgeons, pediatric gastroenterologists and others as needed
- Children's Memorial pediatric specialists, on site 24 hours every day
- CDH registered nurses with pediatric advanced life support certification
- Child life specialists
- Pediatric nutritionists

- Pediatric social workers
- Patient care technicians.

Nursing Staff

- **General organization:** The PICU nursing staff consists of RNs and appropriate ancillary personnel. Nursing assignments and acuity decisions are made by the nursing staff. If parents make a request to you that relates to nursing staffing, please inform the charge nurse.
- **Continuing education of the nursing staff:** An on-going program of education in pediatric intensive care nursing has been the responsibility of the nursing service. In addition, appropriate seminars discussing subjects of pertinence in pediatric intensive care have been and will continue to be organized with physician participation. This will be an effort to maintain and further the critical care skills of nursing personnel in the PICU.

Respiratory Care

The personnel of PICU will work jointly with the Director of Respiratory Therapy so that optimum respiratory care may be provided. The respiratory therapy staffs are responsible for setting up and maintaining the ventilators, delivering respiratory treatments, and assisting with patient care that involves respiratory care (i.e. suctioning). Pediatric Respiratory Therapists rotate through the PICU, DNCC, and the floors.

Physicians

A PL-3 and PL-2 are assigned to the PICU, and they with the Pediatric Critical Care staff and other services will care for all pediatric patients. The PICU is available to all pediatric patients regardless of the service primarily responsible for the child.

Admission and Discharge

Any child requiring pediatric intensive care must be admitted to PICU. This is accomplished by calling the PICU attending physician.

If a bed is available the patient may be admitted. If the PICU is full, and all beds are occupied, then the physician wishing to admit a patient to the PICU must contact the PICU attending.

The critical care attending will then make the disposition regarding discharge of another patient from the PICU after appropriate consultation with the patient's primary service and the PICU nursing staff, or other appropriate disposition.

There are policies in place regarding triage of surgical and medical patients that are used when beds or nurses are scarce. These policies are necessary to insure optimum care for all children who require pediatric intensive care.

Type of Children Admitted to the PICU

- Medical patients from the ED (emergency department)
- The ED will contact the PICU attending. The intensivist is the attending of record medical patients from the floor.
- The floor attending or resident will contact the PICU attending who will decide about transfer, then call the PICU charge RN and resident.

- The intensivist is the attending of record medical patients transported in for outside institutions.
- Cardiac problem child may be admitted from emergency department.
- Immediate need of post- or preoperative pediatric cardiac surgery, with medical consultation.
- Orthopedic problem child.

Routine Procedures

There are preprinted orders for general PICU admitions, CV surgery admitions (Track A and general), and extracorporeal membrane oxygenation (ECMO) admitions. If you use a preprinted order and want to write more things, use regular order paper. There are also preprinted orders for sedation drips, muscle relaxant drips, cardiac patient ventilator weaning. Others are being added on an ongoing basis.

Admitting orders to the PICU should include the following categories:

- Diagnosis
- Attending physician
- Condition
- Vital sign frequency (routine is q2). If you want things documented more frequently, be specific. (hourly is reasonable for sick patients)
- Allergies
- Nursing—specific nursing requirements
- Dressing changes
- Chest tube orders
- CVP/A-line orders
- Nasogastric
- Foley catheter
- Diet/NPO
- IVF (type/rate)
- Medicines
- Drips written in amount/kg/minute (vasoactive) or amount/kg/hour (sedation/narcotic); consult with PICU MD or nursing staff about concentration to order
- Labs—labs wanted on admission as well as lab schedule if needed
- Ventilator settings along with weaning parameters
- Call HO orders. It is best to write these and also to speak with the RN caring for the patient about specific issues you are worried about, to ensure accurate communication.
- There are special order sheets for muscle relaxants, sedation, and PCA. If you are unfamiliar with them, ask the intensivist or the nurse to assist in using them.
- Postoperative cardiac patients and ECMO patients have preprinted orders. These will be completed by the intensivist or the pediatric resident with attending supervision.

Verbal Orders

The verbal orders may be taken only when necessary. These must be written and signed as soon as possible after having been executed.

EMERGENCY PROCEDURES

In the absence of a physician, if a child's condition changes while waiting for the physician caring for the child, the nurse may do the following where appropriate:

- Draw blood gases, electrolytes and hematocrit, and send these to the lab for stat results.
- Call for chest X-ray or other appropriate X-ray.
- Administer oxygen.
- Institute cardiopulmonary resuscitation with Ambu bag and external cardiac massage.
- The PICU attending should be called immediately for any sudden, unexplained change in a patient's condition. In the event of a cardiorespiratory or respiratory arrest where the PICU attending is not immediately available, the Pediatric Code 99 team may be called.
- If an anesthesiologist is needed emergently, the pediatric on call anesthesiology number should be paged. At the present time, the pediatric anesthesiologists are in house 24 hours/day.

Pediatric Critical Care

The critical care specialists in the Children's Memorial at CDH program provide intensive and compassionate care to postsurgical, critically ill or injured children. Recognized by the Illinois Department of Public Health as a Pediatric Critical Care Center, the PICU at CDH offers state-of-the-art technology and equipment in a child-friendly environment. The six-beded, family-centered unit has private patient rooms with sleeping accommodations for parents. For your child's.

Pediatric Resuscitation Course

Pediatric resuscitation courses such as Pediatric Advanced Life Support (PALS) will be offered several times per year. All pediatric nurses are required to complete this course.

Discharge/Transfer Procedures

Decisions regarding transfer of patients from the PICU to the ward will be made in conjunction with the primary service and RN staff. Confirmation of the availability of a ward bed as well as an accepting physician must be made prior to transfer. The PICU attending will contact the receiving attending for medical patients, the residents should contact the receiving resident to give report.

For surgical patients, the surgery service will write transfer orders. For medical patients, the PICU residents write transfer orders. On occasion, the PICU residents can help the flow of patients by writing transfer orders on surgical patients (confirm with surgical service first).

On medical patients, the PICU resident should write a transfer summary prior to transfer to the floor. Any patient discharged from the PICU (including Shriner's patients going back to Shriner's) need a dictated summary.

PHYSICAL SET-UP OF PEDIATRIC INTENSIVE CARE UNIT

Location

The PICU should be located adjacent to (or) within direct access to pediatric emergency room, children wards, radiology department and operating and recovery rooms. It is also desirable for critical units to be close to each other. All these units should be preferably on same floor.

Size

The ideal size of a PICU is not known there are no clear standards (or) methods to determine its size. It is felt that a multi speciality hospital requires about 5% of beds for critical care, out of which 1% should be in ICU.

A unit smaller than risks insufficiency and units large than 16 beds may be difficult to manage. In our set-up a PICU with 6-8 bed may be considered optimum from all considerations. A survey showed that an average PICU in Britain has 6 beds.

Space

The patient care area should have approximately 20 m^2 space available per patient with 3-3.5 meters separating each patient. There must be provision for enough floor space around the hood end of the bed to assemble necessary personnel and equipment for resuscitation. In addition, space should be provided for nursing and clerical activity, equipment, store, doctors duty rooms, nurses locker room, conference room, toilets, offices of nursing supervisor and consultant physician, laboratory, storage area for janitorial supplies, linen and patients belonging and a clean and soiled workroom. An intermediate care area to allow for continuing care of patients, and waiting room for families should also be provided immediately adjacent to the unit.

The total area needed is about three times the size needed for bed alone.

Floor Plan

Floor plan of an optimum sized PICU is shown in Figure 2.33.

Design/Layout

Design/layout of central importance in the design of patient care area is a provision for adequacy of observation and easy access to the patients. A central station for observation, record keeping and charting, preparation of medications and other functions is therefore necessary.

There may be of two kind of design

1. Open ward design: For 4–6 patients
2. Closed room design: Each room serving 1–2 patients.

However in our set-up with shortage of nurses open ward design is suitable. Each room should have adequate shelf space (cabinet) and gowning and handwashing facility. Presence of glass covered windows is helpful in providing adequate light and for patients to maintain day-night orientation. Attractive colorful designs on walls and ceiling may be helpful.

Each bed must be provided with appropriate electrical sockets, illumination, suction, air and oxygen supply outlets. Appropriate air conditioning, heating, ventilation, plumbing and fire safety features must be observed.

Electrical Equipment

- **Electric outlets:** Sixteen to eighteen per bed, for spot light, call bell alarms, monitoring equipments, vacuum, exhaust fan, air conditioning, TV.

- **Special outlets:** Two, for ventilator and portable X-ray machines.
- Earthing all the outlets must be properly earthed, and have earthing circuit breakers to protect against electrocution.
- **Voltage stabilization:** For all the outlets voltage fluctuations may damage sensitive monitoring equipment.

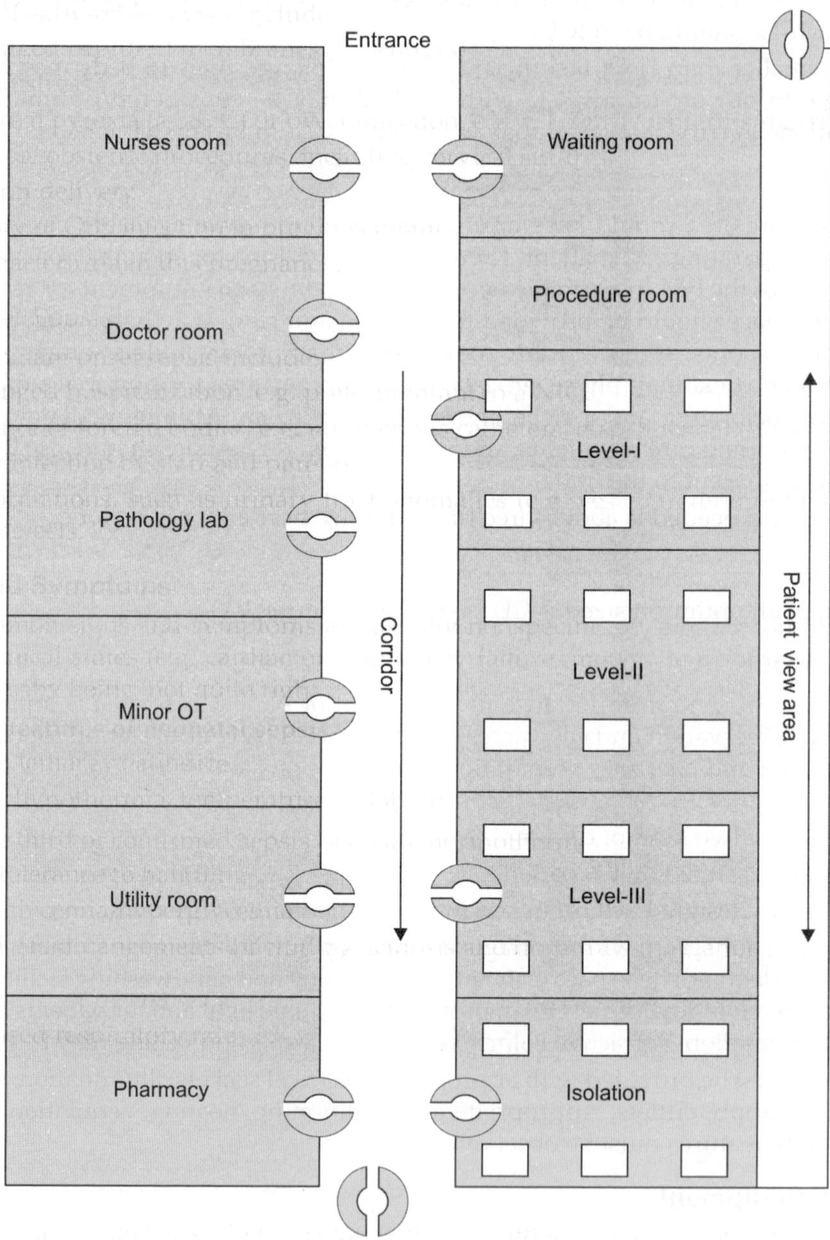

Fig. 2.33: NICU and PICU layout

Illumination (Lighting)

- **Background lighting:** Low intensity lighting below the patients bed level to keep a minimum illumination at all times.
- **General and additional illumination:** During active patient care. For procedures needing extra brightness, additional lights are needed. Full size fluorescent tube lights—fixed in ceilings, four per patient, two for general and two for additional illumination is minimum requirement.
- One spot light to give high level illumination for procedure, examination and treatment. This may be fixed in ceiling (or) may be portable one.

Compressed Air

One outlet per bed, provision of double filtered air at a line pressure of 50–55 psi.

Oxygen Outlets

Two per bed supplied from a central sourced, should be distinct color for identification, alarm for low pressure, and shut-off valve between the main and the outlet to close the flow if needed.

Suction–Vacuum

Two per bed minimum: A third outlet may be desirable, the pressure should be adjustable to varying needs pressure, and shut-off valve between the main and the outlet to close the flow if needed such as nasogastric suction, theracostomy, tube drainage, endotracheal suction, etc.

Physical Environment

- Temperature: Temperature should be between 20 and 25 °C
- Humidity: Humidity should be between 30 and 60%
- Air pressure: Positive air pressure inside as compared to adjacent area
- Air exchange: At least 6 per hour, at least 2 of outdoor air
- Recirculated air must pass through a two bed filter
- Air conditioning system must allow for the above requirements.

PICU PERSONNEL

Physician Staff

Medical Director/Consultant Incharge

The consultant incharge of the PICU should have special training and experience in the care of critically ill children including advanced skill in monitoring and life support techniques. He must be available full time for clinical, administrative and educational activities of the unit.

Activities of Medical Director

- Supervision
- Regular care
- Resuscitation
- Life support measures to all patients

- Quality control and appropriateness of the care
- Coordination of multiple subspecialty services
- Maintenance, calibration and replacement of equipment
- Organization of educational and research activities
- Staff development
- Improvement in standards of care
- Collection of statistical data necessary for evaluation of the unit effectiveness
- Implementation of policies and procedures.

House Staff (Residents)

Around the clock presence of qualified doctor in the PICU is necessary, the doctor should be exclusively designated for the PICU and should not be covering other areas such as the emergency department (or) other wards simultaneously. He must be trained in cardio-pulmonary resuscitation and intubations.

An on-call covers by subspecialist pediatrician's pediatric surgeons and anesthetist.

Nurses

They are the most important staff in any PICU for actual delivery of critical care. It is essential to have high quality, specially trained nurses to provide 24 hours coverage. Therefore, a continuing education program for nurses must be developed within the unit. The nurses who are trained and experienced in PICU should not be changed frequently.

The ideal nurse patient ratio is 1:1 the minimum is one nurse per three patients in the unit at all times.

Qualities of PICU Nurses

They should have basic understanding of commonly encountered clinical conditions and should be trained in resuscitation techniques, respiratory care, electronic monitoring and use of PICU equipment.

They should be able to recognize and interpret changes in patient monitoring data, and result of common laboratory tests, perform vein punctures to obtain blood samples, establish an IV line, and administer drugs and parenteral fluids.

Respiratory Therapist

A person trained in respiratory care with knowledge of ventilation equipment and basic life support has become an important part of ICU team in the developed countries. At least one respiratory therapist should be available round the clock.

Other Members

- A biomedical and laboratory technician.
- A unit clerk: To handle patient and administration paper work.
- A physiotherapist
- A nutritionist
- A social worker: She/he is valuable in sociopsychological evaluation and family support.

Available Services in PICU

Essential Services

- Monitoring.
- Therapeutic (or) diagnostic modalities.

Monitoring

An essential part of successful PICU is the anticipation and treatment of critical problems. Therefore, a PICU must have capability to monitor on continuous basis the following:

- Heart rate and rhythm
- ECG
- Blood pressure (noninvasive and invasive)
- CVP and pulmonary artery pressure
- Cardiac output.

Respiratory function

- Respiratory rate
- Oxygen saturation of hemoglobin (SpO_2)
- Arterial Blood Gases (ABG)
- Inspired oxygen and end-tidal CO_2 monitoring for ventilated children.

Temperature: Including core temperature

Cerebral function

- Intracranial pressure
- EEG
- Evoked potential
- Cerebral blood flow.

Therapeutic (or) diagnostic modalities

Besides the usual facilities available in pediatric wards the following specific services should be available.

- Emergency resuscitation
- Respiratory support
  - Tracheostomy care
  - Mechanical ventilation
  - Tube: Thoracotomy, thoracocentesis
  - Bronchoscopy.
- Cardiac support
  - Defibrillation
  - Temporary cardiac pacing.
- Infusion pumps and pressure infusion devices
- Dialysis–peritoneal/hemodialysis
- Desirable
  - Left heart support
  - Intra-aortic balloon assist

- Extracorporeal membrane oxygenation
- Hyperbaric oxygen.

Support Services

Radio diagnosis and imaging facility

24 hours coverage for portable X-rays of chest, abdomen

- Ultrasound
- CT-scan
- Echocardiography
- Angiography
- Lung scan.

Laboratory services

It is necessary to have 24 hours a day availability of following services.

- Hematocrit, hemoglobin, blood counts.
- Blood glucose, urea and electrolytes.
- Prothrombin time, PTT
- Platelets counts.
- Body fluid analysis (CSF, urinalysis)
- Arterial blood gases.

  Other facilities that should be available are:
- Microbiology
- Blood biochemistry
- Toxicology and drug level measurements.
  - Digoxin
  - Theophylline
  - Aminoglycosides
  - Phenobarbitone.

Centralized O_2, compressed air and suction facility

Blood bank and pharmacy

Physiotherapy and occupational therapy

Transport system

An ambulance team with a nurse and a resident trained in evaluation and stabilization of critically ill patients and resuscitation equipments, drugs and basic monitoring equipments.

Equipment maintenance and care

Services of a biomedical engineer/technician should be available for regular and frequent servicing of equipment to keep it in good working order. For costly equipment regular maintenance contract should be made with the manufacturing firm if possible.

Ancillary services

- Housekeeping related to cleaning, water, electrical, telephone, paging and intercom system.

- Communication–within ICU and outside through telephone, paging and intercom system.
- Computerized record keeping is desirable
- Social services.

EQUIPMENT REQUIRED FOR A PICU

Equipment required for intensive care is costly and needs reliable maintenance.

A list of various equipment required for monitoring and therapeutic (or) diagnosis purposes is given as below:

General Equipment

- Adjustable beds, cribs, incubators
- Emergency resuscitation trolley, laryngoscope and Ambu bag and mask for each bed
- Endotracheal tubes and tracheostomy tubes
- Spot light, suction machine
- Electronic thermometers with low reading facility
- Ophthalmoscope, weighing scale
- Oxygen cylinders and flow meters, humidifiers
- Equipment for venous and arterial access
- BP instrument.

Monitoring Equipment

- Monitor for ECG and heart rate.
- Oscillometric blood pressure (noninvasive), central venous pressure, direct arterial blood pressure, pulmonary artery pressure.
- Respiratory rate and depth with continues wave form
- Oxygen saturation monitor (pulse oximetry)
- Temperature (skin and care temp)
- Cardiac output
- Intracranial pressure monitoring
- Transcutaneous PO_2
- Endtidal PCO_2 measurement
- Simultaneous monitoring of 3 (or) more pressure.

Equipment for Therapeutic and Diagnostic Purposes

- Ventilators with specific capabilities
- Air compressors, air-oxygen blenders, oxygen analyses
- Defibrillators
- Temporary pacemaker.
- **Bronchoscope:** Fiber optic and regular infusion pumps and pressure infusers.

Dialysis Equipment

- Optional
- EEG and cerebral function monitors
- Pulmonary function measuring device.

Intra Aortic Balloon Pump

Note 1: All monitoring equipment should have high and low, visible and audible alarms for heart and respiratory rates and all the pressures. It should be reliable and electrically isolated from the patient.

Note 2: Pediatric ventilators differ from adult ventilator and they should have the following capabilities:

- It should be able to deliver mechanical breaths via a variety of modalities: assist control, synchronous intermittent mandatory ventilation (SIMV), pressure, support ventilation and controlled mechanical ventilation (CMI).
- Facility for providing positive end-expiratory pressure (PEEP).
- Facility for humidification and warming of gases.
- Alarms for oxygen pressure, volumes and apnea.
- Adjustable flow rate and inspiratory/expiratory ratio.
- Control of inspired O_2 concentration.
- Equipment and essential drugs for a pediatric critical care transport team:

Equipment

Respiratory therapy

- Ambu bag/Laerdal bag 250 ml, 50 ml size
- Endotracheal tubes 2.5 – 8.1 mm size
- Laryngoscope with blades for infants and children
- Adhesive tape for stabilization of tubes
- Bag and O_2 mask (all sizes), oxygen tubes and assorted adaptors.
- Oxygen cylinders
- Oxygen saturation monitor
- Desirable portable ventilator.

Cardiovascular care

- ECG monitor (portable)
- Vital sign monitor for respiration, BP and temp with digital readout.
- Cannula and catheters for vascular access/venous ling size 16–24.

Note: All monitors must have a built in battery backup of 3–4 hours.

Drugs: (For IV/IM use)

- Adrenaline
- Sodium chloride, Ringer's lactate, 5% glucose, albumin 5%
- 25% glucose, sodium bicarbonate, potassium chloride

- Salbutamol, calcium gluconate
- Dilantin, diazepam, phenytoin
- Atropine, succamethopium, pancuronium

  Provision of care in PICU or specialized care of child administer in PICU

The Major Components of Care in PICU

- Airway management
- Respiratory support: Oxygen therapy
- Assisted ventilation
- Cardiovascular support
- Neurological evaluation and support
- Renal support.

Airway Management

A stable airway must be established in al the sick children admitted two PICU. It can be maintained by the following ways:

- Oropharyngeal airway
- Endotracheal intubation
- Tracheostomy.

Oropharyngeal airway

Oral airway is used to provide a patent airway when breathing is spontaneous. The airway must be of a size appropriate a child's mandible. The flanged end should protrude from the lips and the curved end should reach the angle of the mandible.

Endotracheal intubation

Endotracheal (ET) intubation is performed when

- Measures to improve oxygenation fail and respiratory failure is imminent
- Prolonged respiratory support is anticipated
- Aspiration is a risk
- Airway obstruction is present.

The size of the endotracheal tube is very important. It should be large enough to provide adequate airway, but small enough to avoid trauma to larynx and glottis region. Proper sized endotracheal tube may be determined roughly by the formula:

$$\text{Orotracheal tube (cm)} = \frac{12 + Age\ (year)}{4}$$

$$\text{Nasotracheal tube (cm)} = \frac{16 + Age\ (year)}{4}$$

Table 2.6: Shows suggested initial size of endotracheal tubes and suction catheters

Age	Endotracheal tube ID (mm)	Tracheotomy tube		Suction catheters
		ID (mm)	Length (mm)	
Newborn term	3.0	3.4	30–40	6
6 months	3.5	3.9	41	8
3 years	4.5	4.8	44	8
5 years	5.0	5.0	46	10
6 years	5.5	5.0	46	10
8 years	6.0	5.0	46	10
12 years	6.5	7.0	67	10

Uncuffed endotracheal tubes are used in small children (under 8 year) to minimize laryngeal injury.

Care of endotracheal tube: All intubated children must receive the following care.

- Humidification of inspired air gases, either through circuit humidifiers (or) mist tent (or) condenser humidifies
- Suctioning and good pulmonary toilet to avoid tube blockage because children have more secretions than adults.
- Sedation and muscle relaxation:

  Sedation is required to prevent excessive movement of the patient and any accidental extubation.

  Sedation may be obtained with:

  Morphine – 0.1 mg/kg IV 4 hourly (or) Diazepam – 0.1 mg/kg IV 4 hourly

  Muscle relaxation can be obtained with:

  Succinylcholine – 1 mg/kg IV for short period of 5-10 minutes (or) Pancuronium – 0.1 – 0.2 mg/kg IV administered 1–2 hourly (for longer period of 30-60 minutes
- Intravenous fluids–To maintain good hydration.
- Nasogastric tube insertion to remove swallowed air and decrease the risk of aspiration

Extubation should be considered when the child no longer has respiratory distress and has minimal tracheal secretions.

Tracheotomy

Indications: It is particularly indicated in presences.

- Upper airway obstruction
- Vocal cord paralysis
- Facial burns (or) Trauma
- Difficult to maintain patency of ET Tube because of secretions, infection, (or) bleeding
- Child who require ventilator support for prolonged period
- Size of tracheotomy tube at various ages are given in Table 2.7.

Table 2.7: Oxygen concentration (FiO_2) delivered through various devices

FiO_2	Device (flow rate/min)
21–50%	Nasal cannula (1–6 L)
35–65%	Simple face mask (6–12 L)
24–40%	Venturimask (Graded 4–12 L)
60–80%	No breathing masks

Respiratory Support: Oxygen Therapy

Indication

Acute respiratory failure is imminent (or) already established. There are two types of respiratory failure

Type I

The type I refers to hypoxemia (low $PaCO_2$) without hypercapnia (high $PaCO_2$) patient with type I respiratory failure require more O_2 in inhaled air.

It can be corrected by an increase in inspired oxygen concentration through mask, nasal prongs, nasopharyngeal catheters, and hood (or) tent, these may provide varying amount of O_2 at different O_2 flow rates.

Type II

The type II respiratory failure refers to hypercapnia (high arterial $PaCO_2$) a dhypoxemia (low PaO_2)

This indicates severe alveolar hypoventilation and patient require assisted ventilation:

Table 2.8: Criteria for initiation of respiratory and ventilator support

Blood gas parameters	Therapy
PaO_2	Increase FiP_2 as needed to maintain PaO_2 > 50 mm/Hg
PaO_2 normal	
PaO_2 < 60 mm 100% O_2	Intubate and add CPAO, increase as tolerated
PaO_2 > 45 mm and pH > 7.2	
PaO_2 > 60 mm Hg in 1% O_2	IPPV, and PEEP starting with 3–5 cm H_2O increase to achieve PaO_2 > 45 mm and pH > 65 mm Hg at FiO_2 of 0.4–1.0 correct pH to > 7.2.
PaO_2 > 60 mm Hg and rising pH < 7.2 Apneic spells	

Assisted Ventilation

Indications for assisted ventilation:

- Serious respiratory depression (or) paralysis causing hypoventilation (or) Apnea.
- Severely distressed cyanosed patient, whose hypoxemia persists inspire of maximal oxygen therapy and sign's of exhaustion appear.
- Children who has reversible disease (such as preemie, aspiration syndromes, pulmonary edema, laryngo tracheitis bronchiolitis, asthma)
- Myocardial failure

- Arterial CO_2 tension ($PaCO_2$) 50 mm Hg (or) more. Arterial O_2 tension ($PaCO_2$) 60 mm Hg (or) less in a fractional concentration of inspired O_2 > 60%
- Very shallow breathing: tidal volume < 3 ml/kg.

Initial evaluation and recording in patient receiving.

Clinical data

- Vital sign's: Respiratory rate, heart rate, blood pressure, core temperature.
- Oxygen saturation.

Laboratory data

- Chest X-ray
- ECG
- Blood counts
- Blood biochemistry: Glucose, Na, K, Cl, urea, creatinine, Ca, PO_4, Mg
- Arterial blood gases
- Coagulation parameters: PT, PTT, Platelet count
- Baseline cultures: Blood, Urine, Oropharyngeal, tracheal suctions.

After recording of patients data proceed as follows.

- Secure an endotracheal tube safely and comfortably measures must be taken to prevent unplanned extubation.
- Connect ventilator tubing to endotracheal tube/tracheostomy tube by appropriate connections.
- Set the desired expiratory and inspiratory ratio and PEEP; avoid negative expiratory pressure.
- Observe degree of excursion of chest wall, the presence of breath sound bilaterally and general response of the child to assess adequacy of ventilation.
- Monitor oxygen saturation and arterial blood gases to ensure satisfactory oxygenation and CO_2 elimination this is the only way to evaluate the efficacy of ventilation.

Saturation of oxygen [(arterial blood) SaO_2] should be allowed to stay below 32 mm Hg. If it is low, it can be elevated by ventilator manipulations (or) introduction if dead space (or) by adding CO_2 to inspired gas mixture. PaO_2 should be adjusted between 75–100 mm Hg. This can be done by increasing total volume and by PEEP.

Monitoring and care of a child on ventilator

When the patient is a ventilator, the following variables should be measured and recorded at least 2–4 hourly to assess proper functioning of ventilator and oxygen delivery demand:

- FiO_2 I:E ratio
- Tidal volume (both inspiratory and expiratory)
- Minute ventilation
- Peak inspiratory pressure and mean airway pressure
- Temperature of inspired gas
- Confirmation of all preset alarms for gas supply airway pressure, apnea and inspired O_2 concentration
- O_2 saturation of hemoglobin

- Heart rate, rhythm and BP
- Temperature.

The following variables must be monitored at interval depending on the clinical condition of the patient and changes in ventilator setting.

- Arterial blood gases and DO_2 calculation.
- Measurement of vital capacity, negative inspiratory force and dynamic compliance.
- Chest X-ray
- Intake and output
- Weight recording
- Blood level of electrolytes; urea and coagulation parameters must be monitored closely
- The cuff the endotracheal tube must be released every 4 hourly for 5 minutes. During this period, deep pulmonary inflation is performed using a bag and 100% oxygen
- The ventilator tubing must be changed every 72–96 hours
- The humidifier fluid must changed daily
- Culture of endotracheal secretions and humidifies fluid must obtained daily to monitor the microbial flora.

Cardiovascular Support

Indication: Low cardiac output

Goal: The goal of cardiovascular support is to achieve reasonable peripheral perfusion as evidenced by warm skin the extremities with palpable peripheral pulses, capillary refill 3–5 seconds, heart rate and blood pressure within normal range for the patient and urine output > 1 m l/kg/hour.

Methods for improving tissue perfusion

- **General support:**
  - The pH should be maintained around acidosis is corrected with sodium bicarbonate 1–2 mEq/kg
  - Hypoglycemia is corrected with a glucose bolus of 0.5–1.9/kg IV using a 25% solution.
  - Hypocalcemia is corrected with calcium chloride solution 10–20 ng/kg IV slowly.
  - Patient in sock should not receive calcium gluconate as liver metabolism which in necessary for converting it to ionized calcium.
- **Correction of hypotension and Hypovolemia:** Hypotension and hypovolemia is corrected with repeated infusion of normal saline, Ringer's lactate (or) plasma 5–10 ml/kg under clinical and BP monitoring.
- **Inotropic support:** To improve the myocardial contractility common inotropic agents available are:
  - Dopamine: 5–20 mg/kg/min.
  - Dobutamine: 5–15 mg/kg/min.
  - Adrenaline: 0.05–10 mg/kg/min.
  - Naradrenaline: 0.05–1.0 mg/kg/min.

- **After load reduction:** Reduction of after load (resistance to forward flow of blood) can be achieved by administration of vasodilators.
  - Sodium nitroprusside: 1–10 mg/kg/min.
  - Nitroglycerine: 0.5–10 mg/kg/min.
- **Neurological evaluation and support:** Assessment of respiratory pattern, heart rate, blood pressure (liability, hypertension) and gradation of sensorium changes. Assess of Intracranial pressure and GCS.

  Management:
  - Control of seizure activity.
  - Cerebral perfusion pressure (It is the difference between systolic blood pressure and the intracranial pressure) must be maintained.
- **Renal support:** Kidneys are one of the vital organs affected by circulatory failure, shock (or) hypoxia, and it is easily reversible by restoration of blood volume.

NEONATAL INTENSIVE CARE UNIT (NICU)

Definition

Neonatal intensive care unit (NICU) equipment includes patient monitoring, respiratory and cardiac support, pain management, emergency resuscitation devices, and other life support equipment designed to care for patients who are seriously injured, have a critical or life-threatening illness, or have undergone a major surgical procedure, thereby requiring 24-hour care and monitoring.

Purpose

An NICU may be designed and equipped to provide care to patients with a range of conditions, or it may be designed and equipped to provide specialized care to patients with specific conditions. For example, a neuromedical ICU cares for patients with acute conditions involving the nervous system or patients who have just had neurosurgical procedures and require equipment for monitoring and assessing the brain and spinal cord.

An NICU is designed and equipped to care for infants who are ill, born prematurely, or have a condition requiring constant monitoring. A trauma/burn ICU provides specialized injury and wound care for patients involved in auto accidents and patients who have gunshot injuries or burns.

Types of Equipment

- Patient monitoring equipment
- Life support and emergency resuscitative equipment
- Diagnostic equipment
- Other ICU equipment.

Description

Intensive care unit equipment includes patient monitoring, life support and emergency resuscitation devices, and diagnostic devices.

Child Monitoring Equipment

Acute Care Physiologic Monitoring System

A comprehensive patient monitoring systems that can be configured to continuously measure and display a number of parameters via electrodes and sensors that are connected to the patient.

These may include the electrical activity of the heart via an ECG, respiration rate (breathing), blood pressure, body temperature, cardiac output, and amount of oxygen and carbon dioxide in the blood. Each patient bed in an ICU has a physiologic monitor that measure these body activities. All monitors are networked to a central nurses, station.

Pulse Oximetry

A monitor the arterial hemoglobin oxygen saturation (oxygen level) of the patient's blood with a sensor clipped over the finger or toe.

Intracranial Pressure Monitor

Intracranial (ICP) measures the pressure of fluid in the brain in patients with head trauma or other conditions affecting the brain (such as tumors, edema, or hemorrhage). These devices warn of elevated pressure and record or display pressure trends. Intracranial pressure monitoring may be a capability included in a physiologic monitor.

Apnea Monitor

A continuously monitors breathing via electrodes or sensors placed on the patient. An apnea monitor detects cessation of breathing in infants and adults at risk of respiratory failure, displays respiration parameters, and triggers an alarm if a certain amount of time passes without a patient's breath being detected. Apnea monitoring may be a capability included in a physiologic monitor.

Life Support and Emergency Resuscitative Equipment

Intensive care equipment for life support and emergency resuscitation includes the following:

Ventilator (Respirator)

An assists with or controls pulmonary ventilation in patients who cannot breathe on their own. Ventilators consist of a flexible breathing circuit, gas supply, heating/humidification mechanism, monitors, and alarms. They are microprocessor-controlled and programmable, and regulate the volume, pressure, and flow of patient respiration. Ventilator monitors and alarms may interface with a central monitoring system or information system.

Infusion Pump

A device that delivers fluids intravenously or epidurally through a catheter. Infusion pumps employ automatic, programmable pumping mechanisms to deliver continuous anesthesia, drugs, and blood infusions to the patient. The pump is hung on an intravenous pole placed next to the patient's bed.

Crash Cart

It is also called resuscitation or code cart. This is a portable cart containing emergency resuscitation equipment for patients who are 'coding.' That is, their **vital signs** are in a dangerous range. The emergency equipment includes a defibrillator, airway intubation devices, a resuscitation bag/mask, and medication box. Crash carts are strategically located in the ICU for immediate availability for when a patient experiences cardiorespiratory failure.

Intra-aortic Balloon Pump

A device that helps to reduce the heart's workload and helps in blood flow to the coronary arteries for patients with unstable angina, myocardial infarction (heart attack), or patients awaiting organ transplants. Intra-aortic balloon pumps use a balloon placed in the patient's aorta. The balloon is on the end of a catheter that is connected to the pump's console, which displays heart rate, pressure, and electrocardiogram (ECG) readings. The patient's ECG is used to time the inflation and deflation of the balloon.

Diagnostic Equipment

The use of diagnostic equipment is also required in the ICU. Mobile X-ray units are used for bedside radiography, particularly of the chest. Mobile X-ray units use a battery-operated generator that powers an X-ray tube. Handheld, portable clinical laboratory devices, or point-of-care analyzers, are used for blood analysis at the bedside. A small amount of whole blood is required, and blood chemistry parameters can be provided much faster than if samples were sent to the central laboratory.

Other ICU Equipment

Disposable ICU equipment includes urinary (Foley) catheters, catheters used for arterial and central venous lines, Swan-Ganz catheters chest and endotracheal tubes, gastrointestinal and nasogastric feeding tubes, and monitoring electrodes. Some patients may be wearing a Posey vest, also called a Houdini jacket for safety; the purpose is to keep the patient stationary. Spenco boots are padded support devices made of lamb's wool to position the feet and ankles of the patient. Support hose may also be placed on the patient's legs to support the leg muscles and aid circulation.

Equipment and Systems

- Common equipment in an ICU includes mechanical ventilator to assist breathing through an endotracheal tube or a tracheotomy opening
- Cardiac monitors including telemetry,
- External pacemakers, and defibrillators
- Dialysis equipment for renal problems
- Equipment for the constant monitoring of bodily functions;
- A web of intravenous lines,
- Feeding tubes,
- Nasogastric tubes,
- Suction pumps,
- Drains and catheters
- A wide array of drugs to treat the main condition(s).
- Medically induced comas, analgesics, and induced sedation reduce pain and prevent secondary infections.

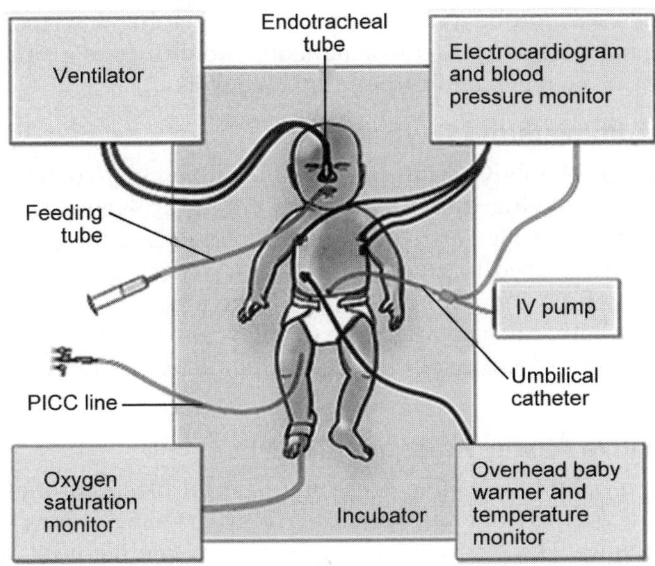

Radiant Warmers and Incubators

Your baby often arrives in the NICU on a radiant warmer (a cart with a mattress on top and a heat source overhead). This helps your baby stay warm, and at the same time, allows easy observation by the NICU staff. It also allows easy access for any procedures or examinations that the staff may need to perform.

- When your baby is stable and having fewer procedures each day, the baby can be moved to an incubator, commonly called an isolate (a large plexiglass box with a mattress inside).
- Some NICUs have warmers with tops that come down and convert the warmer directly into an isolate, so that your baby does not need to be moved from one to the other.
- The isolate helps to maintain a stable body temperature until the baby gets big enough to do this on his own. Babies usually need help staying warm until they reach a weight of about 2,000 grams (4 pounds, 7 ounces).

Monitors for Heart Rate, Breathing Rate (Respiration), and Blood Pressure

The NICU staff must be able to quickly detect any changes in your baby's heart rate, breathing rate, and blood pressure. To do this, they connect your baby to a monitor that displays this information. These instruments are equipped with alarms that sound if there are any abnormalities. This can make the NICU a rather noisy place. An alarm is not always a cause for concern. A baby's movements or crying can trigger an alarm. But, just to be sure, the NICU staff checks each sounding of an alarm to see if there is a problem.

Pulse Oximetry and Transcutaneous Monitors

To assess how well your baby's lungs are working, NICU staff may use a pulse oximeter or a transcutaneous monitor. These devices measure the level of oxygen saturation in your baby's blood; the transcutaneous monitor also measures the carbon dioxide level in the blood. The staff does not need to use needles to get blood for these measurements. Instead, the pulse oximeter uses a probe wrapped around a finger, hand, or toe to read the oxygen level through the baby's skin. The transcutaneous monitor uses a small electrode on the baby's skin to measure oxygen and carbon dioxide levels.

Equipment for Administering Oxygen

There are several ways that NICU staff can administer oxygen to babies who are breathing on their own, but are having difficulty getting enough oxygen. A baby's head can be placed inside a plastic box called an oxyhood. This allows breathing in an oxygen-enriched environment and can be used to give close to 100% oxygen, if necessary. A cannula can also be used to deliver oxygen. This is a small plastic tube with prongs that fit just inside the baby's nose. The baby can sleep with the oxygen cannula in place. The cannula allows for easier feeding, bathing, and performance of other activities than when a baby is using an oxygen hood.

Continuous Positive Airway Pressure (CPAP)

Sometimes, when a baby has trouble breathing, special plastic prongs are placed in the baby's nose to allow delivery of extra pressure to help the baby's lungs stay inflated CPAP, as well as extra oxygen. The pressure may come from a ventilator or from a device using a column of water, called bubble CPAP. CPAP is used commonly for babies with RDS or HMD, either instead of intubation (*see* below), or after an endotracheal tube (*see* below) has been removed. CPAP can also be used to treat babies with apnea of prematurity and bronchopulmonary dysplasia (BPD).

Maintenance of Equipment

Since ICU equipment is used continuously on critically ill patients, it is essential that equipment be properly maintained, particularly devices that are used for life support and resuscitation. Staff in the ICU should perform daily checks on equipment and inform biomedical engineering staff when equipment needs maintenance, repair, or replacement. For mechanically complex devices, service and preventive maintenance contracts are available from the manufacturer or third-party servicing companies, and should be kept current at all times.

TYPES OF PROCEDURES IN THE NEONATAL INTENSIVE CARE UNIT

Nutrition Support

Feeding a Baby through an Intravenous (IV) Line

Not many premature or low birth weight babies can be fed during the first few hours in the NICU, and many sick babies are unable to take anything by mouth for a number of days. To make sure your baby is getting adequate nutrition; the NICU staff starts an IV to administer fluids containing water, glucose, sodium, potassium, chloride, calcium, magnesium, and phosphorus. This kind of nutrition is called **total parenteral nutrition** or **TPN**.

At first, the staff places the IV in a vein in the baby's head, hand, or lower leg. These IV lines often last for less than a day, so a baby may have several IVs placed in the first few days. After a few days, however, most babies need more nutrition than these small IV lines can supply. The staff then inserts a catheter into one of your baby's larger veins so that larger amounts of nutrients can be given.

If a baby is very small or sick, catheters (long IV lines) may be placed in both the umbilical artery and vein. Fluids and medications can be given through the catheter and blood can be drawn for laboratory tests. More concentrated IV fluids can be given through an umbilical line, so babies can get better nutrition. Umbilical lines last longer that smaller IVs, often for a week or more. Umbilical arterial lines can also be connected to a machine that continuously measures a baby's blood pressure.

If a baby is going to need TPN for more than a week to 10 days, doctors often insert another type of line, called a central line, that can remain in place for several weeks, until the baby no longer needs TPN.

Feeding a Baby by Mouth

Feeding by mouth (also called 'enteral nutrition') should be started as soon as possible because it helps a baby's gastrointestinal (GI) tract grow and begin functioning. A very small baby may first need to be fed through a small plastic tube that goes through the mouth or nose and into the stomach. A small amount of breast milk or formula is given through this tube. Often the baby is given a combination of parenteral and enteral feedings at first, because it can take awhile for the GI tract to become accustomed to enteral feedings.

Other Common NICU Procedures

X-rays

X-rays are one of the most commonly performed procedures in the NICU. The most common reason for an X-ray is to examine the baby's chest to see if the condition of the lungs is improving. X-rays are often taken of the baby's abdomen if he is not tolerating his enteral feedings.

Ultrasound

Premature babies are also routinely evaluated by ultrasound. Ultrasound may be used to check for hemorrhage in the brain or for damage to the white matter surrounding the ventricles of the brain (a condition called periventricular leukomalacia). For more information on brain hemorrhage, go to brain problems in the premature baby.

Blood and Urine Tests

- **Blood gases** (the amount of oxygen, carbon dioxide, and acid in the blood)—Blood gas levels can help the staff assess how well a baby's lungs are functioning and how much respiratory assistance may be needed. This test is usually performed on arterial blood. If your baby does not have an arterial catheter in place, a nurse can obtain a blood sample by pricking the baby's heel (a capillary blood gas).
- **Hematocrit and hemoglobin**: These tests provide information about how well a baby is able to carry oxygen through the body.
- **Blood urea nitrogen (BUN) and creatinine**: These substances indicate how well the kidneys are functioning.
- **Chemical salts, like sodium, glucose, potassium, chloride, calcium, phosphorus, and magnesium**: Levels of these salts provide information about different aspects of a baby's medical condition. The nurses also collect a few drops of urine every few hours. The urine is checked for pH level, and for sugar, protein, and blood content. These tests provide information about kidney function and metabolism.

Procedures to Measure Fluids

Nurses measure all the fluids your baby takes in (e.g. by IV and by mouth) and all the fluids that leave the baby's body (e.g. urine output and amount of blood taken for testing). This helps to determine if the fluids are inbalance—i.e.if the baby takes in about the same amount of fluid as leaves his body. The nurses also weigh a baby frequently to determine how much fluid he needs.

Blood Transfusions

Babies in the NICU often require blood transfusions because (1) their blood-forming organs are immature and are not producing enough red blood cells, and (2) they may be losing a lot of blood for various tests.

CONCLUSION

Neonatal intensive care unit (NICU) equipment includes patient monitoring, respiratory and cardiac support, pain management, emergency resuscitation devices, and other life support equipment designed to care for patients who are seriously injured. And it will be reduce the mortality and morbidity rate of the sick children.

LEVEL OF NEONATAL CARE IN NICU AND PICU

Intensive Care

The care given in a special area or intensive care nursery which provides continuous skilled supervision by nursing and medical staff.

Special Care

A care given in a special area of intensive care or in a postnatal ward which provides observation and treatment falling short of intensive care but exceeding normal care.

Normal Care

A care given usually by the mother in a postnatal ward, supervised by a midwife and doctor but requiring minimal medical or nursing advice.

LEVELS OF NEONATAL CARE IN NICU AND PICU

Level I Care

It includes adequate resuscitation at birth (facilities of suction and mouth to mouth or bag and mask ventilation), environmental control of temperature by warming the room, feeding from breast/spoon, bottle feeding should be avoided as far as possible), simple but important aseptic precautions (like handwashing, exclusion of infected individuals and management of milk illnesses). Over 80% of the babies will require this level of care.

This is generally adequate for the term babies weighing above 2000 gm of those who have minor illness. Such a care is provided by the mother under the supervision of basic health professionals including traditional birth attendants and can be instituted at home/ sub center/primary health center.

Level II Care

This level includes ideal resuscitation facilities, clinical and noninvasive monitoring availability of thermoneutral environment, facilities for gavage feeding intravenous infusion, phototherapy, exchange feeding, intravenous infusion, including short-term assisted ventilation.

Such care should be closely supervised by trained nurses and pediatricians. Generally, babies weighing less than 2000 gm, those less than 37 weeks of gestation and those moderately ill require this care.

This type of care should normally available at all teaching hospitals, district/community health centers, Taluk hospitals and nursing homes.

Level III Care

It implies high level of neonatal intensive care including facilities for intensive monitoring (including invasive monitoring), prolonged assisted ventilation and intravenous hyperalimentation.

This will involve availability of central oxygen and suction facilities, servo-controlled incubators/warmers electronic monitoring, etc. Such a care has to be provided by skilled nurses and the specially trained neonatologists.

This type of care is generally needed for babies weighing less than 1500 gm and those less than 34 weeks of gestation and seriously sick infants with organ/system failure. This level of care is required for 3 to 5 percent of the newborn population. Such a facility should be available at all apex institutions, medical college hospitals and regional perinatal centers.

Criteria to Establish the NICU (Level 2 or 3)

- Whatever is the level of neonatal care labor room/birthplace must have adequate facilities for resuscitation temperature control and aseptic technique.
- For every 1000 deliveries, 4 SCNU beds and 5 intermediate care beds are recommended.
- Located as close as possible to the labor room/operation theater.
- The NICU can be in single area or it can be in multiple rooms with a capacity of 2-4 babies each.
- Area for each baby should be 100 sq feet or 10 m^2 with 6 ft space in between two radiant warmers.
- There should be the facilities for maintaining the asepsis.
- Feasibility for adequate sunlight to provide UV rays.
- It should not be on the top floor of the hospital.
- Walls should be of white glazed tiles.
- There should be two layers of glasses on windows.
- There should be abundant open space.
- There should be the provision of good ventilation (12 air changes/hr) AC should have 0.5 micro mm pore size filter.
- Light should be 100 foot candle unit.
- The unit should have an intercom and a direct outside telephone line.
- The unit should be 1 neonatal physician for every 6-10 patients and resident doctors should be present in the unit round the clock.

- The unit should have 1:4 nurse patients ratio.
- The intermediate care beds and 1:1 nurse child ratio for SCNU/NICU.
- The staff should be dedicated, committed and well-trained.
- The unit should have adequate numbers of supportive staffs like ward boys, sweepers and ayas.
- Good laboratory back up is essential.
- Parent should be allowed to the nursery to involve in the care of their baby.

A receptionist area is ideal to control visitation, so that all visitors must go by this area before entering. This area should be monitored by security.

Central Station

- Should provide visibility to all patient areas.
- Should also have ample area to have capacity for all necessary staff functions.
- Patient records should be easily available.
- Adequate space for computer, printers and central monitor is essential.
- Ample space for doctors to write on patient files and space for unit secretarial staff is essential.

At least two telephone lines should be available. A third telephone line dedicated to incoming cells only (toll free number to NICU) to take Critical Care transport request is desirable.

Storage

- Storage for vital supplies should be located within or closely adjoining to each ICU.
- A refrigerator is essential for some pharmaceuticals.
- An area must be provided for storage of large patient care equipment items not in active use.
- An area must be provided for stretchers and wheel chairs.

Clean and Dirty Utility Room

- Clean and dirty utility rooms should be separate rooms.
- Clean utility room should be used for the storage of clean linen.
- Dirty utility room must contain a sink.
- Separate covered bins must be provided for soiled linen and waste material.

An area for emptying and cleaning bed pans and urine bottles. Mechanism of disposal of contaminated waste and adequate disposal of needles and sharp objects needs to be as per standard applicable pollution control guidelines.

Conference Room

A room for ICU physician and staff, for education, discussion of difficult cases, and other necessary meetings related to equal it improvement, is desirable. This room should have a small library facility with ready access to important ICU books, journals, and policy manuals. Stat laboratory with arterial blood gas analysis, electrolytes, blood sugar, blood urea, serum creatinine, PT, PTT, CBC with Gram stain and urine examination facility should be considered adjacent to the PICU. 24 hour availability of on site/in hospital arterial blood gas is essential.

As an alternative to stat lab adjacent to PICU a central main lab facility with a turnaround time of less than one hour for stat lab test results is acceptable.

Equipment

The selection of equipment should be based on following criteria: Cost benefit analysis, accuracy and adaptability for pediatric population. Ease of use for care givers, trouble shooting requirements, proven use on pediatric patients, maintenance requirements and biomedical support of the company and hospital.

Table 2.9: Following is a list of essential and optional equipment for a tertiary level PICU

S. No.	Equipment	Essential	Optional
1	Diagnostic	X	
2	Otoscope/Ophthalmoscope	X	
3	Portable EEG	X	
4	Portable X-ray	X	
5	12 lead portable ECG	X	
6	Blood gas machine	X	
7	Glucometer	X	
8	Portable ultrasound		X
9	Portable echo cardiogram		X
10	Procedural equipment		
11	Emergency cart	X	
12	Emergency drugs	X	
13	Ventilators (Volume/Pressure/Peep Pressure Support, Low Tidal Volume Capacity (30 to 50 mL) with Nebulizer, Humidification and Alarms)	X	
14	Noninvasive ventilator	X	
15	High frequency ventilation		X
16	Nitric oxide (Once licensed)		X
17	Helix		X
18	Micro infusion pumps	X	
19	Defibrillator/Cardioverter	X	
20	Portable suction	X	
21	Pediatric ambu bag	X	
22	Mapleson anesthesia bag with circuit		X
23	Laryngoscope Curved and Straight	X	
24	Endotracheal Tubes (2.5-7)	X	
25	Airway Equipment	X	
26	Pediatric Size Masks	X	
27	Laryngeal Mask	X	
28	Intubating Flexible Scope		X

Contd...

Contd...

S. No.	Equipment	Essential	Optional
29	Nebulizer	X	
30	Oxygen Delivery Devices	X	
31	Rebreather Mask	X	
32	Nasal Cannula	X	
33	Non-Rebreather Mask	X	
34	Oxygen Hood	X	
35	Oxygen Portable Cylinders	X	
36	Nasogastric Tubes	X	
37	Heating and Cooling Blanket		X
38	Over head warmer	X	
39	Bilirubin Light	X	
40	Procedure Light (Portable)	X	
41	Intraosseous Needles	X	
42	Various Size, Multilumen Central Catheters (4.55.5,7R) 8 cm and 16 cm		X
43	Multiple Size (24 22 20) Cannula for IV assess and arterial line	X	
44	Sterile Trays	X	
45	General		X
46	Chest tube		
47	Tracheostomy		
48	Cut Down		
49	Suture Removal		
50	Lumbar Puncture		
51	Bronchoscope with Light Source		X
52	Monitoring Equipment Transducers	X	
53	Doppler		X
54	Rectal Thermometer Probe	X	
55	Glass Thermometer	X	
56	Non-Invasive BP	X	
57	Bed Weighing Scale		X
58	O_2 Analyser	X	
59	Portable Monitor	X	
60	Pulse Oximeter	X	X
61	End Tidal CO_2		
62	Bed side Monitoring of		
63	ECG	X	
64	Respiratory	X	

Contd...

Contd...

S. No.	Equipment	Essential	Optional
65	Temperature	X	
66	Arterial Pressure	X	
67	Non-Invasive Blood Pressure	X	
68	Intra Cranial Pressure	X	
69	Monitors with Arrhythmia Alarms, Heart Rate (High and Low		
70	Monitors with Memory, Trends Printout Feature	X	
71	Miscellaneous		
72	Open Care system	X	
73	Cribs	X	
74	Beds	X	
75	IV Pole	X	
76	Procedural Stool	X	
77	Clocks	X	
78	TV	X	
79	Toys	X	
80	Breast Pump	X	
81	Infant Weighing Machine	X	

Organization and Staffing of NICU and PICU

- Medical Director/Intensivist incharge.
- Preferably a pediatrician must be trained and experienced in critical care of newborn with following:

Responsibilities

Establishing policies and protocols with the help of a group of experts including but not limited to pediatric consultants and subspecialists.

Nursing Director

Administrator

- Laboratory and blood bank representatives. Smooth functioning of PICU with implementation of policies and protocols including admission and discharge criteria.
- Quality assurance and improvement/member of audit committee. Advise administration regarding equipment needs.
- Establishing teaching and training system of staff. Maintaining PICU statistics for mortality and morbidity.

Staffing Requirement

- **Medical:** Round the clock postgraduate level pediatrician in NICU with good airway and pediatric advanced life support skills.

- **Nursing staff:** Ventilated children need one Pediatric/NICU trained nurse by bed side. Very Unstable children (Hypotensive/Hypoxemic patient despite moderate support) may require two nurses by the bed side. Other unventilated/relatively stable patients (Such as postoperative patients and ones admitted for overnight observation may require only one nurse per 2–3 patients.
- **Ancillary support staff:**
  - Physiotherapists
  - Dieticians
  - Technicians
  - Radiographers
  - Respiratory technicians
  - Biomedical engineers
  - Cleaning staff
  - Secretarial/Clerical staff
  - Social worker
  - Nursing director
  - Administrator
  - Laboratory and blood bank representatives.
  - Quality assurance and improvement/Member of audit committee.
  - Advise administration regarding equipment needs.
  - Establishing teaching and training system of staff.
  - Maintaining PICU statistics for mortality and morbidity.

Smooth functioning of NICU with implementation of policies and protocols including admission and discharge criteria.

Low birth weight babies, large size babies, malpresentation, fetal distress, birth asphyxia, birth injuries, neonatal infections, respiratory infections/distress, congenital malformation, Rh/ABO isoimmunization, meconium aspiration syndrome, jaundice/anemia/cyanosis, infant of diabetic mother, chronic maternal diseases, neonatal convulsions, cyanotic heart diseases, tube feeding, total parenteral nutrition, assisted ventilation, cardiopulmonary monitoring, unwell or unwilling mother, babies born by cesarean section, and after forceps.

Any other baby who, need special care/observation, criteria for early discharge from NICU (Before 48 hours). Uncomplicated antepartum, intrapartum and postpartum course, vaginal delivery singleton at 38–42 weeks (AFD). A stable and normal vital sign, physical examination reveals no abnormalities passing urine/stool normally. At least two uneventful, successful feedings no jaundice.

Admission Criteria

Low birth weight babies, large size babies, malpresentation, fetal distress, birth asphyxia, birth injuries, neonatal infections, respiratory infections/distress, congenital malformation, Rh/ABO isoimmunization, meconium aspiration syndrome, jaundice/anemia/cyanosis, infant of diabetic mother, chronic maternal diseases, neonatal convulsions, cyanotic heart diseases, tube parenteral nutrition, assisted ventilation, cardiopulmonary monitoring, unwell or unwilling mother, babies born by cesarean section, and after forceps, any other baby who, need special care/observation.

Criteria for early discharge from NICU (Before 48 hours). Uncomplicated antepartum, intrapartum and postpartum course, vaginal delivery singleton at 38-42 weeks (AFD), a stable and normal vital sign, physical examination reveals no abnormalities, passing urine/ stool normally. At least two uneventful, successful feedings no jaundice. Parents able to feed baby properly, take care of cord and skin, able to recognize abnormal changes in color, behavior, feeding pattern of baby. Mandatory prolonged follow up required:

- Birth asphyxia
- Malpresentation
- LBW
- LFD
- Infant with congenital malformation
- Baby with jaundice/sepsis
- Severe illness
- Maternal psychiatric illness

Ethical Consideration in NICU and PICU

Neonatologist should be the best advocates of their patients and should look after their best interests at all times. Neonatologist should be concerned with saving lives and avoid doing any harm to their patients.

The children's should be taken into confidence while making decisions regarding medical care of their children. Correct distribution of therapeutic measures by balancing medical benefits and burden to the family and society. Every NICU should have written policy to what level of care can be provided, what sort of admissions may be received, what cases may have to be shifted to higher centers. Every NICU should have an ethical committee to look into the dilemmas of ethical practice or to solve Baby Doe Dilemma. When death is imminent the patient should be kept comfortable and the parents should be close at hand or parents should be allowed to be with the baby.

Parent Counseling

In high-risk pregnancies counseling should begin at an early stage. The possible morbidity and adverse outcome will have to be conveyed to both parent in gently and honestly. Parents should be involved in all discussions and decision.

Parents should be allowed to see their baby, touch and handle the baby whenever it is possible. When a baby has to be transferred to a higher center, inform the parent.

In critical condition parents to be encouraged and helped to seek additional medical opinions if they wish.

There must be provision of mother-based neonatal care unit (MNCU) for those babies who need more observation, monitoring and support but do not need the facility of SNCU/ NICU. Must have clean section, septic section, milk preparation room and area for breast-feeding. Equipment in NICU do not necessarily impose the outcome of high-risk neonate. The availability of adequate space, freedom from congestion, maintenances of asepsis and presence of adequate nursing staff are must.

INTEGRATED MANAGEMENT OF NEONATAL AND CHILDHOOD ILLNESS (IMNCI)

Introduction

Over the last three decades the annual number of deaths among children less than 5 years of age has decreased by almost a third. However, this reduction has not been evenly distributed throughout the world. Every year more than 10 million children die in developing countries before they reach their fifth birthday. Seven in 10 of these deaths are due to acute respiratory infections (mostly pneumonia), diarrhoea, measles, malaria, or malnutrition and often to a combination of these illnesses.

In India, common illnesses in children under 3 years of age include fever (27%), acute respiratory infections (17%), diarrhea (13%) and malnutrition (43%) and often in combination (National Family Health Survey). Infant Mortality Rate continues to be high at 68/1000 live births and Under Five Mortality Rate at 95/1000 live births per year. Neonatal mortality contributes to over 64% of infant deaths and most of these deaths occur during the first week of life. Mortality rate in the second month of life is also higher than at later ages. Any health program that aims at reducing Infant Mortality Rate needs to address mortality in the first two months of life, particularly in the first week of life.

Projections based on the 1996 analysis indicate that common childhood illnesses will continue to be major contributors to child deaths through the year 2020 unless greater efforts are made to control them. This assumption makes a strong case for introducing new strategies to significantly reduce child mortality and improve child health and development.

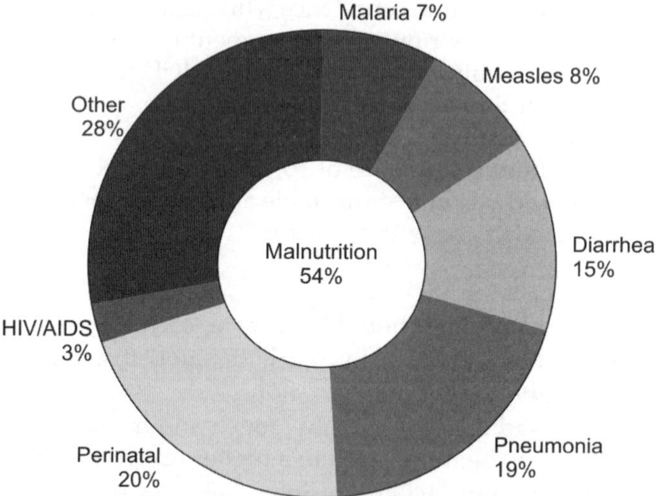

Fig. 2.34: Distribution of 10.5 million deaths among children less than 5 years old in all developing countries, 1999

AN INTEGRATED EVIDENCE-BASED SYNDROMIC APPROACH TO CASE MANAGEMENT

During the mid-1990s, the World Health Organization (WHO), in collaboration with UNICEF and many other agencies, institutions and individuals, responded to this challenge by developing a strategy known as the Integrated Management of Childhood Illness (IMCI). Although the major reason for developing the IMCI strategy stemmed from the needs of curative care, the strategy also addresses aspects of nutrition, immunization, and other important elements of disease prevention and health promotion. The objectives of the strategy are to reduce death and the frequency and severity of illness and disability, and to contribute to improved growth and development. This strategy has been expanded in India to include all neonates and renamed as 'Integrated Management of Neonatal and Childhood Illness (IMNCI)'.

The IMNCI clinical guidelines target children less than 5 years old the age group that bears the highest burden of deaths from common childhood diseases (Figure 2.34).

The guidelines represent an evidence-based, syndromic approach to case management that includes rational, effective and affordable use of drugs and diagnostic tools. Evidence-based medicine stresses the importance of evaluation of evidence from clinical research and cautions against the use of intuition, unsystematic clinical experience, and untested pathophysiologic reasoning for medical decision-making. In situations where laboratory support and clinical resources are limited, the syndromic approach is a more realistic and cost-effective way to manage patients. Careful and systematic assessment of common symptoms and well-selected clinical signs provides sufficient information to guide rational and effective actions.

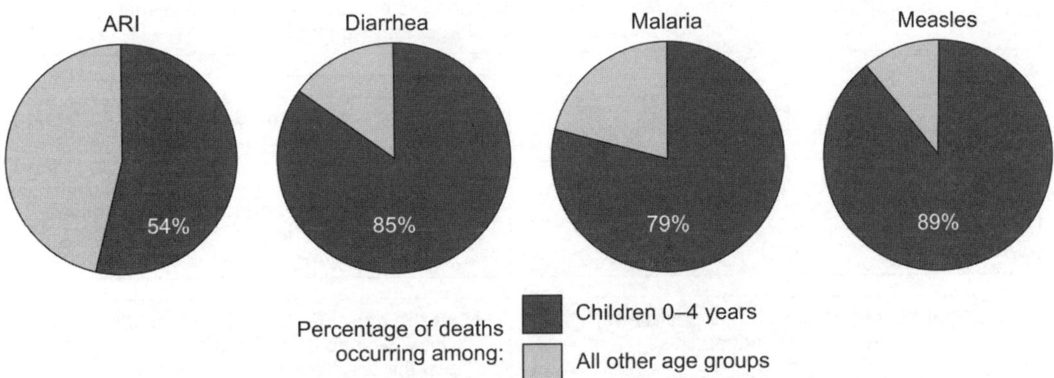

Fig. 2.35: Proportion of global burden of selected diseases borne by children under 5 years (estimated, year 2000)

IMNCI Promotes

- Adjustment of interventions to the capacity of the health system
- Active involvement of family members and the community in the health care process.

Parents, if correctly informed and counselled, can play an important role in improving the health status of their children by following the advice given by a health care provider, by applying appropriate feeding practices and by bringing sick children to a health facility as soon as symptoms arise.

COMPONENTS OF THE INTEGRATED APPROACH

The IMNCI strategy includes both preventive and curative interventions that aim to improve practices in health facilities, the health system and at home. At the core of the strategy is integrated case management of the most common neonatal and childhood problems with a focus on the most common causes of death.

The strategy includes three main components:

- Improvements in the case-management skills of health staff through the provision of locally-adapted guidelines on IMNCI and activities to promote their use
- Improvements in the overall health system required for effective management of neonatal and childhood illness
- Improvements in family and community health care practices
- This document is focused on achieving the first of these components.

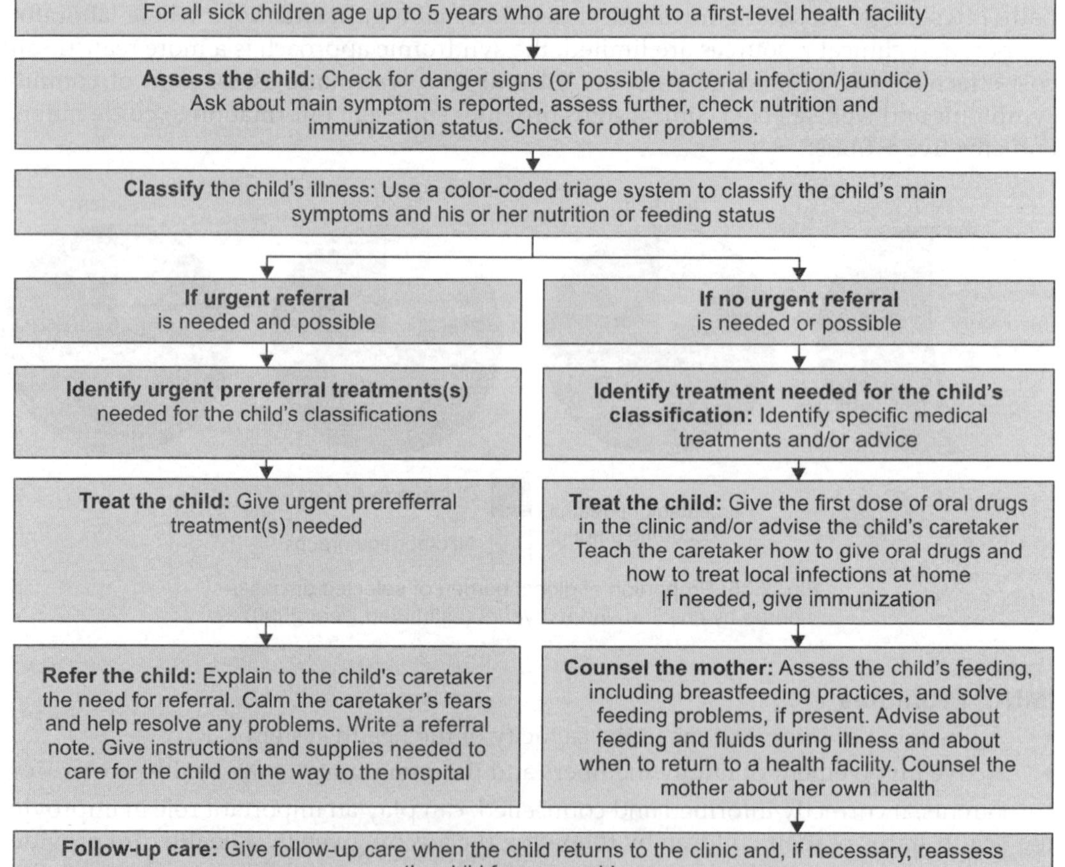

Fig. 2.36: Summary of the integrated case management process

THE PRINCIPLES OF INTEGRATED CARE

Depending on a child's age, various clinical signs and symptoms differ in their degrees of reliability and diagnostic value and importance. Therefore, the IMNCI guidelines recommend case management procedures based on two age categories:

1. Young infants age up to 2 months
2. Children age 2 months up to 5 years.

The IMNCI guidelines are based on the following principles:

- All sick young infants up to 2 months of age 7 must be assessed for 'possible bacterial infection/jaundice'. Then they must be routinely assessed for the major symptom 'diarrhea'.
- All sick children age 2 months up to 5 years must be examined for 'general danger signs' which indicate the need for immediate referral or admission to a hospital. They must then be routinely assessed for major symptoms: Cough or difficult breathing, diarrhea, fever and ear problems.
- All sick young infants and children 2 months up to 5 years must also be routinely assessed for nutritional and immunization status, feeding problems, and other potential problems.
- Only a limited number of carefully selected clinical signs are used, based on evidence of their sensitivity and specificity to detect disease. These signs were selected considering the conditions and realities of first-level health facilities.
- A combination of individual signs leads to an infant's or a child's classification(s) rather than a diagnosis. Classification(s) indicate the severity of condition(s).

They call for specific actions based on whether the infant or child:

- Should be urgently referred to a higher level of care.
- Requires specific treatments (such as antibiotics or antimalarial treatment).
- May be safely managed at home.
  - The classifications are color coded: 'Pink' suggests hospital referral or admission, 'yellow' indicates initiation of specific treatment, and 'green' calls for home management.
  - The IMNCI guidelines address most, but not all, of the major reasons a sick infant or child is brought to a clinic. An infant or child returning with chronic problems or less common illnesses may require special care. The guidelines do not describe the management of trauma or other acute emergencies due to accidents or injuries. They also do not cover care at birth.
  - IMNCI management procedures use a limited number of essential drugs and encourage active participation of caretakers in the treatment of infants and children.
  - An essential component of the IMNCI guidelines is the counselling of caretakers about home care, including counselling about feeding, fluids and when to return to a health facility.

THE IMNCI CASE MANAGEMENT PROCESS

The case management of a sick child brought to a first-level health facility includes a number of important elements Figures 2.37 and 2.38 illustrate the case management process in young infants up to 2 months of age and children 2 months up to 5 years respectively.

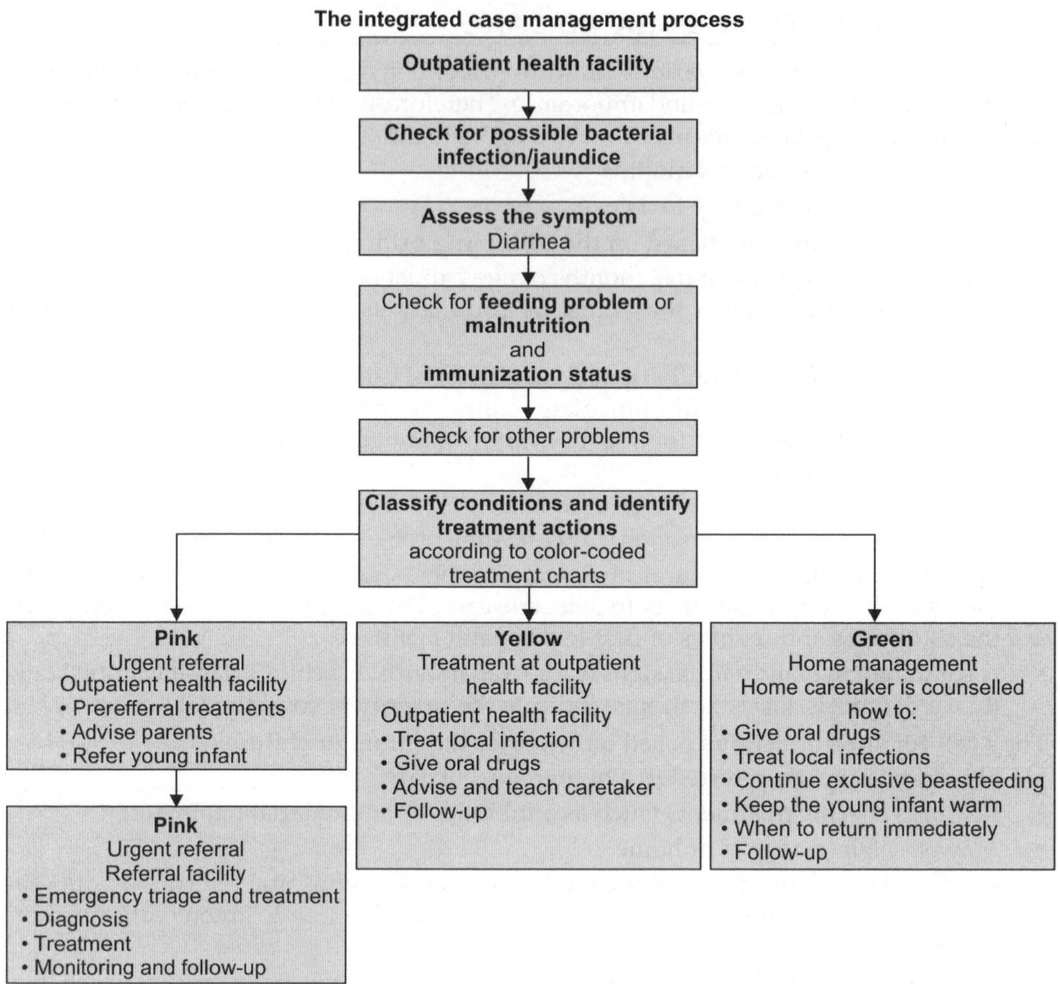

Fig. 2.37: IMNCI case management in the outpatient health facility, first-level referral facility and at home for the sick young infant up to 2 months of age

Outpatient Health Facility

- Assessment
- Classification and identification of treatment
- Referral, treatment or counselling of the child's caretaker (depending on the classification(s) identified)
- Follow-up care.

Referral Health Facility

- Emergency triage assessment and treatment (ETAT)
- Diagnosis, treatment and monitoring of patient progress.

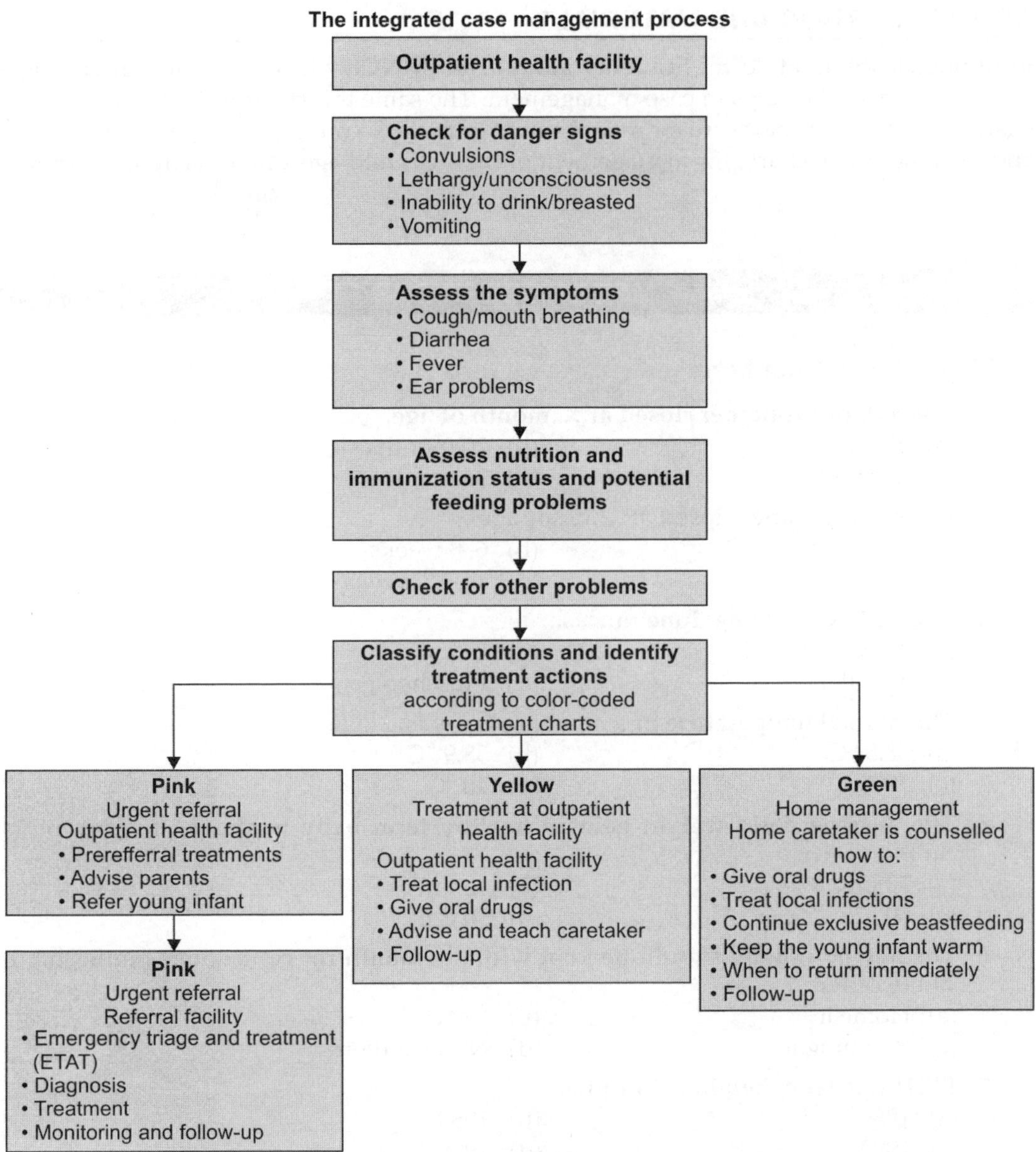

Fig. 2.38: IMNCI case management in the outpatient health facility, first-level referral facility and at home for the sick child from age 2 months up to 5 years

Appropriate Home Management

- Teaching mothers or other caretakers how to give oral drugs and treat local infections at home

Counselling mothers or other caretakers about food (feeding recommendations, feeding problems).

COURSE METHOD AND MATERIALS

In addition to this module, the **Students' module for IMNCI,** you will receive a chart booklet that summarizes the steps in case management. The same information is shown on 5 wall charts. The first two charts are for management of the sick young infant age up to 2 months and the other three charts for management of the sick child age 2 months up to 5 years.

MODEL QUESTIONS

Multiple Choice Questions

1. **The anterior fontanel closed at.....month of age.**
   (a) 18 months (b) 20 months
   (c) 24 months (d) 26 months
2. **Posterior fontanel closed at ....of age.**
   (a) 1–2 weeks (b) 6–8 weeks
   (c) 10–12 weeks (d) 14–18 weeks
3. **The APGAR scoring done in.........**
   (a) Newborn (b) Infant
   (c) Toddler (d) Preschooler
4. **The normal temperature of a newborn baby is...**
   (a) 36.5 °C (b) 38.9 °C
   (c) 39 °C (d) 40 °C
5. **The average daily weight gain in healthy term baby is about ....../day in 1st month of life.**
   (a) 10 gm (b) 30 gm
   (c) 60 gm (d) 90 gm
6. **The newborn baby should be kept with the month for continuous mothering in home called...**
   (a) Home in (b) KMC
   (c) Rooming in (d) None of them
7. **BFHI was launched in.... in India.**
   (a) 1986 (b) 1989
   (c) 1992 (d) 1995
8. **BFHI promote support for the...**
   (a) Breastfeeding (b) Meal
   (c) Education for children (d) All of these
9. **Oral thrush caused by..........**
   (a) Candida albicans (b) Streptococcus
   (c) Both (a) and (b) (d) None of them

10. **Umbilical sepsis also called ....**
    (a) Sepsis (b) Omphalocele
    (c) Omphalitis (d) None of them
11. **Early onset of neonatal sepsis caused before .... of life.**
    (a) 24 hours (b) 72 hours
    (c) 80 hours (d) 100 hours
12. **Facial palsy is also known as ....**
    (a) Poor reflex (b) Brachial palsy
    (c) Bells palsy (d) None of them
13. **Neonatal jaundice is also termed as ....**
    (a) Icterus neonatorum (b) Bilirubin
    (c) Both (a) and (b) (d) None of these
14. **Rh negative mother, who carrying an Rh positive fetus caused...**
    (a) Erythroblastosis fetalis (b) Erythema
    (c) Pyoderma (d) Hypoxia
15. **Small for dates also called ...**
    (a) Newborn (b) LBW
    (c) Infant (d) IUGR
16. **LBW is baby whose birth weight less then ....**
    (a) 3.5 kg (b) 2.5 kg
    (c) 1.5 kg (d) 1 kg
17. **Preterm neonates are born before ...... weeks.**
    (a) 37 (b) 39
    (c) 40 (d) 42
18. **The cause of preterm birth is ....**
    (a) Multipregnancy (b) Eclampsia
    (c) Antepartum hemorrhage (d) All of the above
19. **Except these one is not a characteristic of preterm infant ....**
    (a) Head larger than body (b) Poor reflex
    (c) Crown heel length is 50 cm (d) Hypothermia
20. **The baby born with a gestational age of ...... weeks called post term baby.**
    (a) 33 (b) 36
    (c) 38 (d) 42

Fill in the Blanks

1. BFHI stands for ....
2. BFHI aims..............................
3. BFHI was launched in India in............year.
4. The period from birth to 28 days of life is called as..................
5. Hyperbilirubinemia also known as ....
6. Level of more than ......mg/dL suspected jaundice in baby.
7. Phototherapy works on three principles that is ....,..............and...........

8. Jaundice occurs within 24 hours of birth is called ....
9. Immediately after birth the neonatal assessment is done by ....scoring.
10. Average length of newborn is ....cm.
11. An infant born before ....weeks of gestation called preterm baby.
12. Small for dates also known as.........
13. The weight of baby less than 2.5 kg called as...................

True or False

1. A hospital that conduct a minimum of 150 deliveries can seek the recognition for BFHI.
2. During phototherapy bilirubin absorb light maximally in the range of 420–500 nm.
3. Physiological jaundice develops within 24 hours of birth.
4. Vitamin B is administered at birth to prevent the potential problem of bleeding.
5. Any infant whose birth weight is less than 2500 gm is known as preterm baby.
6. Any neonate born between the age of 37–42 weeks of gestation is known as term baby.
7. Cephalohematoma is the collection of blood in between the periosteum and the flat bone of the skull.
8. Normal body temperature of the newborn is 36.5–37.5 °C.
9. Phototherapy use to treat low birth weight baby.
10. Newborn may lose heat to the environment by conduction, convention, radiation and evaporation.

Short Answer Questions

1. Difference between pathological and physiological jaundice.
2. Phototherapy.
3. Neonatal hypoglycemia.
4. Birth injuries.
5. Low birth weight.
6. Nursing care of newborn baby.
7. BFHI.

Long Answer Questions

1. (a) Define low birth weight. 2
   (b) Write the etiological and classification of low birth weight baby. 5
   (c) Write nursing management of low birth weight baby. 8
2. (a) Define hypothermia. 2
   (b) Write details about prevention and management of hypothermia. 13

ANSWER KEY

Multiple Choice Questions

1. (a)	2. (b)	3. (a)	4. (a)	5. (b)	6. (c)	7. (c)
8. (a)	9. (a)	10. (c)	11. (b)	12. (c)	13. (a)	14. (a)
15. (d)	16. (b)	17. (a)	18. (d)	19. (c)	20. (d)	

Fill in the Blanks

1. Baby friendly hospital initiative.
2. Breastfeeding.
3. 1992.
4. Newborn.
5. Icterus neonatorum.
6. 5 mg/dL
7. Geometric photoisomerization, structural isomerization and oxidation.
8. Icterus jaundice.
9. APGAR.
10. 45–50 cm
11. 37 weeks
12. IUGR
13. LBW

True or False

1. False	2. True	3. False	4. False	5. False	6. True	7. False
8. True	9. False	10. True				

Chapter 3

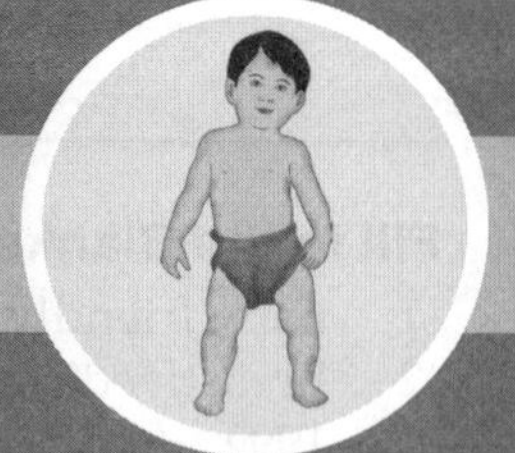

The Healthy Child (Growth and Development)

- **Growth and Development**
  - Principles of Growth and Development
  - Factors Affecting Child Growth and Development
  - The Normal Newborn Reflex
  - Technique of Developmental Assessment
  - Plotting of Growth Chart
- **The Normal Growth and Development of Infant**
  - Breastfeeding and Weaning
  - Immunization
  - The Cold Chain Equipment
- **The Normal Growth and Development of Toddler**
  - Nutritional Counseling
  - Toilet Training and Safety
  - Prevention of Accidents
  - Play Therapy
- **The Normal Growth and Development of Preschoolers**
  - Psychosocial/Emotional
  - Day Care Centers
  - Role of Parents in Sex Education
- **The Normal Growth and Development of School Children (6–12 years)**
  - Growth and Development
  - Rest and Sleep, Physical Exercises and Activity, Dental Health
- **The Normal Growth and Development of Pubescent and Adolescent**
  - Menstrual Hygiene Management
  - Role of Parents in Health Promotion of Adolescents
  - Control of Iron Deficiency Anemia (WIFS Guidelines)

GROWTH AND DEVELOPMENT

Introduction

The child growth and development is refers to the physiological, psychological and emotional changes that occur in child developmental stage between birth to adolescence, as the individual progresses from dependency to independency. It is a continuous process with a predictable sequence yet having a unique course for every child life. The optimal growth and development of children is considered vital to society and so it is important to understand the social, cognitive, emotional, and educational development of children.

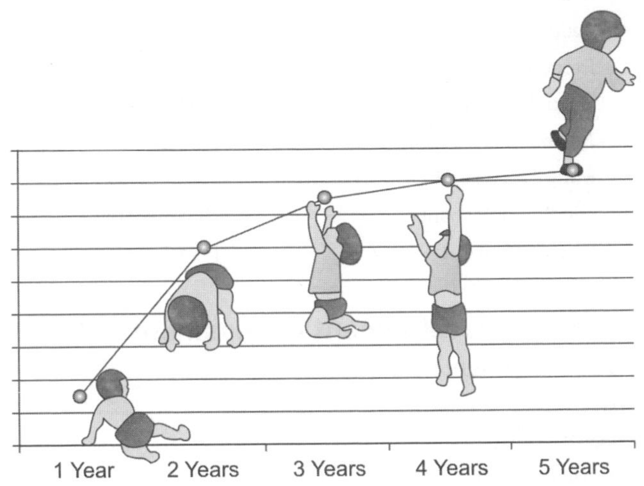

Definition

Definition of Growth

Growth refers to an increase in physical size of the whole or any of its parts and heights can be measured in inches or centimeters and weight measured by pounds or kilograms.

—Marlow

Definition of Development

Development refers to a progressive increase in skill and capacity to function. It causes a qualitative change in the child's functioning. Maturation produces an increase in competence, an ability to function at a higher level depending on the child's heredity.

—Marlow

Definition of Growth and Development

Growth is the progressive increase in the size of a child or parts of a child. Development is progressive acquisition of various skills (abilities) such as head support, speaking, learning, expressing the feelings and relating with other people. Growth and development go together but at different rates.

Stage of Growth and Developmental

S. No.	State	Time period
Prenatal period		
1	Ovum	0–14 days (after conception)
2	Embryo	14 days–8 weeks
3	Fetus	8 weeks–birth (8–40 weeks)
Postnatal period		
1	Newborn	Birth—28 Days
2	Infant	1–12 month
3	Toddler	1–3 years
4	Preschooler	3–5 years
5	School-aged child	6–12 years
6	Adolescent	13–18 years
	Early Adolescent	12–14 years
	Middle Adolescent	15–16 years
	Late Adolescent	17–18 years

Parameters of Growth and Development Assessment of Child

- Physical/biological development
- Motor development
  - Fine motor development
  - Gross motor development
- Sensory development
- Psychosocial development
- Psychosexual development
- Spiritual development
- Intellectual/cognitive development
- Moral development
- Language development
- Play stimulation.

Biological/Physiological Growth

Physical growth refers to an increase in body size (length or height and weight) and in the size of organs. From birth to about age 1 or 2 years, children grow rapidly. After this time, growth slows.

As growth slows, children need fewer calories and parents may notice a decrease in appetite. Two-year-old children can have very erratic eating habits that sometimes make parents anxious. Some children may seem to eat virtually nothing yet continue to grow and thrive. Actually, they eat little one day and then make up for it by eating more the next day.

The National Center for Health Statistics (NCHS) made a massive survey of characteristics of growth, namely length or stature. The children studied were a cross section of cultural, racial, and socioeconomic groups; therefore the findings do not describe any one group.

Length or Height

The pubescent spurt is the only exception to this downward trend in the rate of growth. The yearly increases in stature among children of the same age vary greatly.. The periods of most rapid growth are infancy and puberty.

Weight

Weight is influenced by all the increments in size and is probably the best gross index of nutrition and health. Normal limits vary widely for each year of childhood. Excess weight in relation to the height and pelvic diameter is as abnormal as being underweight. Obesity may result from a glandular deficiency, but it is more likely due to overeating, to a diet containing too much starch and fat and too little protein, or to lack of exercise.

Head Circumference

The circumference of the head is an important measurement since it is related to intracranial volume. An increase in circumference permits an estimation of the rate of brain growth. This measurement has a relatively narrow normal range for a particular age group.

Chest Diameter

The chest measurements increase as the child grows and the shape of the chest changes. At birth the transverse and anterioposterior diameters are nearly equal. The transverse diameter increases more rapidly than does enter posterior diameter—that is, the width becomes greater than the depth.

Abdominal and Pelvic Measurements

The abdominal circumference is not fixed by a bony cage as is the chest; consequently, it is affected by the infant's nutritional state, muscle tone, gaseous distention, and even the phase of respiration.

The pelvic bicristal diameter (the maximal distance between the external margins of the iliac crests) is not affected by variations in posture and musculature and is a good index of a child's slenderness or stockiness.

Physical growth in stature and weight occurs over the 15–20 years following birth, as the individual changes from the average weight of 7½ pounds and length of 20' at full-term birth to full adult size. As stature and weight increase, the individual's proportions also change, from the relatively large head and small torso and limbs of the neonate, to the adult's relatively small head and long torso and limbs.

Mechanisms of Developmental Change

Genetic factors play a major role in determining the growth rate, and particularly the changes in proportion characteristic of early human development.

However, genetic factors can produce the maximum growth only if environmental conditions are adequate. Poor nutrition and frequent injury and disease can reduce the individual's adult stature, but the best environment cannot cause growth to a greater stature than is determined by heredity.

Motor Development

Abilities for physical movement change through childhood from the largely reflexive (unlearned, involuntary) movement patterns of the young infant to the highly skilled voluntary movement's characteristic of later childhood and adolescence of course, older children and adolescents retain some reflex movements in addition to developing voluntary movement. Proceeds to pulling to stand, 'cruising' while holding on to an object, walking while holding an adult's hand, and finally walking independently.

All the older children continue the sequence by walking sideways or backward, galloping, hopping, skipping with one foot and walking with the other, and finally skipping. By middle childhood and adolescence, new motor skill is acquired by instruction or observation rather than in a predictable sequence.

Gross motor development describes the acquisition of increasing mobility and independent locomotion; it precedes fine motor activities. Gross motor activities include turning, reaching, sitting, standing and walking.

Fine motor development evolves as the reflexes give way to the acquisition of motor, dexterity. As the neural tract matures, reflexes disappear and are replaced by purposeful activities.

Mechanisms of Motor Development

The mechanisms involved in motor development involve some genetic components that determine the physical size of body parts at a given age, as well as aspects of muscle and bone strength. Nutrition and exercise also determine strength and therefore the ease and accuracy with which a body part can be moved.

An opportunities to carry out movements help establish the abilities to flex (move toward the trunk) and extend body parts, both capacities being needed for good motor ability. Skilled voluntary movements develop as a result of practice and learning.

Cognitive/Intellectual Development

The capacity to learn, remember, and symbolize information, and to solve problems, exists at a simple level in young infants, who can perform cognitive tasks such as discriminating animate and inanimate beings or recognizing small numbers of objects.

During childhood, learning and information-processing increase in speed, memory becomes increasingly longer, and symbol use and the capacity for abstraction develop until a near-adult level is reached by adolescence.

Mechanisms of Cognitive Development

Cognitive development has genetic and other biological mechanisms, as is seen in the many genetic causes of mental retardation. However, although it is assumed that brain functions cause cognitive events, it has not been possible to measure specific brain changes and show that they cause cognitive change.

Developmental advances in cognition are also related to experience and learning and this is particularly the case for higher-level abilities like abstraction, which depend to a considerable extension on formal education.

Social-emotional Development

New infants do not seem to experience fear or have preferences for contact with any specific people. By about 8–10 months, they go through a fairly rapid change and become fearful of perceived threats; they also begin to prefer familiar people and show anxiety and distress when separated from them or approached by strangers.

The capacity for empathy and the understanding of social rules begin in the preschool period and continue to develop into adulthood. Middle childhood is characterized by friendships with age-mates and adolescence by emotions connected with sexuality and the beginnings of romantic love. Anger seems most intense during the toddler and early preschool period and during adolescence.

Mechanisms of Social-emotional Development

Genetic factors appear to regulate some social-emotional developments that occur at predictable ages, such as fearfulness and attachment to familiar people. Experience plays a role in determining which people are familiar, which social rules are obeyed, and how anger is expressed.

Sexual Development

The development of a child's sexuality after birth is influenced by development in the sexuality after birth is influenced by development in the physical, mental, emotional, and sociocultural areas of living.

Sigmund Freud Psychosexual Development

Prior to the work of Sigmund Freud, a medical doctor in the late 19th century, there was little understanding or acceptance of childhood sexuality. Counter to current thought, Freud believed that sexual feelings do not suddenly emerge during puberty and adolescence. They are present from infancy, he wrote and gradually changes from one form or state to another until adult sexual life is achieved. Psychoanalytic Freudian theory with its stages of psychosexual development (the oral, and phallic, and genital stages) has greatly influenced modern psychiatric thinking. In each stage, instinctual sexual energy (libido) is invested in different biologic areas of the body. These areas determine how the child interacts with other people. Freud's phases of psychosexual development center almost exclusively on the early years of life and include the following:

- **The Oral Stage** (roughly, the period of infancy, the first year of life): During this period, the oral region, or the sensory area of the mouth, provides the greatest sensual satisfaction for the infant.
- **The Anal Stage** (roughly, the toddler period, the second and third years of life): The greatest amount of sensual pleasure for the toddler is obtained from the anal and urethral areas.
- **The Phallic Stage** (roughly, the preschool period—the end of the third year and the fourth and fifth years of life): The site of greatest sensual pleasure is the genital region.

The Oedipal stage occurs in the later part of the phallic period. During this stage the child 'loves' the parent of the opposite sex as the provider of sensual satisfaction. The parent of the same sex is considered to be a rival.

- **The Latency Stage** (roughly, the school-age period from the sixth to twelfth years of life): At the beginning of the latency stage the child has resolved or is resolving the oedipal conflict. During the latency period, children form close relationships with others of their own age and sex.
- **The Pubescent Stage and Adolescence** (roughly, 12 years of age to adulthood): During puberty, secondary sexual characteristics appear in both sexes. The same psychosexual conflicts that occurred during the oedipal period are revived. If children resolve the conflicts they are free to enter into heterosexual relationships as adults.

Language Development

There are four main areas in which the child must attain competence, regardless of the language or dialect spoken. These are referred to as phonology or sounds, semantics or the encoded meanings, syntax or the way in which words are combined and pragmatics or knowledge of how language is used in different contexts.

Mechanisms of Language Development

Although the role of discourse is important in facilitating the child's learning, there is considerable disagreement amongst theorists about the extent to which children's early meanings and expressive words arises directly from adult input as opposed to intrinsic factors relating to the child's cognitive functions. Findings about the initial mapping of new words, the ability to decontextualise words and refine meaning are diverse.

One hypothesis is known as the syntactic bootstrapping hypothesis, referring to the child's ability to infer meaning from cues, using grammatical information from the structure of sentences. Another is the multi-route model in which it is argued that context-bound words and referential words follow different routes; the first being mapped onto event representations and the latter onto mental representations.

In this model, although parental input has a critical role, children rely on cognitive processing to establish subsequent use of words. However, naturalistic research on language development has indicated that preschoolers' vocabularies are strongly associated with the number of words addressed to them by adults.

Theories of Growth and Development

- Ecological systems theory
- Piaget theory
- Vygotsky theory
- Attachment theory
- Erik Erikson theory
- Behavioral theories
- Other theories.

Ecological Systems Theory

It also called 'development in context' or 'human ecology' theory, ecological systems theory, originally formulated by Urie Bronfenbrenner specifies four types of nested environmental systems, with bi-directional influences within and between the systems.

The four systems are:

1. Micro-system
2. Meso-system
3. Exo-system
4. Macro-system.

The Ecology of Human Development has had widespread influence on the way psychologists and others approach the study of human beings and their environments. As a result of this influential conceptualization of development, these environments from the family to economic and political structure have come to be viewed as part of the life course from childhood through adulthood.

Piaget Theory

Jean Piaget was a Swiss scholar who began his studies in intellectual development in the 1920s. Piaget's first interests were those that dealt with the ways in which animals adapt to their environments and his first scientific article about this subject was published when he was 10 years old. As he carried out this intelligence testing, he began developing a profound interest in the way children's intellectualism works.

As a result, he developed his own laboratory and spent years recording children's intellectual growth and attempted to find out how children develop through various stages of thinking.

This led to Piaget develop four important stages of cognitive development:

1. Sensorimotor stage (Birth to Age 2)
2. Preoperational stage (Age 2 to 7)
3. Concrete-operational stage (Age 7 to 12)
4. Formal-operational stage (Age 11 to 14).

Piaget Stages

Sensorimotor: (Birth to age 2)

According to Piaget, when an infant reaches about 7–9 months of age they begin to develop what he called object permanence, this means the child now has the ability to understand that objects keep existing even when they cannot be seen. An example of this would be hiding the child's favorite toy under a blanket, although the child cannot physically see it they still know to look under the blanket.

Preoperational: (age 2 to 7)

During this stage of development, young children begin analyzing their environment using mental symbols. These symbols often include words and images and the child will begin to apply these various symbols in their everyday lives as they come across different objects, events, and situations.

However, Piaget's main focus on this stage and the reason why he named it 'preoperational' is because children at this point are not able to apply specific cognitive operations, such as mental math. In addition to symbolism, children now begin engaging in pretend play where they begin pretending to be people they are not (teachers, superhero's), and they may use different props to make this pretend play more real.

Some deficiencies in this stage of development are that children who are about 3–4 years old often display what is called egocentrism, which means the child is not able to see someone else's point of view, they feel as if every other person is experiencing the same events and feelings that they are experiencing. However, about at seven thought processes of children are no longer egocentric and are more intuitive, meaning they now think about the way something looks instead of rational thinking.

Concrete-operational Stage (ages 7 to 12)

During this stage, children begin developing cognitive operations and begin applying this new thinking to different events they may encounter. Unlike the preoperational stage, children can now change and rearrange mental images and symbols to form a logical thought; an example of this is reversibility in which the child now has the ability to reverse an action just by doing the opposite.

Formal-operational Stage (ages 11 to 14)

The final stage of Piaget's cognitive development defines a child as now having the ability to 'think more rationally and systematically about abstract concepts and hypothetical events'. Some positive aspects during this time is that child or adolescent begins forming their identity and begin understanding why people behave the way they behave.

A personal fable is when the adolescent feels that he or she is unique person and everything they do is unique. They feel as if they are the only ones that have ever experienced what they are experiencing and that they are invincible and nothing bad will happen to them it will only happen to others.

Vygotsky Theory

Vygotsky was a Russian theorist, who proposed the sociocultural theory. During the 1920s–1930s while Piaget was developing his own theory, Vygotsky was an active scholar and at that time his theory was said to be 'recent' because it was translated out of Russian language and began influencing Western thinking.

This technique is called 'scaffolding,' because it builds upon knowledge children already have with new knowledge that adults can help the child learn. An example of this might be when a parent 'helps' an infant clap or roll her hands to the pat-a-cake rhyme, until she can clap and roll her hands herself.

Attachment Theory

Attachment theory, originating in the work of John Bowlby's and developed by Mary Ainsworth, is a psychological, evolutionary and ethological theory that provides a descriptive and explanatory framework for understanding interpersonal relationships between human beings.

Bowlby's observations of close attachments led him to believe that close emotional bonds or 'attachments' between an infant and their primary caregiver is an important requirement that is necessary to form 'normal social and emotional development'.

Erik Erikson Theory

Erikson, a follower of Freud's, synthesized both Freud's and his own theories to create what is known as the 'psychosocial' stages of human development, which span from birth to death, and focuses on 'tasks' at each stage that must be accomplished to successfully navigate life's challenges.

Erikson's eight stages consist of the following:

1. Trust vs mistrust (infant)
2. Autonomy vs shame (toddlerhood)
3. Initiative vs guilt (preschooler)
4. Industry vs inferiority (young adolescent)
5. Identity vs role confusion (adolescent)
6. Intimacy vs isolation (young adulthood)
7. Generativity vs stagnation (middle adulthood)
8. Ego integrity vs despair (old age).

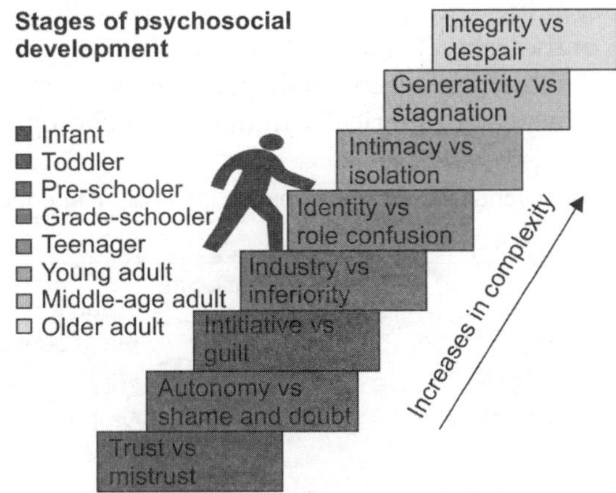

Fig. 3.1: According to Erikson's stages of psychosocial development

Behavioral Theories

John B Watson's behaviorism theory forms the foundation of the behavioral model of development 1925. He wrote extensively on child development and conducted research. Watson also helped bring a natural science perspective to child psychology by introducing objective research methods based on observable and measurable behavior.

Following Watson's lead, BF Skinner further extended this model to cover operant conditioning and verbal behavior. Skinner used the operant chamber, or Skinner box, to observe the behavior of small organisms in a controlled situation and proved that organisms' behaviors are impacted on the environment. Furthermore, he used reinforcement and punishment to shape in desired behavior.

Other Theories

- In accordance with his view that the sexual drive is a basic human motivation, Sigmund Freud developed a psychosexual theory of human development from infancy onward, divided into five stages. Each stage centered on the gratification of the libido within a particular area, or erogenous zone, of the body.
- He also argued that as humans develop, they become fixated on different and specific objects through their stages of development. Each stage contains conflict which requires resolution to enable the child to develop.
- The use of dynamical systems theory as a framework for the consideration of development began in the early 1990s and has continued into the present century.
- Dynamic systems theory stresses nonlinear connections (e.g. between earlier and later social assertiveness) and the capacity of a system to reorganize as a phase shift that is stage-like in nature.
- Dynamic systems theory has been applied extensively to the study of motor development; the theory also has strong associations with some of Bowlby's views about attachment systems. Dynamic systems theory also relates to the concept of the transactional process, a mutually interactive process in which children and parents simultaneously influence each other, producing developmental change in both over time.
- The 'core knowledge perspective' is an evolutionary theory in child development that proposes 'infants begin life with innate, special-purpose knowledge systems referred to as core domains of thought'. There are five core domains of thought, each of which is crucial for survival, which simultaneously prepare us to develop key aspects of early cognition; they are: physical, numerical, linguistic, psychological, and biological.

Table 3.1: Stages of psychosocial, psychosexual, intellectual and moral development

Stage	Age	Tasks	Erikson's psychosocial stages negative counterpart	Freud's psychosexual stages	Significant persons
Infancy	0–12 month	Sense of trust	Mistrust	Oral	Maternal person or substitute
Toddler	1–3 years	Sense of autonomy	Shame and doubt	Anal	Parental persons
Preschool	3–6 years	Sense of initiative	Guilt	Phallic	Basic family
School	6–12 years	Sense of industry	Inferiority	Latency	Neighborhood, school
Early adolescence	Above–12 years	Sense of identity	Identity diffusion	Puberty	Peer groups and out groups, models of leadership
Late adolescence and young adult	16–18 years	Sense of intimacy and solidarity	Isolation	Geniality	Partners in friendship, sex, competition, cooperation

PRINCIPLES OF GROWTH AND DEVELOPMENT

Introduction

There is a set of principles that characterizes the pattern and process of growth and development. These principles or characteristics describe typical development as a predictable and orderly process; that is, we can predict how most children will develop and that they will develop at the same rate and at about the same time as other children.

Although there are individual differences in children's personalities, activity levels, and timing of developmental milestones, such as ages and stages, the principles and characteristics of development are universal patterns.

Principles of Development

Development Proceeds from the Head Downward. This is Called the Cephalocaudal Principle

This principle describes the direction of growth and development. According to this principle, the child gains control of the head first, then the arms, and then the legs. Infants develop control of the head and face movements within the first two months after birth.

In the next few months, they are able to lift themselves up by using their arms. By 6 to 12 months of age, infants start to gain leg control and may be able to crawl, stand, or walk. Coordination of arms always precedes coordination of legs.

Development Proceeds from the Center of the Body Outward

This is the principle of proximodistal development that also describes the direction of development. This means that the spinal cord develops before outer parts of the body. The child's arms develop before the hands and the hands and feet develop before the fingers and toes. Finger and toe muscles (used in fine motor dexterity) are the last to develop in physical development.

Development Depends on Maturation and Learning

The child maturation refers to the sequential characteristic of biological growth and development. The biological changes occur in sequential order and give children new abilities. Changes in the brain and nervous system account largely for maturation.

These changes in the brain and nervous system help children to improve in thinking (cognitive) and motor (physical) skills. Also, children must mature to a certain point before they can progress to new skills (Readiness). For example, a four-month-old cannot use language because the infant's brain has not matured enough to allow the child to talk. By two years old, the brain has developed further and with help from others, the child will have the capacity to say and understand words. Also, a child cannot write or draw until he has developed the motor control to hold a pencil or crayon. Maturational patterns are innate, that is, genetically programmed.

The child's environment and the learning that occurs as a result of the child's experiences largely determine whether the child will reach optimal development. A stimulating environment and varied experiences allow a child to develop to his or her potential.

Development Proceeds from the Simple (Concrete) to the More Complex

Children use their cognitive and language skills to reason and solve problems. For example, learning relationships between things (how things are similar), or classification, is an important ability in cognitive development.

The cognitive process of learning how an apple and orange are alike begins with the most simplistic or concrete thought of describing the two. Seeing no relationship, a preschool child will describe the objects according to some property of the object, such as color. Such a response would be, 'An apple is red (or green) and an orange is orange.'

The first level of thinking about how objects are alike is to give a description or functional relationship (both concrete thoughts) between the two objects. 'An apple and orange are round' and 'An apple and orange are alike because you eat them' are typical responses of three, four and five year olds.

As children develop further in cognitive skills, they are able to understand a higher and more complex relationship between objects and things; that is, that an apple and orange exist in a class called fruit. The child cognitively is then capable of classification.

Growth and Development is a Continuous Process

- As a child develops, he or she adds to the skills already acquired and the new skills become the basis for further achievement and mastery of skills.
- Most children follow a similar pattern. Also, one stage of development lays the foundation for the next stage of development.

  For example, in motor development, there is a predictable sequence of developments that occur before walking.
- The infant lifts and turns the head before he or she can turn over.
- Infants can move their limbs (arms and legs) before grasping an object. Mastery of climbing stairs involves increasing skills from holding on to walking alone.
- By the age of four, most children can walk up and down stairs with alternating feet. As in maturation, in order for children to write or draw, they must have developed the manual (hand) control to hold a pencil and crayon.

Growth and Development Proceed from the General to Specific

In motor development, the infant will be able to grasp an object with the whole hand before using only the thumb and forefinger.

The infant's first motor movements are very generalized, undirected, and reflexive, waving arms or kicking before being able to reach or creep toward an object. Growth occurs from large muscle movements to more refined (smaller) muscle movements.

There are Individual Rates of Growth and Development

- Each child is different and the rates at which individual children grow is different. Although the patterns and sequences for growth and development are usually the same for all children, the rates at which individual children reach developmental stages will be different.
- Understanding this fact of individual differences in rates of development should cause us to be careful about using and relying on age and stage characteristics to describe or label children.

- There is a range of ages for any developmental task to take place. This dismisses the notion of the 'average child'. Some children will walk at ten months while others walk a few months older at eighteen months of age. Some children are more active while others are more passive.
- This does not mean that the passive child will be less intelligent as an adult.
- There is no validity to comparing one child's progress with or against another child. Rates of development also are not uniform within an individual child.
- *For example,* a child's intellectual development may progress faster than his emotional or social development. An understanding of the principles of development helps us to plan appropriate activities and stimulating and enriching experiences for children, and provides a basis for understanding how to encourage and support young children's learning.

Nurses Notes

- Growth and development are continuous, orderly, sequential processes influenced by maturational, environmental, and genetic factors.
- All humans follow the same pattern of growth and development.
- The sequence of each stage is predictable, although the time of onset, the length of the stage, and the effects of each stage vary with the person.
- Learning can either help or hinder the maturational process, depending of what is learned.
- Each developmental stage has its own characteristics. For example, Piaget suggests that in the sensorimotor stage (birth to 2 years) children learn to coordinate simple motor tasks.
- Growth and development occur in the *cephalocaudal direction* that is, starting at the head and moving to the trunk, the legs, and the feet. This pattern is particularly obvious at birth, when the head of the infant is disproportionately large.
- Growth and development occur in the *proximal to distal direction* that is from the center of the body outward. For example, infants can roll over before they can grasp and object with the thumb and second finger. Development proceeds from *simple to complex* or from single acts to integrated acts. To accomplish the integrated act of drinking and swallowing from a cup, for example, the child must first learn a series of single acts: eye-hand coordination, grasping, hand-mouth coordination, controlled tipping of the cup, and then mouth, lip, and tongue movements to drink and swallow.
- Development becomes increasingly differentiated. Differentiated development begins with a generalized response and progresses to a skilled specific response (e.g. an infant's initial response to a stimulus involves the total body; a 5-year-old child can respond more specifically with laughter or fear).
- Certain stages of growth and development are more critical than others. It is known, for example, that the first 10 to 12 weeks after conception are critical. The incidence of congenital anomalies as a result of exposure to certain viruses, chemicals, or drugs is greater during this stage than others
- The pace of growth and development is uneven. It is known that growth is greater during infancy than during childhood. Asynchronous development is demonstrated by rapid growth of the head during infancy and the extremities at puberty.

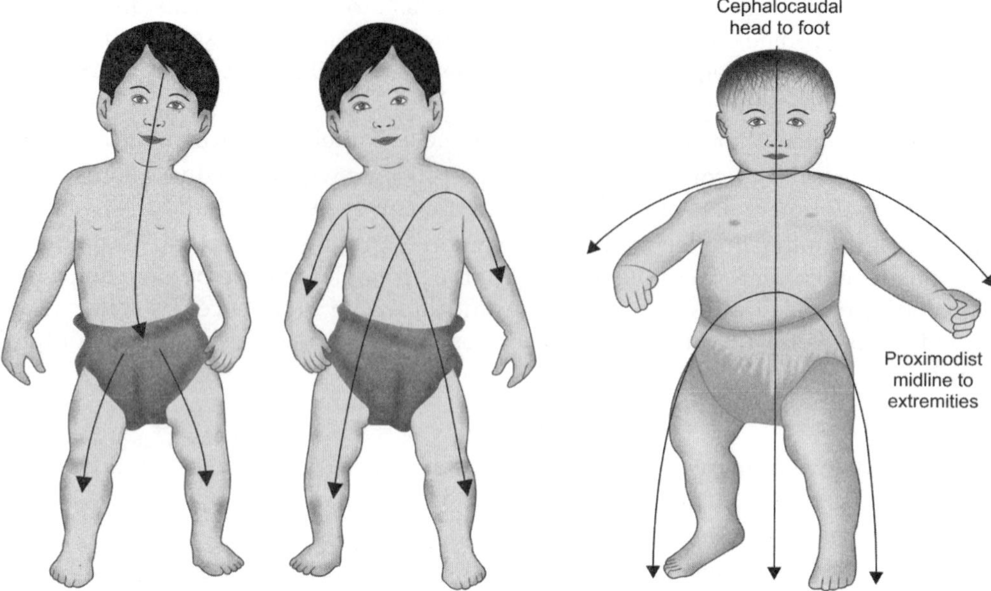

The process of cephalocaudal direction from head down to tail. This means that improvement in structure and function come first in the head region, then in the trunk, and last in the leg region.

Fig. 3.2: Cephalocaudal direction

The process in proximodistal from center or midline to periphery direction. Development proceeds from near to far outward from central axis of the body toward the extremities.

Fig. 3.3: Proximodistal direction

FACTORS AFFECTING CHILD GROWTH AND DEVELOPMENT

Child development can be negatively influenced by a number of risk factors, many of which have been studied in developing countries. They can be broadly grouped under two headings.

1. Hereditary factors
2. Environmental factors.

Prenatal Environment

- Factors related to mothers during pregnancy
  - Nutritional deficiencies
  - Diabetic mother
  - Exposure to radiation
  - Infection with German measles
  - Smoking
  - Use of drugs.

- Factors related to fetus
  - Malposition in uterus
  - Faulty placental implantation.

Postnatal Environment

- External environment
  - Socioeconomic status of the family
  - Child's nutrition
  - Climate and season
  - Child's ordinal position in the family
  - Number of siblings in the family
  - Family structure (single parent or extended family, etc.).
- Internal environment
  - Child's intelligence
  - Hormonal influences
  - Emotions.

Factors Influencing Growth and Development

Growth and development depend on not one but a combination of many factors, all interdependent. The relatively typical pattern of growth and development is influenced by heredity and environment. As will be seen throughout this discussion, heredity determines the extent of growth and development that is possible, but environment determines the degree to which the potential is achieved.

Heredity

- The heredity of a man and a woman determines that of their children. For this reason, the health history of several generations of the families of each of the parents is studied to determine the hereditary traits likely to exist in the child.
- Embryonic life begins with the cytoplasm and the nucleus of the fertilized ovum, genetically determined by both parents.
- Members of families bear physical resemblances to each other, and a high degree of correlation of stature with weight among siblings exists.
- The rate of growth is more alike among siblings than among unrelated persons. Some children are small not because of endocrine or nutritional disturbances but because of their genetic constitution. Before the largeness or smallness of a child is evaluated, the size of the parents should first be observed.

Sex

- Sex is determined at conception. After birth, the male infant is both longer and heavier than the female infant. Boys maintain this superiority until about 11 years of age.
- Girls mature earlier, reach the period of accelerated growth earlier than boys, and are then taller on the average.
- During the prepubertal spurt of growth and thereafter, boys are again taller than girls. Bone development is more advanced in girls than in boys, as shown in roentgenograms of the wrists of infants and young children.

- Advance in osseous development is also demonstrated by the earlier eruption of the permanent teeth in girls.
- The sex of children determines not only their physical attributes and patterns of growth but also the manner in which others react to them. In all cultural groups, family and friends have different attitudes toward and expectations of a child, dependent on the child's gender.

Racial and National Characteristics

Race

Distinguishing characteristics called racial or subracial developed in prehistoric humans. As to height, tall and short examples exist among all races and subraces. Among civilized groups, intermarriage has produced mixed racial types.

Nationality

- Most of them thought about physical characteristics of national groups because the inhabitants of the various nations of Europe tend to be made up of homogeneous subracial groups with specific characteristics.
- Thus we expect children whose forebears and came from the Scandinavian countries to be larger and those of Sicilian ancestry to be smaller than the average American. Yet in America there has been so much intermingling of subracial groups that children with all the typical physical characteristics of any national groups are seldom seen.
- In studying changing characteristics of the American people, one must consider the influence of immigration. Immigrants frequently established themselves in the United States under conditions of extreme poverty.
- Their descendants of the second and third generations make-up the majority of the middle and upper classes, and the lower-income group is now made-up of more recent immigrants.
- Many of the recent immigrant arrivals in the United States are descendants of families in whom short stature is the norm. Even with the influence of good nutrition and environment, these children may not achieve the same height as their peer because of the differences is growth patterns.

Environmental Factors

- Although each human being at birth has a gene-determined physical, mental, and biochemical potential, this potential may not be reached because of the influence of the environment are so interrelated that they are practically inseparable.
- One example of the influence of environment upon potential height is found among the first and second generations of Japanese people in the United States. The children are generally taller than their parents because they had the advantages of better food and better living conditions.
- Another example is the children of Third World countries whose growth and development have been stunted by drought and famine. As food becomes available, many of these children show marked improvement in their physical condition.

Prenatal Environment

Prenatal conditions are part of the environmental climate in which the child develops and should not be forgotten in considering actual development in relation to probable optimal development.

The influence of the intrauterine environment on the child's future development is great, particularly since the uterus shields the fetus from the full impact of external adverse conditions. It is also true that the intrauterine environment itself may be substandard. In such a case, if the fetus has reached the stage of viability, early delivery may make it possible to improve the infant's environment.

Harmful Prenatal Factors

- The fetus may suffer from nutritional deficiencies when the mother's diet is insufficient in quantity or quality, regardless of her socioeconomic standing. Mechanical problems may be present owing to malposition in uterus.
- The mother may suffer from metabolic endocrine disturbances, such as diabetes mellitus, which affect the fetus. If it is necessary for the mother to undergo radiation for cancer or other conditions, the infant may be affected by the treatment.
- The mother may suffer from an infectious disease during gestation. Rubella (German measles) during the first trimester of pregnancy may lead to abnormal development of the fetus. Other infectious diseases may also affect the fetus, but there is less scientific proof of this.
- Toxoplasmosis, syphilis, and herpes during the second and third trimesters adversely influence the fetus. Erythroblastosis fetal is due to Rh incompatibility of the blood types of the mother and the fetus may have a serious influence upon the developing child.
- Most commonly, faulty placental implantation or malfunction may lead to nutritional impairment or anoxia. Research has shown that smoking or the use by the mother of certain drugs such as alcohol and phenytoin may result in prematurity or deformity of the child. If the mother has had good prenatal care, many of these conditions can be prevented or treated, thus ensuring a better prenatal environment for the fetus.

Postnatal Environment

An environment that provides satisfying experiences promotes growth. Since growth and development are interrelated, growth in one area influences and in turn is influenced by growth in all other areas. The most important external and internal environmental factors are discussed next.

External Environment

Cultural Influences

- Groups of human beings create their own cultures, whereas each individual is influenced or shaped by the culture of which he or she is a part. The culture of a group consists of shared ways of behaving, feeling, and knowing.
- The uniformities found in a group may be considered a set of ideals or norms that regulate or govern the particular and recurring activities within the group.
- These values, beliefs, ideas, and practices provide a basis for understanding how people behave in their man-made environment and how these behaviors are passed on from one generation to the next.

- Culture involves both uniformity and organization for diversity in the behavior of its participants: For instance, pregnancy out of wedlock is not sanctioned by many cultures; however, the cultures do provide for a resolution of the problem when it occurs.
- The effect of a particular culture on a child begins before birth because of the manner in which the culture, views and treats the members of the pregnant woman's family. The nutrients are culturally determined.
- The child learns the language of the family and begins to internalize the ideals, traits, and abstractions of the cultural group of which the family is a part. The behaviors expected of the child at each stage of growth and developments are culturally defined.
- The values learned by children are considered 'right' and will be the guideline for their behavior throughout life. Those individuals who have a different set of values are considered 'different' or 'wrong' in their beliefs.
- In the developed countries, where people of many cultural groups live in relatively close proximity, children have an additional cultural problem.
- *For example,* no matter what language is spoken in the home, school children in the United States are expected to communicate in English.
- They may be taught at home to respect their elders and others in authority, but in school they may observe the lack of fair discipline that leads to disrespect and the abuse of teachers by children. Children thus are caught between the ideals and norms of differing cultures.
- They may have to adjust to the predominating culture, but it is hoped that they do not lose their original cultural identity.

Socioeconomic Status of the Family

The environment of the lower socioeconomic groups may be less favorable than that of the middle and upper groups. Parents in unfortunate financial circumstances are less likely to understand the principles of modern scientific child care; they lack money to buy the essentials of health and diet; and often they are unable, unwilling, or unsure of how to obtain medical care and hospital service.

Nutrition

Nutrition is related to both the quantitative and the qualitative supply of food elements—proteins, fats, carbohydrates, minerals, and vitamins. If these essential nutrients are received in the balanced amounts necessary to sustain life, to allow for energy expenditure, and to promote growth and development, a child is well nourished.

The nutritional needs of a child depend on the age, sex, rate of growth, and level of activity. During periods of rapid growth, such as the prenatal period, infancy, puberty, and adolescence, the need from protein and calories is increased. When the metabolic rate is reduced during periods of slower growth, the protein and caloric requirements are likewise reduced. At any age, the caloric intake must be sufficient to cover both the needs for growth and the expenditure of energy.

The effect of inadequate nutrition is especially apparent when the child is growing rapidly. Utilizing a good diet may be impaired by faulty absorption or assimilation of food substances. Causes of under nutrition include:

- An inadequate nutritional intake, both qualitatively and quantitatively.
- Physical hyperactivity or lack of adequate rest.
- A physical illness that causes an increase in nutritional need but at the same time results in poor appetite and poor food absorption.
- An emotional illness that causes decreased food intake or inadequate absorption because of vomiting or diarrhea.

The nutritional requirements of both well and ill children are discussed below.

Climate and Season

Climatic variations influence the infant's health. This is not an important direct factor in the United States, which lies within the Temperate Zone. Summer heat, however, is important when parents may be unable to provide adequate refrigeration of food and extermination of flies and other insects. Infants in such families are prone to suffer diarrhea with subsequent dehydration.

The seasons of the year influence growth rates in height and weight, especially in older children. Weight gains are lowest in spring and early summer and greatest in late summer and autumn. The greatest gains in height among children in the United States occur in the spring. These differences are probably due to seasonal variations in the activity levels of children.

Deviations from Positive Health

These may be caused by hereditary or congenital conditions, illness, or injury and may result in altered levels of growth and development.

Hereditary or congenital conditions may contribute to growth impairment or to an increase in height. Conditions causing shortened stature include various types of dwarfism, Turner syndrome (gonadal digenesis), and XY Turner phenotype (Noonan syndrome), among others. Examples of conditions causing increases in height above normal include Marfan increases in height above normal include Marfan syndrome (arachnodactyly) and Klinefelter syndrome.

Long-term or chronic illnesses of any type may have an adverse effect on growth and development. Certainly, illnesses like cystic fibrosis or malabsorption syndrome an inability to digest and absorb food, may lead to growth retardation. Long-term illnesses, such as congenital cardiac anomalies or chronic infections that are present during rapid growth periods and critical periods of development, have a temporary or permanent delaying effect on the achievement of normal growth and development.

Exercise

Exercise, by increasing the circulation, promotes physiologic activity and stimulates muscular development; fresh air and moderate sunshine favor health and growth.

Prolonged exposure to sunshine, especially in extremely warm areas such as the southwestern United States, however, may cause tissue damage of the skin and even more serious consequences if the child is unprotected from the rays of the sun.

Ordinal Position in the Family

The behavior of parents toward and their expectations of, each child are different, yet predictable, according to the child's position of the family.

The ordinal position of the child has a bearing on the parent-child relationship and the child-rearing practices that are followed. Although birth order alone does not determine intelligence, personality traits, or methods of coping, it does have a significant influence on all of these.

- The first-born child in a family is an only child and receives all the parental attention until the second child is born.
- The parents of the first-born child are usually inexperienced and may know the successive stages of growth and development their child goes through only from may be overly concerned about care-giving.
- The first-born, therefore, may be raised rigidly and with anxiety. The child develops a more anxious, perfectionist personality than do the later siblings and is more conforming, intelligent, an achievement-oriented. The first-born may learn at an early age to control and organize the behavior of others.
- An only child is likely to develop more rapidly intellectually than are children with siblings, because constant companionship with adults is mentally stimulating. An only child may have higher self-esteem than other children but may be more dependent on others. Motor development may be slow, however, because single children do not have older siblings to lead them to various activities and because so much is done for them. When single children are old enough to do things for themselves, parents and other adults may not permit their activities.
- The middle child (or children) many times gets less attention from the parents than does the first-born, especially if their birthdates are close together. Parents of the middle child are more relaxed about their parental roles and stress to the child the values of responsibility and cooperation with other family members.
- The youngest child in a family tends to be more peer-oriented, less intellectually inclined, and less achievement-oriented than the older siblings. The youngest child receives a great deal of love and attention and therefore tends to develop a good-natured, friendly, warm personality and high self-esteem.
- These generalizations apply to many children; however, each child, whether an only child, first-born, second-born, third-born, or last-born, is different. Children deserve all the parental love and respect they can get as individual members of their families to develop their personalities to the fullest extent possible.

Internal Environment

Intelligence

Intelligence is correlated to some degree with physical development that is, the child of high intelligence is likely to be taller and better developed than is the less gifted child. Also, intelligence influences mental and social development. Children who have inherited superior levels of intelligence may be encouraged by their environments to excel, or such intelligence may be wasted because of lack of stimulation. On the other hand, children who are low levels of intelligence can never excel, no matter how enriched are their environments.

Hormonal Influences

There is evidence that all the hormones in the body affect growth in some manner. Although three hormones—somatotropic hormone, the thyroid hormone, and the hormones that stimulate the gonads—are very important, others also influence growth to an extent.

- *Somatotropic hormone (STH) or growth hormone (GH):* The source of this hormone is in the adenohypophysis, the anterior or glandular portion of the hypothesis cerebri. Somatotropic hormone (STH) is utilized largely during childhood. Its major effect is on linear growth in height, because it is essential in the proliferation of cartilage cells at the epiphyseal plates. The growth hormone stimulates skeletal and protein anabolism through the production of somatomedins or intermediary hormones. An excess of the growth hormone causes gigantism; a lack results in dwarfism.
- *Thyroid hormones:* Thyroxin (T_4) and triiodothyronine (T_3). Thyrotrophic hormone (TH), produced by the adenohypophysis, stimulates the thyroid gland to release triiodothyronine (T_3) and thyroxine (T_4). These thyroid hormones stimulate the general metabolism and therefore are necessary for growth and development after birth.
- *Hormones that stimulate the gonads:* The adrenocorticotropic hormone (ACTH), produced by the adenohypophysis, stimulates the hypothalamus, which in turn causes the adenohypophysis to secrete gonad tropic hormones. The gonadotropic hormones stimulate the interstitial cells of the testes to produce testosterone and the interstitial cells of the ovaries to produce estrogen.

Emotions

Relationships with significant other persons, mother, father, siblings, peers, and teachers, among others, play a vital role in the emotional, social and intellectual development of the child. Initially, the caregiver-mother, substitute, or father has the greatest influence on the child.

This person, usually the mother, meets the infant's basic needs and provides the stimulation necessary for the growing child to learn. After the infant learns to trust the mother, trust is extended to other significant persons in the environment.

The mother repeatedly emphasizes socially approved behavior; the child learns early to act in a way that will gain approval from her. For instance, the child learns that it is appropriate to eat with a spoon, but that it is not acceptable behavior to throw the spoon or the food on the floor. This learning is important because it enables the child to be taken outside the home at mealtime and to be given approval by other persons for acceptable behavior.

THE NORMAL NEWBORN REFLEX

Introduction

Reflexes are originating in the central nervous system that is exhibited by normal neonates but not neurologically intact adults, in response to particular stimuli. These reflexes disappear or are inhibited by the frontal lobes as a child moves through normal child development. These primitive reflexes are also called **neonates or newborn reflexes.**

Older children and adults with atypical neurology (for instance, people with cerebral palsy) may retain these reflexes and primitive reflexes may re-appear in adults because of certain neurological conditions including, but not limited to, dementia, traumatic lesions, and strokes.

An individual with cerebral palsy and typical intelligence can learn to suppress these reflexes, but the reflex might resurface under certain conditions such as during an extreme startle reaction. Reflexes may also be limited to those areas affected by the atypical neurology, such as individuals whose cerebral palsy affects only their legs retaining the Babinski reflex but having normal speech; in individuals with hemiplegia, the reflex might be seen in the foot on the affected side only.

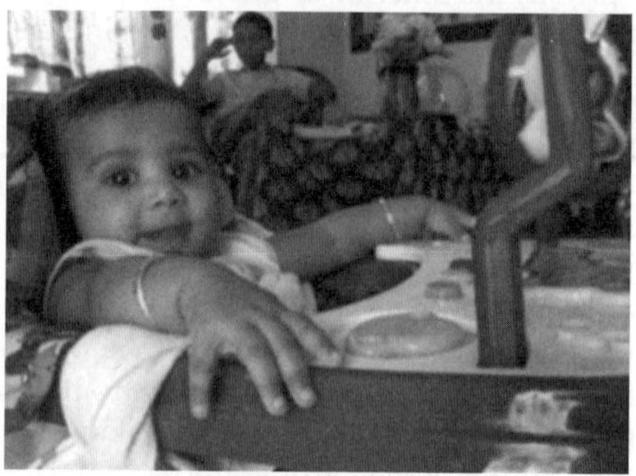

The reflexes are primarily tested with suspected brain injury to test the functioning of the frontal lobe. If they are not being suppressed properly they are called frontal release signs. Atypical primitive reflexes are also being researched as potential early warning signs of autistic spectrum disorders.

Table 3.2: Adaptive value of reflexes

Adaptive value of reflexes	
1	Moro reflex
2	Walking/stepping reflex
3	Rooting reflex
4	Sucking reflex
5	Tonic neck reflex
6	Palmar grasp reflex
7	Plantar reflex
8	Galant reflex
9	Swimming reflex
10	Babkin reflex

Reflexes vary in utility. Some have a survival value. A perfect example would be the rooting reflex, which helps a breastfed infant find the mother's nipple. Babies display it only when hungry and touched by another person, not when they touch themselves. There are a few reflexes that probably helped babies survive during human evolutionary past like the Moro reflex. Other reflexes such as sucking and grabbing help establish gratifying interaction between parents and infants. They can encourage a parent to respond lovingly and feed more competently. They can also help parents comfort their infant because they allow the baby to control distress and the amount of stimulation they receive.

Moro Reflex

The moro reflex commonly seen in 4 days old newborn baby:

- The reflex is initiated by pulling the infant up from the floor and then releasing him
- He spreads his arms
- He pulls his arms in
- He cries (10 seconds).

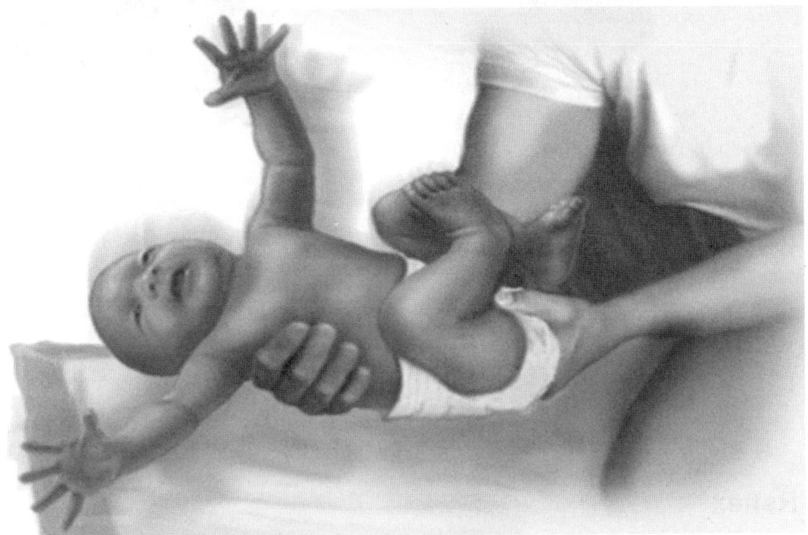

Fig. 3.4: Moro reflex

This is sometimes referred to as the startle reaction, startle response, startle reflex or embrace reflex. It is more commonly known as the Moro response or Moro reflex after its discoverer, pediatrician Ernst Moro.

The Moro reflex is present at birth, peaks in the first month of life and begins to disappear around 2 months of age. It is likely to occur if the infant's head suddenly shifts position, the temperature changes abruptly, or they are startled by a sudden noise.

The legs and head extend while the arms jerk up and out with the palms up and thumbs flexed. Shortly afterward the arms are brought together and the hands clench into fists, and the infant cries loudly. The reflex normally disappears by three to four months of age, though it may last up to six months.

Bilateral absence of the reflex may mean damage to the infant's central nervous system while a unilateral absence could mean an injury due to birth trauma such as a fractured clavicle or injury to the brachial plexus.

Erb's palsy or some other form of paralysis is also sometimes present in such cases. A way to experiment to see if the reflex is present is to hold the infant horizontally on their back and let the head drop slightly or produce a sudden loud sound against the surface. In human evolutionary past, the Moro reflex may have helped the infant cling to his mother while she carried him around all day. If the infant lost its balance, the reflex caused the infant to embrace its mother and regain its hold on the mother's body.

Walking/Stepping Reflex

The walking or stepping reflex is present at birth; though infants this young cannot support their own weight, when the soles of their feet touch a flat surface they will attempt to 'walk' by placing one foot in front of the other. This reflex disappears at six weeks as an automatic response and reappears as a voluntary behavior at around eight months to a year old.

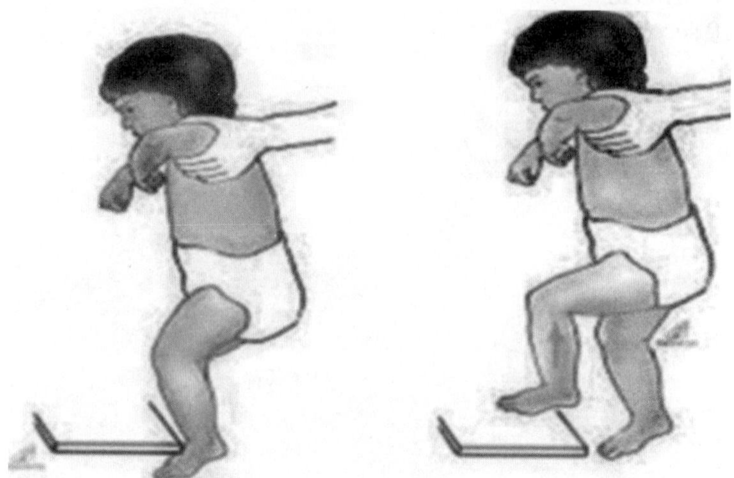

Fig. 3.5: Walking/stepping reflex

Rooting Reflex

The rooting reflex is present at birth and assists in breastfeeding, disappearing at around four months of age as it gradually comes under voluntary control.

A newborn infant will turn his head toward anything that strokes his cheek or mouth, searching for the object by moving his head in steadily decreasing arcs until the object is found. After becoming used to responding in this way (if breastfed, approximately three weeks after birth), the infant will move directly to the object without searching.

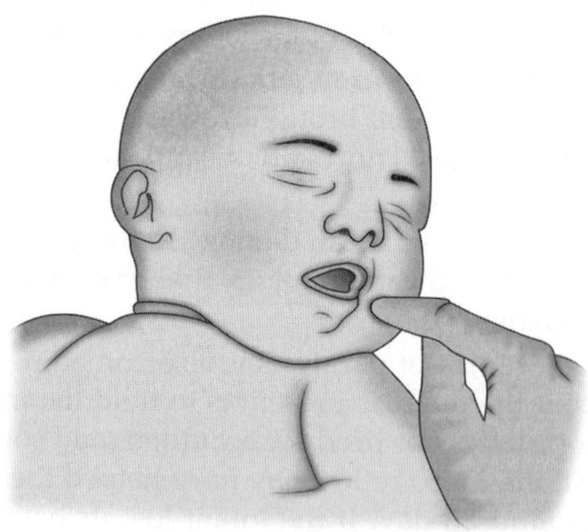

Fig. 3.6: Rooting reflex

Sucking Reflex

The sucking reflex is common to all mammals and is present at birth. It is linked with the rooting reflex and breastfeeding, and causes the child to instinctively suck at anything that touches the roof of their mouth and suddenly starts to suck simulating the way they naturally eat. There are two stages to the action:

1. *Expression:* Activated when the nipple is placed between a child's lips and touches their palate. They will instinctively press it between their tongue and palate to draw out the milk.
2. *Milking:* The tongue moves from areola to nipple, coaxing milk from the mother to be swallowed by the child.

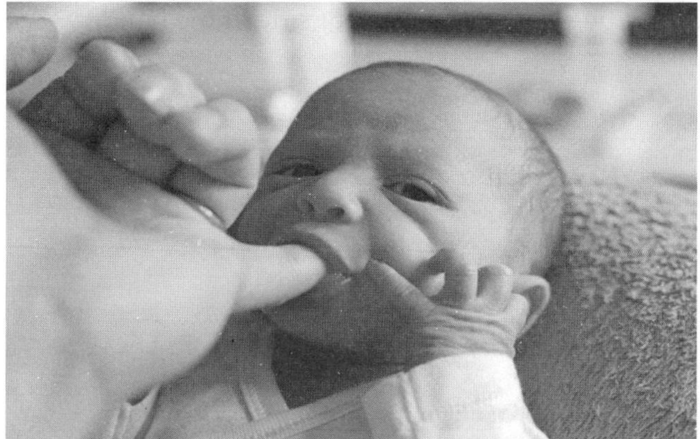

Fig. 3.7: Sucking reflex

Tonic Neck Reflex

Tonic Neck Reflex (Asymmetrical Tonic Neck Reflex)

The tonic neck reflex, or known as asymmetric tonic neck reflex or 'fencing posture' is present at one month of age and disappears at around four months.

When the child's head is turned to the side, the arm on that side will straighten and the opposite arm will bend (sometimes the motion will be very subtle or slight). If the infant is

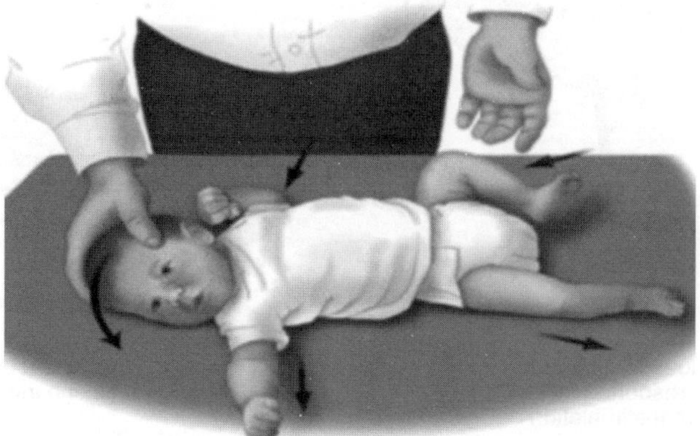

Fig. 3.8: Tonic neck reflex

unable to move out of this position or the reflex continues to be triggered past six months of age, the child may have a disorder of the upper motor neurons.

According to researchers, the tonic neck reflex is a precursor to the hand/eye coordination of the infant. It also prepares the infant for voluntary reaching.

Palmar Grasp Reflex

The palmar grasp reflex appears at birth and persists until five or six months of age. When an object is placed in the infant's hand and strokes their palm, the fingers will close and they will grasp it. The grip is strong but unpredictable; though it may be able to support the child's weight, they may also release their grip suddenly and without warning. The reverse motion can be induced by stroking the back or side of the hand.

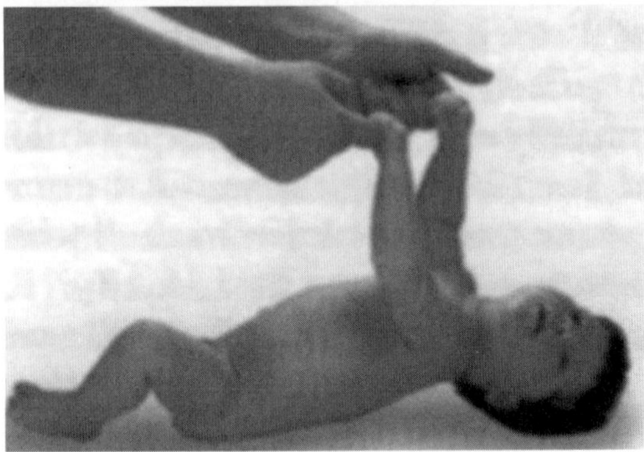

Fig. 3.9: Palmar grasp reflex

Plantar Reflex

A plantar reflex is a normal reflex that involves plantar flexion of the foot (toes move away from the shin, and curl down. An abnormal plantar reflex (Babinski Sign) occurs when upper motor neuron control over the flexion reflex circuit is interrupted.

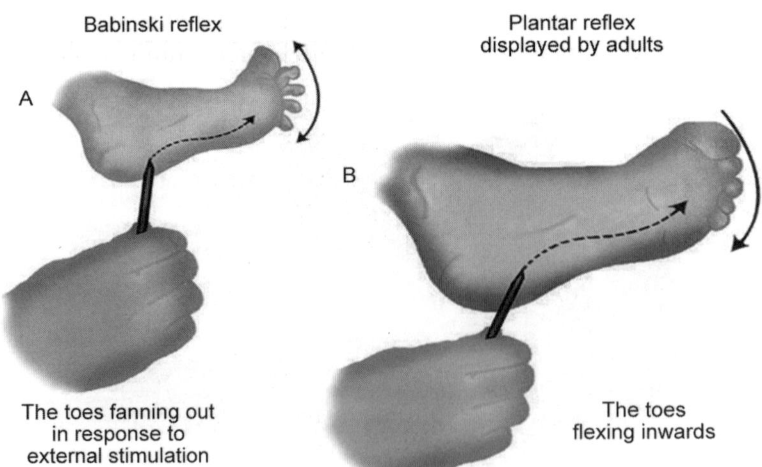

Fig. 3.10: Plantar reflex

This result in a dorsiflexion of the foot (foot angles towards the shin, big toe curls up). This also occurs in babies under ~1 year, because of low myelination of the corticospinal tracts.

As these tracts develop to adult form, the flexion-reflex circuit is inhibited by the descending corticospinal inputs, and the normal plantar reflex develops. Also known as the Babinski reflex, this is a sign of neurological abnormality, e.g. upper motor neuron lesion, in adults.

Galant Reflex

The Galant reflex, also known as Galant's infantile reflex, is present at birth and fades between the ages of four to six months.

When the skin along the side of an infant's back is stroked, the infant will swing towards the side that was stroked. If the reflex persists past six months of age, it is a sign of pathology. The reflex is named after the Russian neurologist Johann Susman Galant.

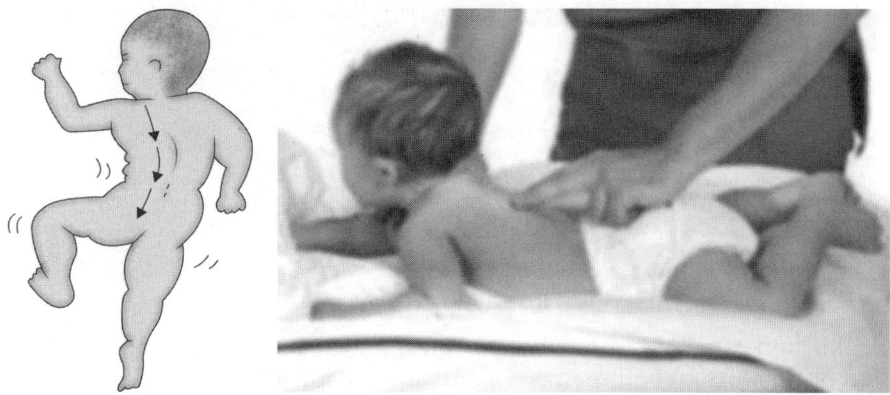

Fig. 3.11: Galant reflex

Swimming Reflex

An infant placed face down in a pool of water will begin to paddle and kick in a swimming motion.

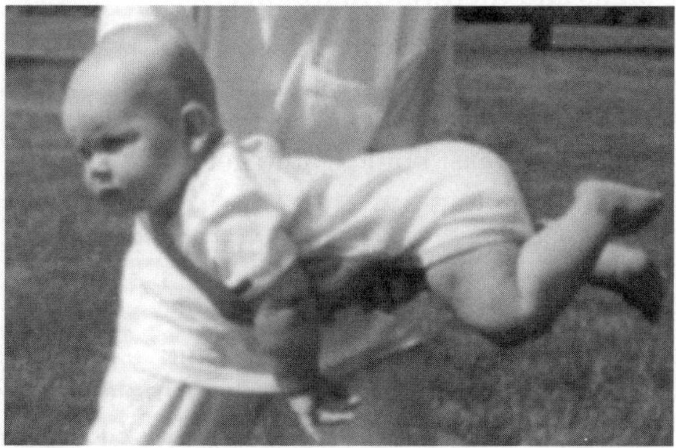

Fig. 3.12: Swimming reflex

The reflex disappears between 4–6 months. Its survival function is to help the child stay alive if it is drowning so a caregiver has more time to save it.

Although the infant will begin to paddle and kick, placing them in water is very risky. They swallow a large amount of water at the same time. It is advisable to postpone swimming lessons in infants until they are at least three months old.

Babkin Reflex

An infant demonstrating the Babkin reflex: he opens his mouth when pressure is applied to both palms (8 seconds).

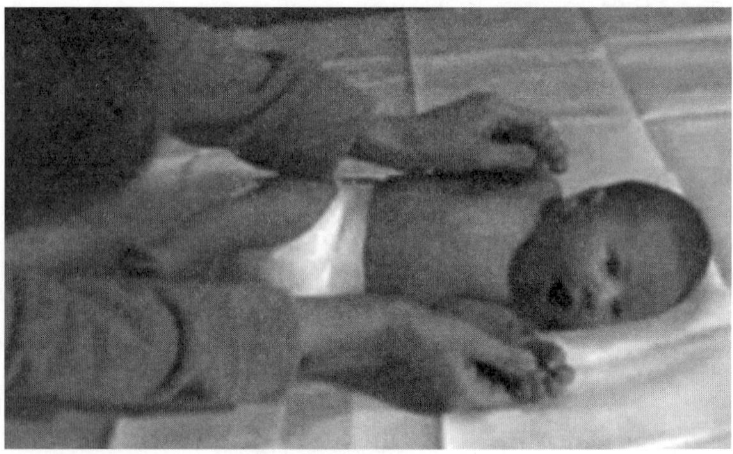

Fig. 3.13: Babkin reflex

The Babkin reflex occurs in newborn babies, and describes varying responses to the application of pressure to both palms. Infants may display head flexion, head rotation or opening of the mouth, or a combination of these responses. Smaller, premature infants are more susceptible to the reflex, with an observed occurrence in a child of 26 weeks gestation. Named for Russian neurophysiologist, Boris Babkin.

Primitive Reflexes

Some frontal release signs and their role in infancy:

- Palmar grasp: Baby naturally grabs objects
- Palmomental reflex: Unknown
- Rooting reflex: Baby finds breast to suckle
- Sucking reflex: Baby sucks breast/bottle teat to get milk
- Snout reflex: Involved in suckling
- Glabellar reflex: May protect eyes in certain situations

Palmomental Reflex

The **palmomental reflex** (PMR) is an example of a primitive reflex. As such it is present in infancy, disappears during maturation of the brain during childhood but may reappear due to processes that disrupt the normal cortical inhibitory pathways. Therefore it is an example of a frontal release sign.

- Marinesco and Radivici in their seminal paper hypothesize that both the afferent (receptive) and efferent (motor) arms of the reflex are on the same side (ipsilateral) to the hand stimulated; however this hypothesis remains unsubstantiated.
- The PMR has been found to be present more frequently in various neurological conditions both localized and diffuse. These include congenital conditions such as Down's syndrome where it is unclear whether the reflex persists throughout life or disappears and then reappears in association with the onset of Alzheimer's disease pathology. The reflex is common in the elderly population and should not be taken as indicative of a demanding process.

Snout Reflex

The **snout reflex** is a pouting or pursing of the lips that is elicited by light tapping of the closed lips near the midline. The contraction of the muscles causes the mouth to resemble a snout.

This reflex is tested in a neurological exam and if present, is a sign of brain damage. Along with the 'suck' and palmomental reflexes, snout is considered a frontal release sign. Frontal release signs are seen in disorders that affect the frontal lobes, such as dementias, metabolic encephalopathy, closed head injuries, and hydrocephalus.

All of these disorders produce diffuse cerebral damage, usually involving many areas and systems in addition to the frontal lobes and pyramidal system, so the frontal release signs are not sufficient for a diagnosis.

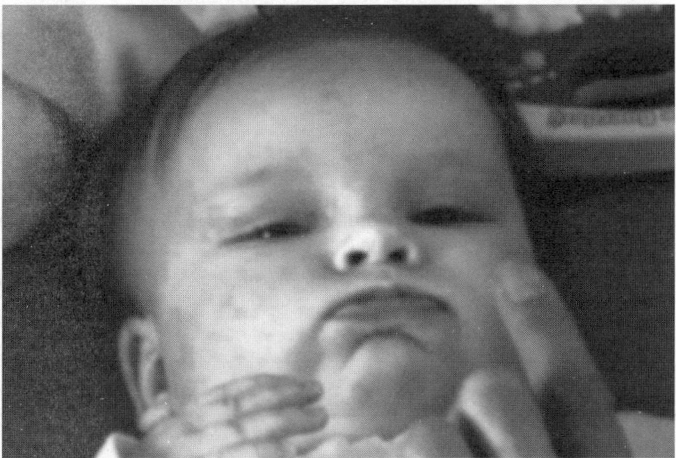

Fig. 3.14: Snout reflex

Glabellar Reflex

Glabellar reflex (also known as the 'glabellar tap sign') is a primitive reflex. It is elicited by repetitive tapping on the forehead. Subjects blink in response to the first several taps. If the blinking persists, this is known as Myerson's sign and is abnormal.

- The afferent sensory signals are transmitted by the trigeminal nerve, and the efferent signals come back to orbicularis oculi muscle via the facial nerve, which in turn reflexly contracts causing blinking.
- Myerson's sign is often seen in patients with Parkinson's disease.

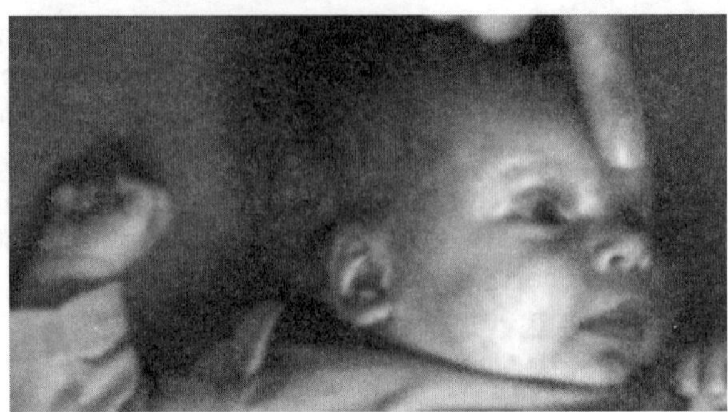

Fig. 3.15: Glabellar reflex

Table 3.3: Neonatal reflexes

Reflex	Stimulation	Response	Duration
Babinski	Sole of foot stroked	Fans out toes and twists foot in	Disappears at nine months to a year
Blinking	Flash of light or puff of air	Closes eyes	Permanent
Grasping	Palms touched	Grasps tightly	Weakens at three months; disappears at a year
Moro	Sudden move; loud noise	Startles; throws out arms and legs and then pulls them toward body	Disappears at three to four months
Rooting	Check stroked or side of mouth touched	Turns toward source, opens mouth and sucks	Disappears at three to four months
Stepping	Infant held upright with feet touching ground	Moves feet as if to walk	Disappears at three to seven months
Sucking	Mouth touched by object	Sucks on object	Disappears at three to seven months
Swimming	Placed face down in water	Makes coordinated swimming movements	Disappears at six to four months
Tonic neck	Placed on back	Makes fists and turns head to the right	Disappears at two months

TECHNIQUE OF DEVELOPMENTAL ASSESSMENT

Introduction

Developmental monitoring and screening can be done by a number of professionals in health care, community, and school settings. However, pediatric primary health care providers are in a unique position to promote children's developmental health. Pediatric primary health care providers have regular contact with children before they reach school age and are able to provide family-centered, comprehensive, and coordinated care.

This care includes a more detailed medical assessment when a screening indicates a child is at risk for a developmental problem. Integrating routine developmental screening into the practice setting can seem daunting. The following are suggestions for integrating screening services into primary care efficiently and at low cost, while ensuring thorough coordination of care.

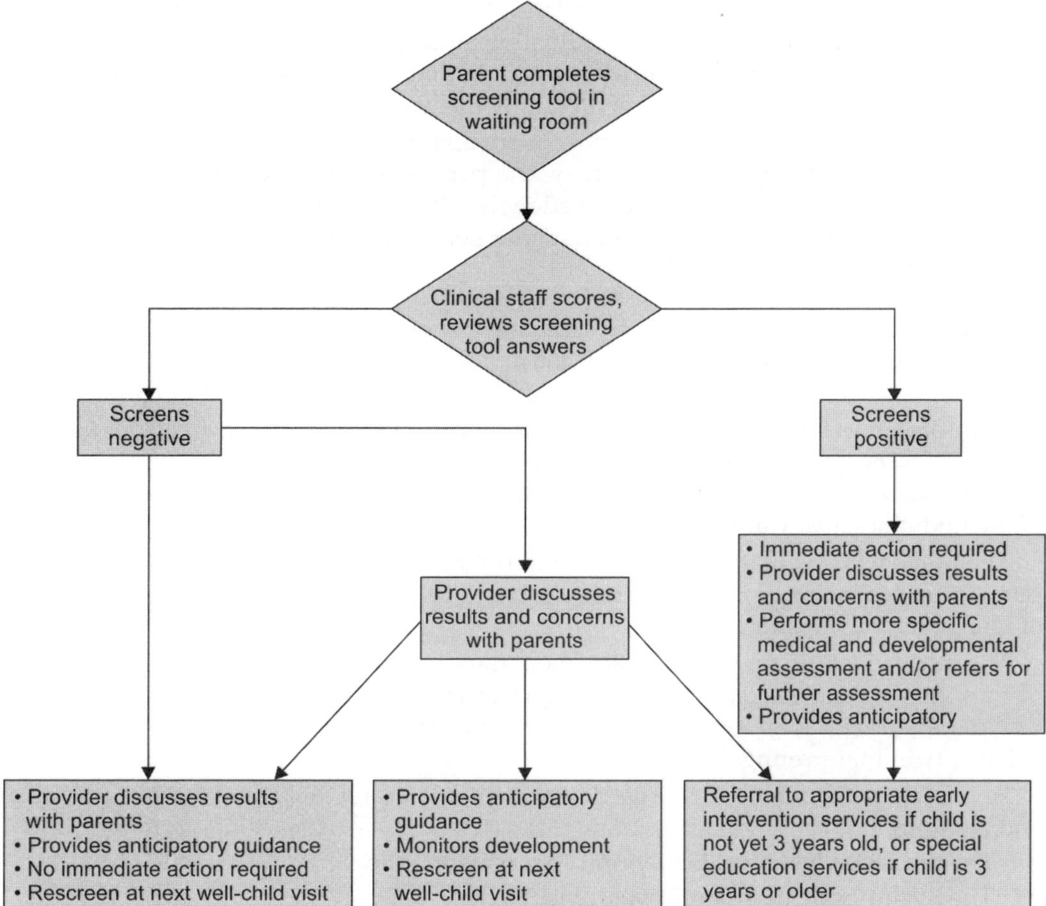

Fig. 3.16: Pediatric developmental screening

Whenever assessing the developmental stages of children, the nurse should look for strengths as well as weaknesses. Too often only the weaknesses are noted, and the child is labeled 'backward' or incorrigible.' Such labeling causes an unfortunate bias in health team members, who may find it difficult to plan nursing intervention for the child on an objective, individualized basis.

- A child who has been labeled may behave 'as expected.' In this way the label applied to become self-fulfilling.
- The label applied to a child, or a parent for that matter, is difficult to erase or change, even when the development of the child or the behavior of the parent improves. Instead of labeling a child or parent, the nurse can make careful and precise observations on positive as well as negative behaviors and evaluate how these can be changed strengthened.
- They can observe their children daily and share their valid data with the nurse. In turn, when the nurse discusses the results of the assessments with the parents, the contributions of the parents, their observations and problem-solving abilities can be highlighted.

- The nurse can then discuss the strengths of their children as well as their weaknesses. Parents can assist in planning and evaluating nursing care practices. They are responsible for themselves and their, children and can participate in making decisions and solving problems pertinent to the care of all family members.
- Developmental assessments of children are do is on a serial basis, because progress or regression can be determined only over a period of time. After the baseline data are determined, comparisons can be made with the results of these comparisons can be made with the results of these comparisons help form a basis for nursing management.

Assessment Tools

The standardized tools can assist nurses in screening developmental changes of children in a systematic manner. Gross motor abilities, fine motor skills, personal-social behaviors, language abilities, and academic abilities can be assessed. Each tool has its advantages and disadvantages.

The nurse must follow the standardized procedure given for using each tool for the results to be valid. The nurse does not give verbal tests to measure the intelligence quotient of a child; these are administered by persons trained to give, score, and interpret the meaning of the findings statistically.

The nurse who evaluates children through standardized assessment tools must use the same format each time for the directions, the same criteria in scoring, and the same method of interpreting the results to others.

The nurse who utilizes various assessment tools in different environments with children of various age and stages of development gradually becomes proficient in their use. Collaboration with a knowledgeable person in learning to use assessment tests increases objectivity in interpreting the results.

Several assessment tools can be used by the nurse to evaluate changes that occur in infants and children.

- The Brazelton Neonatal Behavioral Assessment Scale
- The Bayley Scale of Infant Development
- The Denver prescreening Developmental Questionnaire (PDQ)
- The Denver Development screening examination (DASE)
- The Denver Development Screening Test (DDST), the Development Screening Test (DDST)
- The Development profile, the NCAST Scales.

The Neonatal Behavioral Assessment Scale (Brazelton)

This tool was developed by Dr T Berry Brazelton and associates for the purpose of assessing newborn behavior through the first month of age.

Brazelton—Neonatal behavioral assessment scale	
State 1	Deep sleep, without movements, breathing regularly
State 2	Light sleep, closed eyes, some corporal movement
State 3	Sleepy, eyes opening and closing
State 4	Awake, opened eyes, minimum corporal movement
State 5	Completely awake, strong corporal movement
State 6	Cry

This scale not only documents individual difference in newborn babies and determines how the environment shapes their behavior but also shows how the neonate shapes the environment. In addition, this tool shows the newborn baby gaining mastery over self as progress is made toward the emotional and cognitive developments of the infancy period.

These are important findings because they have an effect on how the infant interacts with caregivers, such as parents and nurses, early in life and can help predict future parent infant interactions. This information can health care team guide parents in the care of their child.

The Brazelton Neonatal Behavioral Assessment Scale can be used to assess normal as well as high-risk neonates, such as premature babies or those from backgrounds of poverty. This tool is valid and reliable when used by experienced examiners on infants from almost all cultural backgrounds. The nurse who uses this tool must be trained in the method of administration and scoring and must be experienced so that the results have high inters corer reliability for the newborn infants is being tested.

Twenty-seven behavioral responses, organized in six categories, are tested in this tool: habituation (the length of time it takes a neonate to reduce response to the stimulation of a light, of sound, and of heel pinpricks); orientation (the time it takes a neonate to focus on and respond to auditory and visual animate or inanimate stimuli); motor maturity (the degree of control of motor activities and motor coordination); variation (the amount of changes in states, color, and activity in the neonate when alert and at peaks of excitement during the testing); self-quieting abilities (how the neonate can console self when upset and how the caregiver intervenes); and social behaviors (the neonate's smiling behavior and response to cuddling by the caregiver).

The Bayley's Scale of Infant Development

This is used to evaluate children between 6 and 30 months of age. It is standardized for all sociocultural groups in the United States. The three general areas like:

- Mental development
- Psychomotor development
- Behavioral development

Specific areas tested include motor development, postural development, attention span to objects and humans, perception, language, object manipulation, understanding commands, and problem-solving.

The Denver Prescreening Developmental Questionnaire (PDQ)

The PDQ identifies those children who need a more thorough screening with the Denver Developmental Screening Test (DDST) (discussed next). It assesses the same four categories as the DDST. It is easy and fairly quick to administer.

The child must be present while the questionnaire is being completed, because on some forms specific tasks must be performed.

The questionnaire consists of 97 questions, divided according to the child's age. The parent is asked to answer the questions from the appropriate age grouping.

After the nurse reviews the answers, the parents have time to ask questions or bring up any concerns they may have. If the child shows a delay in development, a complete Denver Developmental Screening Test is done as a follow-up.

The Denver Developmental Screening Test (DDST)

Developed originally by Franken Burg and Dodd's (1967), this simple, economic, and useful test screens for developmental delays during infancy and the preschool period. On the test, the age divisions are monthly until 2 years of age, and half early from 2 to 6 years of age. The DDST is a screening tool, not a diagnostic procedure. It is a standardized test that is both reliable and valid. It is not an intelligence test or a predictor of future adaptive or intellectual ability.

The DDST provides a developmental profile of the individual child in four areas: personal-social, fine motor-adaptive, language, and gross motor skills. If development in any of these four areas is questionable when compared with normal standards, the child is referred for an in-depth evaluation. Children who have questionable or abnormal scores on the DDST are at risk for developing later problems in school regardless of their intelligence quotients.

- The DDST helps the nurse determine what a child can do at different ages in comparison with other same-aged children and what progress a child is making between tests. Nurses can learn to administer the DDST accurately by following the Test Manual.
- The Manual provides a complete explanation of how each tested activity should be approached demonstrated, and assessed. The nurse should also refer to the manual for the method of test interpretation.
- The nurse should be well trained and supervised for reliability before administering the test on a routine basis. If the nurse improvises when carrying out the test or helps the infant or child performs, the test results will be invalid.
- When using the DDST, the nurse must be sensitive to the individual child's, ways of responding and to the child's strengths and weaknesses.
- The nurse must allow time for the child to, become comfortable both in a new environment and with the examiner before the test is begun.
- The nurse first explains the tasks at the child's level of understanding and then gets the child-to listen and to pay visual attention to each task. If the child seems confused or does not respond, the instructions are repeated to ensure comfort and security.
- The nurse must be aware of the numbers and variety of cues the child gives in.-response to the requests made, the child's interest in the tasks and eagerness to please are important.
- The child's performance may be affected by anxiety, fatigue, shyness, separation from the parent, illness and hospitalization, or a lack of cooperation.
- The parents as well as the child are prepared for the screening. When the DDST is explained, the word 'test' is used as little as possible because of its connotation; the words developmental screening' may be used instead.
- The parents are told that the child will be requested to perform tasks below and above the expected performance level so that the best possible results are attained.
  - *'P' denotes passing of an item*
  - *'F' failing and*
  - *'R' refusal of the child to cooperate.*

- This method of scoring is explained to the parents to relieve their anxiety when tests are administered, the parents must realize that they are not to intervene, and they must be reminded that the child is not expected to perform all tasks.
- The nurse first presents the child's strengths in all areas and second, the weaknesses. The nurse then asks the parents if they agree with the test findings.
- The parents are praised appropriately for the approaches they have used to help their child make constant developmental gains. If there are deficits in the child's performance, the parents are asked, without alarming them, their opinion concerning the developmental delay.
- They may be asked about their goals for their child and given information about what they could do to help with their child's development. Although the nurse does not purposely tell the parents to teach the skills that will help their child pass the screening test, the DDST can be a guide for parents as to what is expected of their child at a particular age level.

General Instruction

- The parent(s) should be told that the purpose is to obtain an estimate of the child's level of development and that the child will not be able to perform all test items.
- The test relies on observations of the child and on report by a parent who knows the child. Direct observation should be used whenever possible. Every effort should be made to put the child at ease.
- The younger child may be tested while sitting on the parents lap in such a way that he or she can comfortably reach the test materials on a table. One or two test materials may be placed in front of the child while the parent is queried regarding personal-social items.
- The first test items chosen should assure the child an initial successful experience. To avoid distractions, it is best to remove all test materials from the table except those required for the test that is being administered.

Steps in Administering the Test

- Draw a vertical line on the examination sheet at the child's chronologic age.
- Place the date of the examination at the top of the age line. For children who were born prematurely, subtract the number of months of prematurely from the chronologic age.
- Adjust the age line appropriately and note the amount of adjustment at the top of the line.
- The items to be administered are those in the Personal-Social, Fine Motor-Adaptive, Language, and Gross Motor sectors through which the child's chronologic age line passes.
- In each sector one should establish age levels at which the child passes all the items and at which all items are failed.
- When a child refuses to do an item requested by the examiner, the parent may administer the item, provided this is done in the prescribed manner.
- If a child passes an item, a large letter 'P' is written on the bar. 'F' designates a failure, and 'R' designates a refusal.
- Note is made of the child's adjustment to the examination (cooperation, attention span, self-confidence) and relationships to parent, to the examiner, and to the test materials.

- The parent reports whether the child's performance was typical. This is recorded.
- For retesting, use the same form, with different colors for each scoring line and age.
- Instructions for administering footnoted items are on the back of the test form.

Precaution

The DDST is not an intelligence test and does not establish a DQ or an IQ. It is a screening instrument for use in clinical practice to identify children whose development may need critical study.

Nursing Child Assessment Satellite Training (NCAST)

Developed by Dr. Kathryn Barnard and her colleagues at the University Of Washington School Of Nursing, the Nursing Child Assessment Satellite Training (NCAST) scales are designed for early finding the diseases and intervention.

Currently, four standardized scales are available to assist the pediatric in assessing both include the Nursing Child Assessment Sleep /Activity (NCASA) Records, used to assess infant states and child behavior; the Nursing Child Assessment Feeding Scale (NCAFS), which assesses infant feeding interactions during the first year of life,

The Nursing Child Assessment Teaching Scale (NCATS), which provides assessment data gathered during a teaching session between child and caregiver; and the Home Observation for Measurement of Environment (HOME), which is valuable tool for assessing the home environment of the infant or child.

Information regarding the NCAST scales and their use can be obtained from NCAST, University of Washington, and Seattle.

The Denver Articulation Screening Examination (DASE)

A Language and speech development can be evaluated through a history of the child's speech development, through observation of the child's verbal ability and speech patterns, and through testing. A child's articulation can be evaluated with the Denver Articulation Screening Examination (DASE).

Language and speech development can be evaluated through a history of the child's speech development, through observation of the child's verbal ability and speech patterns, and through testing. A child's articulation can be evaluated with the Denver Articulation Screening Examination (DASE), a tool that tests the child's ability to imitate word sounds.

This test is easy to administer, since the child is only asked to repeat 30 different sound elements. The person testing the child listens for errors in articulation.

The level of intelligibility is scored in one of four categories: easy to understandable, and cannot evaluate.

The DASE can pinpoint normal variations in the acquisition of speech sounds as well as important delays or abnormalities in speech development. It is emphasized that the SASE in no way evaluates language development.

The Good Enough-Harris Drawing Test

Originally called the good enough Draw-A-Man Test, this revised and re-standardized version of an intelligence test is used for screening children between the ages of 3 and 12 years. Children are requested to make three drawings: a man, a woman, and a representation of the self.

The interpretation of the test results is based on the fact that children generally include more detail in their drawing of the human figure as they become older. This test is as culture-free as is possible, since it does not rely on verbal ability.

The examiner assumes that children of this age have used drawing materials before. The level of fine motor development may be a factor in a child's ability to produce a picture.

The Good enough—Harris Drawing Test is supposedly more accurate than the good enough Draw-A-Man Test but is not as simple to score. The figures a child draws are scored according to standards outlined in the instruction manual.

The Needs of Parents During the Use of Developmental Screening Techniques

Screening tools are used to ascertain an infant's or child's progress in accomplishing appropriate developmental tasks.

They are useful in locating children who have early developmental delays and those who have potential difficulties. Parents can profit from the screening procedures carried out on their children if they are key participants during the entire assessment process. This means that parents must be assisted in gaining the following:

- An understanding of the need for and the process of developmental assessment.
- An understanding of the screening tools and techniques that are to be used.
- An understanding of the need for the assessment to be repeated on a regular basis as their child develops.
- An opportunity to participate in the screening process, if appropriate, and in the discussion of the results.
- An opportunity to ask questions and to have them answered accurately, to discuss any fears or concerns, and to seek assistance in ways of promoting change in their child.
  - A Pediatric Nurses who discuss developmental screening assessments with parents may find that parents need an understanding of the principles of growth and development, given earlier in this chapter, if they are to understand the findings.
  - When discussing this information with parents, the nurse may at times not know the answers to questions they pose. In such a situation, the nurse can simply say, 'I do not know the answer to that question, but I will find out.'
  - When parents ask repeatedly before, during, or after an assessment, 'But is he (or she) all right?,' they are expressing concern about whether they have done everything possible to stimulate their child's development.
  - They have provided various appropriate playthings and experiences based on the child's developmental level and have regulated stimuli from the environment for learning.
  - The nurse must make a point of discussing whether the child is being asked to do either more or less than is possible on the basis of the developmental level and whether opportunities are available to enhance learning.
  - The nurse can also help the parents evaluate how much the child tries to succeed and cooperate, and whether they can truly accept the level of their child's abilities.

- Sharing the results of the developmental screening techniques with parents can assist them in evaluating the status of their children and in coping with the regularities and irregularities of their developmental patterns.
- If a particular child needs further observation and diagnosis because of lags in development, a member of the health care team who recognizes the need can plan for retesting or can assist the parents in their preparation for a more comprehensive developmental evaluation by specialists.

Gestational Age Assessment (Ballard Score)

To determine the approximate gestational age of a newborn, you will assess six neuromuscular and six physical characteristics. This assessment, the New Ballard Score, is appropriate for newborns from 20 to 44 weeks of gestation, with the characteristics to assess varying with the stage of maturity. Each parameter scores from minus 2 to 5, with the cumulative score correlating with a gestational age between 26 and 44 weeks.

Timing of the gestational assessment influences the accuracy of its results. For newborns younger than 26 gestational weeks, perform the assessment sooner than 12 hours after birth. For newborns beyond 26 gestational weeks, perform the examination within 96 hours of birth. Overall, it is best to perform the examination within 48 hours of birth. This assessment information is essential because gestation relates directly to the likelihood of complications during the newborn period. Lower scores correlate with prematurity; higher scores correlate with postmaturity. Commercially printed worksheets are available to use when performing this assessment.

Maturational Assessment of Gestational Age (New Ballard Score)

Name of the child____________________ IP No. ________________

Date/time of birth ____________________Date/time of exam __________

Age when examined ____________________ Sex ________________

Birth weight________________________Length ________________

Head circumference________________ Examiner ________________

Apgar score: 1 Minute __________ 5 Minutes __________

Neuromuscular Maturity

Neuro-muscular maturity sign	Score							Record score here	Score
	–1	0	1	2	3	4	5		Neuromuscular: Physical: Total:
Posture									Maturity rating

Contd...

Contd...

Neuromuscular maturity sign	Score -1	0	1	2	3	4	5	Record score here	Score Neuromuscular: Physical: Total:
Square window (wrist)	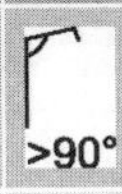 >90°	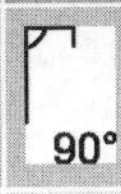 90°	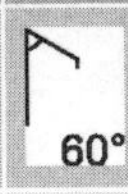 60°	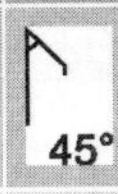 45°	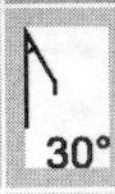 30°	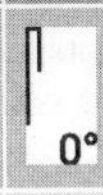 0°			
Arm recoil		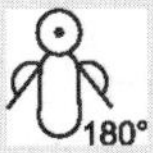 180°	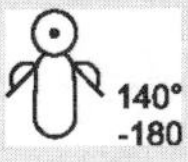 140° -180	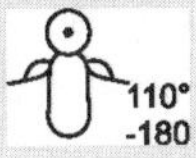 110° -180	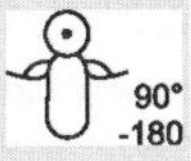 90° -180	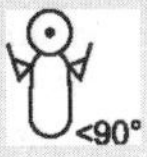 <90°			
Popliteal angle	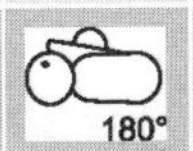 180°	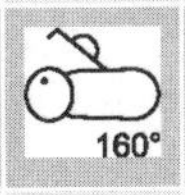 160°	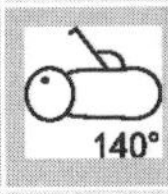 140°	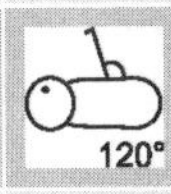 120°	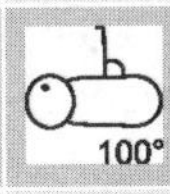 100°	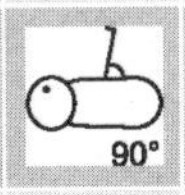 90°	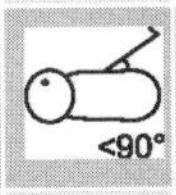 <90°		
Scarf sign									
Heel to ear									
Total neuromuscular maturity score									

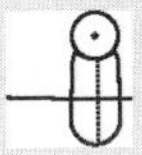

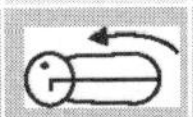

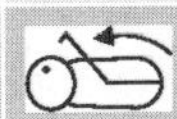

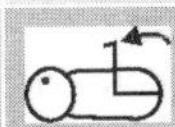

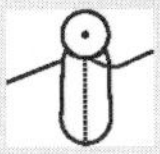

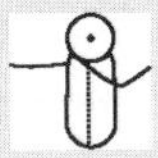

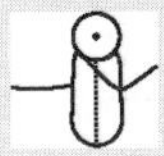

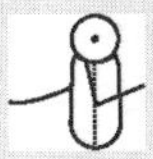

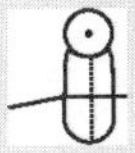

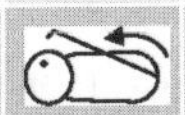

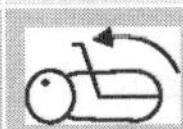

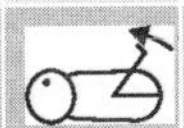

Score	Weeks
–10	20
–5	22
0	24
5	26
10	28
15	30
20	32
25	34
30	36
35	38
40	40
50	44

Physical Maturity

Physical maturity sign	Score –1	0	1	2	3	4	5	Record score here
Skin	Sticky, friable, transparent	Gelatinous, red, translucent	Smooth pink, visible veins	Superficial peeling and/ or rash, few veins	Cracking, pale areas, rare veins	Parchment, deep cracking, no vessels	Leathery, cracked, wrinkled	
Lanugo	None	Sparse	Abundant	Thinning	Bald areas	Mostly bald		
Plantar surface	Heel-toe 40–50 mm: –1 < 40 mm: –2	> 50 mm no crease	Faint red marks	Anterior transverse crease only	Creases ant. 2/3	Creases over entire sole		
Breast	Imperceptible	Barely perceptable	Flat areola no bud	Stippled areola 1–2 mm bud	Raised areola 3–4 mm bud	Full areola 5–10 mm bud		
Eye/Ear	Lids fused loosely: –1 tightly: –2	Lids open pinna flat stays folded	Sl. Curved pinna; soft; slow recoil	Well-curved pinna; soft but ready recoil	Formed and firm instant recoil	Thick cartilage ear stiff		

Contd...

Contd...

Physical maturity sign	Score							Record score here
	–1	0	1	2	3	4	5	
Genitals (male)	Scrotum flat, smooth	Scrotum empty, faint rugae	Testes in upper canal,rare rugae	Testes descending, few rugae	Testes down, good rugae	Testes pendulous, deep rugae		
Genitals (female)	Clitoris prominent and labia flat	Prominent clitoris and small labia minora	Prominent clitoris and enlarging minora	Majora and minora equally prominent	Majora large, minora small	Majora cover clitoris and minora		
						Total physical maturity score		

PLOTTING OF GROWTH CHART

Introduction

It is hard to be 'ethnically correct' when assessing growth in international adoption. Many of the available country-specific growth charts are out-of-date, from a small sample size, drawn from ethnic groups that may not represent the child's ethnicity based on malnourished populations.

In 2006, the WHO (World Health Organization) released new international birth-5yo charts based on 8,500 children from Brazil, Ghana, India, Norway, Oman and the USA. Their unique approach was to select children whose care meets recommended health promotion standards (breastfeeding, standard pediatric care, anti-smoking, etc) so that the charts would represent how children should grow, not necessarily how they are growing. Their big finding was that 'child populations grow similarly across the world's major regions when their needs for health and care are met.'

Definition

The growth monitoring is a screening tool to diagnose nutritional, chronic systemic and endocrine disease at an early stage. It has been suggested that growth monitoring has the potential for significant impact on mortality even in the absence of nutrition supplementation or education.

WHO Growth Charts

- Weight-for-age: 0–5 years
- Height-for-age: 0–5 years
- Head circumference-for-age: 0–5 years

Charts for Premature Infants

- 26 weeks to 1 year chart, for boys and girls
- Fetal-infant growth chart for 22 week– 2 months preterm infants from a meta-analysis of published reference studies
- Charts based on birthweight categories (for when gestational age is unclear)
- LBW (low birthweight) is for birth weights from 1500 g to 2500 g.

- VLBW (very low birthweight) is 1000 g to 1500 g at birth.
  - LBW premature girls
  - LBW premature boys
  - VLBW premature girls
  - VLBW premature boys.

Aims of Growth Chart

Primary Aims

To identify the children with growth deviation, i.e. undernutrition and over nutrition and to identify diseases and conditions that manifest through abnormal physical growth of child.

Secondary Aims

- To discuss health promotion related to feeding, hygiene, immunization and other aspects of the child's health and behavior; education of parents to allay their anxiety about their child's growth.
- To sensitize pediatricians to use growth charts.

Technique of Using the Growth Charts

- At the first visit the child's name, date of birth and other details should be entered on the growth chart and the chart should be explained to the parents. This ensures that they are interested in it and are more likely to keep it properly and bring it at each visit. The growth chart should be kept with the parents in a plastic sleeve.
- Measure the parents and make a note of their heights on the chart. Calculate the child's target height and plot it at 18 years and mark it with an arrow on the growth chart. This represents the child's projected height and his present height percentile can be judged by tracing a line backward from this target height to child's current height. The target range is produced by plotting two points 8 cms above and below the target height and this represents the 3rd and the 97th percentile for that child. Taking those two points above and below the target height 97th and 3rd percentile are constructed by tracing lines backwards to match the current age (Fig. 3.17).
- All the points on the growth chart should be marked only as dots and not circles around the dot.
- The height and weight should be recorded (and head circumference till 3 years) and plotted on the chart. At all subsequent visits join the dot up to the previous dot.
- Remind parents of the time for the next measurement. The group recommends continued use of Tanner staging of sexual maturity rating. For anthropometric measurements standard techniques as described by WHO should be adopted.

Measure the parent's heights and make a note of their heights on the chart. Calculate the child's target height (TH) and plot it at 18 years and mark it with an arrow on the growth chart. This represents the child's projected height and the target range is produced by plotting two points 7.5 cms above and below for a boy and 6 cm above and below for a girl representing the 10th and the 90th percentile for that child). In the example shown above, the 50th percentile for the general population is the 90th percentile for the child measured and the 10th percentile for the child is below the 10th percentile for the population.

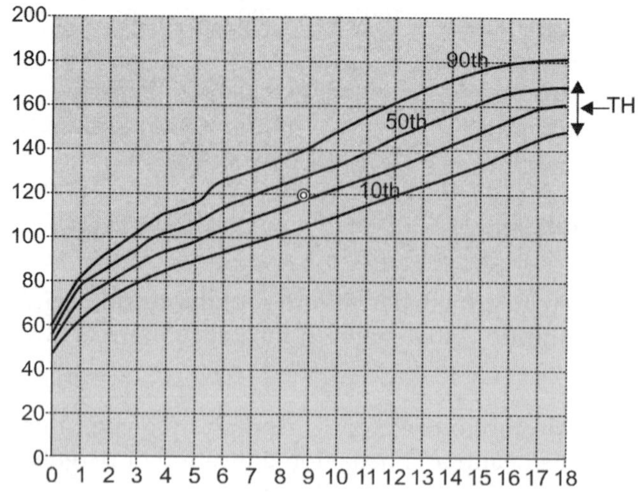

Fig. 3.17: Calculation of target height and target height percentile

Criteria for Referral

First 3 Years

- Length/height, weight or head circumference below 3rd percentile or above 97th percentile on growth chart.
- Crossing of two major percentile lines (upward or downward), e.g. going from above 75th percentile to below 50th percentile on height or weight chart.
- A child below or above mid parental range for height/length (see calculation for target height range in Fig. 3.17).
- Weight loss or lack of weight gain for a month in the first 6 months.
- Absence of weight gain for 2–3 months from 6–12 months of age.
- Micropenis.
- Unilateral or bilateral undescended testis.
- Ambiguous genitals.

3 to 9 Years

- Length/Height below 3rd percentile or above 97th percentile on growth chart.
- Crossing of two major percentile lines (upward or downward), e.g. going from above 75th percentile to below 50th percentile on height or weight chart.
- A child below or above mid parental range for height (See calculation for target height range in Fig. 3.17).
- BMI over the 85th percentile at all ages.
- Rate of growth less than 5 cm/year.
- Girls with axillary, pubic hair growth or breast budding before 8 years and boys with axillary, pubic hair growth, genital growth or and testicular enlargement before 9 years.
- Children with craniospinal irradiation or surgery for brain tumors.
- Micropenis.

9 to 18 Years

- Height below 3rd percentile or above 97th percentile on growth chart.
- Crossing of two major percentile lines (upward or downward), e.g. going from above 75th percentile to below 50th percentile on height or weight chart.
- A child below or above mid parental range for height (Fig. 3.17).
- BMI over the 85th percentile at all ages.
- Arrest at the same stage of puberty for more than 2 years.
- Micropenis.
- Unilateral or bilateral Gynecomastia in boys.
- Hirsuitism and Menstrual irregularities in girls.
- Delayed puberty that is girls with no breast budding by 14 years or no menarche by 15 years and boys with no signs of puberty by 16 years.

Instructions of Using the Growth Chart

- Measure and record weight, length, and head circumference.
- Calculate gestation-adjusted age by subtracting Adjustment for Prematurity in weeks from postnatal age in weeks. Adjustment for Prematurity equals 40 weeks minus GA.

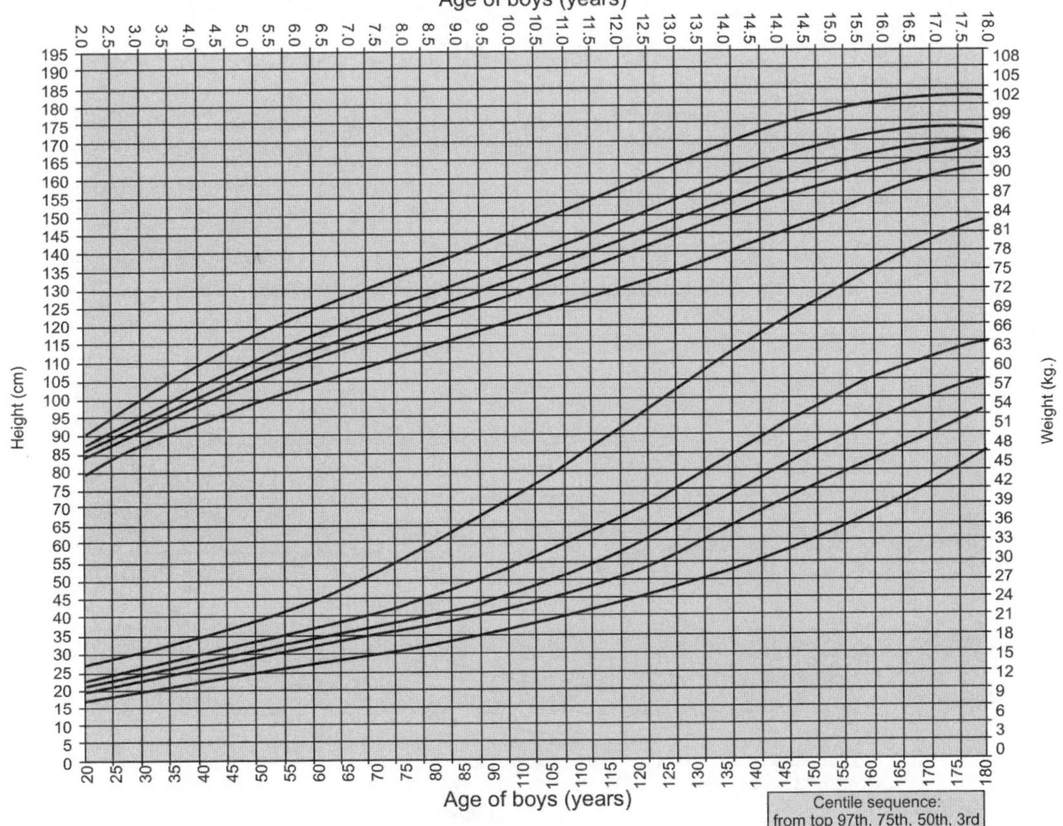

Fig. 3.18: Height and weight for boys 2–18 years

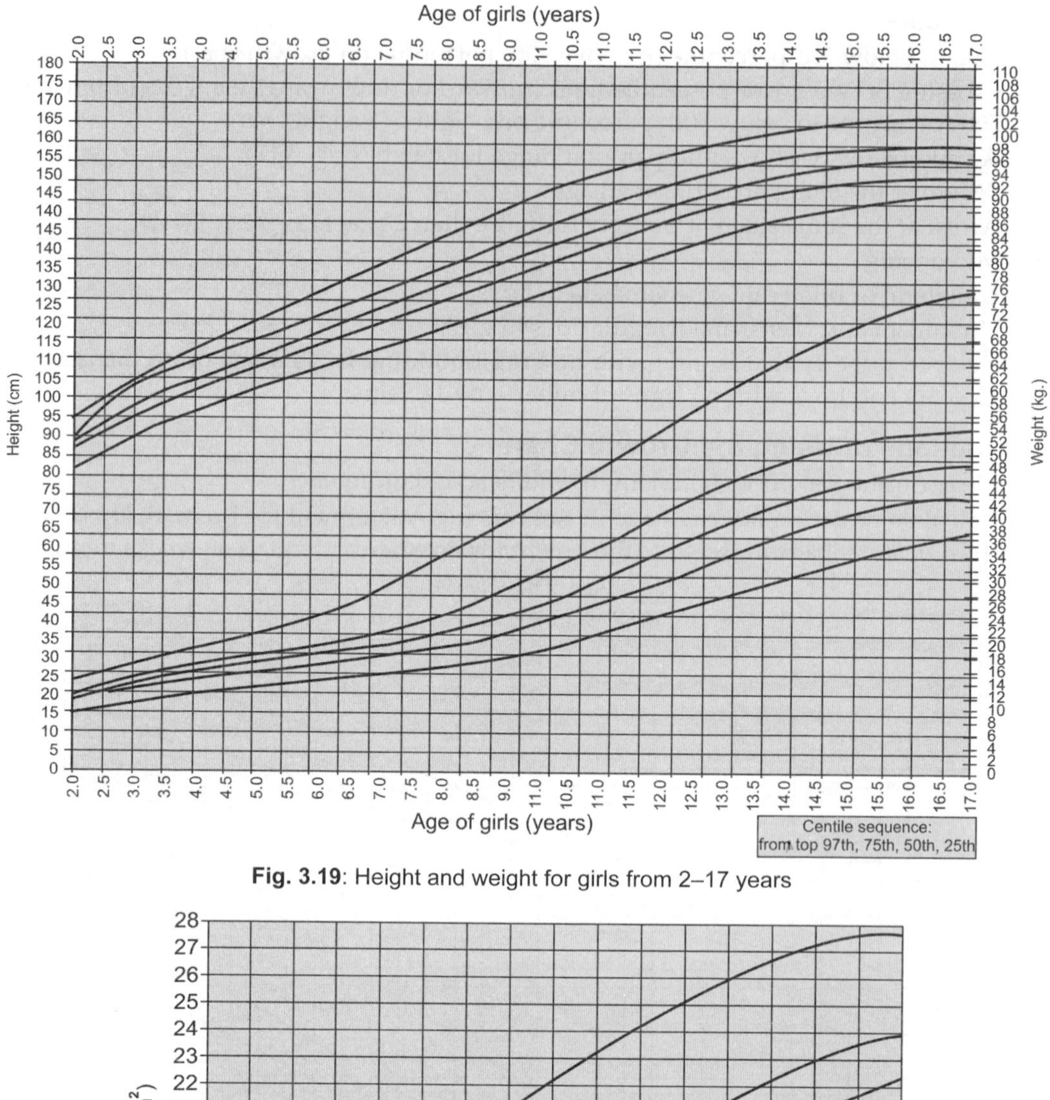

Age of girls (years)

Height (cm)

Weight (kg.)

Age of girls (years)

Centile sequence:
from top 97th, 75th, 50th, 25th

Fig. 3.19: Height and weight for girls from 2–17 years

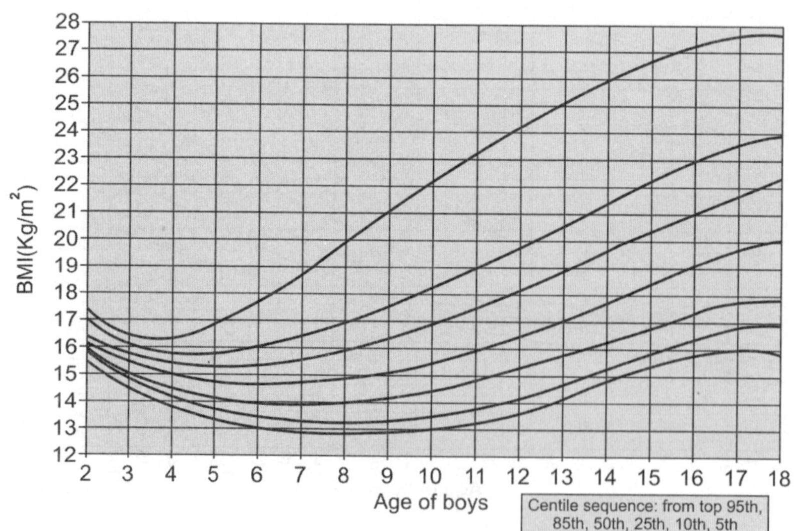

Fig. 3.20: Body mass index for boys 2–18 years

For example, at 12 week postnatal age, an infant born at 30 week GA would be 2 week (0.5 month) gestation-adjusted age.

- Plot data at the gestation-adjusted age on the appropriate graph.
- When possible, plot serial data on the same graph to permit detection of change in growth percentiles with age.

Neonatal Growth and Development

S. No.	Assessment features	Normal value
1	**Anthropometric measurement**	Weight: 2.5–3.5 kg Height: 45–50 cm Head circumference: 33–35 cm Chest circumference: 31–33 cm
2	**Vital signs**	Temperature: 36.5–37 °C Heart rate: 120/140 beats/minute Respiration: 30–60 breaths/minute Blood pressure: 65/41 mm Hg.
3	**Physical appearance**	
	Posture	• Flexion of head and extremities, which rest on chest and abdomen.
	Skin	• Bright red, puffy, smooth vernix caseosa, lanugo, edema around eyes, face, legs, hands, feet, scrotum or labia, magnolia spots.
	Head	
	1. Anterior fontanel 2. Posterior fontanel	• Diamond shaped 2.5–4 cm • Triangular shaped 0.5–1 cm • Flat, soft and firm fontanels
	Eyes	• Lids edematous • Color–gray brown • Absence of tears • Presence of red reflex, corneal and papillary reflex and blinking.
	Ears position	• Top of pinna on horizontal line with outer canthus of eye. • Pinna flexible cartilage present
	Nose	• Nasal potency • Thin and white nasal discharge • Sneezing
	Mouth and Throat	• Intact high pitched palate, frenulum of tongue, frenum of upper lip, suckling reflex, rooting gag and extrusion reflex, absent or minimal salivation, vigorous cry.
	Neck	• Short thick, surrounded by slais folds, tonic neck reflex
	Chest	• Anterioposterior and lateral diameters are equal • Xiphoid process evident • Breast enlargement
	Lungs	• Respiration chiefly abdominal, cough reflex present • Bilateral equal bronchial sound
	(a) Heart	• Apex-4th to 5th intercostals space, s_2 sharper, s_1 low pitch
	Abdomen	• Cylindrical in shape

Contd...

Contd...

S. No.	Assessment features	Normal value
	• Liver	• Palpable 2–3 cm below right costal margin
	• Spleen	• Tip palpable at end of first week of age
	• Kidney	• Palpable 1–2 cm above umbilicus
	• Umbilical cord	• Bluish white with 2 arteries and one vein
	• Femoral pulses	• Bilaterally equal
	• Female genitalia	• Labia and clitoris edematous
		• Urethral meats behind clitoris
		• Vernix caseosa between labia
		• Urination within 24 hours
	• Male genitalia	• Urethral opening at top of glance penis
		• Testis palpable at each scrotum
		• Urination within 24 hours.
		• Pigmented edematous, pendulous scrotum
	Rectum	Spine intact, no opening, masses Trunk incurvation, patent and opening passage of meconium within 48 hours
	Extremities	• Ten fingers and toes
		• Full range of motion
		• Nail beds pink
		• Sole usually flat
		• Symmetry of extremities
		• Equal muscle tone bilaterally
		• Equal bilateral brachial pulses

Neuromuscular System (Reflexes)

S. No.	Assessment features	Normal value
1	Blinking or corneal reflex	Protection of the eye by rapid eye lid closure when the eyes are exposed to bright light.
2	Doll's eye reflex	Turn the neonates head slowly to the right or left side, normally eye do not move.
3	Sneezing and coughing reflex	Foreign substance entering the upper and lower airways, clearing of upper air passages by sneezing and lower air passages by coughing.
4	Rooting reflex	When the cheek or corner of the mouth is stroked, the infants head should turn towards the stimulus and the mouth should be open.
5	Sucking reflex	When touching or stroking the lips with the breast, the mouth opens and sucking movement begin.
6	Swallowing reflex	The passage of food from posterior aspect of the mouth to the stomach.
7	Gagging reflex	When the posterior pharynx is stimulated with food there is an immediate return of undigested food.
8	Extrusion reflex	When substance placed on anterior position of tongue will be expelled out.

Contd...

Contd...

S. No.	Assessment features	Normal value
9	Palmer reflex	When the objects are placed in the newborn's palm, the new born grasps.
10	Plantar reflex	When object touches the sole of the foot at the base of the toes, toes grasp around very small object.
11	Dancing or stepping reflex	Hold neonate in a vertical position with the feet touching a flat, firm surface, there will be rapid alternating flexion and extension of legs.
12	Babinski reflex	Stroking the lateral aspect of the sole of the foot with a relatively sharp object from the heel up toward the little toe and across the foot toward the big toe, there will be fanning of the toes.
13	Tonic neck reflex	Turning the head quickly to one side while the infant is supine, arm and leg on the side the head is turned toward extend. Arm and leg on the opposite side flex.
14	Moro reflex	Sudden jarring or change in equilibrium causes sudden extension and abduction of extremities and fanning of fingers with index finger and thumb forming a 'c' shape followed by flexion and adduction of extremities, legs may weakly flex, infant may cry, disappears after age 3–4 months, usually strongest during first 2 months.
15	Startle reflex	A sudden loud noise causes abduction of the arms with flexion of elbows, hands remain clenched, disappears by age 4 months.
16	Perez reflex	While infant is prone on a firm surface, thumb is pressed along spine from sacrum to neck, infant responds by crying, flexing extremities and elevating pelvis and head lordosis of the spine, as well as defection and urination may occur, disappear by age 4–6 months.
17	Trunk incurvation (Gallant) reflex	Stroking infants back alongside spine causes hips to move toward stimulated side, disappears. By age 4 weeks.
18	Crawl reflex	When placed on abdomen infant makes crawling movements with arms and legs.

THE NORMAL GROWTH AND DEVELOPMENT OF INFANT

Introduction

Normal growth and development is defined as how the infant learns to walk, talk, eat, and interact with others. An infant is 1 month to 1 year old. Babies are called newborns during their first month of life. A newborn sleeps a lot, powerful changes are occurring in the five major areas of development.

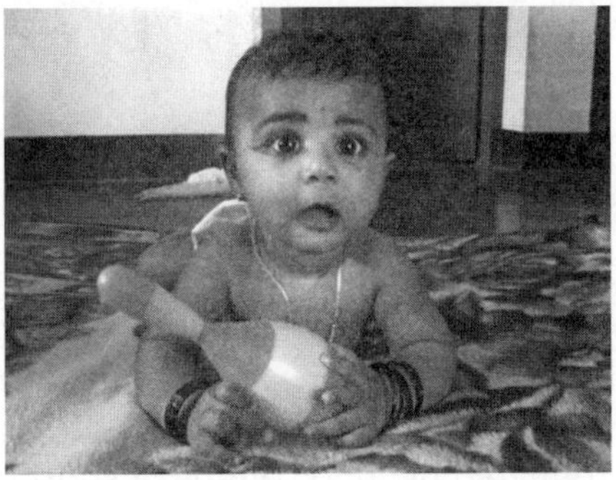

Definition

The Infant child growth and development is defined as it is based on size of the body mass and height of the child. Do not be alarmed if newborn baby loses some weight shortly after birth.

- This weight usually is regained within 10 to 12 days.
- Most newborns gain about 4 oz (113 g) to 8 oz (227 g)
- Height is increasing weekly and grow about 1 inch. (2.5 cm) to 1.5 inch. (3.5 cm) in the first month.

Infant Growth and Development is Usually Divided into the Following Areas

- Physical/Biological development
- Sensory and motor development
  - Fine motor (holding a spoon, pincer grasp)
  - Gross motor (head control, sitting, walking)
- Psychosocial development
- Psychosexual development
- Spiritual development
- **Cognitive/intellectual development:** Cognition is the ability to think, learn, and remember. Newborn's brain is developing rapidly. She promote healthy brain growth every time, she interact in a positive way with the baby.
- **Emotional and social development:** Newborns quickly learn to communicate. They seek interaction with mother and express how they feel with sounds and facial expressions.
- At first, instinctual behaviors, such as crying when uncomfortable, are your baby's ways to signal his or her needs. Soon your newborn starts to subtly communicate and interact with you. For example, baby's eyes will track the adult movements. And his or her face will brighten when you cuddle and talk soothingly. Even at a few days old, baby may try to mimic you sticking out your tongue.
- Language development
- Play stimulation.

Physical Development

An infant's physical development begins at the head, then moves to other parts of the body (for example, sucking comes before sitting and walking).

Newborn to 2 Months

- Child can lift and turn the head when lying on his or her back
- Hands are fisted, the arms are flexed
- Neck is unable to support the head when the infant is pulled to a sitting position.

Primitive Reflexes Include

- Babinski reflex—toes fan outward when sole of foot is stroked
- Moro reflex (startle reflex) extends arms then bends and pulls them in toward body with a brief cry; often triggered by loud sounds or sudden movements

- Palmar hand grasp—infant closes hand and 'grips' your finger
- Placing—leg extends when sole of foot is touched
- Plantar grasp—infant flexes the toes and forefoot
- Rooting and sucking—turns head in search of nipple when cheek is touched and begins to suck when nipple touches lips
- Stepping and walking—takes brisk steps when both feet are placed on a surface, with body supported
- Tonic neck response—left arm extends when infant gazes to the left, while right arm and leg flex inward, and vice versa.

3 to 4 Months

- Better eye-muscle control allows the infant to track objects
- Begins to control hand and feet actions, but these movements are not fine-tuned. The infant may begin to use both hands, working together, to accomplish tasks. The infant is still unable to coordinate the grasp, but swipes at objects to bring them closer
- Increased vision allows the infant to tell objects apart from backgrounds with very little contrast (such as a button on a blouse of the same color)
- Infant raises up (upper torso, shoulders, and head) with arms when lying face down (on tummy)
- Neck muscles are developed enough to allow the infant to sit with support, and keep head up
- Primitive reflexes have either already disappeared, or are starting to disappear.

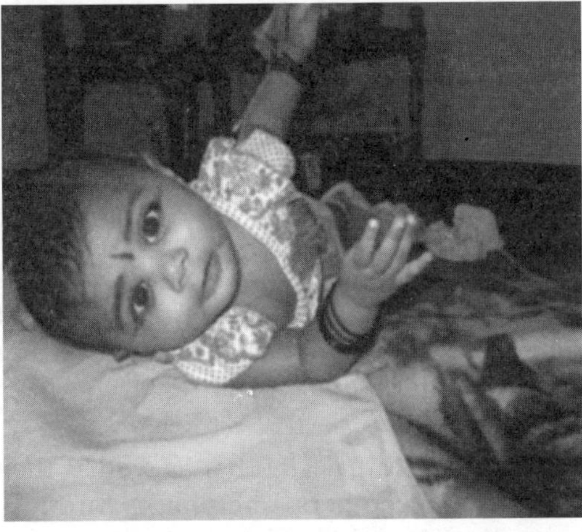

5 to 6 Months

- Able to sit alone, without support, for only moments at first, and then for up to 30 seconds or more
- Infant begins to grasp blocks or cubes using the ulnar-palmar grasp technique (pressing the block into palm of hand while flexing or bending wrist in) but does not yet use thumb
- Infant rolls from back to stomach. When on tummy, the infant can push up with arms to raise the shoulders and head and look around or reach for objects.

6 to 9 Months
- Crawling may begin
- Infant can walk while holding an adult's hand
- Infant is able to sit steadily, without support, for long periods of time
- Infant learns to sit down from a standing position
- Infant may pull into and keep a standing position while holding onto furniture.

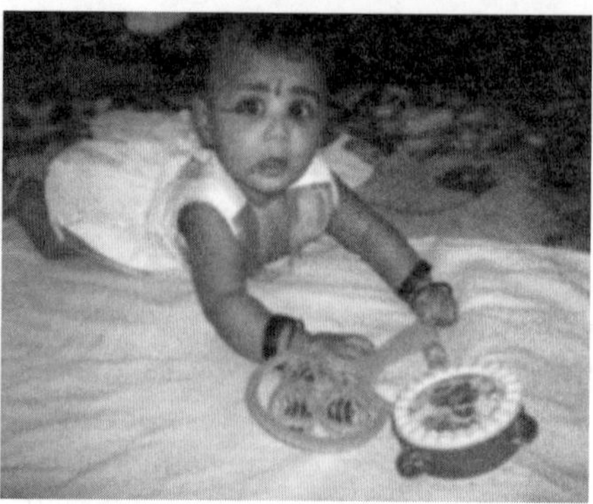

9 to 12 Months
- Infant begins to balance while standing alone
- Infant takes steps and begins to walk alone.

Motor Skills Development

- Motor skills develop as your baby's muscles and nerves work together. Movements are mostly controlled by reflexes, such as the rooting reflex, which is when a newborn's head turns and his or her mouth 'reaches' toward a touch. Hands are tightly fisted when the baby is alert.
- Parents then view their child as they would a blurred photograph from a camera that is out of focus. Spontaneity and enjoyment of the infant by the parents or their substitutes is probably of grater significance to the baby's well-being than the specific procedures used in care giving. If the usual caregiver is a mother who is harassed and overburdened because of her job or the lack of an adequate support system, her care may not be benefited. If parents share care giving, each can spend time with the infant and also provide support to each other.
- Their ability to support and nurture each other as well as their child promotes optimal development of all the family members. The phases through which parent's progress as their child grows are discussed throughout this text.

Sensory Development

- Newborns have all five senses. Newborn quickly learns to recognize parent's face, the sound of their voice, and how they smell. In newborn's sense of touch is especially developed, particularly around the mouth.
- The baby also has a strong sense of smell. After a few days, newborn hears fairly well and responds most noticeably to high-pitched and loud sounds.

- The baby recognizes and prefers sweet tastes to those that are sour, bitter, or salty. Vision is developing quickly but is believed to be the weakest of the senses:
  - Hearing—begins before birth, and is mature at birth. The infant prefers the human voice.
  - Touch, taste, smell—mature at birth; prefers sweet taste.
  - Vision—the newborn infant can see within a range of 8–12 inches. Color vision develops between 4–6 months. By 2 months, can track moving objects up to 180 degrees, and prefers faces.
  - Inner ear (vestibular) senses—the infant responds to rocking and changes of position.

Behavioral Development

Newborn behavior is based on six states of consciousness:

- Active crying
- Active sleep
- Drowsy waking
- Fussing
- Quiet alert
- Quiet sleep.

Healthy babies with a normal nervous system can move smoothly from one state to another. Heart, breathing, muscle tone, and body movements are different in each state. Many bodily functions are not stable in the first months after birth. This is normal and differs from infant to infant. Stress and stimulation can affect:

- Bowel movements
- Gagging
- Hiccupping
- Skin color
- Temperature control
- Vomiting
- Yawning.

Periodic breathing, in which breathing starts and stops again, is normal and is not a sign of sudden infant death syndrome (SIDS). Some infants will vomit or spit up after each feeding, but have nothing physically wrong with them. They continue to gain weight and develop normally.

Other infants grunt and groan while making a bowel movement but produce soft, blood-free stools, and their growth and feeding are good. This is due to immature abdominal muscles used for pushing and does not need to be treated.

Sleep/wake cycles vary and do not stabilize until a baby is 3 months old. These cycles occur in random intervals of 30–50 minutes at birth and gradually increase as the infant matures. By age 4 months, most infants will have one 5-hour period of uninterrupted sleep per day.

Breastfed infants will feed about every 2 hours. Formula-fed infants should be able to go 3 hours between feedings. During periods of rapid growth, they may feed more often.

She should advise the parents no need to give the water to baby. In fact, it could be dangerous. An infant who is drinking enough will produce 6–8 wet diapers in a 24-hour period. Teaching the infant to suck a pacifier or his or her own thumb provides comfort between feedings.

Language Development

The newborn is listening to and absorbing the basic and distinct sounds of language. This process forms the foundation for speech.

A crying is a very important way to communicate. By the baby's third day of life, mothers can tell their own baby's cry from that of other babies. By the first month of life, most parents can tell if their baby's cry means hunger, pain, or anger. Crying also causes a nursing mother's milk to letdown (fill the breast).

The amount of crying in the first 3 months varies in a healthy infant, from 1–3 hours a day. Infants who cry more than 3 hours a day are often described as having colic.

Excessive crying can be due to child abuse. Regardless of the cause, excess crying needs medical evaluation.

0 to 2 Months

- Alert to voices
- Uses range of noises to signal needs, such as hunger or pain

2 to 4 Months

- Coos

4 to 6 Months

- Makes vowel sounds ('oo,' 'ah')

6 to 9 Months

- Babbles
- Blows bubbles ('raspberries')
- Laughs

9 to 12 Months

- Imitates some sounds
- Says 'Mama' and 'Dada', but not specifically for those parents
- Responds to simple verbal commands, such as 'no'.

Safety

A Safety is very important for infants. For example, around age 4–6 months, the infant may begin to roll over. Therefore, be very careful while the baby is on the changing table.

Consider the following important safety tips:

- Be aware of poisons (household cleaners, cosmetics, medications, and even some plants) in your home and keep them out of your infant's reach.
- Do not allow older infants to crawl or walk around in the kitchen while adults or older siblings are cooking. Block the kitchen off with a gate or place the infant in a playpen, highchair, or crib while others cook.

- Do not drink or carry anything hot while holding the infant to avoid burns. Infants begin waving their arms and grabbing for objects at 3–5 months.
- Do not leave an infant alone with siblings or pets. Even older siblings may not be ready to handle an emergency if it occurs. Pets, even though they may appear to be gentle and loving, may react unexpectedly to an infant's cries or grabs, or may actually smother an infant by lying too closely.
- Do not leave an infant alone on a surface from which the child can wiggle or roll over and fall off.
- For the first 5 months of life, always place your infant on his or her back to go to sleep. This position has been shown to reduce the risk of sudden infant death syndrome (SIDS). Once a baby can roll over by himself, the maturing nervous system greatly reduces the risk of SIDS.
- Know how to handle a choking emergency in an infant by taking a certified course through the American Heart Association, the American Red Cross, or a local hospital.
- Never leave small objects within an infant's reach—infants explore their environment by putting everything they can get their hands on into their mouth.
- Place the infant in a proper car seat for every car ride, no matter how short the distance. Use a car seat that faces backwards until the infant is at least 1 year old AND weighs 20 pounds, or longer if possible. Then you can safely switch to a forward facing car seat.
- The safest place for the infant's car seat is in the middle of the back seat. It is very important for the driver to pay attention to driving—not playing with the infant. If an infant needs assistance, safely pull the car over to the shoulder and park before trying to help the infant.
- Use gates on stairways and block off rooms that are not 'child proof'—remember, infants may learn to crawl or scoot as early as 6 months.

Infants Growth and Development Assessment

S. No.	Assessment features	Normal value
1	**Physical/biological development**	**1–6 months**
		Weight:
		• Weight 4.4 ± 0.8 kg: gains above 680 gm, a month during first 6 months, or 150 to 210 gm a week
		Height:
		• 53 ± 2.5 cm (21 ± 1 in); increases about 2.5 cm (1 in) a month during first 6 months
		Dentition:
		• Full set of 20 temporary teeth
		Chest circumference:
		• At birth: 35 cm
		• 3 months: 40 cm
		• 6 months: 43 cm
		• 1 year: 45 cm

Contd...

Contd...

S. No.	Assessment features	Normal value
		Head circumference:
		• Head circumference increases about 1.5 cm (0.5 in) a month during first 6 months.
		– Pulse: 130 ± 20
		– Respirations: 35 ±10
		– Blood pressure: 80/50 ± 20/10
		Posterior fontanel closed:
		• At 6 to 8 weeks of age
		Expected weight calculation formula
		$= \frac{\text{Age in month} + 9}{2}$
2	**Motor development**	**Gross motor:**
		1 month
		• Lies in flexed position, when prone, pelvis is elevated but knees are not beneath abdomen as they were after birth.
		• Head lags when baby pulled from a supine to a sitting position
		2–3 months
		• Symmetric posture of head and body
		• Head in mid position or side
		• Lifts head almost 45 degrees angle
		4–5 months
		• Symmetric body postures predominate
		• Sits with adequate support
		• Lifts head and shoulders at a 90 degree angle
		6–8 months
		• Sits alone briefly if placed in a favorable leaning position on hard surface
		• Holds an arm out back is straight when sitting in high. Chair Pulls to a sitting position
		• Bounces actively when held in standing position
		• Sits alone steadily
		• Pulls self into standing position with help
		9–12 months
		• Raises to a sitting position alone with good coordination
		• Pull self to standing position alone while holding onto furniture
		• Moves from prone to sitting position
		• Makes stepping movements forward when two hands are held
		• Stands erect with minimal support and lifts one foot to take a step
		• Cruises: Walks holding onto furniture

Contd...

Contd...

S. No.	Assessment features	Normal value
		• Stands alone for variable length of time Sits down from standing position alone, Walks in few steps.
		Fine motor:
		1 month
		• Holds hands in tight fists
		• Can grasp an object placed in the hand (palmer grasp reflex) but drops it immediately
		2–3 months
		• Hands may be open
		• Holds a rattle briefly when placed in the hand
		• Hands open or closed loosely
		4–5 months
		• Holds hand predominately open, brings hands together in midline sits with adequate support
		• Plays with fingers, grasps object held near hand
		• Attempts to reach objects with hands but overshoots them
		• Objects are carried to mouth, thumb apposition in grasping occurs between third and fourth months, fingers and clutches clothing
		• Uses thumb in partial opposition to fingers more skillfully
		• Grasps objects with whole hand, either right or left, holds one object while looking at another
		6–8 months
		• Grasps with simultaneous flexion of fingers: Begins to use fingers to feed self
		• Begins to transfer object from one hand to other hand
		• Holds own bottle but may prefer for it to be held
		• Holds 23 toys at once, approaches a toy and grasps it with one hand (ambidextrous) 7 months
		• Holds 2 objects while looking at a third persistently reaches for objects beyond range of grasp, releases objects from hands voluntarily
		• Complete thumb apposition, pincer grasp beginning to develop
		9–12 months
		• Bangs two objects together, pokes objectives with fingers uses thumb and index finger in early pincer grasp
		• Puts nipple in and withdraws it from mouth at will, drinks from cup with some spilling (9-12 months), attempts to use a spoon but spills contents
		• Picks small objects up with index finger and thumb (pincer grasp), Releases an object after holding it brings the hands together
		• Good pincer grasp, picks up small bits of food and transfers them to mouth. Enjoys eating with fingers, attempts to put a small pellet into a narrow-necked bottle but does not succeed, releases one or more objects inside another object or container.

Contd...

Contd...

S. No.	Assessment features	Normal value
3	**Sensory development**	**1–8 months**
		• Visual acuity, 20/200
		9–12 months
		• Visual acuity: 20/100 to 20/50
		• Marked interest in very small
		• Objects: Searches for a lost toy with greater persistence.
4	**Psychosocial development**	***Trust vs mistrust***
		1–2 months
		• A development of sense of trust. Negative counterpart: Mistrust
		• Totally Egocentric
		• Bonding progresses
		• A face orientation, smiling, and vocalization are the evidences of attachment between infant and parents
		• This is the beginning of social behavior
		3–4 months
		• Sense of trust
		• Recognizes and smiles in response to caregiver's (usually the mother's) face.
		• Stops crying when familiar person seen
		• This is the beginning of social behavior
		• Shows interest in new stimuli
		5–6 months
		• Smiles at self in mirror
		• Shows displeasure when toy is lost
		• Recognizes parents and strangers
		• Knows what is liked and disliked
		7–8 months
		• Sense of trust shows increasing fear of strangers
		• Responds socially to own name: Emotional instability
		• Refuses to play with strangers or even accept toys from them
		• Emotional instability still evident: Dislikes changing clothing and diapers
		9–10 months
		• Sense of trust expresses several beginning recognizable emotions such as anger, sadness, jealousy, anxiety, pleasure, excitement, and affection
		• Beginning fears about being left alone, as-when put into the crib, dislikes having face washed so covers face with arms and hands
		• Shows preference for one toy over another

Contd...

Contd...

S. No.	Assessment features	Normal value
		11–12 months
		• Sense of trust shows pleasure when a desired act is accomplished
		• Becomes frustrated when activities are restricted
		• Seeks approval, avoids disapproval
		• Sense of trust theoretically achieved
		• A sense of mistrust predominates: Infant's emotion, such as fear, jealousy, anger, can be more clearly interpreted
		• Responds to requests for affection such as a kiss or a hug
		• Puts arms through sleeves, feet into shoes
5	**Psychosexual development**	**Oral stage (0 to 1 year)**
		• Oral aggressiveness is evidenced by biting and chewing
		• Discover genitalia (7 months)
6	**Spiritual development**	**Undifferentiated (0 to 1 year)**
7	**Intellectual/cognitive development**	**Sensory motor stage (0 to 2 years)**
		Substage I: (birth to 1 month):
		• Infant uses reflexes to begin to make associations between an act and a sequential response: Cannot distinguish self from environment
		Substage II: Primary circular reaction (1 to 4 months):
		• Begins to repeat actions of own body voluntarily (hand to mouth movement permits sucking)
		Substage III: Secondary circular reaction (4 to 8 months)
		• Repeats actions that affect an object to get a response (shaking a rattle)
		• Experiments with old or new responses to produce environmental changes or to reach a goal
		Substage IV: Coordination of secondary schemas (8 to 12 months)
		• Abilities learned earlier are combined and extended to deal with new situations
		• Perceptions of space become refined between 8 to 12 months
		• Problem solving beginning to develop
8	**Moral development**	• **Preconventional morality**
		• **Stage 0 (0–2 years)**
		• The good is what I like and want
9	**Play stimulation**	**Onlooker play 1–3 months**
		• Offer a rattle, pull from supine to sitting position. Hold or dangle toy in front of infant to encourage eye movement. Change patterns of objects from bright and shiny to dull and dark' for further stimulation
		Solitary play (playpen) 4–7 months
		• Place infant when awake where household activities are in progress. Include infant in family's television viewing and activities

Contd...

Contd...

S. No.	Assessment features	Normal value
		• Continue to encourage playing in water and perhaps 'swimming' in shallow tub or pool.
		• Gently push infant from a sitting position to improve balance (8 months)
		8–12 months
		• Continue infant games, including 'pat-a-cake' and 'peek-a-boo,' with appropriate motions
		• Provide opportunities for holding and releasing objects
		• Encourage cruising by placing furniture in a circle. Encourage infant to bounce in a standing position by holding the hands for support
		• Place infant in a jumper seat to encourage standing and jumping
		• Play simple games such as rolling a ball to infant
		• Encourage infant to stand alone by gradually decreasing support (furniture or adult's hands)
		• Encourage infant to walk, eventually holding only one hand

BREASTFEEDING AND WEANING

Introduction

Breastfeeding along is a adequate and sufficient to maintain optimum growth and development of an infant up to the age for 4 to 6 months. It is therefore, necessary to introduce more concentrated energy richer nutritional supplements by this age. Infants also required iron containing food supplements after this age to prevent iron deficiency anemia. **(See the notes on the breastfeeding in unit-II).**

Definition

Weaning or complementary feeding is defined as the process of gradual progressive transfer of the baby from the breastfeeding to the usual family diet. During this process the infant gets accustomed to foods other than mother's milk. Weaning does to mean discontinuity of breastfeeding. Weaning foods are given in addition of breast feed when the amount of breastfeeding is inadequate.

Qualities of Complementary Foods

The weaning foods should be:

- Liquid at starting then semisolid and solid foods to be introduced gradually.
- Clean, fresh and hygienic, so that infections can occur.
- Easy to prepare at home with the available food items and not costly.
- Easily digestible, easily acceptable and palatable for the infants.
- High in energy density and low in bulk viscosity and contains all nutrients necessary for the baby.
- Based on cultural practices and traditional beliefs.
- Well-balanced, nourishing and suitable for the infant.

Principles of Introduction of Weaning Foods

During introduction of weaning foods following principles to be remembered:

- Milk is the main food of infant, so additional feeds should provide extra requirements as per needs of the baby, that must be obtained from good quality food items and should be home made.
- A small amount of new foods to be given in the beginning and gradually the amount of food to be increased during the course of a week.
- New food to be placed over the tongue of the baby to get the taste of the food and to feel the consistency. The baby may spit the food out, but with patience the feed to be given again to get accustomed with it. A single waning food is added at a time.
- There should not be any strict rule for serving new foods, it may be modified. But the foods to be given regularly.
- New foods should be given when the infant is hungry, but never force the child to take the feeds.
- Observe the problems related to weaning process. The infant may have indigestion, pain in abdomen, weaning diarrhea, skin rash, specially in case of food allergy and psychological upset of the baby due to withdrawn from breast milk and sucking. The problems should be managed carefully.
- Weaning should be started between 4 to 6 months of age to all children but breastfeeding to be continued up to 2 years of age of beyond.
- Delayed weaning result in malnutrition and growth failure.

Complementary Feeding at Different Age

Weaning to be initiated with fruit juices, especially the grape juice, which is low in sorbitol. Within one or two weeks new foods to be introduced with suji, biscuit soaked in milk, vegetable soup, mashed banana, mashed and boiled potato, etc. Each food should be given with one or two teaspoons at first for 3 to 6 times per day. Foods should not be over diluted. Within 3 to 4 weeks amounts to be increased to half a cup. Breastfeeding must be continued.

6 to 9 Months

Food items to be given in this period include soft mixture of rice and dal, khichri, pulses, mashed and boiled potato, bread or roti soaked in milk or dal, mashed fruits like banana, mango, papaya, stewed apple, etc. Egg yolk can be given from 6 to 7 months onwards. Curd and khir can be introduced from 7 to 8 months onwards. By the age of 6 to 9 months the infant can enjoy to bite biscuits, piece of carrot and cucumber. The infant can have these foods 5 to 6 times per day and amount of food to be increased gradually. Breastfeeding should be continued.

9 to 12 Months

More variety of household foods can be added. New food items like fish, meat, chicken can be introduced during this period. The infant can eat everything cooked at home but spices and condiments to be avoided. Feeds need not to be mashed but should be soft and well-cooked. Breastfeeding to be continued.

12 to 18 Months

The child can take all food cooked in the family and needs half amount of mothers diet. Number of feeds can be 4 to 5 times or according to the child's need. Breastfeeding to be continued, especially at night.

The weaning period is most crucial period in child important aspect of child rearing and significant approach of preventive pediatrics towards healthy children.

Artificial Feeding

Artificial feeding means to feed the child other than breast milk. It involves the use of breast milk substitutes in the form of liquid milk, i.e. fresh cow's or buffalo's milk or commercially available dried whole milk. It is a form of supplementary feeding.

The main indications for artificial feeding are death or absence of mother, prolonged maternal illness and complete failure of breast milk production. Artificial feeding is given only, if there is no one available as mother surrogate to give breastfeed to the infant or expressed breast milk is not available.

In spite of various attempts to promote the age old breastfeeding practices and superiority of human milk, today artificial feeding and bottle feeding are still in existence and practiced, where they are actually not needed.

Essential Care of Nutritionally Needed in Children

Food is essential for any living organism. Humans, being highly evolved of the animal species, have complex nutritional requirements. Proper nutrition is of essence if a child has to grow optimally and realize its potential. The basic constituents of child's nutrition are water, calories, proteins, carbohydrates, fats, vitamins, minerals and salts.

Water: The total water content of the body is higher in infant than in adults. It constitutes 70 percent body weight in children.

Water content of body compartments	
Intracellular	50 percent
Extracellular	20 percent
Intravascular	15 percent
Interstitial	5 percent

The normal adult value is 60 percent, which is reached by adolescence. Water requirement in the perinatal period varies from 80 ml/kg on the first day to 150 m/mg on the tenth day. Infants require 150 ml/kg fluids daily.

Adults require 50 ml/kg day. Water is absorbed throughout the intestinal tract. Evaporation from lungs and skin accounts for 40–50 percent of water loss and fecal loss for 3–10 percent.

Energy is required for physical activity of daily life. At complete rest energy is spent for basal metabolism. Mothers during pregnancy and lactation and growing children require additional food energy. One gram of carbohydrate or 1 gm of protein gives 4 kcal and 1 gm of fat releases 9 kcal.

Proteins: These are required for the formation of new tissues, to compensate for wear and tear and for specific metabolic functions. They should provide 10 to 15 percent of total caloric needs. Proteins are in the form of amino acids. Nine of the twenty-four amino acids are considered as essential. Deficiency of even one of these can result in negative nitrogen balance.

In children one third of the total intake of protein is utilized for growth, dietary proteins are of animal or vegetable origin. Animal protein is a good source of quality dietary proteins. A mixture of animal and vegetable proteins ensures optimum utilization. During early infancy milk supplies all the protein requirements of a child.

Energy Requirements

Birth–3 months	120 kcal/kg/day
4 Months–6 months	115 kcal/kg/day
7 Months–9 months	110 kcal/kg/day
9 Months–12 months	105 kcal/kg/day
1–2 years	1100 kcal/day
3–4 years	1300–1500 kcal/day
4–5 years	1700 kcal/day
7–9 years	25 kcal/day
10–12 years	2500 kcal/day

Protein Requirements

Birth–3 months	10g/d
4–6 months	12 g/d
7–9 months	18 g/d
9–12 months	19 g/d
1–3 years	16 g/d
4–6 years	20 g/d
7–9 years	25 g/d
10–12 years	30 g/d

A bottle fed infant requires 3.5 gm/kg and a breast fed infant requires 2 gm/kg proteins per day.

Vegetable proteins have low biological value. Cereals are poor in lysine and methionine. Pulses are poor in threonine and methionine and maize in tryptophan. Milk, egg, meat and fish are the dietary source of complete proteins. Cow's milk contains large amount of casein.

Premature infants require more proteins. Boiling, dilution with water, acidification and homogenization of milk reduce the tendency of proteins to form firm coagula in stomach.

Protein Constitution of Common Food Items

Cow's milk	3.5 gm percent
Buffalo's milk	4.3 gm percent
Bengal gram	22.5 gm percent

Contd...

Contd...

Green gram	24.0 gm percent
Lentil (Masur)	25.1 gm percent
Soybean	43.2 gm percent
Egg	13.7 gm percent
Fish	21.5 gm percent
Mutton	18.5 gm percent
Cashewnut	21.2 gm percent
Coconut	4.5 gm percent
Groundnut	26.7 gm percent
Bajra	11.6 gm percent
Rice—Raw	7.5 gm percent
Wheat—whole	11.8 gm percent
Refined wheat flour	10.2 gm percent
Ragi	7.1 gm percent
Maize	11.1 gm percent

Carbohydrates

Provide the greatest bulk of energy and the bulk in the diet. Excess carbohydrates are stored as glycogen in liver and muscle. Carbohydrates spare proteins which are utilized for growth.

Jaggery	95.0 gm percent
Honey	79.5 gm percent
Arrowroot flour	83.1 gm percent
Bajra	67.1 gm percent
Rice (Raw)	76.2 gm percent
Wheat (whole)	71.2 gm percent
Wheat flour	74.1 gm percent
Bengal gram	58.9 gm percent
Green gram	60.7 gm percent
Masur	59.7 gm percent
Potato	22.9 gm percent
Sweet potato	31.0 gm percent
Fresh fruits	15–25.0 gm percent
Human milk	7.0 gm percent
Cow's milk	4.0 gm percent

CHO Constitution of Common Food Items

In sufficient quantity, carbohydrates spare fats for energy purpose. Carbohydrates are consumed in the form of monosaccharides (glucose, fructose, galactose), disaccharides (lactose, sucrose, maltose, isomaltose) and polysaccharides (starch, glycogen, dextrin, cellulose) breastfeed babies receive 10 to 12 gm/kg daily. Children need 12–15 gm/kg of carbohydrates daily. Cane sugar, jaggery, lactose (in milk), and honey are the various forms in which sugars are ingested.

Deficient carbohydrate intake results in under nutrition. Carbohydrates should contribute 45 to 55% of daily caloric needs.

Fats

Fat are a concentrated source of energy in the diet. They should provide 35 to 45 percent of calories per day. Human milk provides about 45 percent of the calories in the form of fat.

Fats play an important role as a vehicle for the absorption of fat soluble vitamins. Triglycerides are the most important lipids. Naturally occurring fats come train saturated and unsaturated fatty acids. These can be synthesized in the body. Polyunsaturated fatty acids can not be synthesized in the body.

These are linoleic and arachidonic acid. These must be available in the diet. They are termed essential fatty acids. At least 3 percent of caloric requirements should be derived from these. Vegetable oils—sunflower oil, corn oil are having sufficient amount of fats, it will fulfill the child physical growth needs.

IMMUNIZATION

Introduction

Immunization is a process of protecting an individual from a disease through introduction of live, or killed or attenuated organisms in the individual system. It is one of the best buys in community health and one of the most cost-effective health interventions.

Immunization against vaccine-preventable diseases is essential to reduce the child mortality, morbidity and handicapped conditions. It is mass means of protecting the largest number of people from various diseases. It gives resistance to infectious diseases by producing or augmenting the immunity. Artificially acquired immunity is developed by the immunization.

Immunity is the security against a particular disease and non-susceptibility to the invasive or pathogenic effects of foreign microorganisms or to the toxic effect of antigenic substances. Acquired immunity can be active or passive.

Active immunity is produced by stimulating immunological defense mechanism through administration of antigen usually prior to natural exposure to infection. Active immunizing agents are known as vaccines.

Passive immunity is produced temporarily by supplying preformed exogenous animal or human antibody to suppress the disease, given soon after or prior to exposure of an infection. It is readymade antibodies. Passive immunity agents are antisera and immunoglobulin.

Vaccine Preventable Diseases

Some infectious diseases can be prevented by vaccines. The diseases against which vaccines are currently available are:

Six killer vaccine preventable diseases, i.e.

1. Poliomyelitis
2. Tuberculosis
3. Diphtheria
4. Pertussis
5. tetanus
6. Measles.

Other vaccine preventable diseases include

- Hepatitis-B
- Mumps
- Rubella
- Hemophilus
- Influenza type B (Hib) infections
- Typhoid
- Meningococcal meningitis
- Japanese encephalitis
- Influenza
- Pneumococcal pneumonia
- Chickenpox
- Rotavirus diarrhea
- Yellow fever
- Cholera
- Malaria
- Hepatitis 'A'
- Plague
- Rabies.

Immunizing Agents

The immunizing agents may be classified as vaccines, immunoglobulin's and antisera.

Vaccines

Vaccines are immunobiological substances which produce specific protection against a given disease. It stimulates active production of protective antibody and other immune mechanisms. Vaccines are prepared from live attenuated organisms, or inactivated or killed organisms, extracted cellular fractions, toxoids or combination of these. More recent preparations are subunit vaccine and recombinant vaccines.

The ideal vaccines should induce permanent immunity, be free of toxic substances, have minimal side effects, not produce disease to the recipient and be easy to administer.

The following immunizing agents are currently used:

Live attenuated vaccines

- Bacterial—BCG, Typhoid (oral), Plague.
- Viral—Oral polio, Measles, Mumps, Rubella, Yellow fever, Influenza.

Killed or inactivated vaccines

- Bacterial—Pertussis, Typhoid, Cholera, Plague, CS Meningitis.
- Viral—Rabies, Hepatitis 'B', Influenza, Salk, Polio, Japanese encephalitis.
- Toxoids-Bacterial—Diphtheria and Tetanus.
- Cellular fractions—Meningococcal and pneumococcal vaccines.
- Combinations:
  - DTP (Diphtheria, Tetanus, Pertussis)
  - MMR (Mumps, Measles, Rubella)
  - DT (Diphtheria, Tetanus)
  - Hib – Heb-B (H. influenza 'B', Hepatitis 'B').

Immunoglobulin

The human immunoglobulin (lg) system is composed of 5 major classes (1gG, 1gM, 1gA, 1gD and 1gE) and subclasses within them. The various classes and subclasses of 1gs represent different functional groups that are required to meet different types of antigenic challenges. All antibodies are immunoglobulin, but it is still an open question whether all immunoglobulin are antibodies.

The WHO recommends that the term 'Gamma globulin' should not be used as a synonym for immunoglobulin.

Two types of immunoglobulin preparations are available for passive immunization. These are normal human immunoglobulin and specific (hyperimmune) human immunoglobulin. They are used in the prophylaxis of viral and bacterial infections and in replacement of antibodies in immunoglobulin. These are:

- Normal Human 1g—Hepatitis 'A', Measles, Rabies, Tetanus and Mumps.
- Specific Human 1g—Hepatitis 'B', Varicella and Diphtheria.

Antisera of Antitoxins

The term 'antisera' is applied to the material prepared in animals originally passive immunity was achieved by the administration of antisera of antitoxins prepared from non-human sources like horses. Human 1g preparations exist only for a small number of diseases. Administration of antisera may have adverse effects like serum sickness and anaphylactic shock due to abnormal sensitivity of the recipient. The current trend is to use the immunoglobulins whenever possible. The important antisera which are still used for passive immunization are:

- Bacterial—Diphtheria, Tetanus, Gas gangrene (also known as clostridial myonecrosis and myonecrosis), Botulism.
- Viral—Rabies.

Table 3.4: IAP immunization schedule 2013

Age (completed weeks/ months/years)	Vaccines	Comments
Birth	BCG OPV 0 Hep-B 1	Administer these vaccines to all newborns before hospital discharge

Contd...

Contd...

Age (completed weeks/ months/years)	Vaccines	Comments
6 weeks	DTwP 1 IPV 1 Hep-B 2 Hib 1 Rotavirus 1 PCV 1	**DTP:** • DTaP vaccine/combinations should preferably be avoided for the primary series • DTaP vaccine/combinations should be preferred in certain specific circumstances/conditions only **Polio:** • All doses of IPV may be replaced with OPV if administration of the former is unfeasible • Additional doses of OPV on all supplementary immunization activities (SIAs) • Two doses of IPV instead of three for primary series if started at 8 weeks and 8 weeks interval between the doses • No child should leave your facility without polio immunization (IPV or OPV), if indicated by the schedule **Rotavirus:** • Two doses of RV1 and three doses of RV5 • RV1 should be employed in 10 and 14 week schedule, instead of 6 and 14 week • 10 and 14 week schedule of RV1 is found to be far more immunogenic than exising 6 and 10 week schedule
10 weeks	DTwP 2 IPV 2 Hib 2 Rotavirus 2 PCV 2	**Rotavirus** If RV1 is chosen, the first dose should be given at 10 weeks
14 weeks	DTwP 3 IPV 3 Hib 3 Rotavirus 3 PCV 3	**Rotavirus** Only 2 doses of RV1 are recommended at present. If RV1 is chosen, the 2nd dose should be given at 14 weeks
6 months	OPV 1 Hep-B 3	**Hepatitis-B:** The final (third or fourth) dose in the Hep B vaccine series should be administered no earlier than age 24 weeks and at least 16 weeks after the first dose.
9 months	OPV 2 Measles	Measles vaccine ideally should not be administered before completing 270 days or 9 months of life
12 months	Hep-A 1	**Hepatitis A:** For both killed and live hepatitis-A vaccines, 2 doses are recommended as of now
15 months	MMR 1 Varicella 1, PCV Booster	Varicella: The risk of breakthrough varicella is lower if given 15 months onwards
16 to 18 months	DTwP B1/DTaP B1 IPV B1 Hib B1	The first booster (4th dose) may be administered as early as age 12 months, provided at least 6 months have elapsed since the third dose. **DTP:** • First and second boosters should preferably be of DTwP • Considering a higher reactogenicity of DTwP, DTaP can be considered for the boosters

Contd...

Contd...

Age (completed weeks/ months/years)	Vaccines	Comments
18 months	Hep-A 2	**Hepatitis A:** For both killed and live hepatitis-A vaccines 2 doses are recommended as of now
2 years	Typhoid 1	**Typhoid:** Typhoid revaccination every 3 years, if Vi-polysaccharide vaccine is used
4 to 6 years	DTwP B2/DTaP B2 OPV 3 MMR 2, Varicella 2 Typhoid 2	**MMR:** The 2nd dose can be given at anytime 4–8 weeks after the 1st dose. **Varicella:** The 2nd dose can be given at anytime 3 months after the 1st dose.
10 to 12 years	Tdap/Td HPV	**Tdap:** It is preferred to Td followed by Td every 10 years. **HPV:** Only for females, 3 doses at 0, 1–2 (depending on brands) and 6 months.

National Immunization Schedule

Immunization schedule should be planned according to the needs of the community. It should be relevant with existing community health problems. It must be effective, feasible and acceptable by the community. Every country has its own immunization schedule.

The WHO, launched global immunization program in 1974, known as Expanded Program on Immunization (EPI) to protect all children of the world against six killer diseases. In India, EPI was launched in January 1978.

The EPI is now renamed as Universal Child Immunization, as per declaration sponsored by UNICEF. In India, it is called Universal Immunization Program (UIP) and was launched in 1985, November, for the universal coverage of immunization to the eligible population.

The Global Alliance for Vaccines and Immunization (GAVI) is worldwide coalition of organization, established in 1999, to reduce disparities in life-saving vaccine access and increase global immunization coverage. GAVI is collaborative mission of Govt, NGOs, UNICEF, WHO and World Bank. The GAVI and Vaccine fund also adopted the objective of introduction of new but under used vaccines in the developing countries, where the diseases like hepatitis-B and H – influenza 'B' *Hib) are highly prevalent.

National Immunization Schedule as recommended by Government of India for uniform implementation throughout the country was formulated. It is shown in Table 3.5. the schedule contents the age at which the vaccines are best given and the number of doses recommended for each vaccine. The schedule also covers immunization of women during pregnancy against tetanus.

Table 3.5: National immunization schedule for infants, children and pregnant women

Vaccine	When to give	Dose	Route	Site
		For pregnant women		
TT-1	Early in pregnancy	0.5 ml	Intramuscular	Upper arm
TT-2	4 weeks after TT-1*	0.5 ml	Intramuscular	Upper arm
TT-Booster	If received 2 TT doses in a pregnancy within last 3 years	0.5 ml	Intramuscular	Upper arm

Contd...

Contd...

Vaccine	When to give	Dose	Route	Site
		For infants		
BCG	At birth or as early as possible till one year of age	0.1 ml (0.05 ml till 1 month age)	Intradermal	Left upper arm
Hepatitis B	At birth or as early as possible within 24 hours	0.5 ml	Intramuscular	Anterolateral side of mid thigh
OPV-0	At birth or as early as possible within the first 15 days	2 drops	Oral	Oral
OPV 1, 2 and 3	At 6 weeks, 10 weeks and 14 weeks	2 drops	Oral	Oral
DPT 1, 2 and 3	At 6 weeks, 10 weeks and 14 weeks	0.5 ml	Intramuscular	Anterolateral side of mid thigh
Hep B 1, 2 and 3	At 6 weeks, 10 weeks and 14 weeks	0.5 ml	Intramuscular	Anterolateral side of mid thigh
Measles	9 completed months-12 months	0.5 ml	Subcutaneous	Right upper arm
Vitamin-A (1st dose)	At 9 months with measles	1 ml (1 lakh IU)	Oral	Oral
		For children		
DPT booster	16–24 months	0.5 ml	Intramuscular	Anterolateral side of mid thigh
Measles 2nd dose	16–24 months	0.5 ml	Subcutaneous	Right upper arm
OPV booster	16–24 months	2 drops	Oral	Oral
Japanese Encephalitis**	16–24 months	0.5 ml	Subcutaneous	Left upper arm
Vitamin-A***				
(2nd to 9th dose)	16 months. Then, one dose every 6 months up to the age of 5 years	2 ml (2 lakh IU)	Oral	Oral
DPT Booster	5–6 years	0.5 ml	Intramuscular	Upper arm
TT	10 years and 16 years	0.5 ml	Intramuscular	Upper arm

*Give TT-2 or booster doses before 36 weeks of pregnancy. However, give these even if more than 36 weeks have passed. Give TT to a woman in labor, if she has not previously received TT.

**JE vaccine, in select endomic districts after the campaign.

***The 2nd to 9th doses of vitamin A can be administered to children 1–5 years old during biannual rounds in collaboration with ICDS.

Immunization of Children

BCG Vaccination

BCG (Bacillus of Calmette and Guerin) vaccine is live attenuated bacterial vaccine produced from 'Dannish – 1331' strain of tubercle bacilli. It produces active immunity to protect the child from tuberculosis. The aim of BCG vaccination is to induce benign artificial primary infection which will stimulate an acquired resistance of possible subsequent infection with virulent tubercle bacilli and thus reduce the morbidity and mortality from primary tuberculosis among risk group.

The presently available and used BCG vaccine is heat stable and in freeze dried form. It should be kept away from direct light and stored in a cool environment below 10 °C (2 to 8 °C). Normal saline is recommended as a diluents for reconstituting the vaccine. The reconstituted vaccine may be used up within 3 hours and then the left over vaccine should be discarded.

The BCG vaccine is administered at birth in institutional deliveries or as soon as possible after birth, or at 6 weeks, if not given at birth. The standard site is the middle of deltoid muscle over the left upper arm, i.e. just above the insertion of the deltoid muscle. If it is injected too high, too forward or too backward, the adjacent lymph nodes may become involved and tender.

The vaccine is given using a special tuberculin syringe in intradermal route. The dose is 0.05 ml in neonates and 0.1 ml in infants.

A satisfactory injection in neonates and 0.1 ml in infants. A satisfactory injection should produce a wheel of 5 mm in diameter. The vaccine must not be contaminated with an antiseptic or detergent. If alcohol is used to swab the skin, it must be allowed to evaporate before the vaccine is injected.

BCG immunization is contraindicated if the child is suffering from generalized eczema, infective dermatosis, hypogammaglobulinemia, immune deficiency conditosis, hypogamma-globulinesmia; immune deficiency conditions and HIV infected children with symptoms of AIDS related complex (ARC) or AIDS. All asymptomatic HIV infected children should receive the BCG vaccine.

The duration of protection is about 15 to 20 years. BCG vaccination is a fundamental component of National Tuberculosis Program and plays a valuable role in preventing severe form of childhood tuberculosis.

Polio Vaccination

Oral polio vaccine (OPV) was first described by Sabin in 1957. It contains live attenuated polio virus of three strains (types 1, 2 and 3). It is administered as trivalent (TOPV) vaccine. The recently available OPV is heat stabilized and can be kept without losing potency at 4 °C for year and for a month at room temperature. The non-stabilized vaccine should be stored at 20 °C in a deep freeze.

The OPV is cheaper, easy to administer, protects the individual child from poliomyelitis and prevents spread of wild pathogenic poliovirus in the community. It induces both humeral and intestinal immunity. The OPV is very safe vaccine without any adverse effects. Rare cases of vaccine associated paralytic polio may occur (one case per million vaccinated child). Vaccine potency can be effectively monitors using vaccine vial monitors (VVM).

OPV is administered with 'zero' dose at birth in institutional deliveries and then 3 doses at one month interval from 6 weeks of age (6 weeks, 10 weeks and 14 weeks). OPV can be given with DTP and BCG at the same time and same day. The dose is two drops or as stated on the label of the vial and given orally. It is very important to complete primary course of

OPV within 6 months. Because most polio cases occurs between 6 months to 3 years. One booster dose is recommended at 16 to 24 months of age.

The contraindications for the administration of OPV include acute infectious disease, fever, diarrhea, dysentery, leukemia, malignancy and corticosteroids therapy.

After vaccination, breastfeeding can be given, if the child is hungry, but hot drinks, hot milk or hot water should be withheld for ½ hour. The OPV should be administered in cool room in the clinic rather than hot, humid and crowded room and the OPV vial should be kept on ice pack.

The problems with OPV are instability of the vaccine at high ambient temperature and frequent vaccine failure even with fully potent vaccines. Failure of 3 dose regimen has been reported and indicates a serous problem in order to overcome this problem, 5 doses of OPV are recommended by Indian Academy of pediatrics in clinic-based programs and 3 doses in community campaigns.

Inactivated (killed) polio vaccine developed by Salk, administered in IM or SC route is expensive and produce short lived immunity which is not recommended in National Immunization Schedule.

DTP (Diphtheria, Tetanus, Pertussis) Vaccination

DTP is a combined vaccine administered for the protection against three diseases, i.e. diphtheria, pertussis and tetanus. DTP vaccine is composed of diphtheria toxoid, tetanus toxoid and killed B. pertussis bacilli. The potency of diphtheria toxoid is enhanced by the pertussis component of DTP vaccine.

There are two types of DTP vaccine, i.e. plain and adsorbed. Absorption is usually carried out on a mineral carrier like aluminum phosphate or hydroxide. Adsorption increases the immunological effectiveness of the vaccine. The WHO recommends that only adjuvant DTP vaccine to be utilized in immunization programs. The plain DTP vaccine can be used as a booster.

DTP/DT vaccines should be stored between 4 to 8 °C temperature and should not be frozen. The vaccines will lose potency if kept at room temperature over a longer period of time.

For primary immunization, DTP vaccine is administered in 3 doses at 4 weeks interval at 6 weeks, 10 weeks and 14 weeks of age. Each dose is 0.5 ml and should be given deep intramuscularly as all vaccines contain mineral carriers or adjuvant. The site of injection for children below one year of age should be lateral aspect of thigh (vastus lateralis muscle). In older children, it may be given in upper and outer quadrant of the gluteus muscle.

DTP vaccine may be given concurrently with OPV. BCG can be given on the same time along with DTP, but the site for the injection should be different.

The booster dose of DTP vaccine is given at 16 to 24 months of age followed by another booster dose of DT (Diphtheria, Tetanus) vaccine at the age of 5 to 6 years, without Pertussis component.

DTP vaccination usually not recommended after 6 years of age. So children above the age of 5 years, who received to primary course of DTP vaccine earlier, should received the primary course of DTP vaccine earlier, should receive only DT as booster at 5–6 years and those who have not received DTP, need only two dose of DT vaccines at 4 weeks interval.

Measles Vaccination

Measles vaccine is live attenuated and tissue culture vaccine, available as freeze dried product. It is safe and effective. Heat stable measles vaccine and its diluting fluid should be stored at 2 to 8 °C temperature to maintain their patency.

The measles vaccine is administered at the age of 9 months, before this age, maternal antibody protects the infants. Single dose of vaccine is given with 0.5 ml amount in subcutaneous route. The freeze dried vaccine should be reconstituted with diluting fluid and must be kept on ice and to be used within one hour. Left over vaccine must be discarded and never used after 4 hours of opening the vial. No booster dose is recommended as the immunity usually appears for long duration.

After the measles vaccination, reactions may develop as fever and rash on 5 to 10 days after immunization and induces a milk measles illness but in reduced frequency and severity. This may found in 15 to 20 percent of vaccines.

The fever may persist for 1–2 days and the rash for 1–3 days. Severe reactions may develop following this vaccination if the recommended temperature is not maintained; and necessary precautions are not followed. Toxic shock syndrome (TSS) may develop with contaminated vaccine or if the same vial is used for more than one session on the same day or next day. The features of TSS are severe watery diarrhea, vomiting and high fever vaccination. This condition may cause death within 48 hours and case fatality rates are high.

Measles vaccine is contraindicated in infants below 6 months of age, acute illness, convulsions, allergy, active tuberculosis, malnutrition, immunodeficiency states, malignancy and immunosuppressive therapy (steroids, antimetabolites, etc).

Measles vaccine can be combined and effectively administered with other live attenuated vaccines such as mumps and rubella. MMR vaccine can be given at the age of 15 months, 3 months following primary measles vaccination. MMR vaccine is not included in National Immunization Schedule.

Hepatitis 'B' Vaccination

Hepatitis 'B' vaccinations is now included in the immunization schedule, in some states of India, as routine vaccine. But due to economical constraints, it is not included as seventh vaccine in the National Immunization Schedule.

Hepatitis 'B' Vaccines are available in two forms: a) plasma derived vaccine and b) RDNA yeast derived vaccine.

Plasma derived vaccine is based on the surface antigen (HBs Ag) which is harvested and purified from plasma of human carriers of hepatitis 'B' virus. It is formalin inactivated subunit viral vaccine. Each 1 ml dose of the vaccine contains 20 mcg of hepatitis surface antigen formulated in an alum adjuvant. The vaccine is safe, effective and cheapest.

The hepatitis 'B' vaccine is given intramuscularly with the 3 doses in general at 0, 1 and 6 months or 4 doses at 0, 1, and 12 months in highly endemic area. The dose of the vaccine is 0.5 ml for the child below 10 years and one ml above 10 years at the same time interval. Antibody response attained after 3 doses. Immunity levels provide protection for about 3 to 5 years. Booster doses may be administered after 3 to 5 years.

Hepatitis 'B' vaccine is given for pre-exposure and postexposure prophylaxis. Examples of postexposure prophylaxis are protection of neonates born to carrier mothers and individuals accidentally, exposed parenterally to HBV infection through transfusion, cuts, injuries and needle sticks.

High-risk children for HVB infections should be immunized with hepatitis 'B' vaccine, e.g. repeated and multiple blood transfusion, (in case of thalassemia, hemophilia), hemodialysis, IV (intravenous) drug users, sexual contact with carriers of HBV, etc.

RDNA or recombinant DNA yeast derived vaccine is an alternate vaccine against hepatitis 'B'. It is genetically engineered vaccine, safe, effective as the plasma derived vaccine and is more cost-effective. It can be given to the newborn and children with one-half of adult dose. Protection appears to be excellent even upto 9 years and booster reimmunization is not routinely recommended.

Typhoid Vaccination

Immunization against typhoid does not give 100 percent protection, but it reduces the incidence and severity of infections. It can be given at any age after one year. Typhoid does not give 100 percent protection, but it reduces the incidence and severity of infections. It can be given at any age after one year. Typhoid vaccine is not now included in National Immunization Schedule. It is recommended to the risk group (school-children, hospital staff), travelers, residents of endemic areas and mela or yatra attendance.

The available injectable typhoid vaccines are: a) monovalent antityphoid vaccine, b) bivalent antityphoid vaccine and c) TAB vaccine.

Monovalent vaccine is prepared from killed S. typhi, as phenol-reserved vaccine and AKD (acetone killed and dried) antityphoid vaccine. Bivalent vaccine contains S. Typhi and S. paratyphi 'A'. the traditional TAB vaccine contained S. typhi, S. paratyphi 'A' and S. paratyphi 'B'. The WHO recommended that the TAB vaccine should be discontinued.

Primary immunization with antityphoid vaccine should consist of 2 doses to subcutaneous injections, each dose of 0.5 ml, at 45 to 6 weeks interval. The children between 1 and 10 years required smaller dose with 0.25 ml. Immunity develops in 10 to 21 days after inoculation and gives protection for about 3 years. So booster dose is needed in every 3 years. This vaccine should be stored at 2 to 8 °C temperature and should not be frozen.

Following typhoid vaccination, local reactions occur as pain, swelling and tenderness at injection site. General symptoms like malaise, headache and fever may occur and usually subside within 36 hours.

Recently oral typhoid vaccines (Typhoral) are available as safe and highly immunogenic. It is developed from live attenuated strains of S. typhi, Ty21a is developed by swiss scientists and 541Ty, by US scientists.

The Ty21a vaccine is used in more than 50 countries including India. It is recommended for the typhoral is given on alternate days, 1, 3 and 5, irrespective of age, one hour before meal with cold milk or water. It gives protection for 3 years and required booster doses (same 3 doses) once every three years. The vaccine should be protected from high and stored at 2 to 8 °C. This vaccine should not be given in immunodeficiency states, immunosuppressive therapy, acute febrile illness, acute intestinal infections and with antimalarial therapy.

Other Available Vaccine

Rabies Vaccines: Rabies or hydrophobia is a fatal disease and transmitted through bite of the infected animal. Incubation period of the disease is long, so postexposure prophylaxis is possible. There are three types of rabies vaccines available for vaccination, i.e.

- Cell-culture vaccines
- Human diploid cell (HDC) vaccines
- Purified chick embryo cell (PCEC) vaccines
- Duck embryo vaccines (DEV)
- Older conventional, nervous tissue (NTV) derived from sheep brain or from suckling mouse brain.

The HDC and PCEC vaccines are recommended as subcutaneous or intramuscular injections on 0, 3, 7, 14 and 30 days for 5 doses and a booster dose on 90 days. These cell culture rabies vaccines can also be given for preexposure prophylaxis.

Hemophilus Influenza Vaccines

H. influenza type 'B' (Hib) is an important cause of meningitis and pneumonia among children below five years of age. At present several Hib vaccines are a available which are sage and effective. The WHO recommends inclusion of Hib vaccine in routine infant immunization programs.

At least four conjugated polysaccharide Hib vaccines are available. Any one of these can be used. Hib vaccine is also available in combination with DTP as DTP – Hib and with DTP and hepatitis 'B' as DTP – HB – Hib.

Routinely, Hib vaccine can be given at the age of 2 months and second dose after 8 weeks along with DTP vaccine. A booster dose is recommended at 12–18 months of age. The dose is 1.5 ml and given in intramuscular route with no known adverse reactions or absolute contraindications except hypersensitivity to the vaccine.

When Hib immunization has not been started by the 7 months of age, only 2 doses are given and only one dose is given to unimmunized children of aged 15 months or more. For the children more than 5 years of age this vaccine is indicated in immune disorder of after spleenectomy.

Combined DTP-HB Vaccines

The combined DTP and hepatitis 'B' vaccines are now available to protect from four disease. It is cost-effective, reduced numbers of visit immunization and has better coverage. It can be given as primary immunization during first 6 months of age with free doses (0.5 ml each dose), intramuscularly at 4 to 6 weeks interval.

Combined DTP-HB-Hib Vaccines

The combined DTP-HB-Hib vaccines protect from five infections in one vaccination. It can be given as 3 dose primary course at 2–4–6 months or 1.5–3-5 months of age.

Hepatitis 'A' Vaccines

Several inactivated and live attenuated vaccines against hepatitis 'A' have been developed. The dose, age and time of the vaccination vary from one manufacturer to other. No vaccine is licensed for children below one year of age. A combined vaccine of inactivated hepatitis 'A' and recombinant hepatitis 'B' vaccine has been licensed.

Varicella Vaccines

Varicella vaccine is live attenuated vaccine for the protection against chickenpox. It is save, well-tolerated but expensive. It is recommended as single dose with 0.5 ml subcutaneously for all age group. Another type of Varicella vaccine can be administered as single dose for the children one year to 12 years and above 13 years as two doses at 6 to 10 weeks interval. If the vaccine is administered within 3 days of exposure to a case of chickenpox, it provides 80 to 90 percent protection.

Influenza Vaccines

Influenza vaccine is prepared from killed virus for protection against influenza type 'A' and type 'B' infections. It can be administered subcutaneously with 0.2 ml of an oily emulsion preparation or 1.0 ml of saline preparation as single dose. It should not be given during acute febrile illness. The vaccine is recommended for children older than 6 months. Previously immunized children should receive 2 doses at 4 weeks interval. Live attenuated vaccine and other newer vaccines for influenza are under trial.

Rotavirus Vaccine

Rotavirus is most common cause of severe diarrhea in infants. Now a tetravalent rhesus rotavirus vaccine (RRV–TV) is available for protection of children below 2 years of age. It is recommended as oral vaccine of 3 doses at an interval of 4 weeks for the infants 6 to 26 weeks of age. No serious adverse effects have been observed.

Cholera Vaccine

Cholera vaccine is whole cell killed vaccine, available for parenterally administration having poor protection (approx. 50%), which lasts for only 3 to 6 months. The available cholera vaccine is administered by subcutaneous injection with two doses at 4 to 6 weeks interval. The dose is 0.2 ml for children below 2 years and 0.3 ml above two years. This vaccination may cause reactions like local pain, Erythema, edema and abscess. Research for developing an improved and more potent oral cholera vaccine is in progress.

Mumps Vaccine

Mumps vaccine is a live-attenuated viral vaccine and gives long immunity with protective value of 75 to 90 percent. It is usually available, combined with measles and rubella vaccines as MMR, a trivalent vaccine. Mumps or MMR vaccine may be given after 12–15 months of age in subcutaneous route. Mumps vaccine is safe and effective.

Rubella Vaccine

Rubella vaccine is also a live attenuated viral vaccine protection against the occurrence of congenital rubella syndrome in offspring. The vaccine is administered to girls between one year of age and puberty. It can also be given to susceptible women of child bearing age provided they are not already pregnant and conception is unlikely in the subsequent 2 months. The dose is 0.5 ml subcutaneously, as single administration. The recommended minimum age is 12 to 15 months, only after maternal antibodies have disappeared.

The adverse reactions after rubella vaccine are transient skin rash, lymphadenopathy and arthralgia, which are usually self-limiting. The vaccine is contraindicated in pregnancy and immunosuppression.

The combined MMR vaccine (Mumps, Measles, Rubella) is now gaining popularity for economical advantage as well as for convenience.

Pneumococcal Vaccine

Currently available polyvalent pneumococcal vaccine can protect children from infection caused by streptococcus pneumonia resulting pneumonia, meningitis, otitis media, bacteremia, etc. The protection efficacy is about 60 percent. The vaccines are not immunogenic in children below 2 years of age. It is indicated in children above 2 years of age and having nephritic syndrome, chronic renal failure, immunosuppressive conditions, malignancy, HIV infection, spleenectomy, etc. The vaccine is given intramuscular or subcutaneously with 0.5 ml amount. Revaccination is recommended for children less than 10 years of age and are at high risk of severe pneumococcal infection. It is given after 3 to 5 years of primary immunization. The adverse reactions may found as anaphylaxis, local painful swelling, fever, GB syndrome, etc.

Meningococcal Vaccine

The vaccine is administered deep subcutaneously in single dose of 0.5 ml, in children older than two years of age. Sound dose is needed after one year if the first dose is given between 2 to 4 years of age. When first dose is given after 4 years of age, than next dose should be administered only after another 5 years. The vaccine may have some adverse reactions like local tenderness, edema and fever.

Japanese Encephalitis (JE) Vaccines

Japanese encephalitis is an important viral disease causing fatal condition in children. Vaccination against JE is significant preventive measure as the specific drugs are not available for treatment.

At present three of JE vaccines are available, i.e. mouse brain derived and inactivated viral vaccine, cell culture derived inactivated vaccine and live attenuated vaccine.

The mouse brain derived JE vaccine is available internationally and stable at 4 °C for at least one year. The vaccine is administered in 2 doses subcutaneously, with 0.5 ml amount to the children of 1 to 3 years age and with 1.0 ml for above 3 years age, at interval of 1–2 weeks. The 3rd dose can be given after 6 months and booster dose every 3 to 4 years. Protective efficacy is about 90 to 95 percent. It is indicated in epidemics and endemics of JE and contraindicated in high fever, diabetes mellitus, liver and heart disease and immunodeficiency states. Live attenuated and cell culture vaccines are used in China.

THE COLD CHAIN EQUIPMENT

The cold chain equipment consist the following:

Walk in Cold Rooms

In the regional level, Vaccines are stored for 4 to 5 districts in the WIC, at recommended temperature upto 3 months.

Deep Freezers

Deep freezer is a top opening cold chain equipment and available as 300 liters or 140 liters capacity. Bit deep freezer (30 ltr) is supplied to all districts and the WIC locations along with ice lined refrigerators (ILR). Deep freezers are used for making ice packs and for storing polio and measles vaccines. A pair of deep freezer and ILR is connected to a common voltage stabilizer. Small deep freezers (140 liter) along with ILR are supplied to PHCs, urban family planning centers and postpartum centers.

Ice Lined Refrigerators (ILR)

ILR is top opening refrigerator. Two types of ILR are available, one with ice tubes (Electrolux) and other with ice packs (vestfrost) as the ice lining. The bottom of the ILR is the coldest part. DTP, DT, TT and diluents should not be kept directly on the floor on the ILR as they can freeze and get denatured. These vaccines should be kept in the basket provided within the ILR.

Temperature of the ILR should be recorded twice a day with the dial thermometer which should be kept inside the ILR, even if there is an inbuilt thermometer. Defrosting should be down at regular interval with alternative arrangement of storing the vaccines. During electric supply transferred to cold boxes and then to alternate storage.

Deep freezer and ILR should be kept in cool room, away from direct sunlight and at least 10 cm away from the wall. They will be kept in leveled and to be fixed through voltage stabilizer. The vaccines should be kept inside the ILR neatly with space in between for air circulation. The ILR should be kept locked and open only when necessary. Do not keep any object on the deep freezer or ILR. Never store any other drugs, drinking water, foods or date expired vaccines or more than one months requirements at PHC level and do not open these equipments unless require.

Cold Boxes

Cold boxes are available at all peripheral health centers. They are used for transporting vaccines and also for storing vaccines during failure of electric supply. Fully frozen ice packs are placed at the bottom and sides of the cold box before placing the vaccines in it. The vaccines should be first packed in cartons or polythene bags, then to be kept inside the cold box. DTP, DT, TT vaccines and diluents should not be kept in direct contact with the frozen ice packs.

Vaccine Carriers

Vaccine carriers are used to carry 16 to 200 vials of vaccines to outreach sites to the sub-centers, village, vaccination clinic or camp. Four fully frozen ice packs are placed for lining the sides of the carriers. DTP, DT, TT and diluents should not be placed in direct contact of frozen ice packs. The carrier must be closed tightly.

Day Carriers

Day carriers are used for nearby areas and only for few hours period with two fully frozen ice packs. It is used to carry small quantities of vaccines, i.e. 6–8 vials only.

Ice Packs

Ice packs are used for cold boxes and vaccine carriers. It is prepared in the deep freezer. Ice pack contains water, filled up to the level marked on the side. No salt is added to it. Leak ice pack should not be used.

At present, household refrigerator and flask are not recommended as cold chain equipments. Cold chain failure is commonly observed at subcenter and village level. So vaccines are not stored at subcenters and supplied for the day of use only. Nurses, especially the community health nurses have to play major role in maintaining cold chain to protect the potency of vaccines. Successful implementation of immunization program depends upon maintenance of vaccine potency at the delivery end of actual vaccination site.

Nursing Responsibilities for Child Immunization

Nursing personnel are mostly responsible for administration of immunization and its related activities. In collaboration with other health team member, the nursing personnel should shoulder the responsibility to organize the immunization session and to ensure the achievement of universal immunization. Administrations of vaccines are the main assignment but other related activities are also vital for success of immunization program.

The nursing responsibilities at various levels can be summarized as follows:

- Motivation of general people about the importance of immunization and its benefits.
- Estimation of beneficiaries of the area and identification of non-participation and intervening reasons for non-acceptance.
- Assessment of problems and reasons for non-acceptance of immunization and intervening to solve the problems
- Information, health education and communication about the immunization session, time, place, available vaccines and other health facilities related to immunization.
- Organization of immunization clinics at different health institutions, immunization camps, outreaches and home based services.
- Arrangement and maintenance of required amount of vaccines and other necessary equipments and materials for the particular immunization center of clinic.
- Maintenance of cold chain system at immunization center or during transportation of vaccines to home or clinics with necessary precautions to preserve the efficacy and potency of the vaccines. Care of cold chain equipments and maintenance of recommended temperature for vaccines are crucial aspects of the success of immunization program.
- Administration of vaccines is important responsibilities of the nurses at all levels of health care. Nurse should follow the basic nursing skills of aseptic techniques and check the vaccine vials or ampoules. Reconstitution of vaccines should be done according to particular institutions with specific diluents. Selection of proper site, positioning of the child, maintenance of six-rights and steps of medication should be followed. Instruction of the vaccine manufacturer of physician's directions or standing orders should be noticed and kept it mind during vaccination.
- Observation of possible reactions after vaccination and providing necessary instructions, about the care of the child following immunization, to the parent and family members.
- Information about the next date of visit to complete the immunization as per schedule and dangers of default.
- Maintenance of immunization card with required informations and next date of visit.
- Maintenance of clinic records, registers, stocks, number of attendance for vaccination, vaccine used, etc.
- Reporting about immunization coverage and problems of the particular area.
- Participating in research activities and new approaches related to immunization program.

- Updating own knowledge and developing skill regarding advancement of immunization practices and changing attitudes.

THE NORMAL GROWTH AND DEVELOPMENT OF TODDLER

Introduction

The normal toddler growth and development are physically, mentally, emotionally, and socially. A toddler is 1 to 3 years old.

Definition

The toddler period extends from age 1 year to 3 years of age. During this time individual emerges from the total dependency of infancy into beginning independence or autonomy. The toddler learned to trust the parents during infancy now can use this trust in exploration and investigation of a world beyond the parent's arms.

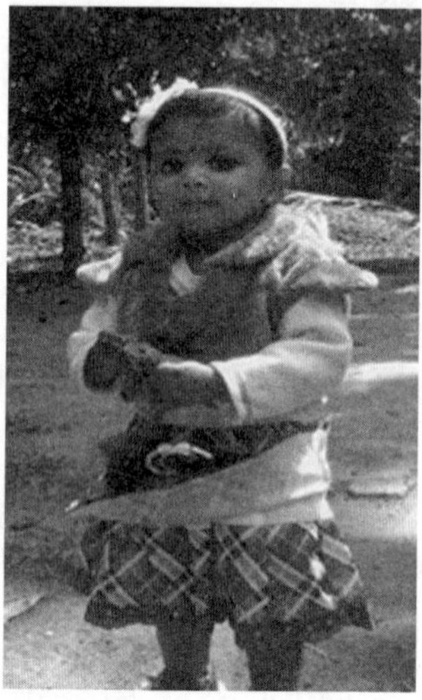

Physical Growth and Development

Biological Growth

Weight

- The toddler's rate of weight gain declines markedly in comparison with that of the infant. Although the toddler gains about 1.8 to 2.7 kg a year, this gain occurs in steps or short spurts rather than being uniform over the months.
- The average weight at 2 years of age is 12 kg. At 2 ½ years of age the child's weight is about four times that at birth. This slowing of weight gain leads to a reduced metabolic rate, which results in a decreased appetite.
- The gain in height is greater than that in weight during the toddler period. Height increases about 10 to 12.5 cm per year and is largely a result of growth in the length of the legs.

Height

- The height at 2 years of age is about 85.0 cm (34 inches). Boys tend to be slightly taller than girls, although this difference is slight.
- The head circumference during the second year increases by 2.5 cm (1 inch). By 2 years of age, the chest circumference exceeds that of the head. The rate of increase in head circumference then decreases so that by 5 years of age, the increase in circumference is less than 1.25 cm 90.5 inch) each year.
- The trunk is long in relation to the length of the legs. As the circumference of the chest increases, the transverse diameter also increases and becomes greater than the antero posterior diameter.
- The abdomen protrudes, making the child appear 'pot-bellied' because of the immature abdominal musculature. The legs are relatively short, but they grow rapidly because of growth at their epiphyseal centers. The legs may appear slightly bowed (tibial torsion) during the second year because of the weight of the rest of the body.
- The feet appear flat; however, arches develop as the muscles are strengthened through exercise. The body begins to assume proportions more like those of the adult.
- As the toddler walks, the chubby appearance of infancy is lost because the musculature is developing.

Dentition

The deciduous (temporary) teeth develop at the approximate times at 2 years, the toddler has about 16 teeth, and at 2 ½ years the full set of 20 temporary teeth has erupted. A discussion on the prevention of caries can be found.

Motor Development

The child muscle grows faster than bone during the toddler period. The size of the muscles, as well as their specificity of movement, increases as a result of use. As the toddler walks, runs, and climbs, the muscles used in these activities increase rapidly in strength.

The hyperplasia of muscle cells, together with a reduction in the production of adipose tissue, results in the child's body assuming a more adult appearance. The principles of motor development, discussed in apply to the development, discussed into the infant. Progression in the gross and fine motor abilities of the toddler is an element.

Gross Motor

- Assumes standing position without help, walks without support at 13 months, wide-based gait
- Loses balance when walking around corners or stopping suddenly
- Kneels without support, creeps up stairs
- Throws small objects repeatedly and picks them up again, but may fall, cannot throw ball without falling.

Fine Motor

- The child builds a tower up to 2–3 cubes
- Opens boxes
- Pokes finger in hole

- Scribbles spontaneously
- Makes line with crayon
- Pats pictures in books and begins to turn pages
- Inserts pellet in narrow-necked bottle.

Sensory Development

- The child have a binocular vision, is fully development by the end of infancy; depth perception does not appear completely until early childhood.
- The toddler cannot determine the distance from the crib or highchair to the floor and must be protected from falling. Visual acuity is 20/40 at 2 years and 20/30 at 2 ½ years of age. Increased visual acuity permits the learning of depth perception and also color discrimination.
- Functional amblyopic ('lazy eye') is usually caused by a child not using the eye to avoid double vision due to strabismus. The child should be referred for treatment as soon as strabismus is assessed, for the younger the child, the better the chance for success.
- The other senses—hearing, taste, smell, and touch continue to develop during the toddler period. The ears of a healthy toddler permit good hearing.
- The taste buds savor the natural flavors of food; toddlers learn what foods they prefer as well as what foods are preferred by those whose cultures they share. When a new food is added to the diet, the toddler may go through the process of smelling, touching, and tasting to determine whether it is liked. The child's decision about a specific food can also be influenced by a caregiver's obvious like or dislike.

Psychosocial (or) Emotional Development

- According to Erikson, the developmental phase to be achieved during the toddler period is a sense of autonomy, toddlers begin to learn that events can be predicted and to some extent controlled.
- As they develop physically and acquire increased motor, language, and cognitive skills, toddlers can gradually separate from the primary caregiver and the environment and begin to develop a self awareness, which can be enhanced through their own successful actions as well as by the approval of significant other persons in their lives.
- When a new developmental milestone becomes evident, parents are proud of their child's accomplishment. This sense of autonomy, or the feeling that the toddler is an independent human being, is pervasive; at the same time, each child recognizes the need to accept and utilize help and guidance from others.

Behavioral Characteristics

Negativism and Temper Tantrums

The toddler period the child begins to separate from the primary caregiver, usually the mother. This beginning emancipation accompanies the attempts to achieve autonomy. At the same time, the toddler exhibits negativism, the propensity to do the opposite of that which is requested or of what one's normal desires would suggest. For example, when the toddler is offered ice cream, the immediate response may be 'No' through the ice cream is eaten quickly.

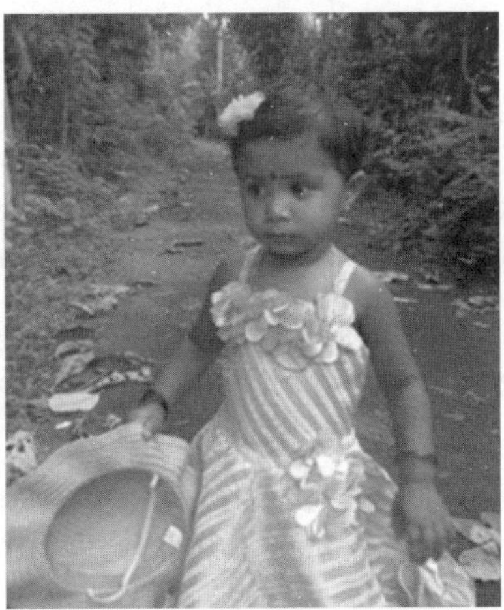

The child focuses attention beyond the primary caregiver; more meaningful relationships are developed with the father and other family members. The child exerts power as an individual through negativism over these family members. The task becomes that of helping the toddler reduce negativistic responses and adjust behavior to the social norm.

Negativism is a behavioral manifestation of frustration when the toddler cannot express autonomy.

Four Developmental Steps in Response to Frustration may be Described

1. The infant's response to the parental 'no' is passive acceptance at this age.
2. The toddler period, this passive acceptance to frustration shifts to active physical aggression or resistance, such as making the body rigid, breath holding biting, kicking, throwing objects, hitting, crying, and full-blown, severe temper tantrums. (This behavior creates a new way for the child to deal with the environment).
3. The older toddler and early preschool child learn to verbalize, the physical aggression is replaced by verbal aggression, the forceful 'No', this form of verbal aggression indicates that the child remembers the often repeated parental 'no' and also that the child is beginning to identify with significant adults.
4. The final step in the response to frustration is the utilization of socially acceptable behavior using alternative goals. Social cooperation is achieved.

Learning self-control or the ability to handle frustration is crucial in the psychosocial development of the toddler and later the preschool child. Culturally acceptable standards of behavior or socialization are achieved as the child acquires self-control through parents establishing and enforcing limits. The methods used by parents to control the child during early childhood become the patterns by which self-control is exerted during later life.

Psychosexual Development

According to Freud, individuals experience sexual sensual pleasure almost from the moment of birth.

This sensuality not only helps children appreciate the concreteness of their own bodies but also appreciate the experiences they have. During the oral period of infancy the child operates primarily on the basis of the intelligences development or instincts, the pleasure principle.

Example: If I want, what I want, when I want it.

During the toddler period, the child begins to operate on the basis of the ego, the part of the psyche that possess consciousness, maintains its identity, and recognizes and tests reality.

The toddler begins to have a conscious sense of self and must deal with the impulses of the id while learning to tolerate frustration and display socially acceptable ways of behaving. As the child is increasingly able to tolerate delayed gratification, behavior becomes based on the reality principle (I will give up an immediate pleasure to gain another pleasure later).

The Anal Stage

This means that the mouth is no longer the major source of sensuous satisfaction. As increased myelination of the nervous system occurs, toddlers begin to obtain sensuous pleasure from the feeling of a distended bladder, from masses of feces in the rectum, and from the release of the contents of these organs. Instead of pleasure, however, pain may be experienced if tension builds up from stretching and spasms of the tissues.

The attitudes of parents concerning feces and urine and their feelings concerning toilet training influence their child's later personality development.

Freud thought that if the toddler believed that the parents were pleased by a gift of a bowel movement, later in life this individual would be generous and giving. Conversely, he felt that if force was used to make the child give up something of value, later in life the individual would have characteristics of possessiveness, frugality, and compulsive cleanliness.

Spiritual Development

During the toddler period, the child has intuitive projective faith that is, a faith derived primarily from the parents or significant others.

The child imitates religious behavior, such as bowing the head in prayer, but does not understand the meaning. Since the toddler is still egocentric and cognitively unable to understand religious concepts, any explanations may be easily misconstrued.

The world of the toddler consists of those concrete things and persons that can be seen and touched; abstract concepts are not understood.

Intellectual or Cognitive Development

According to Piaget (1969), the sensorimotor stage, composed of six substages, occurs during infancy (birth to 1 year) and the early toddler period (1 to 2 years), the first four substages were discussed. Substage V and VI and the preoperational stage are discussed here.

Sensory Motor Stage (Birth to 2 years)

Substage V (12 to 18 Months)

The tertiary circular reaction occurs during this substage. Instead of reproducing accidental events, the child chooses to vary them.

Example: Instead of pulling the same toy, the child varies the play by pulling larger or smaller toys shorter or longer distances. The child seems to try to find new solutions to old problems. Toddler will develop variations of old responses in approaching a new object.

Substage VI (18 Months to 2 years)

The invention of new means through mental combinations occurs during this stage. The toddler shows evidence of the beginnings of mental representations of events.

The child thanks about problems, no longer using only trial and error to solve them. Some solutions to problems may appear in a quick, insightful manner.

Preoperational Stage (2 to 7 years)

The preoperational stage divided into two substages: The Preconceptual phase (2 to 4 years) which is discussed in this chapter, and the intuitive phase (4 to 7 years).

During the preoperational phase the toddler is still egocentric, unable to take the point of view of other people. Because the child's thinking is based on concrete perceptions and on actions in the immediate environment, Piaget labeled this thinking as Preconceptual.

The child used one word to indicate several rather similar persons or actions instead of using a word to identify one class of objects. For example, the toddler for 2 to 4 years of age calls any woman who appears elderly with glasses and white hair by the term used for grandmother.

Moral Development

According to Kohlberg (1975), moral development during the toddler period can be described as being on level Preconventional Morality, which can be divided into 2 stages: 0 and 1 between birth and 3 years, with the second stage spanning from 4 to 7 years.

Stage 0 (birth to 2 years). During Stage 0 the infant and toddler function on the basis of 'The good is what I like and want;' thus egocentric judgment about what the child likes and dislikes occurs.

Stage 1 (2 years to 3 years). During this period of punishment-obedience orientation, the constant cry of harassed caregiver is 'No, No'! The dominant factor in the child's determination of what is right or wrong is the fear of the physical consequences. The child believes,

If I will be mistake for doing it, it must be wrong;
If I will not be mistake, it must be right.

Language and Speech Development

The level of children's comprehension during the toddler period is much greater than the number of words they can speak. They may still use gestures, such as holding out their arms and smiling when they want to be held, even though they may be able to say what they want.

Although approximately four words are spoken at 1 year of age, the child's vocabulary increases to about 300 words at 2 years of age. This increase occurs largely because of the positive interaction between the child and the primary caregiver.

If the mother does not respond when the child speaks, the toddler is not motivated to try to speak further. To a toddler, words have magical powers that should make things happen.

When a toddler says, 'Ma-ma' and points to an object the child means. 'Please give me that.' As the mother gives the object to the child and names it, the child's vocabulary is increased.

The child's first one-word speech is an expression of what is wanted. The use of the word 'bye-bye' has the meaning of 'I want to go outdoors.' Frustration results if the toddler is not understood.

Example

The toddler's idea of an animal is expressed by what the animal does, e.g. a dog barks.

Toddlers who become frustrated in their efforts to express themselves because of their limited vocabulary or who do not get what they want may strike out against the person who they feel is responsible.

The child may express the anger in words, 'I hate you!' Even when toddlers are able to speak, if emotions are too overwhelming to control, putting them into words is not a sufficient outlet. Children may resort to another outlet-crying.

Crying is a distress signal for toddlers as it was for infants and should result in acceptance and understanding from the caregiver. Children should be given help in putting angry feelings into words.

Building Vocabulary

The child builds a vocabulary first on nouns of one syllable ('Ma-ma, Da-da') and then with the use of more difficult nouns relating to objects and people in the environment.

Sentence Making

The child's first attempt at making sentences consists in combing two or more words into and supplementing them with gestures. Early sentences contain nouns and verbs and, later, adjectives and adverbs, e.g. Baby go bye.

Stimulating the Language/Speech

- Listening to the child's utterances
- Recasting the toddler's 2 to 3 word sentences into adult sentences
- Enthusiastic about things that interest the child
- Indirectly correcting the child's use of language by the correct manner of speaking
- Reading and telling stories
- Encouraging the child to interact verbally with other adults and children.

Play and Stimulation

Play during the toddler period stimulates all areas of growth and development. As the child grows, the social importance of play increases.

Cognitive Development

The toddler who plays with various types of toys learns to recognize shapes, sizes, and textures of play materials.

Moral Development

The play develops a very early understanding of moral values. As the parents teach the child not to hurt other children, the difference between right and wrong begins to be appreciated.

Language and Speech Development

Language and speech development are enhanced as the child talks to parents and other persons and pets and toys as well.

Therapeutic Benefits

A play is a psychological development as well as physical value, because negative feelings and tensions can be released in an approved way.

Toddler Growth and Development Assessment

S. No.	Assessment features	Normal value
1	**Physical/biological development**	**Weight:**
		Gain about 1.8–2.7 kg per year
		At 2 years – 12 kg
		2½ years–4 times birth weight
		Height:
		Increases about 10–12.5 cm per year
		Dentition:
		Full set of 20 temporary teeth
		Chest circumference:
		Exceeds head circumference
		Head circumference:
		49–50 cm
		Pulse:
		110 ± 20
		Respirations:
		26–28 per min
		Blood pressure:
		99/64 ± 26/24
		Expected weight calculation formula
		= Age in Year × 2 + 8
2	**Motor development**	**Gross motor:**
		• Walks sideways and backward
		• Moves quickly from place to place
		• Sets self in small chair
		• Climbs on furniture
		• Pulls and pushes toy
		• Kicks large ball without falling
		• Jumps well in place with both feet off floor
		• Rides a walker or pedal car
		Fine motor:
		• Builds a tower of 6–7 cubes
		• Scribbles in more controlled way

Contd...

Contd...

S. No.	Assessment features	Normal value
		• Imitates a circular and horizontal stroke
		• Turns pages of book one at a time
		• Opens door by burning door knob
		• Puts block into hole
		• Eats with spoon, turns spoon in mouth
		• Plays with food
		• Drinks well from a small glass held in one hand
		• Removes most of own clothing
3	**Sensory development**	• Visual acuity: 20/40
		• Accommodation well developed
		• Inserts square object into its appropriate place or hole.
		• Recalls visual images.
		• Identifies various shapes.
4	**Psychosocial development**	**Sense of autonomy vs doubt/shame**
		• Separation anxiety
		• Coping decreased in unfamiliar environment
		• Begins to imitate parents doing house keeping chores
		• Autonomous behavior increasing
		• Begins to have temper tantrums
		• Bedtime retrials begin
		• Beginning of possessiveness
		• Cannot share possessions
		• Beginning to show early signs of individuality and independence.
		• Beginning of possessiveness
		• Cannot share possessions
		• Beginning to show early signs of individuality and independence.
5	**Psychosexual development**	**Anal stage**
		• Obtains sensuous pleasure from the feeling of a distended bladder and release of faces from rectum
		• Pleasure on touching the genitalia
6	**Spiritual development**	**Intuitive projective faith**
		• Imitates religious behavior such as bowing the head in prayer
		• Unable to understand
7	**Intellectual/cognitive development**	**Sensory motor stage**

Contd...

Contd...

S. No.	Assessment features	Normal value
		Substage VI (18–24 months)
		• Invention of new means through mental combinations
		• Concept of object permanence fully developed
		• Can differentiate self from objects
		• Short attention span
		• Begins to think
		Preoperational stage
		Preconceptual phase (2–4 years)
		• Preoccupation with symbols in language, dreams fantasy
		• Very early understanding of past, present and future
		• Increasingly aware of causation while only experiencing the effect
		• Symbolic thought begins
		• Begins causal thinking
8	**Moral development**	***Preconventional morality***
		Stage 0 (0–2 years)
		The good is what I like and want
		Stage 1 (2–3 years)
		If punished for doing it, it is wrong; if not punished, it must be right.
9	**Language development**	**Receptive language:**
		• Recognizes names of various parts of body.
		• Responds to familiar, simple commands.
		• Identifies pictures of familiar objects when named.
		• Enjoys stores with pictures.
		• Obeys 2 commands.
		Expressive language:
		• Says 2–6 words
		• Names familiar pictures or objects
		• Vocalizes wants and points to desired object
		• Shakes head to communicate
		• Use words more than gestures to express desires.
		• Knows about 300 words
		• Uses pronouns 'I', 'me', 'Mine'.
		• Asks 'What's that'?
		• Verbalizes need for drink food and toileting.
10	**Play stimulation**	**Parallel play**
		• Has a favorite toy or transitional object.
		• Little social interaction with other children.

Contd...

Contd...

S. No.	Assessment features	Normal value
		Motor play
		• Large, hollow wooden blocks.
		• Balls
		• Pulls toys
		• Low swing with arms and back
		• Rocking chair
		• Running and chasing games
		Creative play
		• Manipulates play materials such as clay
		• Finger paints
		• Sings songs
		• Brush paints
		• Record player and cords
		• Toys to take apart
		Quit play
		• Sand toys
		• Stuffed animals and dolls to drag, sit upon, hug
		• Enjoys hearing stories illustrated with pictures
		• Takes favorite toy to bed.
		Dramatic play
		• Imitates parental actions in play
		• Enjoys playing with dolls

NUTRITIONAL COUNSELING

Definition

Nutrition counseling is an ongoing process in which a health professional, usually a registered dietitian, works with an individual to assess his or her usual dietary intake and identify areas where change is needed. The nutrition counselor provides information, educational materials, support, and follow-up to help the individual make and maintain the needed dietary changes.

It focus on nutrition is not a new approach to reducing infant mortality. However, nutrition is often inadequately addressed and must be integrated into all reduction and prevention activities. This brief summarizes the impact of nutrition on infant mortality and identifies areas where nutrition interventions can make a difference in reducing infant mortality. This aspect describes the critical role that Pediatric Nurse play in preventing infant mortality.

Purpose

The goal of nutrition counseling is to help the parents to make and maintain dietary changes of child. For a child illness with dietary change may be needed to promote healthier eating, to adopt a therapeutic diet, or to avoid nutrient-drug interactions.

Nutrition counseling is an integral part of treatment for child with parent's eating disorders or chemical dependencies. Persons taking certain drugs, such as monoamine oxidize inhibitors, used to treat depression and anxiety disorders, need to follow diet control to avoid dietary interference with their medication. Many drugs used to treat childhood illness can cause weight gain or loss, so child taking these medications may also benefit from nutrition counseling.

The nutrition counselor and individual work together to assess current eating patterns and identify areas where change is needed. Registered dietitians have met certain education and experience standards and are well qualified to provide nutrition counseling, but nurses, physicians, and health educators also provide nutrition counseling.

Child has special nutritional needs like

- Celiac disease
- Heart disease
- High blood pressure
- High cholesterol
- Allergies
- Diabetes and prediabetic conditions
- Irritable bowel syndrome (IBS)
- Obesity or overweight.

Steps in Counseling

- Assessing dietary habits of child
- Assessing the child body weight
- Identifying child nutritional demands
- Identifying barriers to change needs
- Setting goals
- Finding the support measures
- Maintaining nutritional demands.

Dietary Counseling

Nutritional counseling medically necessary for chronic disease states in which dietary adjustment has a therapeutic role, when it is prescribed by a physician and furnished by a provider (e.g. licensed nutritionist, registered dietician, or other qualified licensed health professionals such as nurses who are trained in nutrition) recognized under the plan.

Thus dietary counseling of parents regarding the child's nutrition may influence, e.g. CHD risk later in life through permanent modification of the child's eating habits and preferences, although food habits are known to be unstable, when children are allowed to choose their meal freely from healthy foods and from foods high in fat, salt and sugar, they tend to choose salty, sugary and fatty foods.

School children between the ages of 10 and 16 years mainly choose their breakfast according to taste preferences, availability and previous habits if given a free choice.

- The dietary counseling focuses on the child's diet and has so far been addressed to the parents.
- In practice, nutrition education for preschool age children is usually delivered via parents, but the impact of such child-oriented nutrition counseling of parents on the food choices made by their children has not been studied in detail.
- Due to the considerable effect of counseling on the food consumption and nutrient intakes of children under school age, and since the children take a more active role in food selection during the preschool period.
- It is important to evaluate the impact of the given dietary counseling on the food choices of preschool-aged children.
- The method used to identify existing food habits of children is based on stacking boxes with food pictures, used for school children aged 10, 13 and 16 years.

Counseling to Antenatal Mother and Newborn Baby

- Inadequate intake of folic acid before and during early pregnancy is associated with an increased risk of spina bifida, anencephaly, and other neural tube defects.
- Folic acid has a protective effect against heart defects. Vitamin B_{12} and folic acid supplementation may have an association with a lower risk of autistic disorder.
  - Some nutritional excesses such as vitamin A, as well as deficiencies in B vitamins, vitamin K, magnesium, copper, and zinc are linked to birth defects.
  - Maternal obesity is associated with increased risk for congenital heart defects, the most common type of birth defect.
  - Maternal diabetes can cause fetal death and congenital anomalies, especially if poorly controlled. In women with pregestational diabetes, poor dietary control of blood sugar during critical periods of organogenesis significantly increases the risk of birth defects, particularly cardiac and neural tube defects.
  - Congenital malformations are reduced among women with phenylketonuria (PKU) if they comply with dietary restrictions during pregnancy, which includes special metabolic formula consumption.

Role of Nurse in Nutritional Counseling

- As nurses and nurse practitioners become more involved with nutritional interventions, the health of child will improve.
- Starting in the community with meaningful nutrition interventions, child outcomes and health can be changed.
- Nursing's staff focus on the childhood disease while that is not a nursing concept, it is often a fact of life. Clients as the complex individuals that they are, the advantage of early nutrition intervention become obvious.
- Taking the step into the role of nutrition educator and researcher is a step forward in autonomy. Being a 'go-to' parental for nutrition education is a big responsibility, but it is also an area that is in great demand.

- Nurses have the physiological knowledge and the education to understand nutrition. The Nutrition Analyzer aids the nutrition educator in recognizing diet deficiencies quickly and easily. Nurses can fill the gap as nutrition educators.
- Using the Nutrition Analyzer tool requires that the nutrition educator evaluate the client's motivation for change.
- There is no amount of dietary information that will help a client unless the information is used to change behaviors. With the eclectic training that nursing education encompasses, nurses are equipped to ascertain a client's readiness for intervention and a path to better health.
- In the area of research, acting on a nursing assumption about nutrition, the nurse can use the Nutrition Analyzer as a research tool to produce evidence-based goals in nutrition.
- The biggest problem for clients is in recognizing that everything entering our gastrointestinal tract affects our health for the good or bad.
- The Nutrition Analyzer is an important tool in the nursing medicine bag and will help nurses provide the counseling and research that are so desperately needed in health care today.

TOILET TRAINING AND SAFETY

Introduction

Toilet training otherwise known as potty training. In order to providing a toilet training to children, the child will takes a dramatic step toward control of his own life. This is often the first real opportunity the child is given to independently manage an activity of daily living. Parents' expectations often exceed the child's abilities or understanding, and the child's frustrations and imperfect attempts at self-control are easily mistaken for willful disobedience.

Definition

The toilet training is defined as children can be using the toilet and they must be able to control their bowel and bladder muscles. Some signs of this control are having bowel movements

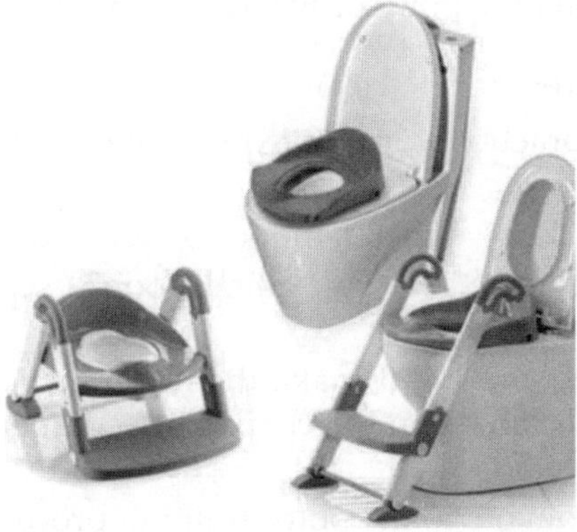

Fig. 3.21: Different types of child toilets

around the same time each day, not having bowel movements at night, and having a dry diaper after a nap or for at least 2 hours at a time. Children must also be able to climb, talk, remove clothing, and have mastered other basic motor skills before they can use the toilet by themselves.

Toilet Training Policy

- Encourage parents to dress children in easy to remove clothing to help children be successful in undressing and dressing.
- When a child is giving the signs of having to use the toilet or tells you they have to use the toilet, take the child in and help undress them and on to the toilet.
- Sit by the child for a few minutes. Try not to push for immediate results. After a few minutes, help the child with the rest of the routine and give praise for the effort or any successes they had.
- Never force a child to sit on the toilet against their will or for long periods of time if they do not want to. This could set up a power struggle and negative feeling toward the toilet training.
- Never punish for accidents. Occasional accidents are normal.
- Clean and change the child immediately.
- Be positive and reassuring that they will be successful.
- Punishment does not make the process go faster and may delay it.
- Supervise children during toilet training.

General Guidelines to Parents

- Advise the parents to follow the simple instructions
- Instruct the parents to use understandable words about the toileting process
- Control the muscles responsible for elimination
- Verbally express a need to help the children
- Advise the parents to keep a diaper dry for atleast 2 hours or more
- Provide the toilet chair and allow the kid sit on it, and then get off the chair (potty)
- Pull down diapers, disposable training pants, or underpants
- Show an interest in using the potty or wearing underpants.

Toilet Training Technique

- Instruct the parents to practice words to express the act of using the toilet ('pee,' 'poop,' and 'potty').
- Ask the child to let you know when a diaper is wet or soiled.
- Identify the child behaviors ('Are you going poop?') so that your child can learn to recognize peeing and toileting.
- Provide a potty chair to child and make them to practice. At first child can sit on it clothed. Then, he or she can sit on the chair with a diaper. And when ready child can go bare-bottomed.
- Set aside some time to devote to the potty-training process.
- Ask the parents do not make the child sit on the toilet against his or her will.

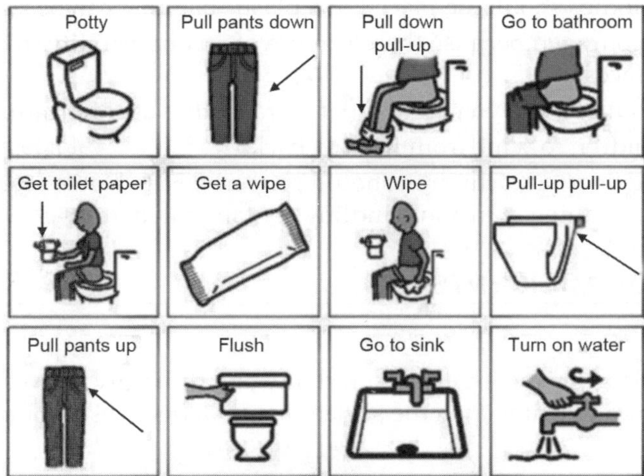

Fig. 3.22: Toilet training technique

- Advise the parents or care taker to establish this routine training. For example, you may want to begin toilet teaching by having your child sit on the potty after waking with a dry diaper, or 45 minutes to an hour after drinking lots of fluid.
- Try to catching the child in the act of toileting. Children often give clear cues that they need to use the bathroom their faces turn red, and they may grunt or squat. And many kids are regular as to the time of day they tend to have a bowel movement.
- The child sit on the potty within 15 to 30 minutes after meals to take advantage of the body's natural tendency to have a bowel movement after eating (this is called the gastrocolic reflex).
- Remove a bowel movement (poop) from your child's diaper, put it in the toilet, and tell your child that poop goes in the potty.
- Make sure the child's wardrobe is adaptable to potty training. In other words, avoid overalls and shirts that snap in the crotch. Simple clothes are a must at this stage and kids who are potty training need to be able to undress them.
- Parents like to let their child have some time during the day without a diaper. If he or she urinates without wearing a diaper, the child may be more likely to feel what is happening and express discomfort.
- Instruct the parents to offer the child for whenever he passed the potty. Keep a chart to track of successes.
- Make sure all of the child's caregivers, including, grandparents, and childcare workers follow the same routine and use the same names for body parts and bathroom acts.

Sanitation and Safety

- Child size toilets or modified toilet seats with step stool are recommended.
- Potty chairs are not recommended to be used in a child care setting because sanitary handling of the potty chairs is difficult.
- The toilet and equipment should be cleaned with soap and water and disinfected with bleach solution (1/4 cup bleach to 1 gallon water) when the seat or area is visibly dirty and at least once daily.

- Wet or dirty clothes should be placed in a plastic bag that can be sealed tightly.
- Rinsing is discouraged because there is more of an opportunity to contaminate hands and other surfaces.
- Each child should have a complete set of extra clothes at child care.
- Encourage children to wipe from front to back.
- Parents or caregivers and children should properly wash hands after toileting, helping with toileting, cleaning area and handling contaminated items.

PREVENTION OF ACCIDENTS

Introduction

Accidents are the largest single cause of mortality and disability between the ages of 1 and 4 years claiming more victims than the six leading fatal diseases combined.

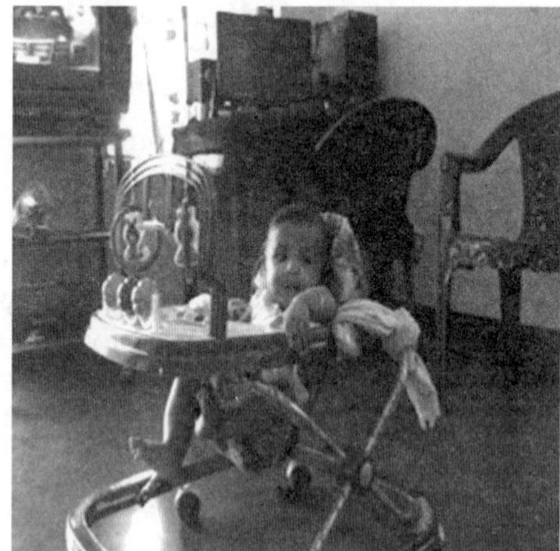

Types of Accidents

- Motor vehicle accidents
- Drowning
- Burns
- Suffocation
- Falls
- Poisoning
- Other types of injuries.

The child can receive the first lesson in cause-and-effect relationships in those activities that are potentially dangerous and can cause pain. The child's knowledge of what can be clone.

Growth, Development and Accidental Injury

The development of gross motor skills enables the toddler not only to move furthermore quickly, by walking, running, climbing, and riding a tricycle but also to pull objects around and to explore areas like pools and pounds without the immediate supervision of an adult.

Improved Fine Motor Control

The smaller muscles of the body are increasingly under voluntary control, the toddler is able to manipulate objects; throw balls and other objects more forcefully; open containers, doors (refrigerator, cabinet, and closet), gates, drawers, and some windows; explore holes and openings with fingers; and pull small parts from toys such as sewn on button eyes from stuffed animals.

Increased Emotional Climate of the Home

In home any sudden change in a child's environment, such as a new baby sitter, moving from one house or apartment to another, or going on vacation, can upset the routine of the home and predispose the child to accidental injury.

The child's hunger and fatigue at a time, when the parents are busy, such as the hour before meals, late in the afternoon, or just before bedtime, can also result in accidental injury.

Tension between the parents can be reflected in their child's behavior and can lead to accidents. If attention is distracted from the child, as on weekends, during the mother's pregnancy, or during illness or death in the family.

The lack of supervision coupled with the toddler's urge to explore can result in serious accidental injury or death.

Prevention of Home Made Accident

The most of the accidents can be prevented by parents who are aware that young children want to explore every nook and cranny in their rapidly expanding world. The parents were to examine their homes at child level; many of these dangers would become obvious. Show all inclusive listing of dangers in the home, may suggest teaching about accident prevention.

Because accidents are the leading cause of death among toddlers and preschoolers, it is essential that the nurse emphasize safety measures to parents.

Although parents would be overwhelmed if the nurse were to attempt to discuss with them every possible cause of accidental injury to their children, the major types of accidents with suggestions for their prevention can be reviewed.

The child-proofing suggestions given for each type of accident are meant as guidelines. Parents should be helped to use their imagination and develop their own methods, tailoring their safety efforts to their home and individual child.

The parents can stay in tune with their child's world is to get down on their hands and knees, crawl around, and try to see the environment as a child might. They also can try to see any potentially dangerous element through a child's eyes.

PLAY THERAPY

Definition

Play therapy is defined as providing opportunities for the child to interact with others in play encourage emotional and social development.

Benefits of Play

All the Children develop their own physical and intellectual abilities during play session. They will be developing the moral values through playing with others. Play can help develop creativity, skill and provide a therapeutic release from stress and tension produced by environmental influences.

Physical Development

It will help the children to develop their muscular and sensory abilities through play. Infants and young children develop their sensory abilities through the tactile, visual, and auditory sensations derived from playing with rattles, balls, and other toys.

Toddlers and preschool children enjoy large-muscle activity such as running, climbing, and exploring the environment. School-age children organize their movements into more complex forms such as roller- or ice-skating, racing, bicycle riding, and skateboarding.

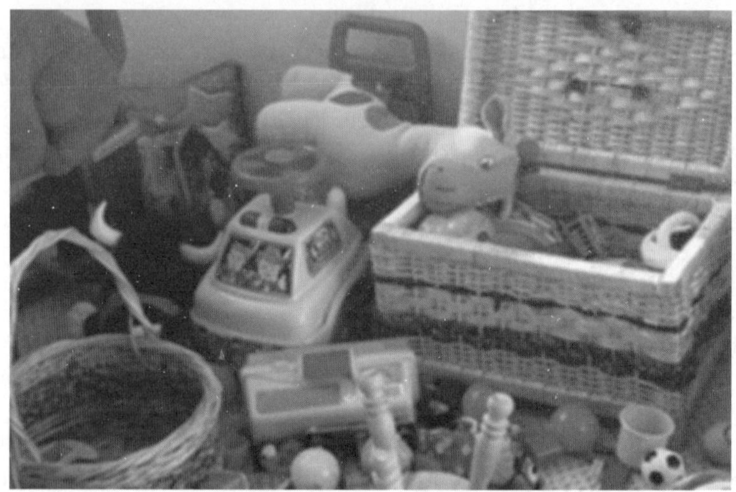

Fig. 3.23: Types of play materials

Intellectual Development

In this age children develop their intellectual abilities through play. They learn the differences in sizes, shapes, colors, textures, numbers, and names of objects. They learn to understand spatial relationships to do abstract thinking, and to engage in problem solving activities.

They can expand their knowledge and increase their language abilities by speaking with others and by being read to by siblings or parents or by reading stories or books on their own. Finally, play helps children distinguish what is real from what is unreal or fantasy, thereby promoting their development into intelligent adults.

Moral Development

They learn moral values from:

- Their parents
- Teachers
- Religious advisers
- Adults and peers.

When children play, cultural values such as honesty, integrity, sportsmanship, and compassion are expected behaviors.

Children also learn to assume responsibility for their own action. Usually more so than adults, a child's peers are impatient with those who do not adhere to the group's values and may ban them from the play group if the faulty behavior continues.

Creative Development

Children develop their creativity largely through play, especially with materials like clay, paper, and finger prints. They are creative in their play with objects such as cardboard boxes representing houses, blocks of wood representing trains, or empty plastic boxes representing guns.

They can be cowboys by roaming through nearby fields or grocery store clerks by handling a few cans of food.

For example: A parents, teachers, or peers who urge children to conform, to play in only one way with a specific toy when it can be used in other ways, stifle creativity. Children are most creative when they are playing alone and will carry their newly discovered abilities into areas of living outside the world of play.

Therapeutic Purpose

Play can provide a release from stress and tension for individuals of all ages. Children especially use play to work through their life experiences in order to understand and master them.

For example: A preschool child who is disturbed by the arrival of a sibling may play with a doll while Mother cares for the new infant.

Children also assume the roles of adults in their environment to lessen their threatening impact. School-age children may assume the role of 'teacher,' and hospitalized children may assume the role of 'nurse' or 'doctor'. During play, children can express their emotions and test out frightening situations in a way that peers and adults can accept.

The children reveal themselves through play. Nurses who carefully observe the play of children can determine needs. Nurses as well as other caregivers must protect children if their play becomes too aggressive and guide them into less destructive types of play activities.

Socialization

The social and emotional development of children is enhanced through play. Parents, other adults, and peers play with children, assisting them in developing their social relationships and in working through problem situations that arise.

Types of Play Behavior

Unoccupied Play Behavior

It indicates no play activity in the usual sense of the world. It represents the lowest extent of social involvement.

The child may move around randomly, crawl under a table, climb on and off a chair, follow another person, or just stand alone fidgeting.

Solitary Independent Play Behavior

It occurs when the child plays alone, independent of other nearby children or adults. Concentrating on a play activity, the child does not acknowledge what others may be doing in the area.

Pretoddlers and toddlers engage in this form of play. As they become more social, interacting with other children, they spend less and less time in solitary play.

Onlooker Play Behavior

It is typical of the child who watches others play but who does not become engaged in their play; the child may sit or stand near other children to hear or see what is going on.

Onlooker behavior differs from unoccupied behavior in that the child is interested in what other children are doing and may communicate with them. Younger children exhibit solitary and parallel play more frequently than onlooker behavior.

Parallel Play Behavior

It is a type of independent activity in which the child plays with toys either similar or identical to those used by other children nearby.

The child plays alongside others but not with them. Children join or leave such a group at will. Children of 2 to 3 years of age typically play in this manner, but parallel play can continue to the later preschool years. Older preschool children engage more frequently in associative or cooperative play.

Associative Play Behavior

The social interaction occurs between or among children, all of them engaging in similar, if not identical, activity. Characteristic activities include leading and following one another using wagons or trains and 'borrowing' and 'lending' of playthings, among others.

Children put forth moderate efforts to control who will and who will not be 'allowed' to participate in play together. No attempts are made to organize the activity or to divide the play tasks, so all engage in basically the same thing. Children play in whatever way they want; conversation concerns the common activity.

The interests of the children lie primarily in the associations with others, not in the play itself. At times, a few children may not participate but may do what draws their attention at the moment.

This type of play is most common among children 3 and 4 years of age. A 2-year-old may tag along but is not totally included in the play group.

Cooperative Play Behavior

It is found in groups of children after the older preschool years. They play with a purpose, whether in making something material, dramatizing a group life situation such as 'playing house,' cooperating to achieve a goal, or engaging in formal game activity such as football or soccer. Children who 'belong' to a group know it, and those who 'do not belong' also know their status.

There are leaders and followers in such their groups. The leaders assign tasks to the other children, either as individuals or in subgroups. Generally, these activities are not duplicated by other subgroups.

The social characters of play become older. Their developing physical, emotional, intellectual, and language skills combine to produce expanding competence in social situations. Children, however, develop these skills at their own rates.

Characteristics of Play Therapy

- Children's play depends to a great extent on their culture and generally the types are handed down from generation to generation through succeeding groups of children.
- Infants engage in social-affective play in their relationships with other people.
- Infants and young children also typically engage in nonsocial experiences or sense-pleasure play by handling articles in the environment or by movements of their own bodies.
- They learn through their play various colors, odors, tastes, and textures by handling sand, mud, water, toys, and food substances.
- Infants and young children also engage in skill play, whereby an action is carried out repeatedly until it is performed well.
- Preschool and school-age children enjoy imitative and dramatic play, through which they learn to identify with the adults in their environments. They can 'pretend' to be anybody they wish and fantasize about adult activities.
- Older school-age children and adolescents also engage in a more sophisticated type of fantasy activity called daydreaming.
- To the infant and toddler a doll is a soft, cuddly object that can be sat upon, dragged around, or thrown on the floor.
- To the preschool or younger school-age child, a doll can be a substitute infant to be cuddled, bathed, and dressed.
- The use made of blocks, drawing materials, and other playthings changes similarly over the years.
- The amount of time children play decreases with age, but the amount of time they use to pursue other interests increases through the years.

Role of Nurse in Selection and Care Play Materials

Play materials helping on the basis of the child's age, personality, abilities, experience, interests, and environment, as well as safety.

While buying playthings, parents or other adults should read the labels for age and safety recommendations. They must consider the child's physical, intellectual, and emotional capabilities.

A child may be very intelligent but not sufficiently coordinated physically to handle a particular toy. For example, shooting games or electrical toys are not advised for young children. In general, the smaller the child, the larger the toy should be.

Toys should be challenging or should offer problem solving opportunities, but children must be old enough to master the skills required to play with them.

Play materials teach new skills and leave room for the children to use their imaginations.

The materials used in making toys should be checked to see that they are sturdy, not flammable, easy to keep clean, and safe.

Parents should dispose of plastic wrappings around toys because of the danger of accidental suffocation.

The wrong toys for the wrong ages can be injurious to children. Toys should have:

- No sharp edges that can cut.
- No sharp points that can puncture. Children should not be allowed to play with adult darts or other equipment having sharp points.
- No propelled objects that can injure eyes. Toys should not be used as missiles or weapons.
- No small parts that can be swallowed or inhaled. The squeakers from some squeeze toys could be picked out and swallowed, and small pellets from stuffed dolls or animals could be inhaled or ingested. For children under 3 years of age, federal regulations define as too small, and therefore dangerous, any toy or part of a toy that is smaller than 1.25 inches in diameter and 2.25 inches in depth.
- No excessive noise, which could damage hearing. Although federal regulations limit the noise levels of toys may still be found that are too noisy for the home.
- No elements that can cause burns. Electrical toys can shock or burn if they are not properly constructed or if they are misused. Only children over 8 years of age should be permitted to use them.
- Play materials with electrical plugs, such as cooking toys, should be avoided unless children are supervised when they are used.
- If toys use electricity, parents should teach children the proper way to unplug them by pulling out the plug, not the cord.
- No toxic paints or other toxic materials. Lead based paints are outlawed in the manufacture but parents still should check the labels of specific toys before purchase.

Children must be Taught

- Parents should explain to children the directions for use and the caution labels.
- To store toys safely where others cannot trip over them, away from traffic areas and stairs. This goal can be achieved by providing an easy-to-reach and attractive storage space for toys.
- A toy box is dangerous; not only can the lid fall on the child's head or the fingers be pinched but also toys are usually in such a jumble that it is difficult to locate a particular plaything.
- A self-locking box for toys must not be used because a child could be trapped inside and suffocate.
- To keep their playthings in good condition. Children can be taught to recognize signs such as loose parts, ragged edges, or rust. Broken toys can expose dangerous sharp edges, pins, wires, or staples. Parents should repair or discard damaged and broken toys.
- To keep the playthings of older brothers and sisters away from younger children.

Observation of the Child at Play

The pediatric nurse is usually in a position to spend more time with children, whether in the home, clinic, hospital, or other community agency, than are other members of the health team. The nurse is thus able to observe their levels of growth and development and their physical and emotional health, as well as their relations with their parents, siblings, and peers.

Children are most unaffected and natural when they are unaware of being watched. They may become self-conscious and react with shyness, embarrassment, or frustration or by showing off, if aware of being observed. Since everything a child does has meaning, the observer should accurately and completely note everything said, every behavior, every action or play activity, and every facial expression, gesture, and movement.

Selection of Play Material

S. No.	Age group	Play items
1	Infants [1–12 months]	• Rattles
		• Soothers
		• Musical toys
		• Blanket
		• Cuddly toys
		• Board books
2	Toddlers [1–3 years]	• Building blocks
	and	• 'Little People' sets (Fisher Price farm, garage, home, etc.)
	Preschool [4–5 years]	• Board books, Lift the Flap books
		• Dolls
		• Trucks and cars (durable and sturdy plastic)
		• Make believe toys such as kitchen utensils, work benches and tools etc. (durable and sturdy plastic such as Little Tykes and Fisher Price brands)
		• Crayons
		• Construction paper
		• Magnadoodles
		• Wooden shape puzzles
		• Interactive toys such as those that light up or make sounds when touched
3	School Age [6–12 years]	• Board games such as Guess Who, Candy Land, Snakes and Ladders, Disney Trivia, Connect Four, Monopoly and Monopoly Jr, Scrabble Jr, etc.
		• Decks of playing cards such as Skip-Bo, UNO, Go Fish, Old Maid, etc.
		• Cuddly Toys
		• Books both early readers and chapter books as well as Look and Find or I Spy books
		• Markers/Crayons/Pencil Crayons
		• Crayola Model Magic
		• Play-doh
		• Craft kits and model kits
		• Small hand held electronic games such as Game boy, and Sony PSP
		• Nintendo, X-box and Play station games that are rated 'E' for everyone. Please no violent games.
		• Journals
		• Lego Kits
		• Puzzles under 100 pieces

Contd...

Contd...

S. No.	Age group	Play items
4	**Adolescents [13–18 years]**	• Board Games such as Monopoly, Life, Scrabble, Risk, Trivial Pursuit, etc.
		• CD's
		• Gift Certificates for music stores or department stores such as Shoppers Drug Mart, The Bay, Sears and Body Shop
		• Art supplies such as sketch books, pastels, more advanced craft kits
		• Word Search and Crossword puzzle books
		• Decks of cards
		• Journals and writing paper
		• Sports items such as new and packaged sports cards, balls, etc.

THE NORMAL GROWTH AND DEVELOPMENT OF PRESCHOOLERS

Introduction

Preschoolers are emerging as creative children who are preparing for their future role in society. These needs may be less frequent or may take a different form from those of the toddler period. Children's needs and preferences should be respected and stability in relationships and in their environment is essential to preschoolers.

Growth and Development

Physical growth and development:

- **Biologic Growth:** Children in the preschool years grow relative slowly: They become taller and thinner with gaining much weight. Starting at age 3 years, the height and weight curves for 3 to 18 years are used.
- **Weight and Height:** The preschooler gains approximately 1.8 kg per year. At age three years, the child weighs an average of 14.4 kg and at age five years, the average weight is 18.3 kg. Growth and height occur at a fairly steady pace.
- The 5-year-old child approximately 110 cm height. Sex-related differences in weight and height are insignificant in the preschool period.

Motor Development

Gross Motor

- **3 years:** Rides tricycle, walks on tiptoe, broad jumps.
- **4 years:** Skips and hops proficiently on one foot.
- **5 years:** Skips on alternate feet, jumps rope.

Fine Motor

- **3 years:** Copies a circle, puts beads on storing.
- **4 years:** Copies a square.
- **5 years:** Copies a triangle crosses vertical lines.

Sensory Development

The child's visual acuity of the normal 3-year-old is approximately 20/20. Depth perception and color vision established before the child enters school. Strabismus or failure in eye muscle coordination may become evident in the preschool years.

The development of the auditory structures is complete by the end of the preschool years. The senses, of taste, smell, and touch continue to develop many preschool children have already acquire 'taste' or preference for foods based on family cultural experience.

PSYCHOSOCIAL/EMOTIONAL

The Sense of Initiative, Erikson identified the sense of initiative as the developmental stage to be achieved in this age group. They learn adult roles from their parents, who serve as role models for behavior. Children enjoy practicing these roles in their play. They begin gradually to learn how to cooperate with their peers and with adults and gain great pleasure from success in their attempts.

Psychosexual Development

The preschooler must learn to function within traditional social values and ideas as instilled by parents and enforced by a system of rewards and punishment. As the child matures, these systems usually work together in harmony and provide a mentally healthy individual.

Freud has Designated this Period as the Phallic Stage

Childhood sexuality reaches a peak during the preschooler periods. During the years from 3 to 6 years, children grow more aware of their sex organs. In addition, both boys and girls experience a period of initial attachment to the parent of the opposite sex and hostility toward the parent of the same sex.

- In the male child encounter the **Oedipus complex** desire their mothers sexually while experiencing an increased hostility toward their fathers.
- In the female child equivalent, the **Electra complex**, girls want their fathers and find their mothers in the way to Children may feel aggression toward parents of the same sex.

The Sexual development is during the Preschool Period, the core gender identity of the' preschooler continues to develop. Fathers have been found to be more active in promotion of their children's gender identity at this time, demonstrating greater discrimination between sons and daughters. Sexual curiosity between boys and girls occurs with importance attributed to the anatomic differences by the sexes. This curiosity may result in exposure of effort to gain knowledge about their differences.

Spiritual Development

Preschool children continue in Fowler's (1974, 1983) stage of **Intuitive-projective Faith**. Children do not follow a religion because they understand it can be expected by their parents. Parents or someone they love influences them to do so, or it offers them some other concomitant pleasure.

Children cannot be kept spiritually neutral. They hear about religion from other children and adults, and they see churches and pictures of religious objects. In the hospital, parents can be involved in the continuing religious training of their children. Their wishes should be considered and sought when questions arise.

Intellectual or Cognitive Development

Preoperational Stage (2 to 7 years)

The preschool child continues in Piaget's Preoperational Stage and spans two substages: The preconception phase—age 2 to 4 years and the intuitive phase.

During the intuitive phase (4 to 7 years), children begin to be able to give reasons for their belief and a rationale for their actions. They are also capable of free associations (stuffed toys are real), fantasies (imaginary playmates, Santa Claus), and illogical meanings that are opinionated. Intuition frees children to experiment regardless of reality.

Preschoolers are precausal thinkers because they are unaware of the causes of natural phenomena or events. They no longer consider all actions emanating from themselves but assume they are caused by persons or a representative being. They cannot conceive of accidents, mechanical forces, or coincidences as causes of these natural phenomena.

Moral Development

According to Kohlberg (1975): A moral growth and development occurs in a specific sequence of developmental stages that are in standard' order. In the preschool period, children are moving from Stage 1 to Stage 2 (4 to 7 years) on Level 1:

Preconventional Morality

The Children in Stage 2 believe 'you do something for me and I will do something for you. They are egocentric and act out to satisfy their own needs.

Language and Speech Development

Most of the preschool children use language in a symbolic way. They not only imitate sounds at this stage but also use words to represent things.

The collective monologue occurs when two or more children are playing together. One child speaks for a long while, but the others do not listen. The child speaking wants the others to listen and is not conscious of their inattention.

Even if others listen, they cannot understand because the child's speech is egocentric, making sense only to the speaker. At the end of the preoperational period language does become truly socialized and communicative.

Learning Language

Preschool children use progressively longer and more complex sentences, and their vocabulary grows rapidly. Between the ages of 2 and 6 years, children learn about 600 words a year, chiefly through the answers given by adults to questions. They also learn by imitating adults and other children with whom they associate. They may acquire words that parents do not want them to use, such as ungrammatical terms slang, or so-called 'bad words.'

Play

The progress that preschool children make in personality development, ability to deal with reality, and control of feelings can be seen in their play. Through play, children learn to express their feelings, whether of anger or love. They develop concern for their playmates;

they are sympathetic with a child who is knocked down or falls. Observation of play provides insight into the child's world.

Play facilitates the development of an optional self-identity by establishment of an imaginary friend, which helps a child work through a particularly difficult time. Activities that promote small muscle development encourage a child's creativity and fine motor skills. Because fantasy dominates the imitative play of the preschooler, the child is able to copy the adult role while acting out adult activities with other children and dolls. Care-taking activities are copied in playing house.

Toward the latter part of the preschool period, a more organized kind of play emerges. The membership of the group changes less frequently. However, it is still neither complex nor stable in its organization. Within such groups the typical child takes temporary roles of leader or follower.

Safety Factors in Selection of Toys

According to the National Safety Council, the age of five years appears to be the most dangerous single year for children to sustain toy or play injuries, Playground equipment, such as merry-go-rounds, swing, and jungle gyms, account for most injuries to the 0 to 7-year-old child.

Safety factors for playground equipment include

- All spaces between moving parts are wide enough not to catch or pinch toes and fingers
- Swing seats should be strong, with rolled, smooth edges, separated a safe distance from each other, and supported by strong chains without open-ended hooks
- All protruding bolt ends should be covered with protective plastic caps
- All sharp, exposed edges should be rounded off
- All equipment must he anchored firmly to the ground
- Frequent checks of the equipment should be done for evidence of wear and tear, and all bolts should be tightened and joints lubricated every several months.
- Whenever purchasing tricycles, the size of the child should be matched to the vehicle's size. Widely spaced wheels and seats close to the ground provide stability. Pedals and handgrips with rough surfaces or tread can prevent the child's hands and feet from slipping. All edges should be checked for sharpness, particularly on or along the fenders.

Adults should choose toys appropriate for the child's age and ability, read the instructions for use before giving a toy to a child; instruct the child in the safe use of the toy; teach the child's proper care and storage of toys; and avoid toys producing extremely loud noises that can damage hearing and toys that have propelled objects that can cause eye injuries.

Preschooler Growth and Development Assessment

S. No.	Assessment features	Normal value
1	Biological development	**Weight**
		• 3 years–14.5 kgs
		• 4 years–16.7 kgs
		• 5 years–18.7 kgs

Contd...

Contd...

S. No.	Assessment features	Normal value
		Height
		• 3 years–95 cm
		• 4 years–103 cm
		• 5 years–110 cm
		Mid arm circumference
		12.5 to 16 cm
		Physical proportions
		• Temperature
		37–37.2 °C (98.6–99 °F)
		• Pulse
		105 ± 15 beats/minutes
		• Respiration
		25 ± 5 beats/minutes
		• Blood pressure
		$\frac{100 \pm 24}{67 + 25}$
		25 ± 5 beats/minutes
2	**Motor developments**	***Gross motor***
		3 years
		Rides tricycle, walks on tiptoe, broad jumps.
		4 years
		Skips and hops proficiently on one foot.
		5 years
		Skips on alternate feet, jumps rope.
		Fine motor
		3 years
		Copies a circle puts beads on storing.
		4 years
		Copies a square.
		5 years
		Copies a triangle crosses vertical lines.
3	**Sensory development**	Visual acuity: 20/20
4	**Psychosocial development**	***Initiative vs guilt***
		3 years
		• Egocentric in thought and behavior.
		• Less dependent on parents but need reassurance and help.
		• Knows own sex.
		4 years
		• Egocentric; separate easily from parents.

Contd...

Contd...

S. No.	Assessment features	Normal value
		• Physically and verbally aggressive
		• Sexually arouse
		5 years
		• Independent and trustworthy.
		• Engages in cooperative play.
5	**Psychosexual development**	***Phallic stage***
		Genitalia are interesting and sensitive area of the body.
		Oedipal complex *(Male)*
		Electra complex (Female)
6	**Spiritual development**	***Intuitive-projective faith***
		Children imitate the religious gestures and behavior of others.
7	**Intellectual (or) cognitive development**	***Preoperational thought***
		Substage I
		Preconceptual (2–4 years)
		• Language acquisition
		Substage II
		Intuitive stage (4–7 years)
		• Problem solution
		• Aware of cultural differences
8	**Moral development**	• Punishment and obedience orientation. (2–4 years)
		• Native instrumental orientation (4–7 years)
9	**Language/speech development**	***Receptive language***
		3 years
		Can obey two prepositional commands
		(i.e. on under)
		4 years
		Understands directives (on, under, in back, in front)
		5 years
		Understands directives (on, under, in back, in front)
		Expressive language
		3 years
		Uses 4 word sentences—asks, why, uses, plurals. Has vocabulary of 800–1000 words.
		4 years
		Uses 3 to 7 word sentences has a vocabulary of 1500 words.

Contd...

Contd...

S. No.	Assessment features	Normal value
		5 years
		Repeats sentence of 12 (or) more syllables. Has a vocabulary of 2100 words.
10	Play stimulation	• Dramatic play—playing like police officer, storekeeper, teacher (or) nurse
		• Cooperative play such as play telephone, music record player, doll house, garden toys, puzzles

DAY CARE CENTERS

Introduction

A day care center otherwise known as creche or nursery. This centers where babies, toddlers, and young children are cared for in a safe and stimulating surrounding. Crèches mostly cater to the children of parents with full-time or part-time jobs. With the increase in the number of nuclear families and working parents, creches and day care centers are being used by many parents.

Definition

Day care centers is defined as it refers to the care provided for infants and toddlers, preschoolers, and school-aged children, either in their own homes, in the home of a relative or other caregiver, or in a center-based facility.

History

These institutions appeared in France about 1840, and the Society crèches was recognized by the French government in 1869. Day care centers were established in most European cities and industrial centers during the second half of the 19th century; the first in Great Britain, for example, was established in 1860. In the United States, the terms day nursery, day-or child-care center, and nursery school are often used interchangeably to identify various types of day care for children and for preschool educational programs.

Types

- **Private day care centers**: These are run by the private management in more than one location or operate as franchises. Standard rules and regulations are followed uniformly all across the centers. Teachers or supervisors take care of the babies with the help of assistants, nannies or ayahs (maids). Centers like this usually have a large number of babies.
- **Private or stand-alone nurseries**: These are run either by an individual or group of individuals. They do not have any branches or other centers. Teachers or supervisors take care of the babies with the help of ayahs or nannies. The number of babies admitted in these nurseries usually depends on the space and staffing.
- **Home-based crèches:** This is the most common form of day care in India. Here, the caretaker runs creche at her own home. Usually, it's only one or two people who handle the babies. They may have an ayah who helps them out. Home based crèche usually have a limited amount of seats. Usually these have just a few babies.

- **Day care centers attached to independent schools**: Some schools have the option of day care for babies. These may be a combined playschool or regular school with older children. They generally have qualified professionals to take care of the babies, along with ayahs.
- **Workplace crèches**: Some companies offer the option of workplace crèches. This option helps working mothers to provide care for the baby in the same premises while they are at work. These are quite uncommon in India but some organizations are now offering this set-up.

Principles

- There is adequate supervision and attention to each child.
- Parents can find out their state's specific day care regulations by contact their state's department of health and human services.
- Caregivers are well-trained and professional.
- Close attention is paid to health and safety issues.
- There are proper hand washing routines and the facility (or home) is clean.
- Caregivers have training in first aid and cardiopulmonary resuscitation [CPR].
- Safety precautions and accident prevention measures are in place.
- Children are encouraged to explore and are exposed to games, songs, and conversation in order to foster language development.
- There are appropriate and sufficient equipment and play materials.
- Parents are welcomed to make unscheduled visits and are encouraged to voice concerns and suggestions.
- Stability of caregivers is recognized as an important component of quality care.

Function of Day Care Centers

A day care centers should be a place where the child is secure and happy while she is away from her home and set up. It should contribute to your child's emotional, social and physical development. Look around and do your homework well so you can find one that is perfect for the child.

- **Physical development activities**: Many of the day care centers will have outside activity areas where the child can play outdoor games. Depending on the age of child. A child may play running and catching games, hide-and-seek games and other such games that include physical activities. This helps child in motor skill development.
- **Social activities**: The biggest advantage of day care centers are that the children will be able to play with other children. There may be separate rooms for different age groups, partly so that the babies are not disturbed by active toddlers. This helps child to develop social skills at a very young age.
- **Creative activities**: Children will be made to paint, listen to stories, play music and be creative. They would enjoy freeplay, in which the children can choose what they would like to do. This way child's creativity gets nurtured.
- **Reading activities**: The day care centers should have picture books, rhyme books and story books in their collections. The teachers or supervisors help the children to read and understand what is given in the books. This helps your child to develop her reading skills.

Role of Parents

An additional concern for parents is that children who attend day care centers especially in center-based environments are more frequently exposed to such as:

- Communicable diseases
- Respiratory illnesses (more frequently experience)
- Ear infections
- Diarrhea
  - The children who are cared for primarily at home.
  - The size of the group, the child is in seems to play a role.
  - Larger groups have higher incidences than smaller groups.
  - In contrast, however children who spend more time in day care miss fewer days of school than their peers who were cared for at home. Finally, parents need to consider who will care for their child if the child is ill, since most day care providers will not accept ill children for fear of infecting other children.

ROLE OF PARENTS IN SEX EDUCATION

Definition

It's defined as sex refers to the biological characteristics of humans as female or male. While these sets of biological characteristics are not mutually exclusive, as there are individuals who possess both, they tend to differentiate humans as males and females. In general use in many languages, the term sex is often used to mean 'sexual activity', but for technical purposes in the context of sexuality and sexual health discussions.

The World Health Organization (2004) defines sexuality as a central aspect of being human throughout life and encompasses sex, gender identities and roles, sexual orientation, eroticism, pleasure, intimacy and reproduction. Sexuality is experienced and expressed in thoughts, fantasies, desires, beliefs, attitudes, values, behavior, practices, roles and relationships.

Concept of Sexuality

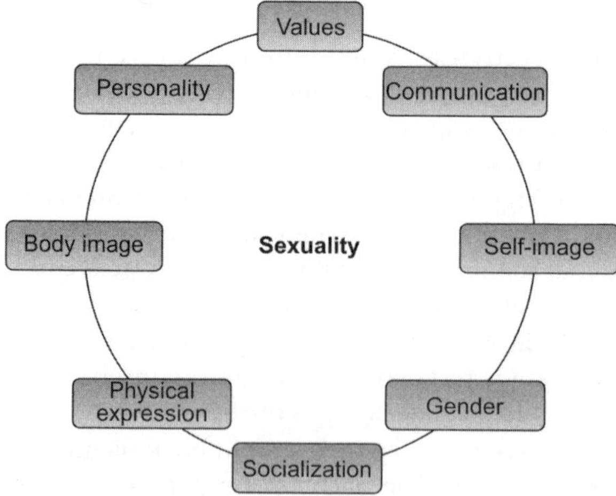

Fig. 3.24: Concept of sexuality in parents

Role of the Parents

Parents of adolescent boys and girls can play an important role in imparting information on sex-related topics especially in the wake of it being sidelined in schools. Most often parents feel shy or embarrassed to educate their children about sex. Parents will be happy to learn about the concrete evidence provided by research about the benefits of parental involvement in discussing these essential facts of life.

Parents are having the major role in sex education, they want to provide the guidance and knowledge their children need to become responsible and happy adults. Parents are sometimes afraid of talking about sexuality with their children because:

- They are uncomfortable talking about reproductive body parts and functions. For many parents, the topic of sex never came up when they were growing up.
- They wonder if talking about sexuality and reproduction will encourage their children to experiment. The fact is young people, whose parents discuss all aspects of sexuality with them, tend to delay becoming sexually active, compared to those parents who do not discuss this topic.
- They are not sure what their children need to know and at what age they need to know it.
- As parents should teach to children many things about sexuality and have been since the day they were born.
- The way they are physically touched by others
- The way their bodies feel to them
- What your family believes is okay and not okay to do
- The words that family members use (and do not use) to refer to parts of the body
- Watching the relationships around them
- Observing male/female roles
- Providing the family perspective
- Supporting the child's level of comfort in discussing sexuality-related issues
- Maintaining an open dialogue with the school about the school-based sexuality education program
- Responding positively and supportively to learning opportunities at home
- Attending a school's parent information meeting
- They are also picking up a great deal from outside the family whenever they watch television, listen to music, and talk with their friends.

THE NORMAL GROWTH AND DEVELOPMENT OF SCHOOL CHILDREN (6–12 YEARS)

Introduction

The school-age child development describes the expected physical, emotional, and mental abilities of children ages 6–12 years. Children ages 6 to 12 years are more independent and physically active than they were in the preschool years. They are also more involved with friends and are learning to think in more complex ways. Progress in the major areas of development physical, intellectual, emotional, and social is gradual. But the changes you will see in your child from one year to the next can be dramatic.

The strength and muscle coordination improve rapidly in these years. Many children learn to throw, hit a baseball, or kick a soccer ball. Some children may even develop skills in more complex activities, such as playing basketball or dancing.

The children's self-esteem, which is their sense of worth and belonging is fragile and can change rapidly depending on what is happening around them. At times, children of this age seem like little adults as they march off to school with backpacks full of responsibilities. But at other times, they can be as unreasonable as toddlers.

The child has come to respect and love that parent, and now identifies with or tries to be like the parent of the same sex. One's social role is learned by imitating that parent's role. The school children learn to think of themselves as persons in their own right and may resent limits that parents continue to impose on their behavior. Furthermore, they dislike shows of affection that may be observed by peers or other adults.

Children of this age often pull away from an adult's embrace and turn their faces from kisses. Parents may be confused and thrown into emotional conflict by the new concepts children bring home, by their efforts at independence, and by the apparent disinterest in parental affection.

GROWTH AND DEVELOPMENT

Biological Growth

Growth during the school years is characterized as gradual in almost all body parts. Coordination and muscle control increase as goes and fine motor skills are perfected.

Weight and Height

Weight and height during the school years show a sex-related difference. Boys tend to gain slightly more weight through 12 years. The yearly height gain is similar in boys and girls, although boys tend to be taller. Black children are slightly larger than white children.

Weight Approximately

17.5–25.5 kg. Gains 3.8 kg yearly.

Height Approximately

110–124 cm (43.5–48.5 in). Gains 1.13 cm yearly.

Pulse

90 ± 15 beats/minute

Respirations

27 ± 3 per minute

Blood Pressure

100/60 ± 16 /10 mm/Hg

Dentition

Starts to lose temporary teeth; Acquires first permanent molars, medial incisors, lateral incisors.

Expected Weight Calculation Formula

$$= \frac{\text{Age in Year} \times 7\text{–}5}{2} \times 100$$

Motor Development

The school child continues to refine previously acquired skills. The child needs regular exercise, approximately 4½ to 6 hours daily to develop normally.

Gross Motor

6 to 8 years

- Rides bicycle without training wheels, runs, jumps
- Climbs steps
- Constantly in motion, clumsy and awkward, coordination improving.

8 to 10 years

- Performs tricks on bicycle-races. Participate in the sports.

10 to 12 years

- Enjoy in all physical activities.

Fine Motor

6 to 8 years

- Knows right from left hand draws a person with 12–16 parts.
- Prints the words
- Lear cursive writing
- Good eye and hand coordination.

8 to 10 years

- Child will use both hands independently.
- Draws a person with 18–20 parts.
- Increase the smoothness and speed in fine motor controls.
- Prints fluently and cursive writing.

10 to 12 years

- Coordination continuous to improve.

Sensory Development

By the time the child reaches the age of 6 years, central acuity should be 20/20, which is the adult level. The accommodative and refractive powers of the eye also reach stability.

From 8 years of age to adolescence, the tendency to myopia (nearsightedness) increases. Some children are able to see near objects but see far objects as a blur. Such children may be labeled school failures since no one understands why they do not achieve. Following visual examination, corrective lenses are indicated.

The sense of taste and smell, fully mature prior to the school years, allows for greater discrimination. Children should be able to identify common solid objects by touch alone. In addition, they should be able to discriminate and locate the application of heat, cold, or a pin prick to the body surface. Specific levels of development can be found.

Psychosocial/Emotional Development

The children when enter the school; they leave the security of home and family. They become players on the larger stage of school and friends. Here, they learn some crucial skills including how to make friends that they can use for the rest of their lives.

Children of this age seem like little adults as they march off to school with backpacks full of responsibilities. But at other times, they can be as unreasonable as toddlers.

The stages children pass through before they are 6 years old are probably the most important for healthy personality development.

Sense of Industry

The sense of industry was introduced by Erikson as the developmental stage to be achieved between the ages of 6 and 12 years. Children desire to engage in tasks in the real world. They are internally motivated to put forth effort on purposeful activity, which will yield a sense of worth.

The social interactions facilitate development of the sense of industry and a child's feeling of competence. Achieving concrete skills and performing well impress others, including peers. Criticism and evaluation by peers assist the child in determining success and competence. If accepted by peers, the resultant sense of power and control leads to a child's positive sense of self.

A sense of inferiority may result if children fail in their attempt to separate psychologically from their primary caregiver, if they are made to feel they must achieve goals that are set too high, or if they place too much emphasis on mastering technical skills and little effort of achieving social skills. Children who lack self-esteem have a poor foundation for mastering the tasks of adolescence and adulthood.

Psychosexual Development

At this age of 6 to 12 years starting of the school-age period the child has emerged from or is in the process of resolving the oedipal situation as described by Freud.

The child slowly moving away from the intense psychosexual upheaval of the genital period, the child moves into a somewhat quieter period, termed latency.

In the latency period it is especially important for the child to have the parent of the same sex in the home for proper identification to occur.

The Latency Period

It starts from school age; this period lasts into early pubescence. The child no longer has the intense erotic fantasizing of the preschool years but is free to develop new interest and social abilities beyond the home grounds.

School-age children become much less egocentric and direct their energies beyond themselves.

During the early latency period children associate with same-sex peers and tend to ignore members of the opposite sex. Girls associate with girls in their play and boys with boys.

Girls may fear boys of the same age and tend to draw apart from them. They may think of boys as 'dirty' or 'messy' persons.

Girls have not traditionally participated in the same kinds of active rough and tumble play as boys, although today girls may be as vigorous in their play as boy's role.

Sexual Developments of Children

At this age of 8 to 11 years, children begin to perceive sex roles in a near-adult fashion. School-age children will continue, as they did during the preschool period to ask questions concerning reproduction but the questions will be more specific.

While the 5-year-old may say 'Daddy put the seed in' as a way of explaining birth, the 7-or 8-year-old may want an explanation about how Daddy did it. Such questioning depends upon alertness, the ability of the child to articulate, and the permissiveness of the parents.

All questions about sex should be answered warmly and directly and with a comfortable attitude by the parents. The extent of information given should be commensurate with the child's age and level of emotional maturity.

Boys and girls should be informed about the reproductive cycle and their respective roles as they approach puberty. Both female and male sexual changes should be discussed by a caring, informed parent. In the single parent home, friends of the opposite sex or a relative can provide information and be available as a support in the family system.

Spiritual Development

In this age of school going children, Fowler (1974–1983) identified school children as being in the *Mythic-Literal Faith stage* with *Piaget's concrete operational stage* by nothing that the ability to think logically helps to order the world with categories of causality, space, and time.

The children are learning many specifics about their religion that will develop into a religious philosophy to be used in their interpretation of the world.

As children reach pubescence, they begin to be less mythical in their thinking, and their beliefs are more controlled by reason. Children at this point may drop their religious affiliations or continue to accept the family's preference.

Intellectual/Cognitive Development

The 6-year-old child is still in Piaget's preoperational stage. Able to understand the abstract, this child begins to learn to read, write, and do arithmetic.

Concrete Operational Stage (7 to 11 Years)

This stage is characterized by considerable growth in thinking, imagination, and language, which allows school-age children to expand and understand their world.

Thinking and Reasoning

School children are no longer limited in their focus on aspects in their environment but are able to explore more facets of objects and situations.

They can solve problems because they can manipulate symbols. Their mental ability permits them to carry on converse and reverse processes. School children can think problems through; therefore, a new world of logical think operations opens before them.

Social Behavior and Language

The language is both a means of communication and a reflection of the child's thinking process. Perceiving how another person feels in a situation, the school-aged child is able to cooperate with peers and adults. Equipped with a rapidly expanding cognitive ability and the ability to communicate it, the child becomes more social in relations with others.

Preparation for School

The preschool child who has attended and adjusted well to nursery school or kindergarten probably will have little difficulty with adjustment to school.

This child will consider school a normal responsibility of childhood. As soon as school starts there is an enforced separation of children from their homes.

They may be frightened by leaving their parents and by the demands of a group of children different from those they have known before.

The parents can take their child to school before school starts to provide an orientation to the physical environment and to meet the teacher. Parents should talk positively about the school experience at all times, but particularly to their child entering school.

Moral Development

The school-age children span three stages in Kohlberg's theory of moral development. Children from 4 to 7 years are in stage 2 or preconventional level.

This is focused on egocentricity. At approximately age 7 years, the child enters the Conventional Level in which correct behavior is that which those in authority will approve and accept.

This level is divided into Stages 3 and 4. In stage 3, orientation to interpersonal relations of mutuality, the child conforms to rules to please others. In addition, the child learns to conform to the group norms. Stage 4, maintenance of social order, is usually identified with the preadolescent. The child looks to the rules and the law for guidance and decision-making.

Language and Speech Development

In this period of development, children show tremendous growth in their ability to use words. They expand their vocabulary by 20,000 to 30,000 words. Their sentence structure and use of grammar continue to improve and the use of adjectives and pronouns increases.

Speech proceeds from egocentric to social. The unique culture of the children is reflected in language acquisition and speech patterns.

REST AND SLEEP, PHYSICAL EXERCISES AND ACTIVITY, DENTAL HEALTH

Play Activity

Play is most importance one in school-age children are increasingly interested in the types of play and work usually associated with those of the opposite sex. For instance, girls may be interested in participating in team sports traditionally reserved for boys. Boys may be interested in learning to bake and cook. This blurring of interests is healthy, because it teaches each sex the value of different types of activities.

It also may make it easier later for members of both sexes to adjust to jobs traditionally filled by one sex. Sharing at this age also may lead to a mutual sharing in fulfilling the responsibilities of marriage.

Purposes of Play

- Play serves as a learning tool for children and their play changes with developmental needs. Fantasy and reality are not mixed as they were during preschool years.
- Daydreams continue but they become secret and are not shared with parents.
- The attention span increases as children have a deeper interest in what they are doing.
- Play becomes more formal, more organized, more competitive, and to a degree less physically active.

- Hobbies are acquired as the child develops an interest in collecting various things, which encourages acquiring facts and knowledge about the world.
- A children participate in more organized sports, they gain experience in 'learning the rules of the game' from parents and peers.
- Through play they learn self-government and self-direction of activities.

The Role of School Health Nurse

- The extended role of the school health nurse practitioner in primary care provides improved health care by identifying and managing many of the health problems of school children. The emphasis is on preserving wellness within the psychosocial milieu of the child and family rather than on curing illnesses.
- The nurse practitioner or school health nurse offers comprehensive well-child care and assesses factors that may produce problems of learning, as well as disease.
- The nurse is a member of the school health team members such as:
  - The principal
  - Teachers
  - School physician
  - Dentist
  - Social worker
  - Psychologist
  - Psychiatrist
  - Guidance counselor
  - Special education staff and school custodian.
- The nurse's responsibility is to develop a relationship with members of the school health team that encourages early case finding and referral and adequate care of children
- The nurse may also serve on the school's curriculum committee to emphasize health concerns. Also, the nurse may sponsor the future nurses' club for young students interested in nursing as a career. Children usually visit the nurse because of acute illness, injury, or for general health evaluation, chronic illness, or behavior.

Health Education

The school going children become increasingly capable of a responsible for self-care activities. Parents need to be aware of the influence they exert on their children related to health care. Children model many of the values, beliefs, and habits of their parents.

Nutrition

Children aged 7 to 10 years require 80 calories per kilogram of body weight. After the age of 11 years through adolescence, boys require more protein whereas girls require more protein and iron. School-age children require 2 to 3 cups of milk 2 to 3 servings of meat or other protein and 4 to 5 servings of fruits and vegetables.

The Calorie Distribution Consists of

- Carbohydrates: 50 percent
- Fat: 35
- Protein: 15.

Eating Habits

- Children in this age group are so busy with school and other activities, they may forget to eat.
- Breakfast is crucial to performance in school and after-school snacks are needed to supplement energy needs.
- Good eating habits and table manners are learned largely through imitation of the adults in the child's environment.
- A friendly atmosphere and enjoyment of the meal are the best aids to stimulate the appetite.
- School children have well-defined food preferences and dislikes, preferring large amounts of sugar and starches while avoiding vegetables and protein foods.
- These years also may signal the appearance of obesity, anorexia nervosa, and bulimia.

Dental Hygiene

- Dental caries resulting from poor nutrition is still a significant problem in the school-age population. During these years, the permanent teeth begin to erupt.
- Adequate amounts of fluoride, vitamins A and D, calcium, ascorbic acid, and phosphorus are necessary for tooth development.
- Raw sugars and candies are common contributors to the development of dental caries. By 7 years of age, the child is capable of assuming responsibility for dental care, including the use of dental floss.
- Dental checkups are recommended every 6 months. Normally 35 per cent of the population visits a dental health educational program into the curriculum.

Sleep and Rest

- The sleep of the school child is rarely quiescent because of fears in the form of night terrors or nightmares prevent peaceful sleep.
- The bedtime hour should be a quiet time when the parents and the child feel greater interdependency.
- It is a good time for confidences questions and answers and discussions.
- The amount needed decreases with age. The 6-year-old may need 11 to 12 hours of sleep, whereas the 12-year-old generally needs only 10 hours.

School Age Children Growth and Development Assessment

S. No.	Assessment features	Normal value
1	**Biological development**	**Weight approximately:**
		17.5–25.5 kg.
		Gains 3.8 kg yearly
		Height Approximately:
		110–124 cm (43.5–48.5 in)
		Gains 1.13 cm yearly

Contd...

Contd...

S. No.	Assessment features	Normal value
		Pulse:
		90 ± 15 beats/minute
		Respirations:
		27 ± 3 per minute
		Blood pressure:
		100/60 ± 16 /10 mm Hg
		Dentition:
		Starts to lose temporary teeth; Acquires first permanent molars, medial incisors, lateral incisors
		Expected weight calculation formula
		$= \frac{\text{Age in year} \times 7 - 5}{2} \times 100$
2	**Motor developments**	***Gross motor***
		6–8 years
		Rides bicycle without training wheels runs, jumps, climbs, hops
		Constantly in motion clumsy and awkward coordination improving
		8–10 years
		Performs Tricks on bicycle-races
		Participate in the sports
		10–12 years
		Enjoy in all physical activities
		Fine motor
		6–8 years
		Knows right from left hand draws a person with 12–16 parts
		Prints the words, lear cursive writing, good eye and hand coordination
		8–10 years
		• Use both hands independently
		• Draws a person with 18–20 parts
		• Increase the smoothness and speed in fine motor controls
		• Prints fluently and cursive writing
		10–12 years
		Coordination continuous to improve
3	**Selfcare development**	***Selfcare***
		• Feeding skills at 6 years, likes to eat with fingers, stuffs food into mouth, talkative while eating. More interested in eating as beginning of meal

Contd...

Contd...

S. No.	Assessment features	Normal value
		• At 7 years, improved table manners, less talking, may bolt food grooming and dressing skills
		• Self-care managed; has a tendency to dawdle in bathtub, Needs to be reminded to wash hands
		• May need some help with dressing
		• Wears whatever is selected by parents
		• Leaves clothes where they are removed, can brush and comb hair
4	**Sensory development**	Visual acuity: 20/20
5	**Psychosocial development**	***Sense of industry vs inferiority***
		6–8 years
		• Continues to be egocentric in though bossy, craves attention
		• Return of temper tantrums: May use verbal, physical attack
		• Uses tensional releases: Wiggling, chewing on hair, nose picking
		• Wants other children to play
		• Jealous of siblings
		• Fears of getting injury to themself
		8–10 years
		• Curious about everything
		• Concerned with relationship
		• Peer-oriented, Reasonable fear
		• Aware of sex role
		10–12 years
		• Confident, self control, respect their parents
		• At the age of 10 years, they will have a short burst of anger able to control anger
		• Hero worship, fear of darkness
		• Know about sexual intercourse
6	**Psychosexual development**	***Latency stage*** *(*6–12 years) • Sexual impulses are repressed • Parents are no longer viewed omnipotent • Privacy becomes more impotent in later school-age child • Ask questions about reproduction • Masturbation reduced
7	**Spiritual development**	***Mythical-literal faith***
		• Learn specifics about their religion.
		• Children at this point may drop their religious affiliation or continue to accept the family performance.

Contd...

Contd...

S. No.	Assessment features	Normal value
8	**Intellectual (or) cognitive development**	***Preoperational thought:***
		Substage 11 (4–7 years)
		Attention span increasing can describe objects in picture, knows their use language acquisition
		6 years
		• Able to understand the abstracts
		• Child beings to learn to read write and do the arithmetic.
		1–11 years (concrete operational stage)
		Thinking, Imagination and language development
		Ordering and seriating:
		Able to arrange things or concrete objects according to the size and relation
		Classification:
		Classify in more complex manner
		Thinking and reasoning:
		They can solve the problems because they can manipulate the symbols
		Time:
		• Child can recall the events that happened in the past; they become aware that things exist over a period of time punctual.
		• Memory spans increasing
		• Ashamed of failure
		• Think about vocation
		• Preoccupied with right and wrong
		At 12 years:
		Ethical sense more realistic than idealistic.
9.	**Moral development**	***Preconventional morality***
		Stage 2 (4–7 years)
		• Instrumental hedonism and concrete reciprocity
		• Children focus on the pleasure motive
		• They consider those actions right that meet their own needs or those of action
		Conventional morality
		Stage 3 (7–9 years)
		Orientation to interpersonal relationship of mutuality
		'Am I a good person?'
		Stage 4 (10–12 years)

Contd...

Contd...

S. No.	Assessment features	Normal value
		We need law and other maintenance of social order, fixed rules and authority
10	**Language, speech development**	***Receptive language***
		6–8 years
		Follow the series of three commends response
		8–10 years
		Follow the suggestion better than commends
		10–12 years
		Follow the suggestion better than request, is obedient
		Expressive Language
		6–8 years
		• Can repeat 10 to 12 words vocabulary of 2500 words
		• Number combination up to 10 develops sense of humor
		8–10 years
		• Begins to use shorter and more compact sentence
		10–12 years
		• Oral vocabulary 7200 words
		• Reading vocabulary 50000 words
		• Use number beyond 100 with meaning
11	**Play Stimulation**	***Competitive play/team play:***
		6–8 years
		• Like rough and tumble play
		• Loves active play
		• Prefers group play
		• Doll play, table game, bicycle, puppets, puzzles, etc.
		8–10 years
		• Prefers companionship
		• Likes to complete
		• Continues to require super vision in play
		• Enjoy the Dramatic play–Playing like police officer, storekeeper, teacher (or) nurse
		10–12 years
		Enjoy large musical activity and outdoor activity; like bicycle, reading, collecting, construction activities
		12 years
		• Enjoys
		• Parties (with supervision)

Contd...

Contd...

S. No.	Assessment features	Normal value
		• Athletic sports
		• Talking on telephone
		• Reading loves stories
		• Solitary play
		• Sex differences notices in play

THE NORMAL GROWTH AND DEVELOPMENT OF PUBESCENT AND ADOLESCENT

Introduction

The development of children ages 12 through 18 years old is expected to include predictable physical and mental milestones. Puberty is the process of physical changes through which a child's body matures into an adult body capable of sexual reproduction to enable fertilization. It is initiated by hormonal signals from the brain to the gonads.

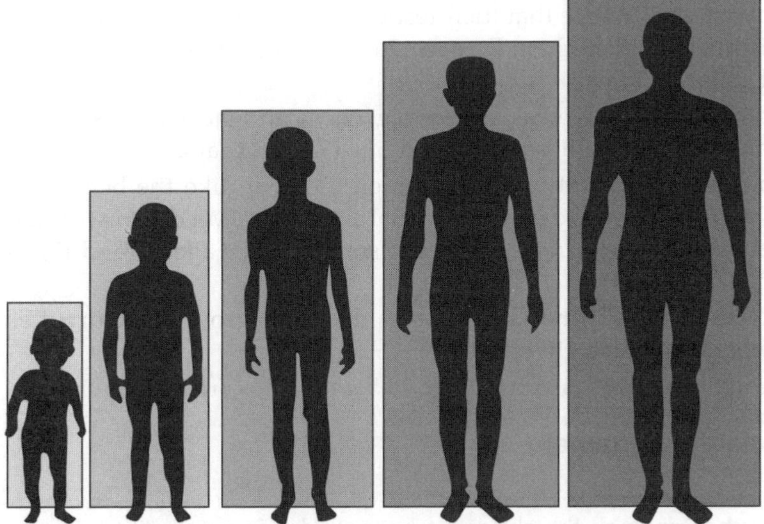

Fig. 3.25: Growth and development of adolescents

Gonads

- Ovaries in a girl
- Testes in a boy.

In response to the signals, the gonads produce hormones that stimulate libido (sexual energy) and the growth, function, and transformation of the brain, bones, muscle, blood, skin, hair, breasts, and sex organs. Physical growth height and weight accelerates in the first half of puberty and is completed when the child has developed an adult body. Until the maturation of their reproductive capabilities, the pre-pubertal physical differences between boys and girls are the external sex organs.

Biological/Physical Development

During adolescence, young people go through many changes as they move from childhood into physical maturity. Early, prepubescent changes occur when the secondary sexual characteristics appear.

Female Children

- Girls may begin to develop breast buds as early as 8 years old. Breasts develop fully between ages 12 and 18.
- Pubic hair, armpit and leg hair usually begin to grow at about age 9 or 10, and reach adult patterns at about 13 to 14 years.
- Menarche (the beginning of menstrual periods) typically occurs about 2 years after early breast and pubic hair appear. It may occur as early as age 9, or as late as age 16. The average age of menstruation in the United States is about 12 years.
- Girls growth spurt peaks around age 11.5 and slows around age 16.

Male Children

- Boys may begin to notice that their testicles and scrotum grow as early as age 9. Soon, the penis begins to lengthen. By age 17 or 18, their genitals are usually at their adult size and shape.
- Pubic hair growth: As well as armpit, leg, chest, and facial hair begins in boys at about age 12, and reaches adult patterns at about 17 to 18 years.
- Boys do not start puberty with a sudden incident, like the beginning of menstrual periods in girls. Having regular nocturnal emissions (wet dreams) marks the beginning of puberty in boys. Wet dreams typically start between ages 13 and 17, with the average at about 14.5 years.
- Boys' voices change at the same time as the penis grows. Nocturnal emissions occur with the peak of the height spurt.
- Boys growth spurt peaks around age 13.5 and slows around age 18.

Psychosocial Development

Puberty

- During pubescence all the children show strides in personality development as well as physical growth. They become increasingly more adaptable, approaching their peer group and problem situation at home and at school with greater confidence.
- They enjoy games that involve not only physical skills but also team cooperation. Although there is a revival of love for the parent of the opposite sex, they argue with parents frequently.
- They are able to assume increasing responsibility in what to the miss reality. Because young teenagers have grown-up in a rapidity moving society, have been influenced to the mass media and have greater communication with an enlarging peer group, their parents may not have the same values that they hold during this period.

- Presents become aware that during pubescence the hostility that previously existed between boys and girls is gradually disappearing.
- These children realize they are inadequate in their initial attempts to be grown-up. There may be a variety of reasons for parental pressure, including their desire that children be popular with both sexes and that they be well accepted in a peer group. Severe pressure of this sort usually does not achieve the positive goal that parents wish.

The Sense of Identity and the Sense of Intimacy

The transition from children to adulthood is not a smooth one. Adolescence is a period of stress for young people and parents alike. The adolescents must learn who they are and must modify their conscience for their adult role in life.

They now question many of the beliefs that they formerly held as certain and true. In addition to this intellectual and emotional upheaval, rapid body growth causes them anxiety, and the cultural pressures of today's world add further stress to their uncertainty.

Adolescents today are faced with many pressures the older generation did not have.

The rapid rate of social change, the threat of nuclear war, the increase in the speed of travel and technologic progress, and the relative ease of access to mind-altering drugs pose problems unknown in previous generations.

Although more adolescents are entering the work force, research has shown that employment does not assist them in their striving for independence (Green berger et al., 1980).

In addition, their support system is not as available because working leads to absence from the family. Since their jobs may not offer much contact with adults, adolescents do not have a model for developing a realistic view of an occupational role. In addition, they may be influenced by their peers to use their earnings for experimentation with alcohol and drugs.

Psychosexual Development

The adolescence the child passes through Freud's genital period of development from approximately 11 to 16 years. Puberty and adolescence are period's development.

The secondary sexual characteristics appear. Masturbation and sexual fantasies are common during this period. Children entering adolescence are not fully sexually matured, yet they are genitally mature and capable of reproduction. Stress results when the adolescent is physically ready for heterosexual genital expression, but denied it.

The heightened sexual tension during adolescence necessitates a mode of expression that usually becomes a pattern for adult life.

Sexual Identity and Roles

Currently our society is sending many signals that may influence a person's sexual identity. What influences whether an individual selects a heterosexual orientation or a homosexual orientation is not fully understood.

Because many children are brought up in the traditional role of male or female, role confusion may result during the adolescent period as the individual makes major decisions regarding sexual orientation, career, education, or marriage. From the beginning, boys are more aware of their genitals and much more aware of genital responsiveness than are girls, Erections occur almost daily. Possession of a penis is the anatomic distinction that makes them clearly men, or male. This awareness is intensified during adolescence by the production of semen in ejaculation.

Spermatogenesis is usually evident by 13 years of age. Overt awareness of sexual feelings is a more diffuse process in the female adolescent and generally occurs at a later age. This awareness is less obviously associated with physiologic changes; learning arises more from the young girl's social and sexual contacts, especially with young men.

Masturbation: Masturbation is a central concern in early adolescence, especially in boys, who almost universally engage in the practice to some extent during the teen years. Girls may do it to a lesser degree, although an increase in recent years has been reported (Godow, 1982).

Boys frequently masturbate in front of a friend, but girls are more private and rarely do. Adolescents should be informed that masturbation is a normal response to an increase in sexual development. Through experience the adolescent learns that masturbation causes sexual excitement and erection of the penis or the clitoris, followed by relief. Masturbation can contribute to a developing sense of mastery over sexual impulses and capacities and helps the adolescent prepare for heterosexual relationships.

Spiritual Development

Adolescents, according to Fowler (1974, 1983) are in the stage of Synthetic-Conventional Faith. In this stage, diverse self-images are integrated into a coherent identity—a deity. Personal and social values evolve to support this identity, and the adolescent is united with other in emotional solidarity.

During this time the adolescent begins to question religious concepts and beliefs of childhood and explores various religious affiliations and cults. This may be a period of conflict for parent and adolescent. A young person without religious ties may be attracted to any new or different religious cult.

Education Concerning Death: Death, a topic that many people would like to ignore, has become an increasingly popular subject for students in high schools. The subject of death may be integrated into various courses in the curriculum or it may be discussed in one special course. The need has arised because students generally have been isolated from the facts of death that used to be learned naturally at home. A variety of books exploring the subject are available for children and adolescents.

Parents also may need help in exploring their feelings and discussing death. Many adults find it difficult to address this topic because of past experiences or unresolved feelings.

Intellectual or Cognitive Development

As a developmental stage, adolescence begins when the achievements of late childhood are integrated into the person and ends when that person is eager to assume the adult role and can do it capably. Many aspects in our culture contribute to the adolescent's growth, including family, peers, school, church, and adolescent heroes.

Formal Operational Stage (11 to 15 Years): Children progress from concrete to formal operations during early adolescence, according to Piaget. Reaching this stage allows adolescents to deal with a problem that does not have a basis in the 'here and now'. Unlike a younger child, adolescents can solve the following problem: 'Tom is shorter than Joe, Tom is taller than Ted. Which boy is the tallest?'

The solution to this problem involves scientific and verbal reasoning. Adolescents can make use of assumptions while thinking, formulating hypotheses, and constructing theories. Adolescents can solve problems that require purely abstract thinking in a flexible manner.

They can have many ideas about a problem simultaneously and can predict a variety of possible solutions. Since adolescents can utilize hypothetical deductive reasoning, they may question and perhaps argue the rules that other impose on them.

They may reject authority if they are not satisfied with the rationale and logic. Adolescents dream and plan into the future, but these dreams and plans may change as they think and learn and their cognitive abilities continue to develop.

Moral Development

According to Kohlberg, reaching a certain age does not mean that a child will progress to the sixth stage (0 to 6 stages) of moral development. However, when adolescents have worked through the preceding stages, achieving the postconventional level of morality will help them face this age group's moral dilemmas, such as sexual behavior, the use of drugs and alcohol, and petty shop lifting.

The postconventional level also has two stages

Stage 5 is characterized by a 'social contract' orientation. The rules or laws established are for the mutual good, mutual cooperation, and mutual development. In addition, values and rights like life and liberty must be upheld in any society even when other values seem to be more important in the culture.

Stage 6, the highest level, is oriented toward decisions of conscience and toward 'universal ethical principles'. These abstract principles pertain to justice, human rights, and the dignity of human beings. It should be recognized that most adolescents' moral codes will continue to develop as they achieve adulthood.

Idealism: As adolescents move toward the adult role, they begin to consider themselves equals of adults and begin to adopt the ideals of adult society.

They use their powers of reflective thinking and abstract ideation to evaluate what the adult world is like and see possibilities for action that lie beyond the constraints of reality. Because what they see is not the ideal, they feel a need to reform the world.

This ability is the basis for the characteristic idealism of adolescents. Adolescents and their peers become involved in the political system and may focus on the plight of the poor. As adolescents mature, they are able to tie their ideals to appropriate social action and to become more tolerant and understanding of society as a whole.

Language and Speech Development

Increasing sophistication of thought is acquired with the development of formal operations. Adolescents continue to learn new words and new concepts, as well as the symbolic organization of their culture. In addition, they learn the relationship between thought and speech.

Vocabulary continues to accrue throughout the life span. Adults should not try to incorporate this slang into their speech because that would take away the purpose of its invention. Language is basic to communication, which is essential to developing and maturing adolescents.

The patterns of communication in a family can facilitate or restrict the move toward independence. Adolescents need parents who can express their needs and desires yet listen to the adolescents' point of view.

Verbal discussions or arguments can foster growth. Adolescents learn to express and defend their desires and wishes while parents also clarify their needs and rules. Interaction is enhanced if there is a give-and-take relationship.

Communication with peers is also invaluable because these relationships provide friends to talk to and to be with. Future committed relationships are arrived at through peer interactions.

These also provide opportunities to discuss the various options that are available as adolescence draws to a close—college, career, marriage.

Play Activity

The parents, school teachers individual interest, cultural and moral attitudes of the community, and the job market affect the play and work interests of the pubescent and adolescent.

In addition, the rapidly changing role of women has resulted in girls' selecting careers other than those historically characteristic of women; teacher, secretary, nurse, social worker, and flight attendant. Women are now successful in all professions medicine, law, publishing, and so on.

They should find satisfaction in knowing that they have done a job well and that they can contribute in some way to society. Adolescents gain great satisfaction from working for a worthwhile cause. Feelings of altruism are well developed at this age, and the individual and group can make valuable contributions to social issues.

Behavioral Development

The sudden and rapid physical changes that adolescents go through make adolescents very self-conscious, sensitive, and worried about their own body changes.

They may make painful comparisons about themselves with their peers. Because physical changes may not occur in a smooth, regular schedule, adolescents may go through awkward stages, both about their appearance and physical coordination.

- Girls may be anxious if they are not ready for the beginning of their menstrual periods.
- Boys may worry if they do not know about nocturnal emissions.

During adolescence, it is normal for young people to begin to separate from their parents and establish their own identity. In some cases, this may occur without a problem from their parents and other family members. However, in some families, the adolescent's rebellion may lead to conflict as the parents try to keep control.

- Their peer group may become a safe haven, in which the adolescent can test new ideas.
- In early adolescence, the peer group usually consists of non-romantic friendships, often including 'cliques,' gangs, or clubs. Members of the peer group often try to act alike, dress alike, have secret codes or rituals, and participate in the same activities.

- As the youth moves into mid-adolescence (14 to 16 years) and beyond, the peer group expands to include romantic friendships.
- In mid to late adolescence, young people often feel the need to establish their sexual identity by becoming comfortable with their body and sexual feelings.
- Through romantic friendships, dating, and experimenting, adolescents learn to express and receive intimate or sexual advances.
- Adolescent child who do not have the opportunity for such experiences may have more difficulty with intimate relationships when they are adults.

Adolescents usually have behaviors that are consistent with several myths of adolescence:

- The first myth is that they are 'on stage' and other people's attention is constantly centered on their appearance or actions.
- This normal self-centeredness may appear (especially to adults) to border on paranoia, self-love (narcissism), or even hysteria.
- Another myth of adolescence is the idea that 'it will never happen to me, only the other person.' 'It' may represent becoming pregnant or catching a sexually-transmitted disease after having unprotected sex, causing a car crash while driving under the influence of alcohol or drugs, or any of the many other negative effects of risk-taking behaviors.

Table 3.6: Tanner's stages of puberty in girls

Tanner stage	Breasts	Pubic hair	Growth	Other	Other
Stage 1	Prepubertal-elevation of papilla only	Prepubertal villus hair only	Basal level: 5 cm to 6 cm per year	Adrenarche	Ovaries grow and enlarge
Stage 2	Breast bud appears under an enlarged areola (mean age 11.2 years)	Sparse hair along labia (mean age 11.9 years)	Accelerated growth: About 7 cm to 8 cm per year	Clitoral enlargement with labial pigmentation	Uterine enlargement
Stage 3	Breast tissue grows beyond areola but without contour separation (mean age 12.4 years)	Hair coarser and pigmented: Spreads across pubes (mean age 12.7 years)	Peak velocity: About 8 cm per year (mean age 12.5 years)	Axillary hair (mean age 13.2 years)	Acne (mean age 13.2 years)
Stage 4	Projection of areola-papilla forms a secondary mound (mean age 13.1 years)	Adult pattern but without spread to medial thigh (mean age 13.4 years)	Deceleration-less than 7 cm per year	Menarche (mean age 13.3 years)	Regular periods (mean age 13.9 years)
Stage 5	Adult breast contour with projection of papilla only (mean age 14.5 years)	Adult with spread to medial thigh but not up linea alba (mean age 14.6 years)	Cessation of growth at around 16 years	Adult genitalia	

Table 3.7: Stages of normal puberty (Tanner's stages) in boys

Tanner stage	Genitalia	Pubic hair	Growth	Other
Stage 1	Prepubertal: Testes less than 2.5 cm	Villus hair only	Basal rate: 5 cm to 6 cm per year	Adrenarche

Contd...

Contd...

Tanner stage	Genitalia	Pubic hair	Growth	Other
Stage 2	• Thinning and reddening of scrotal skin (mean age 11.9 years) • Testes 2.5 cm to 3.2 cm	Sparse growth base of penis (mean age 12.3 years)	Basal rate as above	Reduction in total body fat
Stage 3	• Growth of penis (mean age 13.2 years) • Testes 3.3 cm to 4 cm	Thicker hair: Spreads to mons pubis (mean age 13.9 years)	Accelerated growth: 7 cm to 8 cm per year	• Gynecomastia (Mean age 13.2 years). • Voice break (mean age 13.5 years). • Increase in muscle mass
Stage 4	• Growth of penis and gland with darkening of scrotum (mean age 14.3 years) • Testes 4.1 cm to 4.5 cm	• Adult but no spread to medial thigh (mean age 14.7 years)	• Peak velocity about 10 cm per year (mean age 13.8 years)	• Axillary hair (mean age 14 years) • Voice change (mean age 14.1 years) • Acne (mean age 14.3 years)
Stage 5	• Adult genitalia (mean age 15.1 years) • Testes greater than 4.5 cm	• Adult with spread to medial thigh but not linea alba (mean age 15.3 years)	• Deceleration and cessation (about 17 years)	• Facial hair (mean age 14.9 years) • Muscle mass increases further and beyond Stage 5

Safety

Adolescents become stronger and more independent before they have developed good decision-making skills. A strong need for peer approval may entice a young person to try dangerous feats, or take part in risk-taking behaviors.

Motor vehicle safety should be stressed, focusing on the roles of the driver/passenger/pedestrian, the risks of substance abuse, and the importance of using seat belts. Adolescents should not have the privilege of using cars and recreational motor vehicles unless they can show that they can use these vehicles safely.

Other safety issues are:

- Adolescents who are involved in sports should learn to use equipment and protective gear or clothing. They should be taught the rules of safe play and healthy approaches to activities that require more advanced skills.
- Young people need to be very aware of possible dangers—including sudden death—which may occur with regular substance abuse, and with the experimental use of drugs and alcohol.
- Adolescents who are allowed to use or have access to firearms need to learn how to use them safely, properly, and legally.

If adolescents appear to be isolated from their peers, uninterested in school or social activities, or doing poorly at school, work, or sports—they need to be evaluated.

Many adolescents are at increased risk for depression and potential suicide attempts, because of pressures and conflicts in their family, school or social organizations, peer groups, and intimate relationships.

Adolecents Growth and Development Assessment

S. No.	Assessment features	Normal value
1	**Physical/biological development**	**Weight***:*
		***Early adolescence* (12–13 years)**
		• Male: 38–60 kg
		• Female: 40–60 kg
		Middle adolescence (14–16 years)
		• Male: 50–60 kg
		• Female: 42–64 kg
		Late adolescence (17–21 years)
		• Male: 56–80 kg
		• Female: 48–72 kg
		Height:
		Early adolescence (12–13 years)
		• Male: 154–172 cm
		• Female: 153–167 cm
		Middle adolescence (14–16 years)
		• Male: 164–180 cm
		• Female: 155–169 cm
		Late adolescence (17–21 years)
		• Male: 163–182 cm
		• Female: 156–170 cm
		• Temperature: 36.5–37 °C
		• Heart rate: 60–80 beats/min
		• Respiration: 14–20 breaths/min
		• Blood pressure: 124/74 = 17/16 mm Hg
		Secondary sexual development
		Boys
		• Broadening of shoulders from the age of 13 years
		• Increase in size of breast
		• Increase in size of genitalia
		• Growth of pubic, axillary chest and face hair

Contd...

Contd...

S. No.	Assessment features	Normal value
		• Deepening of voice
		• Production of spermatozoa
		Girls
		• Broadening of hips
		• Developing of breast
		• Increase in size of genitalia
		• Growth of pubic, axillaries hair
		• Attending menarche
		• Menstrual cycle regular
		• Change in vaginal secretion
		• Remaining in permanent in teeth eruptions
		Expected weight calculation formula
		$= \frac{\text{Age in year} \times 7 - 5}{2} \times 100$
2	**Motor developments**	• Refine gross and fine motor skills
		• Clumsiness occurs due to rapid physical growth motor function comparable to adult
		• Eye-hand coordination at adult level possesses manual dexterity
		• Can do the craft works
3	**Sensory development**	Visual acuity: 20/20
4	**Psychosocial development (Erick and erickson)**	Early adolescent (12–13 years)
		Identity vs role confusion 'who am I?'
		Middle adolescent (14–16 years)
		Intimacy vs isolation
		Late adolescent (17–21 years)
		Integrity vs despair
		• Shows mood swings and extremes of behavior experiences sense of loss as begins to separate from parents
		• Peer relationship of greatest importance
		• Daydreams over heroes continues same sex friendships
		• Heterosexual relationship and interests common
		• verbally attacks parents beliefs and values
5	**Psychosexual development**	**Genital stage (12–18 years)**
		• The secondary sexual character will develop

Contd...

Contd...

S. No.	Assessment features	Normal value
		• Masturbation occurs
		• Heterosexual genital Expression but is denied it
		• Sexual tension during this period
6	Spiritual development	***Synthetic conventional faith***
		• Personal and social value evolved to support their identity
		• Explore religious affiliation
7	Intellectual (or) cognitive development	***Formal operational thought*** (11 years–Adulthood)
		• Generates hypotheses
		• Uses the scientific method for problem-solving
		• Expresses concern for education vs. vocational choice
8	Moral development	***Postconventional stage***
		Stage 5 (13 + years)
		• 'The individual conforms to maintain other's respect'
		• Orientation toward decisions of conscience 'Universal ethical principles'
9	Language, speech development	• Fluent in spoken language
		• Uses slang within and outside peer group
		• Uses distinct meanings for words
		• Oral vocabulary 72,000 words
		• Reading vocabulary 50,000 words
		• Continuous to learn new concept
10	Play Stimulation	• Recreational activities
		• Chooses activities according to individual interests
		• Parties, conversation
		• Interest in world affairs
		• Expressive arts, Hobbies crafts
		• Social drinking
		• Engages in organized competitive sports

MENSTRUAL HYGIENE MANAGEMENT

Introduction

Menstruation is a normal biological process and a key sign of reproductive health, yet in many cultures it is treated as something negative, shameful or dirty. The continued silence around menstruation combined with limited access to information at home and in schools results in millions of women and girls having very little knowledge about what is happening to their bodies when they menstruate and how to deal with it. A study from UNICEF revealed that 1 out of 3 girls in South Asia knew nothing about menstruation prior to getting it while 48% of girls in Iran and 10% of girls in India believe that menstruation is a disease (Water Aid 2013, Menstrual Hygiene Matters).

Initiated by WASH United, the first global *Menstrual Hygiene Day* will be celebrated on May 28th around the world with exhibitions, film screenings, workshops and gatherings, all aimed at breaking the silence around menstruation. Menstrual Hygiene Day was created to publicly recognize the right of women to hygienically manage their menstruation wherever they are. By acknowledging that menstruation is a normal human process and a sign of good health, Menstrual Hygiene Day confronts the stigmas attached to menstruation with collective advocacy, education and action.

The Principle

Water, sanitation and hygiene services recognize that users have different needs across the human lifecycle by age, gender and physical ability and explicitly provide for a supportive environment and facilities that cater to these needs. Child friendly, older people, chronically ill, disabled—Menstrual hygiene management is part of every WASH service.

The Goal

By 2050 all schools, workplaces, transport hubs, markets and health care settings have functional facilities for sanitation, hygiene (water, soap), means for menstrual hygiene management (spaces for washing, changing, disposal) that provide privacy and security for users of all ages and differential physical accessibility.

Management

- Engender the definition of acceptable water, sanitation and hygiene services to include menstrual hygiene management. MHM must be one dimension of inclusive design that caters to lifecycle needs – including users by age, puberty and limited or restricted physical access.
- Define menstrual hygiene management holistically such as:
  - Articulation, awareness, information and confidence to manage menstruation with safety and dignity using safe hygienic materials together with
  - Adequate water and agents and spaces for washing and bathing.
  - Disposal with privacy and dignity.
- Menstrual hygiene management is not the production and distribution of sanitary pads or hygiene education on its own. The combination of all three dimensions is essential for ensuring that girls and women are able to break taboos and demand adequate facilities for MHM that suit their needs.
- MHM as a theme must resonate across health, education, adolescent and youth development and life skills programmes and of course WASH, and must be resourced and monitored across all these sectors. Menstruation is associated with puberty. For girls–this is a time of biological flowering that immediately brings with it restrictions, rules, confinement and changed expectations in many cultures.
- The physical manifestations of puberty and the lack of safe, dignified practices to manage menstruation have somehow created a complex, heavy silence around this

important and very positive lifecycle change. The resulting restrictions in self expression, schooling, mobility, freedom and space have far reaching and deleterious impacts on girls and women globally.

- Thus good MHM has to be more than just facilities for washing and disposal, for addressing the practical dimensions without taking on the more strategic dimensions that surround this biological phenomenon with shame, silence and disgust will fail to bring dignity and safety to women.

Steps in MHM

- Choose the best method of sanitation
- Change the pad regularly
- Wash the genitalia regularly
- Do not use soaps or vaginal hygiene products
- Use the right washing technique
- Discard used sanitary product properly
- Beware of a pad rash
- Use only one method of sanitation at a time
  - Two sanitary pads
  - A tampon and sanitary pad
  - A sanitary pad along with a piece of cloth.
- Have a bath regularly.

Complication of Unhygienic Menstrual Practice

Practice	Health risk
Unclean sanitary pads/materials	Bacteria may cause local infections or travel up the vagina and enter the uterine cavity.
Changing pads infrequently	Wet pads can cause skin irritation which can then become infected if the skin becomes broken.
Insertion of unclean material into vagina	Bacteria potentially have easier access to the cervix and the uterine cavity.
Using highly absorbent tampons during a time of light blood loss	toxic shock syndrome (see right)
Use of tampons when not menstruating (e.g. to absorb vaginal secretions)	Can lead to vaginal irritation and delay the seeking of medical advice for the cause of unusual vaginal discharge.
Wiping from back to front following urination or defecation	Makes the introduction of bacteria from the bowel into the vagina (or urethra) more likely.
Unprotected sex	Possible increased risk of sexually transmitted infections (see below) or the transmission of HIV or Hepatitis B during menstruation.
Unsafe disposal of used sanitary materials or blood	Risk of infecting others, especially with Hepatitis B (HIV and other Hepatitis viruses do not survive for long outside the body and pose a minimal risk except where there is direct contact with blood just leaving the body).

Contd...

Contd...

Practice	Health risk
Frequent douching (forcing liquid into the vagina)	Can facilititate the introduction of bacteria into the uterine cavity.
Lack of handwashing after changing a sanitary towel	Can facilitate the spread of infections such as Hepatitis B or Thrush.

Nutrition Guidance

Total nutrient requirements increase during adolescence to support a period of dramatic growth and development. Like infancy, it is a period of increase in both cell number and size. Protein supplies approximately 12 to 14 percent of the recommended basic nutritional requirements. During the growth spurt, needs for calcium, iron, and zinc increase. Boys are more likely to eat foods that meet calcium requirements. Iron deficiency anemia is a problem for both boys and girls due to expansion in blood volume and muscle mass. Zinc is recognized as essential for growth as well as for sexual maturation of the adolescent.

Eating Habits

Meal skipping, a part of the American lifestyle, is a common phenomenon during adolescence. Although breakfast is the meal most commonly missed, adolescence who work and have busy schedules may also miss the evening meal. Snacking becomes a definite part of adolescent food habits. The selection of nutritious and easy-to-prepare snacks can provide a fairly adequate balance of nutrients.

Prevention of Long-term Illnesses

Consumption of fast foods, especially popular with teenagers, results in a diet with increased intake of fat and sodium and low in dietary fiber.

These facts have been implicated with degenerative diseases that are seen in later life. Adolescents should be encouraged to supplement their diets with fresh fruits and vegetables, to increase dietary bulk, and to avoid fried foods, which can increase blood cholesterol levels. The abuse of alcohol is increasing in the adolescent population.

Alcohol causes gastric irritation, decreases food consumption, and alters the metabolism and utilization of some nutrients. Long-term alcohol abuse results in liver damage and cirrhosis.

Anorexia nervosa characterized by a loss of control over dieting behavior, may result in semi-starvation, poor nutritional status, and deficiency disease. Medical complications may occur, and death may be outcome.

Sex Education

Adolescents usually need privacy to understand the changes taking place in their bodies. Ideally, they should be allowed to have their own bedroom. If this is not possible, they should have at least some private space.

Teasing an adolescent child about physical changes is inappropriate, because it may cause self-consciousness and embarrassment.

Parents need to remember that it is natural and normal for their adolescent to be interested in body changes and sexual topics. It does not mean that their child is involved in sexual activity.

Adolescents may experiment with or consider a wide range of sexual orientations or behaviors before feeling comfortable with their own sexual identity. Parents must be careful not to call new behaviors 'wrong,' 'sick,' or 'immoral.'

The Oedipal complex (a child's attraction to the parent of the opposite sex) is common during the adolescent years. Parents can deal with this by acknowledging the child's physical changes and attractiveness and taking pride in the youth's growth into maturity without crossing parent-child boundaries.

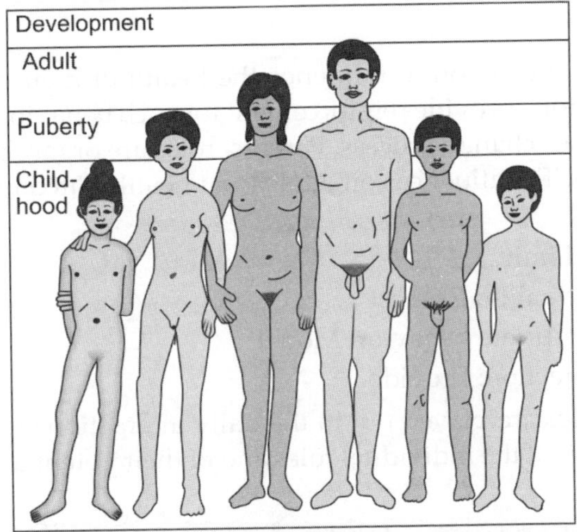

Fig. 3.26: Sexual development of adolescent boys and girls

It is normal for the parent to find the adolescent attractive; especially because the teen often looks very much like the other (same-sex) parent did at a younger age.

It is inappropriate for a parent's attraction to a child to be anything more than an attraction as a parent. Attraction that crosses the parent-child boundaries may lead to inappropriately intimate behavior with the adolescent, which is known as incest.

Characteristics of Effective Sex Education

Experts have identified critical characteristics of highly effective sex education and HIV/STI prevention education programs. Such programs:

- Offer age-and culturally appropriate sexual health information in a safe environment for participants
- Are developed in cooperation with members of the target community, especially young people
- Assist adolescent to clarify their individual, family, and community values
- Assist adolescent to develop skills in communication, refusal, and negotiation
- Provide medically accurate information about both abstinence and also contraception, including condoms

- Have clear goals for preventing HIV, other STIs, and/or teen pregnancy
- Focus on specific health behaviors related to the goals, with clear messages about these behaviors
- Address psychosocial risk and protective factors with activities to change each targeted risk and to promote each protective factor
- Respect community values and respond to community needs
- Rely on participatory teaching methods, implemented by trained educators and using all the activities as designed.

ROLE OF PARENTS IN HEALTH PROMOTION OF ADOLESCENTS

Introduction

Parents are in a unique position to influence the health of their children. Parents set the stage for health behaviors, provide reinforcement for such behavior, and serve as emotional supports in the behavior change process. Parents' roles are organized into five dimensions, each of which has specific influences on adolescent health outcomes:

- Connection: Love
- Behavior control: Limit
- Respect for individuality: Respect
- Modelling of appropriate behavior: Model
- Provision and protection: Provide.

These parenting roles are played out in the daily interactions with adolescents. Parents are usually unconscious of the individual roles and of their potential consequences on health and development.

Strategies for Promotion of Adolescent Health
A = Adoption of healthy life style
D = Develop appropriate IEC strategy
O = Organize adolescent/youth friendly clinic
L = Life skill training, legal support, liaison with peers and parents
E = Educate about sexuality, spirituality
S = Safe, secure and supportive environment
C = Counseling
E = Enable and empower for responsible citizenship
N = Networking for experience sharing
T = Training for income generation, teen clubs

There are three roles

1. Providing support
2. Serving as role models
3. Setting limits.

Providing Support

- Most of children like to be active, but often something more is needed to make it happen. Parents can provide tangible assistance, sometimes called instrumental support, for children to engage in physical activities.

- In order to find a safe place to ride a bike, it might be necessary to drive the child to a park or field.
- Enrolling youth in sport programs or paying for tennis lessons can also aid in the child's quest for an active life. Family support is important for sustaining a child's interest in activity.
- Attending games, watching pickup play in the backyard, asking questions, and generally demonstrating interest add support to the youth's participation in physical activity.

Role Modeling

- Active adults present a consistent and enduring reminder of the role of physical activity in health and happiness. Parents and guardians who participate in exercise or activity have children who are more likely to be active.
- It is not important, however, to be athletic, to engage in any specialized sports, or to be a highly successful performer.
- Regular walking (with the dog or with others), working in the yard, and doing living room calisthenics illustrate the role physical activity plays in the life of an adult. Role modeling was useful, but primarily as a function of support. More active parents tended to provide more support for the physical activities of their children.

Setting Limits

- Parents play important roles in a child's activity level not only through promoting physical activity, but also through their efforts to minimize inactivity. Requiring a child to be active might, in the long run, be an ineffective way to create positive feelings about physical activity.
- It is often easier to set household rules or policies focusing on household objects that create inactivity than to try to force kids to be active. One example is to limit the amount of TV viewing allowed through a TV viewing policy.
- The relationship between inactivity and physical activity seems to be one of opposite behaviors. Decreasing the time spent in sedentary pursuits such as watching TV, playing computer games, or watching videos will surely provide more time for active pursuits.

Adolescents do not grow-up in a vacuum. Both their health and their development are influenced by myriad social and environmental interactions from the immediate (e.g. daily contact with peers, parents, and teachers or physical contact with poison ivy) to the global (e.g. changes in the ozone layer).

The family's significance in this constellation of influences, if not preeminent, is at least major—for it touches the lives of most adolescents on a daily and deeply personal basis. Because parents usually have continuing proximity and can exercise some degree of power over the actions of adolescent family members, they are centrally important to any configuration of social factors shaping adolescent health. From time to time, peers and community may loom larger or smaller among an adolescent's external influences, but the family and parents will remain as constant elements despite fluctuations in their relative importance. Given their ongoing role, if parents and families are to be a positive influence, they need to have accurate and useful information about adolescent development. Using parenting strategies with adolescents that were successful with children may generate conflict that could be avoided through alternative approaches to resolving differences.

CONTROL OF IRON DEFICIENCY ANEMIA (WIFS GUIDELINES)

Introduction

The Ministry of Health and Family Welfare has launched the Weekly Iron and Folic Acid Supplementation (WIFS) Programme to meet the challenge of high prevalence and incidence of anemia amongst adolescent girls and boys. WIFS is evidence-based programmatic response to the prevailing anemia situation amongst adolescent girls and boys through supervised weekly ingestion of IFA supplementation and biannual helminthic control. The long term goal is to break the intergenerational cycle of anemia, the short term benefits is of a nutritionally improved human capital. The programme, implemented across the country both in rural and urban areas.

Features of WIFS

- **Objective** of Weekly Iron Folic acid Supplementation (WIFS). To reduce the prevalence and severity of anemia in adolescent population (10–19 years).
- **Target groups**
  - School going adolescent girls and boys in 6th to 12th class enrolled in government/ government aided/municipal schools.
  - Out of school adolescent girls.
- **Intervention**
  - Administration of supervised Weekly Iron-folic Acid Supplements of 100 mg elemental iron and 500 ug Folic acid using a fixed day approach.
  - Screening of target groups for moderate/severe anemia and referring these cases to an appropriate health facility.
  - Biannual deworming (Albendazole 400 mg), six months apart, for control of helminthic infestation.
  - Information and counselling for improving dietary intake and for taking actions for prevention of intestinal worm infestation.

Table 3.8: Hemoglobin levels to diagnose anemia (g/dl)

Age groups	No anemia	Mild	Moderate	Severe
Children 6–59 months of age	≥ 11	10–10.9	7–9.9	< 7
Children 5–11 years of age	≥ 11.5	11–11.4	8–10.9	< 8
Children 12–14 years of age	≥ 12	11–11.9	8–10.9	< 8
Nonpregnant women (15 years of age and above)	≥ 12	11–11.9	8–10.9	< 8
Pregnant women	≥ 11	10–10.9	7–9.9	< 7
Men	≥ 13	11–12.9	8–10.9	< 8

- **Convergence** with key stakeholder ministries like the Ministry of Women and Child Development and Ministry of Human Resource Development is an essential part of implantation plan of the WIFS programme. Key convergent areas include:
  - Joint programme planning
  - Capacity building of nodal service providers including medical officers
  - Anganwadi worker (AWW)

  - Staff nurses
  - School teachers
  - Monitoring and a comprehensive communication component.
- **Current status:** The programme has been rolled out in all States/UTs. The programme covers 11.2 crore beneficiaries including 8.4 crore in-school and 2.8 crore out of school beneficiaries.

Definition of Anemia

Anemia is a condition in which the number of red blood cells (RBCs), and consequently their oxygen-carrying capacity, is insufficient to meet the body's physiological needs. The function of the RBCs is to deliver oxygen from the lungs to the tissues and carbondioxide from the tissues to the lungs. This is accomplished by using hemoglobin (Hb), a tetramer protein composed of haem and globin. Anemia impairs the body's ability for gas exchange by decreasing the number of RBCs transporting oxygen and carbon dioxide.

Definition of Iron Deficiency

Iron status can be considered as a continuum from iron deficiency with anemia, to iron deficiency with no anemia, to normal iron status with varying amounts of stored iron, and finally to iron overload which can cause organ damage when severe. Iron deficiency is the result of long-term negative iron balance. Iron deficiency anemia (IDA) should be regarded as a subset of iron deficiency, that is, it represents the extreme lower end of the distribution of iron deficiency.

Pathophysiology

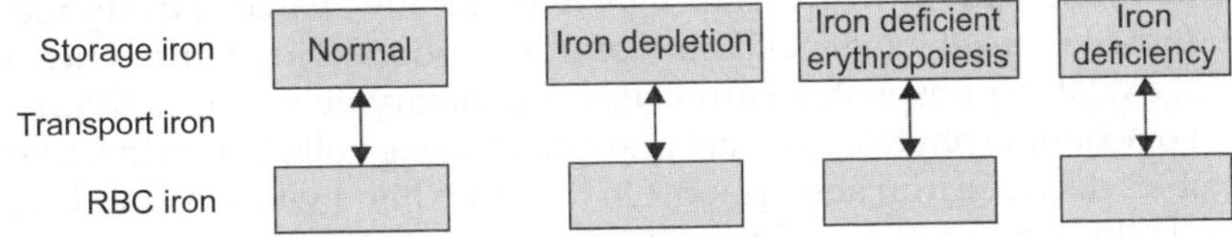

Causes and Risk Factors

Anemia results from one or more of the following process:

- Defective red cell production
- Increased red cell destruction or blood loss.
- Iron is necessary for synthesis of hemoglobin. Iron deficiency is thought to be the most common cause of anemia globally
- Other nutritional deficiencies (including folate, vitamin B12 and vitamin A)
- Acute and chronic inflammation
- Parasitic infections, and inherited or acquired disorders that affect Hb synthesis
- Iron deficiency anemia results in impaired cognitive and motor development in children and decreased work capacity in adults
- In pregnancy iron deficiency anemia can lead to perinatal loss
- Prematurity and low birth weight (LBW) babies

Signs and Symptoms of Anemia

Definitive diagnosis of anemia can only be made by a blood test that measures Hemoglobin (Hb) levels in the blood. The test for Hb is carried out in health centers. However there are some signs that may assist in identifying anemia. They include:

- Whiteness or pallor in the inner rims of the eyelid, tongue, overall skin, nails, palms of the hand
- Soreness of the mouth, with cracks at the corners
- Dizziness, tiredness, fatigue and low energy
- Unusually rapid heartbeat, particularly with exercise
- Shortness of breath and frequent headaches, particularly with exercise
- Lack of interest in play and studies
- Difficulty/inability to concentrate
- Leg cramps
- Lowered resistance to infections.

Prevention and Control of Anemia in Adolescents

Primary prevention of anemia is achieved through well-balanced diet rich in iron and other vitamins and minerals involved in iron absorption or in the production of RBCs/Hemoglobin.

Balanced Diet Rich in Iron

Adolescence is a significant period for physical growth and sexual maturation. Adolescents need to eat a balanced diet, i.e. a diet that provides all nutrients (carbohydrates, proteins, fats, vitamins and minerals) in required amounts and proportions for maintaining health and general well-being. Eating a balanced diet means consuming different types of food items like pulses, chapatti or rice, green vegetables, locally available fruits and milk every day. In our Indian diets, the bioavailability of iron is poor owing to presence of inhibitors like phytates, oxalates, phosphates, carbonates and dietary fibers which interfere with iron absorption. For example phytates in bran, phosphate in egg yolk, tannin in tea and oxalate in some vegetables decrease iron absorption. On the other hand vitamin C and vitamin C rich foods like amla (Indian gooseberry, lime juice, oranges, sprouts, etc. promote iron absorption.

Foods Rich in Iron

- Green vegetables and fruits
- Grains-wheat, jowar, bajra, sprouted pulses, ground nut, sesame, jaggery, dried fruits
- Liver, egg, fish, meat
- Vitamin C rich foods help in absorption of iron. Citrus fruits (oranges, lemon)
- Indian gooseberry (Amla), apple, pear are rich in vitamin C.

Iron Supplementation

In India, the poor absorption of iron and a predominantly vegetarian diet means that despite the consumption of a balanced diet, iron supplementation is required to prevent and control anemia. Anemia among adolescents can be prevented by regular consumption of iron and folic acid tablets once a week, ideally 52 tablets in a year. This is the basis of the WIFS programme launched by the Ministry of Health and Family Welfare Government of India, has the Weekly Iron and Folic Acid Supplementation (WIFS). This programme addresses nutritional anaemia among adolescents (age group of 10–19 years). This programme will be implemented India both rural and urban areas. It will focus on:

- *School Based (Boys and Girls):* School going adolescent girls and boys in government/ government aided/municipal schools from Classes 6th–12th
- *Community Based through the Anganwadi Center (Girls only):* Out of school adolescent girls.

The WIFS programme will also cover married adolescent girls. Pregnant and lactating adolescent girls will be given IFA supplements, according to current guidelines for antenatal and postnatal care through the existing health system of NRHM. Under the WIFS programme for adolescents, IFA supplements are to be distributed free on a weekly basis to the target groups in Categories A and B. In addition to IFA supplements, Albendazole tablets for de-worming are to be administered twice a year, to the same target groups.

Administration of weekly iron-folic acid supplements (WIFS).

One IFA tablet containing 100 mg elemental iron and 500 microgram Folic acid administered on a fixed day through supervised consumption for 52 weeks in a year.

Screening of target groups for moderate/severe anemia and referring these case to an appropriate health facility.

Biannual Albendazole (400 mg) for deworming given six months apart, for control of worm infestation.

Information and counseling for improving dietary intake and for taking actions for prevention of intestinal worm infestation.

Benefits of Iron supplementation:

- Improved concentration in school, and school performance
- Feeling stronger and less tired
- Increased energy levels and output in day to day work
- Increased appetite
- Improved overall capacity to work and earn
- Better sleep
- Improved skin appearance
- Regularization of menstruation
- Building prepregnancy health.

Prevention and Treatment of Hookworm Infestation

Deworming reduces worm load and blood loss and prevents anemia. To prevent hookworm infestation one should maintain personal hygiene and environmental cleanliness. One should use latrine and avoid open air defecation. Regular consumption of Albendazole 400 mg tablet, six months apart, for control of helminthes infestation should be undertaken.

- Personal hygiene and sanitation, food hygiene
- Use of clean drinking water can help protect from various infections and diseases
- Washing hands with soap water before cooking, consuming food, after defecation and after discarding fecal matter of a child is essential to prevent entry of germs into our abdomen
- Keeping personal hygiene
- Preparing and consuming hygienically treated or prepared food.

Additional Interventions

- Fortification of food with iron (salt, flour, rice, biscuits, etc.)
- Prevention of malaria: Clean surroundings, use of insecticide treated mosquito net while sleeping helps keep malaria mosquitoes away from people and greatly reduces malaria
- Early identification and referral: Early identification and referral of suspected cases of anemia constitutes an important measure of secondary prevention of anemia.

Implementing Weekly Iron and Folic Acid Programme through Schools

School-going Adolescents

- The school adolescent population, enrolled in 6th to 12th standard, in rural and urban regions will be reached.
- The programme will be initiated in government schools government aided and municipal schools through the nodal municipal or district education officer.
- Each school will designate one/two teachers as the nodal teachers for WIFS Programme persons.
- The programme in all the schools could be initiated preferably in the month of April after beginning of new session.
- Separate time should also be allotted in the week to provide nutrition and health education (NHE) to the adolescents. The nodal teacher should take the NHE session(s). Guidance and counseling if needed can be provided to the adolescents during these sessions.
- Before the school closes for vacations, the children can be given a complete set of IFA tablets for consumption during the holidays.
- The first dose of deworming tablet, i.e. 400 mg of Albendazole should be administered in month of August and the second dose should be given by February.

Implementing Weekly Iron and Folic Acid Programme through ICDS/AWC

Out-of-school adolescent girls in the age group of 10–19 years (married and unmarried) will be provided IFA and Albendazole tablets free of cost under the 'Rajiv Gandhi Programme Scheme for the Empowerment of Adolescent Girls' (SABLA) through the Anganwadi Centers (AWC). In non SABLA districts, the programme will be implemented through the ICDS mechanism. In the urban areas, the network of AWC in slums and Urban Health Centers will be utilized to provide IFA and Albendazole to adolescent girls (both married and unmarried). AWW will advise the girls that IFA tablets are not taken on an empty stomach and to the extent possible ensure that the girls have eaten a meal prior to taking the IFA tablet.

ANM will undertake quarterly health education session on 'Anemia in adolescent and benefits of IFA supplements' on Village Health and Nutrition Days in convergence with SABLA and will record date and attendance in monthly format. In case a girl complains of uneasiness/any side effects, the AWW will refer her to the ANM. Biannual dose of albendazole for deworming is to be administered during the two fixed months of August and February in year.

Table 3.9: Management of anemia on the basis of hemoglobin levels among adolescents 10–19 years

Level of Hb	Treatment	Follow-up	Indication for referral
Mild anemia (11–11.9 gm/dl)	60 mg of elemental iron daily for 3 months	Follow-up every month Hb estimation after completing 3 months of treatment to assess if Hb estimates are >12 gm/dl	In case of no improvement in Hb levels after 3 months of treatment, adolescent will be referred to DH/FRU for further investigation
Moderate anemia (8–10.9 gm/dl)	60 mg of elemental iron daily for 3 months	Investigate follow-up every 14 days Hb estimation after completing 3 months of treatment to assess if Hb estimates are >12 gm/dl.	In case of no improvement in Hb levels after 3 months of treatment, adolescent will be referred to DH/FRU for further investigation
Severe anemia (< 8 gm/dl)	Refer urgently to DH/FRU	Severely anemic adolescents would be line listed by ANM	
The moderately anemic cases/adolescents with nonresponse to 3 months of iron will need			

Table 3.10: Management of anemia on the basis of hemoglobin levels in children 5–10 years

Level of Hb	Treatment	Follow-up	Referral
Mild anemia (11–11.4 gm/dl)	3 mg of iron/kg/day for 2 months	Follow-up every 14 days Hb estimation after completing 2 months of treatment to assess if Hb estimates are >11.5 gm/dl.	In case the child has not responded to the treatment of anemia with daily dose of iron for 2 months, refer the child to the FRU/DH with F-IMNCI trained MO/pediatrician/physician for further investigation
Moderate anemia (8–10.9 gm/dl)	3 mg of iron/kg/ day for 2 months	Follow-up every 14 days Hb estimation after completing 2 months of treatment to assess if Hb estimates are >11.5 gm/dl	In case the child has not responded to the treatment of anemia with daily dose of iron for 2 months, refer the child to the FRU/DH with F-IMNCI trained MO/pediatrician/ physician for further investigations
Severe anemia (<8 gm/dl)	Refer urgently to DH/ FRU		

Precautions for Oral Therapy

- Intake of doses as per regime, should be taken regularly and must complete the treatment
- Ideally, tablets should be taken on empty stomach for better absorption. In case of gastritis, nausea, vomiting, etc. advise to take one hour after meal or at night
- If constipation occurs, advise to drink more water and add roughage to diet
- IFA tablets should not be consumed with tea, coffee, milk or calcium tablets
- IFA treatment should always supplemented with diet rich in iron, vitamins (particularly Vitamin C), protein, minerals and other nutrients, e.g. green leafy vegetables, whole pulses, jaggery, meat, poultry and fish, fruits and black gram, groundnuts, ragi, whole grains, milk, eggs, meat and nuts, etc.

MODEL QUESTIONS

Multiple Choice Questions

1. **The process of physical maturation resulting an increases in size of the body and variation organ called..........**
   (a) Growth (b) Development
   (c) Health (d) All of the above
2. **Newborn period is from birth to.......... weeks of age.**
   (a) 4 (b) 8
   (c) 10 (d) 12
3. **Infancy is from..........**
   (a) 1 to 12 months (b) 1 to 14 months
   (b) 1 to 18 months (d) 1 to 24 months
4. **1 to 3 years of baby called..........**
   (a) Infant (b) Preschooler
   (c) Toddler (d) Both a and b
5. **The weight of full term neonates at birth is approximately.**
   (a) 1.5 to 2.5 kg (b) 2.5 to 3.8 kg
   (c) 2.5 to 4.5 kg (d) 2.5 to 5 kg
6. **The birth weight become double at the age of ....**
   (a) 2 months (b) 3 months
   (c) 4 months (d) 5 months
7. **The average length of newborn baby is about...**
   (a) 30 cm (b) 40 cm
   (c) 50 cm (d) 60 cm
8. **Which month the head and chest circumference become equal?**
   (a) 5 months (b) 8 months
   (c) 12 months (d) 18 months
9. **The total number of temporary teeth is ....**
   (a) 18 (b) 20
   (c) 26 (d) 30
10. **The psychosexual development describe by ....**
    (a) Henry Fayol (b) Sigmund Freud
    (c) Robert Koch (d) Ergun
11. **Anal stage is from ...age**
    (a) 1–3 years (b) 4–5 years.
    (c) 6–12 years (d) Above 12 years
12. **Toilet training must be started at .... years of age.**
    (a) 1 (b) 3
    (c) 6 (d) 8

13. Play help in the development of children.
(a) Physical
(b) Intellectual
(c) Moral
(d) All of these

14. Bright moving objects are suitable for ...... age group.
(a) Infant
(b) Toddler
(c) Adolescents
(d) None of these

15. Fall and burns is the common accidental problem of which age group.
(a) Infant and toddler
(b) Toddler
(c) Preschooler
(d) None of these

16. Weaning diet should be started about .... of age.
(a) 4 to 6 months
(b) 8 to 9 months
(c) 9 to 12 months
(d) 12 to 24 months

17. The children enjoy competitive sports, games in which age?
(a) Infancy
(b) Preschooler
(c) Newborn
(d) Adolescent

Fill in the Blanks

1. Eruption of teeth in child start from ....months.
2. 1st dose of DPT vaccine should be started at the age of ..weeks.
3. Total number of temporary teeth is ......
4. Toilet training must be started at the age of ......months.
5. Psychosexual stage during toddle is ....
6. ....reflex help in breastfeeding.
7. .... measurement include the head, chest, mid-arm circumference height and weight.
8. ....vaccine given for the protection against chickenpox.
9. The birth weight will be double at the age of ....months.
10. At the age of ....the head circumference and the chest circumference becomes equal to head circumference.
11. Tonic neck reflexes disappear by the age of ....

True or False

1. 1 to 3 years of child called infants.
2. Weaning should be started at the age of 1 year.
3. Immunization should be for the treatment aspect.
4. Sex education should be given to adolescent age group.
5. Helmet and seat belt are comes under the safety measures.
6. 1st dose of DPT vaccine given at age of 11 years.

Short Answer Questions **1 × 5 = 5**

1. Therapeutic play
2. Immunization
3. Prevention of accidents
4. Weaning
5. Nutritional counseling.

Long Answer Questions 1 × 15 = 15

1. (a) Define growth and development.
   (b) What are the factor affecting growth and development?
   (c) Write growth and development of a newborn/infant/toddler/preschooler/schooler/adolescent child.
2. (a) Define immunity.
   (b) Write national immunization schedule.
   (c) Explain cold chain.
3. (a) Define weaning.
   (b) What are the principles of weaning?
   (c) Write weaning at different age group.

ANSWER KEY

Multiple Choice Questions

1. (a)	2. (a)	3. (a)	4. (c)	5. (b)	6. (a)	7. (c)
8. (c)	9. (b)	10. (b)	11. (a)	12. (b)	13. (d)	14. (a)
15. (a)	16. (a)	17. (d)				

Fill in the Blanks

1. 6
2. 6
3. 20
4. 3 years
5. Phallic
6. Sucking
7. Anthropometric measurements
8. Varicella
9. 5
10. 1 year
11. 6 to 8 months

True or False

1. False	2. False	3. False	4. True	5. True	6. False

Chapter 4

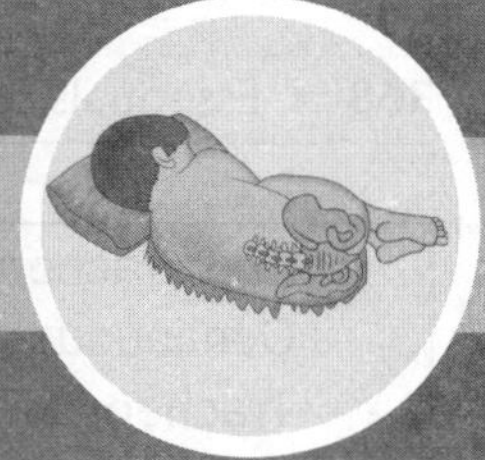

The Sick Child

- **The Sick Child in Hospital**
  - Child's Reaction to Hospitalization
  - Effect of Hospitalization on the Family of the Child
  - Role of Nurse in Care of Hospitalized Child and Family
  - Grief and Bereavement of Children and Family
  - Phases of Grief and Mourning
  - Stages of Grief
  - Grieving Process
  - Parental Bereavement
  - Grief and Developmental Stages
  - Cultural Diversity in Grieving
  - Role of Nurse in Grief and Bereavements
- **Pediatric Procedures**
  - Preparation of Child for Diagnostic Tests and Collection of Specimens
  - Specimen Collection
  - Calculation and Administration of Oral and Parenteral Medication
  - Expected Weight and Height of Normal Children
  - Fluid Calculation
- **Procedures Related to Feeding**
  - Katori and Spoon Feeding
  - Ryle's Nasogastric/Orogastric Tube Feeding
  - Gastrostomy Feeding
- **Procedures Relating to Elimination**
  - Enema
  - Colostomy Irrigation
- **Administration and Analysis of Oxygen Concentration**
  - Airway Management
  - Oropharyngeal Airway
  - Endotracheal Intubation

- Endotracheal Suction
- Continuous Positive Airway Pressure (CPAP)
- Tracheostomy Care
- Steam Inhalation
- Nebulization
- **Other Procedures**
  - Pediatric Advanced Life Support (PALS)
- **Neonatal Advanced Life Support Neonatal Resuscitation Programme (NRP)**
  - Surgical Dressing
  - Lumbar Puncture in Pediatrics
  - Care of Baby Under the Incubator
  - Radiant Warmer
  - Phototherapy Units
  - Umbilical Catheterization
  - Umbilical Vein Catheterization
  - Umbilical Artery Catheterization
  - Kangaroo Mother Care
  - Arterial Blood Gas (ABG)

THE SICK CHILD IN HOSPITAL

CHILD'S REACTION TO HOSPITALIZATION

Introduction

The child sickness is one of the life threatening situations. It will affect the child normal growth and development and family crisis. Child illness characterized by pain, cry, poor feeding, irritability, fear of separation from the parents and family environment, which affect the child emotional status of the child.

Hospitalization is the first crises of children must face. Especially during the early years, children are particularly vulnerable to the crises of illness and hospitalization. Stress represents a change from the usual state of health and environmental routine. Children have limited number of coping mechanism to resolve stressors.

Major stressors of hospitalization include separation, loss of control, bodily injury and pain children reactions to these crises are influenced by their developmental age, their previous experience, will illness separation or hospitalization.

Reaction to Hospitalization

Neonates/Newborns

A newborn baby or neonate is defined as a child under 28 days of age. During these first 28 days of life, the child is at highest risk of dying. It is crucial that appropriate feeding and special care are provided during this period for improvements of child's survival rate and make the strong foundations for a healthy life.

Following reaction to be more common in neonates:

- During hospitalization neonates miss the trust between mother and newborn.
- Deprivation of motor and sensory development.
- Overload of tactile, auditory, kinesthetic, sensory functions.
- Impairment of neonate and parent attachment
- Impairment of neonate ability to respond to their parents and family members.
- Impairment of parents ability to love and care for their baby.
- Risk of physical and psychological disturbances.
- Risk of stress among hospitalized neonate parents and family members.

Infants

Infants are developing the most important attitude of a healthy personality and trust vs mistrust. Trust is established through consistent, living care by a nurturing person. Infants attempt to control their environment through emotional expressions, such as crying or smiling. Inconsistent care and deviations from the infant's daily routine may lead to mistrust and a decreased sense of contract.

Toddlers

Toddlers are striving for autonomy and this goal is evident in most of their behavior, motor skills, play, interpersonal relationships, activities of daily living and communication. When their egocentric pleasures most with obstacles, toddlers react with negativism, especially temper tantrums loss of control also results from altered routines and rituals. Toddlers rely in the consistency and familiarity of daily rituals to provide a measure of stability and control in their complex world of growing and developing.

Toddler's main areas of rituals include eating, sleeping, bathing, toileting and play. Enforced dependency is a chief characteristic of the sick role and accounts for the numerous instances of toddler negatives.

Preschoolers

Preschoolers also suffer from loss of control caused by physical restriction, altered routines, and enforced dependency. However their specific cognitive abilities, which make them feel omnipotent and all powerful also make them feel out of control. This loss of control in the context of their sense of self power is a critical influencing factor in their perception of and reaction to separation, pain, illness and hospitalization.

Preschooler's egocentric and medical thinking limits their ability to understand events because they view all experiences from their own self referenced perspective. Preschoolers preparation thinking means that explanations are understood only in terms of real events.

School-age Children

School-age children may be less concerned with pain than with disability uncertain recovery or possible death. Children with chronic illness are more likely to identify intrusive procedures as stressful, whereas children who are acutely ill are more likely to indicate physical symptoms. Girls tend to express more and stronger feasts than boys. School-age children define illness by a set of multiple concrete symptoms, such as signs of a cold a view the cause as primary germs of bacteria school age children begin to show concern for the potential beneficial and hazardous effects of procedure. Intrusive procedures of an nonsexual nature, such as routine physical examination of the ears, nose, mouth and throat are generally well tolerated.

School-age children verbally communicate about their pain in respect to its location, intensity and description and also use words as a means of controlling their reactions to pain. School-age children will rarely intitate a conversation about their feelings or request someone to stay with them during a lonely or stressful period.

Adolescents

Although the development of body image begins at birth, its relevance is paramount during adolescence. Injury, pain, disability and death are viewed primarily in terms of how each affect adolescents views of themselves in the present. Adolescent's rapidly changing body image during pubertal development often makes them feel insecure about their bodies. Frequently their four of loss of control and body-image change is demonstrated as over confidence. Because of the development of secondary sex characteristics, adolescents are very concerned about privacy. Adolescents typically react to pain with much self control physical resistance and aggression are less likely at this age unless the adolescent is totally unprepared for a procedure.

Common Reaction

Table 4.1: Hospitalized child physiological and psychological reaction

Physiological reactions	Psychological reactions
• Temperature elevations: As response to infections	• Separation anxiety
• Convulsions: Resulted from rise in temperature	• Stranger anxiety
• Immobilization	• Sleep deprivation
• Anorexia, vomiting and diarrhea	• Loss of self control
• Nutritional deficiencies	• Fear of darkness
• Fluid and electrolyte imbalance	• Fear of death
• Inconsistent weight loss	• Sensory overload
• Lack of growth	

Separation Anxiety

The major stress from middle infancy throughout the preschool years for children ages 6 to 30 months is separation anxiety, also called anaclitic depression.

Manifestations of Separation Anxiety in Young Children

- Phase of protest
  - Starting stage (Infancy): Cries, screens
  - Searches for parents eyes: Clings to parent
  - Avoids and rejects with strangers.
- Phase of despair
  - Inactive
  - Withdraws from others

- Depressed, sad mood
- Uninterested in environment
- Uncommunicative
- Regresses to earlier behavior, e.g. thumb sucking, bed-wetting
- Child's physical condition may deteriorate from refusal to eat, drink, or move.

- Phase of detachment
  - Shows increased interest in surroundings
  - Interacts with stranger or familiar caregivers
  - Forms new but superficial relationships
  - Appears happy
  - Behavior represent a superficial adjustable to loss.

Early Childhood

Separation anxiety is the greatest stress imposed by hospitalization during early childhood. If separation is avoided, young children have a tremendous capacity to withstand any other stress. However children in the toddler stage demonstrate more goal-directed behaviors. For temper tantrum refusing to comply with the usual routines of mealtime, bedtime, or toileting or regressing to more primitive levels of development. However temper tantrums, bed wetting or other behaviors may also be expressions of anger or even a physiologic response to stress.

The preschoolers are more secure interpersonally than toddlers, they can tolerate brief periods of separation from their parents and are more inclined to develop substitute trust is other significant adults. Preschoolers may demonstrate separation anxiety by refusing to eat, experiencing difficult in sleeping, crying quietly for their parents, continually asking when the parents will visit or withdrawing from others. They may express anger indirectly by breaking their toys, hitting other children or refusing to cooperate during usual self-care activities.

Later Childhood and Adolescence

The school-age children are better able to cope with separation in general, the stress and often accompanying regression imposed by illness or hospitalization may increase their need for parental security and guidance. Middle and late school-age children may react more to the separation from their usual activities and pears than to the absence of their parents feelings of loneliness, boredom, isolation and depression are common.

School-age children may need and desire parental guidance or support from other adult figures but may be unable or unwilling to ask for it. Cultural expectations to act like a man especially boys who tend to react to stress stoicism, withdrawal, or passive acceptance often the need to express hostile, angry or other negative feelings finds outlets in alternate ways, such as irritability and aggression toward parents withdrawal from hospital personal.

For adolescents, separation from home and parents may be a welcomed and appreciated event. The loss of peer group contact may post a severe emotional thereat because of loss of group acceptance. Deviations within peer groups are poorly tolerated and although group members may express concern for the adolescents illness or need for hospitalization.

Loss of Control

Lack of control increases the perception of threat and can affect children's coping skills. Many hospital situations decrease the amount of control a child feels. The children's needs vary greatly depending on their age, the major areas of loss of control in terms of physical restriction, altered routine or rituals and dependency are discussed for each age-group.

EFFECT OF HOSPITALIZATION ON THE FAMILY OF THE CHILD

Children may react to the stresses of hospitalization before admission, during hospitalization and after discharge.

Parental Reactions

The crisis of childhood illness and hospitalization affects every member of the nuclear family. Parent's reactions to illness to their child depend on a variety of influencing factors. Almost all parents respond to their child's illness and hospitalization with may react with disbelief, especially if the illness is sudden and serious the realization of illness of parents react with anger or guilt of both.

- Fear, anxiety and frustration are common feelings expressed by parents.
- Fear and anxiety may be related to the seriousness of the illness and the type of medical procedures involved.
- Feelings of frustration are often related to lack of information about procedures and treatment.
- Unfamiliarity with hospital rules and regulations.
- Parents eventually may react with some degree of depression.
- Mothers often comment on their feelings of physical and mental exhaustion after all the other family members have adapted to the crisis.

Factors Affecting Parent's Reactions to their Illness

- Seriousness to the threat to the child
- Previous experience will illness or hospitalization
- Medical procedures involved in diagnosis and treatment
- Available support systems
- Personal ego abilities
- Additional stresses on the family system cultural and religious beliefs.

Sibling Reactions

Siblings reactions to a sister's or brother's illness or hospitalization are differ little when a child becomes temporarily ill siblings experience loneliness, fear, worry as well as anger, resentment, jealousy and guild.

Factors Regarding Sibling

- Younger and experiencing many changes
- Cared for outside the home by care provides who are not relatives
- Received little information about their ill brother or sister
- Perceived that their parents to be treating them differently compared with before their sibling's hospitalization.

Altered Family Roles

In addition to the effects of separation on family roles, loss of parenting, sibling and offspring roles may affect each family member differently. One of the most common reactions of parent is specialized and intensified attention toward the sick child. The other siblings may regard this as unfair and intensified attention toward the risk child. The other siblings may regard this as unfair and interpret the parent's attitude toward them as rejection. Ill children may also feel jealousy from other siblings. Rivalry between siblings tends to be greatest in the sibling who is nearest in age to the ill child. Illness may also result in children's loss of status within either family or social group.

Individual Risk Factors

A number of risk factors make certain children more vulnerable than others to the stresses of hospitalization. It has also been noted that rural children exhibit significantly greater degrees of psychologic upset than urban children possibly, because urban children have opportunities to become familiar with a local hospital. The stressors of hospitalization may cause young children to experience short and long term negative outcomes. Common responses include regression, separation, anxiety, apathy, fears and sleeping disturbance especially for children younger than 7 years of age.

Change in the Pediatric Population

The pediatric population in hospital today has changed dramatically over the last two decades. Many of these children are fragile and children with severe injurious or disabilities who have survived because of major technologic advance, yet have been left with chronic is disabling conditions that require often frequent and lengthy hospital stays. The majority of these children are infants and toddlers. The age group are most vulnerable to the effect of hospitalization.

Beneficial Effects of Hospitalization

The most obvious benefit is the recovery from illness, but hospitalization also can present an opportunity for children to master stress and feel competent in their coping abilities. The psychologic benefits need to be considered is maximized during hospitalization.

Defense Mechanism

- *Rationalization:* It is making excuses for questionable behavior.
- *Denial:* Denial is when you refuse to accept or believe the existence of something that is very unpleasant
- *Repression:* Repression is a process of unconsciously forgetting unpleasant and conflicting emotions, desires and experiences.
- *Withdrawal:* When a situation is too difficult and too frustrating, you may physically withdraw in order to protect yourself and self-image. Another form of withdrawal is fantasy or day dreaming.
- *Regression:* To regress in human behavior means to behave in a less mature way.
- *Sublimation:* Sublimation is a process of redirecting the energy produced by unacceptable desires or activities so that they become acceptable.
- *Projection:* Projection is when we pretend that other people have our own undesirable characteristic motives and desires.

- *Identification:* It is the process of finding satisfaction through the behavior and successes of another person or group.
- *Reaction formation:* It is the process of strongly expression the opposite of what one really feels.
- *Intellectualization:* It means to distance oneself from an emotional or threatening situation by talking or thinking about it in intellectual terms.
- *Displacement:* It means to substitute the real object of one's feelings.

ROLE OF NURSE IN CARE OF HOSPITALIZED CHILD AND FAMILY

Preparation for Hospitalization

The rationale for preparing children for the hospital experience and related procedures is based on the principle that fear of the unknown exceeds fear of the know. Therefore decreasing the elements of the unknown results in less fear. Although preparation for hospitalization is a common practice, there is no universal standard or program that is advocated for all setting. The preparation process may be elaborate with tours, puppet shows, playtime with miniature hospital equipment, it may involve the use of books, videos, or films or it may be limited to a brief description of the major aspects of any hospital stay.

Admission Assessment

The nursing admission history refers to a systematic collection of data about the child and family that allows the nurse to plan individualized care. One of the main purposes of the history is to assess the child's usual health habits at home to promote a more normal environment in the hospital. Therefore, questions related to activities of daily living in the nutritional—metabolize, elimination, sleep rest and activity exercise patterns are a major part of the assessment.

After the data are collected, the information must be applied to the nursing process and communication to other staff. Besides taking the nursing admission history, nurse should also perform a physical assessment or obtain the information from the medical examination before planning care.

Preparing Child for Admission

The preparation that children require on the day of admission depends on the kind of prehospital counseling they have received.

Guidelines for Admission

Pre-admission

- Assign a room based on developmental age seriousness of diagnosis
- Prepare roommates
- Prepare room for child and family.

Admission

- Introduce primary nurse to child and family
- Orient child and family to inpatient facilities
- Room: Call light, bed controlled, television

- Unit: Direct to playroom, desk, dining area
- Perform nursing admission history
- Vital signs
- Support child and assist practitioner with physical examination.

Preventing or Minimizing Separation

A primary nursing goal is to prevent separation, particularly is children younger than 5 years of age. Many hospitals have developed a system of family-centered care. The family is considered to be partners in the care of the child. Nurse must have an appreciation of the child's separation behavior. Separation may be equally as difficult for parents, especially when they do not understand the behaviors of separation anxiety. Toddlers and preschoolers have a very limited concept of time. Helping children maintain their usual nonhome contacts also minimizes the effects of separation imposed by hospitalization.

Minimizing Loss of Control

Feelings of loss of control result from separation, physical restriction, changed routines, enforced dependency and magical thinking.

Promoting Freedom of Movement

Younger children react most strenuously to any type of physical reaction or immobilization. Although temporary immobilization may be necessary for some interventions such as maintain an IV line, must physical restriction can be prevented environment factors may also restrict movement.

Maintaining Child's Routine

The daily schedule and loss of rituals are particularly stressful for toddlers and early preschoolers and may increase the stress of separation. The time structure vanishes when the child is hospitalized. One technique that can minimize the disruption in the child's routine is time structuring.

Encouraging Independence

The dependent role of the hospitalized patient imposes tremendous feelings of loss on older children promoting children's control involves maintaining independence and the self concept of self care can be most beneficial.

Preventing or Minimizing Fear of Bodily Injury

Beyond early infancy all children fear bodily injury either from mutilation, bodily intrusion, body image change, disability or birth. In general, preparation for children for painful procedures decreases their fears. Children may fear bodily injury from a great variety of sources X-ray machines, use of strange equipment for examination, unfamiliar rooms or awkward positions can be perceived as potentially hazardous.

Pain Assessment

Pain assessment is critical components in managing pain is multifactorial and include sensory, affective, behavior, cognitive, sociocultural and physiologic components.

Pain Management

Relief of pain is a basic need and right of all children. Effective pain management requires that health professionals be willing to try a number of interventions to achieve optimal results the pain reducing methods.

Nonpharmacologic management: Pain is often associated with fears, anxiety and stress. A number of nonpharmacologic techniques such as distraction, relaxation, guided imagery and extraneous stimulation.

Pharmacologic management: Using pharmacologic methods to control pain requires attention to four rights: Right drug, right dose, right route and right night time.

Right drug: Nonopioids, i.e. non-steroidal anti-inflammatory drugs (NSAIDs).

Providing Opportunities for Play and Expressive Activities

Play is one of the most important aspects of a child's life and one of the most effective tools for managing stress. Play is essential to children's mental, emotional and social well-being. As with their developmental needs, the need for play does not stop when children are ill in the hospital.

Diversional Activities

Almost any form of play can be used for diversion and recreation but the activity should be selected on the basis of the child's age, interest and limitations. Games that can be played alone or with another child or an adult are popular with older children.

Play Materials

Parents of hospitalized children often ask nurses about the types of toys that would be best to bring for their child large number of toys, often confuse and frustrate a small child.

Expressive Activities

Play and other expressive activities provide one of the best opportunities for encouraging emotional expression including the safe release of anger and hostility. Therapeutic play is very effective, nondirective modality for helping children with their concerns and fears and at the same time it often helps the nurse to gain in sights into children's needs and feelings.

Creative Expression

All children desire physical, social, emotional and cognitive benefits from engaging in art in other creative activities, children's need for such activities is intensified when they are hospitalizied.

Dramatics Play

Dramatic play is well-recognized technique for emotional release, allowing children to reenact frightening or puzzling hospital experience.

Nursing Care of the Family

Discharge Assessment

Throughout the hospitalization the nurse should be aware of the need for discharge planning, ad those assessment factors that affect the family ability to provide home care. Discharge

admission to permit sufficient time to assess the family ability to perform care at home and to institute needed teaching. The current nursing shortage has placed more of the burden for caring for children in the home on the parents when often become the child's caregiver supervised by the nurse who acts as a **case manager.**

Discharge planning is also concerned with those treatments their parents or children are expected to continue at home.

Encouraging Parent's Participation

Prevent or minimizing separation is a key nursing goal with the child who is hospitalized, but maintaining parent child contact is also beneficial for the family. A rejection attitude toward parent participation can create barriers to collaborative working relationships. When hospital staffs genuinely appreciate the importance of continued parent child attachment, they foster an environment that encourages parents to stay.

Supporting Family Members

Support involves the willingness to stay and listen to parents verbal and nonverbal messages. Sometimes the nurse does not give this support directly often relatives and friends want to help but do not know how suggesting ways, such as baby-sitting, preparing meals, tending the garden in home, doing laundry or transporting the siblings to school can people others to help lessen the responsibility that burden parents. Support involves an acceptance of cultural, socioeconomic and ethnic valves.

Providing Information

One of the most important nursing interventions is providing information about:

- The disease, its treatment, prognoses and home care
- To child's emotional as well as physical reaction to illness and hospitalization
- The probable emotional reactions of family members to the crisis
- Parents also need to be aware of the effects of illness on the family is strategies that prevent negative change.

Preparing for Discharge and Home Care

Most hospitalizations necessitate some type of discharge preparation often this involve education of the family for continued care and follow-up in the home depending on the diagnose. This may be relatively simple or highly complex preparing the family for home care demands a high degree of competence in planning and implementing discharge instructions. This usually is best accomplished using an interdisciplinary team approach which requires a shift from the multidisciplinary beam approach used during an acute phase of a child's illness. Nurses are the one's responsible for all or some of the discharge teaching, which may be further carried out by the parent as the home caregiver with a nurse acting as resource case manager. All families need to received detailed written instructions about home care, with telephone numbers for assistance before they leave the hospital.

Care of the Child and Family in Special Hospital Situations

Ambulatory/outpatient setting: The ambulatory or outpatient setting provides needed medical services for the child while eliminating the necessity of overnight admission.

- Benefits of ambulatory
- Minimization of the stressors of hospitalization especially separation from the family
- Reduced chance of infection
- Cost savings.

Admission to the ambulatory or outpatient hospital setting usually is for surgical or diagnostic procedures such as insertion of tympanostomy tube; hernia repair, tonsillectomy, etc. waiting is usually inevitable in ambulatory settings. Families frequently report waiting to be the most stressful part of the experience.

Isolation

Admission to an isolation room increases all the stressors typically associated with hospitalization. There is further separation from familiar persons, additional loss of control is added environmental changes which as sensory deprivation and the strange appearance of visitors. When a child placed in isolation, preparation is essential for the child to feel in control.

Emergency Admission

One of the most traumatic hospital experiences for the child and parents is an emergency admission. The sudden onset of an illness or the occurrence of an injury cliques little time for preparation and explanation. Sometimes the emergency admission is compounded by admission to an intensive care unit or the need for immediate surgery. In pediatric population, most visits are for respiratory infections with skin conditions, GI disorders and trauma such as poisoning accounting for the reminder of cases.

Intensive Care Unit

Parents who have a child in as ICU are stressed. The nature and severity of the illness and the circumstances surrounding the admission are major factors especially for parents. The emotional needs of the family are paramount when a child is admitted to an ICU. Critically ill children become the focus of the parents love and parents most pressing need is for information despite the stresses normally associated with ICU admission. A special security develop from being carefully monitored and receiving individualized care.

Health Support Program for Family Members with Hospitalized Child

In Japan it is a common practice for family members to be with patients who are infants with separation anxiety, patients with breastfeeding needs, when preparation periods are needed during hospitalization for home care provides after surgery, or in cases of terminal illness. Family members opt to attend to the patient upon consulting with the patient, other family members and the doctor. However because many hospitals are not equipped to most such family needs, there have been numerous reports of family members developing physical ailments, such as stiff necks, backaches, constipation, and insomnia. Most research has focused on the family member's quality of life or on influences upon other family members.

GRIEF AND BEREAVEMENT OF CHILDREN AND FAMILY

Introduction

Grief is a multi-faceted response to loss, particularly to the loss of someone or something to which a bond was formed. Although conventionally focused on the emotional response to loss, it also has physical, cognitive, behavioral, social, and philosophical dimensions. While the terms are often used interchangeably, bereavement refers to the state of loss, and grief is the reaction to loss.

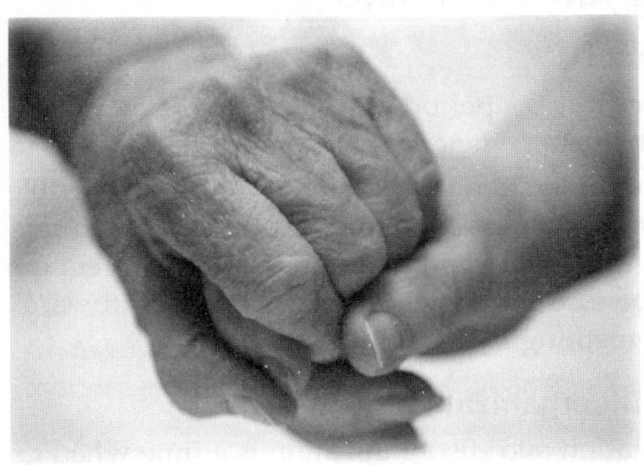

Definition

Grief is a natural response to loss. It is the emotional suffering one feels when something or someone the individual loves is taken away. Grief is also a reaction to any loss.

The grief associated with death is familiar to most people, but individuals grieve in connection with a variety of losses throughout their lives, such as unemployment, ill-health or the end of a relationship.

Loss can be categorized as either physical or abstract, the physical loss being related to something that the individual can touch or measure, such as losing a spouse through death, while other types of loss are abstract, and relate to aspects of a person's social interactions.

Loss

Two categories of loss exist—physical and symbolic losses. A physical loss is the loss of something tangible, and often others recognize physical losses. In contrast, a symbolic loss is the loss of something intangible (divorce, retirement, the development of chronic illness, shattered dreams), which is seldom recognized by others as a loss generating feelings that require processing.

Grief

Grief refers to the process of experiencing psychological, behavioral, social and physical reactions to loss. It is a continuing process involving many changes over time. It is a natural reaction, and its absence may be abnormal and indicative of pathology. It is a reaction to all types of loss, not just death, and it is dependent on an individual's unique perception of loss and does not need social recognition or validation by others (i.e. it is the specific subjective feeling that accompanies a loss).

Mourning

Mourning is the cultural and/or public display of grief through one's behavior. It is the process through which the resolution of grief may be accomplished.

Bereavement

Bereavement is the entire process precipitated by the loss of a loved one through death.

PHASES OF GRIEF AND MOURNING

Avoidance or Protest

Avoidance or protest covers the period during which the news of death is initially received and the time briefly thereafter. Generally, it lasts for a few hours to several days.

It is marked by the understandable desire to avoid the terrible acknowledgment that a loved one is lost, and by a desperate and frantic attempt to reinstitute the relationship with the lost person. Anger and hostility frequently are present during the initial phase of mourning, and may be directed at health care workers or toward oneself, specifically for having failed to do something to avert the loss.

Confrontation and Disorganization

The phase of confrontation and disorganization is a time when grief is experienced most intensely, and reactions to the loss are most acute; it introduces awareness of finality. This is a painful, internal phase when the mourner confronts the reality of the loss and gradually absorbs its meaning.

The most characteristic feature of this phase is preoccupation with thoughts of the deceased while the mourner relives his or her relationship with the lost one. These memories are intrusive and painful, but they constitute the necessary grief work that eventually helps the mourner to relinquish the important attachment.

Accommodation or Reorganization

During the accommodation and reorganization phase, there is a gradual decline in the symptoms of acute grief, and the beginning of social and emotional reinvestment in the world. The deceased or the loss is not forgotten, but the mourner learns to live with the cognizance of the death and its implications in a way that does not preclude a healthy, life-affirming growth. This process, which extends for at least one to two years, indicates the completion of mourning because the person enjoys life again and begins looking toward the future.

STAGES OF GRIEF

The grieving process varies from person to person in terms of the order in which one experiences the stages of grief, as well as the time it takes to go through the stages of grief. People who are grieving do not necessarily progress in order. Some people may start with anger, while others may start with denial. The stages of grieving are not necessarily a onetime experience. However, each step helps with the healing process. Grief is usually divided into five stages:

Denial

Denial is a stage where one can try to believe that the death has not occurred. One may feel numb, or in a state of shock. Denial is a protective emotion when a life event is too overwhelming to deal with all at once.

Anger

Anger is a stage in which you are very upset and angry that this tragedy has happened in your family. One of the best ways of dealing with bursts of anger is to exercise or participate in another type of physical activity. Talking with family and friends, other parents who have lost a child, and the hospital staff, may also be helpful.

Bargaining

Questioning God, asking 'Why my child?' and 'What did we do to deserve this?' are common questions in this stage. Guilt is a primary emotion during this stage. Searching for something that you personally did, which could have contributed to the death, is all part of bargaining. It is important to remember that there is nothing you or your child did which contributed to the death.

Depression or Sadness

This is a stage in which the death of a child can no longer be denied and parents and siblings may feel a profound sense of sadness. This is normal. It may be accompanied by physical changes such as trouble sleeping or excessive sleeping, changes in appetite, or difficulty with concentrating on simple daily activities. It is important to talk about depression with a health care professional such as a social worker, or counselor, or meet with a support group to help you cope with these feelings.

Acceptance

Acceptance is the stage in which you have accepted death and are at a point where your child's death has been incorporated as part of your life. You have made an adjustment to the loss. This does not mean that you will never feel other emotions, but usually families find that they are better able to manage their lives overall on reaching this stage. Some resolution has taken place with the child's death. This may include your religious and cultural beliefs and practices.

GRIEVING PROCESS

Every step of the process is natural and healthy, it is only when a person gets stuck in one step for a long period of time then the grieving can become unhealthy, destructive and even dangerous. When going through the grieving process, it is not the same for everyone, but everyone does have a common goal, acceptance of the loss and to always keep moving forward. This process is different for every person but can be understood in five different steps.

1. **Shock and denial:** Shock is the initial reaction to loss. Shock is the person's emotional protection from being too suddenly overwhelmed by the loss. The person may not yet be willing or able to believe what his mind knows to be true. This stage normally lasts two or three months.
2. **Intense concern:** Intense concern is often shown by not being able to think of anything else. Even during daily tasks, thoughts of the loss keep coming to mind. Conversations with one at this stage always turn to the loss as well. This period may last from six months to a year.

3. **Despair and depression:** Despair and depression is a long period of grief, the most painful and protracted stage for the griever (during which the person gradually comes to terms with the reality of the loss). The process typically involves a wide range of feelings, thoughts, and behaviors. Many behaviors may be irrational. Depression can include feelings of anger, guilt, sadness and anxiety.
4. **Recovery:** The goal of grieving is not the elimination of all the pain or the memories of the loss. In this stage, one shows a new interest in daily activities and begins to function normally day to day. The goal is to reorganize one's life, so the loss is an important part of life rather than its center.
5. **Reactions:** Crying is a normal and natural part of grieving. It has also been found, however, that crying and talking about the loss is not the only healthy response and, if forced or excessive, can be harmful.

Science has found that some healthy people who are grieving do not spontaneously talk about the loss. Pressing people to cry or retell the experience of a loss can be harmful. Genuine laughter is healthy.

PARENTAL BEREAVEMENT

If parental bereavement is analyzed according to the ***six 'R' processes*** of mourning, it is clear that bereaved parents have a number of built-in obstacles to mourning after the loss of a child.

- *Recognizing the loss* because it violates their basic function as parents and defies the laws of nature; often, social negation of the loss exists. With the loss of pregnancies and the deaths of young infants, no dramatic absence is apparent to signal the loss, causing the parents to have difficulty internalizing the fact that the death has really occurred. Recognizing the loss is also made difficult because the neonatal intensive care unit (NICU) exists to save lives with a technical power that is obvious to the parents.
- *Reacting to the separation* not in the least because more secondary losses, especially those relating to the self, take place in this type of bereavement.
- *Recollecting and re-experiencing the deceased and the relationship* is made more difficult for bereaved parents because there is little or nothing concrete to review or remember realistically.
- *Relinquishing old attachments to the deceased and the old, assumptive world* is difficult because an attachment to the deceased fetus or infant also includes attachments to the self as a parent; and also because relinquishing attachments to the old, assumptive world mandates a complete revision of the most fundamental assumptions of being a parent, and fulfilling parental responsibilities and roles.
- *Readjust to the new world without forgetting the old one.* Developing a new relationship with the deceased may be difficult because the parental relationship demands role behaviors that are not as amenable as other relationships to a healthy translation on an intrapsychic plane (i.e. compared with losing a parent, it is more difficult to retrain internally the role 'to mother' than 'to be mothered' because mothering requires more interactive participation).
- Finally, for the sixth 'R', bereaved parents have more difficulty *reinvesting* because reinvesting in a similar relationship is more feasible when the relationship is with a spouse, peer or parent than when the relationship is with a child.

Sibling and Peer Bereavement

The impact of a child's death on their siblings is important to remember and address. Most young children can overcome the trauma of a sibling's death with the necessary support and time. Many children have strong feelings of guilt and blame when their sibling dies. Often the child who has died is idealized after his or her death, leaving feelings of inferiority and neglect for the surviving siblings.

These siblings have often been surrounded by death, illness, and great sorrow from all family members, especially parents, during the dying child's experience. More often, the young siblings of a child with a terminal illness have been protected from some of the experiences associated with the death.

They may not have been allowed to visit the dying child, prevented from participating in the religious or cultural rituals, and possibly, even prevented from attending the funeral. All of these experiences may help with closure and can make a sibling's survivor-guiltless burdensome.

For peers and classmates, the grief process may be experienced in a variety of ways. Many children may not have had an experience with anyone their age dying from an illness or accident. For any age group, review of our own mortality and purpose in life is evaluated. Young children may fear they will die soon also.

They may also have feelings of guilt and blame, similar to the sibling's expression of grief. The peer of a dying child also needs time and emotional support to grieve over his or her loss of a friend, neighbor, and/or classmate. There are many support groups that include nonfamily members and peers in helping work through the grieving process.

Complicated Grief

Prolonged Grief Disorder (PGD), formerly known as complicated grief, is a pathological reaction to loss representing a cluster of empirically-derived symptoms that have been associated with long-term physical and psychosocial dysfunction. Individuals with PGD experience severe grief symptoms for at least six months and are stuck in a maladaptive state. An attempt is being made to create a diagnosis category for complicated grief in the DSM-V. Critics of including the diagnosis of complicated grief in the DSM-V say that doing so will constitute characterizing a natural response as a pathology, and will result in wholesale medicating of people who are essentially normal.

The complicated grief is not synonymous with grief. Complicated grief is characterized by an extended grieving period and other criteria, including mental and physical impairments. An important part of understanding complicated grief is understanding, how the symptoms differ from normal grief.

The Mayo Clinic states that with normal grief the feelings of loss are evident. When the reaction turns into complicated grief, however, the feelings of loss become incapacitating and continue even though time passes.

The signs and symptoms characteristic of complicated grief are listed as 'extreme focus on the loss and reminders of the loved one, intense longing or pining for the deceased, problems accepting the death, numbness or detachment... bitterness about your loss, inability to enjoy life, depression or deep sadness, trouble carrying out normal routines, withdrawing from social activities, feeling that life holds no meaning or purpose, irritability or agitation, lack of trust in others.'

The symptoms seen in complicated grief are specific because the symptoms seem to be a combination of the symptoms found in separation as well as traumatic distress. They are also considered to be complicated because unlike normal grief these symptoms will continue regardless of the amount of time that has passed and despite treatment given from tricyclic antidepressants.

In the study 'Bereavement and Late-Life Depression: Grief and its Complications in the Elderly' six subjects who had symptoms of complicated grief were given a dose of Paroxetine which is a selective serotonin reuptake inhibitor and showed a 50% decrease in their symptoms within a three month period.

The Mental Health Clinical Research team theorizes that the symptoms of complicated grief in bereaved elderly are an alternative of post-traumatic stress. These symptoms were correlated with cancer, hypertension, anxiety, depression, suicidal ideation, increased smoking, and sleep impairments at around six months after spousal death.

A treatment that has been found beneficial in dealing with the symptoms associated with complicated grief is the use of serotonin specific reuptake inhibitors such as Paroxetine. These inhibitors have been found to reduce intrusive thoughts, avoidant behaviors, and hyperarousal that are associated with complicated grief. In addition psychotherapy techniques are in the process of being developed.

GRIEF AND DEVELOPMENTAL STAGES

Death and the events surrounding it are understood differently depending on the age and developmental stage of the child.

Infants

Although infants do not recognize death, feelings of loss and separation are part of a developing death awareness. Children who have been separated from their mothers and deprived of nurturing can exhibit such changes as listlessness, quietness, unresponsiveness to a smile or a coo, physical changes (including weight loss), and a decrease in activity and lack of sleep.

Ages 2–3 Years

In this age range, children often confuse death with sleep and can experience anxiety. In the early phases of grief, bereaved children can exhibit loss of speech and generalized distress.

Ages 3–6 Years

At this age children view death as a kind of sleep; the person is alive, but in some limited way. They do not fully separate death from life and may believe that the deceased continues to live (for instance, in the ground where he or she was buried), and often ask questions about the activities of the deceased person.

The children can acknowledge physical death but consider it as a temporary or gradual event. Death is reversible and not final (like leaving and returning, or a game of peek-a-boo). Children's concept of death may involve magical thinking, i.e. the idea that his or her thoughts can cause actions.

Children may feel that they must have done or thought something bad to become ill or that a loved one's death occurred because of some personal thought or wish. In response to death, children under age five will often exhibit disturbances in eating, sleeping, and bladder or bowel control.

Ages 6–9 Years

It is not unusual for children this age to become very curious about death, asking very concrete questions about what happens to one's body when it stops working. Death is personified as a separate person or spirit: a skeleton, ghost, angel of death, or bogeyman. Although death is perceived as final and frightening, it is not universal. Children at this age begin to compromise, recognizing that death is final and real but mostly happens to the elderly (not to themselves). Grieving children can develop school phobias, learning problems, antisocial or aggressive behaviors, can exhibit hypochondriacal concerns, or can withdraw from others. Conversely, children this age can become overly attentive and clinging.

Boys may show an increase in aggressive and destructive behavior (e.g. acting out in school), expressing their feelings in this way rather than by openly displaying sadness. When a parent dies children may feel abandoned by both their deceased parent and their surviving parent, since often the surviving parent is preoccupied with his or her own grief and is less able to emotionally support the child.

Ages 9 Years and Older

At the time a child is 9 years of age, death is understood as inevitable and is no longer viewed as a punishment. By the time the child is 12 years of age, death is viewed as final and universal.

Examples of Bereavement

Death of a Child

Death of a child can take the form of a loss in infancy such as miscarriage or stillbirth or neonatal death, SIDS, or the death of an older child. In most cases, parents find the grief almost unbearably devastating, and it tends to hold greater risk factors than any other loss. This loss also bears a lifelong process: one does not get 'over' the death but instead must assimilate and live with it.

Intervention and comforting support can make all the difference to the survival of a parent in this type of grief but the risk factors are great and may include family breakup or suicide.

Feelings of guilt, whether legitimate or not, are pervasive, and the dependent nature of the relationship disposes parents to a variety of problems as they seek to cope with this great loss. Parents who suffer miscarriage or a regretful or coerced abortion may experience resentment towards others who experience successful pregnancies. Because of the intensity of grief emotions, irrational decisions are often made.

Suicide

Suicide is a growing epidemic and over the last thirty years there has been national research trying to curb this phenomenon and gather knowledge about who is 'at-risk'. When a parent loses their child through suicide it is traumatic, sudden and affects all loved ones impacted by this child. Suicide leaves many unanswered questions and leaves most parents feeling hurt, angry and deeply saddened by such a loss.

Parents feel they cannot openly discuss their grief and feel their emotions because of how their child died and how the people around them may perceive the situation. Parents, family members and service providers have all confirmed the unique nature of suicide-related bereavement following the loss of a child.

They report a wall of silence that goes up around them and how people interact towards them. One of the best ways to grieve and move on from this type of loss is to find ways to keep that child as an active part of their lives. It might be privately at first but as parents move away from the silence they can move into a more proactive healing time.

Death of a Spouse

Although the death of a spouse may be an expected change, it is a particularly powerful loss of a loved one. A spouse often becomes part of the other in a unique way: many widows and widowers describe losing 'half' of themselves. After a long marriage, at older ages, the elderly may find it a very difficult assimilation to begin anew.

At younger ages as well, a marriage relationship was often a profound one for the survivor. And finally, it must be taken into account as a factor the manner in which the spouse passed away. The survivor of a spouse who died of an illness has a different experience of such loss than a survivor of a spouse who died by, say, an act of violence. The grief, in all events, however, can always be of the most profound sort to the widow and the widower.

Furthermore, most couples have a division of 'tasks' or 'labor', e.g. the husband mows the yard, the wife pays the bills, etc. which, in addition to dealing with great grief and life changes, means added responsibilities for the bereaved. Social isolation may also become imminent, as many groups composed of couples find it difficult to adjust to the new identity of the bereaved, and the bereaved themselves have great challenges in reconnecting with others. Widows of many cultures, for instance, wear black for the rest of their lives to signify the loss of their husband and their grief. Only in more recent decades has this tradition been reduced to a period of two years, while some religions such as Christian Orthodox many widows will still continue to wear black for the remainder of their lives.

Death of a Parent

For a child, the death of a parent, without support to manage the effects of the grief, may result in long-term psychological harm. This is more likely if the adult carers are struggling with their own grief and are psychologically unavailable to the child.

There is a critical role of the surviving parent or caregiver in helping the children adapt to a parent's death. Studies have shown that losing a parent at a young age did not just lead to negative outcomes; there are some positive effects. Some children had an increased maturity, better coping skills and improved communication. Adolescents valued other people more than those who have not experienced such a close loss.

When an adult child loses a parent in later adulthood, it is considered to be 'timely' and to be a normative life course event. This allows the adult children to feel a permitted level of grief. Research demonstrates that the death of a parent in midlife is not a normative event by any measure, but is a major life transition.

Depending on the individual, this transition can impact the child's life in many different ways. One child may evaluate his or her own life more closely, or may look into the child's own mortality. Other children may shut out friends and family while trying to process losing someone with whom they have had the longest relationship with.

An adult may be expected to cope with the death of a parent in a less emotional way; however, the loss can still invoke extremely powerful emotions. This is especially true when the death occurs at an important or difficult period of life, such as when becoming a parent, at graduation, or at other times of emotional stress. It is important to recognize the effects that the loss of a parent can cause, and to address these effects. For an adult, the willingness to be open to grief is often diminished. A failure to accept and deal with loss will only result in further pain and suffering.

Death of a Sibling

The loss of a sibling is a devastating life event. Despite this, sibling grief is often the most disenfranchised or overlooked of the four main forms of grief, especially with regard to adult siblings. However, the sibling relationship tends to be the longest significant relationship of the lifespan and siblings who have been part of each other's lives since birth, such as twins, help form and sustain each other's identities; with the death of one sibling comes the loss of that part of the survivor's identity.

The sibling relationship is a unique one, as they share a special bond and a common history from birth, have a certain role and place in the family, often complement each other, and share genetic traits. Siblings who enjoy a close relationship participate in each other's daily lives and special events, confinde in each other, share joys, spend leisure time together (whether they are children or adults), and have a relationship that not only exists in the present but often looks toward a future together (even into retirement).

Siblings who play a major part in each other's lives are essential to each other. Adult siblings eventually expect the loss of aging parents, the only other people who have been an integral part of their lives since birth, but they do not expect to lose their siblings early; as a result, when a sibling dies, the surviving sibling may experience a longer period of shock and disbelief.

Overall, with the loss of a sibling, a substantial part of the surviving sibling's past, present, and future is also lost. If siblings were not on good terms or close with each other, then intense feelings of guilt may ensue on the part of the surviving sibling (guilt may also ensue for having survived, not being able to prevent the death, having argued with their sibling, etc.)

Loss During Childhood

When a parent or caregiver dies or leaves, children may have symptoms of psychopathology, but they are less severe than in children with major depression.

The loss of a parent, grandparent or sibling can be very troubling in childhood, but even in childhood there are age differences in relation to the loss.

A very young child, under one or two, may be found to have no reaction if a carer dies, but other children may be affected by the loss. At a time when trust and dependency are formed, a break even of no more than separation can cause problems in well-being; this is especially true if the loss is around critical periods such as 8–12 months, when attachment and separation are at their height information, and even a brief separation from a parent or other person who cares for the child can cause distress.

Even as a child grows older, death is still difficult to fathom and this affects how a child responds. For example, younger children see death more as a separation, and may believe death is curable or temporary: in one case, a child believed her deceased mother could be restored with band-aids. Reactions can manifest themselves in 'acting out' behaviors: a return to earlier behaviors such as sucking thumbs, clinging to a toy or angry behavior; though they do not have the maturity to mourn as an adult, they feel the same intensity. As children enter pre-teen and teen years, there is a more mature understanding.

Adolescents may respond by delinquency, or oppositely become 'over-achievers': repetitive actions are not uncommon such as washing a car repeatedly or taking up repetitive tasks such as sewing, computer games, etc. It is an effort to stay above the grief. Childhood loss as mentioned before can predispose a child not only to physical illness but to emotional problems and an increased risk for suicide, especially in the adolescent period. Children can experience grief as a result of losses due to causes other than death.

For example, children who have been physically, psychologically and/or sexually abused often grieve over the damage to, or loss of, their ability to trust. Since such children usually have no support or acknowledgment from any source outside the family unit, this is likely to be experienced as disenfranchised grief.

Relocations can cause children significant grief, particularly if they are combined with other difficult circumstances, such as neglectful and/or abusive parental behaviors, other significant losses, etc.

Loss of a Friend or Classmate

Children may experience a loss during their childhood through the death of a friend or a classmate. This can be especially traumatic if the classmate dies during school. This can happen through sports, illness, bullying and tragically school shootings. Of course a friend or classmate could die off school grounds and it is extremely important to help students cope with their intense feelings and assure them they are not alone.

The schools regardless of where one of the students dies should establish a children's support group to relieve the affects of such a quick loss or traumatic loss and alleviate any other events that may come from this loss.

This type of service has positively impacted students and decreased levels of PTSD and trauma-related anxiety. Caregivers, teachers and professionals can encourage the children to express their feelings through music, art and writing to reduce the re-traumatizing affect of repeatedly bring up the catastrophic event.

Other Losses

The people who become unemployed, such as these California workers, may face grief from the loss of their job, parents may grieve due to loss of children through means other than death, for example through loss of custody in divorce proceedings; legal termination of parental rights by the government, such as in cases of child abuse; through kidnapping; because the child voluntarily left home (either as a runaway or, for children over 18, by leaving home legally); or because an adult refuses or is unable to have contact with a parent.

This loss differs from the death of a child in that the grief process is prolonged or denied because of hope that the relationship will be restored.

Grief may occur after the loss of a romantic relationship (i.e. divorce or break up), a vocation, a pet (animal loss), a home, children leaving home (empty nest syndrome), sibling(s) leaving home, a friend, a favored appointment or desire, a faith in one's religion, etc.

A person who strongly identifies with their occupation may feel a sense of grief if they have to stop their job due to retirement, being laid off, injury, or loss of certification. Those who have experienced a loss of trust will often also experience some form of grief.

CULTURAL DIVERSITY IN GRIEVING

Mourning

Each society specifies manners such as rituals, styles of dress, or other habits, as well as attitudes, in which the bereaved are encouraged or expected to take part.

An analysis of non-Western cultures suggests that beliefs about continuing ties with the deceased varies. In Japan, maintenance of ties with the deceased is accepted and carried out through religious rituals. In the Hopi of Arizona, the deceased are quickly forgotten and life continues on.

Different cultures grieve in different ways, but all have ways that are vital in healthy coping with the death of a loved one. The American family's approach to grieving was depicted in 'The Grief Committee', by T. Glen Coughlin. The short story gives an inside look at how the American culture has learned to cope with the tribulations and difficulties of grief. (The story is taught in the course, The Politics of Mourning: Grief Management in a Cross-Cultural Fiction. Columbia University)

ROLE OF NURSE IN GRIEF AND BEREAVEMENTS

Attaching (Bonding) and Memories

Many actions in the NICU or in the labor and birth area that are taken to facilitate the attachment of the parents with their infant will become memories after a sudden or even an expected neonatal death.

Forming an identity for the baby while he or she is alive is an important part of this process, and can be accomplished by using the infant's correct sex and first name, talking to the parents about what the baby likes and dislikes, and describing his or her personality. Holding should be facilitated where possible.

Parents should be encouraged to bring in toys, siblings' drawings, family pictures and tapes, which may later serve as mementos. Finally, visiting policies should be around the clock, including during bedside rounds. Over 80% of parents who attended bedside rounds learned new facts about their baby or the NICU, which made them feel more comfortable with the health care team, and there were no complaints about a lack of privacy or confidentiality (unpublished data).

Optimize Immediate Interaction with Parents

Bad news should be given by the attending staff physician in a timely and unhurried manner, and in a private area. Both parents, and one parent with another support person who will stay around for some time after the disturbing information has been delivered, should be present.

Whenever possible, the news of impending death should be discussed rather than waiting until death occurs. Parents appreciate and deserve an honest discussion about why their baby died, including a humane overview of the problems, the actions taken and time to allow them to ask questions.

By giving complete and understandable information, there is a smaller chance that parents will feel that health care professionals are hiding something from them. Care providers should be understanding and caring, and it is appropriate for them to express empathy, and to show their feelings and concerns.

During the Dying Process and Afterwards

The present important actions to be taken during and after the death of a baby. Parents need to spend time with their dying or dead baby. The opportunity to spend time with the baby should be offered on several occasions because some parents may need encouragement. One can ask the parents whether they want to be alone, or to have family or a nurse stay with them; some young parents may be frightened because they have no previous experience with death. Privacy, including privacy for the mother, father and baby as a group, is very important at this stage.

This may mean asking additional family members and friends to give the trio some time alone. However, it is important that, at some point, relatives or friends be allowed to see the baby, with the parents' approval. Indeed, these individuals can validate the infant's existence and death, thereby acknowledging the parents' loss and their need for grieving.

Withdrawal of Aggressive Support

The actions that are used to facilitate attachment (bonding) will help to build a relationship of trust and understanding. This rapport will instill confidence when discussions about the withdrawal of aggressive life support need to take place.

In a way, during the infant's stay in the NICU, the health care team enrolls in a relationship of friendship and caring, and engages in a partnership that respects the needs of the parents to come to decisions that are in the best interest of the infant. With such a mindset, statements may be made, such as 'We are doing everything reasonable and possible to help Nina get better, but if she does not respond (by such or such time), we may have to sit down and reconsider what's best for her. And that may include not being so aggressive and letting her go peacefully.

We are not there yet, but I will keep you informed and together we will come to a decision'. Not only does this introduce a way for later conversations, it also starts a thinking process in the parents, who themselves may bring up the issue of withdrawal when they notice that their child is not doing well. The concept of a partnership also takes away the burden of parents feeling that they are responsible for the withdrawal of treatment.

The decision to withdraw life support should never rest with the baby's parents, so they will not feel responsible for their child's death. One can state that everything possible has been done and nothing more can be done. It may be useful to list the problems and the actions taken to solve the problems.

After some kind of statement that 'we should consider withdrawing support', one has to ask the parents what they think and believe. Try to keep the burden of the decision away from the parents by emphasizing that everybody (parents and the health care team) has the best interest of the baby at heart, and is trying to come to the best decision for the infant, even if it will cause pain for those making the decision.

The attending staff physician should state that the team recommends limitation or withdrawal of support rather than asking the parents what they want to be done. Obtaining a second opinion from another neonatologist may be helpful to reach that goal. Several discussions may have to take place the same day or over a few days.

One may advise parents and close relatives to be careful with whom they discuss the exact circumstances of their baby's death because relatively few outsiders will truly understand all the circumstances on which a decision was based without questioning the parents about their agreement to withdraw aggressive support from their baby.

Once the decision to withdraw support is made, explain to the parents precisely how it will happen in practice and offer options so that the parents continue to feel that they are involved in *all* decisions for their baby until the end. Discussions about the duration of survival, sedation, gasping and muscle contractions should take place before extubation. It is advantageous to remove as much equipment, such as intravenous and arterial lines, chest tubes, urinary catheters and monitors, as possible.

It is preferable to dress the infant before the endotracheal tube is removed. Some parents want to hold their baby while he or she is being extubated, and other parents do not. Some parents want to remain at the bedside, which should be screened from other bedsides.

Alternatively, parents and the baby can be brought to a quiet room to spend time together, and to respect privacy and confidentiality. The infant can be bag-ventilated while being carried to a quiet room and extubated while in the parents' arms.

As discussed before, photographs of the infant before and after extubation, and of the parents holding the infant play a large role in the grieving process later on.

Spirituality and Perinatal Loss

Spirituality and perinatal loss is discussed in Cunningham. Spirituality is not just a person's religious affiliation.

To understand spiritual needs better, health care staff should not limit questions to type of religion or to baptism, but include questions about faith, rituals, traditions, and needs while caring for the infant and the family. Parents' personal spiritual beliefs may not be consistent with the caregiver's own faith tradition, and it behooves the health care provider to find out details and specifics of respective parents' needs and wishes.

This clearly implies one cannot impose one's own spiritual values on the family. Finally, the parents' spirituality will influence their emotional, mental and physical responses to bereavement.

The health care provider should take the initiative in assessing the spiritual care of families, keeping respect for people and for their spirituality centrally, along with compromises, empathy and listening. Health care professionals can encourage the presence and participation of the family's clergy, and make them feel a part of the perinatal loss bereavement team.

Table 4.2: Developmental stages of grief

Grief and Developmental Stages	Understanding of Death	Expressions of Grief
Infancy to 2 years	Is not yet able to understand death.	Quietness, crankiness, decreased activity, poor sleep, and weight loss
	Separation from mother causes changes.	

Contd...

Contd...

Grief and Developmental Stages	Understanding of Death	Expressions of Grief
2–6 years	Death is like sleeping.	Asks many questions (How does she go to the bathroom? How does she eat?).
		Problems in eating, sleeping, and bladder and bowel control.
		Fear of abandonment.
		Tantrums
	Dead person continues to live and function in some ways.	Magical thinking (Did I think something or do something that caused the death? Like when I said I hate you and I wish you would die?).
	Death is temporary, not final.	
	Dead person can come back to life.	
6–9 years	Death is thought of as a person or spirit (skeleton, ghost, bogeyman).	Curious about death.
		Asks specific questions.
		May have exaggerated fears about school.
	Death is final and frightening.	May have aggressive behaviors (especially boys).
		Some concerns about imaginary illnesses.
	Death happens to others, it would not happen to Me.	May feel abandoned
9 and older	Everyone will die.	Heightened emotions, guilt, anger, shame.
		Increased anxiety over own death.
		Mood swings.
	Death is final and cannot be changed.	Fear of rejection; not wanting to be different from peers.
	Even I will die.	Changes in eating habits.
		Sleeping problems.
		Regressive behaviors (loss of interest in outside activities).
		Impulsive behaviors.
		Feels guilty about being alive (especially related to death of a brother, sister, or peer).

PEDIATRIC PROCEDURES

PREPARATION OF CHILD FOR DIAGNOSTIC TESTS AND COLLECTION OF SPECIMENS

Introduction

In most of the medical diagnostic procedures create fear and anxiety among the adults and children. Proper preparation help the child feel safe and calm during medical tests.

Some Common Tests

- Blood test
- Urine test
- Sputum test
- Stool test
- X-ray and USG
- CT scan and MRI, etc.

Types of Preparation

Pre-preparation

The pediatric nurse having more responsible to prepare the infant for diagnostic procedure, most of the child will cry and uncooperative for that restraints may be used. The most important way to reduce the infant fear and anxiety use family centered approach. Crying is a normal response to the strange environment, unfamiliar people, restraints and separation from parents. The infant will cry more for these reasons than because the test or procedure is uncomfortable.

- Infants lack the physical control, coordination, and ability to follow commands.
- Restraints may be used during a procedure or other situation to ensure the infant's safety. For example, in order to get clear test results on an X-ray, there cannot be any movement.
- If blood needs to be taken or an IV started, restraints are important in preventing injury to infant. If the infant moves while the needle is being inserted, the needle could damage a blood vessel, bone, tissue, or nerves.
- Health care provider should ensure the safety and comfort of baby. Beside restraints, other measures include medications, observation, and monitors.
- Explain the test or procedures in simple language to child understand, using plain words. When a child is worried or scared, their attention span may be shorter. Try explaining the test or treatment in several sessions, limiting explanations to 10 minutes each.
- The pediatric nurse should use pictures or books, as well as play and toys or dolls, to help explain a test or treatment to younger children. Use videos for older children.
- Answer all questions honestly and in language of the child understands. Try to listen for unasked questions. Offer repeated reassurance that the child is not responsible for being sick.
- Make sure that the child understands the exact body part involved and that the test or treatment will only be done in that area.
- Describe how the procedure will feel and what, if any, may happen afterwards and how long these effects may last.
- Encourage your child to identify their feelings. Teach them that sadness, anger and guilt are normal feelings and to talk about them.
- Tell your child if a procedure will hurt and let them know that it is ok to cry or verbally express any pain.
- Help your child practice the positions or movements that they may need to do during the test or treatment.
- Stress the benefits of the test or treatment and talk about things that the child may enjoy afterwards.

At the Time of Procedures (During the Procedure)

- Allow the child play with safe medical supplies such as a stethoscope or blood pressure cuff.
- Encourage the child to try counting, deep breathing, thinking pleasant thoughts and talking about them and holding hands to help them stay calm.
- Touch the child to help reduce pain or anxiety. Hold their hands or rest a hand on their shoulder.
- Allow school-age children to make choices whenever possible but do not offer choices when no choices exist.
- She should allow the child to do his job or let them play games.
- Permit the child to practice things that are new and scary.
- Have school-age children email, text or call their friends.
- Allow the child go to school or resume school work and activities as soon as possible after the procedure.

Play Preparation

- Play can be a wonderful way to demonstrate the procedure for the child and identify any anxiety child is having or not. Most health care facilities for children use play therapy to prepare children for procedures.
- Most of the children have a favorite toy or important object that can be used to explain the test. It may be less threatening child to express concerns through the object. For example a child may be able to understand a blood test if you discuss how the 'doll might feel' during the test.
- Toys or dolls can also help the nurse explain the procedure to toddler. These visual examples can take the place of unfamiliar words for younger children with a limited vocabulary.
- The pediatric nurse know how the procedure will be done, briefly demonstrate to child will experience on the toy. Show the body positions the child will be in, where bandages and stethoscopes will be placed, how incisions are made, how injections are given, and how IVs are inserted. After your demonstration, allow your child to play with some of the items (except for needles and other sharp objects). Watch your child for clues about concerns and fears.
- The child will probably cry. This is a normal response to a strange environment, unfamiliar people, and separation from you. Knowing this from the beginning may help relieve some of your anxiety about what to expect.

Special Precaution

- The child will probably resist the procedure and may even try to run away. A firm, direct approach from parents and the health care staff may be helpful.
- Give one direction at a time during the procedure, using 1–or 2–word commands.
- Avoid covering the child's face.
- Ask the child's health care provider to limit the number of strangers entering and leaving the room during the procedure, because this can raise anxiety.
- Get the consent from parents if anesthesia can be used to reduce the child's discomfort.

SPECIMEN COLLECTION

Definition

A specimen is a sample of something, like a specimen of blood or body tissue, stool, sputum and CSF that is taken for medical testing or investigation.

Purpose

- Early detection and reporting of suspect cases
- Rapid epidemiological investigation
- Rapid laboratory confirmation of the diagnosis
- Implementation of effective control measures.

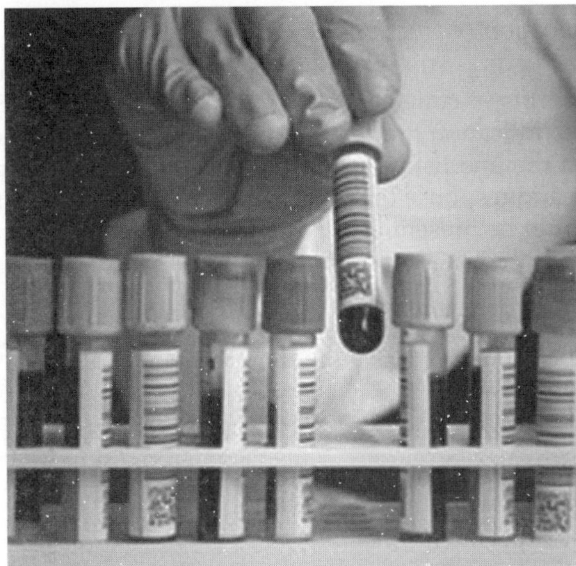

Fig. 4.1: Specimen collection

Role of Nurse

- Advance planning
- Collection of appropriate and adequate specimens
- Correct packaging and rapid transport to an appropriate laboratory
- The ability of the laboratory to carry out the diagnostic tests
- Proper biosafety and decontamination procedures to reduce the risk of further spread of the disease.

Collecting the Specimens

- Stool samples, the health worker should collect the sample, place in cold box and inform WHO Transport to the laboratory should be done as soon as possible.
- CSF the admitting physician should conduct the lumbar puncture and obtain the sample.
- Urine, sputum and Blood samples should be taken by the health worker.

Specimen Collection Procedures

- Investigation should commence as early as possible after a suspected outbreak has been notified.
- Specimens obtained in the acute phase of the disease, preferably prior to administration of antimicrobial drugs, are more likely to yield detectable concentrations of antibody, antigen or infective pathogen.
- Before beginning specimen collection, explain the procedure to the patient and relatives.
- When collecting the specimen avoid contamination and take a sufficient quantity of material (as guided by the laboratory tests).
- Follow the appropriate precautions for safety during collection and processing of samples.

Labeling and Identification of Specimens

In an outbreak investigation the information contained in the case investigation and laboratory request forms is collected along with the specimen. Each child should be assigned a unique identification number by the collection team. It is the link between the laboratory results on the line listing form, the specimens and the patient, which guides further investigation and response to the outbreak. This unique identification number and the patient name should be present on all specimens, epidemiological data forms and the laboratory request and used as a common reference.

Labeling Specimen Container/Slide

The label should be permanently affixed to the specimen container.

It should contain the:

- Patient name
- Unique identification number
- Specimen type and date and place of collection
- Name or initials of specimen collector.

Case Investigation and Laboratory Forms

A laboratory form must also be completed for each specimen. The epidemiological and clinical data gathered in the investigation can later be easily tied to the laboratory results for analysis.

The form includes patient information:

- Name of the child
- Age (or date of birth)
- Gender/sex
- Complete address
- Clinical information
  - Date of onset of symptoms
  - Clinical and immunization history
  - Risk factors, antimicrobial taken prior to specimen collection

- Laboratory information—Acute or convalescent specimen, other specimens from same patient. The form records the date and time when specimen received, name of the person collecting the specimen.

Storage of Specimens

- To preserve bacterial or viral viability in specimens for microbiological culture or inoculation, they should be placed in appropriate media and stored at recommended temperatures.
- These conditions must be preserved throughout transport to the laboratory and will vary according to transportation time. They will differ for specimens and pathogens, depending on their sensitivity to desiccation, temperature, nutrient and pH.
- Many specimens taken for viral isolation are viable for two days if maintained in type specific media at 4–8 °C. Freeze these specimens as directed by expert advice, as infectivity may be altered.
- Specimens for bacterial culture should be kept in appropriate transport media at the recommended temperature.
- This ensures bacterial viability while minimising overgrowth of other microorganisms. With the exception of CSF, urine, and sputum, most specimens may be kept at ambient temperature if the specimen will be processed within 24 hours.
- Longer periods, storage on at 4–8 °C would be advisable with the exception of particularly cold-sensitive organisms, such as Shigella, Meningococcus, and Pneumococcus.
- Longer delays are not advisable as the yield of bacteria may fall significantly. Specimens for antigen or antibody detection may be stored at 4–8 °C for 24–48 hours, or at –20 °C for longer periods. Sera for antibody detection may be stored at 4–8 °C for up to 10 days.
- Although not ideal, sera stored at room temperature may still be useful for antibody testing even after prolonged periods (weeks). Therefore, do not discard sera which have been collected simply because there are no refrigeration facilities available.

Blood Specimen Collection

Definition

Blood and separated serum are the most common specimens. Venous blood can be used for isolation and identification of the pathogen in culture and by inoculation, or separated into serum for the detection of such as:

- Genetic material (e.g. By polymerase chain reaction)
- Specific antibodies (by serology)
- Antigens or toxins (e.g. by immunofluorescence).

The processing of most specimens for diagnosis of viral pathogens, serum is preferable to unseparated blood except where otherwise directed. When specific antibodies are being assayed, it is often helpful to collect paired sera, i.e. an acute sample at the onset of illness and a convalescent sample one to four weeks later. Blood can also collect by finger prick for the preparation of slides for microscopy or for absorption onto special filter paper discs for analysis. Whenever possible, blood specimens for culture should be taken before antibiotics are administered to the patient.

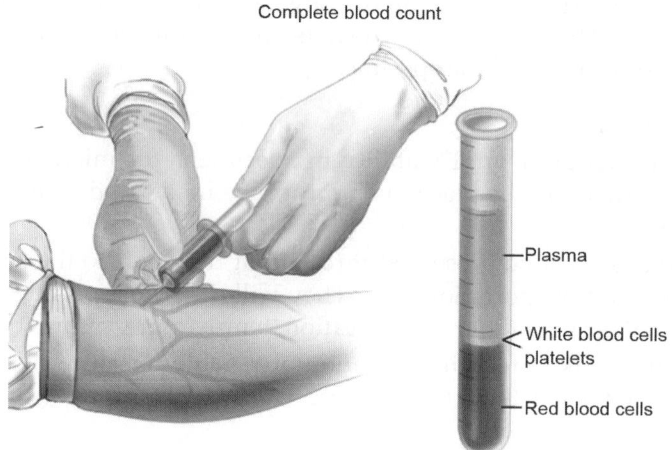

Fig. 4.2: Collection of blood specimen

Materials for Blood Collection

- Clean tray
- Skin disinfection: 70% alcohol (isopropyl alcohol, ethanol) or 10% povidone iodine
- Swabs, gauze pads, Band-aid
- Disposable latex or vinyl gloves
- Tourniquet
- Vacutainer or similar vacuum blood collection devices, or disposable syringes and needles
- Vacutainer or sterile screw cap tubes (or cryotubes if indicated)
- Blood culture bottles (50 ml for adults, 25 ml for children) with appropriate media
- Labels and indelible marker pen.

Procedures

- Place a tourniquet above the venipuncture site.
- Disinfect the tops of blood culture bottles.
- Palpate and locate the vein.
- It is critical to disinfect the venipuncture site meticulously with 10% povidone iodine or 70% isopropyl alcohol by swabbing the skin concentrically from the center of the venipuncture site outwards.
- Let the disinfectant evaporate.
- Do not repalpate the vein again. Perform venipuncture.
- If withdrawing with conventional disposable syringes, withdraw 5–10 ml of whole blood from adults, 2–5 ml from children and 0.5–2 ml for infants.
- Using aseptic technique, transfer the specimen to relevant cap transport tubes and culture bottles. Secure caps tightly.
- If withdrawing with vacuum systems withdraw the desired amount of blood directly into each transport tube and culture bottle.

- Remove the tourniquet. Apply pressure to site until bleeding stops, and apply bandaid.
- Label the tube, including the unique patient identification number, using indelible marker pen.
- Do not recap used sharps. Discard directly into the sharps disposal container.
- Complete the case investigation and the laboratory request forms using the same identification number.

After the Procedures

- Replace the articles
- Provide the comfortable position to child
- Blood specimen bottles and tubes should be transported upright and secured in a screw cap container or in a rack in a transport box.
- They should have enough absorbent paper around them to soak up all the liquid in case of spill.
- If the specimen will reach the laboratory within 24 hour, most pathogens can be recovered from blood cultures transported at ambient temperature.
- Keep at 4–8 °C for longer transit periods, unless it is a cold-sensitive bacterial pathogen.

Cerebrospinal Fluid (CSF) Specimen Collection

Definition

The specimen must be taken by a physician or a person experienced in the procedure. CSF is used to in the diagnosis of viral, bacterial, parasitic, and fungal meningitis/encephalitis. It is a very common procedure in child.

Materials for Collection

Lumbar puncture tray which includes:

- Sterile materials: Gloves, cotton wool, towels or drapes
- Local anesthetic, needle, syringe

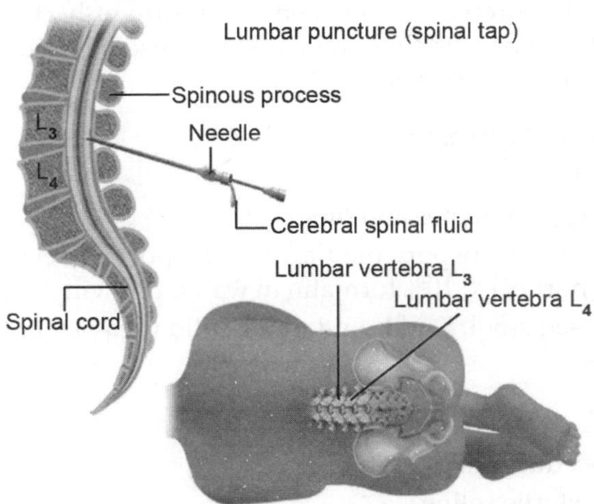

Fig. 4.3: Anatomical position of lumbar puncture

- Skin disinfectant: 10% povidone iodine or 70% alcohol
- Two lumbar puncture needles, small bore with stylet
- Six small sterile screw-cap tubes and tube rack
- Water manometer
- Microscope slides and slide boxes.

Procedures

- As only experienced personnel should be involved in the collection of CSF samples, the method is not described in this document.
- CSF is collected directly into the separate screw-cap tubes.
- If the samples will not be promptly transported, separate tubes should be collected for bacterial and viral processing.

After the Procedures

- In general, specimens should be delivered to the laboratory and processed as soon as possible.
- CSF specimens for bacteriology are transported at ambient temperature, generally without transport media.
- They must never be refrigerated as these pathogens do not survive well at low temperatures.
- CSF specimens for virology do not need transport medium.
- They may be transported at 4–8 °C for up to 48 hours, or at –70 °C for longer periods.

Stool (Fecal) Specimen Collection

Definition

Stool specimens are most useful for microbiological diagnosis in children, if collected soon after onset of diarrhea (for viruses < 48 hours and for bacteria < 4 days), and preferably before the initiation of antibiotic therapy. If required, two or three specimens may be collected on separate days. Stool is the preferred specimen for culture of bacterial, viral and parasitic diarrheal pathogens. Rectal swabs showing feces may also be used from infants. They are not useful for the diagnosis of viruses.

Materials for Collection of Specimen

- Clean tray
- Leak-proof screw cap container and tape
- Appropriate bacterial transport media for transport of rectal swabs from infants Parasitology transport pack: 10% formalin in water, polyvinyl isopropyl alcohol (PVA).
- Collect freshly passed stool, 5 ml liquid or 5 g solid (pea-size), in a container.
- Label the container.

Procedures

- Explained the procedures to parents/child
- Moisten a swab in sterile saline

- Insert the swab tip just past the anal sphincter and rotate gently
- Withdraw the swab and examine to ensure that the cotton tip is stained with feces
- Place the swab in sterile tube/container containing the appropriate transport medium
- Break off the top part of the stick without touching the tube and tighten the screw cap firmly
- Label the specimen tube.

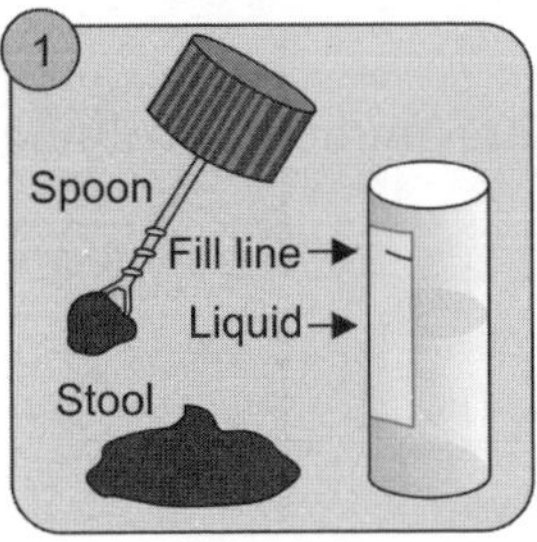

Collect on plastic wrap and transfer to vial until liquid reaches fill line

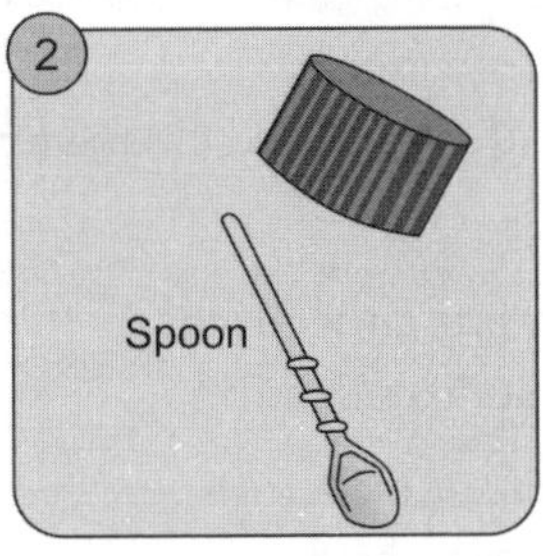

Remove spoon from lid and discard

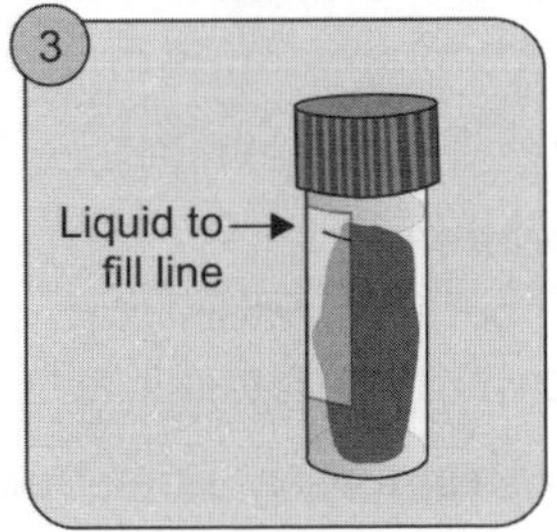

Replace cap on vial tightly and shake for a minute. Place vial in refigerator until ready to ship

Fig. 4.4: Steps in stool collection

After the Procedures

- Replace articles in proper place
- Stool specimens should be transported at 4–8 °C.
- Bacterial yields may fall significantly if specimens are not processed within 1–2 days of collection. Shigellas are particularly sensitive to elevated temperatures.
- Specimens to be examined for parasites should be mixed with 10% formalin or PVA, 3 parts stool to 1 part preservative.
- Transported at ambient temperature in containers sealed in plastic bags.

Respiratory Tract Specimen Collection

Definition

Specimens are collected from the upper or lower respiratory tract, depending on the site of infection.

- Upper respiratory tract pathogens (viral and bacterial) are found in throat and nasopharyngeal specimens.
- Lower respiratory tract pathogens are found in sputum specimens.
- The organisms such as Legionella, culture is difficult, and diagnosis is best based on the detection of antigen excreted in the urine.

When acute Epiglottitis is suspected, no attempt should be made to take throat or pharyngeal specimens since these procedures may precipitate respiratory obstruction. Epiglottitis is generally confirmed by lateral neck X-Ray, but the etiologic agent may be isolated on blood culture.

Materials for Collection

- A clean tray
- Transport media: Bacterial and viral
- Dacron and cotton swabs
- Tongue depressor
- Flexible wire calcium alginate tipped swab (for suspected pertussis)
- Nasal speculum (for suspected pertussis–not essential)
- Suction apparatus or 20–50 ml syringe
- Sterile screw-cap tubes, and wide-mouthed clean sterile jars (minimum volume 25 ml).

Procedures

- Upper respiratory tract specimens collection
- Lower respiratory tract specimens collection

Upper Respiratory Tract Specimens Collection

- Explain the procedures to parents/child
- Hold the tongue down with the depressor
- Use a strong light source to locate areas of inflammation and exudates in the posterior pharynx and the tonsillar region of the throat behind the uvula
- Rub the area back and forth with a Dacron or calcium alginate swab
- Withdraw the swab without touching cheeks, teeth or gums and insert into a screw cap tube containing transport medium
- Break off the top part of the stick without touching the tube and tighten the screw cap firmly
- Label the specimen containers
- Complete the laboratory request form.

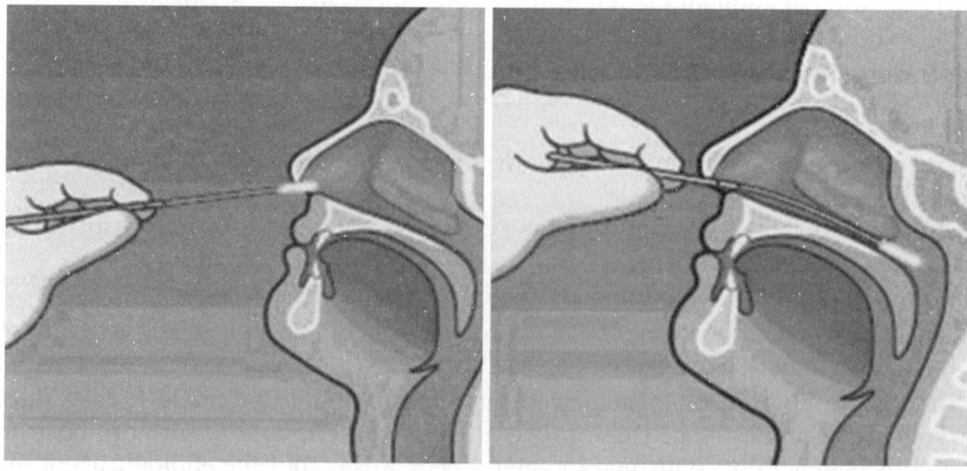

Fig. 4.5: Technique of using *swabs stick*

Method of Collecting Nasopharyngeal Swabs (for Suspected Pertussis)

- Seat the patient comfortably, tilt the head back and insert the nasal speculum.
- Insert a flexible calcium alginate/Dacron swab through the speculum parallel to the floor of nose without pointing upwards.
- Alternately, bend the wire and insert it into the throat and move the swab upwards into the nasopharyngeal space.
- Rotate the swab on the nasopharyngeal membrane a few times, remove it carefully and insert it into a screw cap tube containing transport medium.
- Break off the top part of the stick without touching the tube and tighten the screw cap firmly.
- Label the specimen tube, indicating left or right side.
- Complete the laboratory request form.
- Repeat on the other side.

Lower Respiratory Tract Specimens Collection

Sputum

- Do the chest massage if needed
- Instruct patient to take a deep breath and cough up sputum directly into a wide-mouth sterile container.
- Avoid saliva or postnasal discharge. Minimum volume should be about 1 ml.
- Label the specimen containers.
- Complete the laboratory request form.

After the Procedures

- Replace the articles and provide the comfortable position
- All respiratory specimens except sputum are transported in appropriate bacterial/viral media.
- Transport as quickly as possible to the laboratory to reduce overgrowth by commensal oral flora.
- For transit periods up to 24 hours, transport bacterial specimens at ambient temperature and viruses at 4–8 °C in appropriate media.

Urine Specimen Collection

Definition

Urine has a long, rich history as a source for measuring health and well-being and remains an important tool for clinical diagnosis. The clinical information obtained from a urine specimen is influenced by the collection method, timing and handling. A vast assortment of collection and transport containers for urine specimens are available. Determining which urine collection method and container should be used depends on the type of laboratory test ordered. Infants and small children, a special urine collection bag can be adhered to the skin surrounding the urethral area.

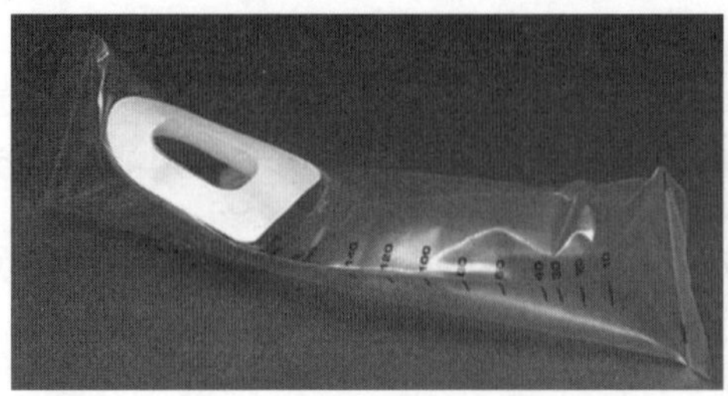

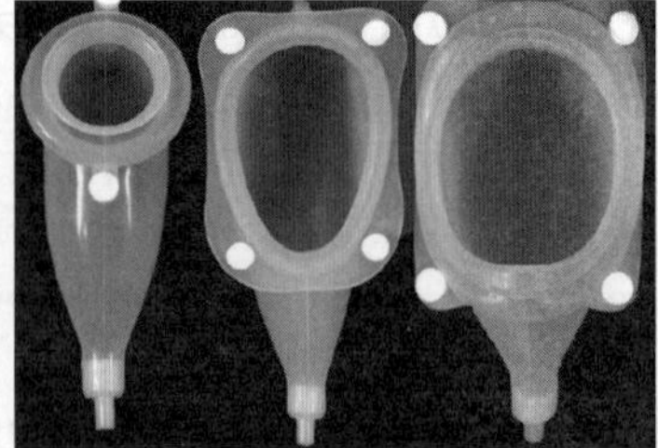

Male type Penile type Female use

Types

- Randomly collected specimens are not regarded as specimens of choice because of the potential for dilution of the specimen when collection occurs soon after the patient has consumed fluids.
- First morning specimen is the specimen of choice for urinalysis and microscopic analysis, since the urine is generally more concentrated.
- Midstream clean catch specimens are strongly recommended for microbiological culture and antibiotic susceptibility testing because of the reduced incidence of cellular and microbial contamination.
- Collection from catheters (e.g. Foley catheter) using a syringe, followed by transfer to a specimen tube or cup. Alternatively, urine can be drawn directly from the catheter to an evacuated tube using an appropriate adaptor.

Material for Collection

- A clean tray
- Sterile plastic cup with lid (50 ml or more)
- Clean, screw-top specimen transport containers ('universal' containers are often used)
- Gauze pads
- Soap and clean water (or normal saline) if possible.

Procedures

- Explain the procedures to parents/child
- Labels and indelible marker pen.
- Give the patient clear instructions to pass urine for a few seconds, and then to hold the cup in the urine stream for a few seconds to catch a mid-stream urine sample.
- This should decrease the risk of contamination from organisms living in the urethra.
- To decrease the risk of contamination from skin organisms, the patient should be directed to avoid touching the inside or rim of the plastic cup with the skin of the hands, legs or external genitalia. Tighten the cap firmly when finished.
- Hospitalized or debilitated patients, it may be necessary to wash the external genitalia with soapy water to reduce the risk of contamination.
- If soap and clean water are not available, the area may be rinsed with normal saline.
- Dry the area thoroughly with gauze pads before collecting the urine.
- Urine collection bags may be necessary for infants.

- If used, transfer urine from the urine bag to specimen containers as soon as possible to prevent contamination with skin bacteria.
- Use a disposable transfer pipette to transfer the urine.
- Label the specimen containers.

After the Procedure

- Replace the articles in proper place and provide comfort position to child
- Transport to the laboratory within 2–3 hours of collection.
- If this is not possible, do not freeze but keep the specimen refrigerated at 4–8 °C.
- Keeping the specimen refrigerated will decrease the risk of overgrowth of contaminating organisms.
- Ensure that transport containers are leak-proof and tightly sealed.

CALCULATION AND ADMINISTRATION OF ORAL AND PARENTERAL MEDICATION

Drug Calculation

Introduction

In children most of the drugs are according to body weight (mg/kg) or body surface area (BSA) (mg/m^2). Care must be taken to properly convert body weight from pounds to kilograms (1 kg = 2.2 lb) before calculating doses based on body weight. Doses are often expressed as mg/kg/day or mg/kg/dose, therefore orders written 'mg/kg/d,' which is confusing, require further clarification from the prescriber.

Chemotherapeutic drugs are commonly dosed according to body surface area, which requires an extra verification step (BSA calculation) prior to dosing. Medications are available in multiple concentrations; therefore orders written in 'mL' rather than 'mg' are not acceptable and require further clarification.

Dosing also varies by indication; therefore diagnostic information is helpful when calculating doses. The following examples are typically encountered when dosing medication in children.

Example 1

Calculate the dose of *Inj. Amoxicillin* suspension in mLs for otitis media for a 1-year-old child weighing 22 lb. The dose required is 40 mg/kg/day divided BID and the suspension comes in a concentration of 400 mg/5 mL.

Step 1. Convert pounds to kg	22 lb × 1 kg/2.2 lb = 10 kg
Step 2. Calculate the dose in mg	10 kg × 40 mg/kg/day = 400 mg/day
Step 3. Divide the dose by the frequency	400 mg/day ÷ 2 (BID) = 200 mg/dose BID
Step 4. Convert the mg dose to mL	200 mg/dose ÷ 400 mg/5 mL = 2.5 mL BID

Example 2

Calculate the dose of *Inj. ceftriaxone* in mLs for meningitis for a 5-year-old child weighing 18 kg. The dose required is 100 mg/kg/day given IV once daily and the drug comes prediluted in a concentration of 40 mg/mL.

Step 1. Calculate the dose in mg	18 kg × 100 mg/kg/day = 1800 mg/day
Step 2. Divide the dose by the frequency	1800 mg/day ÷ 1 (daily) = 1800 mg/dose
Step 3. Convert the mg dose to mL	1800 mg/dose ÷ 40 mg/mL = 45 mL once daily

Example 3

Calculate the dose of *Inj.vincristine* in mLs for a 4-year-old with leukemia weighing 37 lb and is 97 cm tall. The dose required in 2 mg/m^2 and the drug comes in 1 mg/mL concentration.

Step 1. Convert pounds to kg	37 lb × 1 kg/2.2 lb = 16.8 kg
Step 2. Calculate BSA	√16.8 kg × 97 cm/3600 = 0.67 m^2
Step 3. Calculate the dose in mg	2 mg/m^2 × 0.67 m^2 = 1.34 mg
Step 4. Calculate the dose in mL	1.34 mg ÷ 1 mg/mL = 1.34 mL

General Drug Calculation

Formula

Dose = Rate × Concentration

Example:

- You need to administer 800 units/hour of heparin; the label says those 500 ml fluids/25000 units.

  800 = R × 25000/500
  Rate = 800/25000 × 500
  Rate = 16 ml/hour

- You have an order to *Lidocaine* 3 mg/minute label says that 2 gm/500 ml
  What the rate is?

  Dose = Rate × Concentration
  3 × 60 = 180 mg/hours
  180 mg = R × 2000/500
  Rate = 180/2000 × 500
  = 45 ml/hour.

- *Clark's Rule:* Clark's rule uses Weight in Lbs, *never* in Kg.
  Here is the formula: Adult Dose **×** (Weight ÷ 150) = Childs Dose
  Example
  Name of the child: Master XXX, 11-year-old girl/weight 70 lbs
  500 mg × (70 ÷ 150) = Child's Dose
  500 mg × (.47) = Child's Dose
  500 mg × .47 = 235 mg.
  Child's Dose = 235 mg

- *Young's Rule:* Young's Rule uses age. (Which makes it easier to remember, the word young refers to age)
  Here is the formula: Adult Dose **×** [Age ÷ (Age + 12)] = Child's Dose

Example

Name of the child: Master XXXX, 11-year-old girl/70 Lbs

500 mg × [11 ÷ (11 + 12)] = Child's Dose

500 mg × (11 ÷ 23) = Child's Dose

500 mg × .48 = Child's Dose.

Child's Dose = 240 mg

Dosage Based on Weight

Most of the drugs are prescribed based on an adults or childs weight in order to more accurately dose. The calculation is very simple and easy to perform. However, you must pay close attention to whether the dosage has been prescribed per kg or lbs.

Example:

132 lb woman is prescribed Acyclovir 5 mg/kg

First convert lbs to kg

(132 ÷ 2.2) = 60 kg

The prescription calls for 5 mg/kg.

60 × 5 mg = 300 mg

Burns Patients

Brooke Army Formula

- *Colloids:* 0.5 ml × kg body Wt × % TBSA burned
- *Electrolytes:* 1.5 ml × kg body Wt × % TBSA
- *Glucose (5%):* 2000 ml for insensible loss.

Day 1: Half in 1st 8 hrs, remaining half over next 16 hrs.

Day 2: Half of colloids, half of electrolyte all of insensible fluid replacement.

Example: 2-year-old child admitted with 25% burns, how much fluid will be replaced? Weight: 11 Kg

Colloids: 0.5 ml × 11 × 25 = 137.5 ml.

Electrolytes: 1.5 ml × 11 × 25 = 412.5 ml.

Parkland Formula

- In first 24 hrs: The total amount of calculated fluid requirement is = 4 ml of RL × Wt in kg × % TBSA burnt.
- One half amount of calculated fluid is given for first 8 hrs.
- The remaining half of the fluid is given over the next 16 hrs.
- In the next 24 hrs: 2 ml of RL/Kg/% of TBSA.

Example:

8 years old child, Weight of 24 kg. She got burn injury with 50%

4 ml × 24 × 50 = 4800 ml.

First 24 hrs:

First 8 hrs = 2400 ml.

Next 16 hrs = 2400 ml.

Next 24 hrs:

2 ml × 24 × 50 = 2400 ml.

Evans Formula

- *Colloids:* 1 ml × kg body wt × % TBSA burnt
- *Electrolytes:* 1 ml × kg body wt × % TBSA burnt
- *Glucose (5%):* 2000 ml for insensible loss.

EXPECTED WEIGHT AND HEIGHT OF NORMAL CHILDREN

According to 'Ballpark'

- Average birth weight is : 2.5 to 3 kg
- Double the birth weight by the 5 months : 5 to 6 kg
- Triple the birth weight by one year : 7.5 to 9 kg

According to Welch's Formula

Weight

- At birth : 2.5 to 3 kg
- 3–12 month : Age in month + 9/2
- 1–6 years : Age in years × 2 + 8
- 7–12 years : Age in years × 7–5/2

Height

- At birth = 50 cm/20 inches
- At 1 year = 75 cm/30 inches

2 to 12 years:

- Age in year × 6 + 77 (cm)
- Age in year × 2 + 30 (inches)

Example: 1	**Example: 2**
Name of the child: Master Varun	Name of the child: Master Raja
Age : 5 months	Age : 2 years
Sex : Female	Sex : Male
Formula: Age in months + 9/2	**Formula**: Age in years × 2 + 8
$\frac{5+9}{2} = \frac{13}{2} =$ **6.5 kg**	2 × 2 + 8 4 + 8 = **12 kg**

Examples: 3	**Height Examples**
Name of the child: Master Kumar	Name of the child: Master Shiva
Age : 8 years	Age : 5 years
Sex : Male	Sex : Male
Formula: Age in years × 7–5/2	**Formula**: Age in years × 6 + 77 (cm)
$\frac{8+7}{2} = \frac{56-5}{2} =$ **25.5 kg**	= 5 × 6
	= 30 + 77 = **107 cm**

Malnutrition Assessment Formula

$$\frac{\text{Actual weight of the child}}{\text{Expected weight of the child}} \times 100$$

Classification of Nutritional Status

Nutritional status	Expected weight for age	Presence of edema
Normal	More than 80%	No
Under nutrition	60–80%	No
Kwashiorkor	60–80%	Yes
Marasmus	Less than 60%	No
Marasmus and Kwashiorkor	Less than 60%	Yes

Degree of Malnutrition

S. No.	Percentage of malnutrition	Degree of malnutrition
1.	90–95%	Normal
2.	75–85%	1st degree
3.	65–75%	2nd degree
4.	< 65%	3rd degree

FLUID CALCULATION

Introduction

The understanding of the principles of fluid and electrolyte balance is vital for the maintenance of stable internal environment. This is even more essential infants who have less reserves of body water and electrolytes and in newborn babies who may be deficient of the homeostatic mechanism to protect them against the changes related to abnormal losses. Thus, it is important to assess the nature and magnitude of any disturbance in different clinical situations and at different ages because correction of the imbalance is essential for speedy recovery.

- Very young infants are vulnerable to more water loss because of physiological inability of their renal tubules to concentrate.
- Higher metabolic rate and larger surface area compared to total body weight in young infants favor rapid fluid loss. Unless fluids are adequately replaced in the presence of continued loss dehydration and consequences of dehydration are likely to set in.
- Larger turnover is another problem in young infants. An infant exchanges about one-half of his or her ECF every day compared to one-seventh in an adult.
- Thirst mechanism is very effective in older children and adults compared to very young infants. In the presence of excessive water loss, young infants do not express their thirst for fluids effectively when there is a negative balance of intake during water loss.

Fluid Measurement Values

1 ml	15 Drops
1 Liter	1000 ml (1000 × 15 = 15,000 drops)
1 Tablespoon	15 ml
1 Teaspoon	5 ml
1 Ounce	30 ml

Drops Factors

Normal IV set 1 ml = 16 macro drops

Micro volume 1 ml = 60 micro drops

Example

40 ml/hr = 40 × 16

Macro drops = 40 × 16/60 = 12 drops/mts.

Micro drops = 40 × 60/60 = 40 drops/mts.

Formula for Calculation of Daily Fluid Requirements

Method

Body Weight	Fluid/Hour	Fluid/Day
0–10 kg	4 ml/kg/hour	100/kg/day
11–20 kg	40 ml/kg/hour + 2 ml/hour	1000 ml + 50 ml/kg for each kg
Above 20 kg	60 ml/kg/hour + 1 ml/kg/hour	1500 ml + 20 ml for each kg

Notes

- 4 ml/kg/hr for 1st 10 kg
- Adding 2 ml/kg/hour for second 10 kg
- Adding 1 ml/kg/hour for each kg over 20 kg.
- Adding 1st 10 kg 1000 ml/day + (50 ml/each kg/day)
- Adding 1st 20 kg 1500 ml/day + (20 ml/each kg/day)

Examples: 1-hour-based/day-based

Name of the child: Master Raju
Age : 1 year
Actual wt of child: 8 kg
- **Formula**: 4 ml/kg/hour
  = 8 × 4 = 32 ml/hour
- **Formula**: 100 ml/kg/hour
  = 8 × 100 = 800 ml/day

Examples: 2-hour-based/day-based

Name of the child: Master Suresh
Age : 3 years
Actual wt of child: 15 kg
- **Formula**: 40 ml/kg/hour + 2 ml/kg/hour
  = first 10 kg 40 ml/hour (See the Note)
  = 5 × 2 = 10 ml + 40 ml = 50 ml/hour
- **Formula**: 1000 ml + 50 ml/kg for each kg
  = 1000 ml + (50 × 5 = 250 ml)
  = 1250 ml/day

Examples: 1-hour-based

Name of the child: Master Saravanan
Age : 5 years
Actual wt of child: 25 kg
- **Formula**: 60 ml/kg/hour + 1 ml/kg/hour
  = First 20 kg 60 ml/hour (see the note)
  = 5 × 1 = 5 + 60 = 65 ml/hour

Examples: 1-day-based

Name of the child: Master Saravanan
Age : 5 years
Actual wt of child: 25 kg
- **Formula**: 1500 ml + 20 ml/kg for each kg
  = 1500 ml + (20 × 5 = 100 ml)
  = 1600 ml/day

Intravenous fluid (Drops) calculation formula:

$$= \frac{\text{Total volume of fluid (ml)} \times 15 \text{ Drops}}{\text{Total Hours} \times 60}$$

Example

$$\frac{1500 \text{ ml} \times 15 \text{ Drops}}{12 \times 60} = \frac{22{,}500}{720} = 30 \text{ drops/minutes}$$

Hyponatremic Dehydration

Observed sodium volume × 0.6 × wt in kg.

Hypernatremic Dehydration

- Water deficit = Body weight × 0.6 measured Na/Expected Na
- Free water deficit = (observed Na–145) × 4 ml/kg × Body wt.
- Calculating deficit maintenance and total fluids
- Deficit fluid = weight of child × % dehydration × 10.

How to give using IV sets

Normal IV set 1 ml	= 16 macro drops
Micro volume 1 ml	= 60 micro drops
40 ml/hour	= 40 × 16

Macro drops = 40 × 16/60 = 12 drops/minute
Micro drops = 40 × 60/60 = 40 drops/minute.

PROCEDURES RELATED TO FEEDING

KATORI AND SPOON FEEDING

Definition

The breast milk is the ideal feed for the low birth weight babies. Those unable to feed directly on the breast can be feed expressed breast milk (EBM) by gavage or katori-spoon. Feeding with spoon (or a similar device such as paladai) and katori has been found to be safe in small for gestational age (SGA) infants.

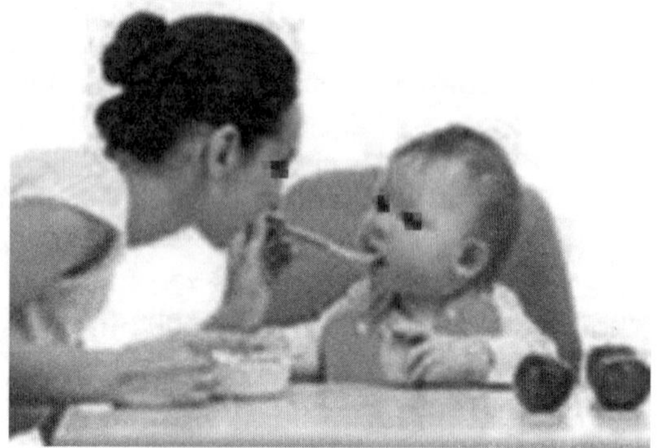

Fig. 4.6: Mother feeding the baby with katori-spoon

Indications

- Small for gestational age infants
- Premature babies who have good swallowing reflex but poor sucking reflux
- Low birth weight baby.

Contraindications

- Extreme LBW babies (< 1000 gm)
- Absent of sucking reflux
- Congenital anomalies (CL/CP)
- Semiconscious/unconscious level.

Table 4.3: Guidelines for the methods of providing fluids and feeding

Age	Categories of newborn baby		
Birth weight (gm)	< 1200 gm	1200–1800 gm	> 1800 gm
Gestational Age (wks)	< 30 weeks	30–34 weeks	> 34 weeks
Initial	• Intravenous fluids • Try gavage feeds	Gavage	Breastfeeding if unsatisfactory, provide katori-spoon feeds
After (1–3 days)	• Gavage	Katori-spoon	Breastfeeding
Later (1–3 wks)	• Katori-spoon	Breastfeeding	Breastfeeding
After (4–6 wks)	Breastfeeding	Breastfeeding	Breastfeeding

Advantages

- This mode of feeding is a bridge between gavage feeding and direct breastfeeding.
- Chances for transmission of infection associated with feeding is less when compare to bottle feeding.
- Best method for stable premature and low birth weight infants.

Disadvantages

- Cannot replace direct breastfeeding advantages
- Delay in development of sucking reflux
- Poor bonding between child and mother
- Oral trauma
- RDS.

Equipment

Sterile tray with sterile cloth containing:

- Sterile bowl/katori (medium) –1
- Teaspoon/paladai –1
- Sterile glass/cup for collecting EBM –1
- Bib –1
- Face towel –1
- Ounce glass/measuring cup –1

Preparation

- Explain the mother why we need to feed through spoon or paladai.
- Assist the mother in expression of breast milk.
- Check the neonatologist's order for feeding amount, frequency and any other precautions.

Procedure

- Arrange all articles nearby baby unit
- Perform handwashing procedure
- Sitting or upright position.
- Measure the required amount of feed and pour into katori.
- Wear the bib around the child's neck.

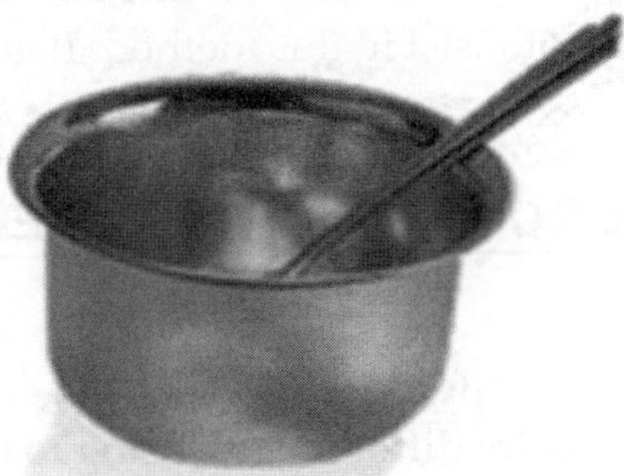

Fig. 4.7: Katori and spoon

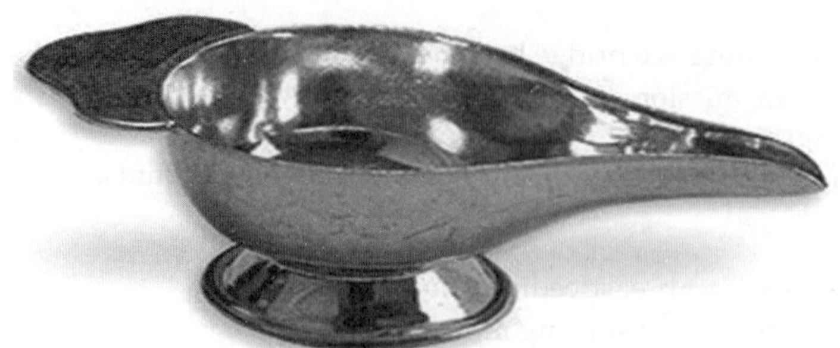

Fig. 4.8: Paladai

- Make the mother to set comfortably and ask the mother to hold baby like cradling.
- The head of the baby should be held at crook of arm of the mother. Ask the mother to support the baby's body with the side of hand.
- Take the milk from the katori with the help of spoon, the spoon should filled just short of the brim with expressed milk.
- Place the spoon or spike of the paladai at the corner of the mouth and milk should be allowed to flow into the infant's mouth slowly, avoiding any spillage.
- The baby would actively swallow the milk.
- This process should be repeated till the required amount has been fed.
- During the procedure, if baby vomit, immediately stop the procedure and report the doctor.
- Maintain intake and output chart after the procedure.

Postprocedure Care

- Wipe the face of the baby with towel
- Remove the bib from the neck
- Burp the child
- Document the procedure in nurse's record with time, amount of feed, any observation made during feeding.

Nurses Responsibilities

- If the infant does not actively accept and swallow the feed, an attempt should be made to wake the infant with gentle stimulation (tactile stimulation).
- If baby is still sluggish, do not insist in this method. It is better to switch back to gavage feeds till the infant is ready.

RYLE'S NASOGASTRIC/OROGASTRIC TUBE FEEDING

Introduction

The nutritional needs of the sick and preterm infant must be met in order to promote survival and better outcome. These needs are different according to the infant's gestation, degree of growth retardation, postnatal age and associated disease.

Bolus feeding has been shown to be more physiological in terms of producing more natural surges in gut hormones. It is usual to start on two hourly feeds, but occasionally babies may need hourly feeds. When on full milk feeds the interval between feeds may be increased to 3 and then 4 hourly depending on the individual infant. Continuous feeds are not indicated in babies with gastric tubes *in situ*.

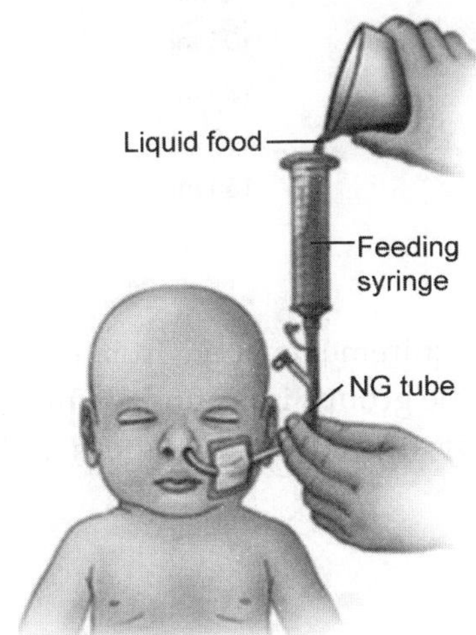

Fig. 4.9: Technique of Nasogastric feeding

Definition

Administration of feed directly into the stomach through a tube passed into the stomach through the nose (nasogastric) or mouth (orogastric).

Purpose for Insertion of a Nasogastric Tube

- Decompression of stomach (to remove fluid and gas)
- To prevent or relieve nausea and vomiting after surgery or traumatic events by decompressing the stomach.
- To determine the amount of pressure and motor activity of GI tract (diagnostic studies).
- To give gastric lavage (to irrigate the stomach in case of active bleeding or poisoning).
- To obtain specimen (gastric contents) for laboratory studies.
- To administer medication.
- To give gastric gavage (feed directly).

Purpose of Administration of Nasogastric Tube Feeding

- To provide adequate nourishment to patients who cannot feed themselves.
- To administer medication.
- To provide nourishment to patients who cannot be feed through mouth, e.g. surgery in oral cavity, unconscious or comatosed state.

Table 4.4: Fluid requirement of neonates (ml/kg body weight)

Day of newborn baby life	Birth weight	
	> 1500 gm	< 1500 gm
1	60 ml	80 ml
2	75 ml	95 ml
3	90 ml	110 ml
4	105 ml	125 ml
5	120 ml	140 ml
6	135 ml	150 ml
7 onwards	150 ml	150 ml

Note

- On the first day the fluid requirements range from 60 to 80 ml/kg.
- The daily increment in all the groups is around 15 ml per kg till 150 ml/kg is reached.
- Adequacy of therapy is indicated by weight pattern in the expected range.

Indications

- Head and neck injury
- Coma
- Obstruction of esophagus or oropharynx
- Severe anorexia nervosa
- Recurrent episodes of aspiration
- Increased metabolic needs: Burns, cancer, etc.
- Poor oral intake or failure to thrive
- Inability to suck
- Respiratory distress.

Contraindications

- Esophageal atresia
- Esophageal fistula
- Esophageal varices.

Equipment

- A sterile tray with tray cloth
- Sterile gloves
- Kidney tray with paper bag
- A bowl with water
- 5–6 French size polyethylene feeding catheter
- Water soluble jelly
- Mackintosh with draw sheet
- Intake output chart

- Syringe (10 ml syringe)
- Stethoscope.

Preparation

- Identification of the right child and explaining the procedure to the parents.
- History collection regarding food allergies, time of last feed, bowl sounds.
- Inspect the child's nose and mouth for any deformities that may interfere with the passage of these.

Procedure

- Arrange the articles nearby the baby unit.
- Performing the handwashing technique
- Wear gloves
- Position the infant supine with the head slightly elevated and with the neck hyper extended so that nose is pointed upward.
- Assist the order child to sitting position if appropriate (fowler position).
- Alternatively have the parents or another person to hold the child to promote comfort and reassurance.
- Place mackintosh and towel across the chest.
- Measure the length of the tube from tip of nose to tip of the ear lobe and to the tip of the xiphoid process and mark with tape.
- For orogastric tube insertion, the tube is measured from the lips to the tip of xiphoid process of sternum.
- Cut the adhesive tape of appropriate size and keep ready to fix the tube.
- Lubricate the tip of the tube about 6–8 inches with water soluble lubricant, using gauze piece.
- Insert the tube through the nostril to the back of the throat aiming back.
- Insert the tube gently and very slowly to nostril and give sips of water to older children for drinking, if newborn or infant give bottle nipple to suck when the tube is inserted.
- Flex the patients head towards the chest after the tube has passed the nasopharynx to reduce the risk of tube entering the trachea.

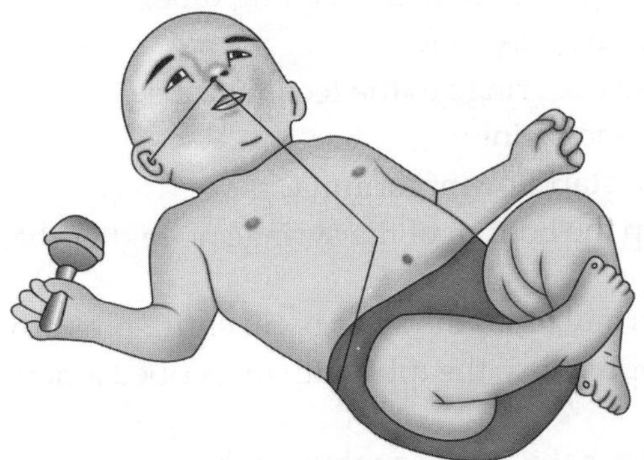

Fig. 4.10: Nasogastric tube measuring technique

- Do not force tube when resistance is met or patient starts to gag, cough, choke or become cyanosed, stop advancing tube and pull tube back, check for position of tube in back of throat with flash light.
- If there is signs of distress such as gasping, cyanosis, coughing pull back the tube for some length and check if patient distress is relieved, if it is relived develops respiratory distress again, immediately remove the tube because the tube may be in trachea.
- Perform one of the following measures to check for the placement of the tube
- Aspirated gastric content because aspirated content indicates that the tube is in the stomach then returns by aspirated contents to the stomach and flush tube with water.
- Place the end of tube in the bowel of water to check for continuous air bubbles indicates that tube is in the respiratory tract.
- If older child ask the speak if she is not able to speak then it means tube is in the trachea.
- Take 2 ml or 5 ml syringe push the air and hear the air entry sound (stethoscope) gargling.
- X-ray may be done.
- Secure tube with tape and avoid pressure on nose. Make sure that mark on the tube is at the nostril.
- Use a piece of tape, split at one end place intact end of tape over bridge of nose. Carefully wrap two ends around tube.
- Secure the tube in check (in neonates). Faster end of tube to gown. It reduces friction on nose when patient moves.
- Make patient comfortable in bed and provide oral hygiene every 4–6 hours to promotes comfort and integrity of oral mucous membrane.

Types of Feeding

Continuous feeding: Given at a slower rate over long period of time and feeding pump is used to administer the solution at a prescribed rate.

Bolus feeding: Before feeding make sure (twice) the NG tube is in stomach.

- It may be helpful to have two people to do. One person can hold and comfort the child while others can feed.
- Make sure, the correct amount of formula and warm to the deserved temperature.
- Check the tube attach a syringe to the feeding tube.
- Check the tube placement as above.
- Clamp the tube attach a syringe to the feeding tube.
- Pour the formula in the syringe
- Unclamp the tube to start flow of formula.
- During feeding keep the bottom of the syringe no higher than 6 inches above the child stomach.
- Continue adding formula into the syringe till entire prescribed amount is given.
- When syringe is empty, flush the tube with prescribed amount of lukewarm water and close the tubing.
- Remove the NG tube. Baby have coughing, wheezing, coughing, skin color, difficulty in breathing, cannot take, the tube is coming out of the mouth.

Postprocedure Care

- Discard the waste, clean and replace re-reusable articles
- Remove gloves and wash hands
- Record type of tube placed, aspirated returns and child intolerance
- Measurement of external tube length after insertion and conformation of placement.
- Administering tube feeding.

Nursing Responsibilities

- Proper positioning must be provided according to age group.
- Application of mummy restraints may be necessary to control the child's movements during the insertion.
- Infant hand may be restrained using a necessary soft restrain to prevent grasp of gavage tube and its removal.
- Sterile equipment should be used.
- Feeding amount should be calculated.
- The flow of feeding should be slow. Do not apply pressure.
- Elevate the reservoir of feed 15–20 cm above the child head.
- Weigh the child daily.
- The feeding formula should be at room temperature.
- Taking care to avoid air entry.

Special Considerations

- Insufflations of air into the tube followed by auscultation are no longer considered reliable in determining tube placement from the pleural space into the upper abdomen, thus giving false impression of tube placement.
- Change the tube after 72 hours/according to child condition or according to institution policy.

GASTROSTOMY FEEDING

Definition

Gastrostomy tubes are feeding tubes placed through the abdomen into the stomach. Gastrostomy tubes are used to provide children formula feeding, liquids, and medicines. These tubes are placed by a Pediatric Surgeon or by a Pediatric Gastroenterologist.

An enteral feeding is when food is put through a tube directly into the stomach or small intestine. This food is usually a liquid form of protein, carbohydrate and fat. It has all the nutrients, vitamins, and minerals to help a child grow and be as healthy as possible.

A gastrostomy tube is placed in two ways:

1. Percutaneously insertion
2. Surgically insertion

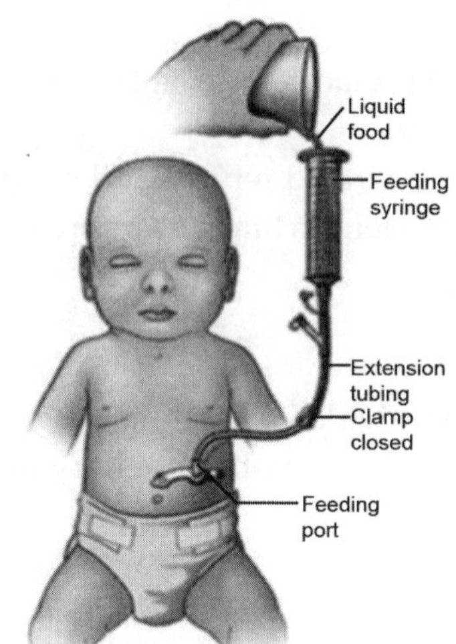

Fig. 4.11: Baby with gastrostomy feeding

Surgically Inserted Gastrostomy Tubes

The surgical inserted gastrostomy tube in the operating room under general anesthesia. This operation is done through a small incision (cut) on the abdomen. The surgeon may place a temporary tube, into the gastrostomy opening. A gastrostomy tube is about twelve inches long, and most of the tube extends out of the abdomen.

After the gastrostomy tube is placed, your child will be remain in the hospital for observation and care. An IV (intravenous line) will be placed in the operating room before the procedure and this will be used to give fluids, antibiotics and pain medications while child is recovering. Feedings are usually started the day after the gastronomy is placed.

Percutaneous Endoscopic Gastrostomy (PEG) Tube

- A PEG Tube, or Percutaneous Endoscopic Gastrostomy tube, is placed in the operating room by the pediatric surgeon. The PEG tube is inserted using an endoscope.
- The endoscope is a small tube with a light and camera on the end that lets the Gastroenterologist see into the esophagus (food tube) and stomach.
- The endoscope allows the doctor to choose the best location in the stomach to place the PEG tube. Once the location is chosen, a small opening is made on the outside of abdomen into the stomach.
- After the opening is made, the top part of the PEG tube is pulled up out of the stomach through this opening.
- The top of the tube rests on the skin and the bottom part of the PEG, which is shaped like bulb, remains inside the stomach. This bulb shape anchors the tube in the stomach and prevents it from coming out.
- After the PEG tube is placed the child will be admitted to the hospital for observation and care. The hospital stay is usually three days.
- Prior to the procedure, an IV (intravenous line) will be placed in the operating room. This will be used to give fluids, antibiotics and pain medication, for one to two days,

as your child is recovering. Feedings will be started through the PEG tube within one or two days.

- The PEG tube which is made of silicone, must stay in the stomach for about three months to allow the tract (hole) to heal between the abdomen and the stomach. The tract must be well healed so it is safe for the gastrostomy tube to be changed.

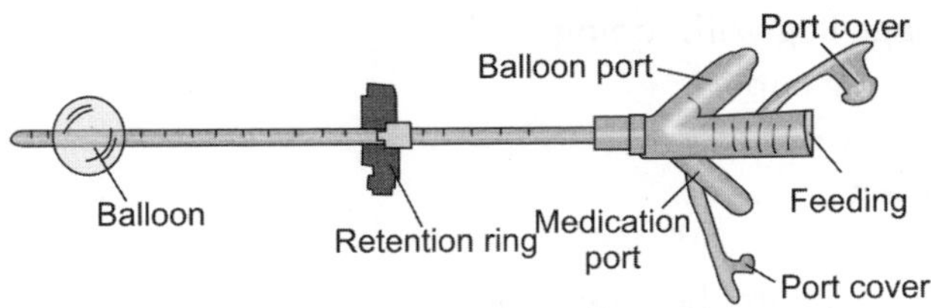

Fig. 4.12: Surgically inserted gastrostomy tubes

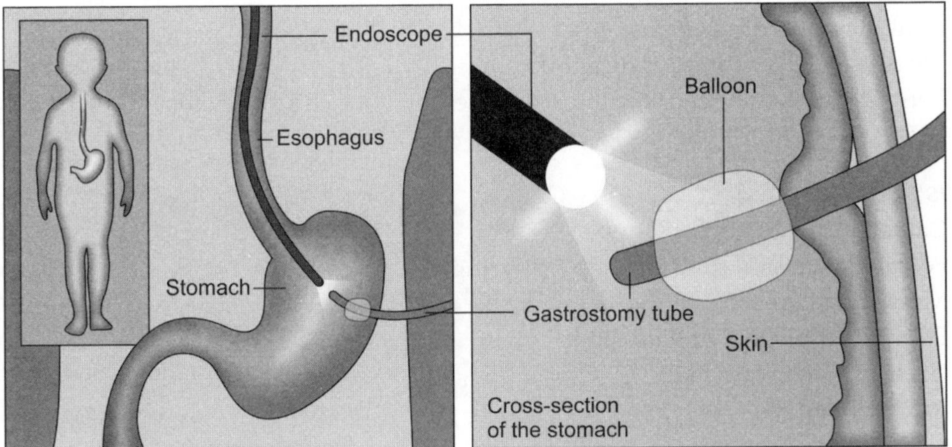

Fig. 4.13: Percutaneous endoscopic gastrostomy (PEG) tube show that different type of gastrostomy tube with insertion methods

Indication

- Congenital abnormalities such as esophageal/choanal atresia or trachea esophageal fistula
- Conditions which require long term feeding
- Esophageal injury/dysmotility
- Child has functioning gastrointestinal tract but is unable to meet his/her total nutritional requirement orally.

Contraindication

- Gross ascites/sever obesity
- Clotting abnormalities
- Gastroparesis

- Esophageal/gastric varices and ulceration
- Complete intestinal obstruction
- Uncontrolled gastroesophageal reflux with a risk of pulmonary aspiration.

Equipment

- Feeding syringe (appropriate to age group)
- Disposable gavage bag with tubing
- IV stand, measuring cup
- Formula, glass of water
- Administration set
- Pair of gloves
- Stethoscope to auscultate the bowel sound.

Feeding by Pump

- Feeding set
- Continuous feeding extension set
- Measuring cup with pouring spout
- Formula or blenderized feeding as ordered by your child's doctor
- Glass of water (optional).

Bolus Feeding

- Catheter tip syringe for G-tube
- Feeding extension tube and slip tip syringe
- Measuring cup
- Formula or blenderized feeding
- Glass of water (optional)
- Rubber band
- Clamp for G-tube
- Safety pin.

Procedures

- Identification of right child
- Explain the procedures to parents and get the consent
- Wash your hands
- Assess gastrostomy site for skin breakdown, irritation or drainage.
- Place the child in a comfortable position. If possible place the child in higher chair or at the table during meal time.
- Insert the syringe tip into the feeding tube.
- Flush tubing with 3–5 ml of water to starting the formula feeding.
- Slowly pour the formula into the syringe.
- Unclamp the feeding tube the feeding rate can be controlled by raising or lowering the syringe.

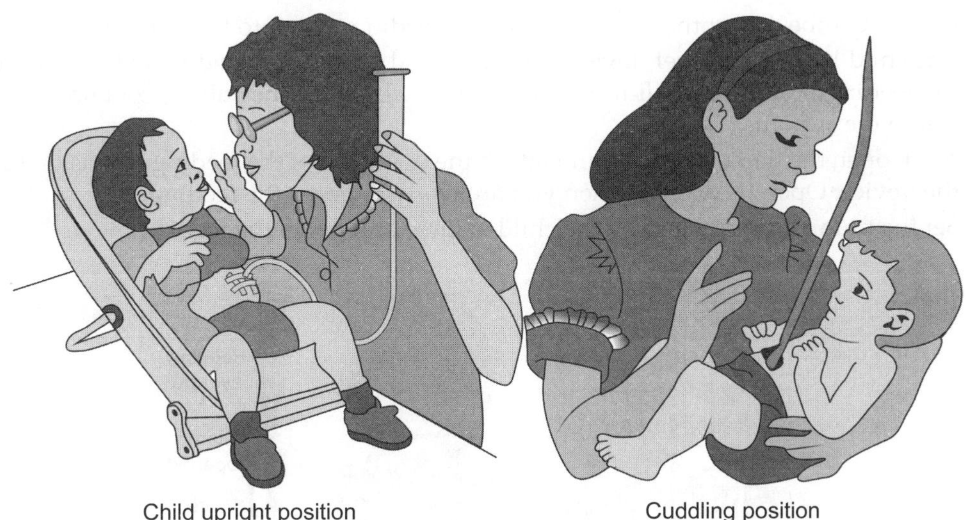

Fig. 4.14: Gastrostomy feeding position

- The feeding should take about the same amount of time as it would take a child drink the formula, about 15–20 minute.
- When all the formula has been given, flush the tubing with water.
- Use formula that is at room temperature. Never microwave formula to bring it to room temperature. Keep opened containers of formula in the refrigerator.
  - This procedure takes about 30 minutes for cold formula to reach room temperature. Measure the amount of formula needed for the feeding 30 minutes before the feeding is due and refrigerate any leftovers promptly.
  - Discard any formula after it has been out of the refrigerator for 4 hours.
  - Any opened blenderized feeding or commercially prepared formula should be thrown out after it has been in the refrigerator for 24 hours.
- Put two or three drops of formula on your wrist before feeding. The formula should feel warm, not hot or cold.
- Assess the patient for allergies to prevent patient from developing localized or systemic allergic responses.
- Auscultate for bowel sound before feeding because it indicate the presence of peristalsis and obesity of gastrointestinal tract to digest nutrients.
- Verify physician order for formula, rate, and frequency.
- Burp the child after each feeding if appropriate.
- Rinse the feeding tube and record the procedures.

Pump Feedings

- Close the clamp on the feeding bag. Pour the formula into the bag. Hang the bag high on a hook. Open the clamp and let the formula flow through the tubing until all of the tubing contains formula. Clamp the system. The nurse will show you how to put the tubing through the feeding pump.

- For the G-tube, insert the catheter tip of the feeding tube into the G-tube.
- The child has a skin level device, you will need to attach a feeding extension tube to the feeding system and fill it with formula. After all of the tubing contains formula, clamp the system.
- Next, open the flap of the tube and attach the open end of the feeding extension tube to the device. Open the clamp when you are ready to begin the feeding.
- Set the pump as instructed by the child's nurse and begin the feeding.

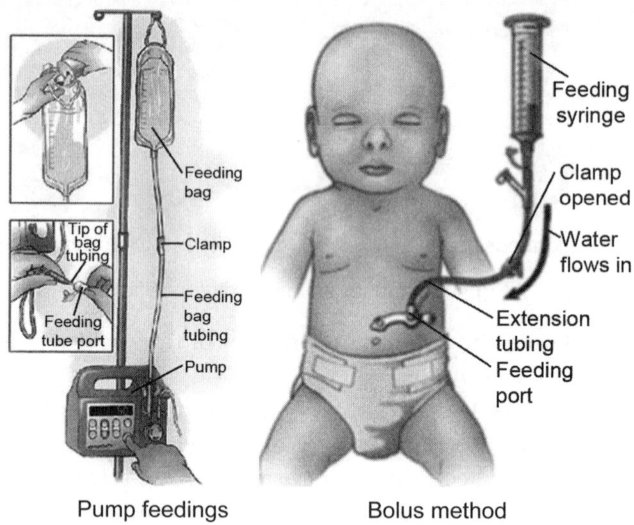

Fig. 4.15: Difference between pump and bolus feeding

Bolus Method

- The child has a skin level device, she will need to attach the extension set to the device and then connect the catheter tip syringe to the extension set. The child has a long G-Tube, connect the catheter tip syringe to the end of the tube.
- Pour the formula into the syringe until it is half full. Filling the syringe full can cause spillage if the child coughs or moves. Next, unclamp the tube or extension tube. Hold the tip of the syringe no higher than your child's shoulders. If the feeding does not start to flow, milk the tube by squeezing it in a downward stroke.

General Feeding Guidelines

(Both Pump and Bolus Method)

- For a gastrostomy feeding, the child's head must be raised. For an infant, you can hold him in the curve of your arm while feeding (cuddling position). If the child is older, you can feed him in a high chair or any seat as long as his head is raised. The child is fed in these positions, hang the feeding set on a hook in the room.
- The feeding should take the same amount of time as a regular feeding or meal, at least 20–30 minutes. If the child cries during the feeding, stop the feeding until the child is quiet. This can be done by clamping or pinching the tube with your finger and thumb.

- Eating is a social time so make the feeding a happy time for the child. If child needs oral stimulation, follow the instructions given to you by child's occupational therapist or nurse, and the way to grow handout for Simulated Feedings.
- After the feeding, add water or air to clear the feeding from the tube. The child's nurse will tell you which to use and how much. If the child has a G-tube, close the clamp on the tube and the feeding system and remove the feeding system.

Cleaning the Equipment

- Wash the syringe, feeding extension tube, feeding set and measuring cup in hot, soapy water. Rinse with hot water and dry. If formula is caked on the syringe or tubing, rinsing with a carbonated beverage before cleaning will help remove the dried formula.
- Change the extension set for the Mic-Key button once a week.
- Change the feeding bag as recommended by your home health care equipment company.

Complication

- Large bowl perforation
- Accidental displacement can result in partial closure of stoma
- Infection
- Occlusion

Nurse's Responsibility

- If the child cannot be fed by mouth, oral stimulation with pacifier can be provided during gastrostomy feeding.
- Encourage oral stimulation by blowing, kissing.
- Disconnect the feeding if the child becomes nauseated. Shows sign of discomfort abdominal distention, vomiting or difficulty in breathing.
- Remember to flush the feeding tube with water between all feeding and medications.

Care of Tube

- First 2–3 days the gastrostomy site should be cleaned 2–3 times/day with half strength hydrogen peroxide. After 2–3 days, the site should be cleaned with mild soap and water.
- Take measure to prevent contamination of feed.

Bathing

- Sponging can be given for first 2–3 days to keep the child's new gastrostomy site dry.
- Showering can be given after two days.
- Clean the site and pat dry after showering.
- Swimming is restricted until the stitch is removed.

Venting the Tube

- Place a 60 cc syringe with the plunger remove into the end of the gastrostomy tube. If the tube is clamped open the clamp.
- Hold the syringe above the child stomach for a few minutes. If the gas is present, you can hear the gas bubbles up through the tube or sometimes even see stomach contents backup into the tube and syringe.

- Once the gas is removed allow the formula to flow slowly back into the stomach.
- Make early referral to speech therapist for children requiring long term feeding.

Accidental Tube Expulsion

If tube comes out cover the site with a clean, dry gauze pad or cloth.

- Once the tube is out, hole will begin to close and may close completely in 4–6 hours.
- So the child should be replaced with new gastrostomy tube immediately and should be checked under X-ray for proper placement.
- Balloon devices should be deflated and reinforced weekly to ensure correct amount of fluid remains in the balloon.

Activity Restriction

- Child should not lift anything heavier and should not participate in vigorous activity for two weeks after surgery.
- The school nurse needs instruction filled by the hospital and signed by doctor.

PROCEDURES RELATING TO ELIMINATION

ENEMA

Introduction

An enema is a technique used to stimulate stool evacuation. It is a liquid treatment most commonly used to help relieve severe constipation. The process helps push waste out of the rectum when child cannot do by own. Other types of enemas are administered to clean out the colon to better detect *colon cancer and polyps.*

Definition

An enema is defined as a liquid that is introduced into the rectum. It flushes out stool (feces) that has built up (impacted) in the bowel. This process is called disimpaction. Disimpaction helps restore the rectum's normal muscle tone. It can also help your child regain the natural urge to defecate.

Purposes

- To relieve constipation fecal impaction.
- To prevent involuntary escape of fecal matter during surgical procedure and delivery.
- To promote visualization of the intestinal tract during the radiographic or instrumental examination.
- To help establish regular bowl functions during a bowl training program.
- Preoperative preparation for bowl surgeries.

Indications

- Constipation
- Hyperthermia
- Bowl surgeries
- Examination of intestinal tract.

Contraindication

- Acute renal failure
- Acute myocardial infarction and cardiac problems
- Appendicitis
- Recent surgical procedures involving lower intestinal tract.
- Intestinal obstruction
- Inflammation and infection of abdomen.

Solution Used

- Hypertonic: Sodium phosphate
- Hypotonic: Tap water
- Isotonic: Physiological saline (one tablespoon salt in 500 ml of tap water.
- Others: 3–5 ml of concentrated soap solution in 1000 ml of water.

Table 4.5: Amount of fluid to be introduced depends upon the size of the child

Age group	Required amount of fluid
Infants	150–250 ml
Toddler	250–300 ml
Pre-schooler and school-age	300–500 ml
Adolescents	500–750 ml
Adult	750–1000 ml

Catheter size: 10–12 Fr and should be inserted only 2–4 inches into the rectum depending upon the size of the child.

- Infants 2.5 cm
- 2–4 years 5 cm
- 4–10 years 7.5 cm
- > 11 years 10 cm
- Temperature of solution 105 °F.

Equipment Needed

- A clean tray containing with sterile dry clothes
- Enema bag or can and tubing with clamp or syringe with rubber tubing.
- Lubricant (liquid paraffin)
- Enema solution
- Rectal catheter
- Gauze pieces in bowl
- Pair of gloves
- Bedpan at the edges
- Kidney tray with paper bag
- Lotion thermometer
- Macintosh with draw sheet.

Position of the Child

- Infant and toddler lie on abdomen with knees bent.
- Older children and adolescent left side with right leg flexed toward chest.

Position for enemas

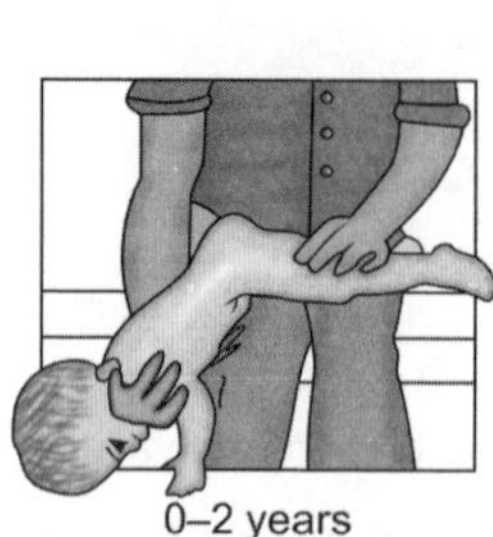

0–2 years

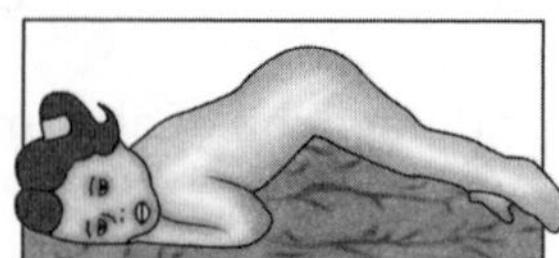

2–12 years

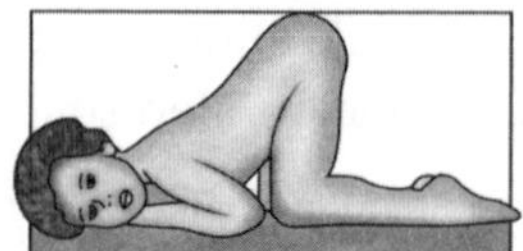

More than 12 years

Positions for using this enema

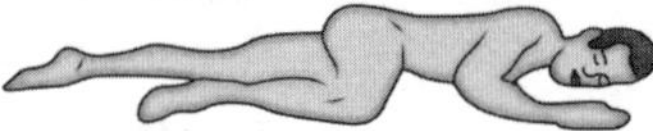

Left-side position: Lie on left side with knee bent, and arms resting comfortably

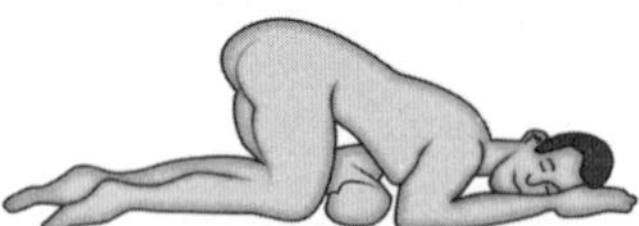

Knee-chest position: Kneel, then lower head and chest forward until left side of face is resting on surface with left arm folded comfortably

Fig. 4.16: According to age group different position for enema procedures

Procedure

- Explain the procedures to parents
- Assess the general status of child—last bowl movement, normal bowl movements, mobility, external sphincter muscles control, abdominal pain and perineal lesion.
- Perform the handwash procedure and apply gloves
- Arrange all the articles nearby child unit
- Provide comfortable positions to child
- Clamp the enema tubing, remove the cap and apply lubricant to the tip of catheter
- Insert the tube into the rectum
- Unclamp the tubing and administer the prescribed volume of enema solution at the rate of about 100 ml per minute

- Remove the catheter gently and put it in kidney tray
- Hold the child buttocks together if enema needed to encourage retention of enema for 5–10 minutes
- Offer bedpan
- In case of ambulatory and older children assist them to go to toilet.

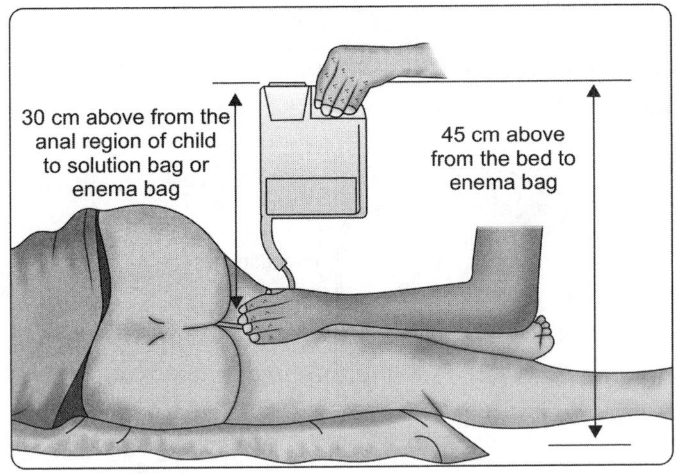

Nursing Responsibilities

- Praise the child for cooperation.
- Make the child comfort.
- Record the procedure in nurse's record.
- Clean and replace the supplies.
- The can should not be held more than 18 inches above the child hip. So that the solution may run slowly by gravity and pressure into the bowl.
- An isotonic solution or physiological saline is used. Tap water alone is not used because of the danger of the fluid shift and overload.
- A cleansing enema can be given 30–40 minutes after the oil retention enema.

COLOSTOMY IRRIGATION

Definition

A colostomy is defined as an opening in the colon. When a part of your large intestine or rectum is removed or is disconnected, the new opening (colostomy) must be made in the colon for waste to leave the body. Colostomy irrigation is a way to regulate bowel movements by emptying the colon at a scheduled time. The process involves instilling water or solution into the colon through the stoma, which stimulates the colon to empty. By repeating this process regularly once a day or once every second day the colon can be trained to empty with minimal to no spillage of stool in between irrigations. Colostomy irrigation also can help avoid constipation.

Equipment

- A clean big tray and sterile cloth
- Enema can and tubing
- Kidney tray
- Sterile gove
- Warm water in a basin
- Bath towel
- Bedpans or pail for collecting the return flow
- Irrigating solution

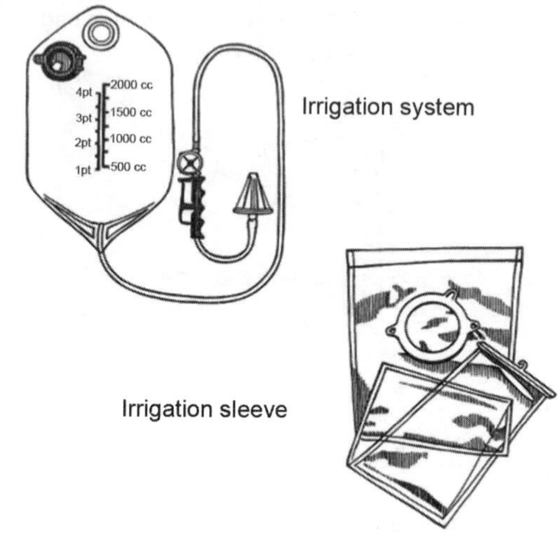

Fig. 4.17: Colostomy irrigation system with sleeve

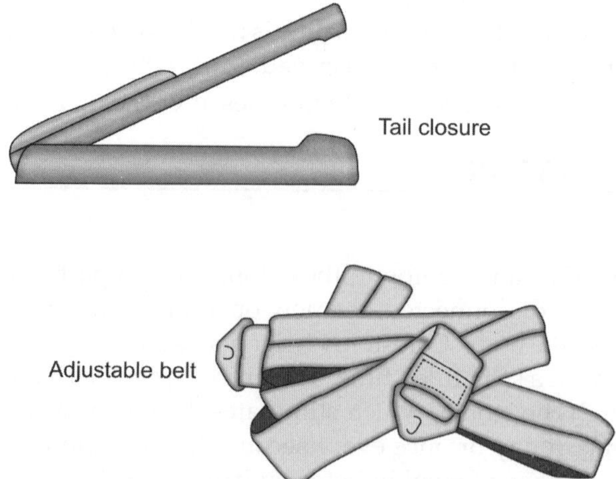

Fig. 4.18: Colostomy irrigation tail closure and adjustable belt

- Soap, extra rubber sheet, small colon tube, plastic apron, colostomy dressing tray, wash cloth
- The plastic cone-shaped piece at end of the tubing fits snugly against the stoma to run water into the colostomy.
- An irrigation sleeve to carry the irrigation output into the toilet.
- A tail closure clip and a belt for extra irrigation sleeve support. (This is optional.)

Procedures

- Explain the procedures to parents
- Assemble your supplies: Irrigator bag, stoma cone, irrigator sleeve, ostomy belt (if needed), water-soluble lubricant (optional), water, and a new pouch or stoma cap.
- Do the handwash
- Provide the comfortable position to child
- Close the regulator clamp on the irrigation tubing and connect the stoma cone tube to the irrigator tubing.
- Fill the irrigator bag with the amount of water recommended by your health care provider. The water should be lukewarm.

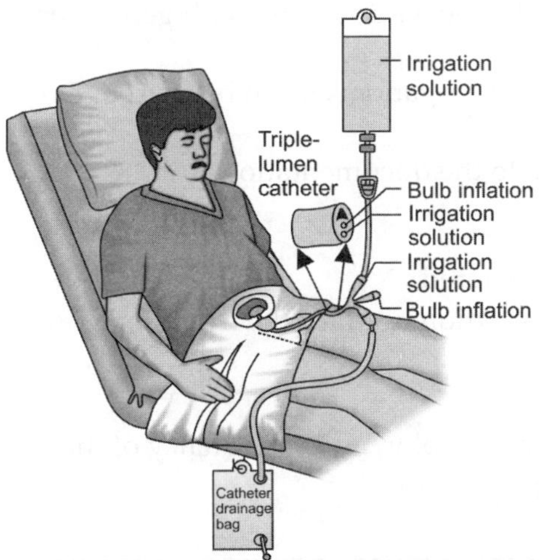

Fig. 4.19: Colostomy irrigation procedure

- Hang the bag at a height where the bottom of the bag is approximately at child shoulder height when you are sitting.
- Open the clamp and allow some water to run out the end of the cone. Close the flow control clamp.
- Remove and discard your existing pouch or stoma cap.
- Attach your irrigation sleeve.
  - If you are using a one-piece irrigation sleeve, a belt will be needed. The belt should be snug enough to create a watertight seal.
  - If you are using a two-piece system, attach the irrigator sleeve to your skin barrier flange.

- Find a comfortable position to sit either on the toilet or next to the toilet. Place the end of the sleeve in the toilet.
- Open the top of the irrigator sleeve. If desired, coat the stoma cone with Hollister Stoma Lubricant. Gently insert the irrigator cone into your stoma as your healthcare provider has instructed you.
- Hold the cone in place and, with your other hand; open the flow control clamp to allow the water to begin to flow into child stoma. Press the cone against the stoma gently, but firm enough to prevent leakage. If water does not flow into the stoma, rotate the angle of the cone until water flows.
- To change the rate of water flow, adjust the flow control. If cramps occur, close the flow control until cramps subside.
- Once all the water is in, remove the cone from your stoma and close the top of the irrigator sleeve. At this time you should have some initial returns of water and stool.
- It usually takes from 30–45 minutes for the bowel to empty.
- When the child bowel is empty, drain the irrigator sleeve into the toilet. Remove the irrigator sleeve and set it aside.
- Clean and dry the child skin and apply a new pouch or stoma cap as usual.
- Clean the child irrigator sleeve and cone with gentle soap. Rinse. Allow the sleeve to air dry.
- The irrigator sleeve and irrigation set can be reused. Do not flush the irrigator sleeve down the toilet.
- After the procedures do the documentation.

After the Procedures

- Time irrigation administered.
- Kind and amount of solution used for the irrigation.
- Dressing applied.
- Condition of the area.
- Results obtained; amount, color, and consistency of the returns.
- Patient's reaction to procedure.

ADMINISTRATION AND ANALYSIS OF OXYGEN CONCENTRATION

AIRWAY MANAGEMENT

Introduction

Airway management is an essential skill for clinicians caring for critically ill or injured patients and is fundamental to the practice of emergency medicine. In emergency medicine practice, rapid sequence intubation (RSI) is the most frequently used and successful means of intubating the trachea. It is employed in approximately 70 percent of all patients requiring intubation in academic emergency departments, and about 82 percent of those without cardiac arrest. Cardiac arrest patients, who are intubated without medications, comprise the bulk of the remaining patients.

Definition

Airway management is the highest priority for clinical care. This is because if there is no airway, there can be no breathing, hence no oxygenation of blood and therefore circulation (and hence all the other vital body processes) will soon cease. Getting oxygen to the lungs is the first step in almost all clinical treatments. The 'A' is for 'airway' in the 'ABC' of cardiopulmonary resuscitation.

Methods

Head Tilt/Chin Lift

The simplest way of ensuring an open airway in an unconscious patient is to use a head tilt chin lift technique, thereby lifting the tongue from the back of the throat. This is taught on most first aid courses as the standard way of clearing an airway.

Jaw Thrust

The jaw thrust is a technique used on patients with a suspected spinal injury and is used on a supine patient. The practitioner uses their thumbs to physically push the posterior (back) aspects of the mandible upwards. When the mandible is displaced forward, it pulls the tongue forward and prevents it from occluding (blocking) the entrance to the trachea, helping to ensure a patent (secure) airway.

Types

- Oropharyngeal Airway
- Endotracheal Intubation
- Endotracheal Suction
- Oxygen Therapy
- CPAP
- Care of Tracheostomy

OROPHARYNGEAL AIRWAY

Definition

The oropharyngeal airway was designed by Arthur E. Guedel (1883–1956). An oropharyngeal airway (also known as an oral airway, OPA or Guedel pattern airway) is a medical device called an airway adjunct used to maintain a patent (open) airway. It does this by preventing

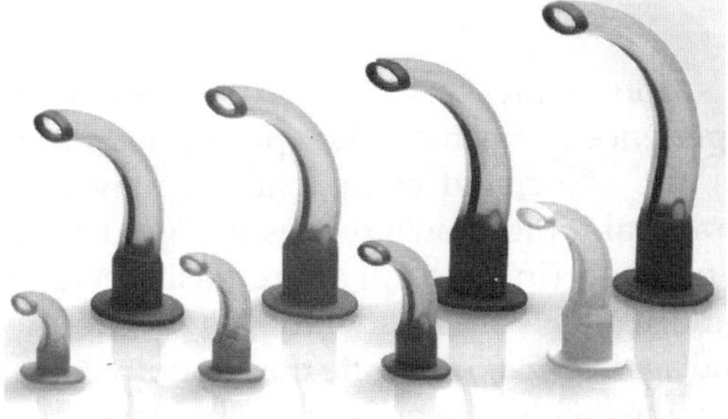

Fig. 4.20: Different sizes of oropharyngeal airways

the tongue from (either partially or completely) covering the epiglottis, which could prevent the patient from breathing. When a person becomes unconscious, the muscles in their jaw relax and may allow the tongue to obstruct the airway; in fact, the tongue is the most common cause of a blocked airway.

Indication

Oropharyngeal airways are usually indicated for unconscious patients, because there is a high probability that the device would stimulate a conscious patient's gag reflex. This could cause the patient to vomit and potentially lead to an obstructed airway.

Procedure

The correct size OPA is chosen by measuring against the patient's head (from the earlobe to the corner of the mouth). The airway is then inserted into the patient's mouth upside down. Once contact is made with the back of the throat, the airway is rotated 180 degrees, allowing for easy insertion, and assuring that the tongue is secured. Measuring is very important, as the flared ends of the airway must rest securely against the oral opening in order to remain secure. An alternative method for insertion, the method that is recommended for OPA use in children and infants, involves holding the tongue forward with a tongue depressor and inserting the airway right side up. To remove the device, it is pulled out following the curvature of the tongue; no rotation is necessary.

Complication

- If the patient has a gag-reflex they may vomit
- When it is too large, it can close the glottis and thus close the airway
- Improper sizing can cause bleeding in the airway.

ENDOTRACHEAL INTUBATION

Definition

Tracheal intubation is the placement of a flexible plastic tube into the trachea to protect the patient's airway and provide a means of mechanical ventilation. The most common tracheal intubation is orotracheal intubation where, with the assistance of a laryngoscope, an endotracheal tube is passed through the mouth, larynx, and vocal cords, into the trachea. A bulb is then inflated near the distal tip of the tube to help secure it in place and protect the airway from blood, vomit, and secretions.

Purpose

Tracheal intubation is a potentially very dangerous invasive procedure that requires a great deal of clinical experience to master. When performed improperly (e.g. unrecognized esophageal intubation), the associated complications may rapidly lead to the patient's death. Consequently, tracheal intubation's role as the 'gold standard' of advanced airway maintenance was downplayed (in favor of more basic techniques like bag-valve-mask ventilation) by the American Heart Association's Guidelines for Cardiopulmonary Resuscitation in 2000, and again in 2005. Despite this, Endotracheal Intubation is still the Gold Standard in airway care and provides the highest level of protection when moving a casualty, against vomits and regurgitation, and from upper airway and maxilofacial hemorrhage.

Indication

Tracheal intubation is performed by practitioners in various medical conditions:

- Comatose or intoxicated patients who are unable to protect their airways. In such patients, the throat muscles may lose their tone so that the upper airways obstruct or collapse and air can not easily enter into the lungs. Furthermore, protective airway reflexes such as coughing and swallowing, which serve to protect the airways against aspiration of secretions and foreign bodies, may be absent. With tracheal intubation, airway patency is restored and the lower airways can be protected from aspiration.
- General anesthesia: In anesthetized patients spontaneous respiration may be decreased or absent due to the effect of anesthetics, opioids, or muscle relaxants. To enable mechanical ventilation, an endotracheal tube is often used, although there are alternative devices such as face masks or laryngeal mask airways.
- Diagnostic manipulations of the airways such as bronchoscopy.
- Endoscopic operative procedures to the airways such as laser therapy or stenting of the bronchi.
- Patients who require respiratory support, including cardiopulmonary resuscitation.

Type of Tubes

Uncuffed tubes (plain tubes) are commonly used in prepubescent children. In cross section the airway in children is circular which makes plain tracheal tube fits better than cuffed tube. Cuffed tubes less than 6.0 mm and not inflated are accepted for use in pediatric but generally in children less than 10 years old cuffed tubes are avoided to minimize subglottic swelling and ulceration.

Size of Tube

Because the airway of a child is narrow, a small amount of edema can produce severe obstruction. Edema can easily be caused by forcing in a tracheal tube that is too tight. (If length of the tube is suspected to be large, immediate changing it to the smaller size is suggestible.) The correct diameter of the tube is that which results in a small leak at a pressure of about 25 cm of water (the tip should be at midtrachea, between the clavicles on an AP chest X-ray). For normally nourished children more than about 2 years old, the following formula to calculate the internal diameter of the tube is likely to be of the correct size.

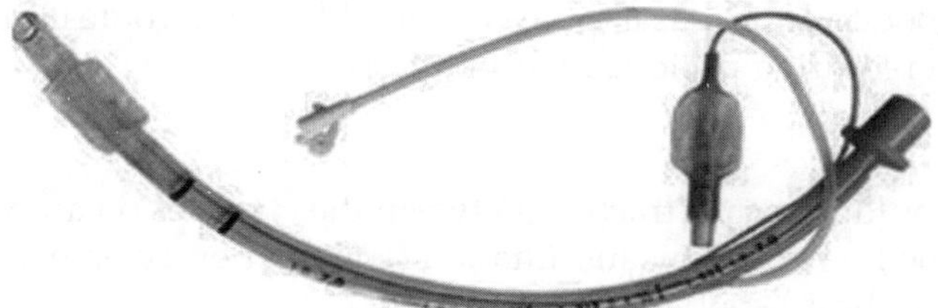

Fig. 4.21: Cuffed endotracheal intubation tube

Formula

Internal diameter of tube (mm) = (age in years ÷ 4) + 4

Procedure

Pediatric Intubation

Most of the general principles of anesthesia can be applied to children, but there are some significant anatomical and physiological differences between children and adults that can cause problems, especially in neonates and children weighing less than 15 kg.

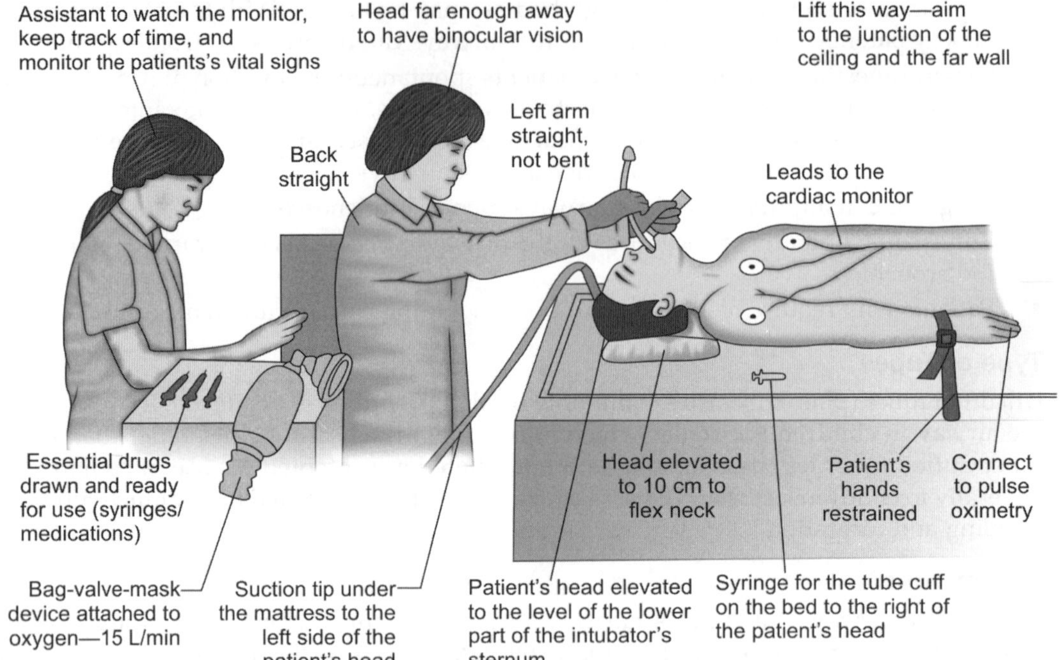

Fig. 4.22: Technique of endotracheal intubation

Route for Intubation

For infants and young children, oral intubation is easier than nasal. Nasal route carries risk of dislodgement of adenoid tissue and epistaxis, but advantages include good fixation of tube. Because of good fixation, nasal route is preferable to oral route in children undergoing intensive care and requiring prolonged intubation.

Position of Tube

The tip of tube should be at midtrachea (between the clavicles on an AP chest X-ray). The position of the tube is checked by auscultation (equal air entry on each side and, in long-term intubation, by chest X-ray).

Rough Idea

Roughly correct tube size can be indicated by Inner Diameter: Can be estimated by the size of the child's little finger. (For neonates, 3 mm internal diameter is accepted while for premature infants 2.5 mm internal diameter may be necessary.)

Length: Can be estimated by doubling the distance from the corner of the child's mouth to the ear canal. Looking from side of the child's head while holding the upper end of the tube level with the mouth can provide an idea of how far into the chest the tube will go.

Management

Observational Methods to Confirm Correct Tube Placement

- Direct visualization of the tube passing through the vocal cords with Laryngoscopy.
- Observe the Clear and equal bilateral breath sounds on auscultation of the chest.
- Absent of breath sounds while auscultation of the epigastric region of the child.
- Equal bilateral chest rise with ventilation.
- Observe the fogging inside the tube.
- An absence of stomach contents in the endotracheal tube.

Instruments to Confirm Correct Tube Placement

Colorimetric end tidal CO_2 detector, waveform capnography, self inflating esophageal bulb, pulse oximetry (patients with a pulse)—delay in fall of saturation, especially if pre-oxygenated, esophageal Detection Device (ODD).

Tube Maintenance

The tube is secured in place with tape or an endotracheal tube holder. A cervical collar is sometimes used to prevent motion of the airway. Tube placement should be confirmed after each physical move of the patient and after any unexplained change in the patient's clinical status. Continuous pulse oximetry and continuous waveform capnography are often used to monitor the tube's correct placement.

ENDOTRACHEAL SUCTION

Introduction

Endotracheal suctioning (ES) is an essential and frequently performed procedure for patients requiring mechanical ventilation. By ES, secretions from the tracheobronchial tree are cleared, guaranteeing optimal oxygenation and avoiding accumulation of secretions, leading to tube occlusion, increased work of breathing, atelectasis, and pulmonary infections.

Endotracheal suctioning may also have adverse effects, such as disturbances in cardiac rhythm, hypoxemia (due to interruption of the mechanical ventilation and subsequently the decay of intrathoracic pressure), microbial contamination of airway and environment, and development of ventilator-associated pneumonia (VAP). The frequency with which ES is performed differs per patient, with reported mean values varying from eight to 17 times per day.

Types

- The single-use/open suction system (OSS)
- The multiple-use/closed suction system (CSS).

The open suction system requires disconnection from the ventilator during ES, which is not necessary when using CSS. Moreover, in contrast to OSS, the closed suction catheter can remain connected to the patient for as long as 24 hours, according to the manufacturer, and thus can be used for multiple ES procedures.

Procedures

The procedures for endotracheal (within the trachea) suctioning are similar to those used for naso and oropharyngeal suctioning with two major differences.

- Endotracheal suctioning, unlike naso- and oropharyngeal suctioning
- Done as an aseptic, or sterile, procedure
- Suctioning the trachea interferes greatly with oxygenation. A high suction pressure and a lengthy suctioning time will greatly decrease the amount
- Apply suction and rotate the catheter to suction the secretions. Suction for only 5–10 seconds at a time. Do not push the catheter in and out against the wall
- The throat as this may injure the mucous membrane
- Withdraw the catheter and clear it by aspirating water through it
- Secretions adhering to the outer surface of the catheter should be removed with moistened gauze
- Repeat the procedure, suctioning around the teeth and gums and under the tongue if secretions have accumulated in these areas
- Suctioning of the mouth, a firm metal suction tip may be used instead of a soft catheter.
- Rigid suction tip to avoid injury to the oral mucosa, e.g. bulb syringe suctioning is used to clear secretions from the nose and mouth of infants
- Grasp the bulb syringe firmly and squeeze the bulb to expel the air
- Very gently, insert the tip into the mouth or nostril of the infant, taking care not to injure the delicate mucosa
- Release the pressure on the bulb. As the air returns into the bulb
- It creates a sucking action that will withdraw the secretions
- When the bulb has inflated, remove the tip from the infant's mouth or nose. Dispose of the secretions into a basin or piece of gauze by squeezing the bulb, forcing out the air and secretions
- Repeat the procedure as necessary.

CONTINUOUS POSITIVE AIRWAY PRESSURE (CPAP)

Definition

CPAP stands for 'continuous positive airway pressure.' CPAP is a treatment that delivers slightly pressurized air during the breathing cycle. This makes breathing easier for persons with obstructive sleep apnea and other respiratory problems.

Indication

CPAP treatment can be highly effective in treatment of obstructive sleep apnea. For some patients, the improvement in the quality of sleep and quality of life due to CPAP treatment will be noticed after a single night's use. Often, the patient's sleep partner also benefits from markedly improved sleep quality, due to the amelioration of the patient's loud snoring.

Given that sleep apnea is a chronic health issue and doesn't go away, ongoing care is needed to maintain CPAP therapy. Based on the study of cognitive behavioral therapy (referenced above), ongoing chronic care management is the best way to help patients continue therapy by educating them on the health risks of sleep apnea and providing motivation and support.

Equipment

- Flow generator (PAP machine) provides the airflow
- Hose connects the flow generator (sometimes via an in-line humidifier) to the interface
- Interface (nasal or full face mask, nasal pillows, or less commonly a lip-seal mouthpiece)
- Provides the connection to the user's airway.

A

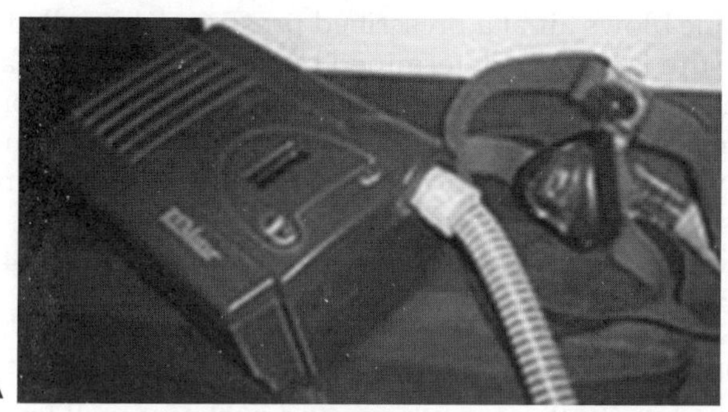

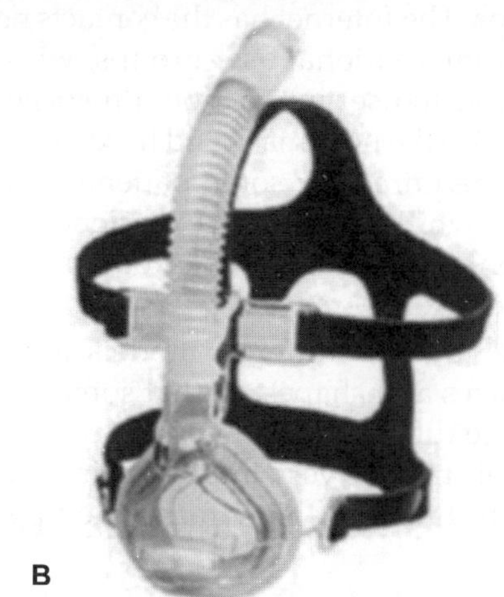

B

Fig. 4.23 A and B: (A) Continuous positive airway pressure (CPAP); (B) Continuous positive airway pressure (CPAP) face mask

Mechanism of Action

Fixed-pressure CPAP (Continuous Positive Airway Pressure)

A continuous positive airway pressure (CPAP) machine was initially used mainly by patients for the treatment of sleep apnea at home, but now is in widespread use across intensive care units as a form of ventilation. Obstructive sleep apnea occurs when the upper airway becomes narrow as the muscles relax naturally during sleep. This reduces oxygen in the blood and causes arousal from sleep. The CPAP machine stops this phenomenon by delivering a stream of compressed air via a hose to a nasal pillow, nose mask or full-face mask, splinting the airway (keeping it open under air pressure) so that unobstructed breathing becomes possible, reducing and/or preventing apneas and hypopneas. It is important to understand, however, that it is the air pressure, and not the movement of the air, that prevents the apneas. When the machine is turned on, but prior to the mask being placed on the head, a flow of air comes through the mask. After the mask is placed on the head, it is sealed to the face and the air stops flowing. At this point, it is only the air pressure that accomplishes the desired result. This has the additional benefit of reducing or eliminating the extremely loud snoring that sometimes accompanies sleep apnea.

The CPAP machine blows air at a prescribed pressure (also called the titrated pressure). The necessary pressure is usually determined by a sleep physician after review of a study supervised by a sleep technician during an overnight study (polysomnography) in a sleep laboratory. The titrated pressure is the pressure of air at which most (if not all) apneas and hypopneas have been prevented, and it is usually measured in centimeters of water (cm H_2O). The pressure required by most patients with sleep apnea ranges between 6 and 14 cm H_2O. A typical CPAP machine can deliver pressures between 4 and 20 cm H_2O. More specialized units can deliver pressures up to 25 or 30 cm H_2O.

Disadvantages and Side Effects

Most factors associated with these machines and parts are well known to manufacturers, suppliers, and end-user groups. The Internet has the contacts needed user and manufacturer web sites, local, national and international user groups, with occasional local face-to-face meetings or other forms of user to user interaction. Prospective PAP candidates are often reluctant to use this therapy, since the nose mask and hose to the machine look uncomfortable and clumsy, and the airflow required for some patients can be vigorous. Some patients will develop nasal congestion while others may experience rhinitis or a runny nose. Some patients adjust to the treatment within a few weeks, others struggle for longer periods, and some discontinue treatment entirely.

PAP manufacturers frequently offer different models at different price ranges, and PAP masks have many different sizes and shapes, so that some users need to try several masks before finding a good fit. These different machines may not be comfortable for all users, so proper selection of PAP models may be very important in furthering adherence to therapy. Every few years, advancing technologies may mean the upgrading of your machine and parts.

Nursing Care and Maintenance

- As with all durable medical equipment, proper maintenance is essential for proper functioning, long unit life and patient comfort.
- The care and maintenance required for PAP machines varies with the type and conditions of use, and are typically spelled out in a detailed instruction manual specific to the make and model.
- Most manufacturers recommend that the end user perform daily and weekly maintenance.

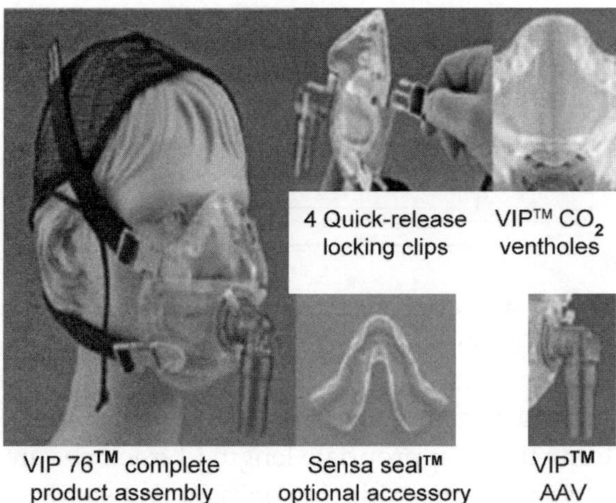

Fig. 4.24: Technique of handling the CPAP face mask

- Units must be checked regularly for wear and tear and kept clean. Poorly connected, worn or frayed electrical connections may present a shock or fire hazard; worn hoses and masks may reduce the effectiveness of the unit.
- Most units employ some type of filtration, and the filters must be cleaned or replaced on a regular schedule. Sometimes HEPA filters may be purchased or modified for asthma or other allergy clients.
- Hoses and masks accumulate exfoliated skin, particulate matter, and can even develop mold.
- Humidification units must be kept free of mold and algae. Because units use substantial electrical power, housings must be cleaned without immersion.

In cold climates, humidified air may require insulated and or heated air hoses. These may be bought ready-made, or modified from commonly available materials (Aluminum foil and bubble-wrap insulation. Noisy machines may be distanced from the sleeper by extension hoses between the machine and the sleeping person.

TRACHEOSTOMY CARE

Introduction

Rubbing of the tracheostomy tube and secretions can irritate the skin around the stoma. Daily care of the tracheostomy site is needed to prevent infection and skin breakdown under the tracheostomy tube and ties. Care should be done at least once a day; more often if needed. Children with new tracheostomy or children on ventilators may need tracheostomy care more often. Tracheostomy dressings are used if there is drainage from the tracheostomy site or irritation from the tube rubbing on the skin.

Equipment

- A clean tray with sterile cloth
- A sterile cotton tipped applicators (Q-tips)
- Gauze and 'unfilled' gauze

- Sterile water
- Hydrogen peroxide (1/2 strength with sterile water)
- Tracheostomy ties and scissors (if ties are to be changed)
- Two sterile cups or clean disposable paper cups
- Small blanket or towel roll.

Procedure

- Wash your hands.
- Explain procedure in a way appropriate for the child's age and understanding.
- Lay your child in a comfortable position on his/her back with a small blanket or towel roll under his/her shoulders to extend the neck and allow easier visualization and trach care.
- Open Q-tips, gauze and regular gauze.
- Cut the tracheostomy ties to appropriate length (if trach ties are to be changed).
- Pour 1/2 strength hydrogen peroxide into one cup and sterile water into the other.
- Clean the skin around the tracheostomy tube with Q-tips soaked in 1/2 strength hydrogen peroxide. Using a rolling motion, work from the center outward using 4 swabs, one for each quarter around the stoma and under the flange of the tube.
- Do not allow any liquid to get into tracheostomy tube or stoma area under the tube.
  Note: Some doctors recommend cleaning with just soap and water in home care, using hydrogen peroxide only to remove encrusted secretions. This is because daily use of hydrogen peroxide might irritate the skin of some children.
- Rinse the area with Q-tip soaked in sterile water.
- Pat dry with gauze pad or dry Q-tips.
- Change the tracheostomy ties if needed (See Changing a Tracheostomy Tube).
- Check the skin under the tracheostomy ties.
- Tuck pre-cut tracheostomy gauze around and under the tube flush to skin.
- Do not cut the gauze or use gauze containing cotton because the child may inhale small particles.
- Use precut tracheostomy gauze or unfilled gauze opened full length and folded into a U shape or use two gauze pads, one placed under each wing of the tube.
- Be sure the dressing does not fold over and cover the tube opening. Change the dressing when moist, to prevent skin irritation.
- Tracheostomy dressings may not be needed for older tracheostomy when the skin is in good condition and the stoma is completely healed and free from rash or redness.
- For tracheostomy tubes with cuffs, check with your doctor for specific cuff orders. Check cuff pressure every 4 hours (usual pressure 15–20 mm Hg). In general, the cuff pressure should be as low as possible while still maintaining an adequate seal for ventilation.
- Monitor skin for signs of infection. If the stoma area becomes red, swollen, inflamed, warm to touch or has a foul odor, call your doctor.
- Check with the doctor before applying any salves or ointments near the trach. If an antibiotic or antifungal ointment is ordered by the doctor, apply the ointment lightly with a cotton swab in the direction away from the tracheostomy stoma.
- Wash your hands after tracheostomy care.

Care of the Inner Cannula

The older children and teens have tracheostomy tubes with an inner cannula. Some inner cannulas are disposable (DIC: Disposable Inner Cannula). These should be changed daily, discarding the old cannula. Check with your equipment vendor regarding disposable cannulas. For the reusable cannulas, the cannula should be cleaned 1 to 3 times a day and more often if needed. Do not leave the inner cannula out for more than 15 minutes.

Equipment

- 1/2 strength hydrogen peroxide
- Sterile water or normal saline
- Two clean or sterile containers (small bowl or cup)
- Inner cannula brush (tracheostomy brush or sterile pipe cleaner).

Procedure

- Wash your hands.
- Explain procedure in a way appropriate for the child's age and understanding.
- Pour 1/2 strength hydrogen peroxide into a bowl or cup and normal saline or sterile water into the other.
- Open the gauze pad
- Remove the inner cannula
- Place the inner cannula into 1/2 strength hydrogen peroxide. Soak it for a few seconds and use the brush to clean secretions on the inside and outside of cannula.
- Place the cannula into normal saline or sterile water solution, soak and rinse.
- Dry off excess water with clean or sterile gauze pad.
- Suction through the outer cannula if needed.
- Replace inner cannula. Be sure the cannula is secure or 'locked' in place in the trach tube.
- Wash your hands.

Cuffed Tracheostomy Tubes

- A cuff is a soft balloon around the distal end of the tube that can be inflated to seal the trachea for children needing ventilator support or to help prevent secretions from entering the lungs.
- Avoid over inflating the tracheostomy tube cuff. The pressure of the cuff against the wall of the trachea can cause damage if it is too high. Two techniques that can be used to help avoid excess pressure are the minimal occluding volume technique and the minimal leak technique.
- Suction the trach tube if needed. After suctioning the tube, suction the mouth and above the trach cuff so that secretions do not go into lungs when cuff is deflated.
- Minimal Occluding Volume Technique: Deflate the cuff, then slowly begin reinjecting air (or sterile water depending on the type of tube) with a luer lock syringe. Place a stethoscope to the side of the child's neck near the trach tube. Inject air into the pilot line until you can no longer hear air going past the cuff. This means the airway is sealed. For children that are totally ventilation dependent, provide breaths with manual resuscitator.

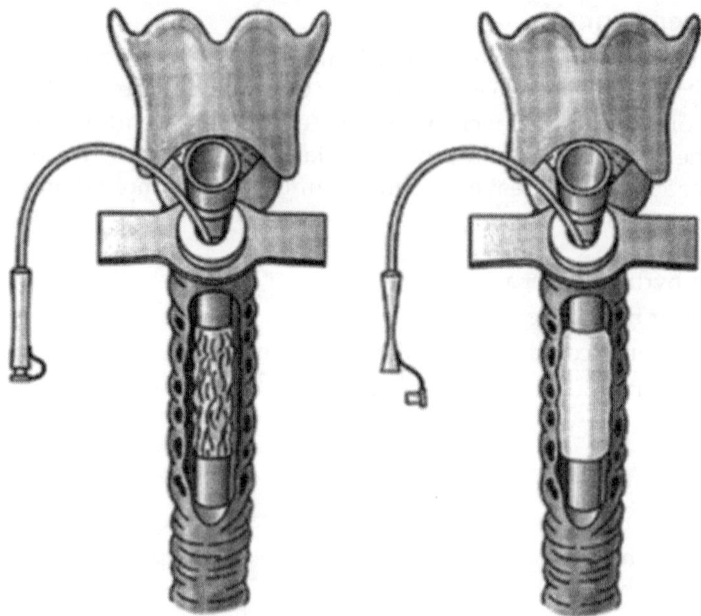

Fig. 4.25: Cuff deflation techniques

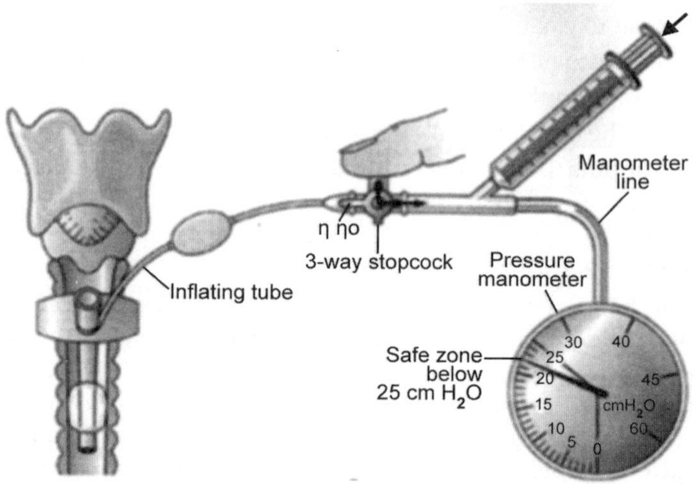

Fig. 4.26: Tracheostomy tube with cuff, pilot inflating balloon and pressure manometer

- Minimal Leak Technique: The same procedure as Minimal Occluding Volume, except that after the airway is sealed, slowly withdraw a small amount (approximately 1 cc), so that a slight leak is heard at the end of inspiration.

Periodic measurements of the cuff volume should be noted and any changes reported to the doctor. A pressure manometer may be used to check cuff pressure on balloons filled with air. Generally, cuff pressure should be below 25 cm H_2O.

STEAM INHALATION

Introduction

The steam inhalation is a common home therapy for upper respiratory tract infections and common cold. The child inhales the steam from heated water, thus bringing heat directly to the tissues of the nose, throat, and bronchial tubes, which may be swollen and painful as a result of infection. Medicines that vaporize are sometimes ordered so that the steam carries their vapor to the tissues.

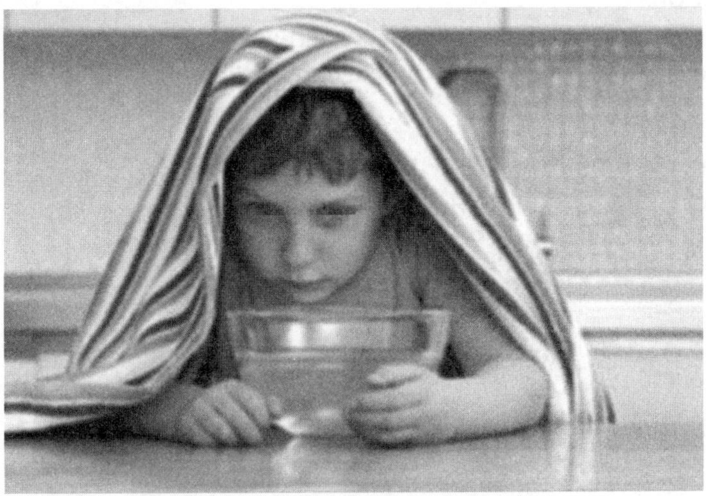

Fig. 4.27: Child with steam inhalation

Definition

A steam inhalation is defined as inhalation of warm, moist air into the mucous membranes and respiratory tract. It will loosen secretions and congestions.

Purpose

- Relieves inflammation and congestion of the mucous membranes of the upper respiratory tract.
- Relieves irritation (throat tickle) by moistening the air.
- Loosens secretions and stimulates expectoration.
- Relieves spasmodic breathing.
- Relaxes muscles and thus relieves coughing.
- Prevents excessive dryness of the mucous membranes.

Mechanism of Action

- Expectorate increase mucus from respiratory tract with hot, wet air
- Steam increase circulation and decrease congestion
- Aromatic oils increase penetration.

Indications

- Dry mucous membrane
- Pharyngitis and laryngitis
- Lung congestion
- Decrease cough
- Sore throat
- Spasmodic breathing.

Contraindications

- Cautious with children (better to have humidifier)
- Congestive heart failure child, it can make breathing more difficult.

Needed Equipment

- Boiling water in a kettle with spout.
- Hot plate of gas stove or local stove using charcoal.
- Vicks Vaporub, ointment or tincture of Benzoin or Camphor oil for good smelling sensation.
- Old newspaper.
- Umbrella.
- Sheets/Blanket.
- Paper Bag.

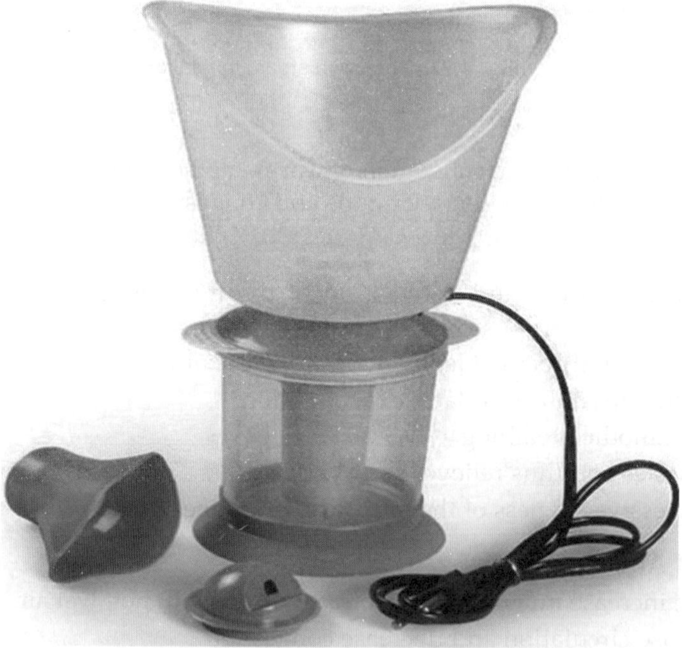

Fig. 4.28: Electronic steam inhalation

Procedure

Steam Inhalation to a Patient in Bed

- Explain the procedures to parents
- Assemble the equipment nearby child unit
- Provide comfortable position to child
- Measure the medication in ordered doctors, water level lower than the top of the kettle to prevent the medicine from staining the inside
- Support the patient's head with the extra pillow, place the extra covering over his shoulders
- Protect his hair with a towel and provide tissues to wipe the patient's face
- Arrange a tent adjust the opened umbrella or frame over the patient's head and shoulders, cover well with the blanket and leave an open air space in front
- Place the kettle with the steaming water on a protected surface at the bedside and fit one end of the funnel over the spout and open top of the kettle and the other end under the tent
- Keep the kettle out of reach of the patient
- Direct the steam toward the top of the tent and away from the patient's face
- Maintain steam in the kettle by changing the water when necessary
- Remain near at hand to give assistance if needed
- Discontinue the inhalation at the time indicated; remove the equipment
- Dry the child face prevents chilling
- The patient should remain quiet in a warm room for about an hour after the treatment
- Document on the daily record the time treatment was given and for how long, the patient's comments, and any improvement noted, such as easier breathing, less coughing, or less hoarseness.

Steam Inhalation to Sitting Position

- Protect the hair and shoulders
- The container with steaming water is placed in a basin at a comfortable height
- The paper sack is inverted over the container
- The patient leans forward and breathes in warm, moist air through the hole in the paper sack.

Inhalations to Babies and Infants

- Fill kettle with water just below the level of the spout and bring the water to boiling point. Add 1 tsp of medication (Vicks or Benzoin) into the boiling water.
- Carry the stove and the kettle with caution near the bedside of the patient, if the patient is unable to stand or sit on the chair or mother lap.
- Open an umbrella over the head of the patient and cover it with a sheet to form a tent.
- With the newspaper make a cylindrical tube direct to the steam into the tent away from the patient's face.
- Treatment time: 30 minutes to one hour, morning and evening, as tolerated.

Precautions

- She should avoid all risks of burning.
- Avoid drafts during time of treatment.
- Close windows near the child.
- Extra care must be observed.
- While doing the procedures should avoid scalding.
- Avoid chilling the patient after treatment.

NEBULIZATION

Definition

A nebulizer changes liquid medicine into fine droplets (in aerosol or mist form) that are inhaled through a mouthpiece or mask. Nebulizers can be used to deliver bronchodilator (airway-opening) medications such as albuterol, Xopenex or Pulmicort (steroid).

A nebulizer is a machine that converts liquid medication into a mist that can be inhaled. Nebulizers are often used in the treatment of asthma and other respiratory illnesses in young children up to age 3 years.

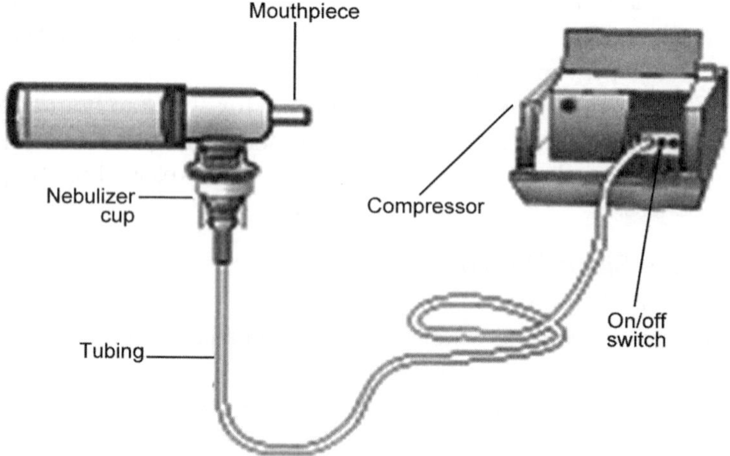

Fig. 4.29: Nebulizer machine

Indication

- Respiratory distress syndrome (RDS)
- Asthma
- Tightness in chest
- Increased or thick secretions
- Pneumonia (congestion)
- Atelectasis.

Needed Equipment

- Clean tray with sterile cloth
- Face mask
- Nebulizer
- Compressor oxygen tank (to drive nebulizer)
- Oxygen tubing
- Normal saline (cc vials)
- Medicine: Glucocorticoids, bronchodilators, antibiotics, mucus hydration agents, and mucolytic agents can be administered via aerosol.

Procedures

- Explain the procedures to parents
- Provide Comfort position to child
- Remove cup portion of the nebulizer
- Draw up prescribed amount of the mediation in the eye dropper/syringe
- Place medication in the medicine cup with 3 cc normal saline
- Return cup to the nebulizer
- Place oxygen tubing on the nipple on the nebulizer and attach other end to the compressor or oxygen tank
- Turn on the compressor or tank until mist is seen coming out of the mouthpiece
- Check the child pulse
- Connect nebulizer to mouthpiece/face mask and allow the child to take slow, deep breaths. If on a ventilator, the nebulizer can be placed in line in the ventilator circuit. To do this, remove the mouthpiece and connect the nebulizer between the dead space tubing and the exhalation valve assembly.
- During the treatment, monitor the pulse. If the pulse increases to more than 20 beats a minute, discontinue the treatment. Otherwise, continue until the medication is used up.

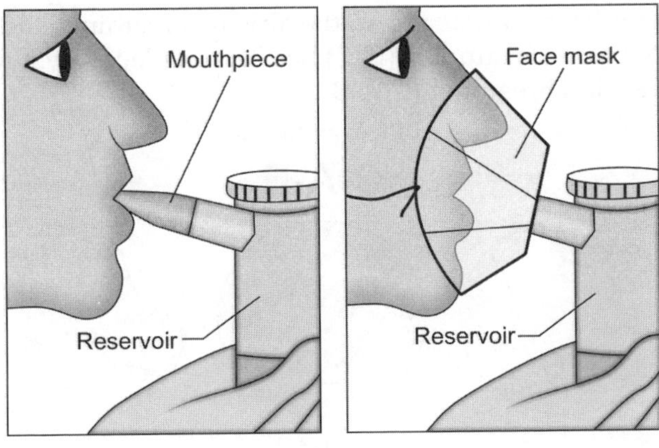

Fig. 4.30: Nebulizer face mask handling technique

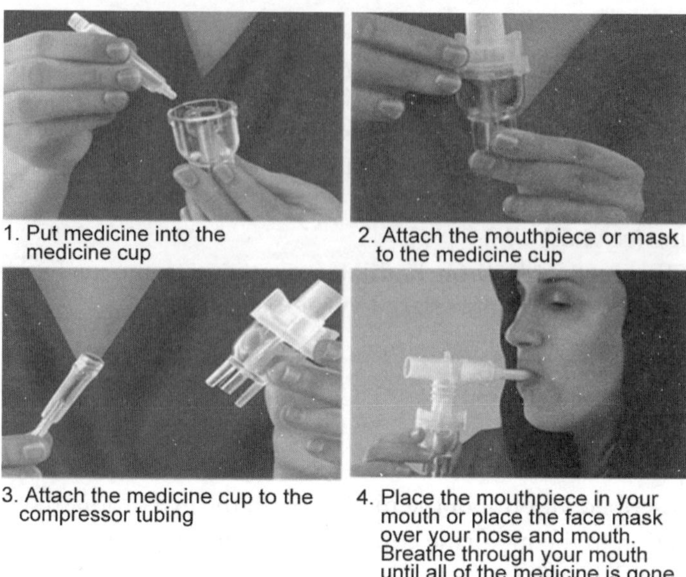

Fig. 4.31: Steps of handling nebulizer

- Following the treatment, use postural drainage, percussion, assisted coughing and/or suctioning, as appropriate.
- After the procedures, do the documentation.

OTHER PROCEDURES

PEDIATRIC ADVANCED LIFE SUPPORT (PALS)

Introduction

Pediatric Basic Life Support

An infant through adults in cardiac arrest, the airway, breathing, and chest compressions (A-B-C) sequence of basic life support (BLS) has been replaced by a new sequence: Chest compressions, airway and breathing (C-A-B).

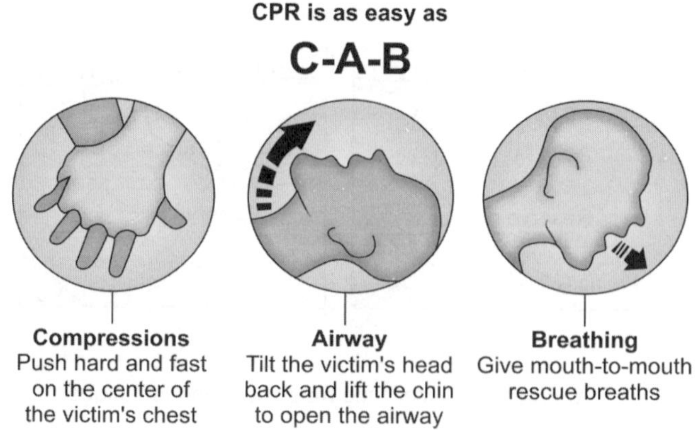

Pediatric Advanced Life Support

Pediatric advanced life support (PALS) usually takes place in the setting of an organized response in an advanced health care environment. In these circumstances, multiple responders are rapidly mobilized and are capable of simultaneous coordinated action. Resuscitation teams may also have access to invasive patient monitoring that may provide additional information during the performance of basic life support (BLS).

NEONATAL ADVANCED LIFE SUPPORT (NALS) NEONATAL RESUSCITATION PROGRAMME (NRP)

Introduction

The latest guidelines on neonatal resuscitation from American Heart Association (AHA) and European Resuscitation Council (ERC) were released in October 2015. There have been slight variations between these guidelines; although they use nearly identical literature for evidence evaluation. We present here the major changes in the recent guidelines and comparison between the ERC and AHA guidelines of 2015.

On October 15, 2015, the American Heart Association (AHA) and American Academy of Pediatrics released new 2015 Guidelines for Cardiopulmonary Resuscitation and Emergency Cardiovascular Care of the Neonate. The guidelines serve as foundation for the Neonatal Resuscitation Program (NRP), 7th edition materials that will be released in Spring 2016 and must be in use by January 1, 2017.

The authors believe that the Indian Academy of Pediatrics and the National Neonatology Forum of India will bring out India-specific recommendations to guide the resuscitation methods to be followed in India. This will ensure that the clinicians practicing resuscitation on a daily basis have some basis for their variance from International Guidelines.

Incidence

Approximately 10% of newborns require some assistance to begin breathing at birth. About 1% requires extensive resuscitative measures. Although the vast majority of newly born infants do not require intervention to make the transition from intrauterine to extrauterine life, because of the large number of births, a sizable number will require some degree of resuscitation.

Definition

Neonatal resuscitation is intervention after a baby is born; it helps the baby to breathe and start the heart beat. Before a baby is born, the placenta provides oxygen and nutrition to the blood and removes carbon dioxide. After a baby is born, the lungs provide oxygen to the blood and remove carbon dioxide.

Neonatal resuscitation is the set of interventions which may be necessary for a midwife to perform at the time of birth to support the establishment of breathing and circulation in the newborn, which can include neonatal intubation and umbilical vein catheterization (UVC).

Neonatal intubation is a procedure performed by midwives to establish access to the trachea, and/or suction meconium, to assist with ventilation of the newborn, immediately after birth.

Umbilical vein catheterization is a procedure performed by midwives to inject medication into the newborn's umbilical vein.

Equipment

• Clean big tray with sterile cloth	• Suction catheter (6,8 fr) – 1
• Sterile glove and mask – 1	• ET tube – 1
• Scissor and adhesive tape – 1	• Inj. Epinephrine – 1
• Cotton ball and gauze	• Inj. Adrenalin – 1
• AMBU bag with reservoir (500 mL + 250 mL) – 1	• Inj. Naloxone – 1
• O_2 face mask- 0,1 size – 2	• Inj. Sodium bicarbonate – 1
• Laryngoscope (0,1 size) – 1	• Bowl medium – 2
• Syringe 1, 2, 5 and 60 mL – 3	• Tray cloth – 1
• IV cannula (24, 26 Gaze) – 2	• Mucous extractor – 1
• NG Tube – 1	• Shoulder roll – 1
• Umbilical cord clamp – 1	• Stethoscope (pediatric) – 1
• Umbilical catheter – 1	

Neonatal Resuscitation Procedures

Steps

- Initial steps of newborn care
- Administration oxygen
- Positive-pressure ventilation
- Endotracheal intubation and laryngeal masks
- Chest compressions
- Medication
- Thermoregulation and stabilization of babies born preterm
- Ethics and care at the end of life.

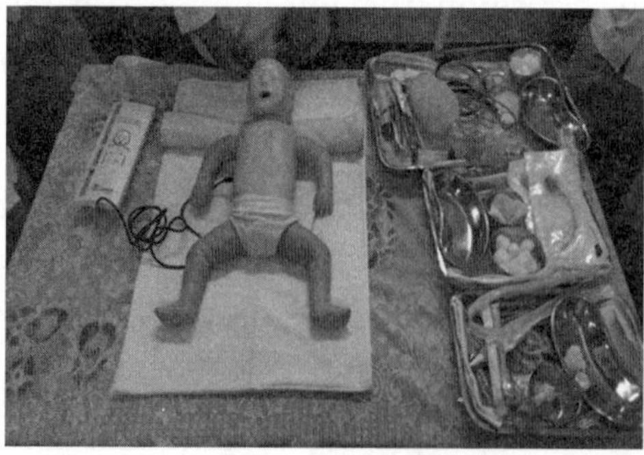

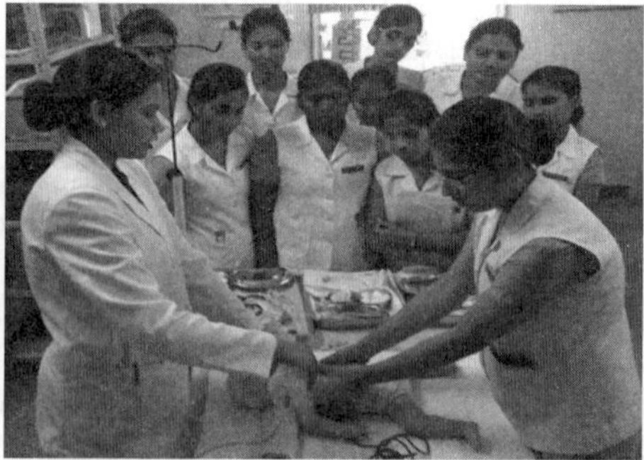

Fig. 4.32: Neonatal resuscitation procedures

Initial Steps of Newborn Care

Non-vigorous newborns with meconium-stained fluid do not require routine intubation and tracheal suctioning; however, meconium-stained amniotic fluid is a perinatal risk factor that requires presence of one resuscitation team member with full resuscitation skills, including endotracheal intubation.

Current evidence suggests that cord clamping should be delayed for at least 30–60 seconds for most vigorous term and preterm newborns. If placental circulation is not intact, such as after a placental abruption, bleeding placenta previa, bleeding vasa previa, or cord avulsion, the cord should be clamped immediately after birth. There is insufficient evidence to recommend an approach to cord clamping for newborns who require resuscitation at birth.

The initial steps of resuscitation are to provide warmth by placing the baby under a radiant heat source, position the head in a 'sniffing' position to open the airway, clear the airway with a bulb syringe or suction catheter, and dry the baby and stimulate breathing.

Administration of Oxygen

- Resuscitation of newborns greater than or equal to 35 weeks gestation begins with 21% oxygen (room air). Resuscitation of newborns less than 35 weeks gestation begins with 21–30% oxygen.
  - If a baby is breathing but oxygen saturation (SpO_2) is not within target range, free-flow oxygen administration may begin at 30%. Adjust the flow-meter to 10 L/min. Using the blender, adjust oxygen concentration as needed to achieve the oxygen saturation (SpO_2) target.
  - Free-flow oxygen cannot be given through the mask of a self-inflating bag; however, it may be given through the tail of an open reservoir.
  - If the newborn has labored breathing or SpO_2 cannot be maintained within target range despite 100% free-flow oxygen, consider a trial of continuous positive airway pressure (CPAP).

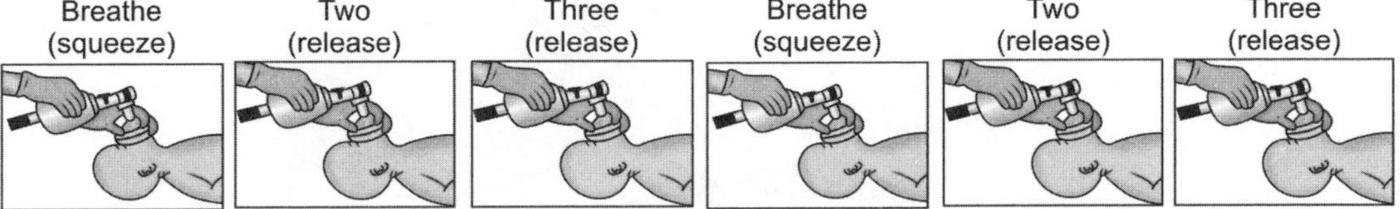

Fig. 4.33: Ambu bag technique

Positive-pressure Ventilation

- After completing the initial steps, PPV is indicated if a newborn is apneic or gasping or the heart rate is less than 100 beats/min. A trial of PPV may be considered if the baby is breathing and the heart rate is more than 100 beats/min but oxygen saturation (SpO_2) cannot be maintained within target range despite free-flow oxygen or CPAP.
- For PPV, adjust the flow-meter to 10 L/min.
- Initial ventilation pressure is 20–25 cm H_2O. When PEEP is used, the recommended initial setting is 5 cm H_2O.
- PPV is required for resuscitation of a preterm newborn, it is preferable to use a device that can provide PEEP. Using PEEP (5 cm H_2O) helps the baby's lungs remain inflated between positive pressure breaths.

- When PPV begins, consider using an electronic cardiac monitor for accurate assessment of the heart rate.
- The most important indicator of successful PPV is a rising heart rate. If the heart rate does not increase, PPV that inflates the lungs is evidenced by chest movement with ventilation. After intubation or laryngeal mask placement, inflation of the lungs is assessed by chest movement and bilateral breath sounds with ventilation.
- When PPV begins, the assistant listens for increasing heart rate for the first 15 seconds of PPV. You are attempting PPV but the baby is not improving and the chest is not moving despite performing each of the ventilation corrective steps (MR. SOPA), including intubation, the trachea may be obstructed by thick secretions. Suction the trachea using a suction catheter inserted through the endotracheal tube or directly suction the trachea with a meconium aspirator.

Endotracheal Intubation and Laryngeal Masks

- Intubation is strongly recommended prior to beginning chest compressions. If intubation is not successful or not feasible, a laryngeal mask may be used.
- Newborns greater than 2 kg and greater than 34 weeks' gestation require a size 3.5 endotracheal tube. The size 4.0 endotracheal tube is no longer listed on the NRP quick equipment checklist.
- The vocal cord guide on the endotracheal tube is only an approximation and may not reliably indicate the correct insertion depth. The tip-to-lip measurement, or depth of the endotracheal tube, is determined by using the 'initial endotracheal tube insertion depth' table or by measuring the nasal-tragus length (NTL).

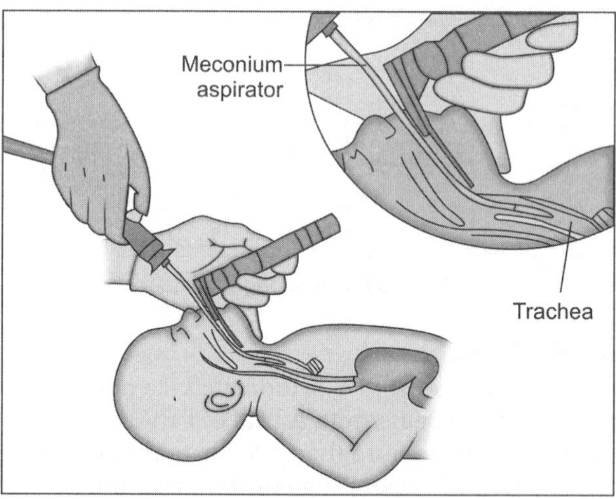

Fig. 4.34: Endotracheal intubation

Chest Compressions

- Chest compressions are indicated when the heart rate remains less than 60 beats/min after at least 30 seconds of PPV that inflates the lungs, as evidenced by chest movement with ventilation. In most cases, you should have given at least 30 seconds of ventilation through a properly inserted endotracheal tube or laryngeal mask.

- Chest compressions are administered with the 2-thumb technique. Once the endotracheal tube or laryngeal mask is secured, the compressor administers chest compressions from the head of the newborn and the person delivering ventilation via endotracheal tube or laryngeal mask moves to the side to make room for the compressor at the head of the newborn.
- An electronic cardiac monitor is the preferred method for assessing heart rate during chest compressions.
- Chest compressions continue for 60 seconds prior to checking a heart rate.

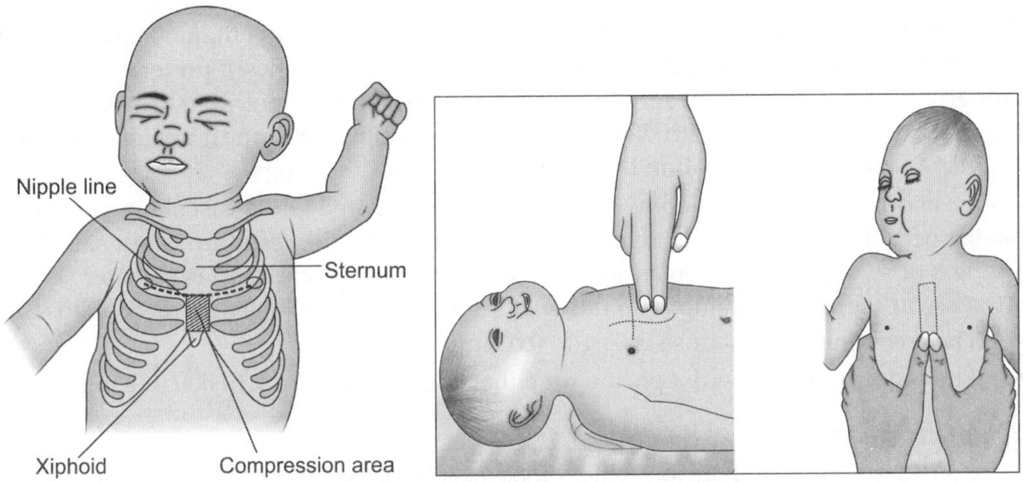

Fig. 4.35: Technique and methods of chest compression

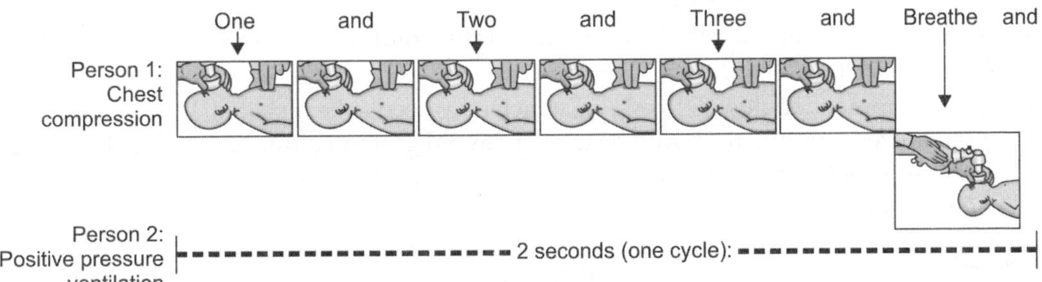

Fig. 4.36: Chest compression coordinating technique

Table 4.6: Initiating chest compressions rationale

Features	Newborn	Infant
Rate of compressions	120/minute	At least 100/minute
Depth of compressions	0.5–0.75 inches	0.5–1 inches
Compression: Ventilation ratio	3:1	5:1
No. of rescuers/staff nurse	2 or more	1 or more
Target heart rate	80/minute	60/minute

Medication

Drugs are rarely indicated in resuscitation of the newly born infant. Bradycardia in the newborn infant is usually the result of inadequate lung inflation or profound hypoxemia, and establishing adequate ventilation is the most important step to correct it. But if the heart rate remains < 60 bpm despite adequate ventilation with 100% oxygen and chest compressions, administration of epinephrine or volume expansion or both, may be indicated. Rarely, buffers, a narcotic antagonist, or vasopressors may be useful after resuscitation.

Epinephrine Administration

Epinephrine is indicated if the newborn's heart rate remains less than 60 beats/min after at least 30 seconds of PPV that inflates the lungs (moves the chest), preferably through a properly inserted endotracheal tube or laryngeal mask, and another 60 seconds of chest compressions coordinated with PPV using 100% oxygen. Epinephrine is not indicated before you have established ventilation that effectively inflates the lungs.

One endotracheal dose of epinephrine may be considered while vascular access is being established. If the first dose is given by the ET route and the response is not satisfactory, a repeat dose should be given as soon as emergency umbilical venous catheter (UVC) or intraosseous access is obtained (do not wait 3–5 minutes after the endotracheal dose).

- The recommended IV dose is 0.01 to 0.03 mg/kg per dose.
- The concentration of epinephrine for either route should be 1:10 000 (0.1 mg/mL).

Volume Expansion

- Consider volume expansion when blood loss is suspected or the infant appears to be in shock (pale skin, poor perfusion, weak pulse) and has not responded adequately to other resuscitative measures.
- An isotonic crystalloid rather than albumin is the solution of choice for volume expansion in the delivery room.
- The recommended dose is 10 mL/kg, which may need to be repeated. When resuscitating premature infants, care should be taken to avoid giving volume expanders too rapidly, because rapid infusions of large volumes have been associated with intraventricular hemorrhage.

Naloxone

- Administration of Naloxone is not recommended as part of initial resuscitative efforts in the delivery room for newborns with respiratory depression. If administration of naloxone is considered, heart rate and color must first be restored by supporting ventilation.
- The preferred route is IV or intramuscular. Given the lack of clinical data in newborns, endotracheal administration of naloxone is not recommended.
- The recommended dose is 0.1 mg/kg, but no studies have examined the efficacy of this dose in newborns. Naloxone may have a shorter half-life than the original maternal opioid; therefore the neonate should be monitored closely for recurrent apnea or hypoventilation, and subsequent doses of Naloxone may be required.

Sodium Bicarbonate

- Sodium bicarbonate should not be routinely given to babies with metabolic acidosis. There is currently no evidence to support this routine practice.

Thermoregulation and Stabilization of Babies Born Preterm

- In preparation for the birth of a preterm newborn, increase temperature in the room where the baby will receive initial care to approximately 23– 25 °C (74–77 °F).
- The goal is an axillary temperature between 36.5 °C and 37.5 °C.
- The anticipated gestational age is less than 32 weeks. Additional thermoregulation interventions, such as plastic wrap or bag and thermal mattress and hat, are recommended. 3-lead electronic cardiac monitor with chest or limb leads provides a rapid and reliable method of continuously displaying the baby's heart rate if the pulse oximeter has difficulty acquiring a stable signal. A resuscitation device capable of providing PEEP and CPAP, such as a T-piece resuscitator or flow-inflating bag, is preferred.
- The anticipated gestational age is less than 30 weeks, consider having surfactant available. Consider administering surfactant if the baby requires intubation for respiratory distress or is extremely preterm.

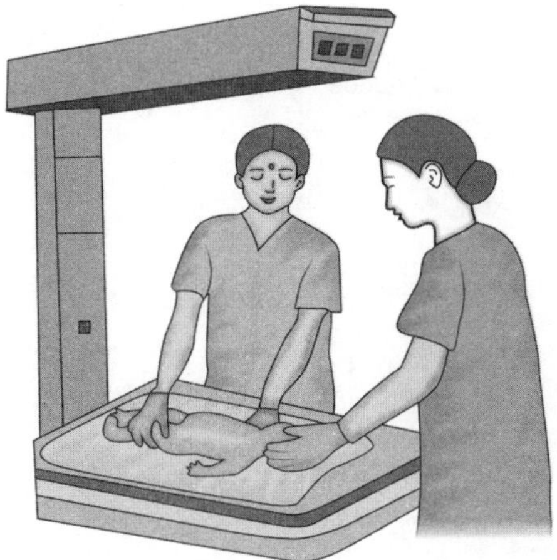

Fig. 4.37: Neonate baby under the radiant warmer

Ethics and Care at the End of Life

- If responsible physicians believe that the baby has no chance for survival, initiation of resuscitation is not an ethical treatment option and should not be offered. Examples include birth at a confirmed gestational age of less than 22 weeks' gestation and some congenital malformations and chromosomal anomalies.
- In conditions associated with a high-risk of mortality or significant burden of morbidity for the baby, caregivers should allow parents to participate in decisions whether resuscitation is in their baby's best interest. Examples include birth between 22 and 24 weeks' gestation and some serious congenital and chromosomal anomalies.

Neonatal Resuscitation Algorithm—2015 update

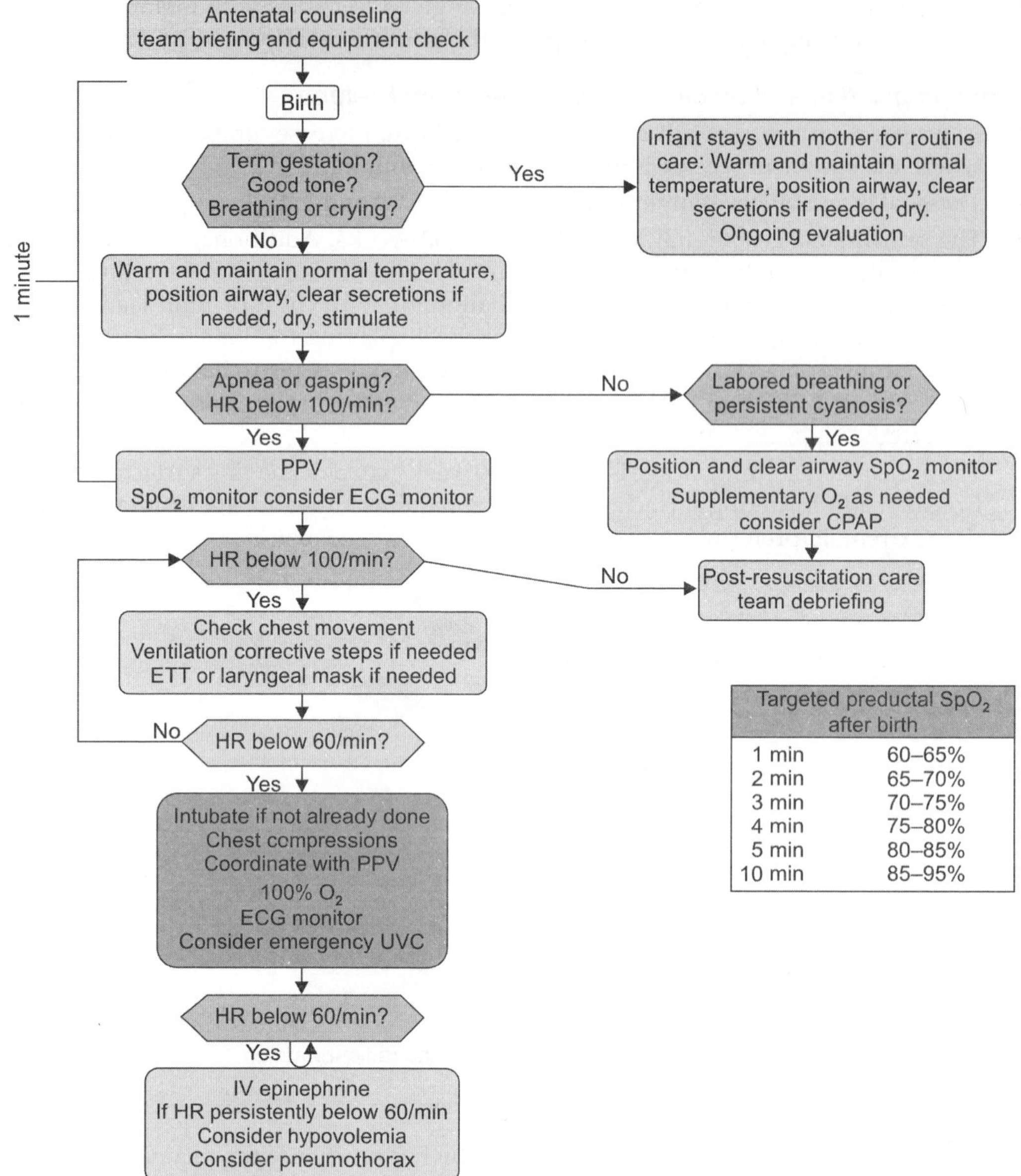

Targeted preductal SpO_2 after birth	
1 min	60–65%
2 min	65–70%
3 min	70–75%
4 min	75–80%
5 min	80–85%
10 min	85–95%

Post-resuscitation Care

Babies who require resuscitation are at risk for deterioration after their vital signs have returned to normal. Once adequate ventilation and circulation have been established, the infant should be maintained in or transferred to an environment in which close monitoring and anticipatory care can be provided.

- It should be noted that central cyanosis is normally present in the first few minutes after birth. Continuous positive airway pressure may be considered, particularly for preterm infants with labored respirations or persistent cyanosis; however, if their cardiorespiratory status fails to improve, oxygen, PPV and intubation should be considered.
- As described in the NRP textbook, post-resuscitation care includes temperature control, close monitoring of vital signs (e.g. HR, oxygen saturation and blood pressure) and awareness of potential complications and provision of the necessary support.
- It cannot be assumed that a baby who has been successfully resuscitated is healthy and requires only routine care; further stabilization may be necessary as a component of post-resuscitation care. For example, the new guidelines provide guidance for the management of newborns considered to be at risk for hypoxic-ischemic encephalopathy.
- Specific recommendations when signs of moderate to severe hypoxic-ischemic encephalopathy are present within 6 hours of age include consideration of therapeutic hypothermia according to an evidence-based protocol, with referral to and follow-up by a regional perinatal center.

Guidelines for Withholding and Discontinuing Resuscitation

Withholding Resuscitation

It is possible to identify conditions associated with high mortality and poor outcome in which withholding resuscitative efforts may be considered reasonable, particularly when there has been the opportunity for parental agreement. A consistent and coordinated approach to individual cases by the obstetric and neonatal teams and the parents is an important goal. No initiation of resuscitation and discontinuation of life-sustaining treatment during or after resuscitation are ethically equivalent, and clinicians should not hesitate to withdraw support when functional survival is highly unlikely.

The following guidelines must be interpreted according to current regional outcomes:

- Low birth weight and congenital anomalies are associated with almost certain early death and when unacceptably high morbidity is likely among the rare survivors, resuscitation is not indicated. Examples may include extreme prematurity (gestational age < 23 weeks or birth weight < 400 g), anencephaly, and chromosomal abnormalities incompatible with life, such as trisomy 13.
- In conditions associated with a high rate of survival and acceptable morbidity, resuscitation is nearly always indicated. This will generally include babies with gestational age 25 weeks (unless there is evidence of fetal compromise such as intrauterine infection or hypoxia-ischemia) and those with most congenital malformations.
- In conditions associated with uncertain prognosis in which survival is borderline, the morbidity rate is relatively high, and the anticipated burden to the child is high, parental desires concerning initiation of resuscitation should be supported.

Discontinuing Resuscitative Efforts

- Infants without signs of life (no heart beat and no respiratory effort) after 10 minutes of resuscitation show either a high mortality or severe neuro developmental disability.
- After 10 minutes of continuous and adequate resuscitative efforts, discontinuation of resuscitation may be justified if there are no signs of life.
- Document the procedures.

Table 4.7: Comparisons of the 2015 neonatal resuscitation guidelines changes with the 2010 guidelines

Resuscitation step	AHA 2010 recommendations	AHA 2015 recommendations	ERC 2015 recommendations	Remarks
Umbilical cord management	No recommendation given	• Delayed cord clamping (DCC) for > 30 • No recommendation for infants resuscitated at birth • Cord milking: Routine use is not recommended	• DCC for ≥ 1 min is recommended • No recom-mendation for infants resuscitated at birth • Cord milking: Routine use is not recommended	Delayed cord clamping recommended, however the minimum wait for clamping is different in both the newer guidelines
Normal temperature of newborn in the delivery room	No temperature range specified	The temperature of non-asphyxiated infants should be maintained between 36.5–37.5 °C	The temperature of non-asphyxiated infants should be maintained between 36.5–37.5 °C	The newer guidelines specifically mention the range of temperature which was missing till now
Interventions to maintain normal temperature	In VLBW (< 1500) preterm babies • Delivery room temperature to 26 °C • Plastic wrap • Exothermic mattress • Radiant heat	In infants < 32 weeks various combinations of following strategies should be used: • Radiant warmers and plastic wrap with a cap • Increased room temperature • Thermal mattress • Warmed humidified resuscitation gases	In infants < 32 weeks various combinations of following strategies should be used: • Radiant warmers and plastic wrap with a cap • Increased room temperature • Thermal mattress • Warmed humidified resuscitation gases	Additional strategies to maintain temperature are recommended for < 32 weeks rather than the weight criteria of < 1500 g. Use of warm humidified resuscitation gases is introduced
Warming of unintentionally hypothermic newborns (i.e. hypothermic after resuscitation)	No recommendation given	Either rapid (0.5 °C/h or greater) or slow rewarming (less than 0.5 °C/h)	No recommendation given	There has always been debate on how to rewarm newborns. The AHA 2015 recommends both methods
Maintaining normothermia in resource limited settings	No specific recommendation	• Covering the newborn in a clean food-grade plastic bag up to the level of the neck and swaddle them after drying • Skin-to-skin contact or kangaroo mother care	For babies born outside hospital setup. • Placement in food grade plastic bag after drying and then swaddling • Skin-to-skin contact care (in > 30 weeks)	AHA has separately introduced recom-mendations for maintaining normal newborn temperature in resource limited countries. The ERC gives similar recommendations for babies born outside ideal delivery environ-ment and thus can be applied to resource-limited countries

Contd...

Contd...

Resuscitation step	AHA 2010 recommendations	AHA 2015 recommendations	ERC 2015 recommendations	Remarks
Clearing the airway when meconium is present	Endotracheal suctioning in non-vigorous babies	• Routine intubation for tracheal suction in non-vigorous babies is not suggested • Initial steps followed by positive pressure ventilation (PPV) should be done as per routine indications	• Routine intubation for tracheal suction in non-vigorous babies is not suggested • Initial steps followed by PPV should be done as per routine indications. For suctioning use of 12–14 FG catheter, connected to a suction source ≤ 50 mm Hg • Routine surfactant is not recommended	This major change has wide implications for developing countries and it puts emphasis on earlier initiation of PPV in on-vigorous babies with meconium stained liquor (MSL)
Assessment of heart rate	No specific recommendation for heart rate measurement	Use of 3-lead electrocardiograpm (ECG) for measurement of the newborn's heart rate	Use of 3-lead (ECG) for measurement of the newborn's heart rate	It is doubtful if this will be utilized in resource-limited settings
Administration of oxygen in preterm infants	No earlier recommendation	• In newborns < 35 weeks of gestation begin resuscitation with low oxygen (21–30%) • Titrate according to the pre-ductal oxygen saturation	• In newborns < 35 weeks of gestation begin resuscitation with low oxygen (21–30%) • Titrate according to the pre-ductal oxygen saturation	A major change for preterms and reducess the complexity for the resuscitation team
Positive pressure ventilation (PPV)	Positive and expiratory pressure (PEEP) with PPV can be used at birth if suitable equipment is available	• Routine application of sustained inflation > 5 seconds is not recommended • Effectiveness of respiratory mechanics monitors and exhaled CO_2 monitors not established • In preterm newborns, along with PPV use approximately 5 cm H_2O PEEP • For PPV: Ventilate at a rate of about 40–60 breaths per minute	• Routine application of sustained inflation > 5 seconds is not recommended • For first 5 positive pressure breaths, maintain the initial inflation pressure for 2–3s. • Effectiveness of respiratory mechanics monitors and exhaled CO_2 monitors not established	Both ERC and AHA latest guidelines also talk about application of sustained inflation in initial few breaths. However, the recommended rate of PPV is different in both the guidelines

Contd...

Contd...

Resuscitation step	AHA 2010 recommendations	AHA 2015 recommendations	ERC 2015 recommendations	Remarks
			• In preterm newborns, along with PPV use approximately 5 cm H_2O PEEP • For PPV—Ventilate at a rate of about 30 breaths per minute allowing 1 second for each inflation	
Spontaneously breathing preterm infants with respiratory distress	Either continuous positive airway pressure (CPAP) or intubation with mechanical ventilation	CPAP is preferred than routine intubation	CPAP is preferred than routine intubation	Most resuscitation terms would be comfortable setting. Initiating it in the delivery room will require a paradigm change
Chest compressions	No specific recommendations were provided for oxygen use during chest compressions. However, it mentained providing 100% oxygen, in newborns with bradycardia even after 90 seconds of resuscitation with lower concentration of oxygen	• Give 100% oxygen with chest compression • Routine use of end tidal carbon dioxide ($ETCO_2$) monitors or pulse oximeters for detection of return of spontaneous circulation is not recommended	Recommended giving 100% oxygen with chest compressions, although mentions lack of evidence for the same	The 2010 AHA guidelines based, AAP-AHA neonatal resuscitation textbook, mentioned 100% oxygen with chest compressions [5], regardless of time of resuscitation, despite not being in the guidelines released in 2010
Induced therapeutic hypothermia	Only under clearly defined protocols and in places with multi-disciplinary care	Recommends use also in resource limited settings (I.e. lack of qualified staff, inadequate equipment)	• Only under clearly defined protocols and in places with multi-disciplinary care • Whole body cooling and selective head cooling are appropriate	Again taking into consideration the emerging evidence from developing countries. AHA recommends therapeutic hypothermia in resouce-limited settings also
Sodium bicrabonate infusion	No recommendation	No recommendation	• During prolonged arrests unresponsive to other therapies • Dosage: 1–2 mmol/kg; slow intravenous injection	Usage of sodium bicarbonate in prolonged arrests does not find any mention in AHA guidelines

Contd...

Contd...

Resuscitation step	AHA 2010 recommendations	AHA 2015 recommendations	ERC 2015 recommendations	Remarks
Prognostic tools	No recommendation given	No recommendation given	Combined Apgar appears to be a better predictor of outcome than routinely used Apgar score. In combined Apgar, the interventions needed to achieve the particular score are scored as well and a combined score is generated [6]	More studies are required to form a universal recommendation
Guidelines for withholding resuscitation	*Not indicated:* Conditions with a almost certain early death and or with high morbidity *Nearly always indicated:* Conditions with a high rate of survival and acceptable morbidity *Borderline:* In conditions with uncertain prognosis in which survival is borderline, and morbidity is high	Prognosis for < 25 weeks consider: • Accuracy of gestational age assessment • Chorioamnionitis • Available facilities • Region-specific guidelines to be followed	*Not indicated:* Conditions with almost certain early death and or with high morbidity *Nearly always indicated:* Conditions with a high rate of survival and acceptable morbidity. *Borderline:* In conditions with uncertain prognosis in which survival is borderline, and morbidity is high. • Comfort and dignity of the baby and family should not be ignored	AHA 2015 introduces regard for region specific guidelines. ERC 2015 mentions fixed criteria similar to AHA 2010

Recommendations that Remain Unchanged

Temperature control	Resuscitation should be performed with temperature-controlling interventions
Clearing the airway when amniotic fluid is clear	Routine suctioning is not recommended
Assessment of need of oxygen therapy	Oximetry should be used to monitor if any neonate needs PPV, with persistent and monitoring of oxygen therapy central cyanosis persists and with the use of supplementary oxygen
Administration of oxygen in term infants	Initiate resuscitation with room air. Supplementary oxygen may be administered to achieve appropriate pre-ductal oxygen saturation
Initial breaths and assisted ventilation	An initial inflation pressure of 20 cm water is adequate; some term babies may require up to 30 to 40 cm water. Rate of giving PPV 40 to 60 per minute

Contd...

Contd...

Endotracheal tube placement	Exhaled CO_2 detection is most reliable
Chest compressions	Coordinated chest compressions and PPV should be done if heart rate < 60 per minute after establishing effective ventilation
Epinephrine	IV dose - 0.01 to 0.03 mg/kg of 1:10 000 epinephrine. For an endotracheal route - 0.05 to 0.1 mg/kg
Volume expansion	Volume expansion when blood loss is known/suspected. Dose - 10 mL/ kg of isotonic crystalloid solution or blood, may be repeated

SURGICAL DRESSING

Introduction

The skin is the largest organ of the body, it cover 16% of body weight. It has several vital functions, which include immune function, temperature regulation, sensation and vitamin production. Skin is a dynamic organ in a constant state of change cells of the outer layers continuously shed and are replaced by inner cells moving to the surface. These guidelines have been developed by a range of clinicians who treat children with skin disorders, breakdowns and wounds; they reflect current research and evidence-based expert opinion.

Principles

- Practice Aseptic Technique procedure
- Wound cleansing should not be undertaken to remove 'normal' exudates
- Cleaning should be performed in a way that minimizes trauma to the wound
- Wounds are best cleaned with sterile isotonic saline or water
- Fluids should be warmed to 37 °C to support cellular activity
- Skin and wound cleansers should have a neutral pH and be nontoxic
- Avoid alkaline soap on intact skin as the skin pH is altered, resistance to bacteria decreases
- Avoid delipidising agents as alcohol or acetone as tissue is degraded
- Antiseptics are not routinely recommended for cleansing and should only be used sparingly for infected wounds.

Needed Equipment

- A clean tray with sterile cloth
- Kidney tray (small size)—1
- Small bowel—2
- Sterile glove—1
- Cotton swabs—1
- Scissor with adhesive tape—1
- Betadine solution—1
- Normal saline solution—1.

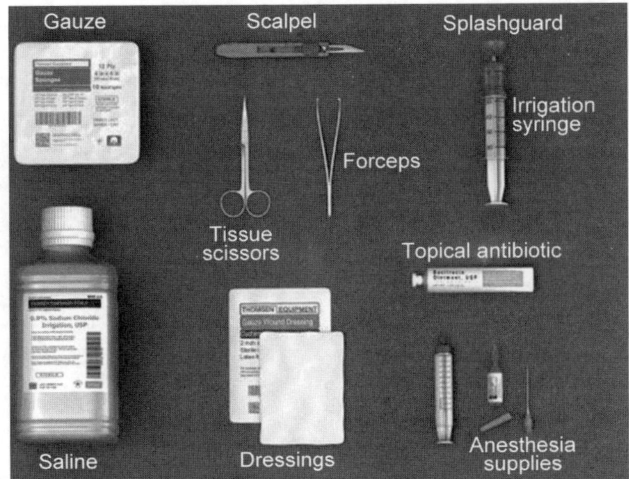

Fig. 4.38: Surgical dressing equipment

Procedure

- Perform sterile wash hands technique before and after dressing.
- Arrange the articles nearby child unit.
- Provide the comfortable position.
- Remove the old dressing and observe the condition of wound.
- Take the cotton swab and soak swab with betadine solution.
- Clean the affected area from the center outwards in a circular pattern.
- Clean only in circular pattern do not use back and forth motion.
- When the betadine solution is dry about 30 seconds, use another cotton swab soaked in the normal saline solution and repeat the procedure, cleaning from the center outwards as diagram indicates.
- Pick up two outer corners of the sterile gauze with your fingers. Do not touch gauze anywhere else to avoid contamination that may cause wound infection.
- Apply adhesive tape around all edges of gauze to keep wound clean and dry.
- It is very important to keep the dressing clean and dry.
- Document the procedure.

Steps in Surgical Dressing

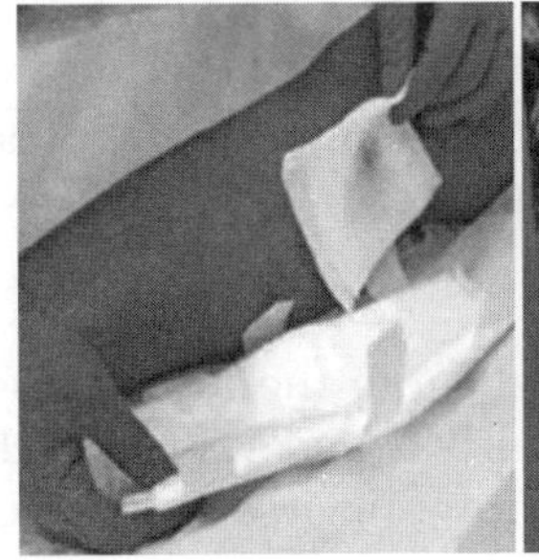

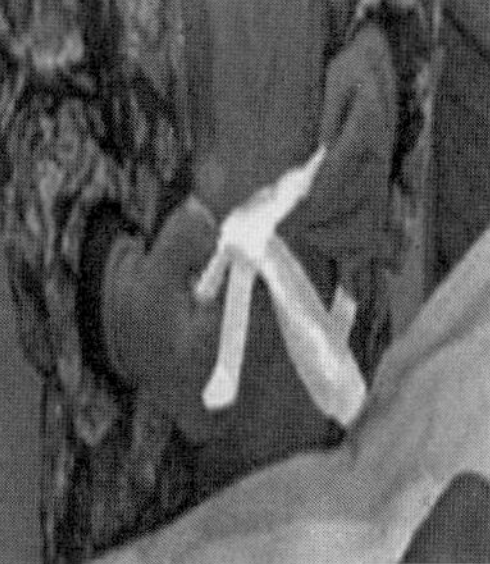

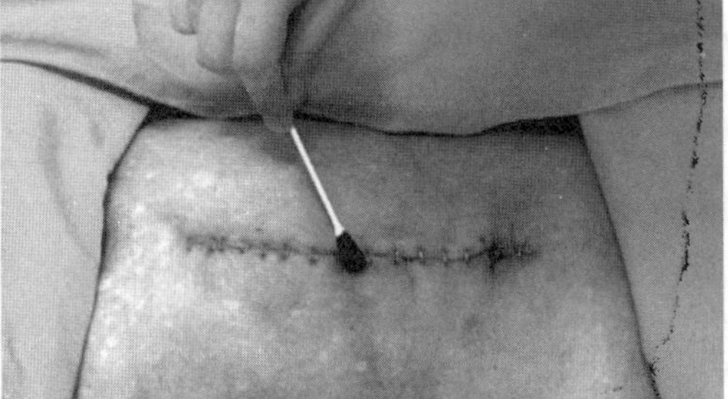

Removing the soiled dressing and inspecting the dressing and wound

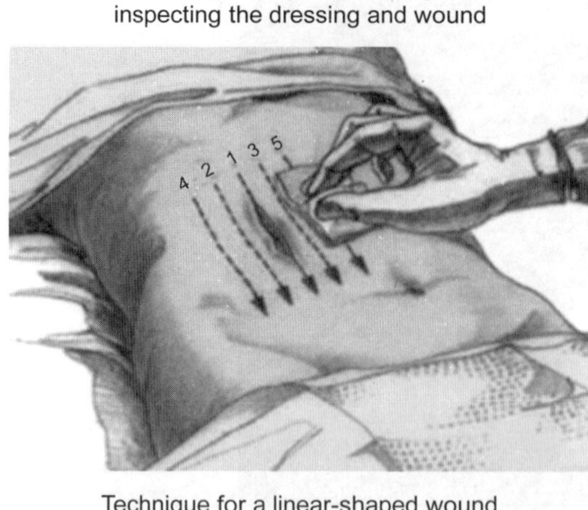

Technique for a linear-shaped wound

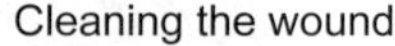

Cleaning the wound

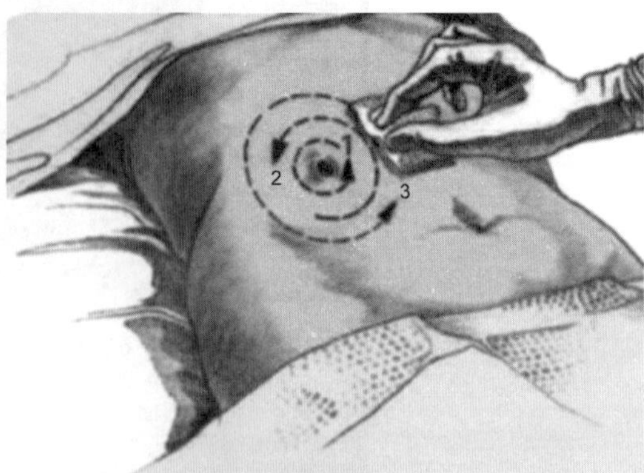

Technique for an open wound

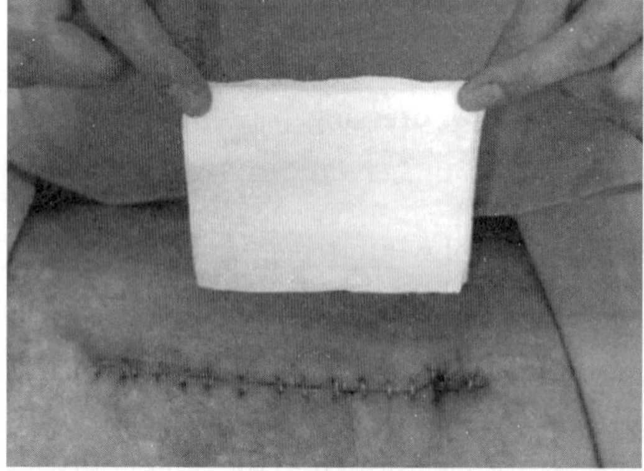

Fig. 4.39: Steps of surgical dressing procedure

LUMBAR PUNCTURE IN PEDIATRICS

Introduction

A lumbar puncture (LP) otherwise called as spinal tap. A lumbar puncture is a medical procedure carried out to obtain a sample of cerebrospinal fluid (CSF). CSF is a clear, colorless liquid that delivers nutrients and 'cushions' the brain and spinal cord or central nervous system.

Definition

A special hollow needle goes through the skin in the lower back, into the lower spine. The CSF comes out through the needle and a few drops are collected and sent to the laboratory.

Indication

Analysis of the cerebrospinal fluid can yield an important insight into the underlying pathological processes CSF can be analyzed for the presence of RBCs and WBCs (with differential), bacteria (Gram stain and other stains, culture and sensitivity), viruses (culture,

PCR), as well as glucose and protein levels. Other more sophisticated tests, such as neurotransmitter levels and metabolic markers may also be performed in certain situation.

- Suspected meningitis or encephalitis
- Suspected subarachnoid hemorrhage, only if CT scan is normal
- Diagnosing or ruling out sepsis in the neonatal period
- Other indications include diagnostic workup of certain malignancies, seizures, metabolic disorders and other neurological conditions (e.g. GBS).

Contraindications

- Coma
- Increased intracranial pressure (ICP)
- Cardiovascular problems
- Respiratory distress
- Suspected cerebral herniation
- Coagulopathy/thrombocytopenia
- Local infection at lumbar puncture site
- Vertebral anomalies.

Complications

- Postdural puncture headache (relatively common)
- Local back pain
- Infection
- Spinal hematoma
- Subarachnoid epidermal cyst
- Apnea
- Transient limp or paraesthesias
- Transient ocular palsy
- Cerebral herniation.

Equipment

- One trained assistant to hold the child
- Sterile gloves
- Sterile drapes and procedure tray
- Skin preparation: Povidone iodine solution (Betadine) or chlorhexidine
- Local anesthetic lignocaine, 2 ml syringe, 25 G needle
- CSF sample tubes (3)
- Spinal needle
- Manometer with stopcock.

Spinal Needles

- 22 G or 25 G beveled spinal needles with stylet (the use of needles without a stylet has an associated risk (rare) of spinal epidermoid tumors)

- Consider 25 G pencil point needles for older children/adolescents (e.g. 25 G 5 cm, 9 cm available in ED at RCH)
  - Pencil-point (blunt) needles reduce the risk of headache in adults, however the evidence is not convincing in children.

Procedures

Lumbar puncture especially pertinent to pediatrics, a topical anesthetic (e.g. EMLA cream) can be applied 30 to 60 minutes before performing the puncture to minimize pain on penetration. Either a sitting or lateral decubitus position can be used for lumbar puncture. Whichever approach is chosen it is important to monitor the patient visually and with pulse oximetry for any signs of respiratory difficulty as a result of assumed position. Have somebody help you hold the patient still to ensure adequate restraint during the procedure.

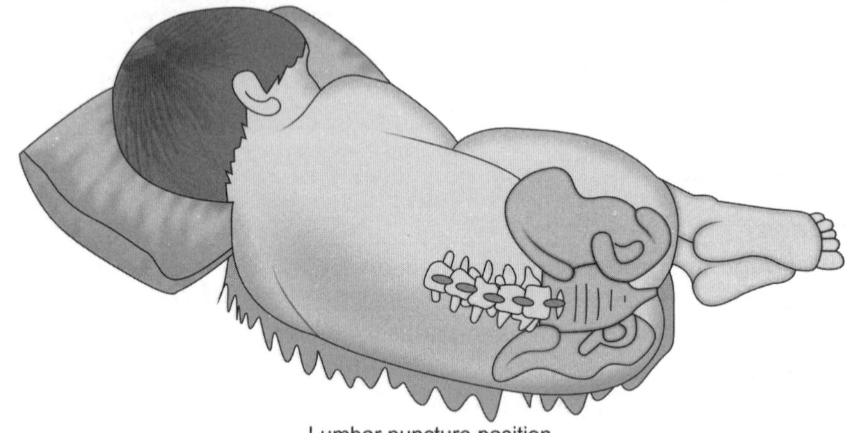

Lumbar puncture position

Fig. 4.40: C-Shape position for lumbar puncture procedures

Preparation

- Explain the procedure to parents and get the legal consent
- Wash hands and aseptically put on sterile gloves
- Prepare the skin with povidone-iodine or chlorhexidine and set up sterile drapes
- Allow adequate time for the skin preparation to dry
- Take the tops off the tubes, ensuring that they remain sterile
- Infiltrate the skin with 1% lignocaine using a 25 G needle.

Position

- Lumbar puncture may be performed with the child lying on their side or sitting up
- Aim for maximum flexion of the spine (curl into fetal position), but avoid over flexing the neck, especially in infants as this may cause respiratory compromise.
- Ask an adolescent to slouch rather than bend from their hips.
- Ensure that the plane of the back is exactly at 90 degrees to the bed (i.e. not leaning towards or away from you). Make sure the hips and shoulders are in line

- Draw an imaginary line between the top of the iliac crests. This intersects the spine at approximately the L3–4 interspace (mark this if necessary)
  - Near L3 at birth, but at L1–2 by adulthood
  - Aim for the L3–4 or L4–5 interspace.

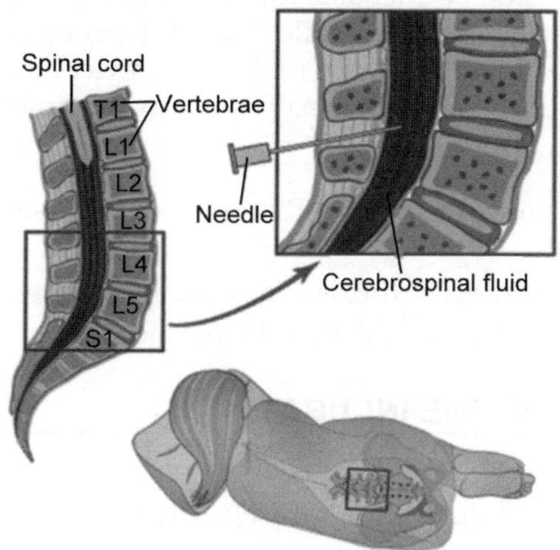

Fig. 4.41: Anatomical view of lumbar puncture procedures

Lumbar Puncture

- Position the needle in the midline with the bevel pointing towards the ceiling (lateral decubitus position) or to the side (sitting).
- Pierce the skin with the needle and pause. Wait for the child to stop wriggling.
- Reorientate (ensure that back is vertical, needle is parallel to the bed and perpendicular to the back). Aim for the umbilicus (i.e. slightly cephalad).
- Advance the needle into the spinous ligament (increased resistance). Continue to advance the needle within the ligament until there is a fall in resistance. Remove the stylet. If CSF is not obtained, replace the stylet and advance the needle slightly then recheck for CSF.
  - An alternative technique is to remove the stylet once the needle is in the ligament and advance very slowly without stylet watching for CSF to flow back. This has the advantage of making it harder to go unintentionally past the subarachnoid space.
  - If the needle meets resistance, withdraw the needle slowly whilst watching for CSF. If none is obtained, replace the stylet, reorient the needle and retry.
  - If blood stained fluid is obtained collect some for culture. If it clears it can be used for a cell count. If it fails to clear another attempt at a different level may be required.
- If CSF is flowing, collect into 2 numbered sterile tubes (5–10 drops each is usually adequate).
- Replace the stylet (this may reduce risk of headache), and remove the needle and stylet.
- Apply brief pressure to the puncture site.
- Send specimens urgently to the lab for microscopy, protein, glucose, culture. (NB CSF glucose estimation is most useful if there is synchronous plasma glucose).

Collecting a Sample

To collect a CSF sample, start with emptying the contents of the manometer into the first collection tube. Once the manometer is empty, detach it and continue with collection straight from the spinal needle. In general, a CSF volume of 1 cc obtained in each consecutive tube (usually up to 4 tubes) should be adequate for most analyses. In the neonate, 2 ml in total can be safely removed and in an older child 3 to 6 ml can be sampled depending on the child's size. When collection is finished, replace the stylet and remove the needle from patient's back. Apply first pressure, then a dressing to the puncture site.

Postprocedure Care

- Cover the puncture site with a band-aid or occlusive dressing (e.g. Tegaderm)
- Replace the articles
- Bed-rest following lumbar puncture is of no benefit in preventing headache in children.
- Monitor the child vitals before and after the procedures.

CARE OF BABY UNDER THE INCUBATOR

Introduction

The neonatal unit provides expert, round-the-clock care for newborn babies who are ill or born prematurely.

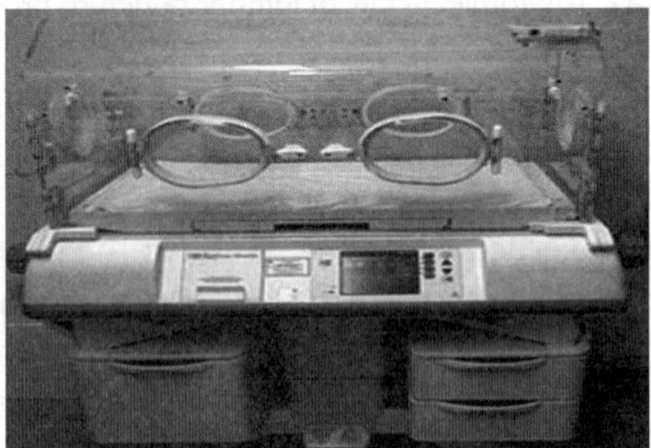

Fig. 4.42: Incubator cum radiant warmer

Premature babies or those born with much less weight than normal find it difficult to adjust to the external environment, immediately after being delivered. These infants stand the risk of catching various infections, and hence they need to be isolated and kept in incubators. Incubators provide intensive care to these babies and maintain suitable temperature and environmental conditions for healthy survival.

Incubator

- It is an equipment to provide optimal condition of temperature, humidity and oxygen for survival of preterm, low birth weight or high risk infants.
- It is important to delay or to prevent cold stress that produces additional hazards to the newborn as hypoxia, hypoglycemia and metabolic acidosis.
- Neutral thermal environment is one that permits the infants to maintain normal core temperature, with minimum oxygen consumption and caloric expenditure.

- Consumption of oxygen is minimal at abdominal temperature '36–36.5 °C', so when abdominal skin temperature is increased or decreased, oxygen consumption increases.

Types of Incubators for Babies and Infants

- Portable and nonportable
- Open box
- Close type
- Double walled
- Servo controlled.

Functions of Incubator

- **Oxygenation:** Providing the required amount of oxygen to the infant via oxygen control valves
- **Observation:** The baby is kept under observation. The incubator provides detailed measurement of respiration, temperature, brain activity, oxygenation, etc.
- **Isolation and protection:** Placing the baby in an incubator isolates it from external infections, noise, and climate. Incubators provide the required warmth and lessen the exposure of newborns to germs and other external factors.
- **Providing required nutrition:** The baby can be provided with the required nutrition inside an incubator through intravenous catheter or NG tube for fast recovery and development.
- **Medicines:** A baby needs regular medication, which can be easily and effectively provided in incubators.

Other Function

- Control temperature
- Humidity and oxygen concentration
- It provides high degree of isolation through slight
- It maintains positive pressure by air circulation
- A client probe to the abdominal skin as a guide in controlling the heater output of unit.

Parts of Incubator

- Incubator lights
- Temperature indicator meter
- Thermostat knob
- Patients prob
- Control point adjust button
- Red line adjust button
- Oxygen inlet
- Ice chamber
- Humidity control
- Humidity chamber
- Portholes and plastic sleeves

- Weighing facility
- Thermometer
- Plexyglass porthole
- Plastic bar
- Storage cabinet.

Note

1. The microfilter pad of the air filter at the rear of the incubator should be changed every three months.
2. Alcohol should never be used to wipe the plexyglass hood.

Indication

- **Premature babies**: Premature babies are weak and underdeveloped. They cannot cope up and sustain the conditions outside the womb, and hence require extra care.
- **Babies with very less weight**: Newborn babies who are underweight are also very weak and susceptible to various diseases. They need a lot of care and vigilance, and thus need to be kept in incubators.
- **Babies suffering from some illness:** Some infants might have infections or ailment that need intensive care and monitoring. Such babies are also kept in incubators for recovery and also to safeguard them from further infections or ailments.

Prepare the Incubator

- Prewarmed to a temperature appropriate to the infant's age, size and condition.
- Use in Air mode and must always be switched on with the motor running if in use for a baby.
- Check and record the incubator temperature hourly.
- Position away from draughts or direct sunlight.
- Do not routinely use on the humidity function while in use for babies in Starship hospital—this function is generally required for premature infants only.

Care of the Baby

Maintaining Temperature

- Prewarming the incubator up to the desired temperature before placing the infant in it.
- For infant weighing less than 1500 gm the incubator prewarmed to 34–36.1 °C.
- For infants weighing more than 1500 gm the incubator prewarmed to 34– 35 °C.
- When infant removed from incubator should be well wrapped in blankets to conserve heat.

Feeding

- The nurse can feed infant inside the incubator through porthole.
- Lift the baby to semi-sitting position for feeding.
- After the feeding burp the baby then place the baby on prone position or on left side after feeding to facilitate getting out of air and to avoid abdominal distension.

Bathing

- Daily skin care involves using of clean water only. Soiled linen is stripped of from the top slowly slipped down to the bottom.
- It is removed through the porthole at the foot end of the incubator.
- Clean linen is placed inside via the porthole at the head end and should be tucked well under the mattress.
- When infant is removed from incubator, the unit should be cleaned before reuse. All water should be removed from reservoirs.

Nursing Care of Infants in Incubator

Principles	Nursing responsibilities
General use	
Physician order should indicate amount of humidity, liter flow of Oxygen and its concentration.	• Observe and record the infant's responses. • Monitor the child reactions like cyanosis, retraction, grunting respiration, or hypothermia. • Give more attention to LBW baby. • At least one vacant incubator should be kept ready. • Don't place incubator on direct sunlight or near radiant warmer.
It is necessary to take body temperature of the infant to determine the amount of external heat required.	• Nurse should record infant temperature every hour until stabilized and then every four hours. • If temperature is elevated or subnormal, the temperature dial of the incubator should be adjusted.
Abrupt changes in the incubator temperature can cause untoward metabolic responses in the newborn that may result in apnea.	• Prewarming to 36.5–37 °C for infants less than 1500 g and to 34–36.1 to infants above 1500 g • The normal range of body temperature for a newborn is not always an exact reading of 98.6 °F/37 °C • Monitor body temperature and respirations
To maintain the atmospheric conditions constant, need not to open during routine care.	• No need of using masks and gowns for caring of infant in incubator. • Use the port holes of the incubator for providing care.
Expose the chest for effective observation of respiration.	• Infant need not be fully clothed, incubator provides stable atmospheric conditions during routine care.
Oxygen	
Oxygen therapy is more effective when interruptions in the oxygen administration are kept to a minimum.	• When the oxygen supply is not centrally located, the oxygen tank must be changed at intervals to ensure continuous therapy. • When the pressure gauge reading falls below 100 lb, the oxygen technician should be notified.
Low oxygen concentration-hypoxia-cause brain damage.	• The oxygen concentration should be checked every hour.
Excessive oxygen concentration damage the optic nerve.	• Incubator care requires organization of nursing care activities to prevent loss of oxygen, warmth and humidity.
Weaning	
Should be gradual process to avoid chilling due to the change from incubator temperature to room temperature.	• Dress and wrap the infant and open all the portholes. • After the incubator cooled, the infant may be removed and placed in a regular basinet.

Contd...

Contd...

Principles	Nursing responsibilities
Terminal cleaning	
Stagnant water harbors virulent pathogens. Thorough cleansing of the unit and removal of the water will prevent the spread of infection.	• When infant is removed from incubator, the unit should be cleaned before reuse. All water should be removed from reservoirs. • Alcohol, ether, or acetone should not be used to clean plastic parts.

RADIANT WARMER

Introduction

Radiant warmer is a mechanical device which is proving heat and maintains the body normal temperature of the baby. This device helps to maintain the body temperature of the baby and limit the metabolism rate. Heat has a tendency to flow in the heat gradient direction that is from high temperature to low temperature. The heat loss in some newborn babies is rapid such as LBW baby, Preterm baby and Hypothermic baby; hence Radiant warmers provide an artificial support to keep the body temperature constant. In certain areas with very cold climate, babies are kept on Radiant Warmer for couple of hours immediately after birth to ensure the baby is stabilized after birth.

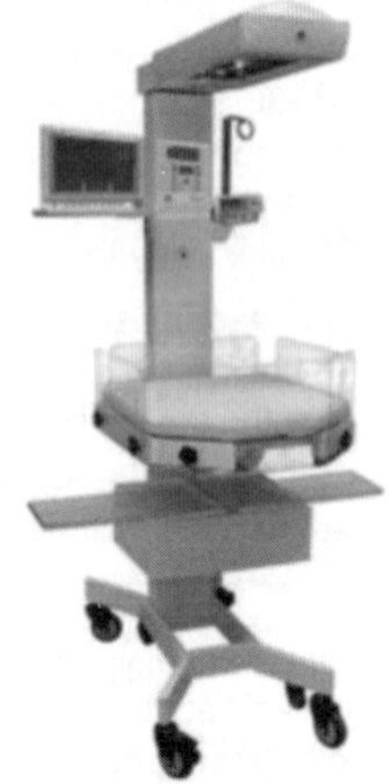

Fig. 4.43: Radiant warmer

Features of Radiant Warmer

Incubator Mode

- Air temperature control
- Baby temperature control
- Integral humidification
- Access doors two
- Access ports up to five.

Radiant Warmer Mode

- Maximum power 450 W
- Manual control
- Baby temperature control.

General Features

- Vertical height adjustment—foot-switch
- Canopy control foot-switch (raise only)
- Finger-switch (raise and lower)
- Mattress rotates—360°
- Electroluminescent control screen
- Four wheel locks X-ray tray
- Sliding storage draw
- Integral scales.

Mechanism of Radiant Warmer

Radiant Warmers can be manual or automatic (servo system—heater output is determined automatically based on skin temperature. The skin temperature is set at 36.5 degree celsius) depending on the mechanism that the manufacturer employs for temperature control. The heat generated and the temperature of the skin can be individually seen but the basic difference between these two models will be the regulation of temperature. The automatic model increases the heat output in small predetermined steps to reach at the desired temperature of the body. The device may seem simple to handle, but it is always recommended to have a proper training and read the manufacturers guidelines for person handling this equipment. It is necessary to regularly clean and disinfect the instrument.

Servo Mode

- Set temperature at 36.5 °C, heater output will adjust automatically to keep baby at set temperature.
- If baby temperature is below the set temperature, the heater output will increase, if baby is at set temperature or higher the heater output will become zero.
- Look for probe displacement when the baby is in servo mode. Check for and ensure proper probe placement every hour.

Manual Mode

- Once connected to mains heater output regulated by knob on front panel.
- The output is displayed as % or bars or bulbs.
- Use maximum (100% output) for rapid warming of bassinet in labor room 10 minutes before delivery.
  - Reduce output to 25–75% after 10 minutes depending on ambient temperature.
  - If left on with heater output > 80% alarm is activated within 15 or 20 minutes later and there after the heater output goes to 40%.
  - If alarm is silenced the heater will kept on for another 15 to 20 minutes as per manufacturers recommendation.

- For low birth weight or sick neonate adjust heater output depending on baby temperature. Never use full (100%) heater output unsupervised.
- Record baby temperature every 2–4 hourly.
- Use this mode only for prewarming, during resuscitation and initial stabilization.

Indication

- Hypothermic baby
- Low birth weight baby
- Preterm baby
- When an infant reaches 1700 to 1800 grams, has no respiratory distress and only occasional apnea, and has been stable in an incubator operated in the air temperature control mode with air temperature 32 °C or less, an attempt can be made to move him to a bassinet.

Role of Nurse in Radiant Warmer

- She should ensure that the temperature of the room is 22 °C.
- Place the warmer away from air currents.
- Clean the mattress and platform, and cover the mattress with clean linen sheet.
- The warmer at least 20 minutes prior to prewarm the linen and mattress so that the baby does not lie on a cold surface initially.
- If baby is in supine position place the skin probe on the right hypochondrium.
- When in prone position, place the probe on the lumbar region of the back. To prevent skin injury.
- Place Tegaderm and fix the probe on it with an adhesive.
- Ensure that the baby's head is covered with cap and feet secured in socks.
- The baby is clothed or covered unless it is necessary for the baby to be naked
- Partially undressed for observation or for a procedure.
- Place only one baby under each radiant warmer.
- Turn the baby frequently while under the warmer, if possible.
- Check the temperature of the warmer and of the room every hour, and adjust the temperature setting accordingly. Record the heater output in each shift (every 6 hours). Any sudden increase in heater output is an early indicator of sickness.
- Move the baby to be with the mother as soon as the baby no longer requires.
- Frequent procedures and treatment: If in servo mode the heater output is < 20%.
- It is safe to shift the baby to mother's side.

Check body temperature in 30 minutes and each hour for four hours; if the axillary or rectal temperature drops to below 36.5 °C, return infant to incubator, reheat on skin temperature servocontrol as described above, then revert to air temperature control; try again in two or three days.

Read Temperature on Display

- High: If baby temperature is below 36 °C
- Medium: If baby temperature is between 36–36.5 °C

- Low: If baby temperature is between 36.5–37.5 °C
- Once the baby's temperature is between 36.5–37.5 °C, switch on the servo mode/skin mode.

PHOTOTHERAPY UNITS

Introduction

Phototherapy has been in use since 1958 and has stood the test of time. Despite the use of phototherapy for over 40 years now, there are still many simple issues, which the treating physician should know. Phototherapy involves exposure of the skin of the jaundiced baby to blue or cool white light of wavelength 400–500 nm.

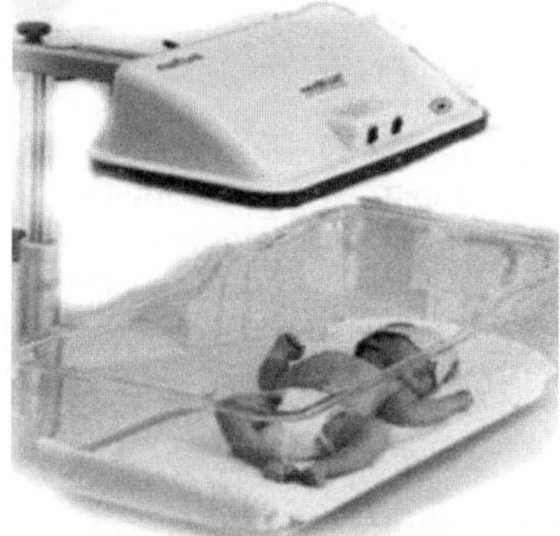

Fig. 4.44: Newborn baby under the phototherapy machine

Detoxification begins immediately by the production of configurational and structural photo-isomers of bilirubin in the skin and precedes the fall in serum bilirubin. Special lamps emitting light predominantly in these wavelengths are considered to be the most effective and specific for administering phototherapy. Its ability to bleach the infant's skin because its blue content is low. Besides, hyperpyrexia and skin burns may occur due to prolonged sunlight exposure.

Definition

Phototherapy (light treatment) is the process of using light to eliminate bilirubin in the blood. Your baby's skin and blood absorb these light waves. These light waves are absorbed by your baby's skin and blood and change bilirubin into products, which can pass through their system.

Types

There are two main types of phototherapy:

- **Conventional phototherapy**: Where your baby is laid down under a halogen or fluorescent lamp with their eyes covered to prevent damage to eyes.
- **Fiber optic phototherapy**: Where your baby lies on a blanket that incorporates fiber optic cables. Light travels through the fiber-optic cables and shines onto your baby's back.

Mechanism of Phototherapy

Phototherapy reduces the serum concentration of bilirubin and the risk of bilirubin toxicity. It has been found to be effective in treating hyperbilirubinemia in hemolytic as well as in nonhemolytic settings. This has dramatically reduced the need for exchange transfusion. Unconjugated bilirubin in skin gets converted into water-soluble photo-products on exposure to light of a particular wavelength (425–475 mm).

These photo-products are water soluble, nontoxic and excreted through the intestine and in the urine. Phototherapy acts upon bilirubin bound in the skin and sub-cutaneous tissue up to a depth of around 2 mm. It takes about 1–3 hours for fresh bilirubin from the blood to re-equilibrate into the tissue. For phototherapy to be effective bilirubin needs to be present in skin, hence there is no role for prophylactic phototherapy.

- **Configurational isomerization**: Here the Z-isomers of bilirubin are converted into E-isomers. The reaction is instantaneous upon exposure to light but reversible as bilirubin reaches into the bile duct. After exposure of 8–12 hours of phototherapy, this constitutes about 25% of total serum bilirubin (TSB), which is nontoxic. Since this is excreted slowly from body, this is not a major mechanism for decrease in TSB.
- **Structural isomerization:** This is an irreversible where the bilirubin is converted into bilirubin. This conversion is directly proportional to the dose of phototherapy. This product forms 2–6% of TSB and is rapidly excreted from the body. Thus this fraction is mainly responsible for phototherapy induced decline in TSB.
- **Photo-oxidation:** This is a minor reaction where photo-products are excreted in urine.

Types of Ultraviolet B (UVB) Phototherapy

UVB phototherapy is highly effective in patients who have moderate to severe psoriasis and thin plaques. Patients usually receive between 2 and 5 treatments per week. During treatment, the skin is exposed to UVB, which is generated from a special lamp or laser to enhance penetration of UVB rays.

An emollient is usually applied before exposure. UVB phototherapy may be combined with another psoriasis therapy, such as calcipotriene, tazarotene, anthralin or coal tar to increase effectiveness. UVB phototherapy proves to have few side effects. There are 2 types of UVB phototherapy:

1. Broadband (3–5 treatments per week)
2. Narrowband (2–3 treatments per week)

Broadband

This UVB therapy has been around for more than 80 years, and it is still highly effective. The biggest drawbacks are that the patient must travel between 3 and 5 times per week to a site that offers this therapy and that broadband light does not reach the scalp and areas where skin folds occur.

Narrowband

This newer form of UVB therapy is called 'narrowband' because it emits a narrower band of UVB wavelengths. Narrowband UVB therapy is proving to be more effective than the traditional broadband therapy. However, it does have the potential to produce severe burning. Like broadband, it is still not known if narrowband UVB therapy poses a long-term risk for development of skin cancer.

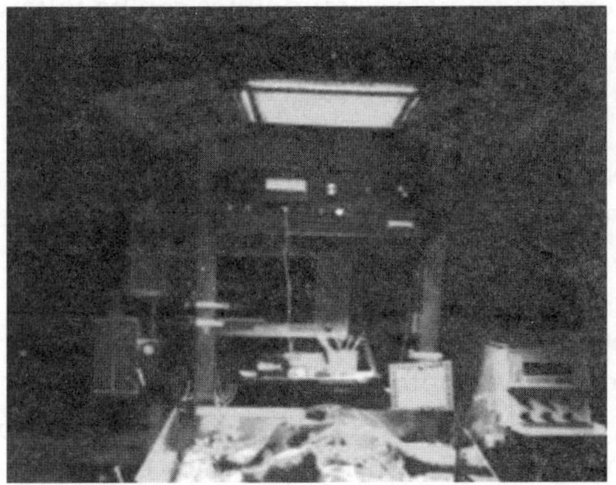

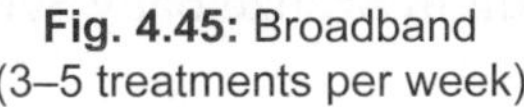

Fig. 4.45: Broadband
(3–5 treatments per week)

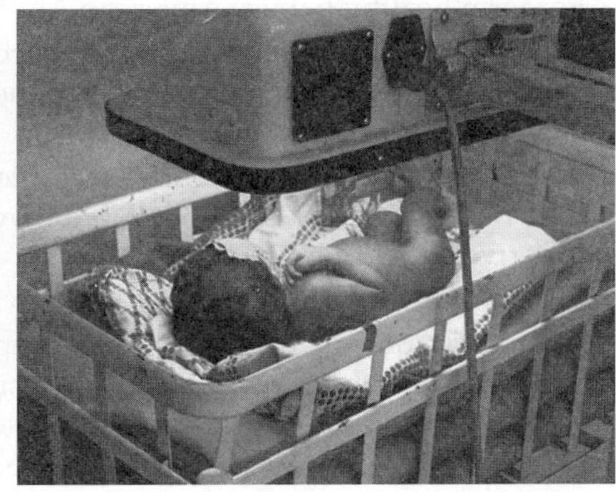

Fig. 4.46: Narrowband
(2–3 treatments per week)

The effectiveness of phototherapy depends upon:

- Area of skin exposed. Body surface area exposed to phototherapy determines the efficacy. Therefore, babies exposed to double surface phototherapy are reported to have faster decline of bilirubin levels.
- Gestational age and birth weight. In premature babies, the light waves penetrate deeper due to thin skin. Extended posture in preterm babies lead to exposure of greater surface area resulting in greater efficacy.
- Postnatal age. If the bilirubin level has already peaked, the effect of phototherapy is greater.
- Light dosage and spectral emission. There is a dose-response relationship, with increasing dosage of light, increasing response to phototherapy occurs.
- Distance of light source from the baby. The effective therapeutic output directed at the patient varies as Inverse Square of the distance. In other words, farther the phototherapy unit is from the patient, lesser will be the irradiance delivered. Keep in mind not to keep the unit too close to the baby, otherwise direct warming can occur.
- The general condition of neonate (well or sick) does not influence the efficacy of phototherapy.

Indications for Phototherapy

Neonatologists hold varying opinions about how much bilirubin is too much for the preterm neonate. Whether some of it actually has a free radical scavenging effect and when a term healthy neonate without hemolysis needs phototherapy are debatable issue. One needs to grasp the overall essence of the matter and not get mired in controversies. Broad guidelines are available which help us deal individual situations.

Simply put, phototherapy should be initiated whenever it appears that bilirubin could reach such levels that can cause bilirubin induced brain damage (BIND).

Each institution must create it's own guidelines. For an individual case, here are a few general guidelines that the pediatrician must be aware of before deciding to start phototherapy:

- For term healthy babies, American Academy of Pediatrics guidelines can be followed.
- Guidelines are provided for very low birth weight babies. As a rough guide, phototherapy is indicated at a level equal to 1% of the body weight (for e.g. 10 mg/dl in a 1000 gm baby or 15 mg/dl in a 1500 gm baby).
- Exchange blood transfusion is warranted when the TSB level is 5 mg/dl higher than the phototherapy level. However, the overall clinical situation needs to be considered to arrive at a proper decision.
- In case of hemolysis, start phototherapy at a lower level.
- Acidosis, asphyxia, hypoglycemia or sepsis makes the blood brain barrier less efficient and more susceptible to BIND. So, consider early phototherapy.
- In case of prolonged jaundice (> 3 week), one should always check fractional bilirubin estimation. Phototherapy is contraindicated in the presence of conjugated hyperbilirubinemia (> 2 mg/dl) because it may result in Bronze Baby Syndrome.

Features of Phototherapy Units

A light source designed to give an irradiance of 6 to 8 μw/cm²/nm in the 400–500 nm range at the surface of baby's skin is desirable. Harmful infrared and ultraviolet radiation should be filtered and light should be focused on the baby. It should preferably be a mobile unit which can be used for babies nursed in cots, incubators or radiant warmers.

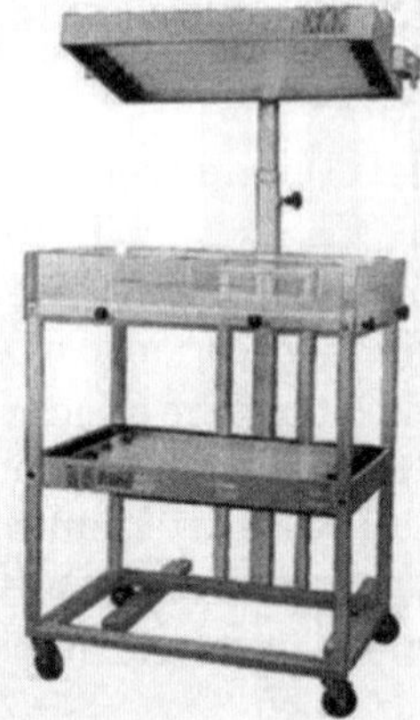

Fig. 4.47: Double surface phototherapy machine

The height should be adjustable, while a few units may be titled on axis. Phototherapy lights may or mounted on the radiant warmers themselves. A standard phototherapy unit consists of 6 to 8, fluorescent tubes (20 watts). To increase the effectiveness, double surface phototherapy is preferred.

- In recent years, halogen bulb spotlight phototherapy units have been available in the market. These can emit a relatively high level of irradiance compared with the conventional fluorescent tubes. Light of relatively narrow spectrum is emitted when a high voltage excites a mixture of halogens. They have a 150 watt, 21V halogen bulb with a specially coated reflector which absorbs infrared waves. A fan continuously cools the heated bulb. Options for varying aperture diameter and different filters are available. Positioning of the light on baby is critically important in determining the spotlight's effectiveness.

- They are most effective when delivered from directly above the infant at a distance of 45–50 cm. This should be measured in a vertical distance from the infant with a tape measure. Directing the light from the side of the crib or allowing the circle of light to move off the infant's largest surface area, e.g. abdomen, significantly reduces the dose delivered. A few halogen spotlights incorporate a dosimeter which depicts how much dose of phototherapy the baby has received. It considers the total irradiance received by the baby and multiplies this by the duration in hours.
- Combination of special blue and white fluorescent lights (2 special blue + 4–6 white fluorescent tubes) The blue tubes have the serial number F20T12/BB to be special phototherapy lights. This combination would deliver 12 μw/cm²/nm should have tubes replaced even though they still appear to be working. Again, directing the light from the side of the infant significantly reduces the dose delivered.
- 6–8 white fluorescent lights (20/40 watt each): These should be positioned above the infant and deliver 6–8 μw/cm²/nm. They also continue to appear effective despite giving minimal irradiance. If the irradiance delivered falls below 6 μw/cm²/nm the tubes need replacement.
- Bile-blanket: The latest phototherapy units are based on the principle of fibreoptics in which an illuminated blanket is wrapped around or placed under the baby which delivers light in the 425 to 475 nm waveband. The pad is cool and can be placed in direct contact with the baby. The unit consists of an illuminator with halogen bulbs which is connected by a fibre optic cord to an illuminator pad (blanket) on which baby lies. It ensures greater surface area of exposure.
- It minimizes infant/mother separation, has less risk for hypothermia or hyperthermia and does not increase insensible water loss. There is no need for occlusive eye patches. The blanket needs cleaning if solid and must be disinfected if used for another baby. The three settings on the unit deliver the following irradiance: low = 7 μw/cm²/nm. It can be used as a sole source of phototherapy or as an adjunct to conventional treatment by laying the infant on the blanket to give 'double phototherapy', i.e. increasing the surface area exposed.

Maintenance Tips for Phototherapy Units

- With flux-meter, measure the blue-green content of light output from the phototherapy equipment and replace the tubes or halogen light sources with new ones if the useful phototherapy output has fallen to two thirds of its original value.
- If a flux-meter is not available, it is better to keep a record of the hours each tube/bulb is used. In a phototherapy unit this facility is in built at an additional cost. Change halogen bulb or tubes every 1000 hours of use or every 3 months whichever is earlier.

Role of the Nurse

- Undress the baby completely. Cover the eyes to prevent damage by bright lights.
- Keep baby at a distance of 45 cm from the source.
- Provide frequent breastfeeding.

- Turn the baby after each feed to expose maximum surface area of baby to light.
- Monitor temperature every two to four hours or more frequently if fluctuation in temperature is noted.
- Record weight daily.
- Ensure that baby passes adequate urine (6–8 times per day).
- During breastfeeding switch off the phototherapy unit.
- Monitor bilirubin levels as per physician order at least one a day or more often.
- Discontinue phototherapy when serum bilirubin returns to a safe value as per unit protocol.
- Monitor clinically for rebound bilirubin rise within 24 hours after stopping phototherapy for babies with hemolytic disorders.
- Keep diaper area dry and clean because skin in this area is prone to break down.

Side Effects

Phototherapy is in use since the last 40 years and has an excellent safety record. The predominant adverse effects of phototherapy include rash, overheating, dehydration and diarrhea. Retinal damage is prevented by shielding the eyes. In vitro studies have suggested that DNA damage may be caused by phototherapy.

Advantages	Disadvantages
• Well-tolerated	• Cannot treat entire body
• See results quickly, sometimes in 2 weeks	• Treatment may be painful
• Fewer treatment sessions and shorter treatment time than with traditional UV therapy	• Darkening of the skin can occur
• Does not damage surrounding healthy skin	• Scarring possible
• Effective on treatment-resistant lesions, such as those that frequently occur on the elbows and knees	
• Most side effects mild: redness, blistering, erosion	

Recently, the effect of phototherapy on cerebral blood flow velocity (CBFV) has been reported. Phototherapy increased mean CBFV in all preterm infants, which returned to pretherapy values after discontinuation of phototherapy only in non-ventilated babies. Even in term babies, phototherapy increased CBFV, which returned to pretherapy level upon discontinuation of phototherapy. In addition, phototherapy influences cytokine production by peripheral mononuclear blood cells.

Phototherapy also has photo-oxidative effects on intravenous lipids, proteins and drugs like amphotericin B. phototherapy has been shown to affect short-term behavior of the term infant, which has been attributed to maternal separation. This least discussed and often overlooked aspect, is the most common side effect. So one should encourage the mother to breastfeed and interact with her baby regularly during phototherapy.

Caution

- Do not use phototherapy without trying to find the cause of jaundice.
- Phototherapy results in dehydration and iatrogenic hyperthermia/hypothermia.

- Blue light may interfere with monitoring of cyanosis. Blue light causes nausea, giddiness and headache, which may disturb the staff.
- In direct hyperbilirubinemia, phototherapy results in Bronze Baby syndrome (green color)

Most of us do not have a flux-meter to measure blue light output of phototherapy unit. We must remember that the phototherapy unit is not just a source of a visual illumination. It is biomedical equipment which needs to be serviced by a trained and knowledgeable person. Ensure that supplier/dealer of phototherapy unit has flux-meter with him and checks the efficiency of the phototherapy unit periodically.

Conclusion

Phototherapy continues to be the preferred method of treatment for neonatal hyperbilirubinemia by virtue of its safety and non-invasive nature. Appropriate use of phototherapy has significantly reduced the need for exchange blood transfusion. It is convenient and inexpensive. Hence, it has been immensely popular even in small hospitals and nursing homes. Any technology which is so easy to use and apparently safe is liable to be overused, at the cost unnecessary hospitalization and separation of the baby from the mother.

UMBILICAL CATHETERIZATION

Introduction

A procedure in which a radiopaque catheter is passed through an umbilical artery to provide a newborn with parenteral fluid, to obtain blood samples, or both, or through the umbilical vein for an exchange transfusion or the emergency administration of drugs, fluids, or volume expanders.

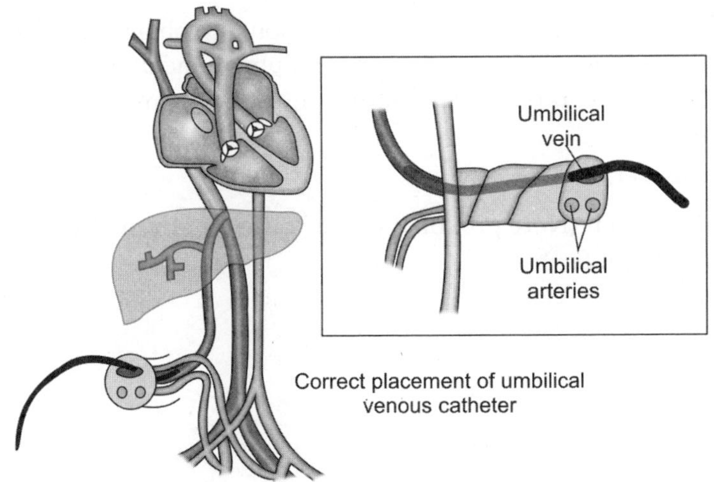

Fig. 4.48: Anatomical view of fetal heart circulation

Types

- Umbilical Vein Catheterization
- Umbilical Artery Catheterization

UMBILICAL VEIN CATHETERIZATION

Introduction

Umbilical vein catheterization may be a life-saving procedure in neonates who require vascular access and resuscitation. The umbilical vein remains patent and viable for cannulation until approximately 1 week after birth. After proper placement of the umbilical line, intravenous fluids and medication may be administered to critically ill neonates when critically ill newborns present to the emergency department, peripheral access is preferred. If this is impossible, umbilical vein catheterization may be attempted.

Indication

- The principal indication for umbilical vein catheterization is to gain vascular access during emergency resuscitation.
- Alternative uses of the umbilical vein may include exchange transfusions and central venous access.

Contraindications

Absolute contraindications to umbilical vein catheterization include the following:

- Omphalitis
- Peritonitis
- Necrotizing enterocolitis.

Equipment

Before initiating the procedure, a radiant warmer should be obtained, and the patient should be connected to a cardiac monitor. Necessary equipment includes the following:

- Personal protective equipment (i.e. sterile gown, gloves, mask)
- Sterile drapes
- Umbilical catheter, 3.5 F or 5 F

5 F—Umbilical catheter. (Note proximal part of catheter attached with stopcock).

- Iris forceps without teeth
- Small clamps
- Scalpel
- Scissors
- Needle holder
- Silk suture (3–0) or umbilical tape
- Intravenous tube—3 way stopcock
- Infusion solution (dextrose 5% in water or 0.9% sodium chloride [NaCl] with heparin 1 U/mL solution).

Position

The newborn should be restrained in a supine position and placed beneath a radiant warmer.

Procedure

- The umbilical cord stump and surrounding abdomen should be sterilized with a bactericidal solution. Sterile drapes should be placed.
- A purse-string suture or umbilical tape is tied around the base of the stump to provide hemostasis and to anchor the line after the procedure.
- Using the scalpel, the cord is cut horizontally, approximately 1.5–2 cm from the abdominal wall. Two thick-walled small arteries and one thin-walled larger vein should be identified. The umbilical vein may continue to ooze blood.
- Hemostasis is achieved through tightening the umbilical tape or suture. The arteries do not usually bleed secondary to vasospasm.
- Forceps are then used to clear any thrombi and dilate the vein.

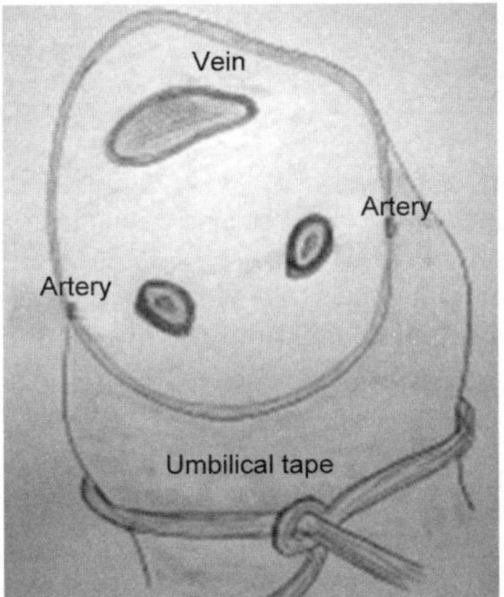

Fig. 4.49: Anatomy of umbilical cord

Dilating the Umbilical Vein and Clearing Thrombus

- A 3.5 F catheter is used for preterm newborns, and a 5 F catheter is used for full-term newborns.
- The catheter should be flushed with preheparinized solution and attached to a closed stopcock.
- The catheter is then grasped 1 cm from its distal tip with the iris forceps and gently inserted, aiming the tip toward the right shoulder. Advance the catheter only 1–2 cm beyond the point at which good blood return is obtained. This is approximately 4–5 cm in a full-term neonate. If resistance is initially met, loosen the umbilical tape or suture and manipulate the angle of approach.
- Do not force the advancement.
- Secure the catheter with a suture through the cord, marker tape, and a tape bridge.
- The position of the catheter must be confirmed radiographically. A properly placed umbilical vein catheter appears to travel cephalad until it passes through the ductus venosus.

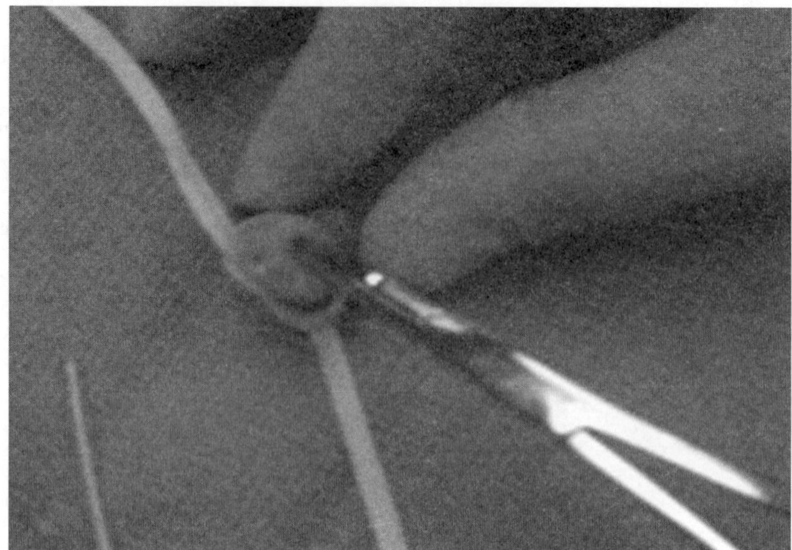

Fig. 4.50: Dilating the umbilical vein and clearing thrombus around cord

- Standardized graphs estimate the length of catheter insertion based on shoulder-to-umbilicus length. Alternatively, the shoulder-to-umbilicus length may be multiplied by 0.6 to determine a length that leaves the tip of the catheter above the diaphragm but below the right atrium.
- In an emergency resuscitation, the catheter is best advanced only 1–2 cm beyond the point at which good blood return is obtained.

Insertion of Umbilical Vein Catheter

- When identifying vessels, remember that the vein is usually located in the 12-o'clock position.
- To ensure an air-free catheter, fill the lumen with infusion solution and close the stopcock until the catheter is in the vein.
- Umbilical vein catheters may be placed in the inferior vena cava above the level of the ductus venous and below the level of the right atrium (10–12 cm). This acts as central venous access, allowing central venous pressure (CVP) monitoring, medication infusions, and the administration of hyperalimentation solutions.
- In an emergency, the catheter is best advanced only 1–2 cm beyond the point at which good blood return is obtained to avoid injecting hyperosmolar fluids into the portal vessels and causing liver necrosis.
- The catheter may be pulled back, but not advanced, once the sterile field is down.
- To avoid air embolism as the catheter is removed, tighten the purse-string suture or tape and apply pressure to the umbilicus.
- Intraosseous access is another option that can be used in neonates. Evidence suggests that intraosseous access may be obtained more rapidly than umbilical vein access.

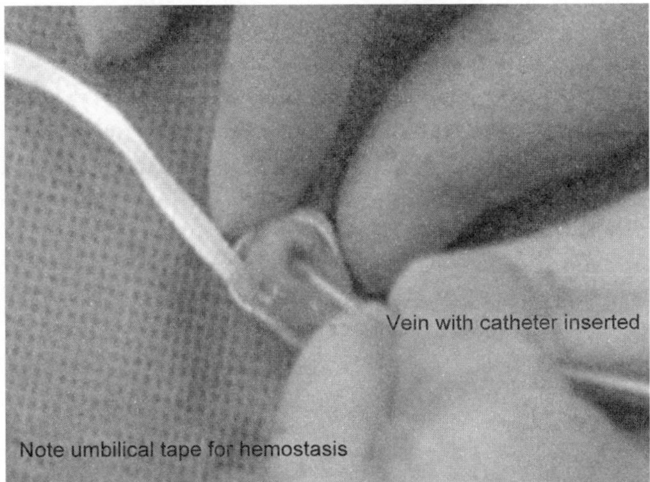

Fig. 4.51: Insertion of umbilical vein catheter

Complications of Umbilical Vein Catheterization

- Infection
- Hemorrhage
- Vessel perforation
- Creation of a false luminal tract
- Hepatic abscess or necrosis
- Air embolism
- Catheter tip embolism
- Portal venous thrombosis
- Dysrhythmia and pericardial tamponade or perforation (if the catheter is advanced to the heart).

UMBILICAL ARTERY CATHETERIZATION

Introduction

The first cannulation of an umbilical artery is attributed to Dr. Virginia Apgar in the late 1950s. Today, umbilical artery catheterization is a common procedure in the neonatal intensive care unit and has become the standard of care for arterial access in neonates. The umbilical artery can be used for arterial access during the first 5–7 days of life, but it is rarely used beyond 7–10 days. The placement of an umbilical artery catheter is easy in principle but often challenging in practice. Umbilical artery catheterization provides direct access to the arterial blood supply and allows accurate measurement of arterial blood pressure, a source of arterial blood sampling, and intravascular access for fluids and medications.

Indication

- Continuous arterial blood pressure monitoring
- Arterial blood gas sampling

- Blood sampling for other laboratory tests and studies
- Exchange transfusion
- Angiography
- Infusion of maintenance fluids when other routes are not available.

Contraindications

- Omphalocele
- Omphalitis
- Cord anomalies
- Peritonitis
- Necrotizing enterocolitis
- Vascular compromise to the kidneys, buttocks, or lower limbs.

Equipment

- Umbilical catheter insertion tray
  - Syringe, 1 mL
  - Syringe, 3 mL (2)
  - Syringe, 5 mL (2)
  - Hypodermic needle, 20 gauge
  - Mosquito hemostat, straight, 5 inch
  - Mosquito hemostat, curved, 5 inch (2)
  - Vessel dilator probe, 5 ½ inch
  - Iris forceps, full curve, 4 inch
  - Iris forceps, half curve, 4 inch
  - Iris forceps, straight, 4 inch, 1 × 2 teeth
  - Straight forceps, smooth
  - Hemostat needle holder, 5 inch
  - Straight Iris scissors
  - Safety scalpel with no. 11 blade
  - Silk suture, 4–0, with curved cutting needle
  - Umbilical tape, 15 inch
  - Measuring tape
  - Drape with 6 cm orifice
  - Gauze pads, 4 × 4 inch (6)
  - Gauze pads, 2 × 2 inch (6)
- Single lumen umbilical artery catheter
  - Catheter, 3.5 F (neonate weight < 1500 g)
  - Catheter, 5 F (neonate weight > 1500 g)
- Stopcock, 3-way
- Additional 5 mL syringes (2)

- Heparinized flush (0.45% sodium chloride plus 1:1 heparin)
- Skin preparation solution (4% chlorhexidine gluconate or povidone iodine)
- Sterile surgical towels (4)
- Surgical mask
- Surgical gown
- Sterile gloves
- Arterial pressure transducer.

Position

- The neonate should be placed in a supine position under a radiant warmer.
- The head of the neonate should be positioned toward the top of the warmer.
- Care must be taken to ensure adequate thermal support during the procedure, especially in neonates with extremely low birth weight.

Procedure

- Before beginning the procedure, restrain the neonate under the radiant warmer using soft arm and leg restraints.
- Prepare the catheter under sterile conditions by connecting the 3-way stopcock to end of the catheter. Connect 1 prefilled 5 mL syringe to each port of the stopcock. Flush the system with heparinized solution (0.45% sodium chloride plus 1:1 heparin). Ensure that no air bubbles are present in the system. Turn stopcock off to catheter.
- An assistant should hold the umbilicus upright with the cord clamp while the physician cleans the cord and an area of surrounding skin (approximately 3–5 cm around cord base) in sterile fashion with 4% chlorhexidine gluconate or povidone iodine solution.

Cleansing the Umbilical Stump

- Drape the neonate's abdomen with sterile towels, allowing adequate exposure to the umbilical cord and base.
- Place the umbilical tape at the base of the umbilicus. Tie a square knot around the base of the cord as close to the abdominal wall as possible. Tighten the knot securely to avoid bleeding after the umbilical stump is cut. Do not over tighten the umbilical tie, as this makes advancement of the catheter past the knot difficult and may impair blood flow to the skin distal to the tie at the umbilical base.

Tying the Umbilical Cord Base

- Cut the umbilical stump to within 1–2 cm of the abdominal wall using a no. 11 scalpel blade. Use a straight cut across with a gentle sawing motion.
- Identify the vessels in the freshly cut cord (a large, single, thin-walled umbilical vein and 2 small muscular arteries). Vessel identification and isolation is made easier by holding the edges of the cord with the curved 5-inch mosquito hemostats.

Identification of the Umbilical Artery

- Isolate 1 umbilical artery and carefully dilate the lumen using curved Iris forceps. Insert the tip of the forceps into the lumen as deeply as possible; then allow the forceps tips to spread open over 15–30 seconds while holding the tips in the vessel lumen.

Remove the Iris forceps tips from the lumen and repeat the dilation procedure. Perform the dilation technique 2–3 times until the lumen of the vessel appears dilated enough to accept the catheter.

- Grasp the end of the catheter, approximately 1 cm from the tip, with the half-curve Iris forceps. Hold the vessel lumen open with the full-curve forceps and gently insert the catheter into the dilated umbilical artery lumen.

Introduction of the Umbilical Artery Catheter into the Vessel

- Once the catheter is advanced into the lumen to a depth of 2 cm, remove the half-curve Iris forceps. If unable to advance catheter to 2 cm, withdraw the catheter and dilate the vessel again.
- Continue to advance the catheter to a depth of 4–5 cm, and aspirate to verify position in the lumen. If blood is easily aspirated, the catheter is within the lumen. Clear the catheter of blood by injecting 0.5 mL of heparinized flush.

Aspiration of Blood into the Umbilical Artery Catheter to Verify Intraluminal Position

- If resistance is met prior to this depth, try to loosen the umbilical tie.
- If a 'popping' sensation is encountered while advancing the catheter, the catheter has likely exited the lumen and created a false tract. If this occurs, remove the catheter and use the second vessel for catheterization.
  - Continue to advance the catheter to the predetermined depth. Once there, again aspirate to verify position in the aorta and flush the catheter. The catheter should draw and flush easily.
- If resistance is encountered in the first 5 cm during advancement, apply gentle steady pressure for 30–60 seconds to allow the vessel to relax.
- If blood is not easily aspirated after insertion, the catheter is likely outside the vessel in a false tract.
  - Once the catheter has been advanced to the predetermined depth, confirm placement with a chest and abdominal radiograph. The catheter tip should lie above the level of the diaphragm between thoracic vertebrae T6 and T9.
- On radiograph, the catheter should be seen entering the umbilical cord and then proceeding inferiorly to connect with the internal iliac artery. The catheter should be seen curving cephalad to enter the aorta and proceeding in a straight line to the left of the vertebral column.
- If the catheter is noted to be in the femoral artery or gluteal artery, pull the catheter back to a depth of 4–5 cm and attempt reinsertion. The femoral and gluteal arteries are not suitable sites for sampling, infusion, or blood pressure monitoring.

Umbilical Artery Catheter Incorrectly Positioned in Left Femoral Artery

- Once correct position is verified on radiograph, secure the catheter in place using a purse-string suture through the umbilical cord stump (not through the skin or vessels). This is done in 2–3 bites through the cord in an in-to-out manner. Secure the catheter to the stump by wrapping the tails of the suture snugly around the catheter and then tying securely with a surgical instrument tie.

- Further secure the catheter by way of a self-made or commercially available umbilical catheter bridge adhered to the abdominal wall.

Tape Bridge Placed to Secure Umbilical Catheters in Place

- Loosen and remove the umbilical tape once the catheter is secured.
- Connect the arterial pressure transducer and verify good arterial wave form.
- To remove the umbilical artery catheter, stop fluid infusion, cut retention suture, and pull the catheter back to a depth of 1–2 cm. Wait at least 5–10 minutes to allow the umbilical artery to constrict before removing the catheter. Use umbilical tape secured around the base of the cord if bleeding occurs. Alternatively, pressure can be applied to the iliac artery to control bleeding. Keep the neonate supine for 30–60 min after umbilical artery catheter removal to allow easy monitoring of bleeding.

Complication

Malpositioned Catheter

- Vessel perforation
- Refractory hypoglycemia (if infusing glucose-containing fluids and catheter tip near celiac axis)
- Peritoneal perforation
- Sciatic nerve damage.

Vascular Accident

- Thrombosis
- Embolism/infarction
- Vasospasm
- Loss of extremity
- Hypertension
- Paraplegia
- Heart failure (from aortic thrombosis)
- Air embolism.

Equipment-related

- Broken catheter
- Transection of catheter.

Other

- Hemorrhage
- Infection
- Necrotizing enterocolitis
- Intestinal necrosis or perforation
  - Vascular accident
  - Infusion of hypertonic solution
- Cotton fiber embolus
- Wharton-jelly embolus.

Role of Nurse in Umbilical Catheterization

- Within 1 hour of insertion of the catheter, the position of the tip is validated by X-ray examination.
- The rate of flow is checked hourly, and the IV bottle is never allowed to empty.
- All connections to the umbilical line are checked every 30 to 60 minutes, and only grounded electric equipment is used on or near the infant.
- At hourly intervals the young patient is repositioned, and the cardiac and respiratory rates are monitored.
- The axillary temperature is taken every 2 to 3 hours, and the pedal pulses are checked every 2 to 4 hours. The condition of the cord is observed every 2 to 3 hours for signs of infection such as redness, edema, or drainage at the catheter insertion site.
- The IV tubing is retaped when required, the cord dressing is changed, and antibiotic or antiseptic ointment is applied as ordered. If the umbilical line is displaced, pressure is quickly applied to the cord with a sterile 4 × 4 inch gauze, and an associate is delegated to notify the physician immediately.
- Fluid intake and output are measured.
- The infant is observed for oliguria or anuria; signs of vasospasm such as blanching, mottling, or darkening of the legs and absence of peripheral pulses; evidence of sepsis, hemorrhage, or oozing at the catheter insertion site; thromboembolism; and abdominal distension and vomiting, which may indicate necrotizing enterocolitis.

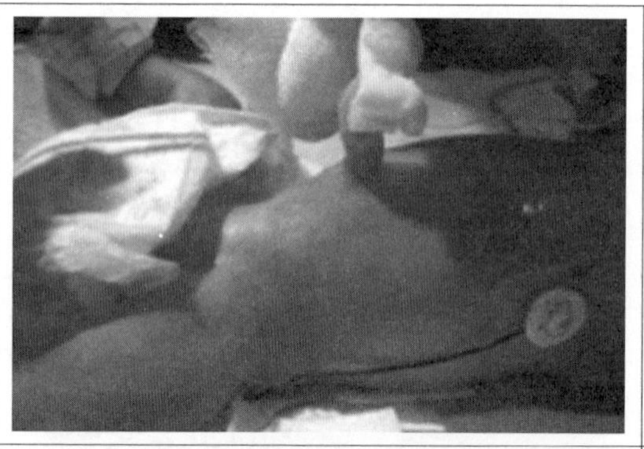

Cleansing the umbilical stump

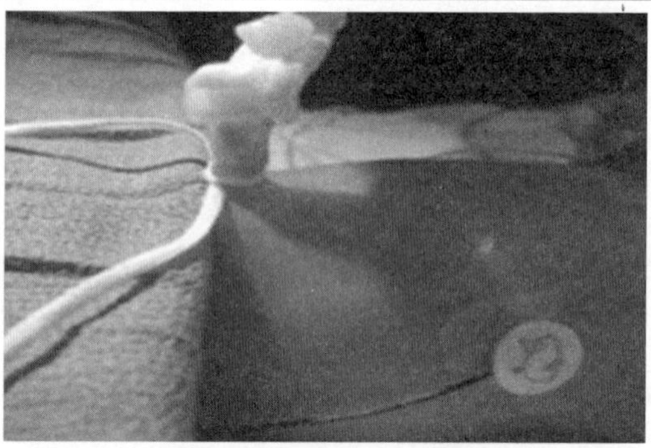

Tying the umbilical cord base

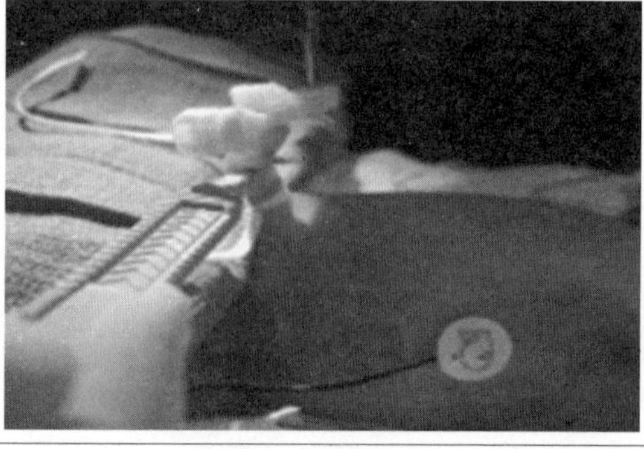

Cutting the umbilical cord

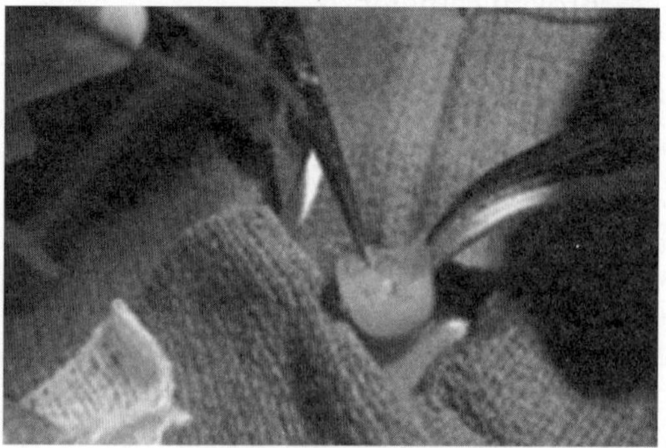

Identification of the umbilical artery

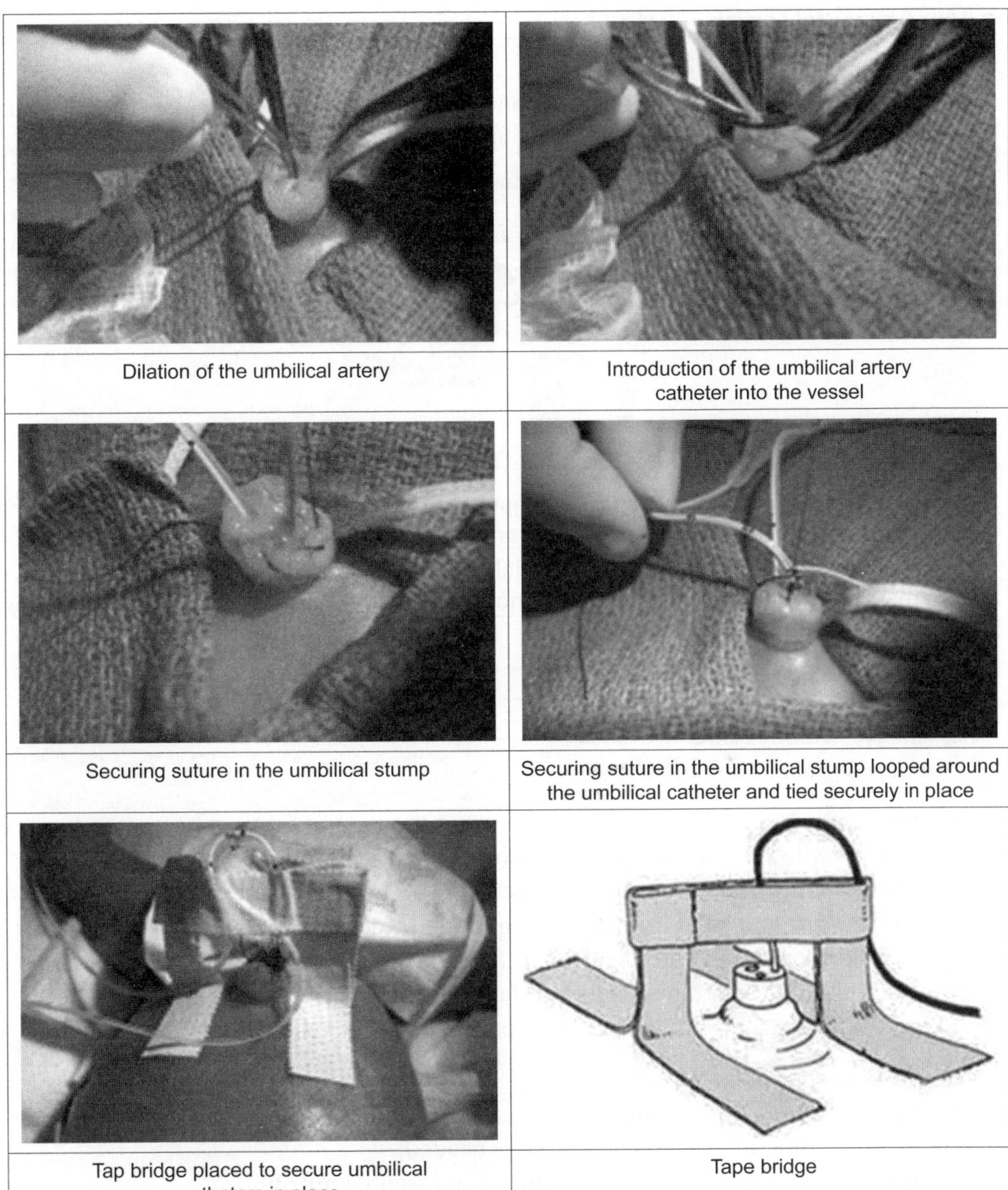

Dilation of the umbilical artery	Introduction of the umbilical artery catheter into the vessel
Securing suture in the umbilical stump	Securing suture in the umbilical stump looped around the umbilical catheter and tied securely in place
Tap bridge placed to secure umbilical catheters in place	Tape bridge

Fig. 4.52: Image view of umbilical catheterization procedures

Interventions

- The nurse provides ongoing care, monitoring the catheterized infant for any signs of complications, which are promptly reported. The family is included in the care of the infant as much as possible.

KANGAROO MOTHER CARE

Definition

Kangaroo mother care is defined as method of caring the preterm and low birth weight infants. It's a universally available and biologically sound method of newborns care.

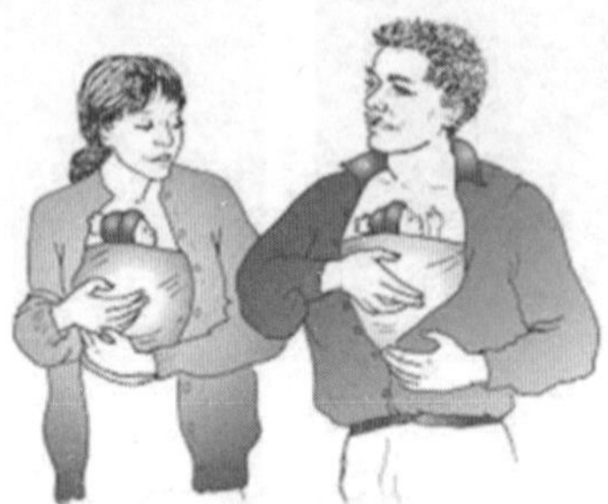

Fig. 4.53: Kangaroo mother and father care

KMC has been shown to prevent infections, promote breastfeeding, regulate the baby's temperature, breathing, and brain activity, and encourages mother and baby bonding.

Kangaroo Mother Care (KMC) is a special way of caring of low birth weight babies. It fosters their health and well-being by promoting effective thermal control, breastfeeding, infection prevention and bonding.

Component of KMC

- Skin-to-skin contact
- Exclusive breastfeeding
- Support to the mother and baby.

Skin-to-skin Contact

- It is between the baby front and the mother's chest.
- The more skin-to-skin contact, the better.
- A diaper is fine and a hat may be used for added warmth.
- Skin-to-skin contact should ideally start at birth, but can be started at anytime.
- Ideally it should be continuous day and night time.
- Skin-to-skin contact is still beneficial to both mother and baby.

Exclusive Breastfeeding

- Exclusive breastfeeding means that for an average mother can express from the breasts or direct suckling by the baby is all that is needed.
- Most of the premature babies need additional essential nutrition.

Support to the Mother and Baby/dyad

Support to the dyad/couplet means that whatever is needed for the medical, emotional, psychological and physical well-being of mother and baby is provided to them, without separating them. This might mean adding modern NICU equipment or providing emotional and psychological support.

Indications for Kangaroo Mother Care

KMC should be started after the baby is hemodynamically stable. Guidelines for practicing KMC include:

- **Birth weight > 1800 g:** These babies are generally stable at birth. Therefore, in most of them KMC can be initiated soon after birth.
- **Birth weight 1200–1799 g**: Many babies of this group have significant problems in neonatal period. It might take a few days before KMC can be initiated. If such a baby is born in a place where neonatal care services are inadequate, he should be transferred to a proper facility immediately after birth, along with the mother/family member. He should be transferred to a referral hospital after initial stabilization and appropriate management, one of the best ways of transporting small babies is by keeping them in continuous skin-to-skin contact with the mother/family member during transport.
- **Birth weight < 1200 g:** Frequently, these babies develop serious prematurity-related morbidity often starting soon after birth. They benefit the most from in-utero transfer to the institutions with neonatal intensive care facilities. It may take days to weeks before baby's condition allows initiation of KMC.

Purpose of Kangaroo Mother Care

Parents

- Enhanced attachment and bonding
- Increased milk volume, doubled rates of successful breastfeeding and increased duration of breastfeeding
- Physiologically her breasts respond to her infant's thermal
- Resilience and feelings of confidence, competence, and satisfaction regarding baby care.

Preterm and Low Birth Weight Infants

- Normal temperature, heart rate, and respiratory rate
- Breast milk is readily available and accessible, and strengthens the infant's immune system
- The maternal contact causes a calming effect with decreased stress and rapid quiescence (Reduced physiologic and behavioral pain responses)
- Increased weight gain
- Enhanced mother-infant bonding
- Positive effects on infant's cognitive development
- Less nosocomial infection, severe illness, or lower respiratory tract disease
- Restful sleep
- Earlier discharge
- Possible reduced risk of sudden infant death
- Normalized infant growth of premature infants
- May be a good intervention for colic
- Possible positive effects in motor development of infants.

Institutions/Hospital

- Shorter hospital stay
- Advanced healthcare technology only used in addition to kangaroo care
- Different monitoring of infants
- More parental involvement, with greater opportunities for teaching and assessing
- Better use of health care dollars.

The Community

- Less morbidity and mortality especially in developing countries
- Opportunities for teaching during pregnancy and follow-up in preparation for postnatal implementation
- Decreased use of financial resources
- Promotion of total family health.

Procedure

Step-1: Kangaroo Positioning

- The baby should be placed between the mother's breasts in an upright position.
- The head should be turned to one side and in a slightly extended position.
- This slightly extended head position keeps the airway open.
- Allows eye to eye contact between the mother and her baby.
- The hips should be flexed and abducted in a 'frog' position; the arms should also be flexed.
- Baby's abdomen should be at the level of the mother's epigastrium.
- Mother's breathing stimulates the baby, thus reducing the occurrence of apnea.
- Support the baby's bottom with a sling/binder.

Step-2: Monitoring

- The babies receiving KMC should be monitored carefully especially during the initial stages.
- Nursing staff should make sure that baby's neck position is neither too flexed nor too extended, airway is clear, breathing is regular, color is pink and baby is maintaining temperature.
- Mother should be involved in observing the baby during KMC so that she herself can continue monitoring at home.

Step-3: Feeding

- The mother should be explained how to breastfeed while the baby is in KMC position.
- Holding the baby near the breast stimulates milk production.
- She may express milk while the baby is still in KMC position.
- The baby could be fed with paladai, spoon or tube, depending on the condition of the baby.

Step-4: Privacy

- KMC unavoidably requires some exposure on the part of the mother.
- This can make her nervous and could be demotivating.
- The staff must respect mother's sensitivities in this regard and ensure culturally-acceptable privacy.
- Standards in the nursery and the wards where KMC is practiced.

Babies must be kept warm and dry. This method can be used continuously around the clock or for short periods per day gradually increasing as tolerated for infants who are compromised by severe health problems. It can be started at birth or within hours, days, or weeks after birth. Proponents of kangaroo care encourage maintaining skin-to-skin contact method for about six weeks so that both baby and mother are established in breastfeeding and have achieved physiological recovery from the birth process.

Promotion of Kangaroo Mother Care

Given the benefits of the kangaroo care method on mothers, babies, families, hospitals, health care workers and society, it is essential that it be promoted and implemented on a wider scale in developed and developing countries (Kennell, 2006). Further research and studies must be done to provide quality information for evidence-based practice in mother-infant care.

Advantages of Kangaroo Care for Mother

- Promotes bonding with the infant
- Increases mom's breast milk supply
- Mom can breastfeed earlier and longer
- Parents actually feel like PARENTS!
- Better prepared for discharge
- More confidence in caring for their infant
- Increased sense of control
- Easier to cope with stress and emotions of having a premature infant.

Advantages of Kangaroo Care for the Baby

- Promotes bonding with the parent
- Parent's heartbeat comforts the infant
- Increases deep sleep patterns
- Shorter hospital stay
- Increases ability to stay warm
- Increases oxygen level
- Reduces pauses in breathing
- Decreases episodes of a slow heart rate
- Breastfeed earlier.

Disadvantages of Kangaroo Care for Baby and Parents

- Limited to stable
- Weight-gaining

- Infants who meet specific hospital guidelines
- Time consuming
- Requires intense commitment.

Discharge Criteria

Generally the following criteria are accepted at most hospital/centers:

- Baby's general health is good and no evidence of infection
- Feeding well, and receiving exclusively or predominantly breast milk
- Gaining weight (at least 15–20 gm/kg/day for at least three consecutive days)
- Maintaining body temperature satisfactorily for at least three consecutive days in room temperature
- The mother and family members are confident to take care of the baby in KMC and should be asked to come for follow-up visits regularly.

Follow-up Care

- Pre-requisite of parents should be continued KMC practice in home.
- Although each unit should formulate its own policy of follow-up.
- In general, a baby is followed once or twice a week till 37–40 weeks of gestation or till the bay reaches 2.5–3 kg of weight. (Smaller the baby at discharge, the earlier and more frequent follow-up visits should be).
- Thereafter a followup once in 2–4 weeks may be enough till 3 months of post-conceptional age.
- Later the baby should be seen at an interval of 1–2 months during first year of life.
- The baby should gain adequate weight (15–20 gm/kg/day up to 40 weeks of post-conceptional age and 10 gm/kg/day subsequently). More frequent visits should be made if the baby is not growing well or his condition demands.

ARTERIAL BLOOD GAS (ABG)

Definition

An arterial blood gas (ABG) defined as a test measures the blood acidity level (pH) and the levels of oxygen and carbon dioxide in the blood from an artery. This test is used to check the child lungs are able to move oxygen into the blood and remove carbon dioxide from the blood.

Blood gas analysis otherwise known arterial blood gas (ABG) analysis, this test which measures the amount of oxygen (O_2) and carbon dioxide (CO_2) in the blood as well as the acidity (pH) of the blood.

- Drawn from artery—radial, brachial, femoral
- It is an **invasive** procedure
- Caution must be taken with patient on anticoagulants.

Arterial blood gas analysis is an essential part of diagnosing and managing the patient's oxygenation status, ventilation failure and acid base balance.

Component/Parameters of ABG Analysis

- pH : [H^+]
- PCO_2 : Partial pressure CO_2
- PO_2 : Partial pressure O_2
- HCO_3 : Bicarbonate
- BE : Base excess
- SaO_2 : Oxygen Saturation

Table 4.7: Normal ABG values

Ideal blood cases			
	pH	pCO_2	pO_2
Preterm	7.28–7.32	35–45	50–80
Term	7.30–7.35	35–45	80–95
*Normal values (1 hr age, not ventilated)			

Acceptable arterial blood gas	
pH	More than 7.2
pCO_2	50–60 mm of Hg
pO_2	50–60 mm of Hg
HCO_3	18–20

- **pH**: The pH measures hydrogen ions (H^+) in blood. The pH of blood is usually between 7.35 and 7.45. A pH of less than 7.0 is called acid and a pH greater than 7.0 is called basic (alkaline). So blood is slightly basic.
- **Partial pressure of carbon dioxide ($PaCO_2$):** This measure the pressure of carbon dioxide dissolved in the blood and how well carbon dioxide is able to move out of the body.
- **Partial pressure of oxygen (PaO_2)**: This measure the pressure of oxygen dissolved in the blood and how well oxygen is able to move from the airspace of the lungs into the blood.
- **Bicarbonate (HCO_3):** Bicarbonate is a chemical (buffer) that keeps the pH of blood from becoming too acidic or too basic.
- **BE**: The base excess is used for the assessment of the metabolic component of acid-base disorders, and indicates whether the patient has metabolic acidosis or metabolic alkalosis. A negative base excess indicates that the patient has metabolic acidosis (primary or secondary to respiratory alkalosis). A positive base excess indicates that the patient has metabolic alkalosis (primary or secondary to respiratory acidosis).
- **Saturated Oxygen (SpO_2):** An oxygen saturation (SpO_2 Sat) values. O_2 content measures the amount of oxygen in the blood. Oxygen saturation measures how much of the hemoglobin in the red blood cells is carrying oxygen (O_2).

Indication

- RDS (Respiratory Distress Syndrome)
- Asthma

- Cystic fibrosis
- Chronic obstructive pulmonary disease (COPD)
- Mechanical Ventilation Requiring Child
- Measure the acid-base level in the blood
- Heart failure
- Kidney failure
- Diabetes mellitus
- Sleep disorders
- Severe infections
- Drug overdose.

Needed Equipment

- A clean tray with sterile tray cloth—1
- Two bowel (small size)—2
- Macintosh—1
- Glove—1
- Kidney tray (small size)—1
- Cotton ball and gauze as required
- Syringe 2 ml and 1 ml—1
- Vacutainer/sample container
- Scissor and adhesive tape.

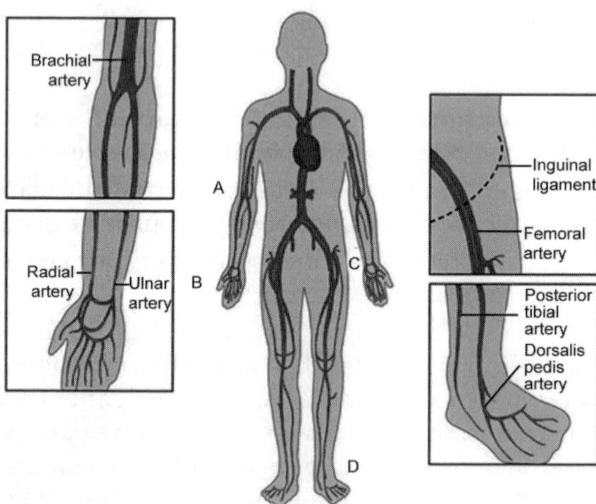

Fig. 4.54: Anatomical view to select the artery for ABG sample blood collection

Preparation

- Explain the procedures to parents
- Get the legal consent from the parents

- Provide the comfortable position to child
- Do the eligibility test (Allen's test)
- Check the any bleeding problems and drug allergic.

Allen's Test

Allen's test is used to evaluate ulnar-artery patency before radial-artery cannulation or radial-artery harvesting for coronary-artery bypass grafting. The diagnostic accuracy of the test is reported to be greatest at a cutoff time of 5 to 6 seconds.

- Instruct the patient to clench his or her fist; if the patient is unable to do this, close the person's hand tightly.
- Using your fingers, apply occlusive pressure to both the ulnar and radial arteries, to obstruct blood flow to the hand.
- While applying occlusive pressure to both arteries, have the patient relax his or her hand, and check whether the palm and fingers have blanched. If this is not the case, you have not completely occluded the arteries with your fingers.

Positive modified Allen test: If the hand flushes within 5–15 seconds it indicates that the ulnar artery has good blood flow; this normal flushing of the hand is considered to be a positive test.

Negative modified Allen test: If the hand does not flush within 5–15 seconds, it indicates that ulnar circulation is inadequate or nonexistent; in this situation, the radial artery supplying arterial blood to that hand should not be punctured.

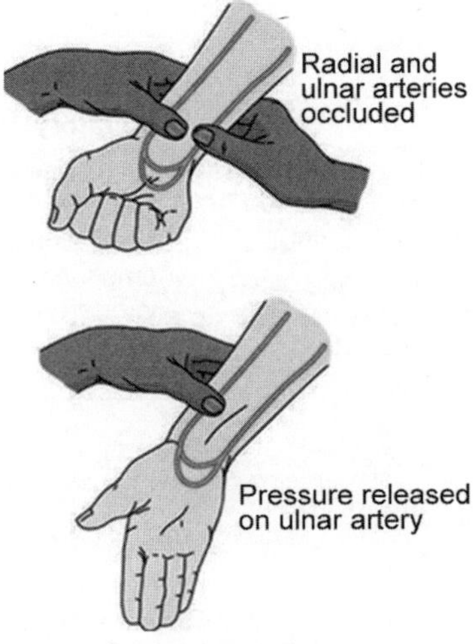

Fig. 4.55: Allen test

Procedures

ABG Specimen Collection

- Perform the handwash procedures.
- Maintain the proper position (supine position).

- Arrange the articles nearby child unit.
- The radial artery at the wrist is the most preferred site of ABG specimen collection as it has adequate collaterals where inadvertent puncture of veins is unlikely.
- When this is not feasible, popliteal, brachial or femoral arteries can be chosen.
- The injection site is cleansed with iodine or alcohol.
- The index and middle finger of the other hand can be used to palpate the artery.
- Heparinized syringe with 22 gauge needle should be held like a pen with 45° angle (with beveled edge of the tip facing downwards) and the artery should be punctured just 2 cm above the wrist crease.
- ABG syringes are the most advantageous where the arterial blood gets filled on its own without any application of suction force and ensure anaerobic collection.
- Presence of air bubbles may increase oxygen values and lower CO_2 values. If ordinary syringes are used, the nozzle should be stoppered immediately and transported to the laboratory by placing on an ice slush or refrigerated to reduce metabolism of red blood cells.
- Estimation should be done immediately otherwise values of oxygen and CO_2 may be altered due to cellular metabolism. Though 0.05 ml of heparin is enough for 1 ml of blood, up to 0.1 ml of heparin may not interfere with blood gas values.
- Excess of heparin should be avoided as it may increase the acidity because of its high hydrogen ion concentration.
- After arterial puncture, the site should be compressed tightly for 3 to 5 minutes to prevent hematoma formation.

Results of ABG Analysis

Respiratory Acidosis	Respiratory Alkalosis
• Respiratory acidosis is characterized by a **lower pH** and an **increased PCO_2** and is due to respiratory depression (not enough oxygen in and CO_2 out). • This can be caused by many things, including pneumonia, chronic obstructive pulmonary disease (COPD), and over-sedation from narcotics. 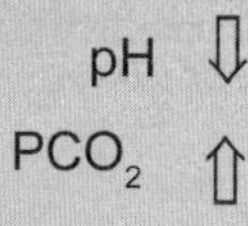 	• Respiratory alkalosis, characterized by a **raised pH** and a **decreased PCO_2**, is due to over ventilation caused by hyperventilating, pain, emotional distress, or certain lung diseases that interfere with oxygen exchange 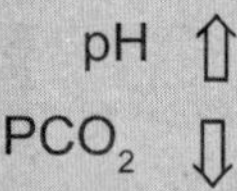
Signs and Symptoms • **Respiratory**: Dyspnea, respiratory distress and/or shallow respiration. • **Nervous**: Headache, restlessness and confusion. If CO_2 level extremely high drowsiness and unresponsiveness may be noted. • **CVS:** Tachycardia and Dysrhythmia	**Signs and Symptoms** • CNS: Lightheadedness, numbness, tingling, confusion, inability to concentrate and blurred vision. • Dysrhythmia and palpitations • Dry mouth, diaphoresis and tetanic spasms of the arms and legs.

Contd...

Contd...

Metabolic Acidosis	Metabolic Alkalosis
• Metabolic acidosis is characterized by a lower pH and decreased HCO_3^- the blood is too acidic on a metabolic/kidney level. • Causes include diabetes, shock, and renal failure. pH ⇩ HCO_3 ⇩	• Metabolic alkalosis is characterized by an elevated pH and increased HCO_3^- and is seen in hypokalemia, chronic vomiting (losing acid from the stomach), and sodium bicarbonate overdose. 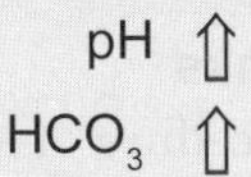 pH ⇧ HCO_3 ⇧
Signs and Symptoms • **CNS:** Headache, confusion and restlessness progressing to lethargy, then stupor or coma. • **CVS:** Dysrhythmia • Kussmaul's respirations • Warm, flushed skin as well as nausea and vomiting	**Signs and Symptoms** • **CNS:** Dizziness, lethargy disorientation, seizures and coma. • **M/S:** Weakness, muscle twitching, muscle cramps and tetany. • Nausea, vomiting and respiratory depression. • It is difficult to treat.

Role of Nurse

- After the blood has been taken, the technician or the patient applies pressure to the puncture site for 10–15 minutes to stop the bleeding, and then places a dressing over the puncture.
- The child should rest quietly while applying the pressure to the puncture site. Health care workers will observe the patient for signs of bleeding or circulation problems.

MODEL QUESTIONS

Multiple Choice Questions

1. **The pediatric setting should be ....**
   (a) Happy (b) Simple
   (c) Serious (d) Happy and attractive
2. **The child reaction to hospitalization like protest, despair, denial and regression present in which age?**
   (a) Infancy (b) Schooler
   (c) Toddler (d) Preschooler
3. **Hospitalization of child is the break in the........... of family.**
   (a) Unity (b) Growth and development
   (c) Punctuality (d) Happiness
4. **The pediatric nurse must be aware about the feeling of ....**
   (a) Child parents (b) Mothers
   (c) Health care team (d) Fathers
5. **The finding of physical examination helps in making ....**
   (a) Diagnosis (b) Planning
   (c) Intervention (d) Rationale

6. **For the examination of back the child should be placed in which position?**
   (a) Sitting (b) Lateral
   (c) Prone (d) Fowler's position
7. **Universal precaution to be followed to prevent infection.**
   (a) Nosocomial (b) Staff
   (c) Communicable (d) Hazards

Fill in the Blanks

1. During procedure of enemas the catheter should be inserted only ....into the rectum depending upon the size of the child.
2. ....feeding is given in child has an upper gastrointestinal tract abnormalities.
3. In the newborn vitamin K is given ....muscle.
4. Restrains are used to ....the child.

True or False

1. Temperature of solution for enema in child in 100 °F or 37 °C .
2. Gastrostomy is used for elimination.
3. LBW stands for low birth weight.
4. Oral feeding, gastrostomy and gavage feeding are the techniques of feeding is the child.

Short Answer Questions

1. Role of nurse in helping child and family during hospitalization.
2. Care of child in incubator.
3. Phototherapy.
4. Oxygen therapy.

Long Answer Questions

1. (a) Define phototherapy.
   (b) Principles of phototherapy.
   (c) Nursing management of the patient with phototherapy.

ANSWER KEY

Multiple Choice Questions

1. (b)	2. (c)	3. (a)	4. (a)	5. (a)	6. (c)	7. (a)

Fill in the Blanks

1. 2-4 inches
2. Gastrostomy
3. Vastus lateralis
4. Immobilized

True or False

1. False	2. False	3. True	4. True

Chapter 5

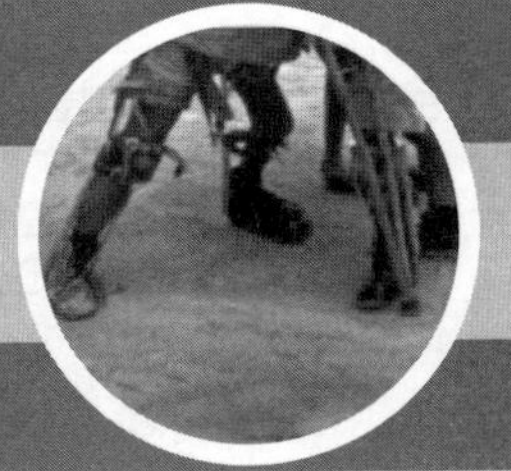

Disorders and Health Problems of a Child

- **Infancy Disorders and Health Problems**
  - Failure to Thrive (FTT)
  - Diarrhea
  - Dehydration
  - Vomiting
- **Childhood Disorders and Health Problems**
  - Communicable Diseases
- **Common Viral Infectious Diseases in Children**
  - Measles
  - Chickenpox (Varicella)
  - Mumps (Parotitis)
  - Poliomyelitis
  - HIV/AIDS
  - Dengue Syndrome
  - German Measles (Rubella)
  - Herpes Simplex Virus (HSV)
  - Varicella-Zoster
  - Guillain-Barré Syndrome
  - Influenza
  - Infectious Mononucleosis
  - Swine Flu (A Big Threat to World)
  - Zika Virus
- **Common Bacterial Infections**
  - Tuberculosis (TB)
  - Typhoid Fever (Enteric Fever)
  - Tetanus
  - Diphtheria

- Whooping Cough (Pertussis)
- Leprosy
- Hospital Acquired Infections (Nosocomial Infections)
- Haemophilus Influenzae (Type-B)
- Meningococcal Infection
- Helicobacter Pylori Infection
- Congenital Syphilis

• **Common Parasitosis in Children**
  - Malaria
  - Lymphatic Filariasis
  - Kala-Azar (Visceral Leishmaniasis)
  - Giardiasis
  - Intestinal Amebiasis
  - Cryptosporidiosis

• **Worm Infestations (Helminthiasis)**
  - Roundworms (Ascariasis)
  - Pinworm or Threadworm (Oxyuriasis)
  - Hookworms (Ancylostomiasis)
  - Tapeworms (Cestodes)

• **Other Disorders**
  - Tonsillitis
  - Otitis Media
  - Child Abuse
  - Breath Holding Spasms
  - Enuresis
  - Encopresis
  - Nail Biting
  - Thumb-Sucking
  - Sleep Disorders (Somnambulism)
  - Teeth Grinding (or) Bruxism
  - Protein-energy Malnutrition (PEM)
  - Helminthic Infections
  - Bites and Stings
  - Pica
  - Tics

• **Adolescent Disorders and Health Problems**
  - Precocious Puberty
  - Gynecomastia
  - Accident/Sports Injuries
  - Poisoning in Children
  - Specific Drugs Poisons and Management

- **Foreign Bodies**
  - Foreign Bodies in the Respiratory Tract
  - Foreign Bodies in the Alimentary Tract
  - Burns
  - Drowning
  - Sports Injuries
  - Obesity
  - Anorexia Nervosa
  - Juvenile Delinquency

INFANCY DISORDERS AND HEALTH PROBLEMS

FAILURE TO THRIVE (FTT)

Introduction

Definition of growth failure related to aberrant care failure to maintain an established pattern of growth and development that responds to the provision of adequate nutritional and emotional needs of the patient. Most cases of FTT are not related to neglectful care giving, although it may be a sign of maltreatment and should be considered during an evaluation for growth failure.

It is a common problem of children from peer socioeconomic group. This term was mentioned as early 1915. Afterwards it was termed as emotional deprivation and as maternal deprivation syndrome by bowl in 1969. Failure to thrive is now used to describe infants and children who without superficially evident cause fail to gain and often lose weight.

Definition of Failure to Thrive

Failure to thrive (FTT) is a sign of inadequate growth resulting from inability or use calories required for growth.

Failure to thrive has no universal definition although one of the more common parameters is a weight (and sometimes height) that falls below the 5th percentile for the child's age. Growth measurements alone are not used to diagnose children with FTT.

Categories of Failure to Thrive

- *Organic failure to thrive:* The result of a physical cause such as congenital heart defects, neurologic lesions, microcephalic chronic renal failure, gastroesophageal, netflix malabsorption syndrome, endocrine dysfunction, cystic fibrosis or acquired immunodeficiency syndrome.
- *Nonorganic failure to thrive:* A definable cause that is unrelated to disease FTT is most often the result of psychosocial factors such as inadequate nutritional information by the parents, deficiency in maternal care is a disturbance in maternal child attachment is a disturbance in child's ability to separate from the parent.
- *Idiopathic failure to thrive:* Unexplained by the usual organic and environmental etiologies but may also be classified.

Factors Lead to Inadequate Feeding

The category of FTT has implied a disturbance in the parent child interaction.

- Poverty:
  - Lack of funds to buy sufficient food
  - May dilute form to extend available supply.
- Health or child rearing beliefs:
  - Use of fad diets
  - Excessive concern with presenting conditions such as:
    - Obesity
    - Hypercholesterolemia (or)
    - Strict use of scheduled feedings.
- Inadequate nutritional knowledge:
  - Cultural confusion of newly arrived immigrant food, who are unaware of appropriate food selection in markets
  - Parents with cognitive impairment.
- Family stress:
  - Overwhelming involvement with another chronically ill child
  - Any number of other stresses (financial, marital, excessive parenting, employment, responsibilities and depression)
- Feeding resistance: Result of nonoral nutritional therapy early in life.
- Insufficient breast milk: Result of a number of different causes–fatigue, illness, poor release of milk, etc. insufficient glandular tissues, and lack of maternal confidence.

Causes of Failure to Thrive

The causes of failure to thrive can be grouped into:

- Environmental (common):
  - Emotional deprivation
  - Child maltreatment
  - Material depression
  - Poverty
  - Poor feeding techniques
  - Improper formula preparation
  - Unusual parental nutritional beliefs.
- Gastrointestinal system:
  - Cystic fibrosis and other causes of pancreatic in sufficiency
  - Celiac disease
  - Other malabsorption syndromes
  - Gastrointestinal reflux.
- Congenital/Anatomic defect:
  - Chromosomal abnormalities, genetic syndromes
  - Congenital heart disease

  - Gastrointestinal abnormalities, e.g. pyloric stenosis
  - Vascular rings
  - Upper airway obstruction
  - Dental caries
  - Congenital immunodeficiency syndromes.
- Infections:
  - HIV
  - Tuberculosis
  - Hepatitis
  - Urinary tract infection
  - Chronic sinusitis
  - Parasitic infection.
- Metabolic causes:
  - Adrenal or pituitary disease
  - Aminoaciduria, organic aciduria
  - Galactosemia.
- Neurological causes:
  - Coeternal palsy
  - Hypothalamus
  - Hypotonic syndromes
  - Neuromuscular disease
  - Degenerative and storage diseases.
- Renal:
  - Chronic renal failure
  - Renal tubal acidosis
  - Urinary tract infection.
- Hematologic:
  - Sickle cell disease
  - Iron deficiency anemia.

Clinical Manifestations of Failure to Thrive

- Growth failure:
  - Below 5th percentile in weight only or weight and height
- Developmental delay:
  - Social, motor, adaptive, language
- Apathy
- Poor hygiene
- Withdrawn behavior
- Feeding or eating disorders such as
  - Vomiting, anorexia, pica.
- No fear of strangers
  - At age when stranger anxiety is normal.

- Avoidance of eye contact
- Wide-eyed gaze and continual scan of the environment (radar gaze)
  - Stiff and unyielding or flaccid and unresponsive
  - Minimal smiling.

Diagnostic Evaluation

- History collection
- Physical examinations
  - Dysmorphic features that may suggest a genetic or teratogenic cause for growth failure
  - Prenatal and postnatal factors
  - Maternal illness during pregnancy
  - Fetal growth problem
  - Prematurity
  - Anthropometric assessment (height, length, head circumference).
- Medical symptoms
  - Vomiting, diarrhea, fever.
- Diet history
  - Lactation problems
  - Improper formula preparation
  - Neurological examination
    - Spasticity or hypotonic
    - Skin disorders
    - Screening for iron deficiency anemia and lead toxicity.
  - Urinalysis
  - Urine culture
  - Serum electrotypes tuberculin test.

Therapeutic Management

Children with failure to thrive need the help of their parents. Sometimes, an entire medical team will work on the case.

In addition to the primary doctor, the team might include a nutritionist to evaluate the child's dietary needs, and an occupational or speech therapist to help the caregiver and child develop successful feeding behaviors and address any sucking or swallowing problems. Occupational and speech therapists are often helpful because of their expertise in the muscular control that is involved in eating.

Treatment of failure to thrive involves treating any disease or disorder causing the problem, specialists such as a cardiologist, neurologist, or gastroenterologist may also be part of the care team.

Particularly in cases of failure to thrive that are thought to be caused by caregivers' or parents' actions, a social worker and a psychologist or other mental health professional may help address problems in the home environment and provide any needed support. In cases of poor nutrition, treatment often can be carried out at home with frequent follow-up visits to the doctor's office or clinic.

The doctor will recommend high-calorie foods and place an infant on a high-calorie formula. More severe cases may call for tube feedings in which a tube is put in that runs from the nose into the stomach.

Liquid nutrition is provided at a steady rate through the tube. Once the tube is in place, the child is usually fed at night to avoid interference with daily activities or limiting the child's desire to eat during the day. (About half of a child's caloric needs can be delivered at night through a continuous drip.) Once more adequately nourished, the child will feel better and will probably start to eat more on his or her own. At that point, the tube can be removed.

A child with extreme failure to thrive may need to be hospitalized to be fed and monitored continuously.

During this time, any possible underlying causes of the condition can be evaluated and treated appropriately. This also lets the doctors see the caregiver's feeding technique and the interaction between caregiver and child during feedings and at other times.

How long treatment lasts varies from case to case. Weight gain takes time, so several months may pass before a child is back in the normal range. Kids who require hospitalization may stay for 10 to 14 days or more to establish satisfactory weight gain, but it can be many months until the symptoms of severe malnutrition are gone.

Failure to thrive caused by a chronic illness or disorder may have to be monitored periodically and treated for even longer, perhaps for a lifetime.

Medical Management

- Revising the malnutrition of the underlying cause
- Provide sufficient calories to support
- Psychosocial and family contributors
- A team approach therapy
- Pediatricians nutritionist
- Developmental specialists
- Nurses, social workers.

Nutritional Management

- May require more than 1.5 times the expected calorie and protein intake for their age for catch-up growth
- Formula feed infants 20 cal/oz to 24 or 27 cal/oz.

Dietary

- Three meals and two snacks each day.
- Increase the number and variety of foods offered.
- Increase energy density of usual foods, such as adding cheese, margarine or cream.
- Limit milk intake to 500 mL per day.
- Avoid excessive intake of fruit juice and squash.

Behavioral

- Offer meals at regular times with other family members.
- Praise when food is eaten, but ignore when not.
- Limit a meal's time to 30 minutes.

- Parents should eat at the same time as the child.
- Mealtime conflict should be avoided.
- The child should never be force-fed.

Prognosis

- As a general rule, if small babies double their birth weight in four months and triple it in a year, they will catch up.
- A systematic review concluded that the long-term outcome of FTT is a reduction in IQ of about 3 points, which is not of clinical significance.
- Related to the cause.

Preventive Management

- Good antenatal care and avoidance of toxins such as illicit drugs, tobacco and alcohol in pregnancy will reduce the risk.
- Parenting classes should lead to a better understanding of the needs of the baby. Nowadays fathers are often involved too and this is to be welcomed.
- An astute midwife or health visitor should detect problems before they become serious.

Nursing Management

- Observation of feeding is very important. Nurse should have careful attention to the following:
  - Maternal (caregiver) attachment during the feeding process, evaluation of signs of maternal attachment (eye contact, vocalizations, interpretation of cues)
  - Evaluation of the child-parent dyad (e.g. conflict over eating related to poor limit setting, lack of discipline, or meal time disruption)
  - The perception of parents and/or caregivers regarding the problem
  - Feeding techniques (forced feeding)
  - A 72-hour diet diary that includes the following can be helpful:
  - Details relative to growth from breastfeeding or bottle-feeding
  - Formula preparation and amounts provided
  - Time and amount of feedings (e.g. 5 oz of Enfamil; one-half jar of strained peaches)
  - Behaviors of infant or child during feeding or nursing.
- Nutritional treatment is based on aggressive feeding to prevent cognitive loss. Most children require 100–120 kcal/kg/day, but this may be increased to achieve catch-up weight gain that is greater than normal. Other dietary instructions should include the following:
- Eliminate empty calories from items such as soda or other high sugar drinks.
- Schedule regular meals and snacks (usually 3 meals and 2 snacks per day). No grazing between meals.
- Offer solids before liquids.
- Consider fortifying calories with extra oils and carbohydrates.
  - Increase protein.
  - Consider vitamin and/or mineral supplements, especially zinc and iron.

- Provide support for the caregiver and offer suggestions for improving the feeding environment, such as the following:
  - Avoid blaming the caregiver.
  - Provide respite for the caregiver.
  - Avoid distractions, such as television, at meal time.
  - Offer a role model for the caregivers.
- Psychosocial evaluation must be detailed and must provide an in-depth look at the functioning of the family and the child in the context of the family. Current and past social history of the family, at a minimum, should address the following:
  - Finances and resources, living and childcare arrangements
  - Abuse and neglect risk factors, including any physical or sexual abuse
  - Domestic or interpersonal violence
  - Substance abuse or addiction
  - Mental health disorder, particularly depression and postpartum depression
  - Eating disorder.

DIARRHEA

Introduction

Diarrhea is a very common problem in children. Diarrhea is frequent, loose, or watery bowel movements (BMs) that differ from a child's normal pattern. Sometimes diarrhea contains blood or mucus. Identifying mild diarrhea may be difficult because in healthy children, the number and consistency of BMs vary with age and diet.

For example, breastfed infants who are not yet receiving solid food often have frequent, loose stools that are considered normal. A sudden increase in number and looseness may indicate diarrhea in these infants. However, having watery stools for more than 24 hours is never normal.

Children with diarrhea may lose their appetite, vomit, lose weight, or have a fever. If diarrhea is severe or lasts a long time, dehydration is likely. Infants and young children can become dehydrated more quickly, sometimes in less than 1 day. Severe dehydration can cause seizures, brain damage, and death.

Worldwide, diarrhea causes 2 to 3 million deaths a year mostly in underdeveloped countries. In the United States, diarrhea accounts for about 9% of hospitalizations for children under 5 years old.

Definition

Diarrhea is defined as increase in frequency and change in consistency of stools, passage of liquids (or) watery stools more than 3 times a day per 24 hours, resulting in excessive loss of fluid and electrolytes in stool.

Diarrhea is the body's way of ridding itself of germs, and most episodes last a few days to a week. Diarrhea often occurs with fever, nausea, vomiting, cramps, and dehydration.

Diarrhea: Loose, watery stools occurring more than three times in one day is a common problem that usually lasts a day or two and goes away on its own without any special treatment.

Diarrhea can be of sudden onset and lasting for less than two weeks (acute) or persistent (chronic).

Types

- *Acute diarrhea:* It is defined as a sudden increase in frequency a change in consistency of stool often causal by infectious agent in the tract. It terminates within a 14 days.
- *Chronic diarrhea:* It is defined as an increase in stool frequency, increased water content with duration of more than 14 days, caused by chronic condition such as malabsorption syndrome, inflammatory bowel disease (IBD).

Subtypes

- *Protracted diarrhea:* It is defined as persistence of diarrhea beyond 2 weeks with attract liquid stool per day with no weight gain weight loss and which the conventional time of treatment has failed.
- *Intractable diarrhea of infancy:* It is a syndrome that occurs on the first few months of life. Persist for longer than 2 weeks with no recognized pathogenesis secretary to treatment.
- *Persistent diarrhea:* It persists for more than 2 weeks, it carries a much higher use for mortality to main nutritional malabsorption.
- *Osmotic diarrhea:* It follows ingestion of absurdly absorbed solute because an inherent character of the solute (magnesium phosphate, alcohol) (or) a small bowel defect (lactose in lactase deficiency). It tends to be waters acidic with reducing substances.
- *Motility diarrhea:* It is associated with increased (writable bowel syndrome) or delayed motility (dentinal pseudo-obstruction).

Mode of Transmission

- Dirty hands
- Contaminated food or water
- Some pets
- Direct contact with fecal matter (i.e. from dirty diapers or the toilet)
- Feco-oral route either by contaminated food (or) water.

Causes of Acute Diarrhea

Gastroenteritis

- *Viral infection:* Mainly rotavirus but others include norovirus, echoviruses and enteroviruses.
- *Bacterial infection:* Suggested by high pyrexia and bloody diarrhea. Common bacterial pathogens include *Shigella* spp, *Salmonella* spp and *Campylobacter* spp.
- *Protozoal infection:* Chronic infections might suggest protozoan's—for example, *Giardia lamblia.*
- *Systemic infection:* For example, urinary tract infection, pneumonia, otitis media, meningitis, septicemia.
- *Antibiotic-associated* and rarely pseudo membranous colitis.
- *Dietary:* Food allergy or intolerance (lactose intolerance, cow's milk protein intolerance); starvation stools.

- *Surgical conditions:* For example, appendicitis; intussusception; partial bowel obstruction, e.g. volvulus, Hirschsprung's disease; Meckel's diverticulum; short bowel syndrome.
- *Malabsorption:* Cystic fibrosis, coeliac disease.
- *Inflammation:* Ulcerative colitis, Crohn's disease.
- *Miscellaneous:* Constipation with overflow, HUS, toddler's diarrhea, hyperthyroidism.

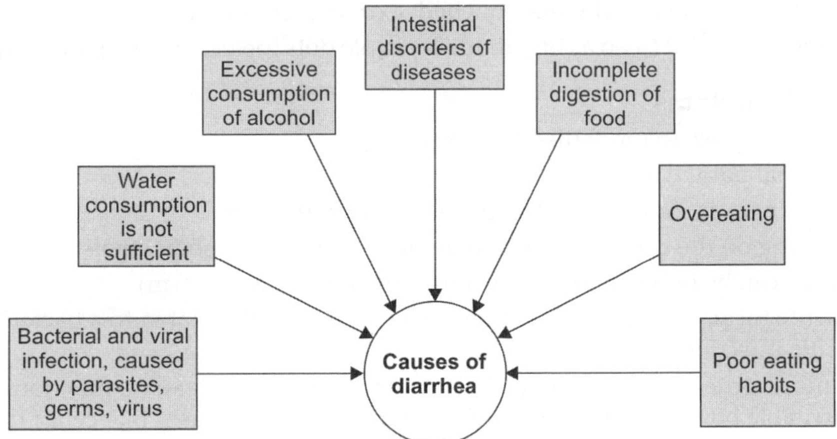

Fig. 5.1: Causes of diarrhea

Causes of Chronic Diarrhea

- Dietary factors, such as lactose intolerance or overconsumption of certain foods
- Infections (particularly those caused by parasites)
- Celiac disease
- Inflammatory bowel disease.

Environmental Factor

- Lack of clean water (or) inadequate water supply
- Lack of sanitary facilities
- Poor personal and domestic hygienic
- Improper food preparation and storage
- Poor wearing practices
- Early stopping of breastfeeding
- Practice of bottle feeding.

Psychogenic Factor

- Tension and excitement
- Fatigue
- Fear and depression.

Warning Signs

Certain symptoms are cause for concern. They include:

- Signs of dehydration, such as decreased urination, lethargy or listlessness, crying without tears, extreme thirst, and a dry mouth
- III appearance
- Blood in stool
- Pain in the abdomen and when touched, extreme tenderness
- Bleeding in the skin (seen as tiny reddish purple dots [petechiae] or splotches [purpura]).

Signs and Symptoms

- Diarrhea may be accompanied by cramping.
- Abdominal pain.
- Bloating, nausea, or an urgent need to use the bathroom.
- Depending on the cause, a person may have a fever or bloody stools.
- Diarrhea can be either acute (short-term) or chronic (long-term).
- The acute form, which lasts less than 4 weeks, is usually related to a bacterial, viral, or parasitic infection.
- Chronic diarrhea lasts more than 4 weeks and is usually related to functional disorders like irritable bowel syndrome or inflammatory bowel diseases like celiac disease.

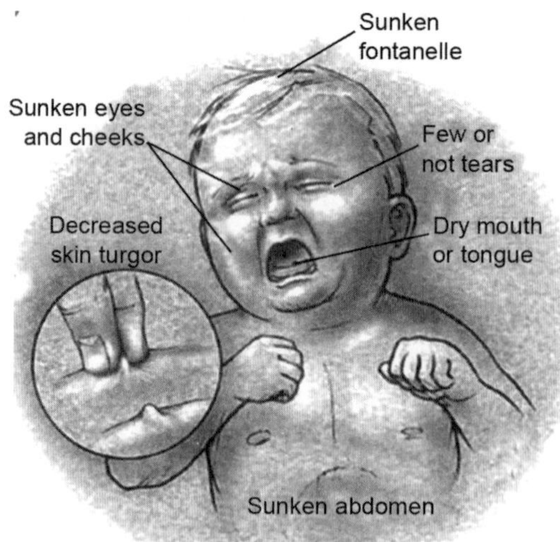

Fig. 5.2: Signs and symptoms of severe diarrhea

General Signs of Diarrhea Include

- Thirst
- Less frequent urination
- Dry skin
- Fatigue

- Lightheadedness
- Dark colored urine.

Signs of diarrhea in children include:
- Dry mouth and tongue
- No tears when crying
- No wet diapers for 3 hours or more
- Sunken abdomen, eyes, or cheeks
- High fever
- Listlessness or irritability
- Skin that does not flatten when pinched and released.

Common signs and symptoms:
- Fever—low grade to high grade
- Anorexia
- Mild to severe vomiting
- Stools are loose may consist maces, play oxblood
- Stool may be greenish (or) yellow
- Irritable and restlessness.

Diagnostic Evaluation
- History collection
- Physical examination
- *Stool culture:* Lab technicians analyze a sample of stool to check for bacteria, parasites, or other signs of disease or infection.
- *Blood tests:* Blood tests can be helpful in ruling out certain diseases.
- *Fasting tests:* To find out if a food intolerance or allergy is causing the diarrhea, the doctor may ask you to avoid lactose (found in milk products), carbohydrates, wheat, or other foods to see whether the diarrhea responds to a change in diet.
- *Sigmoidoscopy:* For this test, the doctor uses a special instrument to look at the inside of the rectum and lower part of the colon.
- *Colonoscopy:* This test is similar to sigmoidoscopy, but the doctor looks at the entire colon.
- *Stool culture:* Including examination for ova, cysts and parasites.
- *Rotavirus antigen tests:* False negative rate is approximately 50% and false positive results occur, particularly in the presence of blood in the stools. Adenovirus (serotype 40 and 41) antigen can be detected by enzyme immunoassay.
- White cell count is usually normal but may be raised in some bacterial infections.
- *Renal function and electrolytes:* Occasionally, a protein-losing enteropathy may lead to a low serum albumin.
- *Other investigations:* It will depend on the individual situation. Further investigations may include endomysial antibodies (celiac disease), intestinal biopsy (celiac disease or inflammatory bowel disease) and sweat test (cystic fibrosis) if indicated, especially if diarrhea persists.

Table 5.1: Signs and symptoms of diarrhea in infants and children

Finding	Mild (3–5%)	Moderate (6–9%)	Severe (≥ 10%)
Pulse	Full, normal rate	Rapid	Rapid and weak
Systolic pressure	Normal	Normal to low	Very low
Respirations	Normal	Deep, rate may be increased	Deep, rapid rate
Oral tissues	Tacky or slightly dry	Dry	Parched
Infant fontanelles (soft spot in skull)	Normal	Sunken	Markedly sunken
Eyes	Normal	Sunken	Markedly sunken
Skin	Normal	Cool	Cool, mottled, blue-tinged hands/feet
Urine output	Mildly reduced	Markedly reduced	Absent
Systemic signs	Increased thirst	Listlessness, irritability	Grunting, lethargy, coma

Management

Most infectious diarrhea is self-limiting and medical care is mainly supportive. The important aspects of management are recognition of more serious causes of diarrhea and adequate oral rehydration at an early stage. Infants under 6 months of age are at greatest risk of dehydration.

The majority of children can be managed safely in the community but there should be a lower threshold for admission to hospital for infants aged under 6 months. Small amounts of fluid given frequently are often tolerated, even when vomiting has been a prominent symptom.

Breastfeeding

Breastfeeding continued use of breast milk has been shown to be beneficial in children with acute diarrhea.

- In treatment of diarrhea, the most important factor is to maintain hydration.
- Racecadotril is an intestinal antisecretory enkephalinase inhibitor. It inhibits the breakdown of endogenous enkephalins and so reduces the hypersecretion of water and electrolytes into the intestine.
- It does not modify the duration of intestinal transit. It is licensed for the complementary symptomatic treatment of acute diarrhea together with oral rehydration (and the usual support measures) when these measures alone are insufficient and it is not possible to treat the cause.

Antibiotic Therapy

Antibiotic therapy is nearly always inappropriate in view of the usual viral etiology but may be required for proven bacterial or protozoal causes of gastroenteritis. When required, antibiotic regimes will be determined by the results of stool culture and sensitivities and local guidelines, e.g. ampicillin—50 to 100 mg/kg/day divided dose loperamide has been shown to reduce the duration of diarrhea but adverse effects are unclear and it should not be prescribed.

Hospitalization

- There is any concern regarding the underlying diagnosis.
- There are signs of dehydration, especially if aged under 6 months.
- There is inability to comply with oral rehydration, e.g. vomiting, poor social circumstances.
- There is a preexisting medical condition which may worsen with diarrhea (e.g. diabetes).

Complications

- Rotavirus infection may lead to dehydration and also to lactose intolerance.
- Bacterial bowel infection may (rarely) lead to infection at other sites, including septicemia, meningitis and osteomyelitis. Infection may also lead to bowel perforation, intussusception, appendicitis or liver abscess. These complications are very uncommon but need to be considered if the child is particularly unwell or not making the expected recovery.
- Other rare complications include HUS and Reiter's syndrome.
- *Giardia* spp. infection may lead to chronic fat malabsorption.
- Carrier states are observed after some infections, e.g. rotavirus and salmonella infections.
- *E. coli* O157 is the most common but not only cause of HUS. It may also cause hemorrhagic colitis.

Prevention

- Food hygiene (storage, handling, cooking).
- Handwashing.
- Appropriate exclusion of children with diarrhea, e.g. from nurseries.
- *Vaccination:* Routine immunization against rotavirus has been administered orally at 2 and 3 months of age.
- It has already made a significant impact. *Salmonella typhi* vaccine is recommended for travellers to countries with a high incidence. *Vibrio* spp. vaccine is available but only protects 50% of immunized persons for 3–6 months and is not indicated for use.

Home Care of Diarrhea

The following are some simple recommendations to help care for children with diarrhea at home.

Dietary Recommendations

There has been much confusion and folklore about optimal foods for children with diarrhea. Fortunately, a number of studies have examined recommendations that are proven to be effective.

Children who are not dehydrated should continue to eat a regular diet and infants who are breastfeeding should continue to do so unless the parent(s) is told otherwise by their clinician. Dehydrated children require rehydration (replacement of lost fluid) and suitable oral rehydration solutions are the most physiologic. After being rehydrated, severely affected children will be able to resume a normal diet.

Specific suggestions for children who are tolerating a regular diet include the following:

- Most children with diarrhea tolerate full-strength cow's milk products. It is not necessary to dilute or avoid milk products, except in children with known allergies to cow's milk.

- Recommended foods include a combination of complex carbohydrates (rice, wheat, potatoes, bread), lean meats, yogurt, fruits, and vegetables. High-fat foods are more difficult to digest and should be avoided.
- The unnecessary restriction of a child's diet to clear liquids or the BRAT diet (bananas, rice, applesauce, toast) results in inadequate intake of nutrients (calories and/or protein). Giving only clear liquids for several days can actually prolong diarrhea (called 'starvation stools').
- Apple, pear, and cherry juice, and other beverages with high sugar content should be avoided. Sports drinks (sample brand name Gatorade) should also be avoided because they have too much sugar and have inappropriate electrolyte levels for the patient with diarrhea. When clear liquids are recommended, the best choices are the commercially prepared oral rehydration solutions for rehydration (sample brand name Pedialyte).

Monitoring for dehydration: Mild dehydration is common in children with diarrhea. Signs and symptoms of mild dehydration include a slightly dry mouth, increased thirst, and slightly decreased urine output (one wet diaper or void in six hours). Common features of moderate or severe dehydration include markedly decreased urination (less than one wet diaper or void in six hours), lack of tears when crying, dry mouth, and sunken eyes.

Oral rehydration therapy: Oral rehydration therapy (ORT) was developed as a safer, less expensive, and easier alternative to intravenous fluids. Oral rehydration solution (ORS) contains glucose (a sugar) and electrolytes (sodium, potassium, chloride) that are lost in children with vomiting and diarrhea. Various rehydration solutions are available. Parents should check with a healthcare provider to determine which solution is preferred. A child who is moderately or severely dehydrated needs to be evaluated by a healthcare provider. If a child refuses to accept ORS because of vomiting and/or becomes moderately to severely dehydrated, as indicated by decreased urination (> 6 hours since passing most recent urine), lethargy, or other features, the child requires professional evaluation and treatment.

ORT does not cure diarrhea, but it does help to treat the dehydration that often accompanies it. ORS can be purchased at most grocery stores and pharmacies in the United States without a prescription. A few widely available brands include Pedialyte, Infalyte, and ReVital, although generic brands are equally effective. Gelatin, tea, rice water, fruit juice, and other beverages are not recommended for use as ORT in children with diarrhea. Parents should not try to prepare ORS recipes at home because the formulas must be exact.

ORS may be given at home to a child who is mildly dehydrated, refusing to eat a normal diet, or has vomiting and/or diarrhea. If needed, ORS can be given in frequent, small amounts by spoon, bottle, or cup over three to four hours. A pediatrician may provide specific instructions for oral rehydration to their patients. One method is described below:

- Parents should first measure out the total amount to be given with a standardized medicine syringe or measuring cup or spoon, rather than a regular cup or spoon.
- A total volume of 5 teaspoons per pound, or 50 milliliters per kilogram, should be given over four hours. For a 20 pound child, this would equal 100 teaspoons; for a 9 kg child, this would equal 450 milliliters.
- The fluid can be given by teaspoonful (approximately equal to 5 milliliters each) every one to two minutes, or as tolerated.
- After the total amount has been given, a normal diet can be resumed.

A child who refuses to drink or vomits immediately after drinking ORT should be monitored closely for worsening dehydration. Children who are not dehydrated may drink ORS after every episode of vomiting to prevent dehydration.

Medications

Medications such as antibiotics and antidiarrheal agents are generally not necessary and could be harmful for infants or children with diarrhea. Rarely, antibiotics may be used in cases of bacterial infection when a specific cause of the diarrhea has been found or is strongly suspected, particularly after recent travel.

Antidiarrheal agents (including Imodium, Pepto-Bismol, and Kaopectate) are not recommended for infants or children, since the benefits do not outweigh the risks. One risk of using an antidiarrheal agent is that it could mask worsening symptoms and delay treatment.

Probiotics

There are 'healthy' bacteria (called probiotics) that may help reduce the duration of diarrhea (by about 12 to 30 hours). Some of these are available in drug stores without a prescription. While it is not unreasonable to use them, their overall benefit is small and they can be expensive.

Preventing spread: Parents with children who have diarrhea should be cautious to avoid spreading infection to themselves, their family, and friends. Care with handwashing, diapering, and keeping sick children out of school or day care until the diarrhea is gone are a few ways to limit the number of people exposed to the infection.

Hygiene measures: Handwashing is an essential and very effective way to prevent the spread of infection. Hands should ideally be wet with water and plain or antimicrobial soap, and rubbed together for 15 to 30 seconds. Special attention should be paid to the fingernails, between the fingers, and the wrists. Hands should be rinsed thoroughly and dried with a single-use towel.

Alcohol-based hand rubs are a good alternative for disinfecting hands if a sink is not available, however, alcohol-based hand rubs do not prevent all types of diarrhea (e.g. *Norovirus, Clostridium difficile*). Hand rubs should be spread over the entire surface of hands, fingers, and wrists until dry, and may be used several times. Hand rubs are available as a liquid or wipe in small, portable sizes that are easy to carry in a pocket or handbag. When a sink is available, visibly soiled hands should be washed with soap and water.

Hands should be cleaned after changing a diaper or touching any soiled item. They should also be washed before and after preparing food and eating, after going to the bathroom, after handling garbage or dirty laundry, after touching animals or pets, and after blowing the nose or sneezing.

Prognosis

- With proper management, prognosis is very good in developed countries.
- Mortality is caused predominantly by dehydration and secondary malnutrition.
- Neonates and young infants are at particular risk of dehydration and malnutrition.

DEHYDRATION

Introduction

Dehydration describes a state of negative fluid balance that may be caused by numerous disease entities. Diarrheal illnesses are the most common etiologies. Worldwide, dehydration secondary to diarrheal illness is the leading cause of infant and child mortality. The first symptom of dehydration appears after fluid loss of about 5% of body weight.

Definition

Dehydration is defined as loss of water and electrolytes in the diarrheal stool results in depletion of ECF volume, electrolyte imbalance (hyponatermia, hypokalemia) and clinical manifestation of dehydration.

Incidence

Diarrheal illnesses in children causes 3 million physician visits, 220,000 hospitalizations (10% of all children who require hospitalization), and 400 deaths per year. On average, North American children younger than 5 years have 2 episodes of gastroenteritis per year.

International

Diarrheal illnesses with subsequent dehydration account for nearly 4 million deaths per year in infants and children. The overwhelming majority of these deaths occur in developing nations.

Mortality/Morbidity

Mortality and morbidity generally depend on the severity of dehydration and the promptness of oral or intravenous rehydration. If treatment is rapidly and appropriately obtained, morbidity and mortality are low. Routine use of hypotonic parenteral fluids in hospitalized children has been associated with hyponatremia and subsequent neurologic complications and death. Monitoring the efficacy and complications of parenteral rehydration with accurate fluid balances and serum electrolytes is crucial.

Age

Children younger than 5 years are at the highest risk.

Causes

Determination of the cause of dehydration is essential. Poor fluid intake, excessive fluid output, increased insensible fluid losses, or a combination of the above may cause intravascular volume depletion. Successful treatment requires identification of the underlying disease state.

Common Causes

- *Gastroenteritis:* This is the most common cause of dehydration. If both vomiting and diarrhea are present, dehydration may rapidly progress.
- *Stomatitis:* Pain may severely limit oral intake.
- *Diabetic Ketoacidosis (DKA):* Dehydration is caused by osmotic diuresis. Weight loss is caused by both excessive fluid losses and tissue catabolism. Rapid rehydration, especially

rapid initial volume resuscitation, may be associated with a poor neurologic outcome. DKA requires very specific and controlled treatment (see Diabetic Ketoacidosis).

- *Febrile illness:* Fever causes increased insensible fluid losses and may affect appetite.
- *Pharyngitis:* This may decrease oral intake.

Life-threatening Causes

- Gastroenteritis
- DKA
- *Burns:* Fluid losses may be extreme. Very aggressive fluid management is required (see Burns, Thermal).
- *Congenital adrenal hyperplasia:* This may have associated hypoglycemia, hypotension, hyperkalemia, and hyponatremia.
- *GI obstruction:* This is often associated with poor intake and emesis. Bowel ischemia can result in extensive capillary leak and shock.
- *Heat stroke:* Hyperpyrexia, dry skin, and mental status changes may occur.
- *Cystic fibrosis:* This results in excessive sodium and chloride losses in sweat, placing patients at risk for severe hyponatremic hypochloremia dehydration.
- *Diabetes insipidus:* Excessive output of very dilute urine can result in large free water losses and severe Hypernatremic dehydration.
- *Thyrotoxicosis:* Weight loss is observed, despite increased appetite. Diarrhea occurs.

Clinical Manifestation

The following should be considered in patients with dehydration:

- Intake of fluids, including the volume, type (hypertonic or hypotonic), and frequency
- Urine output, including the frequency of voiding (last wet diaper), presence of concentrated or dilute urine, hematuria
- Stool output, frequency of stools, stool consistency, presence of blood or mucus in stools
- Emesis, including frequency and volume and whether bilious or nonbilious, hematemesis
- Contact with ill people, especially others underlying illnesses, especially cystic fibrosis, diabetes mellitus, hyperthyroidism, renal disease
- Fever
- Appetite patterns
- Weight loss
- Travel
- Recent antibiotic use
- Possible ingestions

Physical Assessment

A complete physical examination may assist in determining the underlying cause of the patient's dehydration and in defining the severity of dehydration. The clinical assessment of severity of dehydration determines the approach to management. In general, physical signs of dehydration have poor precision and accuracy. Rather than attempting to assign an exact percentage of dehydration, one should attempt to place the child in one of three broad categories.

The determination of dehydration severity should be based on the overall constellation of symptoms. Patients in a given category need not exhibit all the signs and symptoms listed below. Literature reviews have suggested that delayed capillary refill, delayed skin turgor, and abnormal respiratory pattern are the most reliable clinical signs of dehydration in children. Validated clinical dehydration scales may be a useful adjunct to predict need for intravenous fluid and longer stays in the emergency department.

Table 5.2: Clinical findings of dehydration

Symptom/sign	Mild dehydration	Moderate dehydration	Severe dehydration
Level of consciousness	Alert	Lethargic	Obtunded
Capillary refill*	2 s	2–4 s	> 4 s, cool limbs
Mucous membranes	Normal	Dry	Parched, cracked
Tears	Normal	Decreased	Absent
Heart rate	Slightly increased	Increased	Very increased
Respiratory rate/pattern*	Normal	Increased	Increased and hyperpnea
Blood pressure	Normal	Normal, but orthostatic	Decreased
Pulse	Normal	Thready	Faint or impalpable
Skin turgor*	Normal	Slow	Tenting
Fontanel	Normal	Depressed	Sunken
Eyes	Normal	Sunken	Very sunken
Urine output	Decreased	Oliguria	Oliguria/anuria

*Best indicators of hydration status

Table 5.3: Estimated fluid deficit

Severity	Infants (weight < 10 kg)	Children (weight > 10 kg)
Mild dehydration	5% or 50 mL/kg	3% or 30 mL/kg
Moderate dehydration	10% or 100 mL/kg	6% or 60 mL/kg
Severe dehydration	15% or 150 mL/kg	9% or 90 mL/kg

Pathophysiology

The negative fluid balance that causes dehydration results from decreased intake, increased output (renal, GI, or insensible losses), or fluid shift (ascites, effusions, and capillary leak states such as burns and sepsis). The decrease in total body water causes reductions in both the intracellular and extracellular fluid volumes. Clinical manifestations of dehydration are most closely related to intravascular volume depletion. As dehydration progresses, hypovolemic shock ultimately ensues, resulting in end organ failure and death.

Young children are more susceptible to dehydration due to larger body water content, renal immaturity, and inability to meet their own needs independently. Older children show signs of dehydration sooner than infants due to lower levels of extracellular fluid (ECF).

Dehydration can be categorized according to osmolarity and severity. Serum sodium is a good surrogate marker of osmolarity assuming the patient has a normal serum glucose. Dehydration may be isonatremic (130–150 mEq/L), hyponatremic (<130 mEq/L), or hypernatremic (>150 mEq/L). Isonatremic dehydration is the most common (80%).

Hypernatremic and hyponatremic dehydration each comprise 5–10% of cases. Variations in serum sodium reflect the composition of the fluids lost and have different pathophysiologic effects.

- **Isonatremic (isotonic)** dehydration occurs when the lost fluid is similar in sodium concentration to the blood. Sodium and water losses are of the same relative magnitude in both the intravascular and extravascular fluid compartments.
- **Hyponatremic (hypotonic)** dehydration occurs when the lost fluid contains more sodium than the blood (loss of hypertonic fluid). Relatively more sodium than water is lost. Because the serum sodium is low, intravascular water shifts to the extravascular space, exaggerating intravascular volume depletion for a given amount of total body water loss.
- **Hypernatremic (hypertonic)** dehydration occurs when the lost fluid contains less sodium than the blood (loss of hypotonic fluid). Relatively less sodium than water is lost. Because the serum sodium is high, extravascular water shifts to the intravascular space, minimizing intravascular volume depletion for a given amount of total body water loss.

Neurologic complications can occur in hyponatremic and hypernatremic states. Severe hyponatremia may lead to intractable seizures, whereas rapid correction of chronic hyponatremia (>2 mEq/L/h) has been associated with central pontine myelinolysis. During hypernatremic dehydration, water is osmotically pulled from cells into the extracellular space. To compensate, cells can generate osmotically active particles (idiogenic osmoles) that pull water back into the cell and maintain cellular fluid volume. During rapid rehydration of hypernatremia, the increased osmotic activity of these cells can result in a large influx of water, causing cellular swelling and rupture; cerebral edema is the most devastating consequence. Slow rehydration over 48 hours generally minimizes this risk.

Diagnostic Evaluation

Laboratory Studies

No definitive laboratory test for dehydration is available. Laboratory data are generally not required if the etiology is apparent and mild-to-moderate dehydration is present.

With severe dehydration, the following laboratory studies are suggested:

- Serum sodium should be determined because hyponatremia (<130 mEq/L) and hypernatremia (> 150 mEq/L) require specific treatment regimens.
- Potassium may be elevated (e.g. congenital adrenal hyperplasia, renal failure) or low (e.g. pyloric stenosis, alkalosis).
- Chloride may be low in pyloric stenosis (e.g. hypochloremic, hypokalemic, or metabolic alkalosis).
- Poor tissue perfusion in dehydration results in production of lactic acid. Bicarbonate is consumed as lactic acid levels increase. In diabetic ketoacidosis (DKA), ketoacids also consume bicarbonate. Bicarbonate levels can also be reduced because of loss of bicarbonate in diarrheal stools. Low bicarbonate levels have been correlated with increased severity of dehydration in some studies.
- Glucose may be dangerously low because of poor intake or extremely elevated in DKA.
- BUN and creatinine levels may be elevated because of renal hypoperfusion.
- Urine specific gravity may be elevated in patients with dehydration but should not be relied on because it is not an accurate diagnostic test for dehydration. Further caution

should be used in the setting of diabetes insipidus, in which the urine is dilute with low specific gravity, even in patients who are dehydrated.

- Urinalysis may show findings of DKA (e.g. ketones, glucose).
- Electrolyte analysis of any fluid that is lost (e.g. urine, stool, gastric fluid) can be performed to further refine the composition of replacement fluids after providing acute fluid resuscitation.

Procedures

Intravenous Line

If severe dehydration is present, peripheral intravenous line insertion may be difficult. The preferred sites for initial insertion attempts include the basilic and cephalic veins in the antecubital fossa and the saphenous veins near the ankle. Transillumination of the insertion site with a fiberoptic light source may be used to facilitate locating the desired vein.

If peripheral intravenous access cannot be rapidly achieved (< 90 s) in a child with severe dehydration and shock, intraosseous cannulation should be attempted. If the child is not in extremis, more time may be taken to establish central venous access percutaneously (e.g. femoral, subclavian, internal, external jugular).

Intraosseous Line

Intraosseous cannulation can be easily and rapidly achieved in children younger than 6 years. Specially designed intraosseous infusion needles or Jamshidi-type bone marrow aspiration needles may be used. Short large-bore spinal needles may also be used but often bend during placement. The ideal site of insertion is the anteromedial surface of the tibia, 1–3 cm below the anterior tibial tuberosity. Care must be taken to avoid injury to the physeal growth plate.

Orogastric/Nasogastric Tube

An orogastric/nasogastric tube may be inserted to facilitate enteral rehydration in children with mild-to-moderate dehydration. These tubes should be considered to assist in the nutritional recovery of children who are critically ill or severely dehydrated.

Management

Medical Management

Medications such as loperamide, opiates, anticholinergics, bismuth subsalicylate, and adsorbents are not recommended in dehydration because of questionable efficacy and potential adverse effects.

Antiemetic, Serotonin Antagonist

In a recent emergency department study, ondansetron was shown to decrease likelihood of vomiting, increase oral intake, and decrease emergency department length of stay.

Ondansetron (zofran)

Selective 5-HT3-receptor antagonist that blocks serotonin both peripherally and centrally. Prevents nausea and vomiting associated with emetogenic cancer chemotherapy (e.g. high-dose cisplatin), and complete body radiotherapy.

- Adult dose
  - 8 mg PO q1-2h for 3 doses
    Alternatively, 0.15 mg/kg IV q8h for 3 doses or 32 mg IV once
- Pediatric dose
  - Orally dissolving tablets:
    8–15 kg: 2 mg as a single dose
    15–30 kg: 4 mg as a single dose
    > 30 kg: 8 mg as a single dose.

ORT for Mild or Moderate Dehydration

- Mild or moderate dehydration can usually be treated very effectively with ORT.
- Vomiting is generally not a contraindication to ORT. If evidence of bowel obstruction, ileus, or acute abdomen is noted, then intravenous rehydration is indicated.
- *Calculate fluid deficit:* Physical findings consistent with mild dehydration suggest a fluid deficit of 5% of body weight in infants and 3% in children. Moderate dehydration occurs with a fluid deficit of 5–10% in infants and 3–6% in children (see the Table 5.3). The fluid deficit should be replaced over 4 hours.
- The oral rehydration solution should be administered in small volumes very frequently to minimize gastric distention and reflex vomiting. Generally, 5 mL of oral rehydration solution every minute is well tolerated. Hourly intake and output should be recorded by the caregiver. As the child becomes rehydrated, vomiting often decreases and larger fluid volumes may be used.
- If vomiting persists, infusion of oral rehydration solution via a nasogastric tube may be temporarily used to achieve rehydration. Intravenous fluid administration (20–30 mL/kg of isotonic sodium chloride 0.9% solution over 1–2 h) may also be used until oral rehydration is tolerated. According to a Cochrane systematic review, for every 25 children treated with ORT for dehydration, one fails and requires intravenous therapy.
- Replace ongoing losses from stools and emesis (estimate volume and replace) in addition to replacing the calculated fluid deficit.
- An age appropriate diet may be started as soon as the child is able to tolerate oral intake.

Severe Dehydration

Laboratory evaluation and intravenous rehydration are required. The underlying cause of the dehydration must be determined and appropriately treated.

Phase 1 focuses on emergency management. Severe dehydration is characterized by a state of hypovolemic shock requiring rapid treatment. Initial management includes placement of an intravenous or intraosseous line and rapid administration of 20 mL/kg of an isotonic crystalloid (e.g. lactated Ringer solution, 0.9% sodium chloride). Additional fluid boluses may be required depending on the severity of the dehydration. The child should be frequently reassessed to determine the response to treatment. As intravascular volume is replenished, tachycardia, capillary refill, urine output, and mental status all should improve. If improvement is not observed after 60 mL/kg of fluid administration, other etiologies of shock (e.g. cardiac, anaphylactic, septic) should be considered. Hemodynamic monitoring and inotropic support may be indicated.

Phase 2 focuses on deficit replacement, provision of maintenance fluids, and replacement of ongoing losses. Maintenance fluid requirements are equal to measured fluid losses (urine, stool) plus insensible fluid losses. Normal insensible fluid loss is approximately 400–500 mL/m^2 body surface area and may be increased by factors such as fever and tachypnea. Alternatively, daily fluid requirements may be roughly estimated as follows:

- Less than 10 kg = 100 mL/kg
- 10–20 kg = 1000 + 50 mL/kg for each kg over 10 kg
- Greater than 20 kg = 1500 + 20 mL/kg for each kg over 20 kg
  - Severe dehydration by clinical examination suggests a fluid deficit of 10–15% of body weight in infants and 6–9% of body weight in older children. The daily maintenance fluid is added to the fluid deficit. In general, the recommended administration is one half of this volume administered over 8 hours and administration of the remainder over the following 16 hours. Continued losses (e.g. emesis, diarrhea) must be promptly replaced.
  - If the child is isonatremic (130–150 mEq/L), the sodium deficit incurred can generally be corrected by administering the fluid deficit plus maintenance as 5% dextrose in 0.45–0.9% sodium chloride. Potassium (20 mEq/L potassium chloride) may be added to maintenance fluid once urine output is established and serum potassium levels are within a safe range.
  - An alternative approach to the deficit therapy approach is rapid replacement therapy. With this approach, a child with severe isonatremic dehydration is administered 20–40 mL/kg of isotonic sodium chloride solution or lactated Ringer solution over 15–60 minutes. As perfusion is restored, the child improves and is able to tolerate an oral rehydration solution for the remainder of his rehydration. This approach is not appropriate for hypernatremic or hyponatremic dehydration.

Hyponatremic Dehydration

- Phase 1 management of hyponatremic dehydration is identical to that of isonatremic dehydration. Rapid volume expansion with 20 mL/kg of isotonic (0.9%) sodium chloride solution or lactated Ringer solution should be administered and repeated until perfusion is restored.
- Severe hyponatremia (<130 mEq/L) indicates additional sodium loss. In phase 2 management, rehydration is calculated as for isonatremic dehydration. The additional sodium deficit must be calculated and added to the rehydration fluids. The deficit may be calculated to restore the sodium to 130 mEq/L and administered over 24 hours.
- Sodium deficit = (Sodium desired – Sodium actual) × Volume of distribution × Weight (kg)
  - Example: Sodium = 123, weight = 10 kg, assumed volume of distribution of 0.6; Sodium deficit = (130 – 123) × 0.6 × 10 kg = 42 mEq sodium
- A simplified approach is to use 5% dextrose in 0.9% sodium chloride as the replacement fluid. The sodium is closely monitored, and the amount of sodium in the fluid is adjusted to maintain a slow correction (<0.5 mEq/L/h).
- Frequently reassessing the serum sodium level during correction is imperative. Rapid correction of chronic hyponatremia (>2 mEq/L/h) has been associated with central pontine myelinolysis. Rapid partial correction of symptomatic hyponatremia has not

been associated with adverse effects. Therefore, if the child is symptomatic (seizures), a more rapid partial correction is indicated. Hypertonic (3%) sodium chloride solution (0.5 mEq/mL) may be used for rapid partial correction of symptomatic hyponatremia. A bolus dose of 4 mL/kg raises the serum sodium by 3–4 mEq/L.

Hypernatremic Dehydration

- Phase 1 management of hypernatremic dehydration is identical to that of isonatremic dehydration. Rapid volume expansion with 20 mL/kg of isotonic sodium chloride solution or lactated Ringer solution should be administered and repeated until perfusion is restored.
- Varied regimens may be successfully followed to achieve correction of severe hypernatremia (>150 mEq/L). In phase 2 management, the most important goal is to reestablish intravascular volume and return serum sodium levels toward the reference range by not more than 10 mEq/L/24h. Rapid correction of hypernatremic dehydration can have disastrous neurologic consequences, including cerebral edema and death.
- The most cautious approach is to plan a slow correction of the fluid deficit over 48 hours. Following adequate intravascular volume expansion, rehydration fluids should be initiated with 5% dextrose in 0.9% sodium chloride. Serum sodium levels should be assessed every 4 hours. If the sodium has decreased by less than 0.5 mEq/L/h, then the sodium content of the rehydration fluid is decreased. This allows for a slow controlled correction of the hypernatremic state.
- Hyperglycemia and hypocalcemia are sometimes associated with hypernatremic dehydration. Serum glucose and calcium levels should be closely monitored.

Pharmacologic Management

- Antidiarrheal agents are not recommended because of a high incidence of side effects including lethargy, respiratory depression, and coma.
- Routine empiric antibiotics should be avoided and may worsen some specific diarrheal disease states (e.g. hemolytic-uremic syndrome, clostridium difficile).
- Over-the-counter antiemetics are not recommended due to side effects including drowsiness and impaired oral rehydration.
- In an emergency department study, ondansetron has been shown to decrease likelihood of vomiting, increase oral intake, and decrease emergency department length of stay but has not shown significant effects on hospitalization rates or long-term outcomes.
- Dimenhydrinate, although used in Europe and Canada, has not been found to improve oral rehydration.

Table 5.4: Fluid management of dehydrated child

S. No.	Parameters	Isotonic dehydration	Hypertonic dehydration	Hypotonic dehydration
1	Skin			
	• Color	Gray	Gray	Gray
	• Temperature	Cold	Cold or hot	Cold
	• Tongue	Poor	Fair	Very poor
	• Feel	Dry	Thickness	Clammy (Moist)

Contd...

Contd...

S. No.	Parameters	Isotonic dehydration	Hypertonic dehydration	Hypotonic dehydration
2	Mucous membrane	Dry	Pulse	High moist
3	Eyes	Sun lien and soft	Sun lien	Sun lien and soft
4	Anterior fontanel	Depressed	Depressed	Depressed
5	Sensorium	-	Very irritable	Concertos
6	Pulse	Rapid	Moderately rapid	Rapid
7	Blood pressure	Low	Moderately low	Very low

Formula for calculating the IV fluids:

- Macro drips 10 to 20 drops (ml)

$$\frac{\text{Volume of infusion} \times \text{drip factor}}{\text{Time of infusion} \times \text{minutes}} = \text{drops 1 mt}$$

(or)

$$\frac{\text{Total volume of in fluid} \times \text{drip factor}}{\text{Time of infusion} \times \text{minutes}} = \text{drops 1 mt}$$

- Micros drops 60 drips (mt)

$$\frac{\text{Volume of infusion} \times 60}{\text{Time of infusion} \times \text{minutes}} = \text{drops 1 mt}$$

Follow-up Care

- Severe dehydration warrants hospital admission for rehydration, as do hypernatremic or hyponatremic states.
- Inability to tolerate oral rehydration therapy (ORT) may necessitate hospital admission for nasogastric or intravenous fluid therapy.
- ORT may be continued at home if clear instructions are provided for the family and if the family members can be relied upon to carry out the hydration regimen. Close follow-up by the primary physician is recommended.

Complications

Complications may include irreversible shock, sagittal or other venous sinus thrombosis, intractable seizures, and renal failure.

Prognosis

Prognosis is excellent if the child is promptly and effectively treated. However, the child with severe dehydration and hypovolemic shock can have significant morbidity and mortality if treatment is delayed.

VOMITING

Introduction

It is normal for babies and children to vomit occasionally. In most cases, it will last no longer than one to two days and is not a sign of anything serious. The most common cause of vomiting in children and babies is gastroenteritis. This is an infection of the gut usually caused by a virus or bacteria, which also causes diarrhea. The symptoms can be unpleasant but your child will usually start to feel better after a few days.

Persistent vomiting can sometimes cause your child to become severely dehydrated and occasionally it can be a sign of something more serious, such as meningitis.

Definition

Causes of Vomiting

Vomiting can be caused by a number of different problems. The possible causes of vomiting depend upon a child's age.

Newborns and Young Infants

It can be hard to tell if an infant is spitting up or vomiting because some infants reflux forcefully or in large amounts. Your child's doctor or nurse can help to determine the cause and if treatment is needed.

Forceful vomiting in newborns can indicate a serious condition and always requires further evaluation. Potential causes of vomiting in newborns and young infants include a blockage or narrowing of the stomach (pyloric stenosis) or a blockage of the intestines (intestinal obstruction).

Infants can also vomit because of infections of the intestine or other parts of the body. Any young infant (newborn to 3 months) who develops a temperature of 100.4 °F (38 °C) or higher, with or without vomiting, should see a doctor or nurse.

Older Infants and Children

The most common cause of vomiting in older infants and children is infectious gastroenteritis (an infection of the stomach or intestines), usually caused by a virus. Vomiting caused by gastroenteritis usually begins suddenly and resolves quickly, often within 24 to 48 hours. Other signs of gastroenteritis can include nausea, diarrhea, fever, or abdominal pain.

Gastroenteritis can develop after eating contaminated food or putting a contaminated object (or hand) into the mouth. The viruses that commonly cause gastroenteritis are spread easily. Careful hygiene (especially handwashing) can prevent these infections from spreading.

Less commonly, vomiting occurs after consuming improperly stored or prepared foods that contain bacteria or toxins; this is called food poisoning.

Other illnesses can also cause vomiting in older infants and children, including gastroesophageal reflux, peptic ulcer disease, an intestinal blockage (obstruction), cyclic vomiting syndrome, respiratory and urinary tract infections, and others.

Adolescents

Similar to children, the most common cause of nausea and vomiting in adolescents is infectious gastroenteritis. Vomiting usually resolves within 24 to 48 hours in an adolescent with gastroenteritis.

Less common causes of vomiting in adolescents include appendicitis (inflammation of the appendix), induced vomiting (e.g. as seen with bulimia), pregnancy, gastric ulcers (of the stomach), pancreatitis (inflammation of the pancreas), inflammatory bowel disease (e.g. Crohn's disease), and consumption of toxic substances (e.g. overdose).

Common Causes

- Gastroenteritis
- Food allergy or milk intolerance
- Gastroesophageal reflux where stomach contents escape backup the gullet
- Poor bottle feeding advice
- Accidentally swallowing something poisonous
- Congenital pyloric stenosis—a condition present at birth where the passage from the stomach to the bowel has narrowed, so food is unable to pass through easily; this causes projectile vomiting
- A strangulated hernia—your baby will vomit frequently and cry as if they are in a lot of pain; this should be treated as a medical emergency
- Intussusception (where the bowel telescopes in on itself)—as well as vomiting, your baby may look pale, floppy and have symptoms of dehydration.

Diagnostic Evaluation

Most children with vomiting do not need to be seen by a health care provider. However, you should monitor for signs that the child is getting worse or not getting better within 24 hours. If your child has severe or persistent pain or has signs of dehydration, they should be seen sooner.

Warning Signs

- Bile (green) or blood-tinged (red or brown) vomit.
- Any episode of forceful vomiting in a newborn or vomiting that continues for more than 24 hours in an infant or child.
- If an infant refuses to eat or drink anything for more than a few hours.
- *Moderate to severe dehydration:* Dry mouth, no tears when crying, not urinating or having a wet diaper in four to six hours (for babies and young children) or not urinating in six to eight hours (for older children).
- Abdominal pain that is severe, even if it comes and goes.
- Bloody bowel movements.
- Fever higher than 102 °F (39 °C) once or fever higher than 101 °F (38.4 °C) for more than three days.
- Behavior changes, including lethargy or decreased responsiveness.

Management

Infants

If a breastfeeding infant vomits, he or she should continue to breastfeed unless doctor or nurse tells you otherwise. Oral rehydration solutions (e.g. Pedialyte) are not usually needed for infants who exclusively breastfeed because breast milk is more easily digested.

Infant vomits immediately after nursing, you can try to breastfeed more frequently and for a shorter time. For example, breastfeed every 30 minutes for five to 10 minutes. If vomiting improves after two to three hours, resume the usual feeding schedule. If vomiting worsens or does not improve within 24 hours, call your child's doctor or nurse.

Infant drinks formula, initially offer one-half to one ounce of an oral rehydration solution (e.g. Pedialyte) every 15 minutes for two to three hours. If vomiting occurs after drinking, wait 30 minutes and try again. If vomiting improves, resume feeding with full strength infant formula. If vomiting worsens or does not improve within 24 hours, call your child's doctor or nurse.

Older Infants and Children

Older infants and children who vomit can continue to eat, if desired. However, it is common for children to have little or no appetite during a vomiting illness.

- Monitor for signs of dehydration, and do not force the child to eat, especially during the first 24 hours. Encourage the child to drink fluids. The best fluids are the commercially prepared oral rehydration solutions (e.g. Pedialyte). Other fluids, including water, diluted juice, or soda can be given in small quantities.
- Apple, pear, and cherry juice, and other beverages with high sugar content, should be avoided. Sports drinks (e.g. Gatorade) should also be avoided since they have too much sugar and have inappropriate electrolyte levels.
- Recommended foods include a combination of complex carbohydrates (rice, wheat, potatoes, bread), lean meats, yogurt, fruits, and vegetables. High fat foods are more difficult to digest, and should be avoided.
- It is not necessary to restrict a child's diet to clear liquids or the BRAT diet (bananas, rice, applesauce, toast). Although these and similar foods might be recommended to decrease diarrhea, these foods do not contain enough nutrients for a child.

Oral Rehydration Therapy

- Oral rehydration therapy (ORT) was developed as a safer, less-expensive, and easier alternative to intravenous (IV) fluids. Oral rehydration solution (ORS) is a liquid solution that contains glucose (a sugar) and electrolytes (sodium, potassium, chloride), which are lost during vomiting and diarrhea.
- ORS does not cure vomiting, but it does help to prevent and treat the dehydration that can develop because of a vomiting illness.
- A few widely available brands include Pedialyte, Infalyte, and ReVital, although generic brands work equally well, gelatin, tea, fruit juice, rice water, and other beverages are not recommended in children who are dehydrated. Do not try to prepare ORS recipes at home because the formulas must be exact.
- The recommended amount is 5 teaspoons of ORS for every pound of body weight (or 50 milliliters per kilogram). For a 20-pound (9 kg) child, this would equal 100 teaspoons (450 milliliters) of ORS. This amount should be given gradually, spread out over about four hours.
- Measure the solution with a standardized medicine syringe or measuring cup or spoon, rather than a regular cup or spoon.
- Give the fluid by teaspoonful (5 milliliters each) every one to two minutes or as tolerated.

Medicines

Medicines to reduce nausea and vomiting, like antiemetics, might be recommended in certain situations (to reduce the risk of dehydration in children who vomit repeatedly or to reduce motion sickness).

Hygiene Measures

- Handwashing is very effective and the preferred way to prevent the spread of infection.
- Wet your hands with water and plain or antimicrobial soap, and rub them together for 15 to 30 seconds.
- Pay special attention to the fingernails, between the fingers, and the wrists.
- Rinse your hand thoroughly, dry them with a paper towel, and throw away the paper towel.
- Alcohol-based hand rubs are an acceptable alternative for disinfecting hands if a sink is not available. Spread the hand rub over the entire surface of your hands, fingers, and wrists until dry.
- Hand rubs are available as a liquid or wipe in small, portable sizes that are easy to carry in a pocket or handbag. If your hands are visibly dirty, you should wash them with soap and water.

Preventive Measures

The viruses that cause some gastroenteritis are spread through close contact with infected people, says the Centers for Disease Control and Prevention (CDC). The viruses make their way easily from person to person and can be passed around through shared food, water, and eating utensils.

To prevent viral gastroenteritis and the vomiting that often goes with it, the CDC suggests:

- Wash your hands often, including after you use the bathroom or change diapers.
- Use alcohol-based hand rubs when soap and water are not available.
- Disinfect contaminated surfaces with bleach-based cleaners.
- Be sure food is stored, cooked, prepared, and served hygienically.

CHILDHOOD DISORDERS AND HEALTH PROBLEMS

COMMUNICABLE DISEASES

Introduction

A communicable disease such as a cold is a disease that spreads from person to person. Communicable diseases are diseases that you can 'catch' from someone or something else. Some people may use the words contagious or infectious communicable diseases

Children have maturing immune systems and are often in close proximity to one another, such as in day-care centers, classrooms, and on school busses. This makes the transmission of contagious diseases particularly easy and explains, in part, why these diseases are so common in children. Contagious diseases are often caused by the spread of bacteria (such as in scarlet fever) or viruses (such as in chickenpox, measles, hand-foot-and-mouth disease, and quite a few others) in droplets of saliva and mucus, especially when coughing or sneezing. Contagious diseases may also occur by coming in close personal contact with another infected person or even by sharing personal items of an infected person, as in the case with infestation caused by insects (such as with lice and scabies) or a fungal infection (such as in Tinea infections, commonly called 'ringworm').

Definition

A communicable diseases spread from one person to another or from an animal to a person. The spread often happens via airborne viruses or bacteria, but also through blood or other bodily fluid. The terms infectious and contagious are also used to describe communicable disease.

Causes

Common Infectious diseases caused by:

- *Bacteria:* These one-cell organisms are responsible for illnesses, such as strep throat, urinary tract infections and tuberculosis.
- *Viruses:* Even smaller than bacteria, viruses cause a multitude of diseases ranging from the common cold to AIDS.
- *Fungi:* Many skin diseases, such as ringworm and athlete's foot, are caused by fungi. Other types of fungi can infect your lungs or nervous system.
- *Parasites:* Malaria is caused by a tiny parasite that is transmitted by a mosquito bite. Other parasites may be transmitted to humans from animal feces.

Classification

- Common Viral Infectious Diseases
  - Measles
  - Chickenpox
  - Mumps
  - Poliomyelitis
  - HIV/AIDS
  - Dengue syndrome
  - German measles (Rubella)
  - Herpes simplex infection
  - Herpes zoster
  - GBS **(Guillain-Barré syndrome)**
  - Infective mononucleosis
  - Influenza
  - Swine Flu.
- Common Bacterial Infectious Diseases
  - Tuberculosis
  - Typhoid fever
  - Tetanus
  - Diphtheria
  - Whooping cough
  - Leprosy
  - Nosocomial Infection
  - *Haemophilus influenzae* 'B' (Hib)
  - Meningococcal infections

- *Helicobacter pylori* infections
- Congenital syphilis.
- Common Parasites Infectious Diseases
  - Malaria
  - Filaria
  - Kala-azar
  - Giardiasis
  - Amebiasis
  - Worm infestations
  - Cryptosporidiosis
  - Hydatid disease.

Mode of Transmission

Direct Contact

An easy way to catch most infectious diseases is by coming in contact with a person or animal who has the infection. Three ways infectious diseases can be spread through direct contact are:

Person to Person

A common way for infectious diseases to spread is through the direct transfer of bacteria, viruses or other germs from one person to another. This can occur when an individual with the bacterium or virus touches, coughs on or kisses someone who is not infected.

These germs can also spread through the exchange of body fluids from sexual contact or a blood transfusion. The person who passes the germ may have no symptoms of the disease, but may simply be a carrier.

Animal to Person

Being bitten or scratched by an infected animal even a pet can make you sick and, in extreme circumstances, can be fatal. Handling animal waste can be hazardous, too. For example, you can acquire a toxoplasmosis infection by scooping your cat's litter box.

Mother to Unborn Child

A pregnant woman may pass germs that cause infectious diseases to her unborn baby. Some germs can pass through the placenta. Germs in the vagina can be transmitted to the baby during birth.

Indirect Contact

Disease-causing organisms also can be passed by indirect contact. Many germs can linger on an inanimate object, such as a tabletop, doorknob or faucet handle.

When you touch a doorknob handled by someone ill with the flu or a cold, for example, you can pick up the germs he or she left behind. If you then touch your eyes, mouth or nose before washing your hands, you may become infected.

Insect Bites

Some germs rely on insect carriers such as mosquitoes, fleas, lice or ticks to move from host to host. These carriers are known as vectors. Mosquitoes can carry the malaria parasite or West Nile virus, and deer ticks may carry the bacterium that causes Lyme disease.

Food Contamination

Another way disease-causing germs can infect you is through contaminated food and water. This mechanism of transmission allows germs to be spread to many people through a single source. E. coli, for example, is a bacterium present in or on certain foods such as undercooked hamburger or unpasteurized fruit juice.

COMMON VIRAL INFECTIOUS DISEASES IN CHILDREN

MEASLES

Introduction

Measles, also known as rubeola, is a viral infection of the respiratory system. Measles is a very contagious disease that can spread through contact with infected mucus and saliva. The coughing or sneezing of an infected person can release the virus into the air. The virus can live on surfaces for several hours. As the infected particles enter the air and settle on surfaces, anyone within close proximity can become infected with the measles virus.

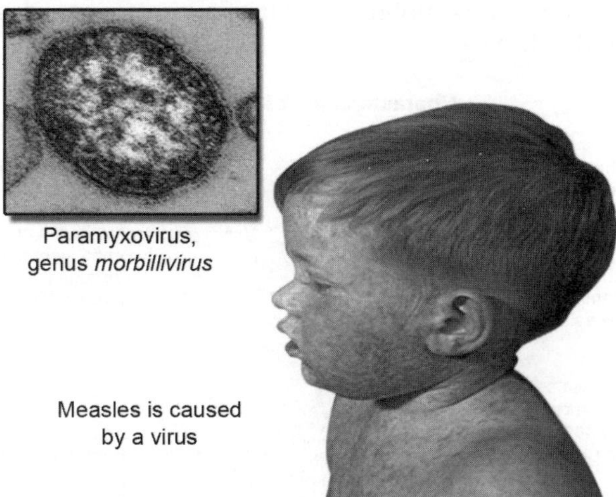

Fig. 5.3: Child with measles

Definition

Measles defined as a highly contagious (easily spread) infection that causes a rash all over your body. It is also called rubeola or red measles.

Measles is a childhood infection caused by a virus. Once quite common, measles can now almost always be prevented with a vaccine. Signs and symptoms of measles include cough, runny nose, inflamed eyes, sore throat, fever and a red, blotchy skin rash.

It is a significant contributor to childhood mortality, especially in the malnourished children below the age of 3 years.

Incidence

Measles is a leading cause of death in children. Of the 139,300 global deaths related to measles in 2010, the World Health Organization (WHO) reports that most of the victims were under the age of 5 (WHO).

Mode of transmission is mainly by droplet infections and droplet nuclei. Portal of entry is the respiratory tract and sometimes through conjunctiva. It can spread directly by air borne route or by indirect contact with fomites.

Measles is highly contagious—90% of people who have not been vaccinated for measles will get it if they are near an infected person. Measles spreads when people breathe in or have direct contact with virus-infected fluid, such as the droplets sprayed into the air when someone with measles sneezes or coughs. A person who is exposed to the virus might not show symptoms until 8–10 days later.

Incubation Period

Incubation period is 10 to 15 days. Measles usually occurs in winter and spring months but may found in all seasons.

Risk Factors for Measles Include

- *Being unvaccinated:* If you have not received the vaccine for measles, you are much more likely to develop the disease.

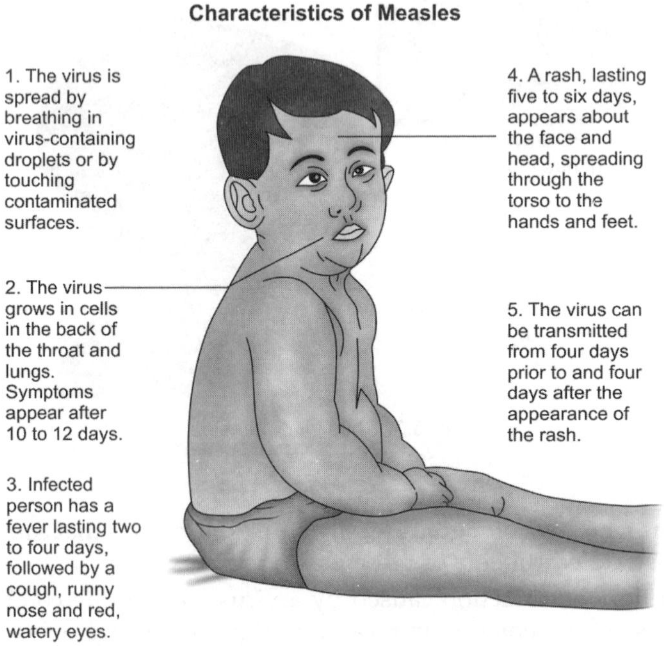

Characteristics of Measles

1. The virus is spread by breathing in virus-containing droplets or by touching contaminated surfaces.

2. The virus grows in cells in the back of the throat and lungs. Symptoms appear after 10 to 12 days.

3. Infected person has a fever lasting two to four days, followed by a cough, runny nose and red, watery eyes.

4. A rash, lasting five to six days, appears about the face and head, spreading through the torso to the hands and feet.

5. The virus can be transmitted from four days prior to and four days after the appearance of the rash.

Fig. 5.4: Characteristics of measles

- *Traveling internationally:* If you travel to developing countries, where measles is more common, you are at higher risk of catching the disease.
- *Having a vitamin A deficiency:* If you do not have enough vitamin A in your diet, you are more likely to contract measles and to have more-severe symptoms.

Clinical Manifestations

Symptoms of measles generally appear within 14 days of exposure to the virus.

Symptoms include:

- Cough
- Fever
- Red eyes
- Light sensitivity
- Muscle aches
- Runny nose
- Sore throat
- White spots inside the mouth.

Clinical features of measles are in three stages:

Prodromal (catarrhal) or preeruptive stage: Commonly it will starts after 10 days of infection and lasts 3 to 5 days.

- Fever
- Malaise
- Coryza
- Sneezing
- Nasal discharge
- Brassy cough
- Redness of eyes
- Lacrimation
- Photophobia.

The important characteristics of this stage are appearance of Koplik's spots. It is Grayish or bluish-white spots, fine tiny grain like papules on a faint red base, smaller than head of a pin.

These spots appear before the appearance of rash. They are found on the buccal mucosa opposite the first and second lower molars. The spots usually disappear a day after the rash appears. Practically the spots are observed in only a small numbers of cases.

Eruptive stage: Commonly it will occur 3 to 5 days after the onset of the disease.

In this stage typical irregular dusky-red macular or maculopapular rash which found behind the ears and face first, then it spreads to neck, trunk, limbs, palms and soles in next 3 to 4 days.

- Fever
- Anorexia
- Malaise
- Cervical lymphadenopathy.

There is fine shedding of superficial skin of face, trunk and limbs, leaving brownish discoloration which may persist for 2 months or more.

Convalescent or postmeasles stage: In this stage symptoms will disappear, fever and rash. But mostly the children remain sick few more days and lost weight.

Pathophysiology

Due to causes organism (virus) enter in the respiratory track epithelium cell which affect in local multiplication and viremia. The infection spreads to reticuloendothelial system and become secondary viremia which produces systemic symptoms. Superficial blood vessels of skin and mucous membrane are affected and formed inclusion bodies. This multinucleated giant cell can be demonstrated in both epidermis and oral epithelium cell.

Diagnostic Evaluation

- History collection
- Physical examination
- Blood test
- Specific sign of Koplik's spot on the inside lining of the cheek.
- ELISA test to detect the presence of measles antibody.

Management

- Acetaminophen to relieve fever and muscle aches
- Adequate rest boost child immune system
- Plenty of fluids (six to eight glasses of water a day)
- Humidifier to ease a cough and sore throat
- Vitamin a supplements.

Postexposure Management

Vaccination

Nonimmunized children, including infants, may be given the measles vaccination within 72 hours of exposure to the measles virus to provide protection against the disease. If measles still develops, the illness usually has milder symptoms and lasts for a shorter time.

Immune Serum Globulin

Pregnant women, infants and children with weakened immune systems who are exposed to the virus may receive an injection of proteins (antibodies) called immune serum globulin. When given within six days of exposure to the virus, these antibodies can prevent measles or make symptoms less severe.

Medications

Antipyretic: The child may also take over-the-counter medications such as acetaminophen (Tylenol, others), ibuprofen (Advil, Motrin, others) or naproxen (Aleve) to help relieve the fever that accompanies measles.

Be caution when giving aspirin to children or teenagers. Though aspirin is approved for use in children older than age 3, children and teenagers recovering from chickenpox or flu-like symptoms should never take aspirin. This is because aspirin has been linked to Reye's syndrome, a rare but potentially life-threatening condition, in such children.

Antibiotics

A bacterial infection, such as pneumonia or an ear infection develops while child has measles, doctor will prescribe an antibiotic.

Vitamin A

The children with low levels of vitamin A are more likely to have a more severe case of measles. Giving vitamin A may lessen the severity of the measles. It is generally given as a large dose of 200,000 international units (IU) for two days. Early detection and management of complications should be done promptly to prevent poor prognosis.

Preventive Measures

Immunizations can help prevent a measles outbreak. The MMR vaccine is a three-in-one vaccination that can protect you and your children from the measles, mumps, and rubella. Children can receive their first MMR vaccination at 12 months (or sooner if traveling internationally), and their second dose between the ages of 4 and 6.

Active immunization with live attenuated measles vaccine is administered 0.5 ml subcutaneously in single dose at 9 to 12 months of age. It provides protection to the susceptible children for the life time. MMR vaccine can be administered for protection against measles along with mumps and rubella.

Isolation

Isolation is most important because measles is highly contagious from about four days, before to four days after the rash breaks out, people with measles should not return to activities in which they interact with other people during this period.

It may also be necessary to keep non-immunized children (siblings) for example away from the infected children.

Vaccination

Make sure that anyone who is at risk of getting the measles who has not been fully vaccinated receives the measles vaccine as soon as possible.

Complications

- *Ear infection:* One of the most common complications of measles is a bacterial ear infection.
- *Bronchitis, laryngitis or croup:* Measles may lead to inflammation of your voice box (larynx) or inflammation of the inner walls that line the main air passageways of your lungs (bronchial tubes).
- *Pneumonia:* Pneumonia is a common complication of measles. People with compromised immune systems can develop an especially dangerous variety of pneumonia that is sometimes fatal.
- *Encephalitis:* About 1 in 1,000 people with measles develops encephalitis, an inflammation of the brain that may cause vomiting, convulsions and rarely coma or even death. Encephalitis can closely follow measles, or it can occur months later.
- *Pregnancy problems:* If you are pregnant, you need to take special care to avoid measles because the disease can cause pregnancy loss, preterm labor or low birth weight.

- *Low platelet count (thrombocytopenia):* Measles may lead to a decrease in platelets—the type of blood cells that are essential for blood clotting.

Prognosis

Prognosis of a well-nourished child with measles is usually good. Measles is self-limiting disease unless it is complicated. Approximately 90 percent of death may occur in severe respiratory and neurological complications. The survivors of post-measles encephalopathy may have neurological deficits as long-term sequel.

CHICKENPOX (VARICELLA)

Introduction

Chickenpox is an infection caused by the varicella virus. It cannot be treated with antibiotics. Treatment is usually to relieve the symptoms.

It is easily spread by either having direct contact with (i.e. touching) the person who has chickenpox, or from fluid droplets in the air when they cough. Fever and a rash are the most common signs of chickenpox. A child with chickenpox is infectious to others from one to two days before the rash first appears until the last blisters have dried up. Children and adults of any age can get chickenpox but it is more common in children.

In children, the first symptom of chickenpox is usually an itchy rash that appears on the head and spreads down to the trunk and other body parts.

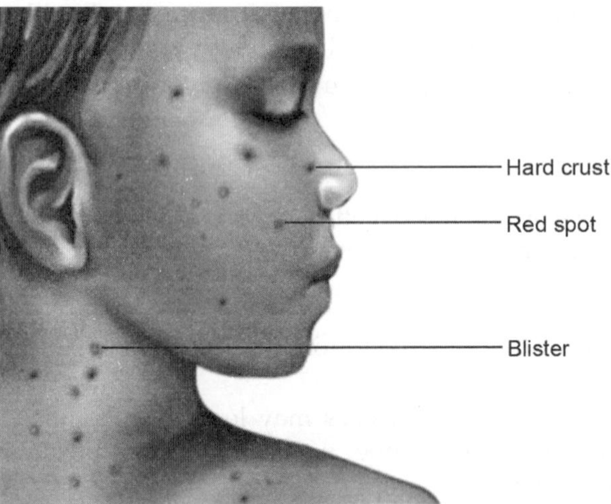

Fig. 5.5: Child with chickenpox

Incidence

Chickenpox is caused by the *Varicella zoster* virus. It can be spread either through person-to-person contact, or through sneezing and coughing. Children can develop chickenpox after being in contact with someone who has shingles (but elderly people cannot get shingles from chickenpox).

Causes

Chickenpox is caused by the herpes varicella-zoster virus. It is spread by droplets from a sneeze or cough, or by contact with the clothing, bed linens or oozing blisters of an infected person. The onset of symptoms is 10 to 21 days after exposure. The disease is most contagious a day or two before the rash appears and until the rash is completely dry and scabbed over.

Mode of Transmission

Chickenpox is easily transmissible from person to person. About 90% of nonimmune household contacts of someone infected with chickenpox will contract the disease.

Transmission of chickenpox occurs via infected respiratory tract secretions, respiratory droplets, and fluid from the blisters. A person is infectious from one to two days before the rash appears to the time the blisters crust over and no longer contain fluid.

The virus can transmit through placental barrier and can infect the fetus. So infection during pregnancy presents risk for fetus and neonates and may cause limb atrophy, skin scaring, microcephaly, neurological and ocular anomalies. Incubation period is usually 14 to 16 days with a range from 7 to 21 days.

Clinical Manifestations

- *Hyperthermia:* 101–102 °F (38.3–38.8 °C)
- Feeling tired and irritable
- Itching
- Rash (Spots)
- Loss of appetite or feeding problems.

The rash usually first appears on the chest, back or face. It then can move to other areas of the body including inside the mouth. At first, the rash looks like small pimples. These later become blisters full of fluid.

Chickenpox causes a red, itchy skin rash that usually appears first on the abdomen or back and face, and then spreads to almost everywhere else on the body, including the scalp, mouth, arms, legs, and genitals.

Two stages of clinical manifestation:

The preeruptive or prodromal phase presents with sudden onset of mild to moderate fever, back pain, shivering and malaise for a short period (about 24 hours). This stage may be overlooked in some cases.

The eruptive stage manifests with rash which can be first sign. It appears usually on the day, the fever starts. The eruptions pass through the stages, i.e. macules, papule, vesicle, pustule and crusts or scabs.

Pathophysiology

Based on causes organism enters to the skin and respiratory tract. The skin lesions found as macules which quickly develop into papules and vesicles with scab and crust formation.

The vesicles are formed in prickle cell layer of skin. Degeneration of cells in the vesicles results in multinucleated giant cells containing intranuclear inclusions. The inclusion bodies and foci of necrosis may be present in esophagus, pancreas, liver, adrenal gland and genitourinary tract. Varicella may cause disseminated interstitial pneumonia, encephalitis, perivascular demyelization.

Diagnostic Evaluation

Chickenpox is usually diagnosed by clinical manifestations. It should be differentiated from other skin lesions like impetigo, herpes urticaria, etc. It is differentiated from smallpox, which is already eradicated. Laboratory investigations are difficult. Virus isolation, antibody test can be done.

Management

There is no specific treatment. Symptomatic and supportive management are essential.

Isolate the infected child because the disease is highly contagious and airborne spread can occur. Isolation is especially important if the hospital also admits patients who are immune-compromised because their exposure to the disease can be serious and even fatal.

Antipyretic Drugs (Acetaminophen)

(Tylenol, Feverall, Tempra, Aspirin-Free Anacin)

Acetaminophen is the drug of choice because it has no association with Reye syndrome. It is available as drops containing 80 mg/0.8 mL; a suspension containing 160 mg/5 mL; a chewable tablet or capsule containing 80 mg; and a tablet containing 160 mg, 325 mg, or 500 mg.

Ibuprofen (Motrin, Ibuprin)

Ibuprofen A is a propionic acid-derivative NSAID. It acts by inhibiting prostaglandin synthesis and also has anti-inflammatory and analgesic properties. It is available as an oral suspension (100 mg/5 mL) and a tab containing 200 mg, 400 mg, 600 mg, or 800 mg.

Acyclovir

Acyclovir is an antiviral agent that acts by inhibiting herpes virus DNA polymerase and terminating viral replication. It reduces the number of lesions and duration of fever if it is started within 24 hours of rash appearance. In young children with uncomplicated varicella, the benefit of acyclovir therapy is only marginal, and its use is not routinely recommended.

Antihistamines

Diphenhydramine (Benadryl)

Diphenhydramine is an antihistamine that has a sedating effect and is effective for pruritus. It is available as a liquid containing 12.5 mg/5 mL, capsule containing 25 and 50 mg, and injection containing 50 mg/mL.

Hydroxyzine (Vistaril)

Hydroxyzine antagonizes H1 receptors in the periphery. It may suppress histamine activity in subcortical region of the CNS. It is a second-line agent useful for pruritus when diphenhydramine is ineffective.

Hydroxyzine may only be given orally or intramuscularly (IM). It is available as a 25- or 50mg capsule; 10 mg/5 mL suspension; 10-, 25-, or 50-mg tablet; or 25-mg/mL and 50-mg/mL for intramuscular injection.

Immune Globulins

Varicella Zoster Immune Globulin, (VariZIG)

Varicella zoster immune globulin (VZIG) contains immunoglobulin G (IgG) varicella-zoster antibodies. It provides passive immunization to exposed individuals at high risk of complications from varicella (e.g. immunocompromised children or adults, pregnant women, newborns of mothers with varicella close to delivery, premature infants, normal susceptible adults, full-term infants < 1 year). Administer by deep IM injection, preferably in deltoid muscle. For neonates or infants, administer IM in anterolateral aspect of thigh.

Varicella Virus Vaccine (Varivax)

The varicella virus vaccine is indicated for children aged between 12 months and 12 years.

Complication

- Inflammation of the lung (pneumonia)
- Inflammation of the brain (encephalitis).

Other Serious Complications

- Reye's syndrome (a very rare condition with brain and liver problems)
- Inflammation of the heart muscle (myocarditis)
- Kidney inflammation (glomerulonephritis)
- Appendicitis
- Ataxia (problem with movements)
- Inflammation of the pancreas (pancreatitis)
- Henoch-Schönlein purpura (a condition that can affect the kidneys)
- Inflammation of the testes (orchitis)
- Inflammation of the joints (arthritis)
- Inflammation of various parts of the eye.

Preventive Measures

The chickenpox vaccine is 99% effective at preventing the VZV infection in Children. Doctors recommend that kids receive the chickenpox vaccine twice when they are 12 to 15 months old, with a booster shot at 4 to 6 years old.

Passive immunity can be provided by Varicella Zoster Immunoglobulin (VZIg) which is quality effective and indicated in the children with leukemia, steroid therapy, susceptible pregnant women and neonates whose mothers develop chickenpox 2 days before and 5 days after delivery.

Prognosis

Chickenpox is usually a self-limiting disease with good prognosis. In case of serious complications like encephalitis especially in immunocompromise children the prognosis may be worse.

MUMPS (PAROTITIS)

Introduction

Mumps is an acute, self-limited, systemic viral infection characterized by the swelling of one or more of the salivary glands, typically the parotid glands. The illness is caused by the RNA virus, rubulavirus. Rubulavirus is within the genus *Paramyxovirus* and is a member of the family paramyxoviridae.

Mumps is a viral infection of the salivary glands, especially the parotid glands that run along the angle of the jaw in front of and below each ear. Children between the ages of 5 and 10 are most likely to contract mumps. Being infected once gives you lifelong immunity.

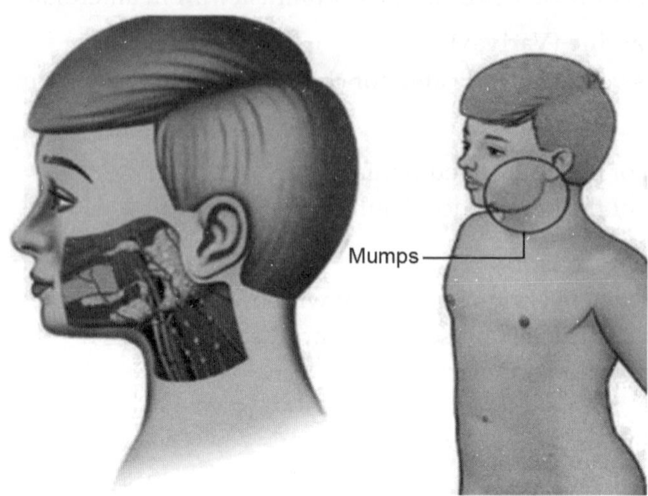

Fig. 5.6: Child with mumps

Definition

Mumps is defined as generalized acute infection caused by a paramyxovirus, usually in children and young adults.

Causes

Paramyxovirus

It is transmitted via the mouth by tiny drops of saliva from talking, sneezing, sharing drinks, kissing, or coughing.

Mode of Transmission

The transmission mode is person to person via respiratory droplets and saliva, direct contact, or fomites. The presence of maternal antibodies typically protects infants younger than 1 year from the disease.

Incubation Period

Mumps has an incubation period of 16–18 days; it can arise 12–25 days after exposure. After this period, **Prodromal symptoms** (such as low-grade fever, malaise, Myalgia, headache, and anorexia) occur; these symptoms can last 3–5 days.

Clinical Manifestations

Mumps is commonly asymptomatic. The initial features are hyperthermia, headache, nausea, malaise, anorexia and sore throat. When child is chewing and swallowing usually get the earaches and pain in behind the ear lobes. Tenderness and pain usually subside within 3 days and swelling disappears within 10 days.

Other Symptoms

- Problem in mastication and swallowing
- Often very high grade fever
- Swollen lymph nodes around the neck
- Inflammation of the mucus lining of the mouth.

Neurological Symptoms

- Aseptic meningitis
- Encephalitis
- Auditory nerve damage
- GBS
- Facial palsy
- Facial neuritis
- Transverse myelitis
- Cerebellar ataxia.

Pathophysiology

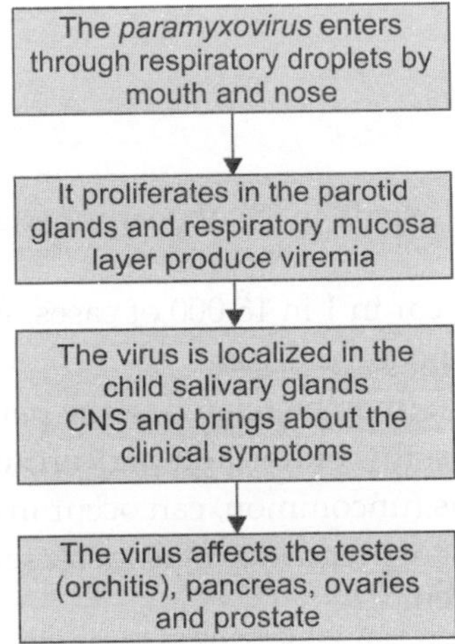

Fig. 5.7: Pathophysiology of mumps

Diagnostic Evaluation

- History collection with consideration of signs and symptoms, questioning of potential contact with other children with mumps.
- Physical examination helps to assess the swelling of the parotid and cheek swollen.
- Blood examination (Determination of antibodies in the blood).
- Identification of the pathogen by smears, saliva, in the cerebrospinal fluid, urine or with a tissue sample if needed.
- Laboratory investigations CBC test.
- CSF study.

Management

There is no any specific treatment for mumps. The symptomatic treatment includes antipyretics and analgesic to treat fever and pain.

Ibuprofen (Advil, Motrin)

This is the drug of choice for patients with mild to moderate pain and fever. It inhibits inflammatory reactions and pain by decreasing prostaglandin synthesis.

Acetaminophen (Tylenol, Aspirin)

This is the drug of choice for pain in patients with documented hypersensitivity to nonsteroidal anti-inflammatory drugs (NSAIDs), with upper GI disease, or who are taking PO anticoagulants. Acetaminophen reduces fever by acting directly on hypothalamic heat-regulating centers, which increases dissipation of body heat via vasodilation and sweating

Measles-Mumps-Rubella (MMR) Vaccine, Live

Live virus vaccine: Combined MMR vaccine is recommended for the prevention of mumps, measles, and rubella. For children, the typical recommended 2-dose schedule is administered at age 12–15 months for the 1st dose and age 4–6 years for the second dose.

Complications

- Orchitis
- Meningitis and encephalitis.

Other Complications

- Oophoritis, which may cause pain in 5% of postpubertal female's child, sterility seldom occurs.
- Profound deafness (in one ear in 1 in 15,000 of cases, which is usually transient).
- Pancreatitis occurs in around 4% of cases.
- Mild upper abdominal pain (may be related to the pancreas in around 50% of cases).
- Neuritis, arthritis, nephritis, thyroiditis and pericarditis have all been reported.
- Transient and mild mastitis (uncommon, can occur in either sex).
- Mumps in the first trimester of pregnancy may increase the rate of spontaneous abortion but the virus is not teratogenic.

Preventive Measures

- MMR vaccine is given in the national immunization programme (Mumps, Measles, Rubella).
- Normal hygiene measures to prevent droplet infection should be instituted in the household of a child who has mumps.
- Children should be excluded from school for five days following onset of parotid swelling.
- Isolation of the affected children.

Nursing Management

- Wet clothes sponging to reduce fever
- Cold compresses around the neck, cheek, testicular

- Motivate warm water consumption
- Strict bed rest for fever and inflammation of the testicles
- The food in the form of boiled and mashed reduces salivary secretion, which improves the swallowing of the child.
- Good oral hygiene with regular gargling with a disinfectant solution.

Prognosis

The most cases can see the full recovery. About 1 in 1,000 people with mumps meningitis develop encephalitis, of whom 1.5% of cases are fatal. Deaths from other causes are rare, more than half the cases arising in men over the age of 19 years.

POLIOMYELITIS

Introduction

Poliomyelitis is an enteroviral infection that can manifest in 4 different forms: Inapparent infection, abortive disease, nonparalytic poliomyelitis, and paralytic disease. Before the 19th century, poliomyelitis occurred sporadically. During the 19th and 20th centuries, epidemic poliomyelitis was more frequently observed, reaching its peak in the mid 1950s.

The worldwide prevalence of this infection has decreased significantly since then because of aggressive immunization programs. Eradication of this disease during the present decade is a top priority for the World Health Organization (WHO).

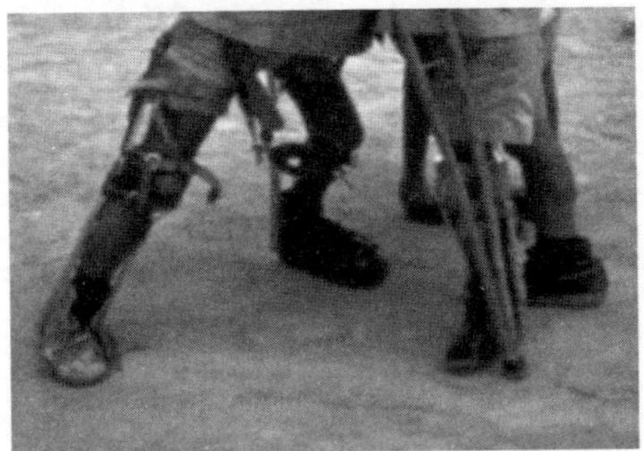

Fig. 5.8: Child with poliomyelitis affected legs

Definition

Poliomyelitis, also called polio, is a highly contagious infectious disease caused by three types of poliovirus. The poliovirus is a virus most recognized for its destruction to the nervous system causing paralysis.

- Type-1 (Burnhide)
- Type-2 (Lansing)
- Type-3 (Leon).

Incidence

- Polio (poliomyelitis) mainly affects children under 5 years of age.
- One in 200 infections leads to irreversible paralysis. Among those paralyzed, 5 to 10% die when their breathing muscles become immobilized.

- Polio cases have decreased by over 99% since 1988, from an estimated 350 000 cases then, to 416 reported cases in 2013. The reduction is the result of the global effort to eradicate the disease.
- In 2014, only 3 countries (Afghanistan, Nigeria and Pakistan) remain polioendemic, down from more than 125 in 1988.
- As long as a single child remains infected, children in all countries are at risk of contracting polio. Failure to eradicate polio from these last remaining strongholds could result in as many as 200 000 new cases every year, within 10 years, all over the world.
- In most countries, the global effort has expanded capacities to tackle other infectious diseases by building effective surveillance and immunization systems.

Mode of Transmission

It is mainly the feco-oral route, directly through contaminated fingers and indirectly through contaminated water, milk, food, flies and articles of daily use. Infection can spreads through droplets in the acute phase of disease when the viruses present in the throat and oropharyngeal secretions.

Poliomyelitis is commonly found in infancy (approximately 50%) and childhood. The most vulnerable age is between 6 months and 3 years. Maternal antibody can protect the infant for first few months of life. Male children are more affected than female. Predisposing factors are intramuscular injection, trauma, operative procedures (e.g. tooth extraction, tonsillectomy), strenuous exercises, etc.

Poliomyelitis is more likely to occur during rainy season. The environmental sources of infections, are contaminated water, food, finger and flies. Overcrowding place, poor sanitation, lack of hygienic practices, urban slum and villages facilitate the exposure of infection.

Incubation Period

Incubation period is usually 7 to 14 days, but may range from 3 to 35 days.

Types of Poliomyelitis

There are three types of polio infections:

- *Subclinical/Asymptomatic poliomyelitis:* Approximately 95 percent of polio cases are subclinical, and patients may not experience any symptoms. This form of polio does not affect the central nervous system (the brain and spinal cord).
- *Nonparalytic:* This form, which does affect the central nervous system, produces only mild symptoms and does not result in paralysis.
- *Paralytic:* This is the rarest and most serious form of polio, which produces full or partial paralysis in the patient. There are three types of paralytic polio: Spinal polio (affects the spine), bulbar polio (affects the brainstem), and bulbospinal polio (affects the spine and brainstem).

Causes

The poliovirus resides only in humans and enters the environment in the feces of someone who is infected. Poliovirus spreads primarily through the fecal-oral route, especially in areas where sanitation is inadequate.

Poliovirus can be transmitted through contaminated water and food or through direct contact with someone infected with the virus. Polio is so contagious that anyone living with a recently infected person is likely to become infected, too. People carrying the poliovirus can spread the virus for weeks in their feces.

Clinical Manifestations

Subclinical/Asymptomatic poliomyelitis

The child does have symptoms, they usually last for 72 hours or less and may include:

- Headache
- Sore, red throat
- Slight fever
- Vomiting
- General discomfort.

Nonparalytic Poliomyelitis

The symptoms of non-aralytic polio may last for a couple of days to a week or two and includes:

- Fever
- Sore throat in the absence of upper respiratory infection
- Headache
- Vomiting
- Fatigue
- Abnormal reflexes
- Problems swallowing and/or breathing
- Back and neck pain and stiffness, particularly neck stiffness with forward flexion of the neck
- Arm and leg pain or stiffness
- Muscle tenderness and spasms.

Paralytic Poliomyelitis

Children with paralytic polio experience the symptoms associated with non-paralytic polio first. Soon after, the following symptoms appear:

- Loss of reflexes
- Severe spasms and muscle pain
- Loose and floppy limbs, sometimes on just one side of the body, this is due to the weakness which results from the involvement of the spine
- Sudden paralysis (temporary or permanent)
- Deformed limbs (especially the hips, ankles, and feet due to prolonged weakness and the lack of appropriate orthopedic bracing.

Full paralysis can eventually develop, but it is rare. Only about one percent of all polio cases will result in a person being permanently paralyzed. Of those patients who experience paralysis, five to 10% will die when the paralysis attacks the muscles that control breathing.

Post-polio Syndrome

The symptoms of postpolio syndrome are:
- Continuing muscle and joint weakness
- Muscle pain that gets worse
- Becoming easily exhausted or fatigued
- Muscle wasting, also called muscle atrophy
- Trouble breathing and/or swallowing
- Sleep related breathing problems (sleep apnea)
- Becoming easily cold
- New onset of weakness in previously uninvolved muscles.

Pathophysiology

The poliovirus is an RNA virus that is transmitted through the oral-fecal route or by ingestion of contaminated water.

Three serotypes are able to cause human infection. The incubation period for poliovirus is 5–35 days.

The viral particles initially replicate in the nasopharynx and GI tract and then invade lymphoid tissues, with subsequent hematologic spread.

After a period of viremia, the virus becomes neurotropic and produces destruction of the motor neurons in the anterior horn and brainstem. The destruction of motor neurons leads to the development of flaccid paralysis, which may be bulbar or spinal in distribution.

Diagnostic Evaluation

Diagnostic procedures for poliomyelitis may include the following:
- History collection
- Physical examination
- Cultures of the throat
- Stool examination
- Urine culture
- Test of polio antibodies levels
- *Lumbar puncture (spinal tap):* A special needle is placed into the lower back, into the spinal canal. This is the area around the spinal cord. The pressure in the spinal canal and brain can then be measured. A small amount of cerebral spinal fluid (CSF) can be removed and sent for testing to determine if there is an infection or other problems. CSF is the fluid that bathes your child's brain and spinal cord.
- Discovering a history of the child not receiving the polio vaccine or not completing the series of polio vaccines.

Management

There is no specific treatment available for poliomyelitis. The prompt symptomatic and supportive management will help the good prognosis. Good nursing care plays vital role for recovery and better outcome.
- Provide bed rest
- Painkillers to relieve headaches, muscle aches, and muscle spasms
- Antibiotics for urinary tract infections

- Portable ventilators to help with breathing
- Physical therapy and/or corrective braces to help with walking
- Heating pads or warm towels to ease muscle aches and spasms
- Physical therapy to treat pain in the affected muscles
- Physical therapy to address breathing and pulmonary problems and then pulmonary rehabilitation to increase the child pulmonary endurance as the acute breathing problems improve
- In advanced cases of leg weakness, when a patient has difficulty walking he or she may need a wheelchair or other mobility device.

Rehabilitation of the paralyzed child should be planned according to the degree of involvement. Corrective splints brace or other orthotic devices may be necessary for the handicapped child. Surgical correction of the deformities may be done in later stages.

Complications

- *Pulmonary complications:* Most important pulmonary complication is respiratory distress. It is a serious life threatening problem and develops due to one or more of the factors, i.e. paralysis of diaphragm and intercostals muscles, obstruction of upper respiratory center or vagus nerve and local lung conditions like pneumonia, atelectassis, pulmonary edema, etc. Respiratory failure may also develop.
- *Cardiovascular problems:* Heart failure, myocarditis, hypertension and cardiac arrest.
- *Gastrointestinal problems:* GI bleeding, perforation, fecal impaction.
- *Urinary problems:* Transient paralysis of bladder, urinary tract infection and renal stone.

Preventive Measures

Polio Vaccine

Presently most of the children receive four doses of inactivated poliovirus vaccine (IPV) at the following ages:

- Two months
- Four months
- Between 6 and 18 months
- Between ages 4 and 6 when children are just entering school

IPV is 90 percent effective after two shots and 99 percent effective after three. It can not cause polio and is safe for people with weakened immune systems, although it is not certain just how protective the vaccine may be in cases of severe immune deficiency. Common side effects are pain and redness at the injection site.

Prognosis

About 5 to 10 percent cases of polio may be complicated with respiratory paralysis. It is not always fatal and many patients may survive with prompt management. Prognosis is generally worse in sudden onset with high fever and in older children. Mortality rate is about 5 to 7 percent and mostly due to respiratory failure. Among survivors, signs of recovery are found in the first few weeks, then recovery slows down during the next 6 months. Recovery may continue slowly up to 2 years. Post-polio residual paralysis may found among survivors of paralytic polio along with bony deformities. Prognosis varies from complete recovery to complete paralysis.

HIV/AIDS

Introduction

AIDS (acquired immunodeficiency syndrome) is a disease that makes it difficult for the body to fight off infectious diseases. The human immunodeficiency virus (HIV) causes AIDS by infecting and damaging part of the body's defenses against infection, its lymphocytes, which are white blood cells in the immune (infection-fighting) system that are supposed to fight off invading germs.

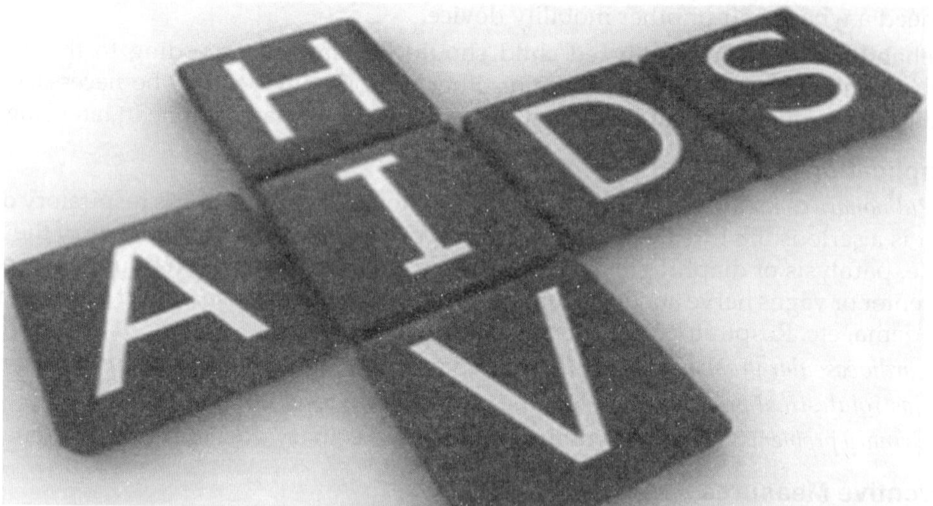

Definition

Children are innocent victim of HIV/AIDS. HIV or human immunodeficiency virus infection leads to AIDS, i.e. acquired immunodeficiency syndrome. It is fatal illness and a pandemic disease with large number of infected children throughout the world. Approximately 0.8 million children, below 15 years of age are infected as estimated by WHO, at the end of 2001. Pediatric AIDS in developing countries comprises 15 to 20 percent of all cases against only 2 percent of the West.

Incidence

Globally, between 2002 and 2013, there was a 58 percent reduction in the number of new HIV infections among the children.

More than 240,000 children were infected with HIV during 2013—700 new infections every day. In addition, millions more children every year are indirectly affected by the impact of the HIV epidemic on their families and communities.

Causes

The human immunodeficiency virus (HIV) is a retrovirus belonging to the family of lentiviruses. Retroviruses can use their RNA and host DNA to make viral DNA and are known for their long incubation periods. Like other retroviruses, HIV infects the body, has a long incubation period (clinical latency), and ultimately causes the signs and symptoms of disease, here AIDS. HIV causes severe damage to the immune system and eventually destroys it by using the DNA of CD4+ cells to replicate itself. In that process, the virus eventually destroys the CD4+ cells.

Mode of Transmission

Mode of transmission is mainly by sexual route in adult. Parent to child transmission is major concern in pediatric HIV/AIDS which include vertical transmission (90%) from infected mother to fetus or from infected mother to child. Transmission may occur in uterus (30–35%), during delivery (60–65%) and also through breastfeeding (1–3%).

Mother-to-child Transmission

The majority of children living with HIV were infected via mother-to-child transmission, during pregnancy, labor, delivery or breastfeeding. However, preventing mother-to-child transmission (PMTCT) is one of the greatest HIV medical success stories. Administrating antiretroviral drugs (ARVs) to mother and child keeps the mother healthy and prevents the risk of HIV passing to the child.

It is vital that children who were infected via mother-to-child transmission receive treatment to keep them healthy. If they are not on antiretroviral treatment (ART), a third of children who are living with HIV will not reach their 1st birthday, and half will not reach their 2nd birthday. This shows that with funding, trained staff and resources, new infections among many thousands of children could be avoided.

Sexual Transmission

There has been a global decrease in the number of young people who report having sex under the age of 15. However, girls under the age of 15 can still marry with their parents consent in 52 countries around the world. This and other cultural norms lead to children becoming sexually active at a young age, or being subjected to sexual violence.

The lower the age of first sex, the higher the lifetime risk of HIV infection. This is because early sexual debut is often associated with older partners, higher rates of coerced sex and lower levels of condom use.

Children Those Who are Injecting Drugs

Global and national figures for the number of children under 15 who inject drugs are limited. This is despite studies reporting that some begin to inject drugs as young as age 10. Children who inject drugs are more likely to share needles and not access harm reduction services, as a result of restrictions due to their age. This makes them more vulnerable to HIV infection.

Children who inject drugs are more likely to be living on the street, orphaned, and out of school. Orphaned and vulnerable children are often marginalized in society, making it difficult to reach them with healthcare and HIV services.

Blood Transfusions

Although very rare today, HIV infection can occur in medical settings. For instance, through needles that have not been sterilized or through blood transfusions where infected blood is used. Between 1987 to 1991, more than 10,000 babies and children were infected with HIV as a result of unsafe medical practices that used contaminated injections and unscreened blood transfusions in Romania.

Incubation Period

Incubation period of HIV infection is uncertain. It may vary from few months to 6 years or more to develop AIDS from HIV infection. It depends upon lifestyle of the infected children and supportive care of the infected child. Natural history of HIV infection is not yet completely understood.

Pathophysiology

The HIV virus is commonly transmitted via unprotected sexual activity, blood transfusions, hypodermic needles, and from mother to child.

↓

The HIV virus replicates inside and kills T helper cells, which are required for all adaptive immune responses.

↓

Depletion of CD4+ lymphocytes in blood and lymph nodes are the important characteristic of AIDS.

↓

Initially asymptomatic phase

↓

A long asymptomatic period may found due to decline in viremia as a result of vigorous cellular and humoral response of the immune system

↓

Opportunistic infections usually occur when CD4+ cell count fall below approximately 200 to 400/ml. death may occur due to infections, cancer

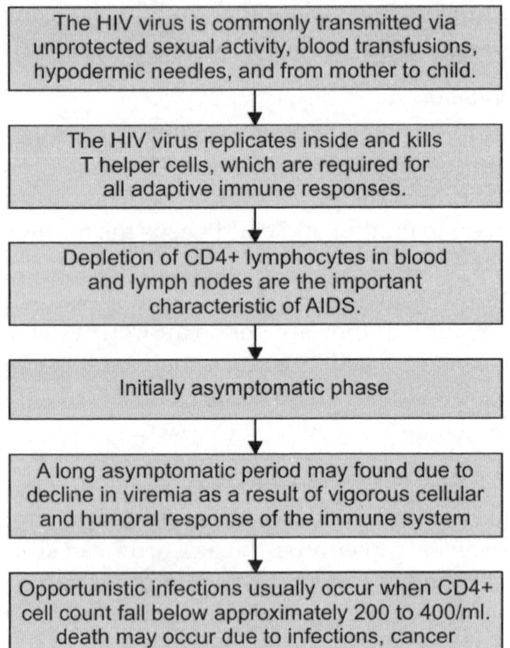

Fig. 5.9: Pathophysiology of HIV infection

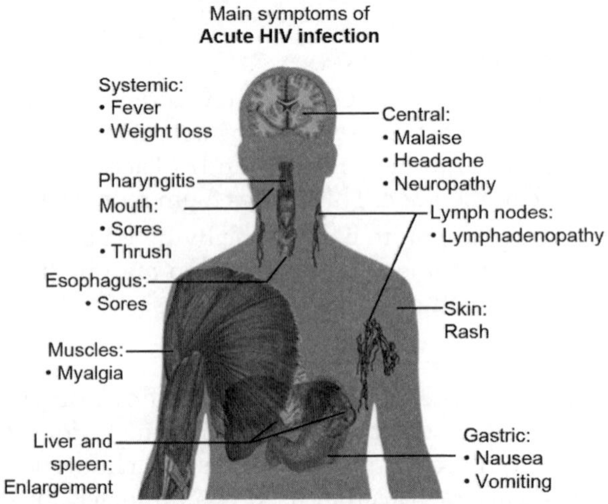

Main symptoms of
Acute HIV infection
Systemic:
• Fever
• Weight loss
Central:
• Malaise
• Headache
• Neuropathy
Pharyngitis
Mouth:
• Sores
• Thrush
Lymph nodes:
• Lymphadenopathy
Esophagus:
• Sores
Skin:
Rash
Muscles:
• Myalgia
Liver and spleen:
Enlargement
Gastric:
• Nausea
• Vomiting

Fig. 5.10: Signs and symptoms of acute HIV infection

Clinical Manifestations

There are no immediate physical signs of HIV infection at birth, if untreated child might appear within 2 to 3 months after a child is born. Children who are born with HIV can develop opportunistic infections, which are illnesses that can develop in weakened immune systems, such as *Pneumocystis jirovicii* pneumonia.

HIV infection has three stages. The first stage is called acute infection or seroconversion and it happens within two to six weeks after exposure or becoming infected. This is when the body's immune system puts up a fight against HIV. The symptoms of acute infection are similar to those of other viral illnesses and are often compared to getting the flu. The symptoms may last a week or two and then completely go away as the virus goes into a nonsymptomatic, or asymptomatic stage.

The initial symptoms of acute HIV infection may include:

- Headache
- Diarrhea
- Nausea and vomiting
- Fatigue
- Myalgia
- Sore throat
- A blotchy red rash that does not itch, usually on the torso
- Hyperthermia

The infants born to mothers with risk factors/HIV infected may present with low birth weight, failure to thrive, microcephaly, hepatosplenomegaly, lymphadenopathy and pneumocystis pneumonia. Recurrent otitis media, chronic sinopulmonary infection, oral thrush, chronic diarrhea, chronic parotid swelling, unexplained anemia, thrombocytopenia and recurrent infection may develop. Cardiac of kidney disease may also found. *Kaposi's sarcoma* is uncommon in childhood AIDS.

Stages of Manifestation (According to WHO)

According to World Health Organization clinical staging system for HIV infection and related disease in children:

- Stage I
  - Mostly asymptomatic
  - Persistent generalized lymphadenopathy.
- Stage II
  - Chronic diarrhea
  - Severe persistent or chronic candidiasis outside the neonatal period
  - Poor weight gain
  - Failure to thrive
  - Persistent hyperthermia
  - Recurrent severe bacterial infections.
- Stage III
  - AIDS
  - Severe failure to thrive
  - Progressive encephalopathy
  - Malignancy
  - Recurrent septicemia or meningitis.

Diagnostic Evaluation

History Collection

- Unusually frequent and severe occurrences of common childhood bacterial infections, such as otitis media, sinusitis, and pneumonia
- Recurrent fungal infections, such as candidiasis (thrush), that do not respond to standard antifungal agents: Suggests lymphocytic dysfunction
- Recurrent or unusually severe viral infections, such as recurrent or disseminated herpes simplex or zoster infection or cytomegalovirus (CMV) retinitis; seen with moderate to severe cellular immune deficiency
- Growth failure
- Failure to thrive
- Muscle wasting
- Failure to attain typical milestones:
- Behavioral abnormalities (in older children), such as loss of concentration and memory, may also indicate HIV encephalopathy.

Physical Examination

Signs and symptoms of child with HIV infection found during physical examination include the following:

- *Candidiasis:* Most common oral and mucocutaneous presentation of HIV infection
- *Oral Thrush* in the posterior pharynx: Observed in approximately 30% of HIV-infected children
- Linear gingival erythema and median rhomboid glossitis
- Parotid enlargement and recurrent aphthous ulcers
- *Herpetic infection with herpes simplex virus (HSV):* May manifest as herpes labialis, gingivostomatitis, esophagitis, or chronic erosive, vesicular, and vegetating skin lesions; the involved areas of the lips, mouth, tongue, and esophagus are ulcerated
- *HIV dermatitis:* An erythematous, papular rash; observed in about 25% of children with HIV infection
- *Dermatophytosis:* Manifesting as an aggressive tinea capitis, corporis, versicolor, or onychomycosis
- *Pneumocystis jiroveci (formerly P carinii) pneumonia:* Most commonly manifests as cough, dyspnea, tachypnea, and fever
- *Lipodystrophy:* Presentations include peripheral lipoatrophy, truncal lipohypertrophy, and combined versions of these presentations; a more severe presentation occurs at puberty
- *Digital clubbing:* As a result of chronic lung disease
- Pitting or nonpitting edema in the extremities
- Generalized cervical, axillary, or inguinal lymphadenopathy.

Laboratory Investigations

- ELISA test (Enzyme-linked immunosorbent assay test) is done for screening test for anti-HIV IgG detection.

- Western blot test is performed as confirmatory test.
- CD4 count—use of CD4 count to assess HIV associated. Immunosuppression is not free from problem, because normal CD4 count is higher in infants and children and they have opportunistic infections at higher levels of CD4 count.
- T cell ratio and T cell growth factors.
- HIV culture and HIV antigen test.
- HIV specific PCR (polymerase chain reaction) to detect viral nuclei acid.
- TLC, DLC, platelet count.
- Quantitative measurement of immunoglobulin levels and circulating immunocomplex testing.

Material antibodies transmitted to fetus or child remains at significant level until 18 months. So IgG antibody tests are not reliable indicators status to a child before 18 months of age.

- An antibody screening test (also called an immunoassay) looks for antibodies-proteins your body makes when it fights invaders like the HIV virus. Most people form antibodies, the test can detect within 3 months after they are infected, but it can take up to 6 months for a few.
- Another test looks for antibodies and a substance made by the virus, called an antigen. It can find HIV in as little as 2 weeks after you have been exposed.
- The RNA test, which looks for the virus itself instead of antibodies, can diagnose HIV about 10 days after exposure. It is expensive, though, and doctors do not usually recommend it as a first screening.

Management

There is no curative treatment of HIV/AIDS. No vaccine is available for prevention of the condition. Preventive measures are the important aspect of management. Children should be protected from contacting the HIV infection from the adult.

Appropriate ART and therapy for specific infections and malignancies are critical in treating children who are HIV positive. Classes of antiretroviral agents include the following:

- Nucleoside or nucleotide reverse transcriptase inhibitors (NRTIs)
- Protease inhibitors (PIs)
- Nonnucleoside reverse transcriptase inhibitors (NNRTIs)
- Fusion inhibitors
- CCR5 coreceptor antagonists (entry inhibitors)
- Chemokines receptor antagonists (CRAs).

Antiretroviral Drugs Therapy

Antiretroviral drugs (ARDs) are used for the treatment of human immunodeficiency virus (HIV) infection and for postexposure prophylaxis (PEP). ARD monotherapy does not produce sustained clinical benefits, such as improved survival. This failure is partly due to the development of drug-resistant variants of HIV. Resistance develops rapidly during monotherapy, and cross-resistance among related drugs is common.

The drugs which can be used for the children are zidovudine, didanosine8, zalcitabine, stavudine and lamivudine as nucleoside analogs. Other drugs like protease inhibitors (ritanavir, indinavir, saquinavir, nelfinavir) and non-nucleoside reverse transcriptase inhibitors (nevirapine, delavirdine) can also be used as antiretroviral combination therapy.

Nursing Management

- Impaired oral mucosa related to stomatitis, or candiasis.
- Risk for infections related to immunodeficiency state.
- Imbalanced nutrition status related to anorexia, pain abdomen and malabsorption.
- Diarrhea and dehydration related to enteric pathogens and infections.
- Hyperthermia related to HIV infection and secondary infections.
- Pain related to advanced HIV disease.
- Impaired growth and development related to HIV infections and CNS involvement.
- Ineffective family coping related to chronic fatal illness of the child.
- Fear and anxiety related to diagnostic and treatment procedures.
- Knowledge deficit regarding transmission of HIV infection, follow-up care, treatment and home care.

Prevention of HIV/AIDS

Prevention of child HIV remains of worldwide importance. Despite much research, there is no vaccine that will prevent HIV infection. Infection can be prevented by never sharing needles. Since most people will eventually become sexually active at some point in their lives, always using condoms for all types of sexual intercourse can drastically reduce the risk of getting HIV.

Child HIV preventive methods are three main routes of transmission listed above. Knowing the facts about HIV and being aware of your status (if you are HIV-positive or HIV-negative) makes it easier to prevent HIV infection.

- HIV awareness education
- HIV testing and counseling.

Preventing the Sexual Transmission of HIV

- Condom use (including female condoms)
- Safer sex education
- Treating sexually transmitted infections
- Male circumcision.

Preventing HIV Transmission Through Blood

- Screening blood products
- Reducing needle sharing
- Stopping needle stick accidents.

Preventing Mother-to-Child Transmission

There are a number of steps to preventing mother-to-child transmission of HIV:

- Testing the mother for HIV at their first antenatal appointment, during their third trimester and after delivery of their baby.
- Treatment should be offered if the mother tests positive.
- The child should be tested when it is born and also offered treatment if HIV positive.

HIV is not spread through:
- Casual contact, such as hugs or handshakes
- Drinking glasses
- Sneezes
- Coughs
- Mosquitoes or other insects
- Towels
- Toilet seats
- Doorknobs.

DENGUE SYNDROME

Introduction

Dengue fever is a tropical disease caused by a virus carried by mosquitoes. The virus can cause fever, headaches, rashes, and pain throughout the body. Most cases of dengue fever are mild and go away on their own after about a week.

Definition

Dengue fever is an illness caused by the dengue virus, which is carried and spread by the *Aedes* mosquitoes. These viruses cause the body to bleed easily and may affect other organ systems.

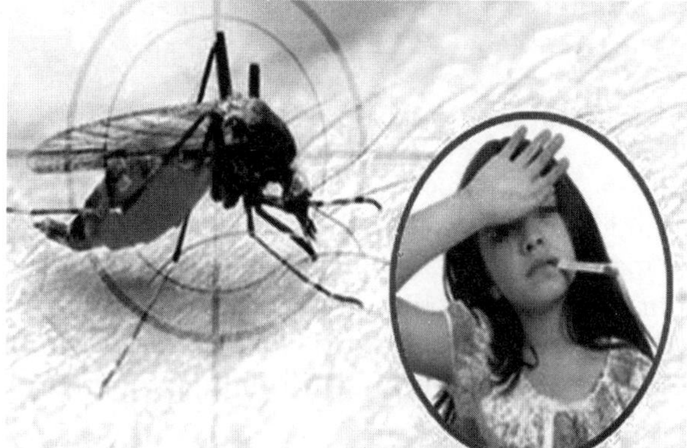

Fig. 5.11: Child with dengue fever

Types

This infection may be found as asymptomatic cases. Symptomatic cases can be presented as:
- Dengue fever (DF)
- Dengue hemorrhagic fever (DHF)
- Dengue shock syndrome (DSS).

Epidemiology

Dengue is endemic in Asia, Southeast Asia, several Southern and Central Pacific Countries and the Americas, with several outbreaks in India. Over 2.5 billion people (more than 40% of the world's population) are now at risk from dengue. WHO currently estimates that 50–100 million dengue infections may be occurring worldwide each year. An estimated 500 000 people with severe dengue require hospitalization annually, a large proportion of whom are children and about 2.5% of those affected die.

Causes

The viruses are transmitted from *Aedes aegypti* and *Aedes albopictus* mosquitoes to humans in a viral cycle that requires both humans and these mosquitoes. There is no human-to-human dengue fever transmission. Once a mosquito is infected, it remains infected for its life span. A human can infect mosquitoes when the human has a high number of viruses in the blood (right before symptoms develop).

The viruses belong to the *Flaviviridae* family and have an RNA strand as its genetic makeup. Virologists term them dengue virus types 1–4 (DENV 1–4). All four serotypes are closely related. However, there are enough antigenic differences between them that if a person becomes immune to one serotype, the person can still be infected by the other three serotypes.

Mode of Transmission

Mode of transmission is through bite of the female Aedes mosquito. This mosquito lives indoor and breeds in stored water. It bites the patient at daytime during viremia and sucks the infected blood. The virus multiplies in the salivary glands of the mosquito. After 3 to 14 days, the infection transmitted to other person by the bites of infected mosquito.

The Incubation Period

The incubation period is about 3 to 15 days with an average of 5 to 7 days.

Clinical Manifestations

Dengue syndrome is clinically presented in three forms. The classical benign form is termed as dengue fever. Two main pathophysiological changes occur in DHF/DSS. Such as:

- Increased vascular permeability that gives rise to loss of plasma from the vascular compartment leading to hemoconcentration, low pulse pressure and other signs of shock
- Disorder in the hemostasis involving thrombocytopenia, vascular changes and coagulopathy.

Dengue Fever

Common signs and symptoms of dengue fever include:

- Hyperthermia possibly as high as 105 °F (40 °C)
- Pain behind the eyes and in the joints, muscles and/or bones
- Severe headache
- Rash over most of the body
- Mild bleeding from the nose or gums
- Bruising easily
- Sore throat
- Anorexia, vomiting.

The condition may be complicated with convulsions, tonsillitis, pharyngitis, rhinitis, diarrhea, lymphadenopathy and hepatosplenomegaly. The child generally will recover within 7 days.

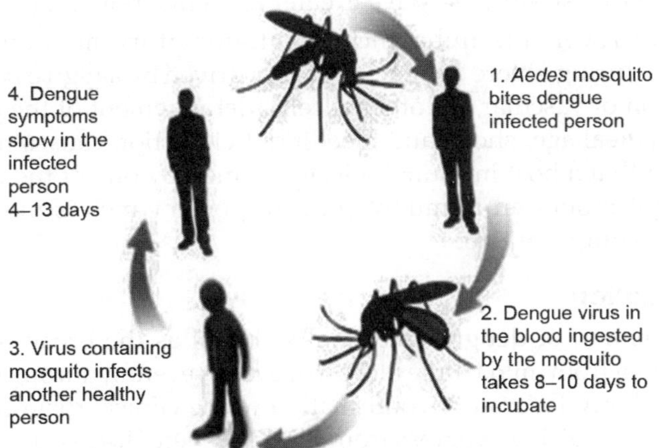

Fig. 5.12: Dengue infection cycle

Dengue Hemorrhagic Fever

Dengue hemorrhagic fever manifested with acute onset of high continuous fever, epigastric discomfort, abdominal pain, and tenderness at right costal margin with palpable liver, moderate to severe thrombocytopenia, hemoconcentration and polyserositis developed. Petechiae, purpura and ecchymosis are present on extremities, axilla, face and palate.

There is easy bruisability and petechiae are also seen on skin and the mucosa. Prolonged bleeding occurs at needle prick and venipuncture site. The patient may be complicated with circulatory failure and shock or may recover spontaneously. Febrile convulsions may occur particularly in infants. Epistaxis, gum bleeding, hematemesis and/or malena may present. The tourniquet (Hess) test usually becomes positive.

Dengue Shock Syndrome

Dengue shock syndrome usually found after 2 to 7 days of dengue fever. The child presents with cold congested blotchy skin, rapid and weak pulse, lethargy, restless and acute abdominal pain before the onset of shock. Hypotension and reduced pulse pressure are found. Fatal outcome may occur if not treated adequately, otherwise complete recovery occurs within 2 to 3 days with prompt management of shock. Good prognosis is indicated by good appetite and adequate urine output.

Pathophysiology

The immune enhancement hypothesis posits that patients with a second infection with a heterologous dengue serotype have a higher risk of developing severe dengue. The existing heterologous dengue antibody recognizes the invading virus and establishes an antigen-antibody complex, which binds to the receptor on the cell membrane of leukocytes.

The virus freely replicates through antibody dependent enhancement. Anti-dengue virus antibodies cross-react with platelets, clotting factors and endothelial cells in humans. Anti-

NS1 antibodies induce apoptosis in endothelial cells and increase vascular permeability, leading to hypovolemia and shock. The selection pressure hypothesis claims that dengue virus varies and mutates as a result of selection pressure as it replicates in humans and/or mosquitoes. Some virus strains also have greater epidemic potential.

A transient and reversible imbalance of inflammatory mediators, cytokines and chemokines occurs during severe dengue, probably driven by a high early viral burden, and leads to dysfunction of vascular endothelial cells, derangement of the coagulation system resulting in plasma leakage, shock and bleeding. Reinfection causes more severe disease and it is suggested that a host immunologically primed by one of the three other types of dengue virus might mount an immunological response which is more florid leading to severe dengue and complications.

Diagnostic Evaluation

Laboratory confirmation of dengue infection is crucial as the broad spectrum of clinical presentations, ranging from mild febrile illness to several severe syndromes, can make accurate diagnosis difficult. Early laboratory confirmation of the clinical diagnosis can be valuable because some patients quickly progress from mild to severe disease and sometimes death.

- History collection and physical examination
- The diagnostic investigations include blood examination, stool examination for occult blood, virus isolation, IgM antibody estimation, etc.
- Blood examination shows raised hematocrit (20% above baseline), thrombocytopenia, leucopenia, lymphocytosis, prolonged prothrombin and partial thromboplastin time. Other common findings are hyponatremia, raised SGPT level and hypoproteinemia.
- Polymerase Chain Reaction (PCR) for detecting viral genomic sequence from Serum or Cerebrospinal Fluid (CSF) samples collected from the patient, which is more expensive and complicated.

Management

There is no specific medicine to treat dengue infection. If child has dengue fever, should use pain relievers with acetaminophen and avoid medicines with aspirin, which could worsen bleeding. Provide more bed rest, allow the child should drink plenty of fluids.

Management of dengue shock and other complications should be done promptly with IV fluid therapy and other supportive measures. Child should be discharged when body temperature becomes normal, for at least 24 hours, urine passed normally, improved appetite, no respiratory distress and stable hematocrit and platelet count.

Prognosis

Dengue fever is self-limiting and benign in nature. Full recovery is possible with appropriate management. In DHF, mortality is about 40 to 50 percent, but intensive care may reduce the mortality to as low as 2 percent.

Preventive Measures

- It is better to avoid stagnant water in flowerpots, buckets, barrels, etc. in and around the house, as these are the favorite places for mosquitoes to lay eggs. Water should be stored in closed containers.

- Bleaching powder may be used in water sources that are not meant for drinking, as it prevents the development of mosquito eggs.
- The female mosquito feeds on blood as it requires the blood protein to produce eggs, hence it is better to use mosquito repellents, even when indoors.
- It is advised to reside in a well screened or air conditioned house. If not, mosquito nets may be attached to the windows.
- Usage of long-sleeved shirts, boots, socks and long pants is advised when outdoors.
- It is healthier to avoid being outdoors during dawn, dusk or early evenings when mosquitoes tend to roam around in the open.
- Mosquitoes are attracted to dark colored clothing hence it is better to wear bright and light colored clothes.
- Avoid strong perfumes, as mosquitoes are drawn towards strong body odors.

Vaccines for Dengue

As all four dengue serotypes cocirculate, vaccines need to be tetravalent. Current candidate vaccines include live attenuated vaccines, chimeric live attenuated vaccines, inactivated or subunit vaccines and nucleic acid-based vaccines.

Live attenuated vaccines are in phase 1 testing. Vaccines in advanced preclinical development include DEN-DEN chimeras, wherein the prM and E protein genes of DEN-1, DEN-3 and DEN-4 have been inserted into the infectious clone of PDK-passaged attenuated DEN-2.

Complications

Primary infections with dengue fever and dengue-like diseases are usually self-limiting and benign. Fluid and electrolyte losses, hyperpyrexia and febrile convulsions are the most frequent complications in infants and young children. Epistaxis, petechiae and purpuric lesions are uncommon but may occur at any stage. In adults and possibly in children, underlying conditions may lead to clinically significant bleeding. Some atypical manifestations have been observed but may be unrecognized and under-reported, although their detection is essential for clinical diagnosis and appropriate management, especially given the global health problems caused by dengue.

- Severe dehydration
- Continuous bleeding
- Low platelets, due to which clotting of blood does not occur
- Blood pressure may go dangerously low
- Enlargement of liver and damage to it
- Bradycardia (heart beating less than 60 counts per minute)
- Damage to brain due to bleeding, seizures or encephalitis
- Damage to the immune system.

GERMAN MEASLES (RUBELLA)

Introduction

Rubella commonly known as German measles or 3-day measles is an infection that mostly affects the skin and lymph nodes. It is caused by the rubella virus. Rubella spreads when people breathe in virus-infected fluid, such as the droplets sprayed into the air when a person with rubella sneezes or coughs, or share food or drink with someone who is infected. It also can pass through a pregnant woman's bloodstream to infect her unborn child.

Definition

Rubella (German measles) is an infection caused by the rubella virus. Although it most commonly occurs in young children, it can affect anyone. The illness is usually mild. However, rubella in a pregnant woman can cause serious damage to the unborn child.

Mode of Transmission

It spread by contact with an infected person, through coughing and sneezing.

Incubation Period

The incubation period for rubella is 14–23 days, with an average incubation period of 16–18 days. This means that it can take 2–3 weeks for a child to get rubella after being exposed to someone with the disease.

The rubella rash usually lasts 3 days. Lymph nodes may remain swollen for a week or more, and joint pain can last for more than 2 weeks. Children who have rubella usually recover within 1 week, but adults may take longer.

Signs and Symptoms

A Red-pink Rash

The rubella rash is typically a red-pink color. It consists of a number of small spots, which may be slightly itchy.

The rash usually starts behind the ears, before spreading around the head and neck. It may then spread to the trunk (chest and tummy), legs and arms. In most cases, the rash will disappear by itself within three to five days.

Swollen Lymph Glands

Lymph nodes, or glands, are small lumps of tissue found throughout the body. They contain white blood cells that help fight bacteria, viruses and anything else that causes infection. If child have rubella, the glands behind the ears, below your skull at the back of child head, and in your neck usually swell. In some cases, this swelling can be painful.

These lymph glands sometimes start to swell before the rash appears and the swelling can last for several weeks after the rash has gone.

Other Symptoms

- A high temperature (fever), which is usually mild (less than 39 °C or 102.2 °F), but can be more severe in adults
- Cold-like symptoms, such as a runny nose, watery eyes, sore throat and cough
- Slightly sore and red eyes (conjunctivitis)
- Aching and painful joints
- Tiredness
- Loss of appetite
- Rash that starts on the face and spreads to the rest of the body
- Low fever (less than 101 degrees).

These symptoms last 2 or 3 days.

Older children and adults have swollen glands and symptoms like a cold before the rash appears. Aching joints occur in many cases, especially among young women.

Serious Problems

- Brain infections
- Bleeding problems.

Diagnostic Evaluation

- History Collection
- Physical Assessment
- Saliva and blood tests.

If rubella is suspected, a sample of saliva from child mouth or a sample of blood from a vein in child arm can be taken and tested for certain antibodies.

- Antibodies are proteins that child body produces to destroy disease-carrying organisms and toxins.
- The IgM antibody will be present if you have a new rubella infection.
- The IgG antibody will be present if you have had the rubella infection in the past, or you have been vaccinated against it.

Management

Rubella cannot be treated with antibiotics because they do not work against viral infections. Unless there are complications, rubella will get better on its own.

Paracetamol or ibuprofen can be used to reduce a high temperature (fever) and treat any aches or pains. Liquid infant paracetamol can be used for young children. Aspirin should not be given to children under 16 years old.

Allow the child to drink plenty of fluids for risk of dehydration. Keeping hydrated will also help reduce discomfort caused by coughing.

Preventive Measures

Rubella can be prevented by the rubella vaccine. Widespread immunization against rubella is critical to controlling the spread of the disease, thereby preventing birth defects caused by congenital rubella syndrome.

The vaccine is usually given to children at 12–15 months of age as part of the scheduled measles-mumps-rubella (MMR) immunization. A second dose of MMR usually is given at 4–6 years of age. As with all immunization schedules, there are important exceptions and special circumstances.

HERPES SIMPLEX VIRUS (HSV)

Definition

The herpes simplex virus, also known as HSV, is an infection that causes herpes. Herpes can appear in various parts of the body, most commonly on the genitals or mouth.

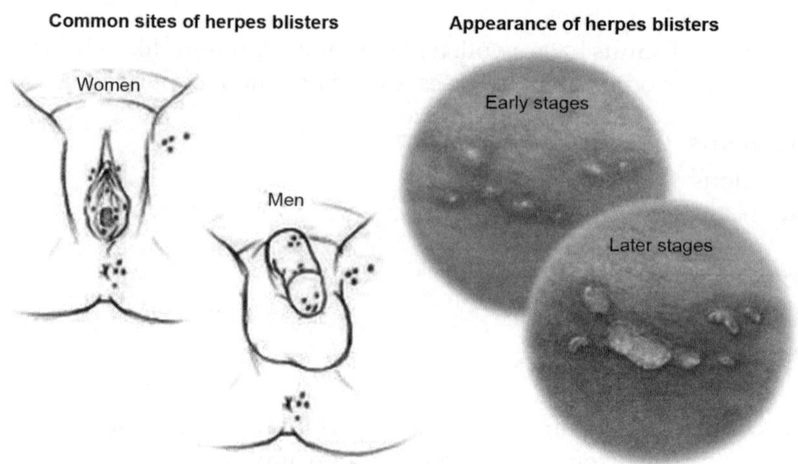

Fig. 5.13: Child with herpes simplex virus

Types

There are two types of the herpes simplex virus:

- **HSV-1**, also known as oral herpes, can cause cold sores and fever blisters around the mouth and on the face.
- **HSV-2** is generally responsible for genital herpes.

Incidence

Worldwide rates of either HSV-1 or HSV-2 are between 60% and 95% in adults. HSV-1 is usually acquired during childhood, rates of both increase as people age, rates of HSV-1 are between 70% and 80% in populations of low socioeconomic status and 40 to 60% in populations of improved socioeconomic status. An estimated 536 million people worldwide (16% of the population) were infected with HSV-2 as of 2003 with greater rates among women.

Causes

The herpes simplex virus is a contagious virus that can be passed from person to person through direct contact. Children will often contract HSV-1 from early contact with an infected adult. They then carry the virus with them for the rest of their life.

HSV-1 Infection

Oral HSV-1 can happen from general interactions such as eating from the same utensils, sharing lip balm, or kissing. The virus spreads more quickly when an infected person is experiencing an outbreak. Additionally, it is possible to get genital herpes from HSV-1 if the individual has had cold sores and performed sexual activities during that time.

HSV-2 Infection

Genital HSV-2 is contracted through forms of sexual contact with a person who has HSV-2. They are transmitted by direct contact with body fluids or lesions of an infected individual. Transmission may still occur when symptoms are not present. It may be spread to an infant during childbirth.

Signs and Symptoms

Clinical Features of Oral HSV-1 Infection

- Abrupt onset of illness
- Fever
- Listlessness or irritability
- Inability to eat and/or drink
- Gingivitis (with markedly swollen, erythematous, and occasionally bleeding gums)
- Increased drooling in infants due to pain on swallowing
- Vesicular lesions on the tongue, buccal mucosa, and palate with extension, at times, to the lips and face (these may rupture and coalesce to form large, ulcerated areas)
  - Tender submandibular or cervical adenopathy
  - In recurrent cases, a prodrome of pain, burning, tingling, and itching.

Clinical Features of Genital HSV-2 Infection

- Genital infection
- Intrauterine and perinatal infection (herpes neonatorum)
- Central nervous system infection
- Infection in immunocompromised hosts
- Other infections: Herpetic whitlow, herpes gladiatorum, keratoconjunctivitis, meningitis, erythema multiform
- In first episodes, severe constitutional symptoms (e.g. fever, malaise, myalgias)
- Initial itching and pain, followed by more troublesome signs and symptoms
- Lesions that evolve from vesicles to pustules to wet ulcers and heal by crusting
- Painful inguinal lymphadenopathy, dysuria, and vaginal discharge
- Paresthesias of the legs and perineum
- Urinary retention.

Herpes Neonatorum

- Skin, eye, and mucous membrane (SEM) disease
- Disseminated infection
- CNS infection.

Diagnostic Evaluation

- History collection
- Physical examination
- Isolation of the virus in tissue cultures (most common confirmation method)
- Histological analysis of scrapings or punch biopsy specimens
- Cytological evaluation
- Serologic testing (only for determining past HSV exposure)
- PCR assay (preferred for CNS infection and possibly valuable for disseminated disease)
- Lumbar puncture and cerebrospinal fluid analysis
- Immunofluorescent microscopy
- Brain biopsy
- *Imaging studies:* Computed tomography (CT-Scan), magnetic resonance imaging (MRI).

Pathophysiology

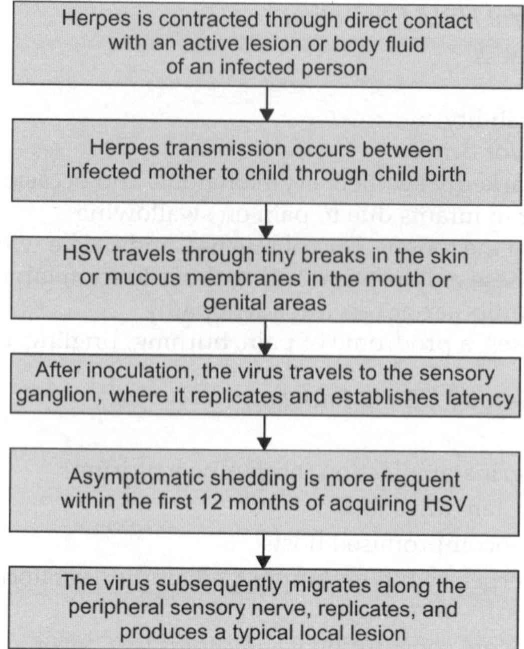

Fig. 5.14: Pathophysiology of HSV infection

Management

There is specific medical treatment for the pediatric HSV infection involves antiviral medications. Antiviral agents used include the following:

- Oral acyclovir
- Oral famciclovir (a prodrug that is converted to penciclovir)
- Oral valacyclovir (a prodrug that is converted to acyclovir)
- IV acyclovir (for encephalitis, neonatal disease, severe infection in immunocompromised patients, occasional cases of severe orolabial or genital disease, and recurrent genital HSV infections).

Inpatient Management

Most of the children with severe HSV:

- Neonates with disseminated or CNS disease
- Older children with encephalitis who may be very ill at hospitalization
- HSV infection in immunocompromised children.

Preventive Measures

Genital HSV infection includes the following:

- Avoid contact with individuals excreting the virus (difficult, because they are often asymptomatic)
- Start oral antiviral therapy at the first symptom or sign of genital HSV disease

- Promote condom use
- Provide appropriate evaluation, counseling, and education.

Prevent transmission of HSV to newborns include the following:

- Reassure women with recurrent disease that risk of neonatal infection is low
- Perform cesarean delivery if a mother has active lesions during delivery.
- Observe infants delivered vaginally by mothers with active genital herpes; follow-up neonates carefully, and immediately institute antiviral therapy if symptoms occur.
- In pregnant women with symptomatic genital herpes, consider antiviral suppressive treatment initiated at 36 weeks' gestation.

VARICELLA-ZOSTER

Definition

Reactivation of varicella-zoster virus (VZV) that has remained dormant within dorsal root ganglia, often for decades after the patient's initial exposure to the virus in the form of varicella (chickenpox), results in herpes zoster (shingles). Although it is usually a self-limited dermatomal rash with pain, herpes zoster can be far more serious; in addition, acute cases often lead to postherpetic neuralgia (PHN).

Causes (Etiology)

Herpes zoster is caused by VZV infection. VZV is an enveloped, double-stranded DNA virus belonging to the Herpesviridae family; its genome encodes approximately 70 proteins. In humans, primary infection with VZV occurs when the virus comes into contact with the mucosa of the respiratory tract or conjunctiva. From these sites, it is distributed throughout the body. After primary infection, the virus migrates along sensory nerve fibers to the satellite cells of dorsal root ganglia where it becomes dormant.

- External exposure to the virus
- Acute or chronic disease processes (particularly malignancies and infections)
- Medications of various types
- Emotional stress.

Risk Factors

Risk factors in children and adults include the following:

- VZV-specific immunity and cell-mediated immunity, which generally declines with age
- Immunosuppression (e.g. by HIV infection or AIDS), immunosuppressive therapy
- Primary VZV infection in utero or in early infancy, when the normal immune response is decreased
- Anti-tumor necrosis factor (TNF)—an agents (may pose an increased risk)
- Immune reconstitution inflammatory syndrome (IRIS)
- Acute lymphocytic leukemia and other malignancies.

Signs and Symptoms

Herpes zoster may begin with a systemic response (e.g. fever, anorexia), symptoms typically include prodromal sensory phenomena along 1 or more skin dermatomes lasting 1–10 days (average 48 hours), which usually are noted as pain or, less commonly, itching or paresthesias.

After the onset of prodromal symptoms, the following signs and symptoms present:

- Patchy erythema, occasionally accompanied by induration, in the dermatomal area of involvement.
- Regional lymphadenopathy, either at this stage or subsequently.
- Grouped herpetiform vesicles developing on the erythematous base (the classic finding).
- Pain in the dermatomal area of involvement may remain the same as in prodrome or may change in character and intensity with the onset of other symptoms; many patients describe the pain as burning, throbbing, or stabbing in nature; it may be severe, mild, constant, rare, or felt as another sensation such as pruritus; the involved area may be tender to palpation.
- Vesicular involution: Vesicles initially are clear but eventually cloud, rupture, crust, and involute, a process that may be greatly accelerated by treatment.
- After vesicular involution, slow resolution of the remaining erythematous plaques, typically without visible sequelae: Note, however, that scarring can occur if deeper epidermal and dermal layers have been compromised by excoriation, secondary infection, or other complications.

Diagnostic Evaluation

Diagnosis of herpes zoster is based primarily on the history and physical findings. In most cases, confirming the diagnosis via laboratory testing has no utility. In select patient populations, however particularly immunocompromised child the presentation of herpes zoster can be atypical and may require additional testing.

Laboratory studies for VZV include the following:

- Direct fluorescent antibody (DFA) testing of vesicular fluid or a corneal lesion
- Polymerase chain reaction (PCR) testing of vesicular fluid, a corneal lesion, or blood
- Smear of vesicular fluid (lower sensitivity and specificity than DFA or PCR).

Management

- Analgesics
- Antiviral drugs
- Steroids therapy.

Analgesics

Oxycodone (OxyContin, Roxicodone)

The oxycodone is a narcotic analgesic that is indicated for the relief of moderate to severe pain. Patients with herpes zoster usually experience pain. Antiviral and steroid therapies provide relatively minor relief of pain, and narcotic analgesics are often needed.

Acetaminophen (Tylenol)

Acetaminophen is indicated for use in child with mild pain or fever. It is the drug of choice for the treatment of pain in patients who reduces fever via direct action on hypothalamic heat-regulating centers, which increases dissipation of body heat via vasodilation and sweating.

Ibuprofen (Advil, Motrin)

Ibuprofen is a nonsteroidal anti-inflammatory drug (NSAID) that is the drug of choice for treatment of mild to moderately severe pain, if no contraindications exist. It inhibits inflammatory reactions and pain, probably by decreasing the activity of the enzyme cyclooxygenase and thereby, in turn, inhibiting prostaglandin synthesis. Ibuprofen is one of the few NSAIDs that are indicated for fever reduction.

Naproxen (Aleve, Naprosyn, Naprelan, Anaprox)

Naproxen another NSAID that is commonly used for the relief of mild to moderate pain. It inhibits inflammatory reactions and pain by decreasing the activity of cyclooxygenase, an effect that results in a decrease of prostaglandin synthesis.

Varicella-Zoster Vaccine (Zostavax)

Zostavax is a lyophilized preparation of the Oka/Merck strain of live, attenuated VZV. It has been shown to boost immunity against herpes zoster virus (shingles) in older patients. It has been shown to reduce the occurrence of shingles by about 50% in individuals older than 60 years, by 64% in those aged 60–69 years, and by 70% in subjects aged 50–59 years. It also slightly reduces pain compared with no vaccination in those who develop shingles. The vaccine is indicated for the prevention of herpes zoster in patients who have no contraindications.

Antiviral Drugs

Acyclovir (Zovirax)

Acyclovir is a synthetic purine nucleoside analogue with in vitro and in vivo inhibitory activity against human herpes viruses, including HSV type 1 (HSV-1), HSV-2, VZV, Epstein-Barr virus (EBV), and cytomegalovirus (CMV). Treatment with acyclovir is indicated in patients with involvement of the first branch of the trigeminal nerve, those who are immunocompromised, or those with increased risk for major complications from a varicella infection (i.e. patients older than 13 years, those receiving long-term corticosteroid or aspirin therapy, and those with chronic cutaneous or pulmonary diseases). Zoster in adolescents may be treated with oral acyclovir if it is initiated within 72 hours of eruption.

Famciclovir (Famvir)

Famciclovir is a prodrug that, once ingested, is rapidly biotransformed into the active compound penciclovir and phosphorylated by viral thymidine kinase. By competition with deoxyguanosine triphosphate, penciclovir triphosphate inhibits viral polymerase. Activity against HSV-1, HSV-2, and VZV has been demonstrated.

Therapy should be initiated as soon as herpes zoster is diagnosed. No data are available on the efficacy of treatment started 72 hours after rash onset. The dosage should be adjusted in patients with renal insufficiency or hepatic disease.

Valacyclovir (Valtrex)

Valacyclovir is an L-valyl ester of acyclovir. It is rapidly converted to acyclovir, which has demonstrated antiviral activity against HSV-1, HSV-2, VZV, and other viruses.

Therapy should be initiated at the earliest sign or symptom of herpes zoster; it is most effective when started within 48 hours of the onset of zoster rash. No data are available on the efficacy of treatment started 72 hours after rash onset.

Complications

Most cases of shingles will heal on their own, with or without treatment, and will not lead to any other problems. In rare cases, shingles can lead to complications, including:

- *Ongoing pain (postherpetic neuralgia):* Damaged nerve fibers in the skin send confused messages to the brain, leading to pain that can go on for a long time after a shingles rash has disappeared.
- *Vision problems:* If shingles happens near or in an eye, it can lead to vision loss.
- *Skin infections:* A shingles rash can become infected with bacteria, leading to impetigo or cellulitis.
- *Nervous system problems:* Shingles on the face can involve different nerves that connect to the brain. This can lead to nerve-related problems such as facial paralysis, hearing problems, and problems with balance. In very rare cases, shingles can lead to encephalitis (inflammation of the brain).

Prognosis

The rash usually resolves within 10–15 days. The prognosis for younger and otherwise healthy patients is excellent. Elderly people have a significantly increased risk of complications.

Herpes zoster rarely causes fatalities in patients who are immunocompetent, but it can be life-threatening in severely debilitated or immunocompromised patients. Disseminated zoster in immunocompromised patients can lead to death from encephalitis, hepatitis, or Pneumonitis.

GUILLAIN-BARRÉ SYNDROME

Guillain-Barré syndrome is a rare but serious autoimmune disorder in which the immune system attacks healthy nerve cells of the peripheral nervous system. This leads to weakness, numbness, and tingling, and can eventually cause paralysis.

Guillain-Barré syndrome is a rare medical condition that affects a person's immune system and nerves. The immune system, which usually keeps a person from getting sick, starts damaging the nerves that are outside of the brain and spinal cord.

Guillain-Barré syndrome (GBS) is a temporary, but often life-threatening, disorder that affects the nerves in the body. GBS can result in muscle weakness, pain, and even temporary paralysis of the facial, chest, and leg muscles. Paralysis of the chest muscles can lead to breathing problems and death if not treated.

INFLUENZA

Definition

Influenza, commonly called 'the flu', is an infection caused by the influenza virus. It affects the nose, throat, lungs and other parts of the body. The flu can be a serious and sometimes life-threatening infection.

Causes

The flu is caused by one of three types of influenza viruses. Types-A and B are responsible for the yearly flu epidemics, and type-C flu virus causes sporadic mild illness.

Mode of Transmission

Flu is highly contagious, particularly when people share close quarters as children do in school classrooms. Flu is spread among children when a child either inhales infected droplets in the air (coughed up or sneezed by an infected person) or when the child comes in direct contact with an infected person's secretions.

A person can be contagious one day before onset of symptoms and 5–7 days after being sick. This can happen, for example, when they share pencils at school or play computer games and share the remotes or share utensils such as spoons and forks.

- **Direct contact** such as kissing, touching or holding hands with an infected person. If you have a virus, you will have germs in your nose, mouth, eyes or on your skin. By touching other people, you can pass on the virus.
- **Indirect contact** means touching something a toy, doorknob or a used tissue that has been touched by an infected person and now has germs on it. Some germs, like the ones that cause colds and diarrhea, can stay on surfaces for many hours.
- Some germs spread **through the air** when a person coughs or sneezes. Droplets from the cough or sneeze may reach another person's nose or mouth.

Signs and Symptoms

- Sudden fever
- Chills and shakes
- Headache
- Muscle aches
- Extreme fatigue
- Dry cough and sore throat
- Loss of appetite.

Children with the flu symptoms:

- Newborns have a high fever
- Children usually have temperatures over 39.5 °C and have febrile seizures (convulsions).
- Stomach upset and pain, vomiting, and diarrhea are common in younger children. Earaches and red eyes are also common.

Diagnostic Evaluation

- History collection
- Physical examination
- Blood test
- Throat culture
- Urine test.

Management

Children recover within seven days without any treatment. Provide adequate bed rest and encourage them to drink lots of fluids and use paracetamol for pain or discomfort.

Do not give aspirin to your child if they have influenza as this can lead to serious side effects.

Antibiotics are not helpful for influenza and will not be prescribed unless your child also has a bacterial infection.

Antiviral medications (such as Tamiflu) are not given to children who have influenza and who are otherwise fit and healthy. This is because they do not usually make a difference to the duration of the illness.

Preventive Measures

The best way to prevent influenza is the influenza vaccine; Good hygiene habits can also reduce the chance of getting influenza or passing it to others.

These include:

- Regular handwashing
- Not sharing cups or cutlery
- Covering your mouth when you cough or sneeze
- Influenza vaccine (the flu-shot).

The influenza vaccine can be given to any child over six months of age to reduce the chance of becoming sick with influenza.

The child has a chronic medical condition; it is strongly recommended that they have an annual influenza vaccination. All household members should also be vaccinated to decrease the chances of your child being exposed to influenza. Because the influenza virus changes (or mutates) slightly from year to year, your child will need a new and updated influenza vaccine at the beginning of each influenza season. Side effects of the vaccine include pain and redness at the site of injection. Less commonly, children may develop fever or aches and pains which last one to two days. The vaccine cannot cause influenza as it contains killed or inactivated influenza virus.

INFECTIOUS MONONUCLEOSIS

Infectious mononucleosis, more commonly known as 'mono', is a viral illness characterized by flu-like symptoms, fatigue and swollen lymph glands. It has long been nicknamed the 'kissing disease' as it is easily transmitted through saliva.

- Mononucleosis is contagious and difficult to prevent.
- Symptoms last about one to two months.
- Once you have had mono, the virus remains inactive in the throat and blood cells for the rest of your life.
- Almost 95 percent of adults have been exposed to the virus.
- Antibiotics do not work; the best treatment is rest and plenty of fluids.

Causes

- Epstein-Barr virus
- Cytomegalovirus.

Mode of Transmission

The Epstein-Barr virus infection is spread via saliva, and has an incubation period of four to seven weeks. The length of time that an individual remains contagious is unclear, but the chances of passing the illness to someone else may be the highest during the first six weeks following infection.

Signs and Symptoms

The infants and young children infected with EBV have no symptoms or only very mild ones. When there are signs and symptoms of mononucleosis, they usually include the following:

- Fever
- Sore throat, including white patches in the back of the throat
- Swollen lymph glands in the back of the neck, groin, and armpit
- Fatigue.

Classic Symptoms

- Chills
- Headache
- Decreased appetite
- Puffy eyelids
- Enlargement of the liver and spleen
- Oversensitivity to light
- Anemia.

Diagnostic Evaluation

The diagnosis of infectious mononucleosis is usually made through a:

- History collection
- Physical examination
- Blood tests.

These tests may include a complete blood count to check for unusual looking white blood cells (atypical lymphocytes). Blood tests can also detect increases in antibodies against EBV.

Management

- Paracetamol (acetaminophen)
- NSAIDs drugs such as ibuprofen
- Prednisone
- Corticosteroid
- Hydrocortisone or dexamethasone
- Acyclovir.

Prevention

It is difficult to prevent the spread of this virus because children who have been infected can spread the virus for the rest of their lives. Youngster should avoid infected saliva by not sharing drinking glasses, water bottles, or eating utensils.

Prognosis

In most of the child with infectious mononucleosis clear up in 1 to 3 weeks (although symptoms, particularly fatigue, can last for several additional weeks in some children). Child with abnormal immune systems can have a more severe infection that further weakens the immune system, resulting in cancers or death caused by liver failure and bacterial infections.

SWINE FLU (A BIG THREAT TO WORLD)

Swine flu (technically called the 2009 H1N1 flu) was a new strain of influenza (flu) that made its debut in the spring of 2009 and reached its peak in late 2009 and early 2010. Symptoms of swine flu are similar to most influenza infections: Fever (100 °F or greater), cough, nasal secretions, fatigue, and headache, with fatigue being reported in most infected individuals.

Definition

Swine flu or swine influenza is a very contagious respiratory disease. It is called swine flu because it regularly affects pigs.

Causes

Influenza A (H1N1) virus.

Mode of Transmission

Swine flu spreads from person to person in the same way as other flu viruses: Through coughing and sneezing of people who are infected. Swine flu is very contagious and spreads easily, particularly in enclosed spaces where there is close contact between infected people and healthy people.

Transmission between the pigs: Direct contact between infected and animals particularly common during animal transport.

Transmission to humans: People who work at poultry and swine, especially those people with intense exposures are at increased risk of zoonotic infection with influenza virus, endemic in these animals and constitute a population of human hosts in which zoonotic and reassortement can occur.

The Incubation Period

The incubation period from exposure to first symptoms is about one to four days, with an average of two days. The symptoms last about one to two weeks and can last longer if the person has a severe infection.

Signs and Symptoms

- Fever
- Sore throat
- Tiredness
- Cough
- Headache
- Muscles and joint pain.

Swine flu can also cause:

- Acute abdominal pain
- Diarrhea
- Vomiting.

Diagnostic Evaluation

- History collection
- Physical examination
- Nose and throat swab
- Blood test.

Management

The first H1N1 vaccine released in early October 2009 was a nasal spray vaccine that was approved for use in healthy individuals ages 2–49. The injectable vaccine, made from killed H1N1, became available in the second week of Oct. 2009. This vaccine was approved for use in ages 6 months to the elderly, including pregnant females.

Treating Swine Flu—Tamiflu

- Tamiflu can reduce the symptoms of Swine Flu illness.
- Their benefits are limited: They usually reduce the time your child is sick by 1 to 1.5 days. They reduce the symptoms, but do not cure the disease.
- For optimal results, antiviral drugs (such as Tamiflu) should be started within 48 hours of the onset of flu symptoms.
- Indications: Severe symptoms OR underlying health problems (HIGH-RISK group).
- For HIGH RISK children, call your doctor at the start of flu symptoms.
- Most patients have mild to moderate symptoms and Tamiflu treatment is not necessary.
- Unnecessary overuse of Tamiflu causes resistant strains of the virus. (8/2009 some resistance has occurred)
- Tamiflu also has side effects: Vomiting in 10% of children.

Preventive Measure

Prevention in Swine

- Facility management (disinfectant and temperature control)
- Herd management (new animals quarantined)
- Vaccination.

Prevention in Humans

Pig to Human Transmission

- Farmers and veterinarians (use face mask, wearing gloves)
- Use of vaccines on swine (research on going).

Human to Human Transmission

- Handwashing with soap and water (or) alcohol based hand sanitizers in order to prevent fomites transmissions.
- Use of respirators by health care workers.
- Social distancing.

ZIKA VIRUS

Introduction

Zika virus (ZIKV) is a member of the virus family Flaviviridae and the genus *Flavivirus*. It is usually spread by daytime-active *Aedes* mosquitoes, such as *A. aegypti* and *A. albopictus*. Its name comes from the Zika forest of Uganda, where the virus was first isolated in 1947. Zika virus is related to dengue, yellow fever, Japanese encephalitis, and West Nile viruses.

It was reported that the Zika virus 2015 after the Pan American Health Organization (PAHO) issued a similar alert about the first confirmed Zika virus infection in Brazil. In a span of months, the virus took hold of the country, bringing an outbreak of cases involving adult neurological abnormalities and birth casualties which are closely linked to the virus. Since then, the virus has continued to extend its territory in Central and South America and the Caribbean.

Definition

Zika virus disease is an emerging viral disease transmitted through the bite of an infected *Aedes* mosquito. This is the same mosquito that is known to transmit infections like dengue and chikungunya. World Health Organization has reported 22 countries and territories in Americas from where local transmission of Zika virus has been reported. Microcephaly in the newborn and other neurological syndromes (Guillain Barré Syndrome) has been found temporally associated with Zika virus infection.

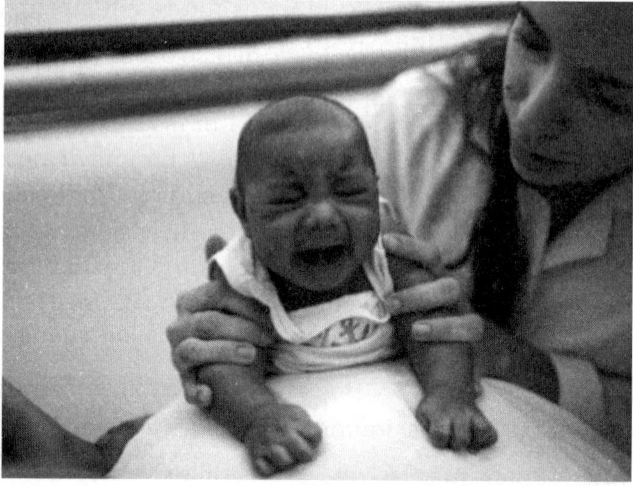

Fig. 5.15: Child with zika virus

Causes

The zika virus is spread by daytime-active mosquitoes. It is primarily spread by the female *Aedes aegypti* order to lay eggs but has been isolated from a number of arboreal mosquito species in the *Aedes* genus such as:

- *Africanus*
- *Apicoargenteus*

- *Furcifer*
- *Hensilli*
- *Luteocephalus*
- *Vittatus* with an extrinsic incubation period in mosquitoes of about 10 days.

Incidence

In 2014, Brazilian health officials reported 147 cases of babies born with microcephaly, a congenital deformation of the skull that compresses the infants' brains. In 2015, some 3,000 microcephaly cases were reported in the country, along with 500 other infections; about a quarter of the 4,000 were detected in the month of December. That represents a twenty-fold year-to-year increase in an extreme birth defect the cause should be identified, preventing it from claiming more babies.

Mode of Transmission

Zika is primarily transmitted through the bite of infected *Aedes* mosquitoes. Mosquitoes become infected when they bite a person already infected with the virus. Infected mosquitoes can then spread the virus to other people through bites. It can also be transmitted from a pregnant mother to her baby during pregnancy or around the time of birth and sexual contact have been reported.

The Zika virus is spread to humans through the bite of an infected mosquito. The virus manifests itself through symptoms of fever, rash, joint pain and conjunctivitis. Only about 1 in 5 people infected will actually exhibit symptoms. For those who do become sick from the virus, the illness is usually mild and self-limited lasting for several days to a week. If an expecting mother becomes infected, the virus may be transmitted to her baby during pregnancy or around the time of birth.

It is important to know that while a mother can transmit it to her unborn baby, it appears that the virus can only be transmitted from one person to another person through a mosquito bite, i.e. a person who is infected may transmit the virus to another person if they were bitten by a mosquito and if then in turn that mosquito were subsequently to bite another person.

Incubation Period

The incubation period is typically 3–12 days. There is no specific therapy for Zika virus infection and acute symptoms typically resolve within 4–7 days. Use paracetamol for pain and fever if needed.

Signs and Symptoms

Symptoms of the Zika virus (symptoms may last for 2 to 7 days).

- Low-grade fever
- Arthralgia, notably of small joints of hands and feet, with possible swollen joints
- Myalgia
- Headache, retro-ocular headaches
- Conjunctivitis
- Cutaneous maculopapular rash.

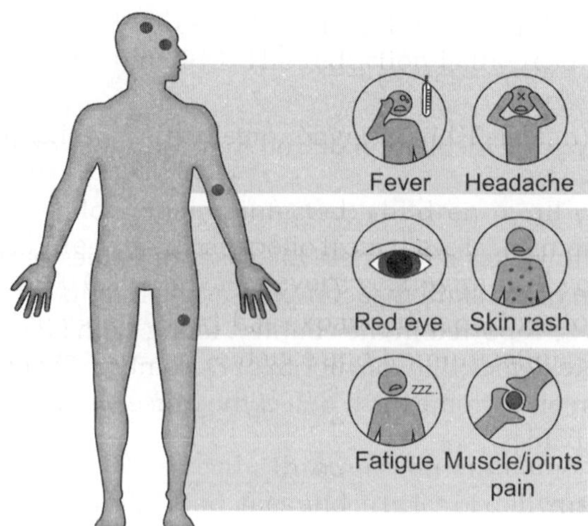

Fig. 5.16: Symptoms of the zika virus

Diagnostic Evaluation

Infection with Zika virus may be suspected based on symptoms and recent history (e.g. residence or travel to an area where Zika virus is known to be present). Zika virus diagnosis can only be confirmed by laboratory testing for the presence of Zika virus RNA in the blood or other body fluids, such as urine or saliva. Reverse-transcriptase PCR (RT-PCR) can be used to detect the Zika virus during the first 1 week (in blood) to 4 weeks (in urine) of the illness. This RT-PCR test is currently performed in Wellington at ESR.

Treatment

The common flu, individuals are advised to rest, remain hydrated and to take medicines such as Paracetamol or Acetaminophen to relieve pains and spikes in temperature. Nb. Individuals are advised against taking aspirin and other non-steroidal anti-inflammatory drugs (NSAIDs) like ibuprofen and naproxen. Aspirin and NSAIDs should be avoided until dengue can be ruled out to reduce the risk of hemorrhage/bleeding, (Centre for Disease Control, 2016).

Nursing Management

Assessment

- Follow the universal precaution and use the PPE (Personal protective equipment).
- Isolate the infective client.
- Assess the general condition of the clients.–(vitals, find out the specific signs and symptoms).
- Collect the information like any recent overseas travel of prenatal client during or within two weeks of travel.
- Assess the fluid and electrolyte status of the client.–(maintain the intake and output chart).
- Assess the nutritional status of the client (24-hours menu recall).
- Coping status of the clients.
- Assess the client knowledge on zika virus treatment and follow-up care.

Intervention

Nursing interventions should also include thorough travel assessment, education, and provision of comfort measures, safety and pain management. The nurses should make every effort to use available resources to deliver and incorporate bereavement support to the patients and their families.

- Provide symptomatic nursing care to elevate the symptoms.
- Maintain the normal fluid and electrolyte status.
- Provide comfort rest and sleep to client.
- There is no antiviral treatment for the Zika virus.
- Supportive care should be given for any symptoms such as rest, antipyretics, pain management and fluids.
- Patient Health Education As per CDC:
  - Pregnant patients or patients who want to get pregnant to avoid visiting countries with high incidence of Zika virus.
  - If any patients need to travel teach them how to avoid getting mosquito bites such as using bed nets, window and door screens, staying in air-conditioned rooms and not exposing skin.

Sexual Transmission of Zika Virus

There is only limited information available about the risk of sexual transmission of Zika virus, but the risk is considered to be low when compared to the risk of transmission from infected mosquitoes.

- *All the men's:* Who have travelled to a Zika-affected area and have a pregnant partner should abstain from sexual activity (oral, vaginal, and anal) or use condoms for the duration of the pregnancy, whether they have symptoms or not.
- *All the men's:* Who have travelled to a Zika-affected area and have a partner who is at risk of becoming pregnant should abstain from sexual activity (oral, vaginal, and anal) or use condoms, whether they have symptoms or not.
- International advice about how long to abstain varies:
  - At least four weeks (WHO)
  - 3-months (Australian Department of Health)
  - 6- months (ECDC and Public Health England).

Nursing Diagnosis

According to NANDA nursing diagnoses few nursing diagnosis are:

S. No.	Nursing diagnosis	S. No.	Nursing diagnosis
1	Risk for Ineffective Relationship	7	Hopelessness
2	Ineffective protection	8	Disturbed body image
3	Fatigue	9	Stress overload
4	Activity intolerance	10	Decreased intracranial adaptive capacity
5	Deficient knowledge	11	Risk for impaired parenting
6	Readiness for enhanced knowledge	12	Disabled family coping

Contd...

Contd...

S. No.	Nursing diagnosis	S. No.	Nursing diagnosis
13	Ineffective coping	22	Compromised family coping
14	Grieving	23	Defensive coping
15	Complicated grieving	24	Disabled family coping
16	Risk for impaired attachment	25	Ineffective coping
17	Interrupted family processes	26	Grieving
18	Ineffective relationship	27	Readiness for enhanced power
19	Risk for ineffective relationship	28	Powerlessness
20	Risk for ineffective activity planning	29	Risk for sudden infant death syndrome
21	Anxiety	30	Social isolation

Preventive Measures

- Advise the client to prevent mosquito breeding around houses.
- Advise the client to use mosquito repellents to protect you from mosquito bites.
- Non-essential travel to the affected countries in the Latin American region and the Caribbean should be deferred/cancelled.
- Pregnant women or women who are trying to become pregnant should defer/cancel their travel to the affected areas.
- All travellers to the affected countries/areas should strictly follow individual protective measures, especially during the day time to prevent mosquito bites (use of mosquito repellant cream, electronic mosquito repellants)
- Advise to use of mosquito nets and dress that appropriately covers most of the body parts).
- Persons with co-morbid conditions (diabetes, hypertension, chronic respiratory illness, immunity disorders, etc.) should seek advice from the nearest health facility, prior to travel to an affected country.
- Travellers who complain of fever within two weeks of return from an affected country should report to the nearest health facility.
- Pregnant women who have travelled to areas with Zika virus transmission should mention about their travel during ante-natal visits in order to be assessed and monitored appropriately.
- Advise the patient this zika virus also spread through sexual intercourse.

Preventive Measures (Baby or Child)

- Do not use insect repellent on babies younger than 2 months of age.
- Dress your child in clothing that covers arms and legs.
- Cover crib, stroller, and baby carrier with mosquito netting.
- Do not apply insect repellent onto a child's hands, eyes, mouth, and cut or irritated skin.

Conclusion

Nowadays our nursing professional has facing so many challenges while providing health care to the patients so they need to update their knowledge and skill towards betterment of patient's health care. The Zika virus is a mild disease and most people with the virus do not have symptoms. However, the recent rise in the spread of Zika virus in Brazil has been accompanied by an unprecedented rise in the number of children being born with unusually small heads identified as microcephaly. In addition, several countries, including Brazil, reported a steep increase in Guillain-Barré syndrome a neurological disorder that could lead to paralysis and death. Evidence is growing that Zika virus causes both microcephaly and Guillain-Barré syndrome.

COMMON BACTERIAL INFECTIONS

The most common bacterial infections among children are skin infections (including impetigo), ear infections, and throat infections (strep throat). These and many other less common bacterial disorders are treated similarly in adults and children and are discussed elsewhere in the book. Other infections occur at all ages but have specific considerations in children. Several severe bacterial infections are preventable by routine immunization early in childhood.

Types of common bacteria:

- Diphtheria
- Infection with *Haemophilus influenzae* type b (meningitis, epiglottitis, some severe eye infections, and occult bacteremia)
- Infection with *Streptococcus pneumoniae* (pneumonia, meningitis, occult bacteremia, and ear infections)
- Infection with *Neisseria meningitidis* (meningitis, sepsis, and occult bacteremia)
- Pertussis
- Tetanus.

Classification of bacterial infectious diseases:

- Tuberculosis
- Typhoid fever
- Tetanus
- Diphtheria
- Whooping cough and leprosy
- *Haemophilus influenzae* 'B' (Hib)
- Meningococcal infections
- *Helicobacter pylori* infections
- Toxic shock syndrome
- STDs/RTIs
- Congenital syphilis.

TUBERCULOSIS (TB)

Introduction

Tuberculosis (TB) is infective disease caused by *mycobacterium* which primarily affects the lungs. In some cases the intestines, kidneys, bone marrow, brain, spine, and stomach can also be affected. World Health Organization (WHO) estimates in 2013 revealed that up to 80,000 children die from TB each year and children account for over half a million new cases annually. It should be noted that the estimated deaths only include those in human immunodeficiency virus (HIV)-negative children. In fact, the actual burden of TB in children is likely higher, especially given the challenge in diagnosing childhood TB.

Definition

Tuberculosis is a specific infectious chronic disease caused by *'Mycobacterium tuberculosis'*. The disease primarily affects the lungs causing pulmonary tuberculosis. It can also affect meninges, intestine, bones, joints, lymph glands, skin and other tissues of the body.

Causes

Tubercle bacilli belongs to the Actinomycetales and family Mycobacteriaceae. *Mycobacterium tuberculosis* is the most common cause of this disease; other rare causes include *M. bovis* and *M. africanum*. The acid-fast characteristic of the *mycobacterium* is their unique feature. *M. tuberculosis* is an aerobic, non-spore-forming, nonmotile, slow-growing bacillus with a curved and beaded rod-shaped morphology. It is a very hardy bacillus that can survive under adverse environmental conditions. Humans are the only known reservoirs for *M. tuberculosis*.

Mode of Transmission

The TB bacterium is spread through the air when an infected person coughs, sneezes, speaks, sings, or laughs and mainly droplet infection and droplet nuclei during coughing and sneezing in sputum positive patient of pulmonary tuberculosis. Nasopharyngeal secretions also may transmit infection. Extra pulmonary tuberculosis and sputum negative cases contribute in minimal transmission of infection. Transplacental transmission may occur causing congenital tuberculosis.

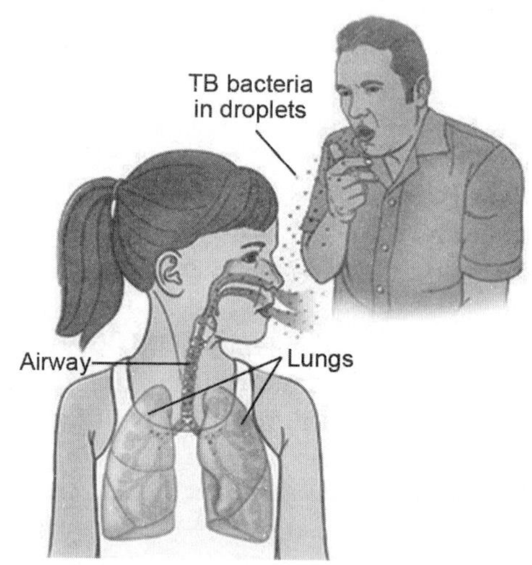

Fig. 5.17: Mode of transmission of TB infection

Incubation Period

Incubation period may be weeks, congenital tuberculosis. It depends upon host parasite relationship, closeness of contact, extent of disuse and sputum positivity of the source cases. Average incubation period is 3–8 weeks.

Incidence

In India from an average of one percent in the under 5 age group, the infection index climbs to above 30 percent at the age of 15 years. The risk factors of tubercular infection are inherited susceptibility inter current infections like measles, pertussis and malnutrition.

Tuberculosis is a social disease. There are so many social factors which contribute to the occurrence and spread of this disease. These factors are poor housing, poor ventilation, overcrowding, air pollution, less sunshine, population explosion, undernutrition, poor quality life style, lack of education and health awareness, large families, early marriages and poor economy.

Pathophysiology

The child is infected from an open case of tuberculosis. The common mode of entry of tubercle bacilli is inhalation. Occasionally the organism may enter by ingestion and rarely through abraded skin. Majority (95%) of the primary tuberculosis occur in the lungs. The tubercle bacilli reach the finest bronchioles and alveoli where they are taken up by phagocytes. Bacilli multiply and set up a pathological lesion tubercle, a central area of caseation and necrosis lesion tubercle surrounded by a ring of small round of lymphocytes. A number of such tubercle may merge to form the primary focus, also described as Ghon focus. The primary focus may be found in any portion of the lungs, but is often found sub pleurally in the lower part of upper lobe of right lung. The infection spreads to the regional lymph nodes through the involved lymphatic. The regional glands become enlarged and caseous and may be associated with pleural reaction to form primary complex. The Ghon focus usually shows slow healing with calcification and fibrosis. The primay complex may be reactivated, following reinfection especially at the time of puberty.

The primary infection afterwards may spread through the lymphatics and the blood steam and carried in different parts of the body, i.e. meninges, peritoneum, bone, joints kidney, spleen, liver, lymph glands, etc. Tuberculous meningitis and military tuberculosis are more likely to occur. Local spread may cause pleural effusion, atelectasis, obstructive emphysema and endobrochial segmental tuberculosis.

Congenital tuberculosis may occur from transplancental transmission or the fetus inhaling bacilli from liquor amnii as a result of the tuberculosis focus in the plancenta. This condition is characterized by enlargement and caseation of the glands at pecta hepatic and disseminated tubercles throughout the liver. This comprise the primary complex and formation of tubercles. Scatterly through the lungs, spleen, brain, meninges and other viscera.

Signs and Symptoms

In children:

- Fever (Hyperthermia)
- Unintended weight loss
- Poor growth

- Sweating at night
- Cough
- Swollen glands
- Chills.

In adolescents:

- Cough more longer than 3 weeks
- Productive cough
- Pain in the chest
- Blood in their sputum
- Weakness and fatigue
- Swollen glands
- Unintended weight loss
- Decrease in appetite
- Fever (Hyperthermia)
- Chills or night sweats.

Diagnostic Evaluation

Tuberculosis (TB) is a disease that is spread through the air from one person to another. There are two kinds of tests that are used to determine if a person has been infected with TB bacteria: Tuberculin skin test and TB blood tests. The diagnosis of tuberculosis is done based on history of illness with special emphasis on history of exposure to infection in family or in neighbors. Clinical examination, radiology and laboratory investigations help to confirm the diagnosis.

- History collection
- Physical assessment
- Mantoux tuberculin test
- Blood test
- Chest X-ray.

The laboratory investigations should include isolation of AFB by bacteriological examination, histopathology, immunodiagnosis and other supportive investigations.

The effective confirmatory investigation is the bacteriological isolation of the AFB. Sputum examination or laryngeal swab or peritoneal fluid in abdominal TB and CSF study in CNS involvement are very useful to confirm the diagnosis.

The recommended Mantoux test, the dosage of 0.1 mL or 5 tuberculin units [TU] of purified protein derivative (PPD) should be injected intradermally into the volar aspect of the forearm using a 27-gauge needle. A detergent called Tween 80 to prevent loss of efficacy on contact and adsorption by glass stabilizes the PPD. A wheal should be raised and should measure approximately 6–10 mm in diameter.

Always read the test 48–72 hours after administration. Measure the amount of induration and not erythema. This should be measured transverse to the long axis of the forearm.

BCG test is performed by intradermal injection with BCG vaccine in the left deltoid region. An induration of more than 5–6 mm after 3 days of injection is accepted as positive reaction.

Blood examination for ESR shows elevation during active phase of the disease, though the test has no diagnostic value.

Radiology is an important diagnostic approach of childhood tuberculosis. X-ray and CT scan of the affected part help in diagnosis of tuberculosis.

Management

As a result based TB classified in two TB-related conditions exist: Latent TB infection and TB disease. Both latent TB infection and TB disease can be treated.

Treatment for Latent TB Infection

Child with latent TB infection has TB bacteria in their bodies, but they are not sick because the bacteria are not active, child with latent TB infection do not have symptoms, and they cannot spread TB bacteria to others. However, if TB bacteria become active in the body and multiply, the person will go from having latent TB infection to being sick with TB disease. For this reason, people with latent TB infection are often prescribed treatment to prevent them from developing TB disease.

Because there are less bacteria in a child with latent TB infection, treatment is much easier.

Four drugs regimens are approved for the treatment of latent TB infection. The medications used to treat latent TB infection include:

- Isoniazid (INH)
- Rifampin (RIF)
- Rifapentine (RPT)

Treatment for TB Disease

TB bacteria become active (multiplying in the body) if the immune system can not stop them from growing. When TB bacteria are active, this is called TB disease. TB disease will make a person sick. Children with TB disease may spread the bacteria to people with whom they spend many hours.

TB disease can be treated by taking several drugs for 6 to 9 months. The first-line anti-TB agents that form the core of treatment regimens include:

- Isoniazid (INH)
- Rifampin (RIF)
- Ethambutol (EMB)
- Pyrazinamide (PZA).

Regimens for treating TB disease have an initial phase of 2 months, followed by a choice of several options for the *continuation phase* of either 4 or 7 months (total of 6 to 9 months for treatment.

Treatment completion is determined by the number of doses ingested over a given period of time. Although basic TB regimens are broadly applicable, there are modifications that should be made under special circumstances (such as people with HIV infection, drug resistance, pregnancy, or treatment of children).

DOTS (Directly observed therapy short-term) is now practiced in India, under Revised National Tuberculosis Control Programme. Who recommended antitubercular treatment regimens have also produced cure rates approaching 100 % when drug-taking has been fully supervised. WHO has recommended 6 months regimen, 8 months regimen and 12 months regimen depending upon the child's condition for the treatment of childhood tuberculosis.

Drug resistant cases should be managed on the basis of type of resistance which can be primary, natural, acquired, initial or multidrug type of resistance. Relapse cases and defaulter cases need special attention for management.

Baby born to the mother with tuberculosis, diagnosed in 3rd trimester or during delivery should be considered as special condition. Breastfeeding must be continued. BCG vaccination should be given at birth. Chest X-ray to be done to detect the lung condition and drug therapy to be started depending upon the findings.

Steroid (prednisolone) can be used as anti-inflammatory agent in the treatment of tuberculosis. The indications are TB meningitis, military tuberculosis, renal tuberculosis, precardial or pleural effusion, endobronchial tuberculosis or segmental lesion and in extremely ill patients or terminally ill children. It is administered with the dose of 1–2 mg/kg/day during first 6 weeks of infection and can be continued for 1–3 months.

Surgical interventions may be need though number of surgery has greatly reduced. The common indications for surgical interventions are pleural effusion, bronchiectasis, cavity formation ascites, cold abscess, pott's spine, CNS tuberculosis with hydrocephalus, GI bleeding and for diagnostic approaches (biopsy, bronchoscopy).

Supportive nursing measures should include general nursing care and drug compliance. All drugs should be administered in a single daily dose on an empty stomach. The drugs are safe if used in the recommended dosage schedule. Supervised drug therapy is essential in home based management. Hepatotoxicity may be found in malnourished children or in disseminated disease. Avoidence of defaulter, assessment of any adverse effects and complications are very important. Good diet with balanced intake of protein and vitamins are essential. Fresh air, sunshine, hygienic measures, necessary rest and ambulation should be promoted. Follow-up regular interval even by home visit and involvement of family members in continued care are essential part of management.

Prognosis

Prognosis of tuberculosis depends upon age, duration of infection, type of disease, site of infection, nutritional status, living condition, socioeconomic status, intercurrent infections resistance to drugs, early diagnosis, continuation of treatment and facilities available.

Prognosis is worse in military tuberculosis, TB meningitis, chronic pulmonary tuberculosis, TB with malnutrition and drug resistant cases.

Adequate treatment facilities with antitubercular drugs and improvement of BCG vaccination help to bring the declining trends of mortality and mortality pattern with increased life span of tuberculosis patient.

Preventive Measures

Vaccination

The Bacilli Calmette-Guérin (BCG) vaccine is available for the prevention of disseminated TB. BCG is a live vaccine prepared from attenuated strains of *M. bovis*. The major role of BCG vaccination is the prevention of serious and life-threatening disease such as disseminated TB and TB meningitis in children. The BCG vaccine does not prevent infection with *M. tuberculosis*.

- Avoiding contact with those who have the active TB disease.
- Using medications as a preventive measure in high-risk cases.
- Maintaining good living standards.

Early detection of tuberculosis patients with prompt and adequate treatment help to prevent spread of infection. Completion of treatment schedule, prevention of defaulter cases, identification and treatment of relapse cases are important aspect of prevention of the disease.

Chemoprophylaxis should be given to high risk infants and children especially in household contact, BCG adenitis and baby born to mother with tuberculosis.

Sources of infection need adequate treatment after tracing them out. Familial and extra familial contacts should be find out from the school teacher, food venders, domestic servants and visitors.

Health education is the most important aspect of prevention of tuberculosis. The informations and explanation should include mode of transmissions and explanation should include mode of transmission, early symptoms, treatment facilities, regularity of treatment, home care, methods of coughing and sneezing, disposal of sputum, prophylaxis of contact and BCG vaccination. Health education should also include hygienic living with good housing, improved environmental sanitation, better living condition, well ventilation, avoidance of dampness, overcrowding and indiscriminate spitting, prevention of malnutrition, promotion of balanced diet, intake of boiled milk, family support, acceptance of family based treatment of tuberculosis patient and rehabilitation of them.

TYPHOID FEVER (ENTERIC FEVER)

Introduction

Typhoid fever is a serious and sometimes life-threatening infection that mostly affects people in developing countries, where clean water and other sanitation measures are hard to come by. The disease usually causes symptoms that include a high fever, a stomach ache, and achiness. It can be cured with antibiotic.

Definition

Typhoid fever is a bacterial infection caused by *Salmonella typhi*. The illness is characterized by prolonged typical continuous fever for 3 to 4 weeks with prostration, relative bradycardia and involvement of spleen and lymph nodes.

The term enteric fever indicates both typhoid and paratyphoid fever. This condition may found as epidemics, endemics and sporadics. In India, typhoid fever occurs in endemics. It is found all over the world where water supplies and sanitation are substandard. The disease is uncommon in developed countries.

Incidence

The incidence of typhoid fever is highest in 5–19 years of age group. Most of the cases are found among males, but carriers are more in females. The disease is found throughout the year but more in summer and rainy season with increased number of cases are recorded.

Pollution of drinking water supply, open airway defecation and urination, poor food hygiene practice and personal hygiene, health ignorance, illiteracy and poor socioeconomic conditions are important contributing factors.

Causes

Typhoid fever is caused by bacteria called *Salmonella Typhi* (*S.Typhi*), which are related to the bacteria *salmonella* that cause food poisoning. *S. Typhi* typically lives in humans and is shed through a person's feces (stools) or urine.

Risk Factors

Typhoid fever remains a serious worldwide threat especially in the developing world affecting an estimated 22 million people each year, according to the Centers for Disease Control and Prevention. The disease is endemic in India, Southeast Asia, Africa, South America and many other areas.

Worldwide, children are at greatest risk of getting the disease, although they generally have milder symptoms than adults do.

- High risk to get typhoid fever those who are living in endemic area
- Work as a clinical microbiologist handling Salmonella typhi bacteria
- Have close contact with someone who is infected or has recently been infected with typhoid fever
- Weakened immune system children such as who are undergone corticosteroids therapy and diseases such as HIV/AIDS
- Drink water contaminated by sewage that contains *S. typhi*.

Mode of Transmission

Typhoid fever is communicating by drinking or eating the bacteria in contaminated food or water. Child with acute illness can contaminate the surrounding water supply through stool, which contains a high concentration of the bacteria. Contamination of the water supply can, in turn, taint the food supply. The bacteria can survive for weeks in water or dried sewage.

Transmission is mainly feco-oral route or urine oral routes. Infection takes place directly through soiled hands contaminated with stool or urine of infected patients or carriers.

Indirect transmission occurs by the ingestion of contaminated water, food, milk or through flies. Vegetables grown in the sewage firm and washed in contaminated water promote the transmission.

Typhoid bacilli may survive for about 7 days in water, one month in ice or ice cream and 70 days in soil irrigated with sewage under moist or cold condition. Food provides shelter to the bacilli, where they can multiply or survive for sometimes. The bacilli grow rapidly in milk without changing the taste and appearance.

Incubation Period

Incubation period is usually 10–14 days with a range of 3 days to 3 weeks depending upon the dose of bacilli ingested. It is shortest if food-borne and longest in waterborne.

Signs and Symptoms

The common signs and symptoms appear in 7 to 14 days after finding the disease. Some children may not become sick for as longer as 2 months after exposure.

The symptoms of typhoid fever may range from mild to severe, depending on factors such as the age, health, and vaccination history of the infected person and the geographic location where the infection originated.

Signs and symptoms of typhoid fever may include:

- A persistent fever that rises gradually to 39 to 40 °C (102 to 104 °F)
- Headache
- Sore throat
- Anorexia
- Tiredness
- Restlessness
- Stomach pain
- Constipation
- Diarrhea
- A temporary rash with raised pink spots on the stomach or chest.

Pathophysiology

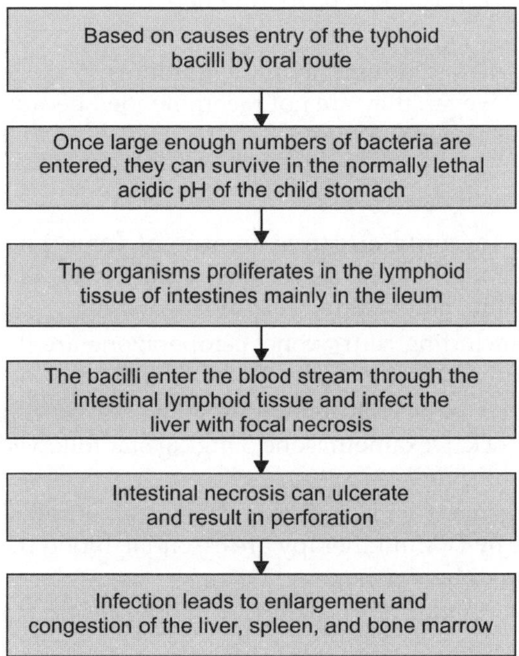

Fig. 5.18: Pathophysiology of TB infection

Diagnostic Evaluation

The following laboratory investigations may be down to support the diagnosis.

- History collection/physical examination
- Routine blood examination: It shows normal or low WBC count. Eosinophils may be low or completely absent.
- Widal test is positive, 60 percent in 2nd week and 80 percent in third week.
- Bone marrow culture is highly sensitive (90%) for diagnosis of typhoid fever.
- CBC count with differential
  - CBC count is often 10,000–15,000/µL in simple gastroenteritis.
  - Child with enteric fever commonly have anemia, thrombocytopenia, or Neutropenia.
- Blood cultures
  - Isolation of *Salmonella* from cultures of stool, blood, urine, or bone marrow is diagnostic
  - Cultures of rose spots and/or bone marrow aspirate may be positive in enteric fever even when stool culture findings are negative for *Salmonella.*
- *Stool examination:* Stool may be Hemoccult positive and may have positive findings for fecal polymorphonuclear cells.
- *Biochemistry*
  - Electrolyte tests may reveal metabolic acidosis or other abnormalities consistent with dehydration.
  - Child with enteric fever may have mild hepatitis.
- Serologic tests
  - Tests for *Salmonella* agglutinins (febrile agglutinins, Widal test) may suggest infection with *S. typhi;* however, they are not recommended because of the number of false-positive and false-negative results.

Management

Antibiotic therapy is the only effective treatment for typhoid fever in children is chloramphenical 50–100 mg/kg/day in 4 divided doses for 10–14 days. Other drugs which can be sued are Ampicillin, amoxicillin, Cotrimoxazole, etc.

The cephalosporin including ceftriaxone, cefoperazone are the drug of choice (50–100 mg/kg/day) in single or two divided doses IV for 5 to 10 days.

Corticosteroid is given to the children with severe toxic state, prolonged illness, altered mental function and shock. Dexamethasone 3 mg/kg stat followed by 1mg/kg 6 hourly for another 8 doses is administered.

Symptomatic management with antipyretics, hydrotherapy and maintenance of fluid and electrolyte balance by IV fluid therapy are essential. Blood transfusion may be needed in intestinal perforation or hemorrhage.

Nutritious diet to be provided. Early detection of complications and prompt management promote better prognosis.

Surgical management may be required in intestinal perforation and gallbladder infection in chronic carrier's stages.

Nursing Management

Nursing care is important for better prognosis.

- Provide adequate bed rest
- Provide the skin care for avoid skin damage
- Maintain the good oral and dental hygiene and frequent mouth care with antiseptic mouth wash
- Provide adequate fluid intake or IV fluid therapy
- Administration of prescribed medications proper time
- Provide tepid sponge to reduce the fever and continuous monitoring of child condition are important aspects of nursing measures
- Isolation of infected child and care of bladder and bowel are essential
- Prevention of constipation or care during diarrhea
- Prevention of urinary retention, observation for frank or occult blood in stool and careful disposal of stool and urine are important
- Diet should be planned with adequate calories, protein, iron and vitamins by liquid or semisolid food
- Assessment and recording of vital signs and drug effects or any features of complications should be emphasized
- Parental involvement in child care during the hospitalization and necessary instructions to parents for continuing child care at hospital and home level.

Complications

Complications of *Salmonella* infection

- Nontyphoidal salmonellosis
  - Bacteremia
  - Meningitis
  - Pneumonia
  - Endocarditis/pericarditis
  - Osteomyelitis (most common in patients with sickle cell anemia)
  - Hepatic/Splenic abscess.
- Typhoid fever (Enteric Fever)
  - Intestinal perforation and severe hemorrhage (occurs in 1–10% of children)
  - Toxic encephalopathy and cerebral thrombosis
  - Hepatitis, pancreatitis, arthritis, and myocarditis.

Other Common Complication

- *Abdominal cavity:* Intestinal perforation, GI bleeding, hepatitis, cholecystitis, peritonitis, gastroenteritis, urinary tract infection, liver abscess, fatter liver, pancreatitis.
- *Neurological system:* Encephalopathy, meningitis, hemiplegia, transverse myelitis, GB syndrome, psychiatric problems like depression, schizophrenia.
- *Hematologic system:* Hemolytic anemia, bone-marrow depression.
- *Cardiovascular system:* Toxic myocarditis, pericarditis, endocarditis, venous thrombosis.

- *Respiratory system:* Pneumonia, bronchitis, empyema, pulmonary infarction, pleurisy.
- *Miscellaneous:* Parotitis, bed sores, otitis media, tonsillitis, alopecia, chronic osteomyelitis, supportive arthritis, superficial abscesses.

Preventive Measures

Health education is the most significant method of controlling this disease by increasing awareness about safe water, food hygiene, food handling, handwashing, kitchen hygiene, personal hygiene, sanitary sewage disposal, control of flies, hazards of contaminated food and water and mode of transmission of the disease, etc.

- *Safe drinking water:* Boil or disinfect any water that will be used for drinking, washing or preparing food, making ice, or brushing teeth. Allow the child to drink only hot water.
- *Hygienic food preparation:* Fully cook all food, and avoid food from street vendors and food stored or served at room temperature. Instead, serve packaged foods or meals that are freshly cooked and served steaming hot.
- *Food habit:* Avoid raw, unpeeled fruits and vegetables that may have been washed with contaminated water, especially lettuce and fruits like berries that cannot be peeled. Bananas, avocados, and oranges make better choices, but make sure peeled or not.
- *Personal hygiene:* Wash with soap and clean, warm water, especially after kids use the bathroom or before they eat or prepare food. If no soap and water are available, use an alcohol-based hand sanitizer.

Three types of vaccines are available

1. Whole cell vaccine
2. Vi-vaccine
3. Oral vaccine.

Whole cell vaccine: Vaccine is given with two doses of SC injection with 0.5 ml for the children more than 10 years of age and 0.25 ml for young children. It has 70 percent efficacy and side effects of fever, malaise, local pain and swelling.

Vi-vaccine: It is given as a single dose with 0.5 ml SC or IM. It has 70–80 percent efficacy for five years. Dose may be repeated after 5 years. No side effects observed for this vaccine. It is not given to children below 2 years of age.

Oral vaccine (typhoral): It is available as a capsule and recommended for children older than 6 years on three alternate day (one capsule each on day 1, 3 and 5). Efficacy is 70–80 percent with 3 to 5 years immunity.

Prognosis

Prognosis varies as follows:

- Nontyphoidal salmonellosis
  - Prognosis of child with simple gastroenteritis is excellent except for very young infants or child with debilitating diseases.
  - The prognosis for *Salmonella* meningitis or endocarditis is poor.
- Typhoid fever (enteric fever)
  - Therapy with antibiotics has decreased the mortality rate to 1%; however, prognosis depends on the extent of complications from the disease.
  - Relapse is common after therapy for enteric fever.

TETANUS

Introduction

Tetanus, also called as lockjaw, is a serious but preventable disease that affects the muscles and nerves. It typically arises from a skin wound that becomes contaminated by a bacterium called *Clostridium tetani*, which is often found in soil.

Tetanus is acquired through exposure to the spores of the bacterium *Clostridium tetani* which are universally present in the soil. The disease is caused by the action of a potent neurotoxin produced during the growth of the bacteria in dead tissues, e.g. in dirty wounds or in the umbilicus following nonsterile delivery.

Definition

Tetanus is defined as an acute infectious diseases cause by *Clostridium tetani*, sometimes fatal, disease of the central nervous system, which usually enters the body through an open wound. Tetanus bacteria live in soil and manure, but also can be found in the human intestine, animal saliva.

Tetanus is one of the leading causes of neonatal death. Neonatal tetanus considered as a killer disease second only to measles among the six-killer vaccine preventable diseases.

Incidence

Neonatal tetanus is particularly common in rural areas where most deliveries are at home without adequate sterile procedures. In 2000, WHO estimates that neonatal tetanus killed about 200 000 babies.

It is common at periods of life when an individual is more exposed to trauma (childhood, adolescent). The number of neonatal tetanus is declining mainly due to significant increase in immunization coverage of pregnant women with tetanus toxoid.

Causes

The causative agent of tetanus is clostridium tetani, a gram-positive, anaerobic, spore bearing organism. The spores are highly resistant to injurious agent, boiling, phenol, cresol, etc.

The Mode of Transmission

Tetanus is not transmitted from person to person. A person usually becomes infected with tetanus when dirt enters a wound or cut. Tetanus germs are likely to grow in deep puncture wounds caused by dirty nails, knives, tools, wood splinters, and animal bites. Women face an additional risk of infection if a contaminated tool is used during childbirth or during an abortion.

A newborn baby become infected through the contaminated knife, razor, or other instrument used to cut the umbilical cord, if dirty material is used to dress the cord, or contaminated hands of the medical team who delivering the baby.

Infants and children may also contract tetanus when dirty instruments are used for circumcision, scarification, and skin piercing, and when it dirt, charcoal, or other unclean substances are rubbed into a wound.

Types of Tetanus

Generalized Tetanus

The generalized tetanus is the most common type of tetanus in children. The onset of this condition is usually sudden with rapid progression of muscle spasm and cramps. The initial feature is the 'lock jaw' or trismus due to stiffness of the masseters which make the difficulty in opening mouth.

This condition followed by generalized muscle spasms, precipitated by external stimuli like touch, loud sounds, bright light, etc. Other features are difficulty in swallowing, restlessness, irritability, headache, neck rigidity, spasms of facial muscles (risus sardonicus), spasms and rigidity of muscles of neck make the body arch backward like a bow (opisthotonos position) and constant spasm of the muscles in extremities and abdomen.

Localized Tetanus

The localized tetanus is manifested with pain, constant rigidity and muscle spasm in the region of injury. It may be associated with otitis media. This condition may recover fully within a few weeks or may progress to generalized tetanus.

Cephalic Tetanus

The cephalic tetanus is very rare variety and manifested as paralysis of one or more cranial nerves (usually 7th cranial nerves) with gradual spastic symptoms of whole body.

Neonatal Tetanus

The neonatal tetanus develops due to unhygienic delivery or contamination of umbilicial stump, manifestations usually occurs between 2 days and 2 weeks of age. The neonate presents with unexplained crying, refusal of feeds and apathy. On forceful feeding, reflex spasm of masseters and pharyngeal muscles leads to trismus (lock jaw), dysphasia and choking.

It is followed by spasms of limbs, generalized rigidity and opisthotonos. Reflex laryngeal spasm may lead to apnea and cyanosis. Continued spasm may cause to pyrexia, tachypnea, tachycardia, acidosis and dehydration. Superadded infections are common.

Pathophysiology

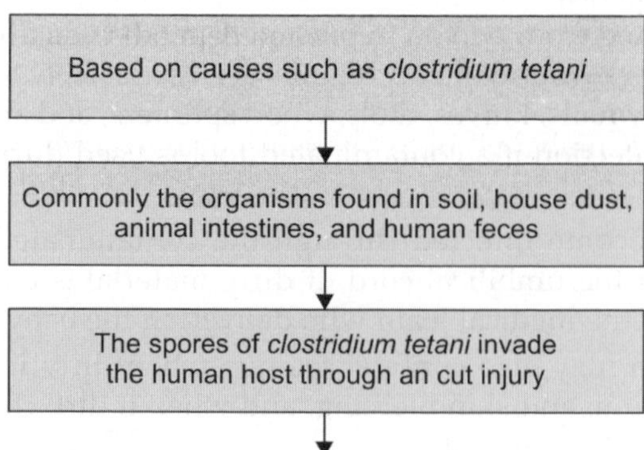

Contd...

Contd...

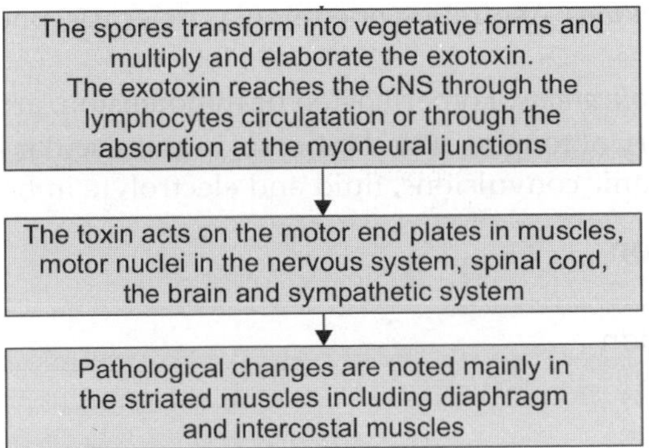

Fig. 5.19: Pathophysiology of tetanus

Signs and Symptoms

Common symptoms of tetanus:

- Stiffness of the jaw (also called lockjaw)
- Stiffness of the abdominal and back muscles
- Contraction of the facial muscles
- Convulsions
- Tachycardia
- Fever
- Sweating
- Painful muscle spasms near the wound area (if these affect the larynx or chest wall, the person may can not able to breathe)
- Trouble swallowing.

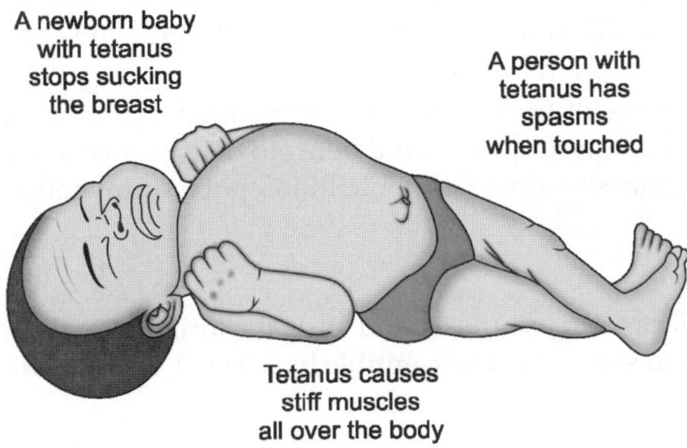

Fig. 5.20: Specific signs and symptoms of tetanus

Complications

- *Respiratory complications:* Aspiration pneumonia, atelecasis, pneumothorax, mediastinal emphysema.
- *Cardiovascular complications:* Hypertension or hypotension, arrhythmia, myocardititis.
- *Miscellaneous:* Injury of tongue or oral mucosa, intramuscular hematoma and vertebral fracture during titanic convulsions, fluid and electrolyte imbalance, malnutrition.

Diagnostic Evaluation

- History collection
- Physical examination
- Blood examination
- CBC
- Biopsy (necrotic tissue).

Management

Antimicrobials are used to decrease the number of vegetative forms of C *tetani* (the toxin source) in the wound. For years, penicillin G was used widely for this purpose, but it is not the current drug of choice. Metronidazole (e.g. 0.5 g every 6 hours) has comparable or better antimicrobial activity and penicillin is a known antagonist of gamma-aminobutyric acid (GABA), as is tetanus toxin. Metronidazole is also associated with lower mortality.

The goals of medical managements are to stop toxin production within the wound, to neutralize unbound toxin, and to control disease manifestations. Drugs used to treat muscle spasm, rigidity, and tetanic seizures include sedative-hypnotic agents, general anesthetics, centrally acting muscle relaxants, and neuromuscular blocking agents.

Antibiotics are used to prevent multiplication of *Clostridium tetani,* thus halting production and release of toxins. Antitoxins are given to neutralize unbound toxin.

Penicillin G

Penicillin G is a bactericidal antibiotic that binds to and inhibits penicillin-binding proteins, which are transpeptidases that cross-link peptidoglycans, the final step in bacterial cell wall synthesis. Inhibition of cell wall synthesis and autolytic enzyme activation are responsible for its bactericidal action on dividing bacteria.

A 10- to 14-day course of treatment is recommended. Large intravenous (IV) doses of penicillin may cause hemolytic anemia and neurotoxicity. Cardiac arrest has been reported in patients receiving massive doses of penicillin G potassium. child with renal failure are particularly at risk.

Doxycycline

Doxycycline inhibits protein synthesis and thus bacterial growth by binding to 30S and possibly S0S ribosomal subunits of susceptible bacteria. A 10- to 14-day course of treatment is recommended.

Erythromycin

Erythromycin is a bacteriostatic agent that inhibits protein synthesis by binding to the 50S subunit of bacterial ribosomes. It is not the drug of choice for tetanus but may be used when the drugs of choice cannot be administered for some reason.

Clindamycin

Clindamycin is a bacteriostatic agent that binds to the 50S ribosomal subunit. It is not the drug of choice for tetanus and may be used only if the drugs of choice cannot be used.

Tetracycline

Tetracycline is a bacteriostatic agent that inhibits protein synthesis. It is not the drug of choice for tetanus and may be used only if the drugs of choice cannot be used.

Vancomycin

Vancomycin is a bactericidal agent that inhibits cell wall and RNA synthesis. It is not the drug of choice for tetanus and may be used only if the drugs of choice cannot be used.

Vaccines

The human tetanus immunoglobulin 500 to 3000 IU should be given intramuscular immediate on admission to hospital. It is safest and most effective treatment without any complications. Antitetanic Serum (ATS) can be administered after skin test with 30,000 to 1,00,000 IU, IM or IV.

Nursing Management

- The nurse should clean the wound with soap water
- A course of tetanus antitoxin injections
- A tracheostomy (a breathing tube inserted surgically in the windpipe) in severe cases with respiratory problems
- Medications to control spasms
- Antibiotics
- Hospitalization
- Suctioning of or pharyngeal secretions, comfortable positioning, oxygen therapy, IV fluid therapy
- Hygienic measure and constant monitoring with recording of vital signs are important essential measures. Initially oral feeding should be avoided and nasogastric tube feeding should be given
- Administration of medications should be done following specific precautions (e.g. skin test for penicillin)
- Care of wound or injury or umbilical stump or ear discharge need special attention. Special care to be taken for tracheostomy and for mechanical ventilation.
- Pyridoxine therapy may give gratifying results in neonatal tetanus with conventional regimen.

Prognosis

The prognosis is dependent on incubation period, the time from spore inoculation to first symptom, and the time from first symptom to first tetanic spasm.

- In general, shorter intervals indicate more severe tetanus and a poorer prognosis
- Children usually survive tetanus and return to their predisease state of health.
- Recovery is slow and usually occurs over 2–4 months
- Some child remain hypotonic status
- Clinical tetanus does not produce a state of immunity; therefore, child who survive the disease require active immunization with tetanus toxoid to prevent a recurrence.

The total score indicates disease severity and prognosis as follows:

- 0 or 1: Mild tetanus; mortality below 10%
- 2 or 3: Moderate tetanus; mortality of 10–20%
- 4: Severe tetanus; mortality of 20–40%
- 5 or 6: Very severe tetanus; mortality above 50%.

Preventive Measures

Provide active immunization to pregnant women with tetanus toxoid. The infants and children with DPT, DT, and TT are the best definite method of prevention. In case of child with open wound, both active immunization with T. Toxid and passive immunization with tetanus immunoglobin should be given.

Antitetanic serum (ATS) is not usually used as prophylactic purpose. Thorough wound cleaning with antiseptic lotion is also very important measures. Increasing awareness about the clean and aseptic delivery, safe care of umbilical cord and improvement of immunization status of mothers and children are significant preventive measures to reduce neonatal and childhood tetanus.

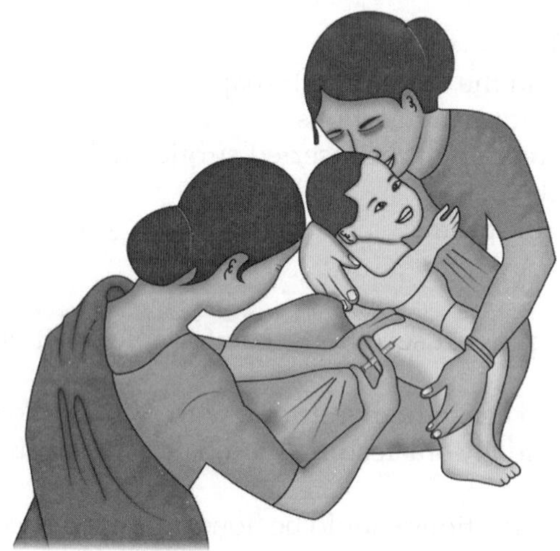

Fig. 5.21: TT vaccination to child

DIPHTHERIA

Definition

Diphtheria is caused by the bacterium *Corynebacterium diphtheriae*. This germ produces a toxin that can harm or destroy human body tissues and organs. One type of diphtheria affects the throat and sometimes the tonsils. Another type, more common in the tropics, causes ulcers on the skin. —*WHO*

Diphtheria is an acute infectious bacterial disease caused by *Corynebacterium diphtheriae*. The disease is characterized by inflammation of epithelial surface, formation of a membrane in the upper respiratory tract and presence of severe toxemia due to the effect of powerful exotoxin.

Causes

The causative agent of diphtheria is a gram-positive, nonmotile bacteria named as Corynebacterium diphtheriae. It has no invasive power but produces powerful exotoxin.

Mode of Transmission

The diphtheria bacterium can enter the body through the nose and mouth. However, it can also enter through a break in the skin. It is transmitted from person-to-person in close contact by aerosol route (breathing in respiratory secretions or droplets that contain diphtheria bacteria from an infected person coughing, sneezing, or laughing). After being exposed to the bacteria, it usually takes two to four days for symptoms to develop.

- The disease can be transmitted directly from skin lesions or through contaminated objects (utensils, care articles, toys, etc.) portal of entry is mainly respiratory tract.
- Other routes of entry are cut injury, wounds, ulcers, and occasionally through eye, genitalia, middle ear, etc.
- Diphtheria affects mainly the children of one to five years of age. It can be found even in preschool and school children. Infants of the immune mothers are protected for few weeks or months of life.
- The disease occurs in all seasons but found more in winter or in autumn.

Incubation Period

Incubation period is 2 to 6 days.

Types

- Respiratory diphtheria
- Skin (cutaneous) diphtheria.

Pathophysiology

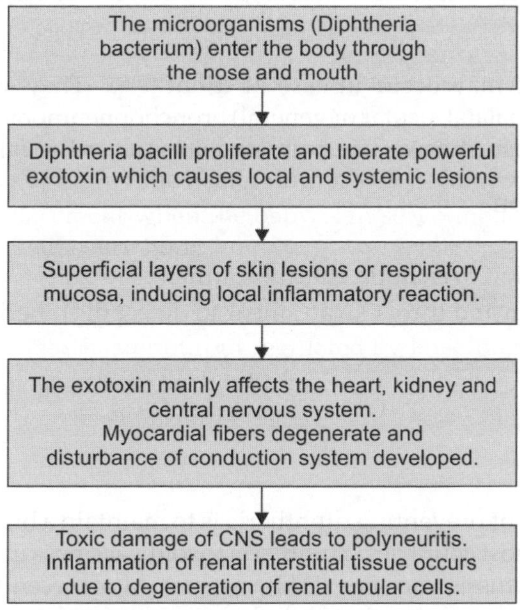

Fig. 5.22: Pathophysiology of diphtheria

Signs and Symptoms

Respiratory Diphtheria

The child is infected with diphtheria, the bacterium usually multiplies in the throat, leading to respiratory diphtheria. A membrane may form over the throat and tonsils, causing a sore throat. Other common symptoms of respiratory diphtheria may include:

- Breathing difficulty
- Low grade fever
- Husky voice
- Stridor (a shrill breathing sound heard during inspiration, or breathing in)
- Enlarged lymph glands of the neck
- Increased heart rate
- Nasal drainage
- Swelling of the palate (the roof of the mouth).

Untreated children may die from asphyxiation when the membrane obstructs breathing. Other complications of respiratory diphtheria are caused by the diphtheria toxin released in the blood, leading to heart failure.

Skin (Cutaneous) Diphtheria

This type of diphtheria, the symptoms is usually milder and may include yellow spots or sores (similar to impetigo) on the skin.

Diphtheria toxin spreads through the bloodstream and can lead to potentially life-threatening complications that affect other organs, such as the heart and kidneys. The toxin can cause damage to the heart that affects its ability to pump blood or the kidneys' ability to clear wastes. It also can cause nerve damage, eventually leading to paralysis.

Complications

Various complications may occur in case of diphtheria. They are mainly myocarditis, paralysis (pharyngeal, palatal, ocular or general) bronchopneumonia, nephritis, polyneuritis, hepatitis, vasomotor disturbances like hypotension and cardiac failure.

Diagnostic Evaluation

- History collection
- Physical examination to exclude clinical features
- Throat examination and throat swab smear to detect diphtheria bacilli
- Blood culture
- Tissue culture.

Management

Diphtheria Antitoxin

The most effective way of preventing diphtheria is to maintain a high level of immunization in the community. In most countries, diphtheria toxoid vaccine is given in combination with tetanus toxoid and pertussis vaccines (DTP vaccine). More recently, some countries have been using a combination vaccine that includes vaccines for diphtheria, tetanus, pertussis, vitamin A (Hep-B), and sometimes *Hoemophilus influenzae* type b (Hib). Approximately every ten years, booster doses of the adult form of the vaccine, tetanus-diphtheria toxoids vaccine (Td), may be needed to maintain immunity.

Antimicrobial therapy is indicated to halt toxin production, treat localized infection, and prevent transmission of the organism to patient contacts. *C diphtheriae* is usually susceptible to various agents in vitro, including penicillin, erythromycin, clindamycin, rifampin, and tetracycline.

Penicillin G Procaine

Long-acting parenteral penicillin (IM only) to treat moderately severe infections caused by penicillin G-sensitive microorganisms.

Penicillin G Benzathine

The drug should administered only IM. A tissue depot is created at the site of IM injection and slowly releases active drug into the systemic circulation. Penicillin serum concentrations are lower but more prolonged with the benzathine form than with the procaine form.

Erythromycin

Inhibits bacterial growth, possibly by blocking dissociation of peptidyl tRNA from ribosomes causing RNA-dependent protein synthesis to arrest.

Nursing Management

- Isolation of infected child and provide bed rest for 2–3 weeks
- Provide easily digestible diet with high calorie
- Drug therapy with antipyretics and sedative. In case of seriously ill patient, IV fluid
- Provide oxygen therapy
- Nasogastric tube feeding may be needed for maintenance of fluid electrolyte and nutritional requirements.
- Frequent removal of oropharyngeal or nasal secretion is essential. Tracheostomy may be required in respiratory obstruction. Mechanical ventilation may be needed in case of respiratory failure.
- Cardiac complications should be detected early by close monitoring and necessary management should be initiated promptly.

Prognosis

Prognosis depends upon the type of child illness, respiratory tract diphtheria; the fatality rate can be set at 10–15%. The prognosis depends on multiple factors, including the virulence of the organism, the patient's age and immunization status, the site of infection, and the timing of administration of the antitoxin. In most diphtheria-related deaths due to complications, mechanical obstruction and cardiac causes are important factors initiation of specific therapy and available treatment facilities. Among survivor permanent cardiac damage and paralytic sequelae may found children.

Preventive Measures

The most effective way of preventing diphtheria is to maintain a high level of immunization in the community. In most countries, diphtheria toxoid vaccine is given in combination with tetanus toxoid and Pertussis vaccines (DTP vaccine). More recently, some countries have been using a combination vaccine that includes vaccines for diphtheria, tetanus, pertussis, vitamin A (Hep-B), and sometimes *Hoemophilus influenzae* type b (Hib). Approximately every ten years, booster doses of the adult form of the vaccine, tetanus-diphtheria toxoids vaccine (Td), may be needed to maintain immunity.

All close contacts need to have Schick test and throat swab culture before administering chemoprophylaxis. Passive immunization with ADS may be given to the carriers with negative Schick test and positive culture with unknown immunization status.

Complications of Diphtheria

Diphtheria leads to potentially life-threatening complications, such as breathing difficulties and problems with the heart and nervous system.

- Respiratory failure
- Myocarditis
- Nervous system complications
- Paralysis of the diaphragm
- Bladder problems
- Malignant diphtheria.

WHOOPING COUGH (PERTUSSIS)

Introduction

Whooping cough (pertussis) is an infection of the respiratory system caused by the bacterium *Bordetella pertussis* (*B. pertussis*). It is characterized by severe coughing spells, which can sometimes end in a 'whooping' sound when the person breathes in.

It mainly affects infants younger than 6 months old before they are adequately protected by immunizations, and kids 11 to 18 years old whose immunity has started to fade.

Definition

Whooping cough is defined as acute bacterial infections of the respiratory tract. It is a lethal disease manifested as an insidious onset of mild fever with irritating cough which gradually becomes paroxysmal with the characteristic inspiratory whoop.

Causes

The causative agent of whooping cough is *'Bordetella pertussis'*, a non-motile rod shaped gram-negative bacillus. Other microorganisms which may cause pertussis like mild illness are Bordetella parapertussis, Bordetella bronchiseptica, Haemophilus hemolyticus and adenovirus.

Pertussis, a respiratory illness commonly known as whooping cough, is a very contagious disease caused by a type of bacteria called *Bordetella pertussis*. These bacteria attach to the cilia (tiny, hair-like extensions) that line part of the upper respiratory system. The bacteria release toxins, which damage the cilia and cause inflammation (swelling).

Mode of Transmission

The mode of transmission is mainly droplet infection and direct contact. Pertussis is a very contagious disease only found in humans and is spread from person to person. Child with pertussis usually spread the disease by coughing or sneezing while in close contact with others, who breathe in the pertussis bacteria. Many infants who get pertussis are infected by older siblings.

Incubation Period

Whooping cough is highly infectious when the 'cold-like' symptoms occur in the early stages. Without treatment, a person is infectious for the first 3 weeks of coughing. With appropriate antibiotic therapy, the person is no longer infectious to others 5 days after starting antibiotics.

Incubation period of the disease is about 7 to 14 days but not more than 3 weeks.

Risk Factors

- The disease is more common in female children.
- Pertussis cases more common in winter and spring season.
- Overcrowding place
- Poor sanitation
- Low socioeconomic data.

Signs and Symptoms

Pertussis (whooping cough) can cause serious illness in infants, children and adults. The disease usually starts with cold-like symptoms and maybe a mild cough or fever. After 1 to 2 weeks, severe coughing can begin. Unlike the common cold, pertussis can become a series of coughing fits that continues for weeks.

In infants, the cough can be minimal or not even there. Infants may have a symptom known as 'apnea.' Apnea is a pause in the child's breathing pattern. Pertussis is most dangerous for babies. About half of infants younger than 1 year of age who get the disease are hospitalized. Learn more about pertussis complications.

- *Catarrhal stage:* Onset of the disease is usually insidious with symptoms of rhinitis, sneezing, Lacrimation, fever and irritating cough. Initially, cough is usually disturbing at night and later both in night and day time.
- *Paroxysmal or spasmodic stage:* In this stage there is rapid paroxysmal, explosive and repeated series of cough in expiration followed by a sudden deep violent inspiration with crowing sound or whoop. The whoop sound is produced due to rushing of air through half open glottis during inspiration. Sometime whoop may be present with or without cyanosis and apnea.
- *Convalescent stage:* During this stage severity of paroxyms decreases and the interval between paroxyms increases. Child general condition and appetite improve. Habit pattern of cough may persist for weeks or months. This stage may be prolonged due to pulmonary and other complications.

Early symptoms can last for 1 to 2 weeks:

- Runny nose
- Low-grade fever (generally minimal throughout the course of the disease)
- Mild, occasional cough
- Apnea-a pause in breathing (infants).

The traditional symptoms of pertussis appear and include:
- Paroxysms (fits) of many, rapid coughs followed by a high-pitched 'whoop'
- Vomiting (throwing up)
- Exhaustion (very tired) after coughing fits.

The coughing fits can go on for up to 10 weeks or more. In China, pertussis is known as the '100 day cough.'

Pathophysiology

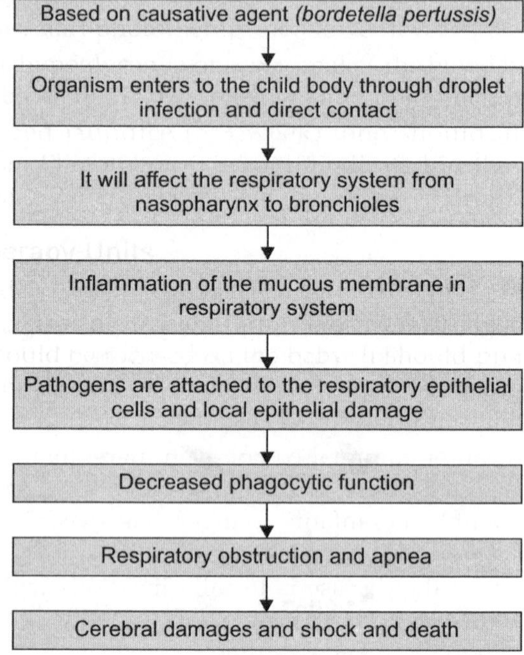

Fig. 5.23: Pathophysiology of *Bordetella pertussis*

Diagnostic Evaluation

Diagnosis is most accurately made by PCR (polymerase chain reaction) testing in a pathology laboratory of mucus from the nose and throat, combined with clinical history, although blood tests are still used in some places.
- History of typical signs and symptoms
- Physical examination
- Laboratory test which involves taking a sample of secretions (with a swab or syringe filled with saline) from the back of the throat through the nose
- Blood test
- ELISA test
- Chest X-ray helps to detect atelectasis or emphysema.

Management

The whooping cough is highly infectious when the 'cold-like' symptoms occur in the early stages. Without treatment, a person is infectious for the first 3 weeks of coughing. With appropriate antibiotic therapy, the person is no longer infectious to others 5 days after starting antibiotics.

- The child with severe illness required compulsory hospitalization and child need bed rest, antibiotic therapy, Symptomatic treatment and supportive care.
- Antibiotics should be started by early diagnosis in the catarrhal stage to prevent severity and spread of infection. The drug of choice is erythromycin 40 to 50 mg/kg/day in 4 divided doses for 2 weeks orally. Other antibiotics like roxythromycin, azithromycin and clarithromycin for 5 to 7 days also give good results.
- In case of severe paroxysmal cough, bronchodilator (Salbutamol, albuterol) should be administered by nebulization; otherwise 0.3 to 0.5 mg of Salbutamol per kg/day in three divided doses may be given.
- Betamethasone (0.75 mg/kg/day) may be useful in severe coughing paroxysms. Pertussis immunoglobin may be helpful in the first week of disease to reduce whoop.
- Complications of pertussis should be detected as early as possible and prompt specific management should be initiated.

Nursing Management

- The nurse should isolate the infected child from others.
- Provided supplementary oxygen administration to prevent hypoxia and cerebral anoxia.
- Do the frequent suctioning for removal of secretions.
- Provide comfortable positioning to relieve respiratory discomfort.
- Maintenance of fluid and electrolyte balance to prevent alkalosis and dehydration.
- Provide well-balanced diet by small frequent well-tolerated food, minimal gentle handling during care, avoidance of precipitating factors of cough, close and continuous observation and recording for complications and child's condition.
- Administration of prescribed medications on time.
- Psychological support to parents and child, hygienic measures, parental involvement in child care and related health teaching to the parents are important aspects of nursing care.

Prognosis

Prognosis depends upon age of child and presence of complications. Most of the deaths occur below the age of one year. Mortality rate is higher in malnourished children and with the presence of ARI. The associated complications obviously influence the immediate outcome and sequelae. The high morbidity and mortality is related to nature of complications.

Preventive Measures

Active immunization is the best measure for prevention of pertussis. DPT should be administered with 3 doses from 6 weeks of age at one month interval. A booster dose is given after one year of 3rd dose or at 16–24 months of age.

Pertussis vaccine should be given to a child with history of convulsion associated with progressive neurological manifestations. Encephalopathy may develop following pertussis vaccine.

Other preventive measures are isolation of infected case, disinfection of secretions and contaminated articles and chemoprophylaxis of contact cases.

Complications

Complications of pertussis include the following:

- *Respiratory complication:* Atelectasis, bronchopneumonia, bronchiectasis, emphysema, pneumothorax, pneumomediastinum, flaring up of pulmonary tuberculosis and hemoptysis.
- *Neurological complications:* Encephalopathy, intracranial hemorrhage, persistent seizures, blindness, deafness, mental subnormality, etc.
- *Miscellaneous:* Alkalosis due to persistent vomiting, epistaxis, subconjunctive hemorrhage, rectal prolapse, hernia (umbilical and inguinal), otitis media, frenularulcer, growth failure and malnutrition.

LEPROSY

Introduction

Leprosy condition was described above 3000 years ago and is still associated with stigma. The causative pathogen, *Mycobacterium leprae,* was first described in 1873, when Gerhard Armauer Henrik Hansen discovered it while examining lymph nodes and other tissues obtained from patients with leprosy. Although significant progress was made during the 20th century in the treatment and eradication of this disease, the World Health Organization (WHO) estimates that the worldwide prevalence is still in the area of 10–12 million cases.

Neuromuscular symptoms associated with this disease are occasionally the first to be observed. Patients may also present with a history of chronic nasal discharge, which is frequently observed in individuals with lepromatous leprosy who have upper airway compromise. The hallmark clinical findings in leprosy are hypopigmented skin lesions with loss of sensation. These lesions are observed more frequently in the cooler areas of the body, such as the nose and earlobes.

Definition

Leprosy is a chronic infectious disease caused by *Mycobacterium leprae*. It affects peripheral nerves, skin, muscles, eyes, bones, testes and internal organ.

Causes

Leprosy is a chronic granulomatous disease caused by infection with *M leprae*. The exact mechanism of *M leprae* transmission remains unknown; however, direct human-to-human contact, contact with respiratory secretions from infected individuals, and vertical transmission have been considered the most likely routes of transmission.

The major portal of exit is the discharge from nasal mucosa during sneezing or blowing. The bacilli can also exit through ulcerated or broken skin of positive cases or though hair follicles of infant skins. Among household contact of lepromatous cases, 4 to 12 percent is expected to show signs of leprosy within 5 years.

Risk Factors

Although the majority of cases of leprosy are sporadic, the greatest risk factor for leprosy is household contact with patients with untreated disease.

The relative risk of infection is 8 to 10 fold higher among household contacts of patients with lepromatous leprosy and 2 to 4 fold higher for contacts of patients with tuberculoid leprosy

- Animal reservoirs of leprosy include nine-banded armadillos (15% of which are thought be to infected in the wild in Louisiana and Texas), chimpanzees, and mangabey monkeys.
- Exposure to insect vectors and soil containing *M. leprae* also have been suggested as possible modes of transmission.

Incidence

The World Health Organization (WHO) reports that the current prevalence of leprosy is less than 1 case per 10,000 persons in all countries except for Brazil, Mozambique, Madagascar, Tanzania, and Nepal, where the prevalence exceeds 2 cases per 10,000 persons.

Modes of Transmission

The modes of transmission are mainly droplet infection and contact transmission. Contact transmission may occur between infectious child and healthy but susceptible person, by direct skin to skin contact or indirect contact with contaminated soil and fomites (contaminated cloths and linen). Bacilli may also be transmitted via breast milk from lepromatous mother or by insect vectors or by tattooing needles.

Incubation Period

Incubation period is 3 to 5 years or more for lepromatous cases. The tuberculosis leprosy is having shorter incubation period.

Classification

There are various classification of leprosy. The Indian classification includes five types. It is clinic-bacterial classification includes five types.

1. *Indeterminate type:* These types of leprosy with one or two vague hypopigmented macules and definite sensor impairment. These lesions are smear negative.
2. *Tuberculoid type:* These cases are manifested with one or two well defined lesions which may be flat or raised, hypopigmented, erythematous and are anesthetic. These lesions are also smear negative.
3. *Borderline type:* These cases are found with four or more lesions, which may be flat or raised, well or ill defined, hypopigmented, erythematous and with sensory impairment or loss. These lesions are bacteriological may or may not be positive. It can degenerate from borderline tuberculoid to borderline lepromatous, if left intreated.
4. *Lepromatous type:* These cases are presented with diffuse infiltration or numerous flat or raised, poorly defined, shiny, smooth, symmetrically distributed lesion. These lesions are smear positive.
5. *Pure neurotic type:* These cases are having nerve involvement without any skin lesion. These lesions are smear negative.

Clinical Manifestations

- Hypopigmented patches
- Partial or total loss of cutaneous sensation in the affected body parts
- Presence of thickened nerves and presence of leprosy bacilli in the nasal smear or skin.
- Presence of nodules or lumps in the skin of face or ears
- Planter ulcer, loss of fingers and toes, nasal depression, loss of eye brow, glove and stocking anesthesia of hands and feet, contracture of medial tow fingers from ulnar involvement, foot drop, claw toes and other deformities are found.
- High fever
- Arthralgia
- Adenopathy
- Orchitis.

Diagnostic Evaluation

- History collection
- Physical examination
- Bacteriological examination of skin smear, nasal smear or nasal blows or nasal scraping is important diagnostic approaches
- A biopsy from the edge of the skin or nasal lesion confirms the clinical diagnosis.
- Monoclonal antibody test
- ELISA test and radio immune essay.

Management

The drugs that are more frequently used in the treatment of leprosy include rifampin, dapsone, clofazimine, ofloxacin, minocycline, and clarithromycin. Multidrug therapy is required in all cases to prevent antimicrobial resistance. Prolonged therapeutic regimens have traditionally been recommended in the treatment of leprosy; however, recommendations by the World Health Organization (WHO) now focus on regimens with shorter duration both for tuberculoid (TT) or Panucibacillary (PB) leprosy and for lepromatous (LL) or Multibacillary (MB) leprosy.

The drugs that are more frequently used in the treatment of leprosy include rifampin, dapsone, clofazimine, ofloxacin, minocycline, and clarithromycin. Multidrug therapy is required in all cases to prevent antimicrobial resistance.

Antitubercular Agents

A multiple drugs to which *Mycobacterium tuberculosis* is susceptible. Guidelines for preventing the transmission of *M tuberculosis* are available. In addition, the therapy must be taken regularly and continued for a sufficient period.

Rifampin

Rifampin, also called rifampicin, inhibits RNA synthesis in bacteria by binding to the beta subunit of DNA-dependent RNA polymerase, which, in turn, blocks RNA transcription.

Dapsone

Dapsone is a competitive para-aminobenzoic acid (PABA) antagonist. It prevents formation of folic acid, causing bacterial growth inhibition.

Clofazimine

Clofazimine binds preferentially to mycobacterial DNA. It was discontinued from the US market in 2005 but is now available as an orphan product.

Antibiotics Therapy

The antimicrobial therapy must be comprehensive and should cover all likely pathogens in the context of the clinical setting. Antibiotics with efficacy against mycobacteria are used.

Ofloxacin

The Ofloxacin is a pyridine carboxylic acid derivative with broad-spectrum bactericidal effect.

Minocycline

Minocycline treats infections caused by susceptible gram-negative and gram-positive organisms, in addition to infections caused by susceptible Chlamydia, Rickettsia, and Mycoplasma species.

Clarithromycin

Clarithromycin inhibits bacterial growth, possibly by blocking dissociation of peptide RNA from ribosomes, causing RNA-dependent protein synthesis to arrest. Treatment with clarithromycin for 56 days has been demonstrated to be effective in eliminating more than 99.9% of M leprae present before treatment.

Prognosis

Childhood leprosy is self healing. Adequate treatment should be given to prevent complications and promote healing. Prognosis is usually good with prompt initiation of treatment by early diagnosis. The long-term complications are neural involvement, reactive episodes and deformities of face, hands and feet.

Preventive Measures

The nurse should isolate the infectious child, adequate treatment of affected individual by MDT, chemoprophylaxis of the contact person with dapsone, immunoprophylaxis by BCG vaccine and screening (individual or mass) of susceptible population (school children, household contacts) are important preventive measures.

Adequate treatment of infectious patient with MDT is most significant measure because it can turned the patient to noninfectious with dapsone therapy for 90 days or with rifampicin for 3 weeks. Local (nasal) application of rifampicin (drops or spray) may destroy all bacilli within 8 days.

HOSPITAL ACQUIRED INFECTIONS (NOSOCOMIAL INFECTIONS)

Introduction

Hospital-acquired infections are caused by viral, bacterial, and fungal pathogens; the most common types are bloodstream infection (BSI), pneumonia (e.g. ventilator-associated pneumonia [VAP]), urinary tract infection (UTI), and surgical site infection (SSI).

Hospital acquired infections (HAI) are those infections which in developed within the hospital or produced by cross infections from one patient to another, from doctors, nurses, visitors, attendants or other hospital staff during hospital stay.

Incidence

The incidence of central line-associated BSI and VAP declined significantly between 2007 and 2012 in critically ill pediatric client, according to a national cohort study of patients admitted to 173 neonatal intensive care units (NICUs) and 64 pediatric intensive care units (PICUs). No change was observed, however, in the rate of catheter-associated UTI.

In the NICUs, the rate of central line-associated BSI decreased from 4.9 to 1.5 per 1000 central-line days during the study period; in the PICUs, the rate fell from 4.7 to 1.0 per 1000 central-line days. The rate of VAP decreased from 1.6 to 0.6 per 1000 ventilator days in the NICUs and from 1.9 to 0.7 per 1000 ventilator days in the PICUs.

Causes of HAI in Children

- Hospital delivery without aseptic technique.
- Congenital or intrauterine infections from mothers.
- Intravenous procedures.
- Neonatal resuscitation, assisted ventilation and any respiratory procedures like suctioning, endotracheal intubation, etc.
- Nonjudicious use of broad spectrum antibiotics.
- Delayed initiation of oral feeding and arterial feeding.
- Surgical interventions and inappropriate wound management.
- Invasive procedures, care in PICU/NICU and use of unsterile articles.
- Inadequate isolation technique of infected patients and malpractice related to barrier nursing.
- Infections among hospital staff.
- Poor hospital environment laden with microorganisms, i.e. hospital dust, line, bed cloths, furniture, etc.

Risk Factors

The responsible factors of hospital acquired infections are immunocompromised children, long hospital stay, lack of handwashing practices, preterm or LBW baby, serious illness, corticosteroid therapy, use of indwelling catheter, care in ICU, etc.

Mode of Transmission

There are different routes of transmission of nosocomial. The common routes of spread of cross infection such as:

- *Contact spread:* There are two routes of contact transmission, i.e direct or indirect routes. Organisms may spread directly from contaminated hands of doctors and nurses to the susceptible host or from other patients by physical contact. Indirect contact may occur through feeding articles, syringe and needles, suction equipments, venous or arterial catheters, renal dialysers, contaminated linen, bed pans, sputum cups, etc.

- *Vehicle spread:* Contaminated inanimate vehicle serves as the vector for transmission of infectious agent to different individuals, e.g. contaminated food and water, blood and its products, IV fluids, etc.
- *Vector-borne spread:* Both external and internal vectors can spread infections. External vectors are flies which transmits diseases like Shigela and Salmonella. Internal vectors are mosquitoes which are responsible for biological transmission.
- *Air-borne spread:* Droplets released during coughing and sneezing by the infected persons and hospital dusts are important route of dissemination of infections from the source to the victim.

Signs and Symptoms

Risk factors for catheter-associated BSI in neonates include the following:

- Catheter hub or exit-site colonization
- Catheter insertion after the first week of life
- Duration of parenteral nutrition
- Extremely low birth weight (< 1000 g) at catheter insertion
- Disruption of catheter dressings
- Pediatric ICU: Neutropenia, prolonged catheter dwell time (> 7 days)
- Percutaneous placed central venous lines, frequent manipulation of lines.

Risk factors for neonates include the following:

- Gestational age of less than 32 weeks
- 5-minute Apgar scores below 5
- Shock, disseminated intravascular coagulation
- Prior intralipid use
- Parenteral nutrition, central venous line placement
- H2 blocker administration
- Intubation
- Hospital stay longer than 7 days.

Risk factors for VAP in pediatric patients include the following:

- Reintubation
- Genetic syndromes
- Immunodeficiency, immunosuppression
- Prior BSI.

Risk factors for hospital-acquired UTI in pediatric patients include the following:

- Bladder catheterization
- Prior antibiotic therapy
- Cerebral palsy.

Management

Treatments for nosocomial infections depend on the infection type. If the infection occurs at the site of a catheter or other inserted line, the line should be removed immediately. Antibiotics can combat symptoms of many infections. A healthy diet, fluid intake, and rest can encourage natural healing processes and prevent dehydration.

The Medical treatment includes symptomatic treatment of shock, hypoventilation, and other complications, along with empiric broad-spectrum antimicrobial therapy.

Management of BSI may include the following:

- Line removal as appropriate
- Antibiotic therapy covering gram-positive and gram-negative organisms, started empirically and then tailored according to specific susceptibility patterns
- Antifungal therapy as appropriate
- Antiviral therapy as appropriate
- Prevention through use of catheter disinfection caps.

Management of pneumonia includes the following:

- Initial empiric broad-spectrum antibiotic therapy, later streamlined on the basis of identified organisms and susceptibilities, with attention to the risk of multidrug-resistant (MDR) pathogens
- Antiviral medications against influenza for symptomatic patients and patients with immunodeficiency or chronic lung diseases to limit morbidity and mortality.

Management of UTI includes the following:

- Removal of indwelling catheters if possible
- Empiric antibiotic and antifungal therapy.

Management of SSI includes the following:

- Surgical debridement
- Antibiotic therapy.

Prevention and Control Measure of HAI

The Healthcare Infection Control Practices Advisory Committee (HICPAC) has developed a guideline for isolation precautions to prevent transmission of infectious agents in healthcare settings.

Standard precautions are to be applied to the care of all patients in all healthcare settings regardless of the suspected or confirmed presence of an infectious agent. This is the primary strategy in preventing transmission of infectious agents among patients and healthcare personnel.

Role of the Staff Nurse

Implementation of patient care practices for infection control is the role of the nursing staff. Nurses should be familiar with practices to prevent the occurrence and spread of infection, and maintain appropriate practices for all patients throughout the duration of their hospital stay.

The senior nursing administrator is responsible for:

- Participating in the Infection Control Committee
- Promoting the development and improvement of nursing techniques, and ongoing review of aseptic nursing policies, with approval by the Infection Control Committee
- Developing training programs for members of the nursing staff
- Supervising the implementation of techniques for the prevention of infections in specialized areas such as the operating suite, the intensive care unit, the maternity unit and newborns
- Monitoring of nursing adherence to policies.

The nurse in charge of a ward is responsible for:

- Maintaining hygiene, consistent with hospital policies and good nursing practice on the ward
- Monitoring aseptic techniques, including handwashing and use of isolation
- Reporting promptly to the attending physician any evidence of infection in patients under the nurse's care
- Initiating patient isolation and ordering culture specimens from any patient showing signs of a communicable disease, when the physician is not immediately available
- Limiting patient exposure to infections from visitors, hospital staff, other patients, or equipment used for diagnosis or treatment
- Maintaining a safe and adequate supply of ward equipment, drugs and patient care supplies.

The nurse in charge of infection control is a member of the infection control team and responsible for:

- Identifying nosocomial infections
- Investigation of the type of infection and infecting organism
- Participating in training of personnel
- Surveillance of hospital infections
- Participating in outbreak investigation
- Development of infection control policy and review and approval of patient care policies relevant to infection control
- Ensuring compliance with local and national regulations
- Liaison with public health and with other facilities where appropriate
- Providing expert consultative advice to staff health and other appropriate hospital programs in matters relating to transmission of infections.

HAEMOPHILUS INFLUENZAE (TYPE-B)

Introduction

Haemophilus influenzae is gram-negative coccobacillus. Some strains of *H. influenzae* possess a polysaccharide capsule, and these strains are serotype into 6 different types (a-f) based on their biochemically different capsules. The most virulent strain is *H. influenzae* type b (Hib). Some *H. influenzae* strains have no capsule and are termed nonencapsulated *H. influenzae* or non type able *H. influenzae* (NTHi).

Haemophilus influenzae type B (Hib) vaccine is given to children under 5 years old to protect them against certain serious infections, such as meningitis and pneumonia. *Haemophilus influenzae* type B vaccine causes the body to make antibodies against a certain bacteria or germ called *Haemophilus influenzae* type B.

Definition

Haemophilus influenzae is a nonmotile gram-negative rod-shaped bacterium. *H. influenzae* can cause serious invasive disease especially in young children. Invasive disease is usually caused by encapsulated strains of the organism.

Incidence and Causes

- The most virulent strain is *H. influenzae* type B (Hib), which accounts for more than 95% of *H. influenzae* infections in children and half of infections in adults.
- Hib may cause bacteremia, meningitis, cellulitis, epiglottitis, septic arthritis, pneumonia, pleural or gallbladder empyema, endophthalmitis, urinary tract infection, abscesses, cervical adenitis, glossitis, osteomyelitis and endocarditis.
- Nonencapsulated and non-type able *H. influenzae* strains cause mucosal infections, including:
  - Exacerbations of chronic bronchitis
  - Otitis media
  - Conjunctivitis
  - Sinusitis
  - Bronchitis
  - Pneumonia.

Risk Factors/Mode of Transmission

- Hib bacteria are carried in the nose and throat without showing any signs of infection.
- Hib is spread through coughing, sneezing or close contact with an infected person.
- Hib infections are uncommon in patients older than 6 years. However, the frequency of Hib infections is increased in patients with, spleenectomy, sickle cell disease, malignancies and congenital or acquired immunodeficiency.

Signs and Symptoms

The symptoms of Hib-B depend on the specific disease based on causes.

Meningitis

It is an inflammation and swelling of the tissues that cover the brain and spinal cord. Until a vaccine became available, it occurs most often in children between the ages of 6 months and 5 years. Symptoms include a fever, a decrease in appetite, an increase in crying or irritability, seizures, excessive sleepiness, and vomiting. In children older than 2 years, there may be additional symptoms such as a headache, a stiff neck, and back pain.

Epiglottitis

This condition is rare but serious inflammation in the throat, affecting the epiglottis (a flap of tissue at the back of the throat) and occurring most often in children 2 to 4 years of age. The child's first symptoms will probably be a severe sore throat and fever (typically a temperature greater than 101 °F [38.3 °C]), followed by a raspy or harsh sound called stridor during breathing. As the epiglottis becomes swollen, it can make swallowing difficult, trigger drooling, and may block normal breathing. Some children with Epiglottitis have choked to death.

Other Hib Infections

This bacterial infection will affect the different area of the body

- *Joints:* Arthritis
- *Bones:* Osteomyelitis

- *Skin of the face:* Cheek or around the eye
- *Lungs:* Pneumonia
- *Heart:* Pericarditis
- Signs of infections in these areas include fever, swelling, pain, and redness along with a drastic decrease in energy and activity.

Diagnostic Evaluation

- History collection
- Physical examination
- Gram stain: Small, gram-negative, pleomorphic coccobacilli with polymorphonuclear cells.
- Bacterial or other relevant body fluid cultures.
- Slide agglutination with type-specific antisera is used for serotyping *H. influenzae*.
- Cerebrospinal fluid (CSF) features in meningitis: Pleocytosis with a predominance of neutrophils, decreased CSF glucose levels, increased CSF protein, detectable capsular antigen in 90% and a positive CSF Gram stain result in 80%.
- CT scan: May be required, particularly to identify a possible subdural effusion, in patients with meningitis, to exclude raised intracranial pressure, if there are focal neurological findings or failure of expected improvement with appropriate antibiotics.
- Chest X-ray: Hib pneumonia tends to cause more pleural and pericardial involvement compared with other bacterial pneumonias. Community-acquired pneumonias due to non-typeable *H. influenzae* are characterized by alveolar infiltrates in patchy or lobar distributions.
- Other investigations will depend on the site of infection, e.g. echocardiogram if pericarditis is suspected, joint aspiration for septic arthritis.

Management

Management includes treating all aspects of the infection, including fever, dehydration and any other specific interventions such as oxygen therapy in respiratory tract infections. Serious *H. influenzae* type b (Hib) infections are best treated with an intravenous third-generation cephalosporin until antibiotic sensitivities become available. In Malawi, Africa, intramuscular ceftriaxone was compared with intravenous ceftriaxone and was not found to increase the mortality rate. This may be important in developing countries where the intravenous route may not be possible.

Antibiotics and Supportive Care

- Azithromycin
- Cefotaxime (Third-generation cephalosporin with gram-negative spectrum)
- Chloramphenicol
- Erythromycin
- Meropenem.

Prognosis

The prognosis of meningitis depends on age at presentation, duration of illness prior to antimicrobial therapy, CSF capsular polysaccharide concentration, and the rapidity with which it is cleared from the CSF, blood, and urine. Dexamethasone administered concurrently or shortly before the initial administration of antibiotics decreases the likelihood of hearing loss associated with Hib meningitis.

Complications

The most common complications is meningitis include seizures, cerebral edema, subdural effusion or empyema, inappropriate secretion of antidiuretic hormone syndrome, cortical infarction, cerebritis, intracerebral abscess, hydrocephalus, and cerebral herniation. Protracted fever is not uncommon, with approximately 10% of children remaining febrile for at least 10 days.

- Complications of orbital cellulitis include subperiosteal or orbital abscesses.
- Complications of pneumonia include empyema and pericarditis.
- Complications of otitis and sinusitis include mastoiditis and parameningeal abscess.

MENINGOCOCCAL INFECTION

Definition

Meningococcal infection is caused by bacteria (germ) called meningococcus, and can cause serious infections including:

- *Meningitis:* An infection of the covering of the brain and spinal cord.
- *Septicemia:* A serious infection of the blood.
- Infections in other parts of the body, such as in the joints.

Meningococcal meningitis can be fatal or cause great harm without prompt treatment; as many as one out of five people who contract the infection have serious complications. According to the Centers for Disease Control, about 15% of those who survive are left with disabilities that include deafness, brain damage, and neurological problems.

HELICOBACTER PYLORI INFECTION

Introduction

The *Helicobacter pylori* (Hp) is a gram-negative bacillus responsible for one of the most common infections found in humans worldwide. Warren and Marshall first cultured and

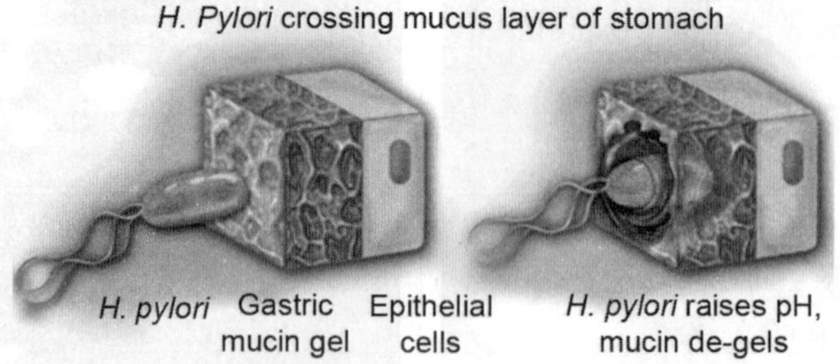

Fig. 5.24: Structure of *H. pylori*

identified the organism as *Campylobacter pylori* in 1982. By 1989, it was renamed and recognized to be associated closely with antral gastritis (gastric and duodenal ulcers in adults and children). In recognition of this crucial discovery, they were awarded the Nobel Prize for medicine in 2005. By the early-to-mid 1990s, further evidence supported a link between chronic gastritis of *H. pylori* infection in adults and malignancy, specifically gastric lymphoma and adenocarcinoma.

Definition

Helicobacter pylori is a bacterial infection of the stomach that is usually acquired in the early years of life. Its transmission is related to living conditions, particularly crowding. The clinical implications of *H. pylori* infection in children are unclear; although *H. pylori* is classed as a grade I carcinogen in adults.

Incidence

These bacteria are found worldwide, but especially in developing countries, where up to 10% of children and 80% of adults can have laboratory evidence of an *H. pylori* infection usually without having symptoms.

Signs and Symptoms

The mostly *H. pylori* infections are 'silent' and produce no symptoms. When the bacteria do cause symptoms, they are usually either symptoms of gastritis or peptic ulcer disease.

In child, symptoms of gastritis may include nausea, vomiting, and frequent complaints about pain in the abdomen. *H. pylori,* which used to be called *Campylobacter pylori,* can also cause peptic ulcers (commonly known as stomach ulcers). In older children and adults, the most common symptom of peptic ulcer disease is a gnawing or burning pain in the abdomen, this pain often gets worse on an empty stomach and improves as soon as the person eats food, drinks milk, or takes antacid medicine.

Diagnostic Evaluation

- History collection
- Physical examination
- USG
- Endoscope
- Blood tests
- Stool tests
- CT scan.

Management

Antibiotics therapy

- Amoxicillin
- Clarithromycin
- Omeprazole
- Esomeprazole.

CONGENITAL SYPHILIS

Definition

Congenital syphilis is an infectious disease caused by *Treponema pallidum,* which belongs to the Spirochaetaceae family. The genus name, *Treponema,* is derived from the Greek term for 'turning thread.' Pathogenic members of this genus include *T. pallidum, T. pertenue,* and *T. carateum.*

Signs and Symptoms

- Failure to gain weight or failure to thrive
- Fever
- Irritability
- No bridge to nose (saddle nose)
- Rash of the mouth, genitals, and anus
- *Rash:* Starting as small blisters on the palms and soles, and later changing to copper-colored, flat or bumpy rash on the face, palms, and soles
- Watery fluid released from the nose.

Symptoms in older infants and young children may include:

- Abnormal notched and peg-shaped teeth, called Hutchinson teeth
- Bone pain
- Blindness
- Clouding of the cornea
- Decreased hearing or deafness
- Gray, mucus-like patches on the anus and outer vagina
- Joint swelling
- Refusal to move a painful arm or leg
  - Saber shins (bone problem of the lower leg)
  - Scarring of the skin around the mouth, genitals, and anus.

Diagnostic Evaluation

The placenta will be examined for signs of syphilis. A physical examination of the infant may show signs of liver and spleen swelling and bone inflammation.

A routine blood test for syphilis is done during pregnancy. The mother may receive the following blood tests:

- Fluorescent treponemal antibody absorbed test (FTA-ABS)
- Rapid plasma reagin (RPR)
- Venereal disease research laboratory test (VDRL)

An infant or child may have the following tests:

- Bone X-ray
- Dark-field examination to detect syphilis bacteria under a microscope
- Eye examination
- Lumbar puncture.

Management

The management of congenital syphilis includes administration of IV penicillin G aqueous and IM penicillin G procaine for 10–14 days. Either penicillin regimen is considered adequate to manage congenital syphilis.

Complications

- Blindness
- Deafness
- Deformity of the face
- Nervous system problems.

COMMON PARASITOSIS IN CHILDREN

A parasite is an organism, or small animal, that lives in or on and takes its nourishment from another organism. A parasite cannot live by itself. Parasites include fleas, lice, and worms. A parasitic disease includes:

- Protozoa (single-cell organisms such as malaria)
- Helminthes (worms)
- Arthropods (such as scabies).

Types of common parasitosis infection:

- Malaria
- Filaria
- Kala-azar
- Hydatid disease
- Giardiasis
- Amebiasis
- Worm infestations
- Cryptosporidiosis.

MALARIA

Introduction

Malaria is a common mosquito-borne disease in India. It is characterized by fever, chills and sweating. Malaria can be a serious illness in children, especially those under five years old children.

Definition

Malaria is defined as an infectious diseases caused by parasites. It is passed from person to person by mosquitoes. The infection leads to chills, fever, and other flu-like symptoms. If left untreated, malaria can be deadly. Children are most at risk for malaria.

Malaria is defined as a protozoal disease caused by arthropod borne infection with malarial parasite (plasmodium), which is transmitted by infected female anaphylactic mosquito.

Causes

Malaria is caused by *Plasmodium* species, which are protozoal blood parasites. The following four species can infect humans:

1. *Plasmodium vivax*
2. *Plasmodium falciparum*
3. *Plasmodium malariae*
4. *Plasmodium ovale*.

Incidence

Children under five years of age are one of most vulnerable groups affected by malaria. There were an estimated 660 000 malaria deaths around the world in 2010, of which approximately 86% were in children under five years of age.

Malaria occurs all year round, but the number of cases more in during monsoon season.

Malaria is widespread in India and most common in Maharashtra, Gujarat, Rajasthan and Karnataka. The hilly regions of the north and the north-eastern part of the country have fewer cases.

Mode of Transmission

Mode of transmission is mainly vector transmission by female anaphylactic mosquito. Direct transmission may occur accidentally by hypodermic, IM or IV injection or blood transfusion. Anyone having malaria should not be accepted as blood donor until three years afterwards. Congenital malaria rarely may occur to the newborn from an infected mother.

Incubation Period

Incubation period varies depending upon the types of parasite.

- *Plasmodium vivax:* 14 days (8–17 days)
- *Plasmodium falciparum:* 12 days (9–147)
- *Plasmodium malariae:* 28 days (18–4 days)
- *Plasmodium ovale:* 17 days (16–18 days).

Signs and Symptoms

Symptoms of less than five years children:

- Hyperthermia (fever)
- Shivering
- Cold
- Anorexia
- Vomiting
- Sleeplessness
- Stomach pain
- Hypothermia (instead of a fever)
- Tachyponea.

Symptoms of more than five years children's:

- They are similar to flu-like symptoms
- A high fever, sometimes in 48-hour cycles of shivering and then extreme sweating

- Headaches
- Chills
- Nausea and vomiting
- General body pain
- Loss of appetite.

Diagnostic Evaluation

- History collection
- Physical examination
- Laboratory investigations include
  - Peripheral blood smears examination (thick and thin film) to detect presence of malarial parasite and its type
  - Routine blood examination for Hb% (usually low), WBC count (shows leucopenia) bilirubin and gammoglobin level (both raised)
  - Fluorescent antibody technique to detect species specific antibody (IgG)
  - Bone marrow examination.

Management

The malarial infected children should treat with antipyretics and adequate fluid therapy, orally or with IV fluid. Anticonvulsive drugs and steroids may be needed. Blood transfusion may be required in severe anemia. Other complication should be detect and to be managed accordingly.

Malaria can be severe in pregnancy. This is a major problem because many antimalarial drugs are considered unsafe during pregnancy.

Indications for immediate hospitalization include the following:

- Intractable vomiting
- Dehydration
- Seizures
- Impaired consciousness or coma
- Repeated convulsions
- Difficulty in breathing
- Severe pallor (indicating severe anemia)
- Hypoglycemia (blood glucose < 2.5 mmol/L, or 3 mmol/L in malnourished children)
- Oliguria or anuria
- Shock
- Hyperparasitemia
- Bleeding diathesis.

Antimalarial Drug Therapy

Blood schizonticides are the first-line drugs for the treatment of malaria.

Chloroquine

This drug is effective against the erythrocytic forms of the parasite and is the drug of choice for P vivax, P malariae, and P ovale malaria, against which it is gametocidal as well. It is not effective against hypnozoites.

It is very effective against sensitive strains of P falciparum. However, P falciparum resistance to Chloroquine is now widespread in Africa and Asia, and it should not be depended on in severe malaria. Resistance to this drug in P vivax has also been reported, but resistance is currently rare.

Chloroquine can be used as a suppressive prophylactic agent, with the advantage of once-weekly dosing. It is available as tablets that contain 300 mg of the base and injections that contain 40 mg base/mL.

Quinine

Quinine is a blood schizonticidal drug and is still the drug of choice for severe and complicated malaria in most parts of the world. It is gametocidal for P vivax and P malariae but not for P falciparum. It is available as tablets containing 260 mg and as injections containing 300 mg/mL. Spreading resistance among P falciparum strains to this drug make quinine less reliable in certain parts of Asia and Africa.

Quinidine

A stereoisomer of quinine and a blood schizonticides drug, quinidine is as effective as quinine against blood schizonts but has significantly more cardiac toxicity. This agent is used if quinine is not readily available. It is available as tablets of quinidine sulfate containing 200 mg. The injectable preparation is not always available.

Primaquine

Primaquine is the only drug in clinical use that destroys hypnozoites of P vivax and P ovale and so is used for the radical cure of the relapsing malarias. It is also gametocidal against all four species of human plasmodia and is used to render patients noninfectious. Primaquine has a very weak effect against erythrocytic forms of P vivax and cannot be used to terminate an acute attack.

It has no activity against erythrocytic forms of P falciparum. This drug can be administered to patients on chemoprophylaxis after they have left the endemic area. It is not to be used until erythrocytic forms have been destroyed by another drug.

Primaquine is an effective and fairly safe drug for chemoprophylaxis. Since it acts on the liver forms, it need not be taken before entering a malarious area or for more than 3 days after leaving it. This is an advantage for people making sudden or short trips.

Mefloquine

Mefloquine is useful for the treatment of multidrug-resistant P falciparum infections. It is effective against blood schizonts but has no activity against hypnozoites and gametocytes. Its long half-life makes it suitable for use as a prophylactic drug, and it is the recommended drug in areas where drug resistance is common (chiefly Africa and Asia). Not having a parenteral preparation limits mefloquine's usefulness for severe and complicated malaria.

Mefloquine may cause adverse neuropsychiatric reactions, which may be difficult to identify in children; monitor for symptoms, especially in nonverbal children. The drug is available as tablets containing 250 mg.

Tetracycline

Tetracycline is an antibiotic with action against blood schizonts of all species of malaria. Its action is slow and it is used in combination with another drug, such as quinine, in areas where resistant P falciparum is common. It is available as capsules containing 250 mg and 500 mg.

Clindamycin (Cleocin)

This is an antibiotic that acts against *P. falciparum*. Clindamycin has been found to be very effective in combination with quinine, even against malaria acquired in areas where drug resistance is common. Used in combination, it shortens the duration of fever and improves cure rates. This is an important drug for use in children, because tetracyclines are contraindicated. It is available as capsules containing 75 mg, 150 mg, and 300 mg and as granules that, after reconstitution with water, contain 75 mg/5 mL.

Complications

Severe complications include:

- Severe anemia
- Seizure
- Shock
- Kidney failure
- Brain damage
- Coma.

Nursing Management

- Provide adequate bed rest, skin care
- Provide tepid sponge to reduce the fever
- Encourage the child to drink more amount of fluid
- Provide the well balanced diet and hygienic measures
- Psychological support and involvement of the parent with necessary instructions are important aspect of care.

Prognosis

Prognosis is generally good with early diagnosis and prompt treatment. With the presence of complications, outcome may vary. Malnutrition and other associated problems may also be found.

Preventive Measures

Malaria is a potentially fatal illness. People planning to travel to an area with malaria should see their physician before travel, preferably at least six weeks before departure. Travelers should use mosquito precautions and take medications to reduce the risk of disease.

Mosquito precautions include wearing light, protective clothing and using window screens and bed nets when available. The mosquito that spreads malaria is active between dusk and dawn. Insect repellants should be used and should contain DEET. Room sprays may be used to reduce the mosquito population in sleeping areas.

Several medications are available to prevent malaria. The choice of medication used for prophylaxis depends on the area of the world that is being visited and the drug-resistance pattern in that area. In general, the medications are started before travel, taken while in the malarias area, and continued for a period of time after leaving the area.

Other ways to protect against malaria:

- Use mosquito net
- Use insect repellents
- Wear protective clothing like long sleeves and pants
- Stay indoors from dusk to dawn
- Use air conditioners where available, instead of opening windows
- Control the mosquito breeding place.

LYMPHATIC FILARIASIS

Introduction

Lymphatic filariasis, a common parasitic infection in tropical countries, causes lymphedema of limbs, hydrocele and acute attacks of dermato-lymphangio-adenitis. In lymphatic filariasis, repeated episodes of inflammation and lymphedema lead to lymphatic damage, chronic swelling, and elephantiasis of the legs.

Lymphatic filariasis is a global problem. It is major public health problem in India. The problem increased every year due to gross mismanagement of the environment. The disease is endemic all over India both in urban and rural areas.

Definition

Lymphatic filariasis is commonly known as elephantiasis, is a neglected tropical disease. Infection occurs when filarial parasites are transmitted to humans through mosquitoes. Infection is usually acquired in childhood causing hidden damage to the lymphatic system.

Causes

The mosquitoes of the genera *Aedes, Anopheles, Culex*, or *Mansonia* are the intermediate hosts and vectors of all species that cause lymphatic filariasis.

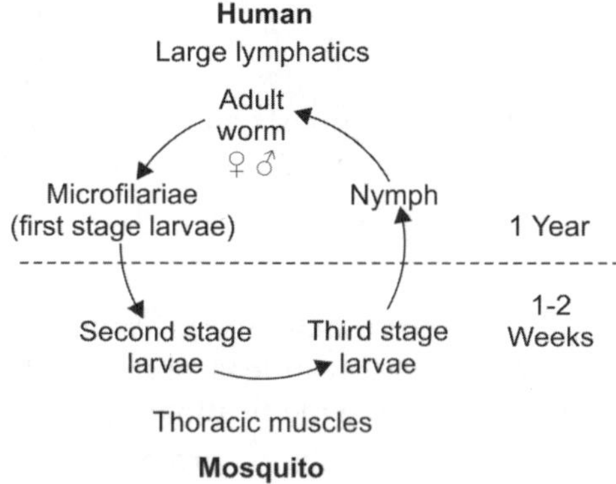

Fig. 5.25: Life cycle of *Wuchereria bancrofti*

Elephantiasis occurs in the presence of microscopic, thread-like parasitic worms such as *Wuchereria bancrofti*. Infections usually begin when people are children. Three types of worms cause the disease and damage the lymphatic system:

- *Wuchereria bancrofti*
- *Brugia malayi*
- *Brugia timori*

All the types are transmitted by infected mosquitoes

Poor drainage system promotes profuse vector breeding in polluted water. Inadequate sewage disposal and lack of town planning also facilitates the breeding of the vector mosquitoes. The common breeding places are soakage pits, poorly maintained drains, septic tanks, open ditches, burrow pits and cesspools.

Incidence

Lymphatic filariasis is caused by infection with nematodes of the family Filarioidea: 90% of infections are caused by *Wuchereria bancrofti* and most of the remainder by *Brugia malayi*.

Mode of Transmission

It is transmitted by mosquitoes. When a mosquito with infective stage larvae takes a blood meal, the parasites are deposited on the person's skin, from where they enter the body through the skin. These larvae then migrate to the lymphatic vessels and develop into adult worms over a period of 6–12 months, causing damage to and dilatation of the lymphatic vessels.

Signs and Symptoms

Lymphatic filariasis infection involves asymptomatic, acute, and chronic conditions. The majority of infections are asymptomatic, showing no external signs of infection. These asymptomatic infections still cause damage to the lymphatic system and the kidneys as well as alter the body's immune system.

Lymphatic filariasis can be described in four stages:

1. Asymptomatic microfilaremia
2. Asymptomatic amicrofilaremia
3. Acute stage of manifestation
4. Chronic obstructive lesions.

Asymptomatic Microfilaremia

In this condition child with microfilaremia are generally asymptomatic, although those with heavy microfilarial loads may develop acute and chronic inflammatory granulomas secondary to splenic destruction; passage of cloudy, milk like urine may denote chyluria.

Asymptomatic Amicrofilaremia

In this stage an important source of infection in the community. These carriers are usually detected by night blood examination and their blood is positive for amicrofilaremia.

Acute Stage

In this stage child had a filarial fever, delirium, lymphangitis, lymphadenitis, lymphedema of the various parts of the body and epididymoorchitis in male. There is acute inflammation of lymph glands and vessels. This episode can recur frequently even 10 times a year and subsides spontaneously over 7 to 10 days in each episode.

Chronic Stage

This stage usually develops 10–15 from the onset of first acute attack. Fibrosis and obstruction of lymph vessels lead to permanent structural damage and manifested as elephantiasis, hydrocele, chyluria and lymphedema.

In chronic Bancroftian filariasis, elephantiasis may affect the legs, scrotum, arms, penis, vulva and breasts. The prevalence of chyluria is usually very low.

Diagnostic Evaluation

- History collection
- Physical assessment
- Blood test
- Urine test
- Chest X-ray.

Management

The medical management of a filarial infection should be specific and based on the microfilariae isolated or antigenemia detected.

Mass drug administration reduces the transmission of filarial infection and disease morbidity by decreasing the burden of microfilaremia, resulting in suboptimal levels for transmission by disease vectors.

Anthelmintics Drugs

- Mebendazole
- Albendazole is a broad-spectrum anthelmintic.

Antibiotic Therapy

Doxycycline is a broad-spectrum, synthetically derived, bacteriostatic antibiotic in the tetracycline class. This agent is almost completely absorbed, concentrates in bile, and is excreted in urine and feces as a biologically active metabolite in high concentrations.

Prognosis

Prognosis of filarial depends upon phase of disease during initiation of treatment, available treatment facilities and presence of complications.

Preventive Measures

Prevention includes giving entire communities medicine that kills the microscopic worms and controlling mosquitoes. Avoiding mosquito bites is another form of prevention. The mosquitoes that carry the microscopic worms usually bite between the hours of dusk and dawn. If you live in an area with lymphatic filariasis.

Prevention of filariasis can be best done by mosquito control through antilarval measures, environmental management, sewage disposal, use of mosquito nets and increasing community awareness about mosquito control measures.

Mass treatment with DEC in endemic area with annual single dose or use of DEC medicated salt as a special from of mass treatment can be used for filarial control. Common salt medicated with 1 to 4 gm of DEC per kg is used. Diagnosis of clinical cases of filarial and appropriate treatment to reduce the morbidity is also an important control measures along with reduction of transmission and interruption of transmission cycle.

KALA-AZAR (VISCERAL LEISHMANIASIS)

Introduction

Kala-Azar or visceral leishmaniasis is a group of protozoal diseases caused by *Leishmania donovani* transmitted to man by the bite of female phlebotomine sandfly.

The most important form found in Indian population is kala-azar or visceral leishmaniasis. It is a chronic infection of the reticulendothelial system characterized by irregular fever of long duration, hepatosplenomegaly, malnutrition, anemia and progressive emaciation. It is also termed as black sickness due to characteristic grey pigmentation of skin, seen in some patient.

Definition

Visceral leishmaniasis, also known as kala-azar, is characterized by irregular bouts of fever, substantial weight loss, swelling of the spleen and liver, and anemia.

Causes

Leishmaniasis is a disease caused by protozoan parasites of the *Leishmania* genus. The parasite migrates to the internal organs such as liver, spleen (hence 'visceral'), and bone marrow, and, if left untreated, will almost always result in the death of the host. Signs and symptoms include fever, weight loss, fatigue, anemia, and substantial swelling of the liver and spleen.

Incidence

The causative agent of kala-azar is *L. donovani,* a intracellular parasite. There are at least 19 different *Leishmania* parasites which cause human infections. The life cycle of the parasite is completed in two different host, a vertebrate (human) and an inset (sandfly). In human, it occurs in an amastigote form called 'Leishmania bodies' (LD) and in insect as flagellated promastigote. The parasite lives in the reticulendothelial system of human host.

Indian kala-azar is considered as a non-zoonotic infection with man as a sole reservoir. There is a variety of animal reservoirs, e.g. dogs, jackals, foxes, rodents and other mammals.

Mode of Transmission

The mode of transmission of kala-azar is from person to person by the bite of female phlebotomine sandfly, P. argentipes, which is a highly anthropophilic species. Transmission of kala-azar also may occur by blood transfusion or contamination of bite wound or by contact when the insect is crushed during the act of feeding. Cutaneous leishmaniasis is transmitted by P. papatasi and P. sengenti.

The Incubation Period

The incubation period in man is ranging from 10 days to 2 years with an average of 1 to 6 months. Kala-azar can occur in all age groups including infants. The peak age is 5 to 9 years. Males are affected twice than female.

Signs and Symptoms

The clinical manifestations of childhood VL are more or less same as in the adults. Prolonged fever with anorexia and loss of appetite are the major presenting features. Marked enlargement of the spleen and liver (spleen larger than liver) with moderate to severe anemia, pancytopenia and hair changes occur.

Cough and hemoptysis may be due to co-infection of pulmonary tuberculosis. Bacterial infection (pneumonia, septicemia, otitis media, urinary tract infections and skin infections) is a common complication. Bacterial super infection is one of the major complications leading to death in children with VL. Parasitic infestations of the gut are very common in pediatric VL patients.

Organism entering in the human host the parasite carried by the blood circulation to distant organ like liver, spleen, bone marrow and causes marked hyperplasia of reticulendothelial cells which produces clinical features.

The disease is characterized by gradual or insidious onset of intermittent or irregular prolonged low grade fever, which may have double rise in a day.

The child may have

- Headache
- Vomiting
- Malaise
- Toxic features
- Acute enlargement of spleen, bone marrow.

In infant, the disease is manifested as acute onset with high fever, rigors and vomiting. It is often severe and fatal.

Complications

The common complications of kala-azar are pneumonia, dysentery, cancrum oris (gangrenous stomatitis), gingivitis, sever hemorrhage (epistaxis, gum bleeding), agranulocytosis and malnutrition.

- Secondary bacterial infection, including pneumonia and tuberculosis
- Septicemia
- Disfigurement of nose, lips, and palate (e.g. cancrum oris)
- Uncontrolled bleeding
- Splenic rupture
- Late stages: Edema, cachexia, and hyperpigmentation
- Metastatic lesions in the nasopharynx with tissue destruction.

Diagnostic Evaluation

A presumptive provisional clinical diagnosis is made on the basis of presenting clinical features and history of living in an area endemic for VL.

Routine blood examination reveals leucopenia, moderate to severe anemia and thrombocytopenia. Urine examination may reveal mild proteinuria. Stool examination may reveal presence of ova, cyst or different intestinal protozoa or helminths.

Liver function tests may show hypoalbuminemia, normal or mild hyperbilirubinemia with or without raised liver enzymes like serum glutamate oxaloacetate transaminase (SGOT), serum glutamate pyruvate transaminase (SGPT) and alkaline phosphatase. Serum urea and creatinine levels are usually normal.

Clinical features are important clue for diagnosis of kala azar. The conformity tests are blood and bone marrow examination for presence of LD bodies, or demonstration of parasite LD bodies in the aspirates of the spleen, liver, bone marrow, lymph nodes or the skin (in case of CL).

Management

Sodium antimony gluconate (stibogluconate) has been the drug of choice for over past 50 years. Initially the dosage was 10 mg/kg per day deep IM for 7 days. With the appearance of significant unresponsiveness to the drug, the currently recommended dosage is 20 mg/kg body weight per day for 30 days.

Pentamidine isothionate, though effective is relatively toxic. The dosage is 3 mg/kg body weight per day given slowly intravenous on alternate days for 5 doses.

Pentamidine isothionate, though effective is relatively toxic. The dosage is 3 mg/kg body weight per day given slowly intravenous on alternate days for 5 doses.

Paramomycin 15 mg/kg body weight per day for 21 days has recently been found to be highly effective for the treatment of VL in adults and has to be administered by the intramuscular route. The efficacy of the drug in children is yet to be demonstrated.

Prognosis

With adequate treatment 90% cases can be cured. Untreated cases may have fatal outcome in 2 years. Some cases are said to have spontaneous cure (about 13 to 20%). Emergence of drug resistance (both primary and secondary) may be related to delay in diagnosis and inadequate treatment. Relapse and complications are common.

Preventive Measures

Primary prevention of kala azar can be done by control of source of infection and vector sandlfy eradication. Early detection and treatment of all cases should be done internsively. The reservoir of infection (e.g. patients of post kala azar dermal leishmaniasis) should be treated with repeated course of drug therapy.

Vector (sandfly) plays an important role in disease transmission. High incidence of VL is reported during premonsoon season that coincides with vector abundance and increased man-vector contact due to sleeping habits of children in open space in summer. The vectors are found in abundance in peridomestic vegetations around the households during the period, which are usually not covered by insecticide spray operation. Resistance to DDT by the vectors is also a matter of concern.

Sanitarily measures for elimination of breeding places (i.e. cracks of mud or stone walls, rodent burrows, removal of firewood, bricks or rubbish around houses), location of cattle sheds and poultry at a fair distance from human dwellings and improvement of housing and general sanitation are important. Dog and rodent control are also useful to prevent animal reservoir.

Advice the parents do not allow the child sleeping on floor. Using fine mesh bed nets and insect repellents also very helpful. Health education should be given to provide information about preventive measures. There are no drugs for personal prophylaxis.

GIARDIASIS

Introduction

Giardiasis is an infective diseases that affects the digestive tract (stomach and intestines), is caused by a microscopic parasite called *Giardia lamblia*. The parasite attaches in the lining of the small intestines. It interferes with the body's absorption of fats and carbohydrates from digested foods.

Giardiasis is an intestinal infestation with a protozoal flagellate, i.e. *Giardia lamblia*. It is commonly found in children with malnutrition and immune deficiency conditions. It is considered as an important cause of morbidity in infancy and childhood and even leading to the fatal outcome, if not treated appropriately.

Definition

Giardia infection (giardiasis) is an intestinal infection caused by a microscopic parasite that is found worldwide, especially in areas with poor sanitation and unsafe water. Giardia infection is marked by abdominal cramps, bloating, nausea and bouts of watery diarrhea.

Causes

Giardia parasites live in the intestines of people and animals. Before the microscopic parasites are passed in stool, they become encased within hard shells called cysts, which allows them to survive outside the intestines for months. Once inside a host, the cysts dissolve and the parasites are released.

Giardia infection is far more common in children than it is in adults. Children are more likely to come in contact with feces, especially if they wear diapers, are toilet training or spend time in a child care center. People who live or work with small children are also at higher risk of developing giardia infection.

Giardia infection is a waterborne infection and can be caused by parasites found in backcountry streams and lakes, as well as in municipal water supplies, swimming pools, whirlpool spas and wells.

Mode of Transmission

Eating Contaminated Food

Giardia parasites can be transmitted through food—either because food handlers with giardiasis do not wash their hands thoroughly or because raw produce is irrigated or washed with contaminated water. Because cooking food kills giardia, food is a less common source of infection than water is, especially in industrialized countries.

Person-to-Person Contact

You can contract giardiasis if your hands become contaminated with fecal matter—parents changing a child's diapers are especially at risk. So child care workers and children in child care centers are at high-risk, where outbreaks are increasingly common. The giardia parasite can also spread through anal sex.

Contaminated Water

The most common way to become infected with giardia is after swallowing contaminated water. Giardia parasites are found in lakes, ponds, rivers and streams worldwide, as well as in municipal water supplies, wells, cisterns, swimming pools, water parks and spas. Ground and surface water can become contaminated from agricultural runoff, wastewater discharge or animal feces. Children in diapers and people with diarrhea may accidentally contaminate pools and spas.

Pathology

The infection is transmitted by the ingestion of cysts through contaminated water, food or directly form person to person contact. Each cyst liberates four trophozoits an colonize in the duodenum and jejunum. They attach to the brush border of the intestinal epithelial cells and multiply. The powerful sucking disk of the trophozoite cuases mechanical irritation and damage to the microvilli of the small intestinal mucosa, resulting in deficiency of disaccharidases in the enterocytes.

Pancreatic damage may occur which can cause extra intestinal steatorrhea, poor tryptic activity and deficiency of enterokinase secretion. Fat malabsorption may occur due to bacterial over growth in the duodenum and upper jejunum and deconjugation of bile salts liberating bile acids. There is reduction of secretary IgA in duodenal aspirates and depressed 'T' cell functions.

Signs and Symptoms

It usually appears one to two weeks after exposure and may include:

- Watery, sometimes foul-smelling diarrhea that may alternate with soft, greasy stools
- Fatigue or malaise
- Abdominal cramps and bloating
- Belching gas with a bad taste
- Nausea
- Weight loss.

Other symptoms include:

- Abdominal cramps
- Large amounts of intestinal gas
- An enlarged belly from the gas
- Loss of appetite
- Nausea and vomiting
- Sometimes a low-grade fever.

Sometimes, after acute (or short-term) symptoms of giardiasis pass, the disease begins a chronic (or more prolonged) phase. Symptoms of chronic giardiasis include:

- Periods of intestinal gas
- Abdominal pain in the area above the navel (belly button)
- Poorly formed, 'mushy' bowel movements

Diagnostic Evaluation

Giardial infection is usually diagnosed when giardia is found in your stool (feces) after a stool sample is sent to the laboratory. Ideally, three stool specimens from different days should be examined because of potential variations in the excretion of the giardia in your stools.

- History collection
- Physical examination for presence of clinical features and
- Stool examination help in diagnosis
- Endoscopic brush cytology and intestinal biopsy are useful diagnostic method
- Fecal antigen ELISA test help to detect the parasite in stool
- Antigiardia antibody titers, especially IgM, elevation indicates acute infection.

Management

The drugs commonly used for treatment of G. lamblia in children include metronidazole, quinacrine, furazolidone and paromomycin. Furazolidone, a nitrofuran compound available in liquid form, is more acceptable and tolerable in young children than the other agents. Cure rates range from 80 to 100 percent but, in older children, are usually lower with furazolidone than with metronidazole and quinacrine.

Adverse effects of furazolidone include nausea and/or vomiting (approximately 7 percent of patients), hemolysis secondary to glucose 6-phosphatase deficiency and nitrofuran sensitivity reactions. Furazolidone is administered at 6 to 8 mg per kg per day in three to four divided doses for seven to 10 days.

The specific treatment includes metronidazole therapy, 15 mg/kg per day in 3 divided doses for 10 days or tinidazole 50–75 mg/kg a single dose or 20 mg/kg/day in divided dose for 5 days. Furazolidone 6–8 mg/kg/day in 3 divided doses for 7 to 10 days is also effective. Other drugs like mepacrine, secnidazole, albendazole or ornidozole, also can be used for the treatment of this condition.

Preventive Measures

The Preventive measures protect the child and family from giardiasis:

- Advice the parents should use safe drinking water only.
- Wash raw fruits and vegetables well before you eat them.
- Wash the children hands well before you taking food.
- Encourage the children to wash their hands after every trip to the bathroom and especially before eating. If someone in family has giardiasis, wash your hands often as you care for him or her.
- Advice the child and parents should wash their hands well after handling anything in 'touch tanks' in aquariums, a potential source of giardiasis.
- Breastfeeding appears to protect infants from Giardia intestinal infection. Breast milk contains detectable titers of secretory IgA, which is protective for infants, especially in developing countries.

Complication

Giardia infection is almost never fatal in industrialized countries, but it can cause lingering symptoms and serious complications, especially in infants and children. The most common complications include:

- *Dehydration:* Often a result of severe diarrhea, dehydration occurs when the body doesn't have enough water to carry out its normal functions.
- *Failure to thrive:* Chronic diarrhea from giardia infection can lead to malnutrition and harm children's physical and mental development.
- *Lactose intolerance:* Many people with giardia infection develop lactose intolerance the inability to properly digest milk sugar. The problem may persist long after the infection has cleared.

INTESTINAL AMEBIASIS

Introduction

Gastrointestinal amebiasis is an infection of the large intestine caused by microscopic one-celled parasites commonly known as amebas (*Entamoeba histolytica*). Because these parasites live in the large intestine, they travel in the feces of infected people, and can contaminate water supplies in places where sanitation is poor.

The parasite can contaminate fruits and vegetables grown in areas where human feces are used as fertilizer. They can be transferred on the dirty hands of infected people who do not wash their hands often or correctly.

The route of entry of the infection is by contaminated food and water or by food handlers, or direct contact with infected stools. Rodents, flies and cockroaches also can transmit the infection by carrying cysts and contaminating food and drink. Asymptomatic human cyst carriers are the principal reservoirs of infection. It is found in about 15 percent of Indian population.

Definition

Amebiasis is an intestinal parasitic illness which is caused by a single-celled microscopic parasite called *Entamoeba histolytica*. Parasites are micro or macroorganisms which live or depend on other living organisms for their survival or food or both.

Causes

The causative agent of amebiasis is *E. hystolytica*. It exists in two forms—vegetative (trophozoite) and cystic forms. Trophozoites dwell in the colon where they multiply and encyst. The cyst are excreted in stool the trophozoites are short lived outside the human body.

Amebiasis is frequently a household infecting. When an individual in a family is infected, others in the family may also be affected. It is more closely related to poor sanitation and socioeconomic status. The use of night soil for agricultural purposes favors the spread of the disease.

Epidemic water borne infections may occur, if there is heavy contamination of water supply (sewage seepage). Raw contaminated vegetables especially from fields irrigated with sewage polluted water can readily spread infection. Hand to mouth transmission may occur directly by contaminated hands and finger nails with viable cyst.

Pathophysiology

The causative organism *Entamoeba histolytica* enters the child body in trophozoite form which excyst in the small intestines and float in the intestinal contents.

After that it will carried out large intestine and invade the intestinal mucosa resulting tissue destruction in the form of inflammatory response and ulceration. They mainly settle in the colon due to slow passage of colonic contents.

The infection can reach the liver through the portal circulation and may cause amebic liver abscess, usually found in right lobe of the liver, the liver abscess may be single or multiple with chocolate colored, viscid, usually sterile and nonpathogenic contents.

The abscess may regress or rupture or disseminate. The condition can be complicated by transdiaphragmatic rupture liver abscess which may cause amebic emphysema and pulmonary amebiasis.

The infection may cause amebic hepatitis or may spread to lung, brain, genitourinary system or skin. In swimmers, the free living amebae in the water, can cause meningoencephalitis through olfactory neuroendothelium.

Signs and Symptoms

- Amebic dysentery
- high fever
- severe abdominal pain
- 10 or more episodes of diarrhea daily. Typically, this diarrhea is watery or contains blood and mucus.

When amebas spread to the liver and cause liver abscess:

- Fever
- Nausea
- Vomiting
- Pain in the upper right portion of the abdomen
- Weight loss
- Enlarged liver.

It is possible for a person to develop symptoms of an amebic liver abscess without ever having had the diarrhea typical of infection.

Complications

Intestinal amebiasis may be completed with amebic liver abscess, amebic hepatitis, intestinal obstruction, intussusceptions, performation of the colon, peritonitis, rectal ulcer, rectal fistula, rectal prolapsed, chronic colitis and extraintestinal amebiasis including involvement of lungs, brain, spleen and skin. Amebiasis carries substantial morbidity and mortality. It is a potentially lethal disease. Reinfection is very common.

Diagnosis

History of illness and clinical examination help in diagnosis. Laboratory investigations is useful to confirm the diagnosis and plan of management. Examination of fresh specimens of stool for 3 consecutive days sample is performed to detect E. hystolytica, cysts or trophozoites in stool sample. Smear from ulcerated area of the rectal mucosa may be examined to detect the infection.

Sigmoidoscopy followed by aspiration of mucosal lesions or biopsy is valuable in symptomatic patients. Examination of aspirate of liver abscess may be performed to confirm the complicated condition. Chest X-ray, liver scan or USG abdomen help to diagnose liver abscess and lung complications. Blood examination shows leukocytosis, anemia and increased alkaline phosphatase in chronic intestinal amebaisis. Serological tests (ELISA, IHA, CIE) can be done to detect extraintestinal amebiasis.

Management

Gastrointestinal amebiasis is treated with nitroimidazole drugs, which kill amebas in the blood, in the wall of the intestine and in liver abscesses.

These drugs include metronidazole (Flagyl) and tinidazole (Tindamax, Fasigyn). Metronidazole usually is given for 10 days, either by mouth or directly into the veins (intravenously).

To kill amebas and cysts confined to the intestine, three drugs called luminal drugs are available: iodoquinol (Diquinol and others), paromomycin (Humatin) and diloxanide furoate (Furamide). One of these drugs is used along with metronidazole when gastrointestinal symptoms are present. In people who pass amebas in their stools without having symptoms of amebiasis, the luminal drugs alone can clear the amebas from the bowel.

These drugs may be given in combination of diloxanide furoate. Metronidazole is given as 20–50 mg/kg per day in three divided doses for 10–14 days after meal, tinidazole 50–60 mg/kg/day in three divided dose for 3 days and diloxanide furoate 20 mg/kg/day in three divided doses for ten days, for intestinal infections. These drugs are effective for elimination of both trophozoites and cyst.

Other drugs recommended for treatment of amebiasis are imidazole, ornidazole, secnidazole and paromomycin.

Treatment of complications should be done accordingly. Liver abscess should be done accordingly. Liver abscess should be treated as like as intestinal amebiasis and aspiration to be done in case of failure to respond to medical therapy.

Preventive Measures

Amebiasis is prevented by eradicating fecal contamination of food and water through improved sanitation, hygiene, and water treatment. In nonendemic areas, disease transmission can be reduced by early treatment of carriers.

Prevention of amebiasis at present requires interruption of the fecal-oral spread of the infectious cyst stage of the parasite. Because cysts are resistant to low doses of chlorine or iodine, in developing countries water must be boiled before it is safe to drink, and raw vegetables must be washed with soap and then soaked in vinegar for 15 min before they can be eaten. Since amebiasis often spreads through a household, it is prudent to screen family members of an index case for intestinal *E.* histolytica infection.

Safe disposal of human excreta and sanitary practice of washing hands after defecation and before eating are crucial aspects in the prevention of amebiasis. Protection of water supply from fecal contamination is equally important. Practice of water filtration and boiling are more effective than chemical treatment of water against amebiasis.

Prognosis

Drug treatment can cure amebiasis within a few weeks. However, because medication cannot keep you from getting infected again, repeat episodes of amebiasis may occur if you continue to live in or travel to areas where amebas are found. Among children in developing countries, especially infants and those younger than 5, gastrointestinal amebiasis can be fatal. Worldwide, amebiasis is the third most common cause of death from parasitic infections.

CRYPTOSPORIDIOSIS

Introduction

Cryptosporidium is the one of the parasitic infection. It is a living organism that can be lives in or on another organism. It can infect the bowels (intestines) and cause 'cryptosporidiosis'. This is a form of bowel infection called gastroenteritis, which leads to diarrhea and being vomiting. Infection can occur in child and adult and its spread by contact with soil, water, food or surfaces that have been contaminated by infected stools (feces) containing the parasite.

Definition

The cryptosporidiosis is defined as it is a diarrheal disease caused by microscopic parasites, *Cryptosporidium,* that can live in the intestine of humans and animals and is passed in the stool of an infected person or animal. Both the disease and the parasite are commonly known as 'Crypto.' The parasite is protected by an outer shell that allows it to survive outside the body for long periods of time and makes it very resistant to chlorine-based disinfectants.

The Mode of Transmission

The *Cryptosporidium* parasite may be transmitted person-to-person. Infection is also spread:

- *Direct contact:* It most commonly spread by drinking or swimming in contaminated water and eating uncooked food (such as fruits and vegetables) contaminated with *Cryptosporidium.*
- *Indirect vontact:* When hands will touch the objects and surfaces are contaminated with feces of infected people or animals (cows and other domestic animals).
- *Others:* Feco-oral route from person to person or through contaminated water and food. *Cryptosporidium* resides in the jejunum and may invade the colon and the biliary tract.

The Incubation Period

The incubation period of the disease is 2 to 7 days. The infection is presented with acute watery diarrhea, vomiting and abdominal cramps, which usually recovers in 10 to 14 days spontaneously. The disease can be complicated with loss of weight, malnutrition cholecystitis, pancreatitis, papillary stenosis and persistent diarrhea.

Signs and Symptoms

The symptoms of cryptosporidiosis with child usually develop about 7 days (can range from 2 to 10 days though) after being exposed to crypto parasite, including:

- Watery diarrhea
- Stomach cramps
- Nausea
- Vomiting
- Fever
- Dehydration and weight loss.

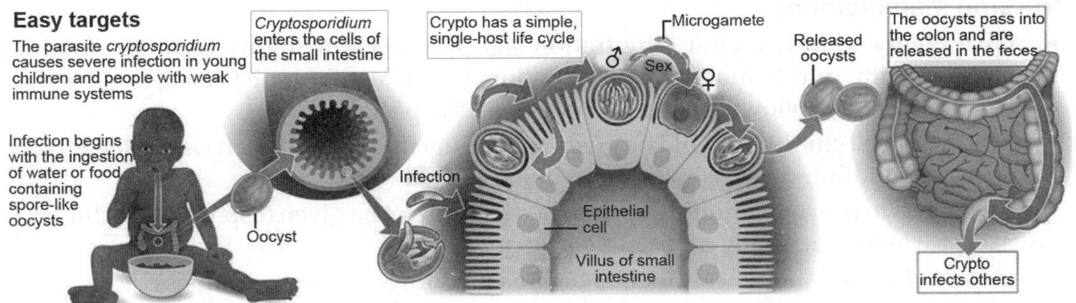

Fig. 5.26: Pathophysiology of cryptosporidiosis

Pathophysiology

Risk Factors

- Children who attend day care centers, including pre-schooler children
- Child health care workers
- Parents of infected children
- People who take care of other child with cryptosporidiosis
- Drinking unfiltered, untreated water
- Child who drink from untreated shallow, unprotected wells water
- Including swimmers, who swallow water from contaminated water sources
- Child who handle infected cattle
- Adult who exposed to human feces through sexual contact.

Diagnostic Evaluation

The infection is diagnosed by examining a specimen of feces under a microscope or by detecting *Cryptosporidium* in a fecal sample using a PCR (polymerase chain reaction) test in a pathology laboratory.

- History collection
- Physical examination
- Blood test
- Stool examination
- PCR (polymerase chain reaction) test.

Management

There is a treatment for crypto though. Alinia (nitazoxanide) is a prescription medication that is approved to treat diarrhea caused by the parasites cryptosporidium parvum and Giardia lambia, another parasite, in children who are at least 12 months old.

Symptomatic management by fluid electrolyte balance, adequate nutrition and antiemetics are useful. The cause of immunosuppression or immune deficiency condition should be treated for better prognosis. Hygienic measures to be followed.

Nursing Management

- Give plenty of fluids. Oral rehydration solution (ORS) is highly recommended for children with mild to moderate dehydration. It is available at pharmacies and should be administered following the instructions on the packaging.
- Mildly unwell children should be given their usual fluids more often carbonated (fizzy) drinks or undiluted juice should be avoided.
- Medicines to prevent vomiting or diarrhea should not be given (especially in children), except where specifically advised by a doctor.
- Breastfed babies should continue to be breastfed throughout their illness.
- Children on formula or solid diets should restart their normal diet (including full strength lactose containing milk) following rehydration with oral rehydration solution.
- Children, who are hungry or ask for food should be given small portions of their usual foods, but avoid foods high in sugar or fat.

Preventive Measures

Wash hands thoroughly with soap and water, paying attention to the backs of your hands, wrists, between fingers and under fingernails. Always wash your hands (even if you are wearing gloves):

- Before and after tending to someone who has Cryptosporidium infection
- Before preparing, handling or eating food
- After using the toilet
- After gardening
- After changing nappies or assisting children with sing the toilet
- After coming into contact with animals, their feces, or their environments.
  - Do not consume untreated ice or drinking water when travelling in countries where the water supply might be unsafe.
  - Avoid eating uncooked foods when travelling in countries with minimal water treatment and sanitation systems.
  - People who have diarrhea should not use swimming pools or spa pools for 14 days after the symptoms have stopped.
  - Infant and children who are not toilet trained should wear tight fitting waterproof pants or swimming nappies in swimming pools and changed regularly in the change room.
  - Avoid touching farm animals, especially young calves and lambs.
  - Wash (with safe water) and/or peel all raw fruits and vegetables before eating.

WORM INFESTATIONS (HELMINTHIASIS)

The worm infestation in children is very commonly seen in India. The common worm infestations are Threadworm, Roundworm and Hookworm. The child suffering from worms usually presents with the following symptoms. Helminthic infestations in children are a major public health problem caused by ineffective disposal of human excreta.

The common helminthes found in adult or sexual forms in the human body are

- Roundworms (*Ascaris lumbricoides*)
- Pinworms or threadworms (*Enterobius vermicularis*)
- Hookworms (*Ancylostoma duodenale* and *Necator americanus*)
- Tapeworms (*Taenia saginata* or *Taenia solium*).

Classification

Three group of worms:

1. Nematodes
   - Round worms
   - Pinworms
   - Hookworms.
2. Cestodes (Tapeworms)
3. Trematodes (fish worms or flukes)

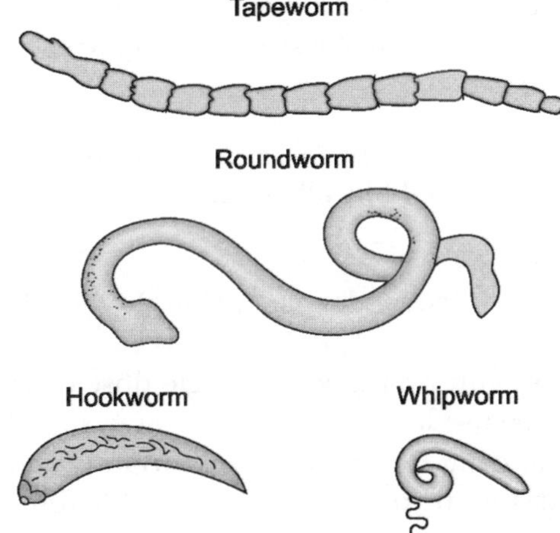

ROUNDWORMS (ASCARIASIS)

Definition

Ascariasis is the name of an infection caused by the roundworm Ascaris lumbricoides. When a worm lives inside the human body, the condition is called a parasitic infection.

Roundworms can live inside the small intestine for up to two years. The worms are about as thick as a pencil and can grow to be about 13 inches long. They reproduce very quickly. Female roundworms may lay more than 200,000 eggs every day; these eggs leave the body through bowel movements.

Mode of Transmission

The mode of transmission is feco oral route by ingestion of infective foods or soil or drink or by contaminated hands and fingers. The period of communicability is continued until all fertile female worms are destroyed and stools are negative of roundworm eggs. Incubation period is about 2 months.

Signs and Symptoms

- Stomach pain
- Vitamin deficiencies
- Pica, sleeplessness, irritability
- Urticaria
- Coughing
- Loss of appetite
- Fever
- Wheezing
- Worms in the stool
- Weight loss or failure to grow.

Diagnostic Evaluation

History collection and physical assessment, stool examination: Child passes the stool Snakelike worm or vomiting is important diagnostic criteria. Clinical examination and stool examinations: Worm eggs are useful to confirm the diagnosis.

Management

The roundworms can be easily treated by taking a medication that kills the worms in about three days. Medications can be used like albendazole, mebendazole.

Anthelmintics Drugs

- Albendazole (15 mg/kg) or mebendazole (100 mg) twice daily for 3 days irrespective of patient's age.
- Levamisole single dose with 2.5 mg/kg or single dose of pyrantel pamoate 10 mg/kg body weight may also be used.
- Piperazin cirtae is ideal drug for eradication of roundworm infestation. It is given in dose of 100–150 mg/kg for one or two days at night before sleep in the form of syrup or tablets or granules.
- The drug paralyses the worms, so the child should pass stools within 12 hours of intake of piperazine.

Preventive Measures

The most important measure of protection against Ascariasis is the safe and sanitary disposal of human waste. Sanitary disposal of human excreta, reduction of fecal contamination of the soil, provision of safe drinking water, food hygiene, good personal hygiene, improving habits of handwashing before eating and after defecation, avoidance of open field defecation are important means of prevention.

Provide special attention to be taken for foods such as salads and vegetables or raw food items to prevent spread of infestation. Avoidance of pica and playing on contaminated soils and dusts are also effective measures.

Health education to the general public create a awareness about the use of sanitary latrines, improvement of personal and environmental hygiene and changing of behavioral patterns especially on preventive measures are significant aspect of prevention.

PINWORM OR THREADWORM (OXYURIASIS)

Pinworm infections (also known as 'seatworm infection,' 'threadworm infection,' 'enterobiasis,' or 'oxyuriasis') are contagious.

Pinworm is an intestinal infection caused by tiny parasitic worms. One of the most common roundworm infections, pinworm infections affect millions of people each year, particularly school-age children.

It is very common parasitic infestations of infants and young children. The worm does not multiply inside the human body. The gravid female travels to the perianal region at night to lay eggs causing perianal itching. Each egg measures 30–60 mm and matures after 6 hours in a larva, which can survive for about 20 days.

Pinworms eggs are carried under fingernails contaminated during perianal scratching or through contaminated clothing, bed linen and dust to infect the human host by autoinfection. Man is only natural host or definitive host of pinworms.

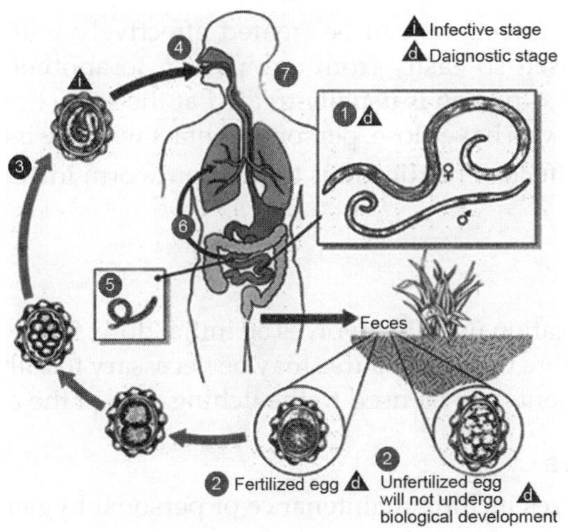

Fig. 5.27: Pathophysiology

Pinworm infection occurs most often in school-age children, and the microscopic eggs are easily spread from child to child.

Signs and Symptoms

The infected child may present with common general symptoms like Anorexia, loss of weight, teeth grinding, abdominal pain, nausea, vomiting and diarrhea.

- Itching of the anal or vaginal area
- Insomnia, irritability and restlessness
- Intermittent abdominal pain and nausea
- Pinworms often cause no symptoms.

Pruritus is the important feature. It occurs due to crowding of gravid females at the anus which produce intense pruritus. Scratching may cause secondary infection. In female child, vulvogaginitis may be found. The infected child may also present with irritability, restlessness, sleep disturbances, enuresis and masturbation. Rarely the condition may be complicated with appendicitis and salpingitis.

Diagnostic Evaluation

- History of passage of worms and other features are diagnostic
- Physical examination
- Routine stool examination to detect the pinworm eggs, because eggs are generally not passed in the stool. Eggs can be demonstrated by examination of early morning perianal swab, before the child has passed stool.
- Use the Cellophane-tape or transparent scotch tape technique can be done to detect the eggs. Eggs can be demonstrated in finger nail dirt in about 1/3 of cases.

Management

Medical Management

Most of the pinworm infections can be treated effectively with oral medication. Since pinworms can be passed so easily from one person to another, everyone living in the household of an infected person is usually treated at the same time to prevent reinfection. Caregivers and others who have close, personal contact with the individual are also treated.

The common and effective medications to treat pinworm infection are:

- Mebendazole
- Albendazole
- Pyrantel pamoate.

One course of medication usually involves an initial dose, followed by a second dose two to three weeks later. More than one course may be necessary to fully eliminate the pinworm eggs. Creams or ointments can be used to the itching skin in the area around the anus.

Preventive Measures

The preventive measures include maintenance of personal hygiene, careful handwashing with soap and water after defecation and before meal, keeping short nails, cleaning nails with soap and old tooth brush, treatment of all infected family members, wearing of tight pants to the children, laundering of infected clothing, etc.

- Encourage the child to wash your hands with warm water and soap after using the toilet. Be especially careful after bowel movements and changing diapers. Do the same before preparing food and eating.
- Advice the parents to keep their children fingernails short and clean.
- Discourage children's habits such as nail biting or scratching that could spread pinworm eggs.
- Encourage the children for daily bath in the morning to remove pinworm eggs that may have been deposited overnight.
- Change the children underwear and clothing daily.
- Use hot water in the washing machine, followed by a hot dryer, to launder bedding, clothing, and towels that may contain pinworm eggs.
- Advice the parents to keep their home well lit during the day because the eggs are sensitive to sunlight.

HOOKWORMS (ANCYLOSTOMIASIS)

Hookworm infection is a condition caused by roundworms that affects the small intestine and lungs. Hookworms are small (less than 0.5 inches long) parasitic worms that can cause infections in the small intestines.

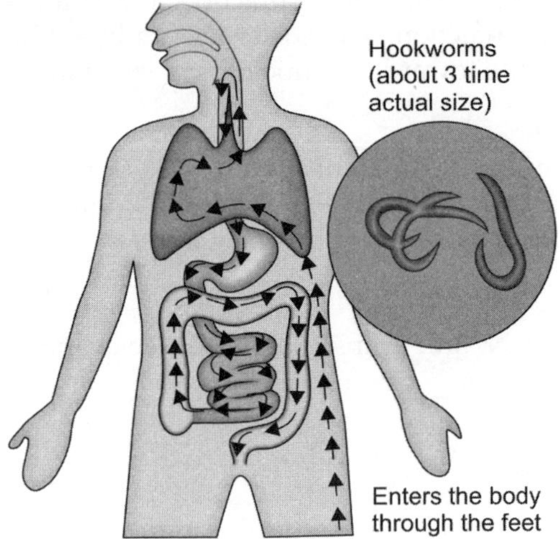

Fig. 5.28: Child with hookworm infection

The major species of hookworms associated with infections in humans are *Ancylostoma duodenale* and *Necator americanus*. They get their name from the teeth ('hooks') or cutting plates in their mouths by which they attach themselves to the intestinal wall.

Causes

The organisms that have been shown to cause hookworm disease include the following:

- *N. americanus* is the globally predominant human hookworm and is the only member of its genus known to infect humans. It is a small, cylindrical, off-white worm; adult males measure 7–9 mm, and adult females measure 9–11 mm.
- *A. duodenale* is more geographically restricted than *N. americanus* and is one of several anthropophilic members of the genus *Ancylostoma*. It primarily infects humans and is responsible for classic hookworm disease.

  A. duodenale resembles *N. americanus* in appearance but is somewhat larger, with adult males measuring 8–11 mm and adult females measuring 10–13 mm.
- *A. ceylonicum* primarily infects canines and felines but can cause milder classic hookworm disease in humans.
- *A. braziliense* is a canine and feline hookworm that, in humans, causes cutaneous larva migrans, or creeping eruption, a self-limiting condition characterized by serpiginous burrows formed as the larvae migrates through the epidermis.
- *A. caninum* is a canine hookworm that mainly causes eosinophilic enteritis in humans (though it also causes cutaneous larva migrans in a minority of cases).

  Eggs are passed in the feces and on warm, moist soil they hatched larva after 1–2 days. Newly hatched larva mouths twice in the soil and become infective, thus able to penetrate skin within 5 to 10 days.

It is common in agricultural areas. Damping the agricultural waste, sandy or friable soil with decaying vegetation is suitable for survival of the larvae. Moisture and rainfall are favorable environmental factors.

Direct sunlight can kill the larvae. Soil pollution by open field defecation, using same place for defecation, going barefoot, farming practices using untreated sewage are significant factors causing spread of infection. The social factors like illiteracy, ignorance and low standard of living contribute towards the hookworm infestations.

Mode of Transmission

Mode of transmission of hookworm infective larvae is usually by skin penetration in barefooted individual. The worm may also transmit by oral route with direct ingestion of infective larvae via contaminated fruits and vegetables.

The Incubation

The incubation period for N. americans is about 7 weeks and for A. duodenale, it varies from 5 weeks to 9 months.

Signs and Symptoms

- Abdominal discomfort
- Cough
- Diarrhea
- Intestinal cramps
- Fever
- Gas collection in the intestine
- Itchy rash
- Loss of appetite
- Nausea, vomiting
- Malena
- Pale color skin.

The infected child may be complicated with malabsorption, malnutrition, growth retardation, gross hypochromic anemia with hypoproteinemia causing edema even anasarca and cardiac failure.

Diagnostic Evaluation

- History collection
- Physical examination
- Complete blood count (CBC) with differential
- Stool examination.

Management

Anthelmintic drugs effective against hookworms include pyrantel pamoate and benzimidazoles (e.g. albendazole, mebendazole). Benzimidazoles are the most convenient and effective drugs for treating hookworm.

- Albendazole 10 mg/kg single dose or 5 mg/kg daily for 3 days orally. It has 80–100 percent effectiveness.

- Mebendazole (100 mg twice daily for 3 days) or pyrantel pamoate or Bephenium hydroxynaphthoate (alcopar) or Levimisole.

Preventive Measures

The preventive measures include maintain the personal hygiene, avoiding contact of contaminated soil by using foot wear, use of sanitary latrine for the sanitary disposal of feces to prevent soil pollution, change in farming practices that is not to use raw feces or untreated sewage as fertilizer and improving use of health facilities for diagnosis and treatment. Community involvement through health education is an important aspect of prevention of hookworm infestations.

Complications

- Iron deficiency anemia caused by loss of blood
- Nutritional deficiencies
- Severe protein loss with fluid buildup in the abdomen (ascites).

TAPEWORMS (CESTODES)

Introduction

Tapeworms are flat worms that live in a children digestive tract. Tapeworms are cestodes commonly found in children as port tapeworm (*Taenia solium*) and beef tapeworm (*Taenia saginata*). Other tapeworms are dwarf tapeworms (*Hymenolepis nana*) and zoonotic cestodes (*Echinococcus granulosus* and *Echinococcus multilocularis*). Man gets *T. Solium* and *T. saginata* infestations through ingestion of cysticerca in contaminated food and echinococcus through ingestion of eggs. *Diphyllobothrium latum* infection occurs through ingestion of cyst in fresh water fish.

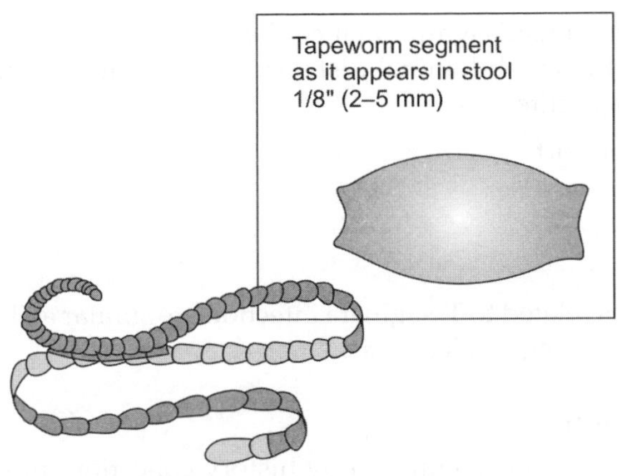

Fig. 5.29: Structure of tapeworms

Morphology

T. Saginata

- Usually less than 5 m long but can grow up to 25 m; 12 mm broad.
- The head, called the scolex, is pear-shaped.
- It has no hooks and no neck.
- It has four suckers in the head.
- The body is long and flat with several hundred segments called proglottids-hermaphroditic, egg-producing sections.
- Each proglottid is 18 × 6 mm with a branched uterus.
- Eggs are round and yellow-brown in color.

T. Solium

- It has a variable size and can be up to 7 m long; it has a neck and a long flat body.
- The scolex is globular in shape.
- There are four suckers and hooks.
- Proglottids are 5 × 10 mm and also have branched uteri.

Mode of Transmission

- The consumption of infective cysticerci in improperly cooked meat of infected port (pig) or beef
- Ingestion of unwashed raw vegetables, food and water contaminated with eggs
- Reinfection by regurgitation of eggs from the small intestine by retroperistalsis (rare).

Clinical Manifestations

The infected children remain asymptomatic. The symptomatic children may present with headache, abdominal pain, abdominal distension, recurrent diarrhea and growth failure inspite of voracious appetite.

- Abdominal discomfort
- Loss of appetite
- Loss of weight
- Malnutrition.

The clinical features related to T. saginata infection are similar as T. solium with exception of less chance of developing cysticercosis.

Diagnostic Evaluation

The diagnosis of tapeworm is confirmed by history collection, physical examination and stool examination for eggs or examination of proglottids or motile segments passed in the stools. Neurocysticercosis is diagnosed by CT scan or MRI. CSF examination and blood for ELISA test are supportive to confirm the condition.

Management

Management of both tapeworms can be done with praziquental 10 mg/kg in a single dose. Other drugs which can be used are mepacrine, niclosamide, albendazole or mebendazole. For neurocysticercosis, praziquental (PZQ) 50 mg/kg/day in 3 divided dose for 2 to 3 weeks or albendazole 15 mg/kg/day in three divided doses for 28 days can be administered.

- Albendazole (Albenza)
- Paromomycin (Humatin)
- Praziquantel (Biltricide)
- Niclosamide (Niclocide)
- Mebendazole (Vermox).

Symptomatic and supportive treatment should be provided depending upon the presence of symptoms and complications. Surgical interventions may be needed in symptom-producing cysticercosis.

Preventive Measures

- Inspect meat thoroughly before cooking
- Adequate handling of food, e.g. freezing or cooking
- Cysticerci do not survive temperatures of < 10 °C and > 50 °C.
- The World Health Organization (WHO) advocates the periodic treatment of tapeworms such as *T. solium* in endemic areas with albendazole. This can prevent neurocysticercosis at a later stage
- Health education messages should include adequate cooking of meat, thorough washing of raw vegetables and fruits, proper housing and feeding of pigs, prevention of pollution of food, water and solid with human feces and improving handwashing practices.

Hydatid Disease (Echinococcosis)

Hydatidosis otherwise called as cystic Echinococcosis (CE) is a parasitic infection of the liver and other organs by the flatworm Echinococcus granulosus. Hydatidosis is the most frequent cause of liver cyst in the world.

The ingested ova borrow through the intestinal mucosa and travel to the liver through the mesenteric vein. A few ova may pass the liver and get trapped in the lungs. Synchronous pulmonary and hepatic hydatid disease may occur in 4% to 25% of cases. Hydatid cyst can be seen in other organs, for example heart, pancreas, spleen, CNS.

Hydatid disease in man is caused mainly by infection by the larval stage of the dog tapeworm Echinococcus granulosus. It follows accidental ingestion of tapeworm eggs excreted in the feces of infected dogs.

Risk Factors

- Feeding dogs with raw offal
- Allowing dogs play with children's
- Poor hygiene (both animal and personal)
- Regular close contact with dogs.

Eggs are ingested by the man and larvae are hatched in the intestines, penetrate mucosa and are carried to the target organs. The important target organs are liver and lungs where larvae develop into characteristic unilocular or multilocular cyst, known as hydatid cyst. It can also occur in kidney, eyes, bones, spleen, peritoneum and brain. It takes several years to grow the hydatid cyst. It is more common where sheep and cattle are raised.

Clinical manifestations varies on the site and number of cysts. Large cyst may cause pressure symptoms (e.g. jaundice in liver cyst). Lung cyst may present with chest pain, hemoptysis and respiratory distress.

Diagnostic Evaluation

- Ultrasound for abdominal cysts with fine-needle aspiration
- Chest X-ray
- Serological exam
- Western blot assay for antigens is highly specific
- Serological diagnosis can be difficult from brain and eye cyst fluid samples
- USG, CT scan, ELISA test.

Management

Management is done with albendazole therapy 15 mg/kg/day in 3 divided doses for 14 to 28 days for four courses with 15 days drug free interval in between two courses with 15 days drug free interval in between two courses. Surgical removal of the large solitary cyst may be required after albendazole therapy.

Preventive Measure

Dog owners should practice good hygiene when handling their animals:

- It is important to wash the hands after handling dogs
- Avoid contact with dog feces
- Prevent dogs from soiling the immediate environment
- Prevent dogs from roaming or having access to raw sheep meat or viscera
- All sheep carcasses should be disposed of correctly and immediately
- All dogs, especially those in rural endemic areas should be treated at six-weekly intervals with a wormer containing Praziquantel.
- Vegetables, salads and fruit should be thoroughly washed before consumption.

OTHER DISORDERS

TONSILLITIS

Introduction

Tonsillitis is an inflammation of the tonsils and surrounded tissue, that both sides of the posterior throat. They help in the immune system to protect the body from infections that may enter the body through the mouth. When the tonsils become infected they become enlarged and red, yellow or white coating tonsils.

Tonsil infections may be contagious, and can spread from person to person by contact with the mouth, throat, or mucous of someone who is infected. Tonsillitis symptoms include a sore throat, fever, swollen glands in the neck, and trouble swallowing.

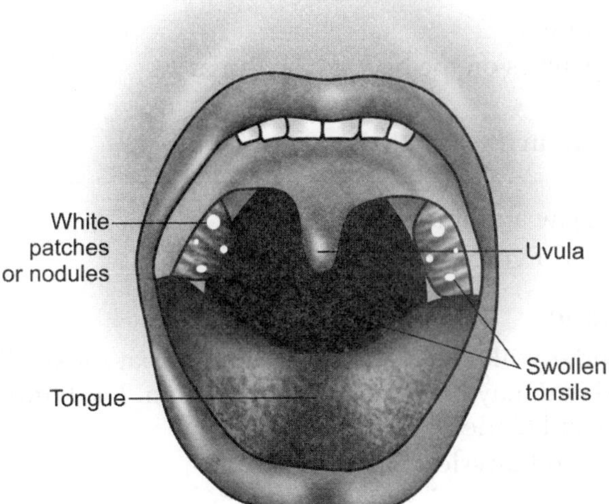

Fig. 5.30: Child with tonsillitis

Definition

Tonsillitis is defined as an inflammation of the tonsils characterized by sore throat and fever.

Types

There are two main types of tonsillitis:

1. Acute tonsillitis can either be bacterial or viral in origin. Subacute tonsillitis is caused by the bacterium Actinomyces.
2. Chronic tonsillitis can last for long periods of time if not treated, and is mostly caused by bacterial infection and will show pus on the tonsils.

Causes of Tonsillitis

There are three common causes of tonsillitis:

- *Group A streptococcus:* Which are common bacteria that cause throat infections in 1 in 5 people, including adults. Many people have no symptoms but they can still transmit the bacteria. Group A streptococcus can also cause strep throat. It is also capable under some circumstances of causing more serious illness, such as rheumatic fever.
- *Various respiratory viruses:* Especially cold and flu viruses, account for most cases of tonsillitis. These infections can be sometimes milder than bacterial infections, but it is often difficult to tell the difference between a viral and bacterial infection.
- *Infectious mononucleosis:* It caused by the Epstein-Barr virus, can also produce symptoms of tonsillitis, especially in children.

Signs and Symptoms

- Fever and sore throat
- Painful/difficulty in swallowing
- Nausea, vomiting, or abdominal pain

- Cough or hoarseness
- Runny or stuffy nose
- Yellow or white patches on the back of the throat
- Bad breath
- Rash on the body or in the mouth
- Ear pain
- Tenderness of the jaw and throat
- Voice changes, loss of voice.

Diagnostic Evaluation

The health care provider will look in the mouth and throat for swollen tonsils. The tonsils are usually reddened and may have white spots on them. The lymph nodes in the jaw and neck may be swollen and tender to the touch.

- History collection and physical examination
- Rapid strep test
- Throat swab culture
- Blood test (CBC).

Pathophysiology

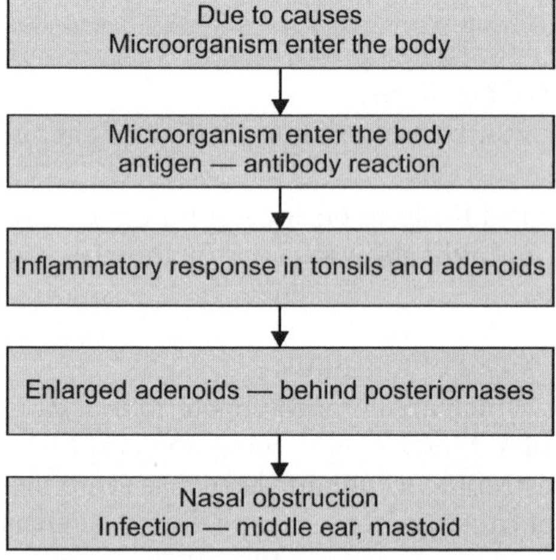

Fig. 5.31: Pathophysiology of tonsillitis

Management

Treatments of tonsillitis consist of pain management medications and lozenges. If the tonsillitis is caused by bacteria, then antibiotics are prescribed, with penicillin being most commonly used. Erythromycin and Clarithromycin are used for patients allergic to penicillin. Chronic cases may indicate tonsillectomy (surgical removal of tonsils) as a choice for treatment. Additionally, gargling with a solution of warm water and salt may reduce pain and swelling.

The antibiotics may be given once as a shot, or taken for 10 days by mouth. If antibiotic pills are used, they must be taken for the entire amount of time prescribed by the doctor. DO NOT stop taking them just because the discomfort stops, or the infection may not be cured. Rest to allow the body to heal. Fluids, especially warm (not hot), bland fluids or very cold fluids may soothe the throat. Gargle with warm salt water or suck on lozenges (containing benzocaine or similar ingredients) to reduce pain.

Such as acetaminophen (Tylenol) or ibuprofen may be used to reduce pain and fever. Do NOT give a child aspirin. Aspirin has been linked to Reye syndrome. Some people who have repeated infections may need surgery to remove the tonsils (tonsillectomy).

Surgical Management

- *Tonsillectomy:* Surgical removal of the palatine tonsils.
- *Adenoidectomy:* Surgical removal of the adenoids who have hypertrophied adenoids that obstruct nasal breathing.

Complications

An abscess may develop lateral to the tonsil during an infection, typically several days after the onset of tonsillitis. This is termed a peritonsillar abscess (or quinsy). Rarely, the infection may spread beyond the tonsil resulting in inflammation and infection of the internal jugular vein giving rise to a spreading septicemia infection (Lemierre's syndrome).

In chronic/recurrent cases (generally defined as seven episodes of tonsillitis in the preceding year, five episodes in each of the preceding two years or three episodes in each of the preceding three years), or in acute cases where the palatine tonsils become so swollen that swallowing is impaired, a tonsillectomy can be performed to remove the tonsils. Child whose tonsils have been removed is certainly still protected from infection by the rest of their immune system.

- Blocked airway from swollen tonsils
- Dehydration from difficulty swallowing fluids
- Kidney failure
- Peritonsillar abscess or abscess in other parts of the throat
- Pharyngitis-bacterial
- Poststreptococcal glomerulonephritis
- Rheumatic fever and related cardiovascular disorders.

Prognosis

Tonsillitis symptoms usually improve 2 or 3 days after treatment starts. The infection usually is cured after treatment is completed, but some people may need more than one course of antibiotics. Complications of untreated strep tonsillitis may be severe. Children with tonsillitis related to strep throat or pharyngitis should generally be kept home from school or day care until they have been on antibiotics for 24 hours. This helps reduce the spread of illness.

Nursing Management

- Providing comfort and minimizing activities or interventions that precipitate bleeding.
- Soft liquid diet.

- Cool mist vaporizer keeps the mucus membrane moist during periods of month breathing.
- Warm salt water gargles.
- Analgesic/Antipyretic drugs Acetaminophen.
- Opioid and nonpaid tablets.

Nursing Diagnoses

- Ineffective breathing pattern related to inflammatory process
- Ineffective airway clearance related to increased secretions.

OTITIS MEDIA

Introduction

Ear infections otherwise also called otitis media, it is a most common problem in children. About 50 percent of infants have at least one ear infection by their first birthday. Ear infections can cause pain in the ear, fever, and temporary hearing loss and general signs such as loss of appetite and irritability. Some children get better without specific antibiotic treatment but most young infants benefit from use of an antimicrobial agent.

Definition

Ear infection is also known as acute otitis media (otitis = ear, media = middle ear). Otitis media is an infection of the middle part of the ear. It is most often develop after a viral respiratory tract infection, such as a cold or the flu. These infections can cause swelling of the mucous membranes of the nose and throat, and diminish normal host defenses such as clearance of bacteria from the nose, increasing the amount of bacteria in the nose.

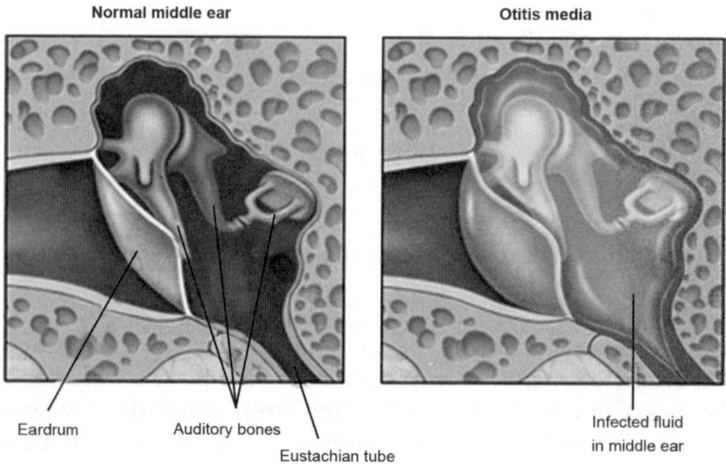

Fig. 5.32: Anatomical difference between normal and otitis media ear

Types

- Acute otitis media (AOM)
- Otitis media with effusion (OME)

- Chronic suppurative otitis media
- Adhesive otitis media.

Causes

Acute otitis media (AOM) is a common problem in early childhood; 2/3 of children have at least one episode by age 3, and 90% have at least one episode by school entry. Peak age prevalence is 6–18 months.

- Viral (25%)
- Streptococcus pneumonia (35%)
- Nontypeable strains of *Haemophilus influenzae* (25%)
- Moraxella catarrhalis (15%).

Risk Factors

- Boys are more vulnerable than girls to develop acute otitis media.
- Children with older siblings at school or nursery are exposed to infections that may be brought home.
- Use of a dummy increases risk. Presumably the sucking and swallowing opens the Eustachian tube and puts the middle ear at risk.
- Children who suffer with many colds or respiratory infections are more likely to develop OME.
- Parental smoking is thought to be associated with an increase in both acute and chronic otitis media.

Signs and Symptoms

- Otalgia
- Otorrhea
- Headache
- Fever
- Irritability
- Hearing loss
- Tinnitus
- Vertigo
- Loss of appetite
- Vomiting
- Diarrhea.

Diagnostic Evaluation

Pneumatic otoscopy remains the standard examination technique for patients with suspected OM. In addition to a carefully documented examination of the external ear and tympanic membrane (TM), examining the entire head and neck region of patients with suspected OM is important.

- *Color:* A normal TM is a translucent pale gray; an opaque yellow or blue TM is consistent with middle ear effusion (MEE)

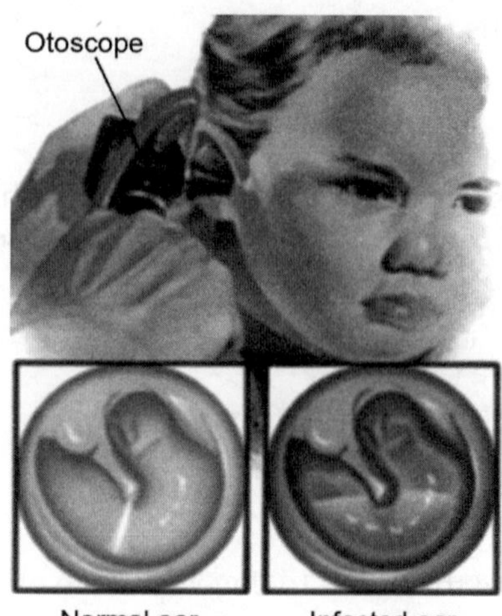

Fig. 5.33: Examination of ear by using otoscope

- *Position:* In AOM, the TM is usually bulging; in OME, the TM is typically retracted or in the neutral position
- *Mobility:* Impaired mobility is the most consistent finding in patients with OME
- *Perforation:* Single perforations are most common
  - Culture of discharge from an ear may be indicated in chronic or recurrent perforation or if grommets are present.
  - Audiometry should be performed if chronic hearing loss is suspected; however, not during acute infection.
  - CT or MRI may be appropriate if complications are suspected.

Management

This condition most of the children resolve spontaneously. Antibiotics provide a small reduction in pain beyond 24 hours in only about 5% of children treated. The modest benefit must be weighed against the potential harms related to antibiotic use, both for the individual patient (adverse effects) and at a population level (resistance pressure). It has been shown that not using antibiotics for otitis media is acceptable to parents if the reasons are explained clearly.

Pain is often the main symptom, so adequate analgesia is very important analgesia guideline.

- Paracetamol 20–30 mg/kg for 2–3 doses/day should be given if pain is significant.
- Short-term use of topical 2% lignocaine drops applied to the tympanic membrane has been shown to be effective for severe acute ear pain.
- Decongestants.
- Antihistamines.
- Corticosteroids have not been shown to be effective in AOM.

The flow-diagram provides a recommended management scheme:

>12 months old, mildly unwell, immunocompetent

Yes → Analgesia consider no antibiotics for first 24–48 hours

No → Analgesia amoxycillin 15 mg/kg/dose TDS for 5 days Give parent handout

Symptoms resolving

No → Analgesia amoxycillin 15 mg/kg/dose TDS for 5 days Give parent handout

Yes → Advise parents to seek medical review if ear symptoms, hearing difficulty or persistent irritablity after 2–3 months (to check for persistent effusion) Give parent handout

Symptoms improved by 48 hours

Yes → Advise parents to seek medical review if ear symptoms, hearing difficulty or persistent irritablity after 2–3 months (to check for persistent effusion) Give parent handout

No → Review consider alternative diagnosis If none, switch to Amoxycillin/clavulanic acid 22.5 mg/kg/dose BD for 5 days

Surgical Management

Tympanostomy tubes in the ears help to prevent recurrent ear infections.

Complications

- Most cases of AOM will resolve spontaneously with no sequelae.
- Perforation of the eardrum in not uncommon and progression to chronic suppurative otitis media may occur.
- Labyrinthitis, meningitis, intracranial sepsis or facial nerve palsy are very rare and occur in less than 1 in 1,000.
- Recurrent episodes may lead to scarring of the drum with permanent hearing impairment, chronic perforation and otorrhea, cholesteatoma or mastoiditis.
- In a small child with a high temperature there is a risk of febrile convulsions. This is discussed more fully in its own article.

Prevention

In recurrent (either three or more acute infections of the middle ear cleft in a six-month period, or at least four episodes in a year) strategies for managing the condition include the assessment and modification of risk factors where possible, repeated courses of antibiotics for each new infection and antibiotic prophylaxis.

CHILD ABUSE

Introduction

Children are all societies in the process of their normal are often neglected, abused intentionally or otherwise by their parents. The norms of child nearing differ culturally with wide differences between conservative and advanced society's child abuse and neglect is a significant community problem.

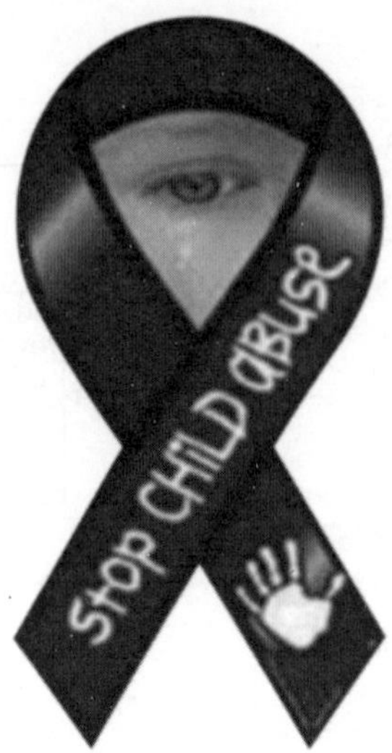

Definition

Child abuse has been broadened to include any problem resulting from lack of reasonable care and protection of child and adolescents by their parents, guardians or care takers.

According to Patricia L Howland the distinction between child abuse and child neglect lies primarily in the element of deliberateness.

In the broad sense, most researchers and authorities agree on the basic issue of child abuse resulting from parental misuse or exploitation of the rights of parents and other guardians to control and discipline children under their care and which are detrimental to the child's health and well-being.

Epidemiology and Incidence

- Child abuse and neglect involves about 1 to 2% of children in the United States.
- The prevalence of abuse is approximately 700 new cases per 1,000,000 populations.
- In the developed countries of the west the incidence of bettered child ranged from 250 to 300 cases reported per 1 million populations.
- In India the first case of battered baby syndrome was described in 1967.

Factors Leading to Child Abuse

Recent research on child abuse has tended to more away from considering the influence of a single factor such as:

- Personality disorder
- Mental illness
- Poverty towards looking at the effect of a whole group of predisposing or risk factors
- Child abuse can happen in any family at all levels of society

- The exact etiology of child abuse is not known, it is thought to be due to interaction of 3 primary factors.
- Sociocultural belief
- The child's and parental factors

Sociocultural Factors

Though there is a wide variation in socioculture belief of the developing and developed countries it is found that the basic factors leading to child abuse are:

- Values and norms of discipline and physical punishment
- Family structure—number of members in family, joint or nuclear family system, socioeconomic status, etc.
- Family and situational stresses—poverty, unemployment's, alcohol abuse, isolation
- Parent child relationship puncture child rearing style, excess or uncounted children role reversal.

Types of Child Abuse

Emotional Abuse

Emotional abuse refers to the psychological and social aspects of child abuse; it is the most common form of child abuse.

Many parents are emotionally abusive without being violent or sexually abusive; however, emotional abuse invariably accompanies physical and sexual abuse.

Some parents who are emotionally abusive parents practice forms of child-rearing that are orientated towards fulfilling their own needs and goals, rather than those of their children.

Their parenting style may be characterized by overt aggression towards their children, including shouting and intimidation, or they may manipulate their children using more subtle means, such as emotional blackmail.

Emotional abuse does not only occur in the home. Children can be emotionally abused by teachers and other adults in a position of power over the child.

Children can also be emotionally abused by other children in the form of 'bullying'. Chronic emotional abuse in schools is a serious cause of harm to victimized children and warrants ongoing active intervention.

Neglect

Complaints of neglect constitute a significant proportion of notifications and referrals to child protection services.

However, there is no single definition of child neglect in Australia. It is generally understood that 'neglect' refers to a range of circumstances in which a parent or caregiver fails to adequately provide for a child's needs.

Physical Abuse

Physical abuse has been a normal aspect of domestic life in Australia for a long time. Physical assaults that would be serious criminal offenses if committed by one man against another—for instance:

- Hitting
- Slapping
- Striking with an object.

When committed by a man against his wife and child, or by parents against their children. Today, incidents of domestic violence committed against both women and children remain at epidemic proportions, although there is increasing recognition within the Australian community of the prevalence and harms of violence against women and children.

Whilst community attitudes to violence against women and children have changed for the better, Australian policymakers have failed to outlaw physical assaults against children by caregivers.

According to the 2007 report of the Global Initiative to End All Corporal Punishment of Children, Australia is one of a number of countries that has failed to prohibit violence against children, and has failed to commit to legislative reform. In particular, the legal defenses of 'reasonable correction' and 'reasonable chastisement' are still available to adults who are charged with violent offenses against children in many jurisdictions.

Family Violence

Family violence, or domestic violence, usually refers to the physical assault of children and women by male relatives, usually a father and husband/partner.

In these situations, a man uses violence to control his partner and children, often in the belief that violence is a male prerogative ('I'm a guy, I can't control myself'), or that his victims are responsible for his behavior ('You bought it on yourself').

Whilst women may also be perpetrators of family violence, they are usually 'fighting back' against a physically abusive partner, and it is unusual for violent women to inflict the same scale of harm as violent men.

Sexual Abuse

Sexual abuse describes any incident in an adult engages a minor in a sexual act, or exposes the minor to inappropriate sexual behavior or material. Sexual abuse also describes any incident in which a child is coerced into sexual activity by another child.

A person may sexually abuse a child using threats and physical force, but sexual abuse often involves subtle forms of manipulation, in which the child is coerced into believing that the activity is an expression of love, or that the child bought the abuse upon themself. Sexual abuse involves contact and noncontact offences.

Signs of Child Abuse

You can become aware of child abuse by recognizing the signs. Here are 10 signs that can help.

1. *Unexplained injuries:* Visible signs of physical abuse may include unexplained burns or bruises in the shape of objects. You may also hear unconvincing explanations of a child's injuries.
2. *Changes in behavior:* Abuse can lead to many changes in a child's behavior. Abused children often appear scared, anxious, depressed, withdrawn or more aggressive.
3. *Returning to earlier behaviors:* Abused children may display behaviors shown at earlier ages, such as thumb-sucking, bed-wetting, fear of the dark or strangers. For some children, even loss of acquired language or memory problems may be an issue.

4. *Fear of going home:* Abused children may express apprehension or anxiety about leaving school or about going places with the person who is abusing them.
5. *Changes in eating:* The stress, fear and anxiety caused by abuse can lead to changes in a child's eating behaviors, which may result in weight gain or weight loss.
6. *Changes in sleeping:* Abused children may have frequent nightmares or have difficulty falling asleep, and as a result may appear tired or fatigued.
7. *Changes in school performance and attendance:* Abused children may have difficulty concentrating in school or have excessive absences, sometimes due to adults trying to hide the children's injuries from authorities.
8. *Lack of personal care or hygiene:* Abused and neglected children may appear uncared for. They may present as consistently dirty and have severe body odor, or they may lack sufficient clothing for the weather.
9. *Risk-taking behaviors:* Young people who are being abused may engage in high-risk activities such as using drugs or alcohol or carrying a weapon.
10. *Inappropriate sexual behaviors:* Children who have been sexually abused may exhibit overly sexualized behavior or use explicit sexual language.

Clinical Manifestations

- Physical
  - Bruises, hematoma, fracture
  - Head injury, visceral injury.
- Nutritional
  - Failure to thrive, marasmus
  - Stunting
  - Deprivation of varying severity.
- Sexual abuse
  - Rape, incest, fondling.
- Behavioral abuse
  - With drawl
  - Aggressiveness.
- Emotional abuse
  - Depression
  - Extremely low self-esteem
  - Passive, withdrawn
  - Apathetic.
- Non accidental poisoning
- Substance abuse
- Neglect
- Exploitation
  - Sexual, e.g. prostitution
  - Labor industries work
  - Kidnapping.

Diagnostic Evaluation

- Careful history collection
- Physical examination of child
- Medical attention at different hospitals
- Appropriate radiological investigations.

Management

- Physical injuries and abnormalities are appropriately treated
- Rehabilitation
- Family members need counseling and support
- General education, social coarseness and changes in attitudes and imperilments in socioeconomic conditions are imported.

BREATH HOLDING SPASMS

Introduction

Breath holding spell is common in children under six years of age. Breath holding spells can happen after the child has a fright, a minor accident, is frustrated or gets very upset. Breath holding is often called a 'spell' or an 'attack' and is most common in toddlers.

Breath holding spells or breath holding spasms is a benign involuntary phenomenon seen in children between 6 months and 6 years of age. Either due to pain, fear or in anger frustration the child cries and then holds the breath.

Definition

Breath holding spells are brief periods of children stop breathing for up to 1 minute. These spells often cause a child to pass out (lose consciousness). Breath holding spells usually occur when a young child is angry, frustrated, in pain, or afraid.

Types

There are two main types of breath holding:

1. Cyanotic spells
2. Pallid spells

Cyanotic spells are the most common variety though some children may present with both the varieties (mixed)

Cyanotic spells: They are often provoked by an upsetting situation, in anger or in frustration. The child usually cries or screams loudly and then the cry gradually becomes noiseless as child open the mouth and holds the breath in expiration for about 20–30 sec (apnea). The child turns blue (cyanotic) and then the child may again start breathing or may proceed to lose consciousness. Sometimes, fits or seizure like activity may follow the loss of consciousness. The entire episode may last less than one minute and the child generally regains full activity within a few minutes.

Pallid spells: They are usually seen following a painful or fearful experience. The child becomes pale and often loses consciousness within a single gasp or cry.

Causes

It is more common in 2 months old and up to 2 years old can start having breath holding spells. Most children stop having breath holding spells by the times they are 6–8 years old. Some children have severe spells. They usually stop by the time the child is 6–8 years old.

Children can have breath holding spells when they are responding to:

- Fear
- Pain
- Traumatic event
- Being startled or confronted.

Breath holding spells are more common in children with:

- Genetic conditions, such as Riley-Day syndrome or Retts syndrome
- Iron deficiency anemia
- A family history of breath holding spells (parents may have had similar spells when they were kids).

Signs and Symptoms

Breath holding spells most often occur when a child becomes suddenly upset or surprised. The child makes a short gasp, exhales and stops breathing. The child's nervous system slows the heart rate or breathing for a short amount of time. Breath holding spells are not thought to be a willful act of defiance, even though they often occur with temper tantrums.

Symptoms can include:

- Blue or pale skin
- Crying, then no breathing
- Fainting or loss of alertness (consciousness)
- Jerky movements (short, seizure-like movements)
- Normal breathing starts again after a brief period of unconsciousness
- The child's color improves with the first breath. This may occur several times per day or only on rare occasion.

Management

- No treatment is usually needed.
- Iron drops or pills if the child has an iron deficiency.

If the child has been diagnosed with breath holding spells take the following steps:

- During a spell, make sure the child is in a safe place where he or she will not fall or be hurt.
- Place a cold cloth on the child's forehead during a spell to help shorten the episode.
- After the spell, try to be calm.
- Avoid giving too much attention to the child, as this can reinforce the behaviors that led to the spell.
- Avoid situations that cause a child's temper tantrums. This can help reduce the number of spells.
- Ignore breath holding spells that do not cause the child to faint.
- Ignore the spell in the same way you ignore temper tantrums.

ENURESIS

Introduction

The word enuresis is derived from a Greek word (enourein) that means 'to void urine.' It can occur either during the day or at night (though some restrict the term to bedwetting that occurs at night). Enuresis can be divided into primary and secondary forms.

- The prevalence at age 5 years is 7% for males and 3% for female
- At age 10 years, it is 3% for male, 2% females.

Types

- Nocturnal enuresis (bedwetting)
- Diurnal enuresis
- Mixed enuresis.

Causes

- Faulty or defects in toilet training
- Overactive bladder
- Feeling of shame and guilt, fear and nightmares
- Emotional atmosphere
- Organic causes.

This can be related to enuresis caused by anatomical defect of the urinary tract, urinary tract infection, neurologic deficit or diabetes insipidus.

Signs and Symptoms

- Overactive bladder or dysfunctional voiding
- Cystitis
- Constipation
- Neurogenic bladder
- Sleep-disordered breathing
- Urethral obstruction
- Major motor seizure
- Ectopic ureter
- Juvenile diabetes mellitus or diabetes insipidus.

Management

- The home conditions, socioeconomic status and habits of the family should be found out
- Child parent relations should be explored. Analysis of the time of bed—wetting frequency and relation to sleep should be done.
- Restriction of fluid intake in the evening and helping the child in developing the habit of passing urine before going to bed.
- Toilet training should be given to the child to increase capacity of the bladder.

ENCOPRESIS

Definition

Encopresis refers to passage of feces into inappropriate place at any age when bowel control should have been established.

Encopresis indicates a more serious emotional disturbance than enuresis and is less common (around 1% of school-age children).

Causes

- Anatomic abnormality
- Emotional disturbances
- Improper toilet training
- Stress in school activity
- Over protection of parents
- Fear related to toilet
- Poor parent child bonding.

Signs and Symptoms

- Withhold defecation
- Distended abdomen
- Diarrhea related to irritation of GI tract
- Tensed feeling
- Aggressiveness.

Diagnostic Evaluation

- History of bowel elimination
- Physical examination
- Details about pattern of current toilet practice.

Management

Management is primarily with behavioral techniques. Establishing regular bowel habits (e.g. make the child to sit in toilet for atleast 10 minutes in a day). Psychiatric assistance can be provided to treat unresolved psychic conflicts. Reestablish a pattern of bowel elimination.

NAIL BITING

The habit is often a way to ease anxiety or to keep at least one part of the body occupied while the mind lacks interest. Frustration and loneliness are additional emotional triggers that can lead to nail biting. Some research suggests genes may play a role.

Biting fingernails can also be a symptom of a psychological condition, such as obsessive-compulsive disorder (OCD). People who wash their hands several times in a row or check the front door locks compulsively may also bite their nails as part of the same spectrum of behaviors. Many children who are nail biters also have other psychiatric disorders, such as attention deficit hyperactivity disorder (ADHD), oppositional defiant disorder (ODD), separation anxiety disorder, or bed-wetting.

Regular nail biting that causes severe damage to the nail and surrounding skin can be considered a form of self-mutilation, similar to cutting and related behaviors.

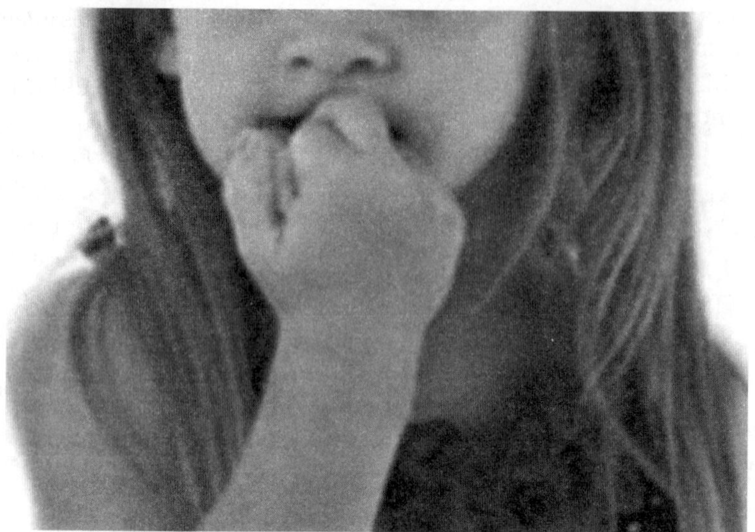

Fig. 5.34: Child with nail biting

Preventive Measures

Try to Tackle the Habit Early

Try to identify if the child is developing a nail biting habit at an early stage. Just like any other habit once it becomes established it will be a lot harder to break.

Identify Triggers

It could be boredom, or stress or a particular time of day. Ask the older child to write down in a diary when they notice they are nail biting. Ask them to note down what they were doing at the time and if anything springs to mind as to what triggered the biting.

Increase Awareness

One of the biggest problems is that it is a subconscious habit. A lot of the time a child will not even notice when they start to bite. Raise the consciousness of their nails. To do this you could try taking photos of their nails every day for a week or two. She can compare the photos and look for any progress or otherwise. Anything that helps someone to think about their nails on a more regular basis can help.

Start to Protect a Nail Campaign

Select a nail and make it the one nail that cannot be bitten. I would suggest you take a nail that is already badly damaged. Watch it grow! This should help your child to feel they are making progress. Once the nail becomes reestablished select another nail to become its protected partner.

Make Them Taste Foul

There are many liquids you can buy that cover the nail with a foul tasting coating. You do need to ensure that this is reapplied on a regular basis. This is one of the most popular methods used to try to break the habit.

Substitute Another Activity

In case the problem is stress or boredom related try another activity that uses the hands. The first one that springs to mind is squeezing a rubber stress ball. You need to be careful if you select substitute activities as many of these have the potential to develop into irritating habits themselves.

Increase Calcium Intake

In case calcium deficiency does play a role in your child's nail biting problem then increase the amount of calcium in their diet. High levels of calcium can be found in leafy green vegetables, nuts and seeds, dairy products and dried fruit.

Hypnotherapy

In older children you can also try hypnotherapy, but I would be very wary when searching for a suitably qualified hypnotist, especially as children are involved. I would try all other tips before embarking on this one.

THUMB-SUCKING

Introduction

Babies have a natural urge to suck. This urge usually decreases after the age of 6 months. But many babies continue to suck their thumbs to soothe themselves. Thumb-sucking can become a habit in babies and young children who use it to comfort themselves when they feel hungry, afraid, restless, quiet, sleepy, or bored.

It is normal in early infancy. It makes the older child appear immature and may interfere with normal alignment of teeth. Like any other rhythmic patterns. It can be seen as a way to securing extra self-nurturance. Emotional insecurity, feeling of isolation and boredom or stress causes thumb-sucking. Encourage child to relieve anxiety and fear. Use reward techniques when obeyed (appreciation, praising of child). If child cooperates cover the thumb using bitter edible substances.

In rare cases, thumb-sucking after age 5 is in response to an emotional problem or other disorder, such as anxiety.

Management

- *Positive reinforcement:* Praise the child or provide small rewards such as an extra bedtime story or a trip to the park, when he or she is not thumb-sucking. Place stickers on a calendar to record the days when the child successfully avoids thumb-sucking.
- *Identify triggers:* If the child sucks his or her thumb in response to stress, identify the real issue and provide comfort in other ways, such as a hug or reassuring words. Mother might also give the child a pillow or stuffed animal to squeeze.

- *Offer gentle reminders:* If the child sucks his or her thumb without thought rather than as a way to get your attention gently remind him or her to stop. Do not scold, criticize or ridicule the child. To spare embarrassment in front of others, you might alert your child to the thumb sucking with a special hand signal or other private cue.

Complication

Thumb-sucking in children younger than 4 is usually not a problem. Children who suck their thumbs often or with great intensity around age 4 or 5, or those who are still sucking their thumbs at age 6, are at risk for dental or speech problems.

Prolonged thumb-sucking may cause the teeth to become improperly aligned (malocclusion) or push the teeth outward. This usually corrects itself when the child stops thumb-sucking. But the longer thumb-sucking continues, the more likely it is that orthodontic treatment will be needed.

SLEEP DISORDERS (SOMNAMBULISM)

Introduction

A substantial portion of children have struggle around bed time (insomnia). Sleep difficulty may be a reflection of parental strife of underlying anxiety disorder such as separation anxiety disorder.

Different types of parasomnias and their management:

- Narcolepsy
- Nightmares
- Night terrors
- Sleep walking (or) somnambulism.

Night Terrors

The childhood night terrors are sudden, partial arousal associated with emotional outbursts, fear, and motor activity. Occurring most often among children ages between 4–8 years during NREM sleep, the child has no memory of night terrors once fully awake. If child experiences night terrors, make sure he or she is comfortable but do not wake the child. In extreme cases, night terrors may require medical intervention.

Somnambulism (Sleep Walking)

Somnambulism is most common among 8–12 years children. Typically, the child sits up in bed with eyes open but unseeing or may walk through the house. Their speech is mumbled and unintelligible. Take safety precautions (e.g. using a first floor bedroom), but keep efforts to intervene to a minimum. Awakening the child on a regular schedule can reduce or eliminate episodes of sleep walking.

Nighttime Bedwetting (Enuresis)

This type of bedwetting is a common sleep problem in children ages 6–12 years, occurring only during NREM sleep. Primary enuresis (the child has never been persistently dry at night) is associated with a family history of the problem, developmental lag, or lower bladder capacity, and is unlikely to signal a serious problem. Secondary enuresis (a recurrence of bedwetting after a year or more of bladder control) is more likely to be associated with emotional distress. Interventions include use of reinforcement and responsibility training (such as keeping a dry night chart), bladder control training, conditioning (e.g. bedwetting alarms), and sometimes medication. In the case of secondary enuresis it might be most helpful to determine any source of emotional stress and address it directly. (For example, if a child starts wetting the bed at night following parents' separation or divorce, providing counseling to address loss issues might help alleviate bedwetting.)

Sleep-onset Anxiety

Sleep-onset anxiety refers to difficulty falling asleep because of excessive fears or worries. The problem may be caused by stressful events or trauma or because of ruminating on more commonplace issues of the day. This type of sleep problem is most common among older elementary school children. Intervention strategies include reassurance, calming bedtime routines, and, in some cases, cognitive-behavioral therapy, which is designed to help children develop effective coping strategies to address their worries.

Obstructive Sleep Apnea

Although more common in adults, 1–3% of children experience difficulty breathing because of obstructed air passages. Symptoms include snoring, difficulty breathing during sleep, mouth breathing during sleep, or excessive daytime sleepiness. In children this type of sleep disturbance is usually not serious, but most children benefit from removal of the tonsils and adenoids. When this is not effective, the condition can be treated (by a physician) with a procedure known as nasal continuous positive airway pressure (CPAP).

Narcolepsy

Narcolepsy is a rare but potentially dangerous, neurologically based genetic condition that may include sudden sleep attacks (irresistible urges to sleep), sleep-onset paralysis, or sleep-onset hallucinations. It affects 1 of every 2,000 adults and may first appear in adolescence. If this disorder is suspected, refer to the child to a sleep specialist. Treatment may include ensuring a full 12 hours of sleep per night or more, scheduled naps, or medication.

Delayed Sleep-phase Syndrome

It is a disorder of sleep (circadian) rhythm that results in an inability to fall asleep at a normal hour (e.g. sleep onset may be delayed until 2–4 am) and results in difficulty waking up in the morning. Symptoms include excessive daytime sleepiness, sleeping until early afternoon on weekends, truancy and tardiness, and poor school performance. Treatment might include light therapy (exposure to very bright light in the morning), chronotherapy (gradually advancing the child's sleep schedule 1 hour per night until a normal routine is achieved), maintaining a consistent sleep schedule, or a short course of sedative medication to help achieve a new schedule.

TEETH GRINDING (OR) BRUXISM

It results from tension originating in unexpressed anger or resentment. It is an involuntary act usually occurs during sleep among school going children. It may create problems in dental occlusion. Helping the child to find ways to express resentment may relieve the problem. Correction of dental surfaces and counseling the child for stressors and encourage to verbalize the unexpressed angers will minimize the bruxism. Teach the child to clench teeth for 5–10 seconds and relax for several times in a week will be beneficial in reducing stressors.

PROTEIN-ENERGY MALNUTRITION (PEM)

Introduction

The World Health Organization (WHO) defines malnutrition as 'the cellular imbalance between the supply of nutrients and energy and the body's demand for them to ensure growth, maintenance, and specific functions.' The term protein-energy malnutrition (PEM) applies to a group of related disorders that include marasmus, kwashiorkor and intermediate states of marasmus-kwashiorkor.

The term marasmus is derived from the Greek word *marasmos*, which means withering or wasting. Marasmus involves inadequate intake of protein and calories and is characterized by emaciation. The term kwashiorkor is taken from the Ga language of Ghana and means 'the sickness of the weaning.' Williams first used the term in 1933, and it refers to an inadequate protein intake with reasonable caloric (energy) intake. Edema is characteristic of kwashiorkor but is absent in marasmus.

Definition

Protein-energy malnutrition (PEM) is a potentially fatal body-depletion disorder. It is the leading cause of death in children in developing countries.

Types of PEM

Primary PEM results from a diet that lacks sufficient sources of protein. Secondary PEM is more common, where it usually occurs as a complication of AIDS, cancer, chronic kidney

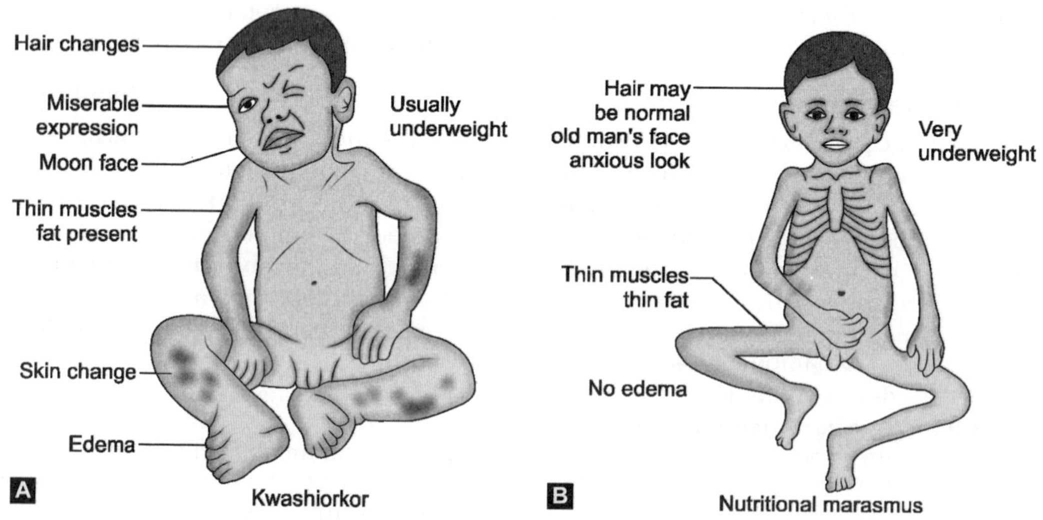

Fig. 5.35A and B: (A) Kwashiorkor; (B) Marasmus

failure, inflammatory bowel disease, and other illnesses that impair the body's ability to absorb or use nutrients or to compensate for nutrient losses. PEM can develop gradually in a child who has a chronic illness or experiences chronic semi-starvation. It may appear suddenly in a patient who has an acute illness.

- Kwashiorkor, also called wet protein-energy malnutrition, is a form of PEM characterized primarily by protein deficiency. This condition usually appears at about the age of 12 months when breastfeeding is discontinued, but it can develop at any time during a child's formative years. It causes fluid retention (edema); dry, peeling skin; and hair discoloration.
- Marasmus, a PEM disorder, is caused by total calorie/energy depletion rather than primarily protein calorie/energy depletion. Marasmus is characterized by stunted growth and wasting of muscle and tissue. Marasmus usually develops between the ages of six months and one year in children who have been weaned from breast milk or who suffer from weakening conditions such as chronic diarrhea.

Causes of Protein Energy Malnutrition

- PEM is purely due to dietary deficiency, it is termed as the primary type. This begins at the fetal stage and continues into infancy and childhood. Nearly 25% of the pediatric hospital beds in India are occupied by children suffering from malnutrition and around 80% of hospitalized children are malnourished to some extent. Hence, this contributes to the infant mortality ratio in a big way.
- Secondary malnutrition arises due to a serious illness like tuberculosis, cancer or inability of the body to absorb nutrients, e.g. in bowel disease like ulcerative colitis, metabolic syndromes and long standing gastroenteritis.
- Dietary factors contributing to PEM are inadequate breastfeeding by the mother due to inability of mother's body to make milk due to inadequate nutrition, stopping breastfeeding early in case of working mothers and inadequate supplementation of other foods, ignorance of weaning and weaning foods, inverted or cracked nipples in mother causing difficulty in breastfeeding. Another important reason is nipple confusion when the baby is switched from breast to the artificial nipple and bottle. Formula milk may not be well tolerated leading to diarrhea.
- Problems in the mother such as mental or psychiatric illnesses, postnatal depression (severe cases), poor maternal health like anemia and having too many children in quick succession or having twins may lead to the mother producing not enough milk to meet the demand of the infants.
- Traditional methods which are harmful to the baby may be practiced in villages and rural areas such as not offering colostrum (the fluid that comes out of the nipple in the first few hours after delivery) which is very healthy and boosts the baby's immune system and withholding breast milk when the baby has diarrhea. Even in remote areas, health professionals should conduct antenatal classes for mothers-to-be and educated them.
- All kinds of infections in the baby such as oral ulcers, gastroenteritis, food poisoning, diarrhea and serious conditions such as congenital heart or kidney disease may cause inability to suckle which causes malnutrition. Thus, infection and malnutrition is a vicious cycle as one contributes to the other.

- Low socioeconomic status of the people coupled with the desire to have more children (especially boys) is the social malady that many uneducated people suffer from.

Signs and Symptoms

Kwashiorkor

- Children appear smaller than their age
- Skin is pale, dry and flaky, hair turns reddish
- Muscles are limp and undeveloped
- Children frequently have digestive problems
- Fluid retention in the body causes a distended abdomen, swollen hands and ankles
- Edema
- Very thin limbs, liver may be enlarged
- Children lack enthusiasm and look unhappy.

Marasmus

This condition is generally seen in infants less than one year old. It occurs due to a deficiency of proteins, carbohydrates and fats. Marasmus is the childhood equivalent of starvation in adults and is more serious than Kwashiorkar.

Symptoms of Marasmus

- A large face over a shrunken body
- Eyes are sunken, cheeks are hollow giving a prematurely aged look
- Edema is absent, abdomen is curved inwards
- Skin is dry, loose and wrinkled due to loss of fat below the skin
- Hair may be normal or dry, thin and light colored
- Muscles are wasted and have poor tone
- Bones are prominent due to absence of fat around them.

Diagnostic Evaluation

Physical examination is performed, and these areas assessed:

- Eating habits and weight changes
- Body-fat composition and muscle strength
- Gastrointestinal symptoms
- Presence of underlying illness
- Developmental delays and loss of acquired milestones in children
- Nutritional status.

Assessment of nutritional status by:

- Comparing height and weight to standardized norms
- Calculating body mass index (BMI)
- Measuring skinfold thickness or the circumference of the upper (mid) arm.

Management

PEM children treatments are designed to provide adequate *nutrition*, restore normal body composition, and cure the condition that caused the deficiency. Tube feeding or intravenous is used to supply nutrients to patients who cannot or will not eat protein-rich foods.

Children with severe PEM, the first stage of treatment consists of correcting fluid and electrolyte imbalances, treating infection with *antibiotics* that do not affect protein synthesis, and addressing related medical problems. The second phase involves replenishing essential nutrients slowly to prevent taxing the patient's weakened system with more food than it can handle. Physical therapy may benefit patients whose muscles have deteriorated significantly.

Prognosis

Children can lose some of their body weight without side effects, but losing more than 40 percent is usually fatal. Death usually results from heart failure, an electrolyte imbalance, or low body temperature. Patients with certain symptoms, including semiconsciousness, persistent diarrhea, *jaundice*, and low blood sodium levels, have a poorer prognosis than other patients. Recovery from marasmus usually takes longer than recovery from kwashiorkor. The long-term effects of childhood malnutrition are uncertain. Some children recover completely, while others may have a variety of lifelong impairments, including an inability to properly absorb nutrients in the intestines, as well as mental retardation. The outcome appears to be related to the length and severity of the malnutrition, as well as to the age of the child when the malnutrition occurred.

Prevention

Breastfeeding a baby for at least six months is considered the best way to prevent early-childhood malnutrition. Talking to a doctor before putting a child on any kind of diet, such as vegan, vegetarian, or low-carbohydrate, can help assure that the child gets the full supply of nutrients that he or she needs.

Every child being admitted to a hospital should be screened for the presence of illnesses and conditions that could lead to PEM. The nutritional status of patients at higher-than-average risk should be more thoroughly assessed and periodically reevaluated during extended hospital stays.

Parental Education

Protein-energy malnutrition is fairly easily treated. If, however, it occurs for a prolonged period, it can have very serious and permanent health consequences. It is important to ensure that children are getting a healthy and balanced diet. Children should not be put on weight loss or other special diets without first consulting a pediatrician.

HELMINTHIC INFECTIONS

Definition

Helminthic infections are among the most common infections worldwide and affect the poorest and most deprived communities. They are transmitted by eggs present in human feces which in turn contaminate soil in areas where sanitation is poor.

Types

- The main species that infect people are the roundworm (*Ascaris lumbricoides*)
- The whipworm (*Trichuris trichiura*)
- Hookworms (*Necator americanus* and *Ancylostoma duodenale*).

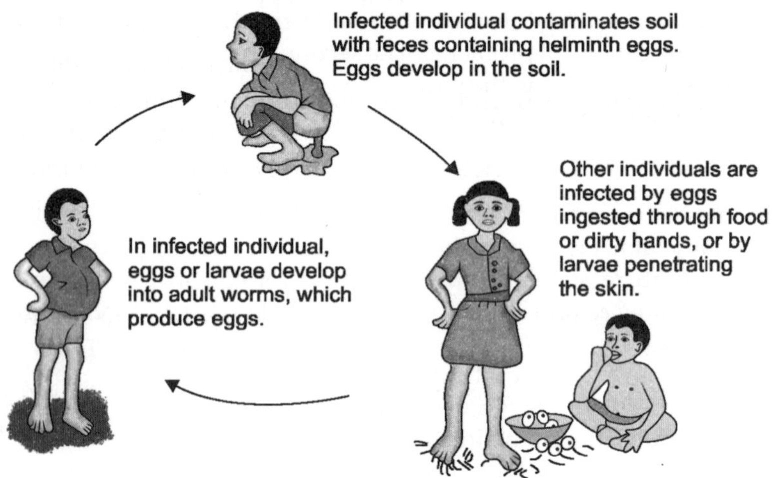

Fig. 5.36: Mode of transmission

Mode of Transmission

The helminths are transmitted by eggs that are passed in the feces of infected people. Adult worms live in the intestine where they produce thousands of eggs each day. In areas that lack adequate sanitation, these eggs contaminate the soil:

- Eggs that are attached to vegetables are ingested when the vegetables are not carefully cooked, washed or peeled
- Eggs are ingested from contaminated water sources
- Eggs are ingested by children who play in the contaminated soil and then put their hands in their mouths without washing them.

Signs and Symptoms

Child with light infections usually have no symptoms. Heavier infections can cause a range of symptoms including intestinal manifestations (diarrhea and abdominal pain), general malaise and weakness, and impaired cognitive and physical development. Hookworms cause chronic intestinal blood loss that can result in anemia.

Management

The WHO recommended medicines—albendazole (400 mg) and mebendazole (500 mg)—are effective, inexpensive and easy to administer by nonmedical personnel (e.g. teachers). They have been through extensive safety testing and have been used in millions of people with few and minor side effects.

BITES AND STINGS

Introduction

Most insect bites and stings are not poisonous but the bites of some insects such as wasps, bees and some spiders can be harmful. If a child is bitten and it is possible to save the insect, this may help with treatment if it is poisonous.

Insect bites and stings are common and usually only cause minor irritation. However, some stings can be painful and trigger a serious allergic reaction.

Signs and symptoms of insect bites and stings:

- *Poisonous stings and bites* mostly cause pain where the bite is. There is a red and swollen area around the bite.
- *Non poisonous bites* usually only cause pain and swelling around the bite at first, followed later by itching. They do not usually cause reactions away from the area of the bite unless the bite becomes infected by scratching.
- *Allergic reactions* can be caused by some insects (bees, wasps and jumper ants).
  - Common symptoms include hives, itching, stomach cramps, coughing, wheezing, difficulty breathing and swallowing, and fainting.
  - The most dangerous symptoms are breathing difficulties or drop in blood pressure (shock). Either of these can be fatal. Anaphylaxis is rare, but may be preventable and is treatable if responded to quickly.
  - A child who has severe reactions to bite or stings may need to carry an Epipen (a syringe containing adrenaline). Anyone who cares for that child (e.g. at school or child care) needs to know how to use it.

Management

- Wash the bite and sting site.
- A cold pack or ice pack can help with pain and swelling from bites.
- Rest and raise an arm or leg that has been stung to help stop swelling.
- Antihistamines may help reduce itchiness and other local symptoms (e.g swelling) if needed—ask your chemist.
- Paracetamol educe the pain (paracetamol or ibuprofen).
- If the pain is very strong and/or does not settle down within a few hours immediately admitted in the hospital.

Preventive Measures

Bee Sting

- Remove the stinger. Do not pull it out as this causes more venom to be injected. Use a blunt knife (or similar object) to scrape the stinger out.
- Child will be having more pain and swelling where the sting occurred. Ice or a cold pack usually eases the pain and the pain lasts a few hours or less.
- The child has a more severe reaction, refer to hospital.

Insect Repellents

- Children's clothing can be soaked in insect repellent.
- Use insect repellent containing 10% to 20% DEET (diethyl toluamide) or picardin on the skin, where it is not covered by clothing. Most personal spray or roll-on insect repellents from your supermarket or chemist are about this strength. Check the label or ask the chemist if unsure.
- Test on a small area of skin first to be sure there is no reaction.
- Avoid using repellents on babies and toddlers. Keep them inside if there are biting insects outside.
- Wash off insect repellent before going to bed unless there are still mosquitoes around.
- Keep repellent away from eyes and mouth and any parts of the hands that may touch eyes and mouth.
- Do not use more insect repellent than you need—it should last 4–6 hours, depending on what you are doing (e.g. swimming washes it off and you may need to apply it more often).
- Household insect sprays and electric vaporisers containing pyrethrin are safe for children (when sprayed into the air, not onto the skin).

European Wasps

- European wasps are black and yellow with colorless wings that fold alongside the body. They are about the same size as bees, but bees are more orange in color, and bees do not fold their wings.
- Native wasps look different and are not environmental pests although they can sting.
- Native wasps build their nests using mud, while European wasps build their nests of paper-like material.
- European wasp nests are always in dark places such as underground or inside walls.
- Nests of native paper wasps are also built of paper-like material but are out where you can see them, in trees or under the eaves of houses.
- Sweet foods and meats attract European wasps to picnic areas, barbecues and school yards. They may crawl into the openings of soft drink cans and bottles.

European Wasp Stings

- The biggest danger from European wasps is when their nests are disturbed. Children should be warned not to disturb their nests.
- A European wasp can sting many times, not just once like a bee.
- Wasp stings cause very painful red lumps which can be several centimeters across. After a few days the site becomes itchy. It usually gets better after a week or so.
- To reduce the pain from a sting site apply ice.
- Wasps are attracted to food and drinks. If they are not noticed, they can sting a person in the mouth or throat which can cause breathing problems.
- Drinking from glass containers not straight from a can and using a straw lessens the risk of swallowing a wasp.
- If stung in the mouth or throat, or if there is a reaction in any part of the body away from the sting, or if there are a lot of stings get medical treatment urgently.

Fleas

- Fleas are small, brown, wingless insects about 1.5 mm to 4 mm in size. They have long hind legs to enable them to jump up to 2 meters.
- Fleas breed in the fur of animals and feed off their blood. The dark 'spots' that you sometimes see around fleas are undigested blood that the fleas have eaten and passed.
- Flea eggs fall off animals and can collect around animal bedding and resting places.
- Larvae (baby fleas) feed off food scraps, animal and human skin scales and flea poo. Adult fleas feed off blood and they sometimes bite people as well as animals.
- Flea bites on people are usually found on the lower legs and feet.
- People and animals often become sensitive to the bites, causing intense itching.
- If fleas get onto a child, stand her in a bath with clothing on, then gradually remove clothing. The fleas will jump into the water and drown.

Prevention and Control of Fleas

- Regularly vacuum floors and any areas where animals rest or sleep.
- Wash animal bedding in hot water regularly. Treat with insecticides if necessary.
- Treat animals for fleas and keep pets out of the house if there is an outbreak.
- Animals with fleas should also be treated for tapeworm.
- If fleas are persistent, you may have to treat floors and animal bedding with insecticide.
- A pest control operator or your local council can give advice in difficult cases.

Jellyfish

- Jellyfish can give painful stings, usually causing a rash.
- For stings in *Southern waters,* a cold pack is most useful. Ice should not be used. Vinegar is not recommended. Reactions away from the sting (anywhere else in the body) in sensitive people need urgent medical attention.
- *Box Jellyfish* which are found in northern Australia are extremely dangerous and the seas, even puddles left by the tide, are not safe for children.
  - The official 'stinger' season for the Northern Territory is from 1 October until 1 June. However stings have been recorded in all months of the year.
  - If someone is stung by a Box jelly fish—remove him from the water, douse the sting area in vinegar, apply a cold pack, keep the person still. Get medical help urgently.

Caterpillars

- Hairy caterpillars, including 'spitfires' can cause severe itch if the hairs get into the skin and then break off.
- Wash clean and apply a cold pack to reduce the itch.

Centipedes

- Centipedes may bite if you touch them. Bites are hardly ever serious but cause severe burning pain. The area around the bite may feel numb.
- Use an ice pack or a cold pack for the pain and raise the arm or leg where the bite is to help prevent swelling. Seek medical help, if the bite becomes infected, e.g. gets very red, swollen, or oozes pus.

Scorpions

- Scorpions will sting if disturbed. Stings are hardly ever serious in Australia but they can cause severe pain, swelling and redness.
- Use an ice pack or a cold pack for the pain and raise the arm or leg where the bite is to help prevent swelling. Seek medical help, if the pain and swelling are severe.

Ants

- Nearly most of all kinds of ant can bite or sting the children.
- Ant bites can hurt for some hours and be red and swollen.
- Sometimes ant bites can cause allergic reactions (any reaction that is away from where the bite is) and need immediate medical attention.

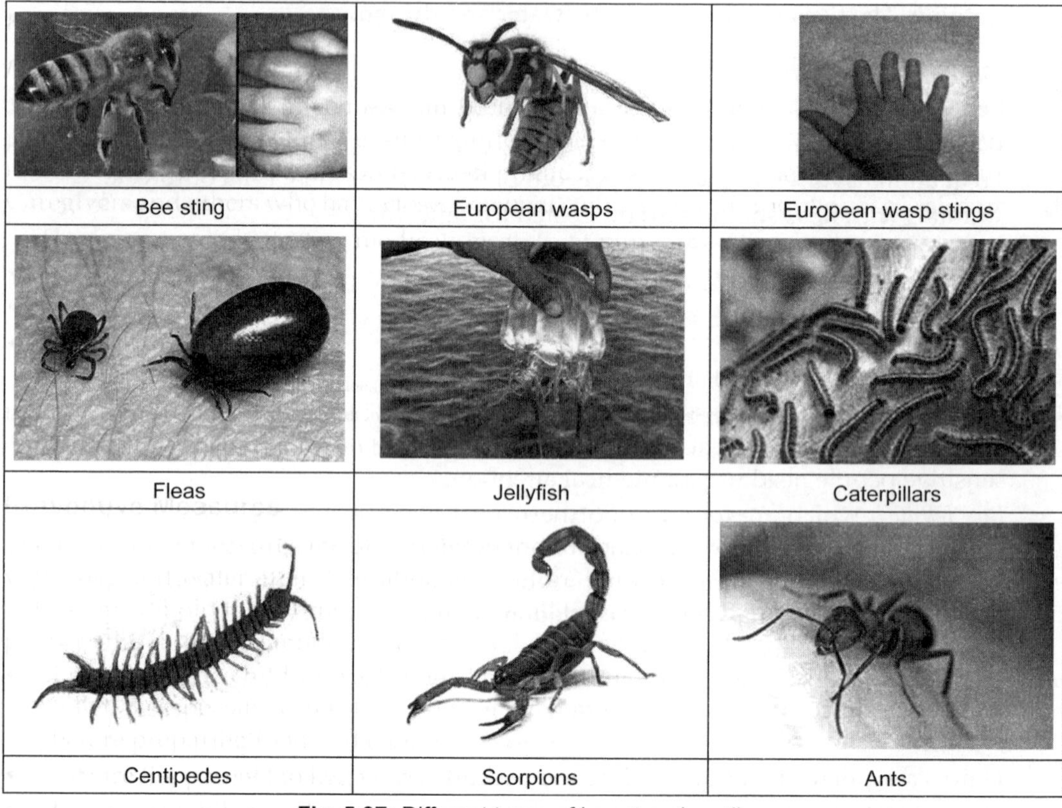

Fig. 5.37: Different types of insect and reptiles

PICA

Definition

This disorder involves repeated or chronic ingestion of nonnutrient or nonedible substances. This may include:

- Charcoal, clay, wool, ashes, paint.
- Earth, the age of onset is usually 1–2 years. Pica after the second year of the life needs investigation.

Causes of Pica

The causes of pica are not fully understood. It happens more often when children have some major problems such as:

- Intellectual disability: People with severe disability are more likely to develop the habit
- Autism
- Neglect or abuse: Pica can sometimes happen when children are not being properly cared for.

Some children who have this habit have low levels of iron or zinc in their bodies. Low zinc levels may lead to changes in the senses of taste and smell. Adults with low zinc levels have reported that food has odd and unpleasant tastes. Things which are not food may taste better if zinc levels are low.

Psychological Theories of Pica

- Mental retardation
- Family disorganization
- Poor supervision
- Low socioeconomic status.

Nutritional Theories of Pica

The deficiencies of such substances as iron and zinc produce creating for substances like ice or dirt. These theories do not have much support. Children with pica are at increased risk for lead poisonings and parasitic infestations.

Signs and Symptoms

- Complaints of abdominal pain
- Pallor, anemic, slow in motor and mental development, neurological deficit
- Deviant behaviors.

Complications

- Bezoar (a mass of indigestible material trapped inside the body, usually in the stomach)
- Infection
- Intestinal blockage
- Lead poisoning
- Malnutrition.

Management

Pica can be treated with a combination of education and guidance, family counseling and behavior modification involves behaviors, the environment, and family education.

- One form of treatment associates the pica behavior with negative consequences or punishment (mild aversion therapy).
- Then the person gets rewarded for eating normal foods.
- Nutritional and emotional needs to be met.
- Supplementary with iron to treat iron deficiency anemia.
- Regular meal pattern can be implemented.

TICS

Definition

Tics involve repetitive movement of muscle group that have no apparent useful function and represent discharges of tension originating in emotional and physical states. Parts of the body most frequently involved are muscles of face, neck, shoulders, trunk and hands.

Types of tics are motor and vocal tics.

- Motor tics involve repetitive motor movements, e.g. grimacing, blinking, stamping, jumping, tongue protrusion.
- Vocal tics involve repetitive vocalizations and sounds, e.g. sniffing, coughing, barking, throat clearing.
- Tics that involve movements are called **motor tics** and those that are sounds are called **vocal tics**. Tics can be either **simple** or **complex**:
  - Simple motor tics involve a single muscle group.
  - Complex motor tics usually involve more than one muscle group.
  - Complex vocal tics involve more meaningful speech (such as words) than simple vocal tics.
  - Complex motor tics are not as rapid as simple motor tics and can even look like the person is performing the tic on purpose.

These short-lasting sudden movements (motor tics) or uttered sounds (vocal tics) occur suddenly during what is otherwise normal behavior. Tics are often repetitive, with numerous successive occurrences of the same action. For instance, someone with a tic might blink his eyes multiple times or twitch her nose repeatedly.

Motor tics can be classified as either simple or complex. Simple motor tics may include movements such as eye-blinking, nose-twitching, head-jerking, or shoulder-shrugging. Complex motor tics consist of a series of movements performed in the same order. For instance a person might reach out and touch something repeatedly or kick out with one leg and then the other

Causes

- Tics may be caused by extreme stress.
- Some medications including Ritalin, Dexedrine, and Adderall (stimulants), or Tegretol may cause them.
- On rare occasions infections that involve the brain (encephalitis) may be associated with tics.
- Other genetic and metabolic disorders, mostly those that affect the basal ganglia may be associated with tics or with tic-like phenomenon.
- Streptococcal infections have been associated with the development of tics and obsessive-compulsive behaviors.
- Pediatric autoimmune neuropsychiatric disorders associated with streptococcal infections, is a known entity in which the antibodies to the streptococcal bacteria attack the basal ganglia causing the above-mentioned symptoms.
- Tics must be differentiated from chorea. Chorea is a movement disorder that unlike tics, cannot be reproduced by an observer, is more difficult to suppress, and is incorporated into voluntary movements. Rarely, some seizures may be brief and rapid imitating tic disorders.

Common Motor Tics

- Nose wrinkling
- Head twitching
- Eye blinking
- Lip biting
- Facial grimacing
- Repetitive or obsessive touching
- Kicking
- Jumping.

Common vocal tics include:

- Coughing
- Throat clearing
- Grunting
- Sniffing
- Barking
- Hissing.

Management

- *Behavioral Therapy:* The best-known behavioral treatment for tic disorders is a form of cognitive-behavioral therapy (CBT) called habit reversal training. A child is taught to recognize the premonitory urge that precedes an oncoming tic, and to identify the situations that may trigger the tics. The child and therapist develop a 'competing' response an action the child performs when he feels the urge that is incompatible with the tic, and less noticeable to others. For example, a child whose tic involves sniffling his nose may do a breathing exercise instead. Children may also be taught relaxation techniques to decrease the frequency of the tics.
- *Pharmacological:* There are a variety of medications commonly prescribed to help control the symptoms of tic disorder, and an experienced professional should closely monitor any course. Doctor prescribes neuroleptic medications, which appear to help control tics by blocking the brain's dopamine neurotransmitters. For example, drugs such as haloperidol, pimozide or clonidine can be used.

ADOLESCENT DISORDERS AND HEALTH PROBLEMS

PRECOCIOUS PUBERTY

Introduction

Precocious puberty is when a child's body begins changing into that of an adult (puberty) too soon. Puberty that begins before age 8 in girls and before age 9 in boys is considered precocious puberty.

Puberty includes rapid growth of bones and muscles, changes in body shape and size, and development of the body's ability to reproduce.

Definition

Precocious puberty is defined as appearance of physical and hormonal signs of pubertal development at an earlier age than is considered to normal age.

Causes

The onset of puberty is normally triggered by the hypothalamus (the area of the brain that helps control pituitary gland function). It signals the pituitary gland (a pea-sized gland near the base of the brain) to release hormones that stimulate the ovaries (in girls) or testicles (in boys) to make sex hormones.

Sometimes, precocious puberty stems from a structural problem in the brain (such as a tumor), brain injury due to head trauma, an infection (such as meningitis), or a problem in the ovaries or thyroid gland that triggers the onset of puberty ahead of schedule but this usually is not the case.

Signs and Symptoms

In girls, the telltale signs of precocious puberty include any of the following before 7 or 8 years of age:

- Breast development
- Pubic or underarm hair development
- Rapid height growth—a growth 'spurt'
- Start of menstruation (her period)
- Acne
- 'Mature' body odor.

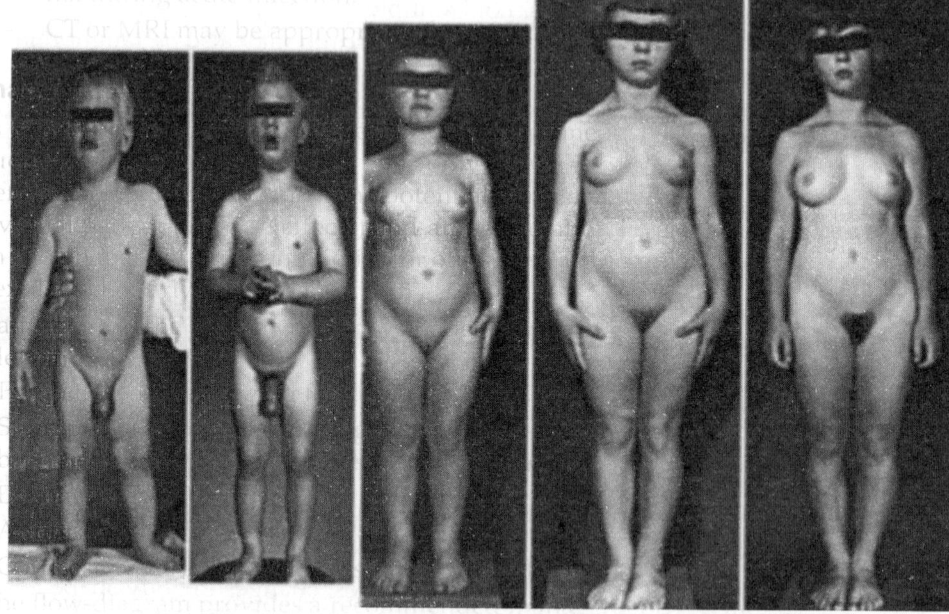

Fig. 5.38: Anatomical difference between male and female precocious puberty

In boys, the signs of precocious puberty before 9 years of age include:

- Enlargement of the testicles or penis
- Pubic, underarm, or facial hair development
- Rapid height growth—a growth 'spurt'
- Voice deepening
- Acne
- 'Mature' body odor.

Diagnostic Evaluation

- *A physical exam:* To evaluate any changes in the body.
- *A family history:* To find out if early puberty might run in the family.
- *Blood tests:* Which check a child's hormone and sometimes thyroid test.
- *X-rays:* Usually of the hand and wrist, to check a child's bone age. This is a way of seeing how quickly he or she is growing.
- Ultrasounds
- *Image study:* Imaging and scanning tests such as CT scans, MRIs (magnetic resonance imaging), and ultrasound studies can help rule out specific causes of precocious puberty, such as a tumor in the brain, ovary, or testicle.

Management

The goal of treating it is to stop or even reverse sexual development and stop the rapid growth and bone maturation that can eventually result in adult short stature.

There are two possible approaches to treatment:

1. Treating the underlying cause or disease, such as a tumor
2. Lowering the high levels of sex hormones with medicine to stop sexual development from progressing.

Treatment of a related health problem can stop the precocious puberty. But in most cases, no other disease is triggering the condition, so treatment usually involves hormone therapy to stop sexual development.

The currently approved hormone treatment is with drugs called LHRH analogs—synthetic hormones that block the body's production of the sex hormones that cause the early puberty. Dramatic results are usually seen within a year of starting treatment with an LHRH analog, which is generally safe and usually causes no side effects in kids.

GYNECOMASTIA

Introduction

Gynecomastia is a benign enlargement of the male breast (usually bilateral but sometimes unilateral) a proliferation of the glandular component of the breast (see the image below). It is defined clinically by the presence of a rubbery or firm mass extending concentrically from the nipples. Gynecomastia should be differentiated from pseudogynecomastia (lipomastia), which is characterized by fat deposition without glandular proliferation.

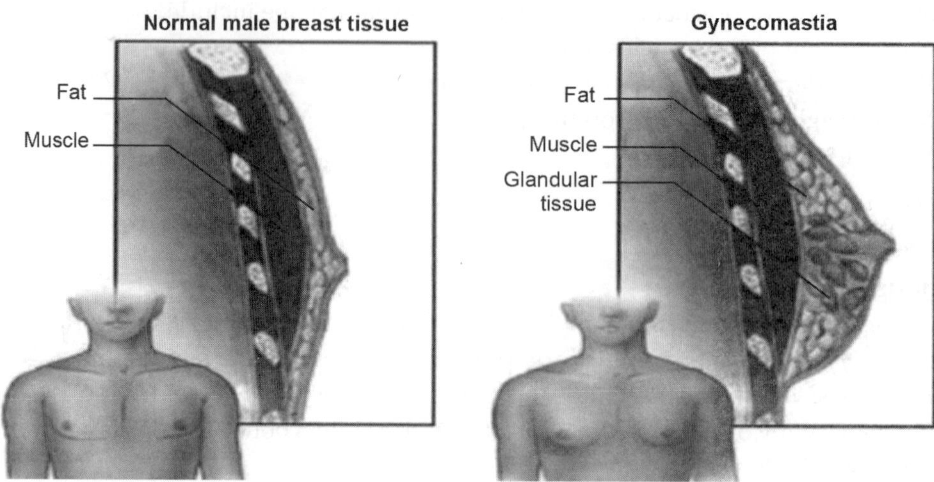

Fig. 5.39: Anatomical difference between male normal and gynecomastia breast

Definition

Gynecomastia is defined as overdevelopment of the male breast. In response to too much estrogen (a female hormone) or too little testosterone (a male hormone), the glandular tissue of the breast swells and forms a breast bud (enlarged breast). Gynecomastia can occur in babies, teen boys and older men.

Classification of gynecomastia with four grades of severity:

1. *Grade I:* Minimal hypertrophy (< 250 g) without ptosis
2. *Grade II:* Moderate hypertrophy (250–500 g) without ptosis
3. *Grade III:* Severe hypertrophy (> 500 g) with grade I ptosis
4. *Grade IV:* Severe hypertrophy with grade II or grade III ptosis

Causes

- *Newborns:* Gynecomastia is caused by estrogen from the mother. Breast buds are common in baby boys. Breast buds tend to go away gradually by 6 months of age, but they can last longer in some babies.
- *Preteen boys:* Gynecomastia can also be caused by an estrogen-producing tumor. Breast buds are common during puberty. The buds may last up to 2 years, but they tend to go away within the first year.
- *Teen boys:* Gynecomastia is caused by the hormonal changes of puberty. Gynecomastia occurs in many boys during early puberty to middle puberty. It usually goes away within 6 months to 2 years.
- *Adult males:* Gynecomastia is usually caused by another condition, such as liver or lung cancer, cirrhosis of the liver, overactive thyroid, or by hormone problems, such as cancer of the pituitary gland, adrenal glands, or testicles. Alcohol, marijuana, methamphetamine, and heroin use also may cause gynecomastia.

Certain medicines also cause gynecomastia including:
- Steroids, such as prednisone or dexamethasone
- Medicines used to treat ulcers (such as cimetidine)
- Medicines used to treat epilepsy (such as phenytoin)
- Digitalis and other heart medicines
- Chemotherapy drugs
- Antiandrogen drugs (such as flutamide, cyproterone, and spironolactone)
- Antianxiety and antidepressant medicines (such as diazepam and tricyclic antidepressant).

Signs and Symptoms

- Age of onset and duration of the condition
- Any recent changes in nipple size and any pain or discharge from the nipples
- History of mumps, testicular trauma, alcohol use, or drug use
- Family history of gynecomastia
- History of sexual dysfunction, infertility or hypogonadism.

Diagnostic Evaluation

Laboratory tests:
- Serum chemistry panel
- Free or total testosterone
- Luteinizing hormone (LH), estradiol, and dehydroepiandrosterone sulfate levels
- Thyroidstimulating hormone (TSH) and free thyroxine levels.

Imaging studies:
- *Mammography:* Indicated if one or more features of breast cancer are apparent upon clinical examination, followed by fine-needle aspiration or breast biopsy as appropriate.
- *Testicular ultrasonography:* Indicated if the serum estradiol level is elevated and the clinical examination findings suggest the possibility of a testicular neoplasm.
- *Breast ultrasonography* (though the positive predictive value of imaging in males is low).
- *CT:* Gynecomastia is often reported on CT scans.

Management

General managements:
- There is no treatment is required for physiologic gynecomastia
- Pubertal Gynecomastia resolves spontaneously within several weeks to 3 years in most patients; breasts larger than 4 cm in diameter may not regress completely
- Identifying and managing an underlying primary disorder often alleviates breast enlargement
- The patients with idiopathic Gynecomastia or with residual Gynecomastia after treatment of the primary cause, medical or surgical treatment may be considered
- If medical therapies are used, they should be tried early in the condition's course.

Pharmacologic agents:
- Clomiphene
- Tamoxifen
- Danazol (less frequently used).

Surgical Management
- *Reduction mammoplasty:* Considered in cases of macromastia, long-standing Gynecomastia, or failed medical therapy, as well as for cosmetic reasons
- *Plastic surgery:* Gynecomastia or excessive sagging of the breast tissue from weight loss
- Endoscopic subcutaneous mastectomy, without skin excision.

Surgical complications:
- Sloughing of tissue due to a compromised blood supply
- Contour irregularity
- Hematoma or seroma formation
- Permanent numbness in the nipple-areolar area.

ACCIDENT/SPORTS INJURIES

Introduction
Accident or sports injuries are commonly classified based on 'intentionality'. Most road traffic injuries, poisoning, falls, fire and burn injuries, and drowning are unintentional. Intentional injuries include interpersonal violence (homicide, sexual assault, neglect and abandonment, and other maltreatment), suicide, and collective violence (war). Evidence suggests that some children and adolescents are more vulnerable to certain types of accident/sports injuries.

Types
- Poisoning
- Foreign bodies
- Drowning
- Burns
- Sports injuries.

While road traffic accidents, interpersonal violence and sports injuries tend to affect older children and adolescents. In addition, injuries tend to be more prevalent in boys.

Causes/Risk Factors
In the rural areas:
- Farming activities
- Pesticide poisoning
- Drowning.

In the urban areas:
- Road traffic accident/injuries
- Linked to gadgets
- Electrical appliances
- Falls or poisonings
- Household chemicals and pharmaceuticals ingested by small children.

Social factors:
- Family stress
- Critical life events (e.g. Hospitalization or chronic disease of a parent, or change of residence)
- Home and school construction
- Furnishing materials can lead to unintentional injuries
- Poisoning may result from exposure to chemicals unsafely used or stored
- Intentional injuries resulting from child maltreatment
- Poor parenting skills
- Marital conflict
- Lack of social support systems for families
- Urban transport services.

POISONING IN CHILDREN

Introduction

Ingestion of toxic substances is a common problem in the pediatric age group. The inherent curiosity and tendency for exploration in children contributes to the high incidence of accidental poisoning in children below five years. The poisoning in children could occur due to diverse causes and could be classified as accidental, homicidal or suicidal. Whereas in a majority of cases poisoning is accidental, there are occasional instances of homicidal and suicidal poisoning. Erroneous administration of over dosage of drugs by the parents or by the medical staff is also frequent. Poisoning is usually seen in children less then 6 years of age, being more common between 1 and 3 years.

Most cases of poisoning are from substances available in the home environment. Ingestion or exposure occurs chiefly because of improper storage. Toxic substances are often stored in containers meant for food. Common substances that account for poisoning are listed.

Types of Poisoning

Chemical Poisoning

- Household cleaners
- Bleach
- Detergents
- Fuel (Kerosene, paraffin)
- Cosmetics, medicines, paints.

Households Poisoning

The house hold poisoning could either be a nontoxic ingestion or toxic ingestion.

- Nontoxic ingestion:
  - Nonedible product
  - Cosmetics, candles, chalk
  - Erasers, ball-point pen, ink
  - Lubricants, etc.

- Toxic ingestion:
  - Soap and detergents
  - Shampoos, bleaches
  - Disinfectants, deodorizers
  - Acids and alkalis
  - Cosmetics, Nail polish remover
  - Disk batteries, Naphthalene
  - Tobacco product, Pica.

Certain Medications are Become Poisoning

- Aspirin, iron, paracetamol
- Insecticides
- Hydrocarbons
- Kerosene oil
- Solvents, polish varnish, detergents.

Pattern of Accidental Poisoning

- Kerosene and other hydrocarbons
- Poisonous plants and seeds
- Household medicines (opium, lithium, belladonna compounds)
- Food poisoning, venomous bites and stings
- Miscellaneous—lead pencils, matches, cigarette, and mercury of thermometer.

Causes of Poisoning

- *Age:* 40% of all cases accidental poisoning 2 years (Toddler)
  - 12% (1 year child) age group
  - 20% 3 year ages group
  - More active male–child
- *Large families:* In large families the mother is often too occupied with household works, is easily fatigued and often caviled in storage of potentially poisonous things.

Small accommodation:

- There is like storage factory
- Over crowded houses
- To greater risk of poisoning.

Environment:

- Lead poisoning
- Workshops for repair of old automobile
- Lead storage batteries
- Printing presses, insecticides, medicines, kerosene.
- Rural or urban area:
  - Rural—chemical, plant, self, animal
  - Urban—chemical, rare in others.

Grading of Poisoning

None	0	No symptoms or sign, vague symptom judged not to be related to poisoning
Minor	1	Transient and spontaneously resolving symptoms
Moderate	2	Pronounced or prolonged symptom
Severe	3	Severe or life threatening symptoms

Signs and Symptoms and Management

Poison	Signs and symptoms	Management
Arsenic (Rat Poison)	Abdominal pain, vomiting, bloody diarrhea, cardiovascular collapse	Gut decontamination (stomach wash), supportive care, medicine (dimercaprol 3/5 mg/kg/dose IM every 4 hours for additional 2 days and every 12 hours for up to 7 additional days
Phenol	Local burns, nausea, vomiting, bloody diarrhea, convulsion's pulmonary edema, cardiorespiratory depression	Dilution with water or milk, then give activated charcoal and olive oil 30 ml stat and 10 ml every hourly
Camphor	Nausea, vomiting, epigastric pain, muscular irritability, seizures	Gut decontamination. Charcoal activation
Naphthalene	Nausea, vomiting, hemoglobinuria, pain, jaundice, acute tubular	Gut decontamination, forced alkaline dieresis, blood transfusion for necrosis
Copper sulfate	Burning pain in mouth and throat, vomiting, watery or bloody diarrhea, hemolysis, jaundice, collapse, convulsions	Water, milk, egg white per oral, gut decontamination, BAL, (See doses given in arsenic poisoning) or penicillamine 100 mg/kg/day (max 1 gm) PO divided use dose should not exceed 10 mg/kg/day
Castor seeds, chandrajyoti seeds	Violent vomiting, abdominal pain, bloody diarrhea	IV fluids, gut decontamination, blood transfusion if required
Yellow and white oleander seeds	Dysphagia, burning in throat, vomiting, abdominal pain, diarrhea, varying degree of heart block, muscular twitching, drowsiness, lock jaw with white seeds	Gut decontamination, treatment for heart block, IV fluids and other

Diagnostic Evaluation

The diagnosis and treatment of poisoning depends upon the type of poisoning and its severity, the latter depends on the amount of substance ingested and the age of the patient. A good detailed, urgent management and life-saving measures take precedence.

Examination

Vital parameters of respiration, pulse, BP and temperature, and level of consciousness are assessed. A thorough systematic examination is done particularly observing the pupillary size, oral cavity, breath odor, skin color, sweating, and any marks of injury, pigmentation, secretions from oral nasal orifices and abdominal examination for peristaltic activity and urinary retention.

Management

Laboratory Investigations

The laboratory investigations are carried out to estimate the serum levels of the drugs and poisons. Serial estimation of the level of the drugs or poisons is essential to predict the prognosis and for assessing the effectiveness of intervention. Estimation of the blood levels of glucose, bicarbonate, urea creatinine, electrolytes and transaminase may be necessary to determine the toxicity of various drugs.

Radiological interventions do not have much role in poisonings. Plain radiograph of the abdomen may be useful to look for unabsorbed medications, or metals like iron, lead, etc.

First Aid Management

- Surface decontamination of poisons absorbed through the skin.
- Emesis, other than substances for which emesis is contraindicated; vomiting is effective if induced within 30 min of ingestion. Emesis can be induced with syrup of ipecac or tickling the posterior pharyngeal wall.
- Patients should be transported to the nearest medical care facility if poisoning is suspected.

Treatment

The initial treatment consists of managing the airway breathing and circulation. If the child is stupors or comatose, it is better to take care of the airway by inserting an appropriate size endotracheal tube so airway is secured and chances of aspiration minimized. In comatose patients, a bolus of 2 ml/kg of 25% dextrose may be given. In adolescents and malnourished children, a thiamine dose of 50 to 100 mg is intramuscularly or intravenously to avoid precipitating acute Wernicke's encephalopathy.

Preventive Measures

Childhood poisoning is an avoidable calamity. Poisonous substances should be kept away from the reach of the children by ensuring their proper storage. Poisonous substances and drugs should be kept in childproof containers and locked away.

SPECIFIC DRUGS POISONS AND MANAGEMENT

Acetaminophen (Paracetamol)

Acetaminophen is a commonly prescribed medication in children and easily available over the counter. Either due to wrong interpretation of the prescription or due to self-medication over dosage may result. An adolescent is much more likely to be symptomatic than a child of less than 6 years for similar blood drug level.

Paracetamol is rapidly absorbed on oral administration. Over dosage leads to hepatic glutathione depletion resulting in production of acetamidoquinone which combines with the liver macromolecules and causes hepatocellular damage. These changes are reversible.

Clinical Features

Initially there is nausea, vomiting, malaise and diaphoresis. The liver enzymes SGOT, SGPT levels are increased. In severe cases, a prolongation of prothrombin time and increase in serum bilirubin levels may occur. Rarely fulminant hepatic failure may develop. Where history of paracetamol ingestion is not forthcoming, Reye's syndrome, infective hepatitis, idiosyncrasy to medications or consumption of other drugs like carbon tetrachloride may be considered.

Management

A child has consumed only a small quantity, the child can be safely observed at home. If there is alteration of consciousness he or she needs to be admitted. Investigations at admission and follow-up are measurement of blood SGOT, SGPT, bilirubin, prothrombin time and creatinine.

The general measures should be instituted following admission to the hospital. Gastric lavage and installation of activated charcoal can be done since it adsorbs paracetamol. The specific antidote is n-acetylcysteine.

Salicylates

Salicylate poisoning was common but with awareness of its potential association with Reye's syndrome, aspirin usage has become less frequent.

Clinical Features

Initial clinical features of toxicity include vomiting, dehydration and increase in the respiratory rate. Further stages are characterized by hyperpnea, restlessness, delirium and convulsions; lethargy, drowsiness and coma may supervene. Chief biochemical features include metabolic acidosis, hypoglycemia and ketonemia. The urine ferric chloride test may be positive. Serum salicylate levels may be elevated. There may be evidence of metabolic acidosis, elevated liver enzymes and prolonged prothrombin time.

Treatment

Stomach wash should be done with normal saline or weak sodium bicarbonate solution. Activated charcoal (1 g/kg) adsorbs aspirin well. Forced alkaline diuresis may be used to enhance excretion. A suitable infusion fluid is N/5 saline to which sodium bicarbonate is added at the rate of 1–2 mEq/kg every 1 to 2 hours so that the urine pH is maintained above 7.5 to 8.

Vitamin K may be administered if prothrombin time is prolonged. Supportive management of renal and hepatic failure is necessary. Hemodialysis results in satisfactory salicylate clearance. Patients with prolonged seizures, severe hypoglycemia or visceral bleeding have poor outcome.

Iron

Iron is an important toxicologic hazard because of its easy availability and brightly colored formulations. Ingestion up to 25 mg/kg of elemental iron does cause any problems. Higher ingestions are potentially serious.

Clinical Features

The first symptoms of iron poisoning are gastrointestinal the child manifests with symptoms of nausea, vomiting, diarrhea and pain in abdomen with onset within 30 min to 6 hours of ingestion. Subsequently the patient improves with abatement of symptoms. Gastrointestinal losses, increased capillary permeability, metabolic acidosis and myocardial dysfunction lead to circulatory shock characterized by hypoperfusion and hypotension.

Thrombocytopenia and hypoprothrombinemia may also occur. Hepatocellular necrosis or hepatic failure is an important cause of mortality. The corrosive effect iron lead to scarring chiefly in the prepyloric region or in the duodenum leading to gastrointestinal obstruction.

Laboratory Investigations

Serum iron levels may be elevated; levels exceeding 400 μg/dl within 4 hours of ingestion are associated with toxicity. Levels above 1000 (μg/dl are usually fatal. Blood glucose levels may initially be elevated, metabolic acidosis is frequent. Tablets or capsules may be seen as radiopaque shadows on a plain radiographic film.

Treatment

Ingestion up to 25 mg/kg need not be treated unless symptomatic. Symptoms suggestive of significant ingestion include lethargy, obtundation, hypoperfusion, oliguria, tachycardia and tachypnea. Children with serum iron more than 500 μg/dl or more than 300 μg/dl with laboratory abnormalities should receive specific therapy. All other patients otherwise receive general measures for poison treatment.

Emesis is induced with syrup of ipecac if seen within 1–2 hours of ingestion. Lavage is indicated even if emesis has been induced since emesis alone may not lead to significant removal of the iron tablets. One hundred ml of milk of magnesia or 100 ml of 5 percent sodium bicarbonate solution can be left in the stomach to protect the denuded gastric mucosa and ionize the residual iron to prevent its absorption.

The child may require treatment with intravenous fluids and inotropic drugs. Acidosis, electrolyte disturbances and hypoglycemia need to be managed appropriately. Occasionally surgery in the form of gastrostomy has been used when lavage has not been successful and radiological localization indicates presence of a large number of tablets. Hemodialysis is not required, as glomerular filtration is effective in clearing the desferrioxamine-iron complex but may be used in case of renal failure.

FOREIGN BODIES

FOREIGN BODIES IN THE RESPIRATORY TRACT

Introduction

Aspiration of foreign bodies into the respiratory passages is encountered quite commonly in children and presents as a surgical emergency with features of acute airway obstruction.

The larynx in relatively narrower than the trachea. Hence, only those foreign bodies which can go across the vocal cords and larynx can enter the trachea and bronchus. The larger ones either get entrapped at the level of the local cords or slip down into the esophagus.

The trachea bifurcates into the right and left main bronchi at the carina. In neonates the angles of bifurcation is almost equal. However, with growth the bronchi bifurcate at unequal angles and the configuration becomes similar to that in adults by 10–12 years, i.e. the right main bronchus is almost in line with the trachea and the left main bronchus takes off at an acute angle. Thus in hunger children foreign bodies may be found with equal frequency in the right and left bronchi but in older children the foreign bodies find their way into the right main bronchus more easily.

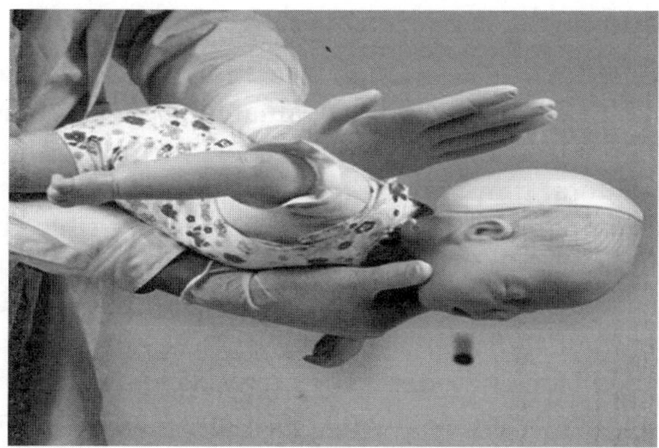

Types of Foreign Bodies

- Seeds
- Nuts
- Other vegetable foreign bodies, e.g. peanuts, sunflower seeds, sater melon seeds, castor seeds, pieces of treated betel nut, etc.

It causes a severe inflammatory reaction because of various chemical components of the vegetable matter. The resultant edema further compromises the lumen and the mucosa bleeds easily on touch. With a long standing foreign body exuberant granulation tissue develops around it leading to complete obstruction, collapse an bronchiectasis.

More often than not foreign bodies cause partial obstruction with a ball valve like mechanism leading to air trapping and obstructive emphysema. Pneumomediastinum and pneumothorax secondary to obstructive emphysema.

Signs and Symptoms

The most common presentation is history of sudden choking and coughing while playing or feeding followed by wheezing, paroxysmal coughing with or without fever and evidences of respiratory distress. The classical clinical trial of cough, sneeze and unilateral restriction of air entry is highly suggestive of foreign body in the airways.

Complications of long standing foreign bodies in the respiratory tract viz. repeated pneumonia, lung abscess, atelectasis and bronchiectasis is a less common mode of presentation. The exact clinical picture may vary with the site of foreign body enlodgement.

- *Larynx:* The onset is dramatic. There is sudden choking, aphonia and stridor or violent inspiratory efforts. Death follows rapidly at impaction is complete.
- *Trachea:* Foreign bodies between the larynx and carina give rise to spasmodic paroxysmal coughing and wheezing. A characteristic thud can be appreciated on auscultation with a freely mobile foreign body. Hoarseness, hemoptysis, cyanosis and dyspnea may be preset. Sometimes after the initial acute discomfort the child presents with a laryngotracheobronchitis or a bronchiolitis type of clinical picture.
- *Bronchus:* The large majority of inhaled foreign bodies find their way into one of the bronchi. There is a variable degree of tachypnea, cough and wheezing. Auscultation reveals restriction of air entry on the side of foreign body enlodgement. Prolonged impaction may lead to pneumonitis and bronchiectasis.

Diagnostic Evaluation

The diagnosis of foreign body inhalation is based on clinical features. Investigations are required to localize the foreign body and to evaluate the effect on the respiratory tract.

- *X-ray:* A plain anteroposterior X-ray of the chest including the neck and diaphragm usually suffices; a lateral film may be required if the foreign body is suspected to be in the larynx. Radio-opaque foreign bodies are easily visible collapse, consolidation, pneumonic patches. Pneumomediastinum and pneumothorax are also easy to discern. Bronchiectasis changes may develop with long standing of foreign bodies.
- *CT scan and ventilation/perfusion scintigraphy:* It is not required in the emergency evaluation of inhaled foreign bodies. They may have a role in the evaluation of long standing foreign bodies to assess the physical and functional state of the underlying lung. In very acute cases the patient may have to be rushed to the operation theater for a diagnostic-cum-therapeutic bronchoscopy.

Management

Home Management

Home remedies viz hanging the child upside down, thumping over the back. Grouping with fingers in the pharynx, backflows, chest thrusts, etc. may produce sustained pressure to facilitate expulsion of the foreign body but are fraught with danger because such maneuvers often cause the foreign body to get-impacted more firmly and hence are not recommended. However, a large air flow and increased expel the foreign body by either subdiaphragmatic pressure or by encircling the patient in the prone position from behind with clasped hands while pushing and kneading the abdominal contents sharply up into the epigastria towards chest.

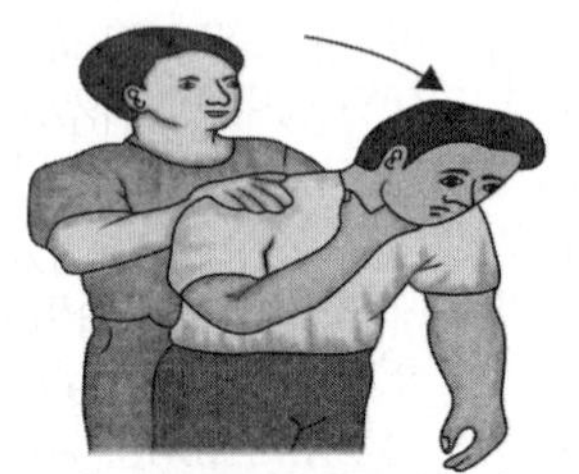

1. Lean the person forward slightly and stand behind him or her.

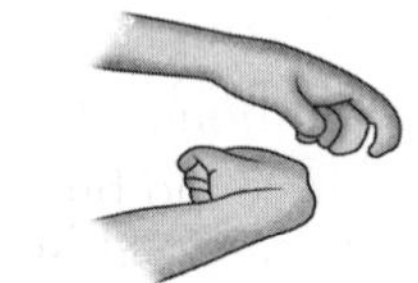

2. Make a fist with one hand.

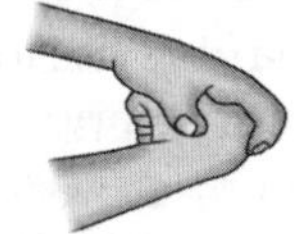

3. Put your arms around the person and grasp your fist with your other hand near the top of the stomach, just below the center of the rib cage.

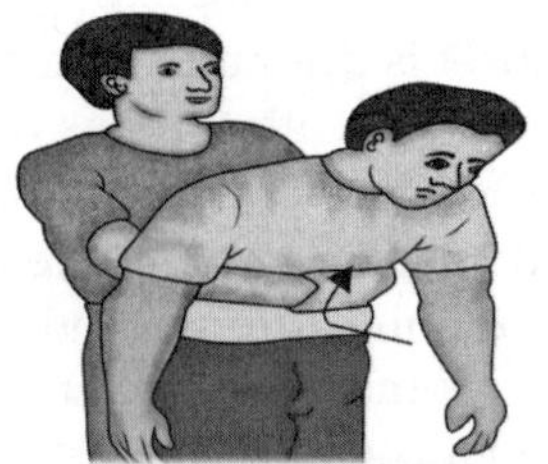

4. Make a quick, hard movement, inward and upward.

Fig. 5.40: Heimlich maneuver

Children

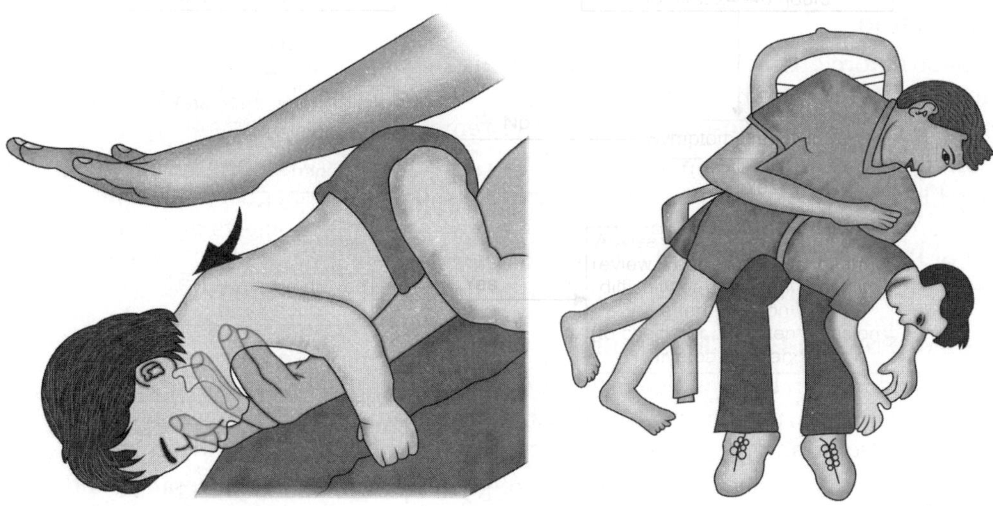

Hospital Management

The confirmed diagnosis is established or strongly suspected; bronchoscopy should be done as soon as possible. Unnecessary delay may worsen the lung condition and there is potential risk of dislodgement and impaction at the larynx to cause immediate death.

Bronchoscopy is performed under general anesthesia with or without muscle relaxant. A local anesthetic spray over the larynx greatly helps in reducing postbronchoscopy laryngospasm. A rigid ventilating bronchoscope laryngospasm. A rigid ventilating bronchoscope of appropriate size with a fiberoptics light is currently the instrument of choice. An array of foreign body forceps is available for extraction. After negotiating the larynx, the endoscope should be advanced under vision so as to avoided pushing the foreign body into the smaller bronchi. After sighting the foreign body it should be grasped with a suitable foreign body, it should be grasped with a suitable forceps and withdrawn along with the sheath as a single unit. Following the extraction, the endoscope should be reintroduced to ensure that there is no residual foreign body and also to clear the air passages or secretions under vision.

After the bronchoscopy some children persist with mild to moderate paroxysmal cough which can be effectively treated with humidification and parenteral steroids. A sort course of antibiotics and chest physiotherapy is necessary. Postoperatively an X-ray of the chest is always done to ensure that there is no pneumothorax and that the lung fields are equally ventilated. The child can be discharged after 24 hours of the bronchoscopy if there are no other contraindications.

A large vegetable foreign body, especially castor seeds, may swell up after being lodged and may be impossible to withdraw through the larynx. A tracheotomy may be performed to facilitate the removal. Decannulation of temporary tracheostomy can be easily done within a week. Impacted long standing foreign bodies in the bronchus require thoracotomy and removal by bronchotomy. Bronchiectasis needs pulmonary resection of the parts involved. Postoperative hospital stay may be as long as 10 days in such cases.

FOREIGN BODIES IN THE ALIMENTARY TRACT

Introduction

Ingestion of foreign bodies, like inhalation, is also a fairly common occurrence. The majority of ingested foreign bodies are spontaneously passed in the stool. However, those that do not do so may need endoscopic or operative removal.

The digestive tract has many naturally occurring narrow areas where foreign bodies can get lodged. At least three such sites are found in the esophagus; (i) at or just below the cricopharyngeus, where the vast majority of the swallowed objects are found' (ii) at the level of the aortic arch and (iii) at the cardioesophageal junction and the ileocecal valve. Sometimes a foreign body may get lodged in the ampulla of rectum.

Types of Foreign Body Materials

An ingested foreign body which is usually an inert metallic (e.g. coin) or plastic (e.g. small parts of toys) object, may get impacted at any of the naturally occurring areas of constriction but it may also bring to light a pathological stricture by obstructing the lumen.

In the alimentary tract, impaction of a foreign body may result in ulceration and pressure necrosis. Sharp objects may perforate any part of the gut.

The advent of button cells or batteries had added to the long list of ingested foreign bodies. These are small mercury or alkaline cells and following impaction their chemical components may leak out and cause focal liquefaction necrosis with resultant mediastinitis/ peritonitis or the absorption of toxic material, e.g. mercury may give rise to poisoning after absorption.

Table 5.5: Most common esophageal foreign bodies

- Coins
- Disk batteries
- Buttons
- Rings
- Lockets
- Hairclips
- Meat chunks

Signs and Symptoms

The initial episode of foreign body ingestion may resemble that of foreign body inhalation but the coughing is not severe and there is minimal choking and gagging. This is usually followed by dysphasia, drooling of saliva and retrosternal/epigastric discomfort if the oreign body gets impacted in the esophagus.

The foreign bodies which go beyond the esophagus are usually asymptomatic and are passed out in the stool spontaneously within 4–5 days. Impaction in the alimentary tract will present with features of intestinal obstruction. Perforation, depending on the site, will lead to mediastinitis, empyema or peritonitis.

Diagnostic Evaluation

The foreign body is suspected to be impacted in trachea esophagus then a plain antero-posterior and lateral X-ray of the neck and chest is all that is necessary in the emergency.

The abdomen should be included in the anteroposterior X-ray if the foreign body is suspected to have passed into the stomach or beyond. The progress of an ingested foreign body should be monitored by fluoroscopy or repeated plain X-ray every 24–48 hours. Perforations by the foreign body can also be diagnosed on the plain X-ray by the findings of pneumothorax or free air in the peritoneum but if empyema has resulted from the perforation then a CT scan is also required to assess the condition of the underlying lung.

Esophagoscopy or barium studies: Foreign bodies like bezoars do not present as emergencies and various imaging modalities, e.g. Ultrasonography, barium studies and CT scans may be necessary for the diagnosis.

Management

Impaction of an ingested foreign body rarely threatens life. Eating food which provides bulk, e.g. mashed potatoes or bananas may help in forcing a foreign body down the esophagus into the stomach. Fishing for the foreign body in the pharynx with one's finger is not a good idea because even small children can bite hard! Children with impacted or symptomatic foreign bodies should be referred to a well-equipped center for endoscopy.

Esophagoscopy in children is always performed under general anesthesia to avoid compromise of the respiratory tract during the procedure. The foreign body is visualized as preferably extracted; it may be pushed down into the stomach if it cannot be gripped adequately with a foreign body forceps. Retrieval of a button cell through an endoscope is often unsatisfactory because of inability to grip it properly hence open surgical removal is much more reliable.

The catheter is passed beyond the foreign body, the balloon is inflated so as to block the lumen of the esophagus and it is then gently pulled up. The foreign body is then spat out or it can be retrieved from the mouth of the patient.

Preventive Measures

- Accidents due to foreign bodies are common in infants and toddlers due to their natural curiosity to explore the environment and due to carelessness and lack of awareness on the part of the attendants.
- Children must be constantly supervised and watched. Nuts and seeds should not be offered to infants and young children.
- Objects like safety pins, buttons, glass beads, coins, tablets and toys with removable small parts or those with sharp edges should be kept away from toddlers and young children.
- Preschool children with food in their mouths should not be triggered to laugh or cry as they can readily get choked.
- A foreign body in the airway and sometimes in the alimentary tract can be a life-threatening emergency requiring immediate treatment. It is, therefore, important that the public and primary health care workers should be educated in the methods of dealing with such exigencies.
- Blunt force is responsible for the majority of serious injuries in children. High energy impact produces more multisystem injuries, related to patient size and momentum.
- Age-based differences in cognition, size and vital signs present special challenges. Priorities of pediatric evaluation and stabilization are identical to those in adults except

for the following important differences which include airway management, vascular access, definition and recognition of shock, fluid requirements, medication dosages, equipment needs and importance of the family unit.

BURNS

Introduction

Burns are common and serious childhood injury causing prolonged effect, one forth of burns cases are below 10 years of age and about 65% of burnt children are below 5 years of age.

Definition

Burns are the tissue injury caused by the contact with heat, flame, chemical, electrical and radiation.

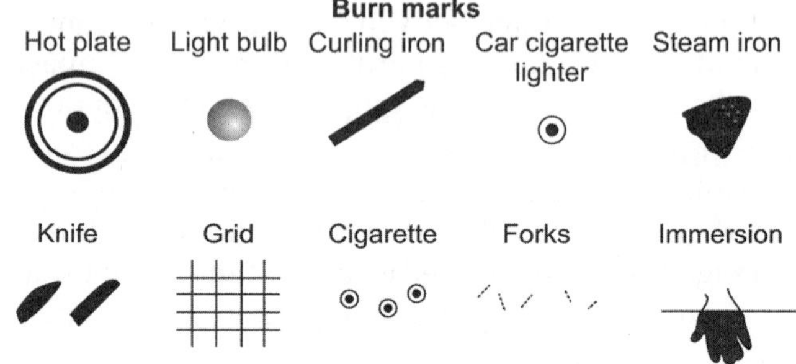

Fig. 5.41: Common instruments to get childhood burns

Types

- *Electrical burns:* It is common in toddler and adolescents when playing with electrical outlet, extension cord, touching high tension wires, etc.
- *Open flame burns:* It is common during playing with lighter or at kitchen near stove or over of gas line.
- *Chemical burns:* It is also common in children out of curiosity they handle household cleansing chemical, acids etc. and get injured.

Causes

The first step in helping to prevent child from being burned is to understand these common causes of burns:

- Scalding is the most common problem (from steam, hot bath water, tipped-over coffee cups, hot foods, cooking fluids, etc.)
- Contact with flames or hot objects (from the stove, fireplace, curling iron, etc.)
- Chemical burns (from swallowing things, like drain cleaner or watch batteries, or spilling chemicals, such as bleach, onto the skin)
- Electrical burns (from biting on electrical cords or sticking fingers or objects in electrical outlets, etc.)
- Overexposure to the sun.

Pathophysiology (Based on Systems)

Hemodynamic Changes

Burns
↓
Decreased Fluids level in the body
↓
Fluids shift from intravascular to extra vascular compartment due to increased capillary permeability
↓
Decreased cardiac output
↓
Hypovolemia and shock
↓
Swelling and edema of burnt area

Cellular Responses

Burns
↓
Cellular elements of blood destroyed
↓
Hemolysis
↓
Anemia
↓
Burn injury
Rise in WBC and phagocytosis are impaired
↓
Decreased plasma proteins and immunoglobin
↓
Vulnerability to get infections
↓
Decreased platelet count with abnormal platelet function and decreased in fibrinogen level
↓
Blood coagulation problems

Renal Function

Hypovolemia and decreased cardiac output
↓
Decreased renal blood flow and decreased FGR
↓
Tubular necrosis and renal failure

Stress Response

Burns injury
↓
Evaporative fluid loss
↓
Hypermetabolic state
↓
Negative nitrogen balance and loss of protein
↓
Increased tissue catabolism
↓
Release of alpha adrenergic agent, cortisol and catecholamine

GI Function

Burns injury
↓
Sympathetic nervous system stimulation
↓
Decreased peristalsis movement
↓
Paralytic illus
↓
Ischemia of gastric mucosa
↓
Duodenal and gastric ulcers
↓
Occult bleeding and hemorrhage

Immune Response

Burns
↓
Decreased immunoglobulin (IgA, IgG, IgM) and serum albumin)
↓
Decreased immunity
↓
Infection and wound sepsis

Classification of Burns in Children

According to Depth of Burn Injury

Superficial burns (partial thickness burns)

- *Superficial partial thickness burns:* Burns injury involves epidermis and superficial layer of dermis is up to papillary dermis. The wound usually heals and regenerates in less than 2 weeks period of burns.
- *Superficial deep dermal burns:* Burn injury involves beyond papillary dermis and takes more than 2 weeks time for healing.
- *Full thickness burns:* Burn injury involves all layer of skin and sometimes underlying tissues are also destroyed. It needs skin grafting.

According to Extent of Burn Injury

First Degree Burns

Superficial burns manifested as pink to red discolored area with slight edema pain may present up to 48 hrs and relieved by cooling within 5 days epidermis peels off, pink skin may persist for a week, no scar develops healing takes place spontaneously within 10–15 days, if not infected.

Second Degree Burns

Superficial second degree burns are presented as pink or red discoloration of the area with blister formation, weeping and edema. Superficial skin layers are destroyed wound becomes moist and painful and takes several weeks to heal, scaring may develop.

Second degree deep dermal burns are manifested as mottled white and red area become pale on pressure. Wound takes several weeks to heal and scar may develop.

Third Degree Burns

It includes destruction of epithelial cells even fat, muscles and bone. Eschar (dead tissue) develops as leathery devitalized tissue, which must be removed. Granulation tissue develops and grafting is required if the burnt area is larger than 3–5 cm. Grafting is done after wound debridement.

First degree and second degree burns are included in partial thickness burns. The third degree burns is considered as full thickness burns.

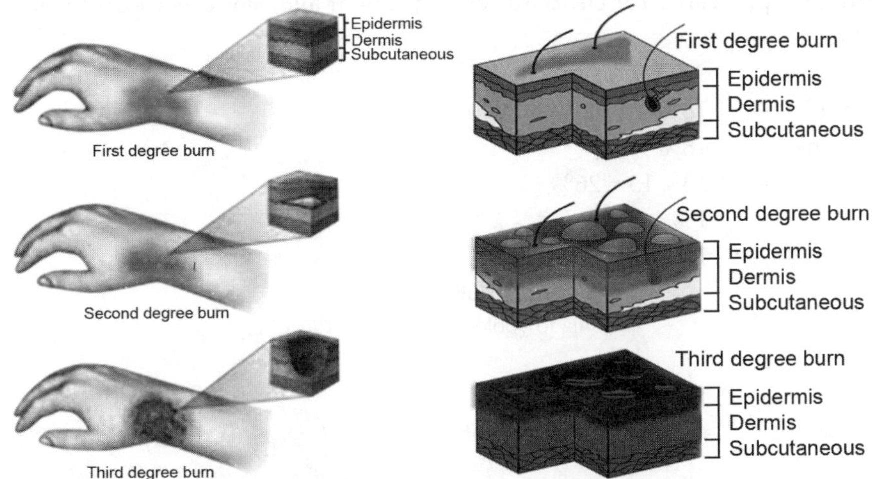

Fig. 5.42: Types of burn injury

According to Severity of Burn Injury

It depends upon total area injured, depth of injury, location of injury, age, general health of the child presence of additional injury and level of consciousness.

- Minor burns:
  - 10% of total body surface area (TBSA) burnt with first and second degree burns.
- Moderate burns:
  - 10–20% TBSA burnt and second degree burns
  - 2–5% TBSA burnt and third degree burn, but not involving eyes, ears, feet, hands, face, genitals.
- Major burns:
  - 20% or more TBSA burnt and second degree burns.
  - All burns involving face, eyes, ears, feet, hands and genitals.

Estimation of Extent of Burns Surface Area

The extent of burns is expected as the amount of surface area burnt in relation to total body surface area. Various methods are used to calculate the burnt area.

A convenient, easy and quick method of estimation of surface area in pediatric burns is Rule of five (Lynch and Blocker, 1963).

Area	Age 0–5 yrs	Age 5–10 yrs	Age 10 yrs onwards
Head and neck	20%	10%	–
Trunk – front	20%	20%	20%
Trunk – back	20%	20%	20%
Upper limbs	10 × 2 = 20%	10 × 2 = 20%	10 × 2 = 20%
Lower limbs	10 × 2 = 20%	15 × 2 = 30%	15 × 2 = 30%

Rule of nine is applicable for child above 10 years of age, same as like adults.

Head and neck — 9%
Arms — 9% + 9%
Anterior trunk — 18%
Posterior trunk — 18%
Legs — 13 + 13 = 26%
Perineum — 1%
Total — 100%

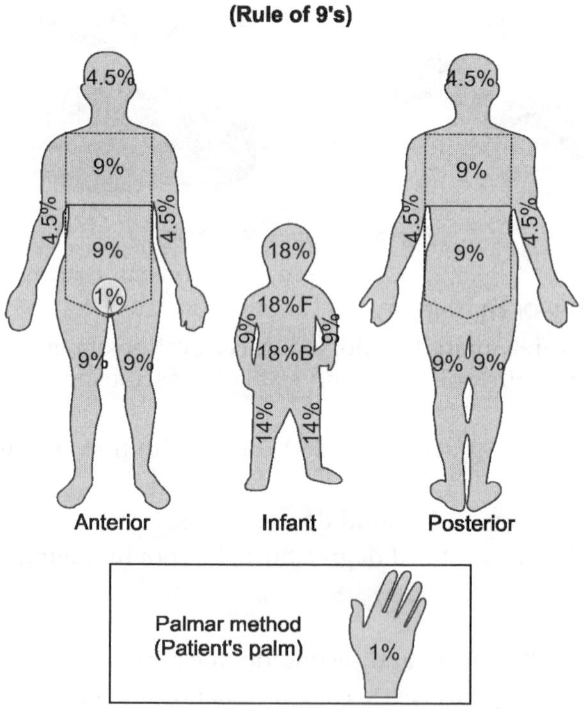

(Rule of 9's)

Fig. 5.43: Using rule of nine to calculate the burns

Signs and Symptoms

The clinical features of burn injury are manifested depending upon the degree of burns.

- Symptoms of shock usually appear soon after burns.
- Pallor, cyanosis, prostration, poor muscle bone, failure to recognize familiar people, rapid pulse, low blood pressure and abnormal temperature.

- Inhalation injury causes inflammation of edema of the glottis, vocal cords and upper trachea leading to upper airway obstruction. The child usually presents with dyspnea, tachypnea, hoarseness, strider, chest retractions, nasal flaring, restlessness, cough and drooling.
- Symptoms of toxemia develop after burns within one to two days. The patient usually manifested with fever, vomiting, edema, decreased urinary output, prostration, rapid pulse, glycosuria and unconsciousness.

Management

Management of burns injury includes first aid measures, assessment of extent of burns, fluid replacement, metabolic support, care of wound and use of topical antibiotics. Wound closure, prevention of infections and other complications, psychological support, malnutrition support and rehabilitation are also major aspects of burn management.

Minor burns can be managed at home with maintenance of aseptic techniques. Moderate burns should be managed at general hospital.

First Aid Measures

- Immediate remove from heat source
- In case of open flame, the child should help to lie flat on the ground and roll on the floor.
- Fire should be extinguished by pouring water.
- Avoiding pouring of water over the burnt area, once the fire has been extinguished.
- The child should be wrapped in clean sheep to prevent heat loss.
- Oral fluid, (ORS) should be given, if the child is thirsty and able to drink.
- Oropharyngeal secretion to be removed and airway to be kept patient. The child to be turned to one side and respiration to be checked.
- Transfer to hospital to be arranged promptly.
- Avoiding use of pain killer and sedative. Blister should not be peeled off and should be allowed to spontaneous collapse.

1. *Initial assessment:* Assessment of ABC helps to initiate resuscitative measures on the basis of priority needs. Level of consciousness and vital signs to be evaluated quickly. Extent and depth of burn injury to be assessed promptly to start fluid replacement especially percentage of total body surface burnt. Presence of additional injury and general health of the child (specially body weight) to be examined quickly.
2. *Subsequent assessment:* Fluid replacement is done promptly on the basis of TBSA burnt and body weight of the child.

Brooke Army Formula

- Colloids: 0.5 ml × kg body weight × % TBSA burned.
- Electrolytes: 1.5 ml × kg body weight × % TBSA
- Glucose (5%): 200 ml for insensible loss.

Day 1: Half in 1st 8 hours, remaining half over next 16 hours.

Day 1: Half of colloids, half of electrolyte all of insensible fluid replacement.

Parkland Formula

- In first 24 hrs: The total amount of calculated fluid requirement is = 4 ml of RL × wt in kg % of TBSA burnt.
- One half amount of calculated fluid is given for the first 8 hrs
- The remaining half of the fluid is given over the next 16 hrs
- In next 24 hrs: 2 ml of RL/% of TBSA.

Evans Formula

- Colloids: 1 ml × kg body wt × % TBSA burnt.
- Electrolytes: 1 ml × kg body wt × % TBSA burnt.
- Glucose (5%): 200 ml for insensible loss.

Day 1: Half for 1st 8 hrs, remaining half over next 16 hrs

Day 2: Half of previous days colloids + electrolytes, all of insensible fluid replacement.

Additional Measures

- Airway management is important
- Tetanus prophylaxis
- Sedative and analgesics to be given
- Systemic antibiotics.

Nutritional Support

According to Davies Formula

- Protein requirement should be 3 gm/kg body wt plus 1 gm% of TBSA.
- Calorie requirement should be 60 kcal/kg body wt plus 35 kcal/% of TBSA.

Wound Management

- Burn wound should be done daily or twice daily as cleaning of wound with debridement or hydrotherapy.
- Tight clothing and ornament should be removed and hair can be removed around the wound.
- Wound should be cleaned with normal saline.
- Dead and loose skin should be remove
- Blisters may be managed by pricking and draining the fluid.
- Wound should be covered with antibacterial ointment.
- Hydrotherapy is used to facilitate cleansing and debridement of the burned area.
- The commonly used topical agent for burns wound is silver sulfadiazine, silver nitrate and mefenide acetate cream.
- In surgical excision of nonviable tissue, the wound should be covered by biological dressing, i.e. oxen graft, allograft or autograft.
- Grafting should be done to avoid formation of hypertrophic scars reading to contracture and deformities.

Treatment for Burns

Typically, a burn that covers more than 10% of the total body surface area (TBSA) of a child is considered to be a critical burn, except for first degree burns. A quick way to estimate the TBSA of a burn is to approximate how large the burn is an compared to the palm of palm of a child's hand (don't include the fingers), which represents about 1% of TBSA.

Most serious burns, including second degree burns that cover more than 10% of the total body surface area (TBSA) of a child, third degree burns that involve more than 5% of TBSA, or burns that involve the face, genitals, hands, feet or that cross a joint or totally encircle an extremity, should be referred to a specialized burn center.

- Heat damages the cells of the skin releasing chemicals that stimulate nerves and cause pain.
- If the burn is very large or very deep, bacteria may invade and cause infection.
- First degree or superficial burns heat naturally. Deep second degree and full thickness burns require skin grafting for rapid healing and minimum scarring and generally require hospital care.
- In addition supportive therapy like fluid, bold infusion and pain medication is required. In some patients, the burn may lead to intolerable and excruciating pain for which even IV morphine may be required.
- The first degree burns and open wounds, topical creams like silver sulfadiazine and bacitracin may be applied. Often dressing may be applied.

Nursing Management

Nursing Diagnosis

- Decreased cardiac output related to hypovolemia and increased metabolism
- Impaired gas exchange related to exposure of burn in front trunk region of the body
- Pain related to burn wound
- Fear and infections related to alterations of skin integrity
- Risk for infections related to alterations of skin integrity
- Potential to injury of gastric mucosa related to stress response and deceased gastic motility
- Impaired physical mobility related to pain and contracture
- Nutrition less than body requirements, related to poor appetite and burn injury
- Altered parenting related to crisis situation.

Nursing Intervention

- Promoting and supporting cardiac output by continuous monitoring of features, and electrolytes values.
- Administering IV fluid therapy, oxygen therapy, maintaining warmth, humidified environment, strict recording of fluid intake, measuring output of urine are important measured to cardiac function
- Reliving pain and discomfort by comfort measures, use of bed cradle, administering analgesics and sedatives as prescribed, providing relaxation and diversion, emotional support and expansion, etc.

- Reducing fear and anxiety by allowing parents to stay with child by allowing him to be verbalize feeling
- Preventing infections by aseptic wound care, administering prescribed antibiotics, change of position, maintaining general cleanliness and assessing signs of infections.
- Proving adequate nutrition by high calories, high protein diet with vitamin and mineral supplementation and offering small frequent feeding and enteral feeding if required.
- Preventing negative body image by reassurance referring for skin grafting and cosmetic surgery, motivation to accept to changed image and use of special clothing's image and use of special clothing, seeking advice from child psychologist and cosmetic specialist.
- Local infection: Penicillin or erythromycin (or by an antimicrobial effective against the bacterial flora of the buccal cavity and venom of local snakes)
- A booster dose of tetanus toxoid should be given.

DROWNING

Introduction

Drowning ranks second most common cause of accidental death in children. Most cases involved children. Most cases involved children who are helpless in water such as inadequately attended in or near swimming pools. Nurses often have difficulty in relating to the parents if obvious neglect has precipitated the accident and subsequent problems.

The article describes the essential highlights of drowning and an interesting case report of an eight year old schooler and four year old preschooler who presented with near drowning and was successfully managed by the team in the department of Pediatric Emergency Service and the Intensive Care Unit of the Christian Medical College, Vellore.

Drowning is a life threatening emergency that results in either a slow or rapid replacement of fluid in the lungs. This is turn causes gasping and aspiration which leads to cardiopulmonary arrest due to asphyxia in 4 to 6 minutes. In order to save the life of children prompt action and meticulous care is necessary to prevent the mortality related to drowning.

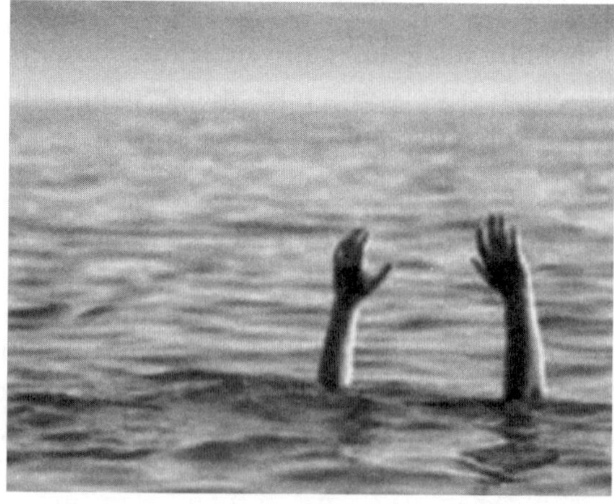

Incidence

Drowning occurs more than 4 times in males than in females. Highest rate is seen among children between 2 to 3 years of age. A study done by Anuradha Bose (2000) in Vaniyambadi block, served by the Community Health Department of Christian Medical College and Hospital, Vellore, reveals that there were a total of 288 deaths in the age group between 1 to 12 years and drowning was the single largest cause of death in this group with a total of 58 deaths.

Clinical Manifestation

Clinical manifestations are directly related to the degree of consciousness following rescues and resuscitation.

Diagnostic Evaluation

Investigations: After drowning history collection, physical examination, Chest X-ray, Arterial Blood Gas, X-ray spine, suction tip for culture and sensitivity, toxicology screening, ECG to document normal functions.

Management

The adjuvant line of treatment should be started and carried out simultaneously. This consists of keeping the child warm, intracardiac administration of stimulant like adrenaline or calcium chloride or birth, and delivering 100% oxygen, gastric and tracheal intubation and suction, defibrillation, administration of sodium bicarbonate to correct the acidosis and electrolyte replacement to correct electrolyte imbalance. Supportive therapy includes postural drainage, steroids and antibiotics are given only for specific indications.

Complications

The common complications that could result from near drowning are:
- Aspiration pneumonia that occurs approximately 48 to 72 hours after the episode.
- Bronchospasm
- Alveolar: Capillary membrane damage
- Atelectasis
- Abscess formation
- Hyaline membrane disease that occur after aspiration of fluid
- Hypoxia and death.

Prognosis

The prognosis is good if the drowning occurred in less than 5 minutes. Severe neurological impairment and death occurs for more than 10 minutes of drowning.

Prevention

- Cover the water tubs and water tanks
- Adequate supervision of infants small children
- Parents with pools should know cardiopulmonary resuscitation.

Nursing Management

Nursing Diagnosis

Ineffective airway clearance related to accumulation of fluid during drowning secondary to spasm of larynx.

Interventions

- Positioned the child in fowlers or according to the condition
- Gave chest physio every 2 hourly followed by oral and tracheal suctioning
- Administered oxygen
- Monitored vital signs of RR [56 b/mt], heart rate [124 bt/mt], BP [103/58 mm Hg], increased CVP
- Administered 2 hourly, nebulizer, and injection Dexamethasone 8 hourly.

Nursing Diagnosis

Impaired breathing pattern related to trachea bronchial obstruction, hypoxia, hypoxemia, secondary to drowning, emphysematous changes in the accumulation space.

Interventions

- Positioned the child with head end elevation of 30–40 degrees
- Cleaner the airway by oral and nasal suctioning
- Started the child on Oxygen 10 L/minute, as the respiratory rate was increased to 58/mt, child was electively intubated with ET tube No 5 and fixed at 14 cm with the setting of FI02 100% rate 30/mt, P/P 15/3
- Administered antibiotics as ink. Cefotaxime q6h and injection Gentamicin q12h
- Kept the child on NPO and started on Iv fluids
- Documented the care provided.

Nursing Diagnosis

Decreased cardiac output related to impaired contractility, decreased oxygenation, and alteration in heart rate, rhythm, and conduction secondary to drowning.

Interventions

- Assessed HR, BP, breath sounds JVP, capillary refill, skin color and peripheral pulses
- Connected the child on ECG monitor
- Compared the vital signs at every shift
- Administered medication as ordered like digitalis, diuretics, vasodilators and inotropic agents
- Maintained the optimal fluid balance
- Placed the child in semifowlers to reduce preload and ventricular filling
- Administered humidified oxygen
- Organized nursing care to allow rest periods
- Provided explanations as appropriate to allay anxiety.

Nursing Diagnosis

Fluid volume excess related to aspiration of water, fluid shift from the interstitial to intravascular space secondary to prolonged submersion in fluid medium.

Interventions

- Checked weight daily
- Calculated and administered IV fluid as accurate per the order
- Monitored strict intake and output chart
- Connected the child on cardiopulmonary monitor
- Administered sodium bicarbonate to correct metabolic acidosis
- Prepared for central line placement
- Provided passive exercises
- Elevated edematous extremities.

Nursing Diagnosis

Hyperthermia related to exposure to cold environment, inactivity, secondary to near drowning.

Interventions

- Assessed temperature every 2 hourly
- Monitored electrolytes and peripheral perfusions
- Removed extra clothing
- Exposed the child under the fan
- Gave the child under the fan
- Gave tepid sponging
- Administered antipyretic 10 ml/kg
- Administered antibiotic on time.

Nursing Diagnosis

Actual infection related to aspiration of contaminated water secondary to inability to keep self above the water level.

Intervention

- Suctioning was done to remove secretions
- Monitored temperature, heart rate and respiratory rate every 2 hourly
- Notified the physical about the temperature, knee pain and X-ray was taken and magnesium sulfate dressing done over the knee
- Administered antibiotics as per order
- Positioned the child every 2 hourly
- Encouraged postural drainage and chest physiotherapy to promote drainage
- Advised parents to but balloons to provide breathing exercises.

Nursing Diagnosis

Knowledge deficit related to near drowning child's critical status. Admission to pediatric intensive care unit and home care.

Intervention

- Assessed the educational statue and level of understanding of the parents about child's illness and treatment
- Established a good rapport with the parents
- Encouraged expression of feeling about condition and treatment
- Reassured and supported the family
- Allowed for questions and answered honestly as possible
- Included family in child's care
- Retreated the importance of supervision, emergency management follow-ups and home care.
- Advised him to come for review after 10 days.

Conclusion

Accidental drowning can be decreased if children are given training in swimming skills at a younger age. Children must swim under supervision. The personal flotation devices (PFDs) should be made available in swimming pools and its use can be encouraged.

SPORTS INJURIES

Introduction

The adolescents who participate in organized sports have increased over the last few decades. In particular, the number of young women participating in sports has grown very rapidly. With this increase has come a corresponding increase in sports injuries. Forty percent of all pediatric injuries are sports related. Estimates put this number at 4.4 million injuries per year. Overall, male and female injury rates are becoming equal.

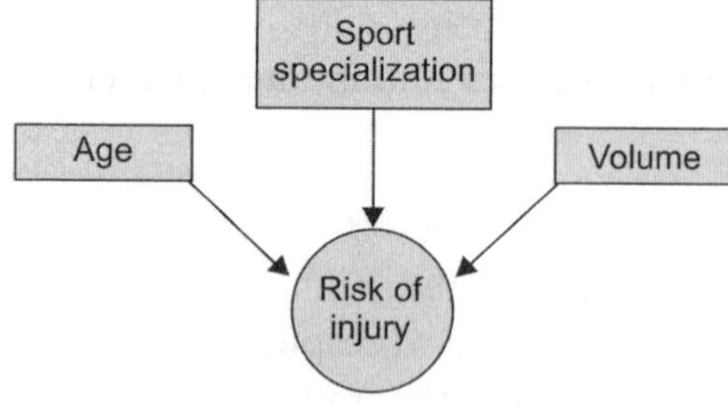

Fig. 5.44: Risk of sports injury

Types of Injuries

Two types of trauma:

1. Micro (due to repetitive trauma)
2. Macro (due to a single traumatic event).

Injuries

- *Fracture:* A fracture through the growth plate can be a very serious injury that can stop the bone from growing properly. These fractures should be treated by an orthopedist, as some will require surgery.
- *Anterior knee pain:* Anterior knee pain, or patella femoral syndrome, is often passed off as growing pains. Causes of this pain include overuse, muscle imbalance, poor flexibility, poor alignment, or, more commonly, a combination of these. Anterior knee pain is one of the most difficult adolescent knee injuries to sort out and treat. Accurate diagnosis and treatment depends on finding a musculoskeletal specialist with a special interest and expertise in this difficult area.
- *Patellar instability:* Patellar (kneecap) instability can range from partial dislocation (subluxation) to dislocation with fracture. Partial dislocation can often be treated conservatively. Dislocation with or without fracture is a much more serious injury and usually will require surgery.
- *Knee ligaments and the menisci (cartilage between the leg bones):* They have greater blood supply and are more elastic in adolescents than in adults. As adolescents near the end of bone growth, their injuries become more adult-like and the adolescents become more susceptible to meniscal and anterior cruciate ligament (ACL) injuries.
- *Medial collateral ligament (MCL) injury:* This injury results from a lateral blow to the knee. Pain is felt on inner side (medially) of the knee. MCL injuries respond well to protective bracing and conservative treatment.
- *Anterior cruciate ligament (ACL) injury:* This injury is most commonly caused by a non – contact twisting or deceleration mechanism which results in excessive hyperextension or interval rotation forces on the anterior cruciate ligament. Non-contact injuries of the ACL are becoming more common than contact injuries. Adolescent females are at high risk. Combination injuries with MCL or menisci are common. Surgical reconstruction is needed if the adolescent wishes to continue participating in 'stop-and-start' sports.

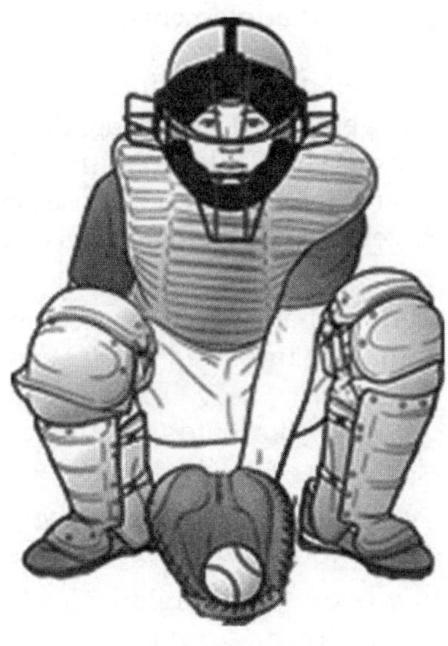

- *Meniscal injury:* An injury to the meniscus, the crescent-shaped cartilage between the thigh bone (femur) and lower leg bone (tibia). These injuries usually result from twisting. Swelling, catching, and locking of the knee are common. Nearly all of these types of injuries will require arthroscopic surgery.

Preventive Measures

There are several strategies that coaches, parents, and athletes can follow to prevent sports injuries.

- Child should proper physical condition to play a sport (a pre-participation sports physical examinations can be very useful in screening for potential problems)
- They should know and abide by the rules of a sport
- Wear appropriate protective gear (e.g. shin guards for soccer, a hard-shell helmet when facing a baseball pitcher, a helmet and body padding for ice hockey)
- Child should know how to correctly use athletic equipment (e.g. correctly adjusting the bindings on snow skis)
- Always warm-up before playing
- Stay hydrated
- Avoid playing when very tired or in pain.

OBESITY

Introduction

The emerging epidemics of obesity, cardiovascular disease (CVD) and diabetes form the crux of this phenomenal change. Among these entities, obesity has become a colossal epidemic causing serious public health concern and contributes to 2.6 million deaths worldwide every year. Obesity is an independent risk factor for CVD. Obesity is associated with an increased risk of morbidity and mortality as well as reduced life expectancy. The last two decades of the previous century have witnessed dramatic increase in health care costs due to obesity and related issues among children and adolescents.

Definition

The children and adolescents overweight and obesity are defined as using age and sex specific normograms for body mass index (BMI). Children with BMI equal to or exceeding the age-gender-specific 95th percentile are defined obese. Those with BMI equal to or exceeding the 85th but are below 95th percentiles are defined overweight and are at risk for obesity related co-morbidities.

Obesity is defined as a condition of abnormal or excessive fat accumulation in adipose tissue, to the extent that health may be impaired (WHO consultation on obesity, 2000).

Causes

- Genetic
- Neuroendocrine
- Metabolic
- Psychological
- Environmental
- Sociocultural factors are clearly evident in childhood obesity.

Diagnostic Evaluation

Body weight is reasonably correlated with body fat, but is also highly correlated with height. Therefore, weight adjusted for height squared [body mass index (BMI in kg/m^2)] is a useful index to assess overweight and is a fairly reliable surrogate for adiposity. It is calculated easily from weight and height and it correlates with other measures of body fatness in children and adolescents.

BMI as of now appears to be the most practical way of measuring and comparing obesity for clinical and epidemic-logical purposes.

- As per WHO classification (for adults)
- BMI > 25 = overweight and BMI > 30 = Obesity.

Management

Obesity-clinic/Individual Approach

Management of established obesity in children needs a concerted and a sustained effort from a team of experienced health professionals. Treatment is more likely to be successful in children than adults.

Goals of Therapy: Approach to Therapy

- *Medical goal:* Medical goal should be resolution of complications and co-morbidities such as hypertension and hyperlipidemia.
- *Behavioral goal:* Achievement of healthy eating and activity patterns rather than achievement of ideal body weight.
- *Weight goal:* Weight maintenance rather than weight loss (unless moribund obesity) in young children–'Let the child grow into his weight'. Prolonged weight maintenance will allow a gradual decline in the BMI as the child grows in height.

The principles of therapy are generally same as in prevention:

- Reduced calorie intake
- Increased activity levels
- Decreased sedentary behavior
- Family involvement
- Behavioral changes.

Infants and Young Children

- Mothers should prevent excess weight gain in pregnancy; control diabetes or impaired glucose tolerance in pregnancy.
- Promote exclusive breastfeeding for six months.
- Avoid adding sugars, starches or oils to feeding formulas.
- Assure appropriate micronutrient intake especially of iron, calcium and vitamins.
- Monitor growth with weight for height and BMI.
- Discourage 'accelerated crossing of centiles'.
- Make clear differentiation of 'catch-up growth' from accelerated weight gain. Catch up growth should be associated with gain in height proportional to weight gain.
- Instruct mothers to accept the child's appetite and not to force feed.
- Instruct families that 'fat infants make fat adults'.

Children and Adolescents

The fat rebound age (5–8 years) and adolescence are particularly high risk periods for accumulating fat. Strategies for prevention include:

- Promote active lifestyles including at least one hour of vigorous 'play' per day. Limit TV and other sedentary activities to < 2 hr/day. Physical activity is as important, if not more than didactic lessons.
- Promote sensible eating: Increase fruit and vegetables and restrict energy dense sweets and soft drinks. Impart health education skills to make healthy food choices, e.g. early home cooked dinners to avoid TV snacking. Substitute soups/salads/baked foods for wafers, chocolates/fried foods.
- Modify environments to promote physical activity, e.g. safe roads for cycling, jogging.
- Celebration should be in the form of outdoor play/picnics rather than fast food joint parties.
- Educate about the evils of alcohol/tobacco to adolescents.

Health education

School-based Programs

Schools are probably the ideal medium of intervention as they are central to children's lives and information can be relatively quickly dissipated through this education.

Aspects to be considered are:

- Training of teachers in lifestyles, nutrition and activity.
- Introduction of ideal school meals or provision of canteens offering only healthy options based on Indian foods.
- Introduction of 'nutrition and physical education' in school curriculum. These activities should become compulsory and/or a 'scoring subject' with marks to be added to total grades. Only then will parents/students give the required attention and time to this in this competitive world of academics!
- After school games (supervised/unsupervised) to be encouraged. Opening up of school playgrounds on weekends and holidays.
- Obese children should not be teased, targeted or bullied or isolated.
- Involve parent associations.
- School health checkups should monitor BMI along with height and weight annually.

Complication of Obesity

Systems	Problems
Cardiovascular	• High blood pressure • Early onset of atherosclerosis • Left ventricular hypertrophy
Endocrine	• Insulin resistance • Diabetes mellitus (NIDDM) • Menstrual abnormalities • Polycystic ovarian syndrome (PCOS)

Contd...

Contd...

Systems	Problems
Gastrointestinal	• Gallstones • Nonalcoholic steatohepatitis (NASH) • Hepatic fibrosis • Cirrhosis
Neurological	• Pseudotumor cerebri
Orthopedic	• Slipped capital femoral epiphysis • Tibia Vara • Osteoarthritis
Psychosocial	• Obsessive concern about body image • Expectation of rejection • Progressive withdrawal • Low self esteem • Depression
Pulmonary	• Increased bronchial hyperactivity • Asthma exacerbation • Obstructive sleep apnea • Pickwick an syndrome • Pulmonary embolism
Renal	• Increased sensitivity to sodium • Decreased natriuresis • Proteinuria • Focal segmental glomerulosclerosis (FSGS)

ANOREXIA NERVOSA

Introduction

Anorexia nervosa (AN) is a severe eating disorder characterized by a distorted normal body image that leads to restricted eating, over exercise and other behaviors that prevents a person from gaining weight or maintaining a normal body weight.

The rapid physical changes that occur at this time lead adolescents to become preoccupied with their body image. Adolescents may become preoccupied with themselves, uncertain about their appearance, compare their bodies with those of other teens, and become increasingly interested in sexual anatomy and physiology.

Definition

Anorexia nervosa is defined as an eating disorder in which the children intentionally limits or avoid the intake of food because of a strong drive for thinness and an intense fear of gaining weight, etc. The resulting progressive weight loss and nutritional imbalance can lead to serious complications, including death.

Incidence

The diagnosis of anorexia nervosa has become more common over the past 20 years. Approximately 90 percent are women between 12 and 25 years of age. Initially found mostly in upper-and middle-class families, anorexia nervosa is now known to affect both sexes and span all ages, socioeconomic, ethnic, and racial groups.

Risk Factors/Causes

These factors are sometimes divided into:
- Predisposing factors
- Precipitating factors
- Perpetuating factor.

Causes

- Genetic factors
- Obsessions and anxiety
- Gastrointestinal problems
- Endocrine problems
- Cardiovascular problems.

Types

- *Restrictive type:* This type of anorexia nervosa is severely limits the intake of food and usually compulsively overexercises.
- *Binge/Purge subtype:* An individual eats in binges and then induces vomiting and/or takes large amounts of laxatives or other cathartics (medications, through their chemical effects, that serve to increase the clearing of intestinal contents).

Signs and Symptoms

- Dry skin that when pinched and released, stays pinched
- Dehydration
- Abdominal pain
- Constipation
- Lethargy
- Dizziness
- Fatigue
- Intolerance to cold temperatures
- Emaciation
- Development of lanugo (fine, downy body hair)
- Yellowing of the skin
- Loss of menstrual periods in girls
- Persons with anorexia nervosa may also be socially withdrawn, irritable, moody and depressed. The symptoms of anorexia nervosa may resemble other medical problems or psychiatric conditions.

Diagnostic Evaluation

- History collection
- Physical examination

- Malnutrition assessment
- Child's behavioral assessment
- Psychological test
- Blood test (CBC)
- GI-USG scan
- Barium meal X-ray.

Management

Specific treatment for anorexia nervosa will be based on condition of child:

- Individual therapy
- Behavioral therapy
- Antidepressants drugs
- Family therapy
- Therapies or medications for medical problems.

Complication

Medical complications that may result from anorexia include the following:

- Cardiovascular
  - While it is difficult to predict which patients with anorexia nervosa might have life-threatening heart problems that result from their illness, the majority of hospitalized patients with anorexia nervosa have been found to have low heart rates.
  - Heart muscle damage that can occur as a result of malnutrition or repeated vomiting may be life threatening.
  - Arrhythmias (tachycardia, bradycardia or irregular heartbeat).
  - Hypotension (low blood pressure).
- Electrolytes
  - Electrolyte abnormalities are common, especially in those who purge
  - Abuse laxatives or diuretics, or drink excessive amounts of fluid
  - Electrolyte abnormalities may also develop during re-feeding
  - Electrolyte abnormalities can cause abnormal heart rhythms
  - Brain swelling, or other complications that can be life threatening.
- Hematological
  - Patients will have mild anemia (low red blood cell count).
  - Leucopenia (low white blood cell count) occurs in up to 50 percent of anorexic patients.
- Gastrointestinal (stomach and intestines)
  - Decreased peristaltic movement
  - Restricted eating and severe weight loss
  - Improved eating and associated weight gain often help to restore normal intestinal motility or movement.
- Renal
  - Restrict fluid intake or drink excessive amounts of fluid
  - Limited fluid intake can cause dehydration and highly concentrated urine

- Excessive fluid intake can cause dilute urine, and also may lead to electrolyte abnormalities
- Polyuria (increased production of urine)
- Renal changes usually return to normal with the restoration of normal weight.

• Endocrine
- In females, amenorrhea (cessation of the menstrual cycle for at least three consecutive months when otherwise expected)
- Amenorrhea may precede severe weight loss and continue after normal weight is restored.
- Reduced levels of growth hormones are sometimes found on anorexic patients and may explain growth retardation sometimes seen in anorexic patients.
- Normal nutrition usually restores normal growth and menstrual cycles.

• Skeletal
- Increased risk for skeletal fractures (broken bones)
- Decreased bone mineral density
- Increased fracture risk exists.

JUVENILE DELINQUENCY

Introduction

Juvenile delinquency refers to criminal acts performed by juveniles. Most legal systems prescribe specific procedures for dealing with juveniles, such as juvenile detention centers.

There are a multitude of different theories on the causes of crime, most if not all of which can be applied to the causes of youth crime. Youth crime is a major issue and is an aspect of crime which receives great attention from the news media and politicians.

Crime committed by young people has risen since the mid-twentieth century, as have most types of crime. The level and types of youth crime can be used by commentators as an indicator of the general state of morality and law and order in a country, and consequently youth crime can be the source of 'moral panics'. Theories on the causes of youth crime can be viewed as particularly important within criminology.

This is firstly because crime is committed disproportionately by those aged between fifteen and twenty-five. Secondly, by definition any theories on the causes of crime will focus on youth crime, as adult criminals will have likely started offending when they were young.

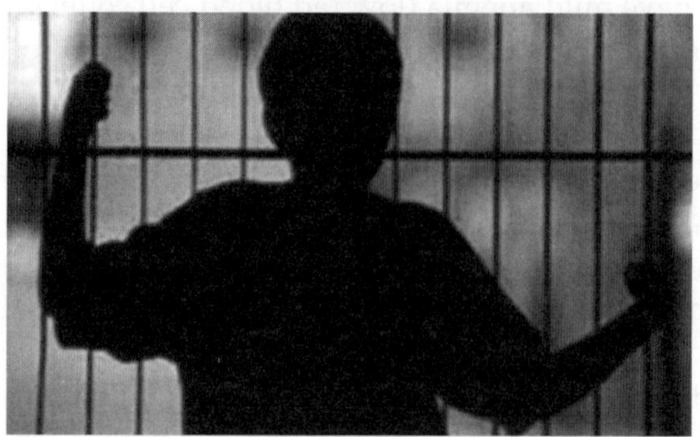

A Juvenile Delinquent is one who repeatedly commits crime; however these juvenile delinquents could most likely have mental disorders/behavioral issues such as schizophrenia, post traumatic stress disorder, conduct disorder or bipolar disorder.

Definition

Children often test the limits and boundaries set by their parents and other authority figures. Among adolescents, some rebelliousness and experimentation is common. However, a few children consistently participate in problematic behaviors that negatively affect their family, academic, social, and personal functioning. These children present great concern to parents and the community at large.

The prevention of delinquency requires identifying at-risk individuals and their environments before delinquent activity and behavior occur, and then removing such risk factors or strengthening resistance to the risk factors already present. The most logical starting place for prevention efforts is the family.

Causes

Social Disorganization

Current positivist approaches generally focus on the culture. A type of criminological theory attributing variation in crime and delinquency over time and among territories to the absence or breakdown of communal institutions (e.g. family, school, church and local government) and communal relationships that traditionally encouraged cooperative relationships among people.

- *Family:* Almost all research workers have accepted that families of delinquents are characterized by discords, desertions and divorces. Such families have been pointed out as one of the main causes of delinquency.
- *Peer group:* To those in sore need of a substitute for family love and group-belongingness, the peer group or the gang presents itself as a kind of close knit unit that will solve the purpose.
- *Neighborhood:* The immediate environments of a child also affect the trend he will adopt in connection with his personality. It has been seen that more delinquents come from slums and thickly populated areas.
- *Educational curriculum:* Although schools and educational institutes are playing an increasingly important role in the training and upbringing of future citizens, they are also contributing towards many cases on juvenile delinquency. Delinquents are typically nonbookish and nonacademic individuals who take studies like a burden. When they fail in exams and get scolded by their family, they tend to indulge themselves in delinquent acts.
- *Poverty and democracy:* Poverty and democracy are also the major contributing factors towards juvenile delinquency. People indulge themselves in delinquent acts in order to meet and satisfy the primary wants of their life. Democratic orders also increase delinquency.

Merton suggests five adaptations to this dilemma:

1. *Innovation:* Individuals who accept socially approved goals, but not necessarily the socially approved means.
2. *Retreatism:* Those who reject socially approved goals and the means for acquiring them.

3. *Ritualism:* Those who buy into a system of socially approved means, but lose sight of the goals. Merton believed that drug users are in this category.
4. *Conformity:* Those who conform to the system's means and goals.
5. *Rebellion:* People who negate socially approved goals and means by creating a new system of acceptable goals and means.

A difficulty with strain theory is that it does not explore why children of low-income families would have poor educational attainment in the first place. More importantly is the fact that much youth crime does not have an economic motivation. Strain theory fails to explain violent crime, the type of youth crime which causes most anxiety to the public.

Subcultural

- Related to strain theory is subcultural theory. The inability of youths to achieve socially valued status and goals results in groups of young people forming deviant or delinquent subcultures, which have their own values and norms.
- Within these groups criminal behavior may actually be valued, and increase a youth's status. The notion of delinquent subcultures is relevant for crimes that are not economically motivated. Male gang members could be argued to have their own values, such as respect for fighting ability and daring.
- However it is not clear how different this makes them from 'ordinary' non-lawbreaking young men. Furthermore there is no explanation of why people unable to achieve socially valued goals should necessarily choose criminal substitutes.
- Sub-cultural theories have been criticized for making too sharp a distinction between what is deviant and what is 'normal'. There are also doubts about whether young people consciously reject mainstream values.

Risk Factors

Individual Risk Factors

Individual psychological or behavioral risk factors that may make offending more likely include intelligence, impulsiveness or the inability to delay gratification, aggression, empathy, and restlessness.

Children with low intelligence are likely to do worse in school. This may increase the chances of offending because low educational attainment, a low attachment to school, and low educational aspirations are all risk factors for offending in themselves.

Children who perform poorly at school are also more likely to truant, which is also linked to offending.

Mental Disorders

Conduct disorder usually develops during childhood and manifests itself during an adolescence life.

Juvenile delinquents who have reoccurring encounters with the criminal justice system are sometimes diagnosed with conduct disorders because they show a continuous disregard for their own and others safety and property. Once the juvenile continues to exhibit the same behavioral patterns and turns eighteen, he is then at risk of being diagnosed with antisocial personality disorder and much more prone to become a serious criminal offender.

One of the main components used in diagnosing an adult with antisocial personality disorder consists of presenting documented history of conduct disorder before the age of 15. These two personality disorders are analogous in their erratic and aggressive behavior.

This is why habitual juvenile offenders diagnosed with conduct disorder are likely to exhibit signs of antisocial personality disorder as they mature. Once the juveniles reach maturation their socially unacceptable behavior has grown into a life style and they develop into career criminals. 'Career criminals begin committing antisocial behavior before entering grade school and are versatile in that they engage in an array of destructive behaviors, offend at exceedingly high rates, and are less likely to quit committing crime as they age.'

Quantitative research was completed on 9,945 juvenile male offenders between the ages of 10 and 18 in the 1970s. The longitudinal birth cohort was used to examine a trend among a small percentage of career criminals who accounted for the largest percentage of crime activity.

The trend exhibited a new phenomenon amongst habitual offenders. For this study habitual offenders were youth who experienced more than five police encounters.

Family Environment

Family factors which may have an influence on offending include; the level of parental supervision, the way parents discipline a child, parental conflict or separation, criminal parents or siblings, parental abuse or neglect, and the quality of the parent-child relationship.

Children brought up by lone parents are more likely to start offending than those who live with two natural parents, however once the attachment a child feels towards their parent(s) and the level of parental supervision are taken into account, children in single parent families are no more likely to offend than others.

Conflict between a child's parents is also much more closely linked to offending than being raised by a lone parent.

Delinquency Prevention

Delinquency prevention is the broad term for all efforts aimed at preventing youth from becoming involved in criminal, or other antisocial, activity. Increasingly, governments are recognizing the importance of allocating resources for the prevention of delinquency.

Because it is often difficult for states to provide the fiscal resources necessary for good prevention, organizations, communities, and governments are working more in collaboration with each other to prevent juvenile delinquency.

With the development of delinquency in youth being influenced by numerous factors, prevention efforts are comprehensive in scope. Prevention services include activities such as substance abuse education and treatment, family counseling, youth mentoring, parenting education, educational support, and youth sheltering.

Untreated Mental Disorders

Once the juvenile offender reaches maturation, he is likely to continue exhibiting maladaptive behaviors and increases his risk of being cycled through the criminal justice system as an adult offender.

Due to the small population of habitual adult and juvenile offenders attributing for the large percentage of violent crimes (i.e. murder and aggravated assault) the criminal justice system should supervise the small population of career criminals in an effort to prevent the spawning of serious violent offenders.

The majority of violent offenders exhibit characteristics of antisocial personality disorder and exhibit it no later than age 15. Antisocial personality disorder is a common diagnosis for a serial killer. Authors Alvarez and Bachman found that one similarity among serial killers was their prior criminal convictions.

In this case conduct disorder can become a probable constituent to serial murder if not diagnosed and treated, before it fully develops in adulthood as antisocial personality disorder. Both conduct disorder and antisocial personality disorder are categorized as personality disorders under the DSM-IV-TR and share extremely similar definitions as explained above in 'Mental Disorders'.

Some of the common characteristics include consistent violation of societal norms, aggressive behavior towards people and a disassociation to the emotion of empathy.

These traits are also common amongst serial killers and if the maladaptive behaviors are not treated, they have the potential to conceive a person that fantasizes about killing several victims and then fulfills their impulsivity when they are no longer capable of suppressing it.

Act of delinquency may include:

- Running away from home without the permission of parents
- Habitual behavior beyond the control of parents
- Spending time idly beyond limits
- Use of vulgar languages
- Wandering about rail roads, streets market places
- Visiting gambling centers
- Committing sexual offences
- Shop-lifting
- Stealing
- Juveniles may do such activities singly or through a gang.

Role of nurse in prevention of juvenile delinquency

- Accept the delinquent as a person in his own right, and give affection and security.
- Watch for the signs of maladjustment; early treatment may prevent this maladjustment from taking a delinquent trend.
- Providing the child with a variety of experiences like music and dance, art and craft, etc.
- Attempt to build-up a stable system of moral and social values.
- Reject the delinquent behavior without rejecting the delinquent.
- Encourage the child to talk about and admit the existence of antisocial tendencies.
- Change the conditions of home, school and community that seem to give rise to such behavior.
- Give a potential delinquent some post of special responsibility, such as task of preventing other children from committing delinquent acts.
- Once a delinquent act has been detected, never pass it over. Make clear to the child that he has done something wrong, but do not punish him harshly.
- Minimize the chances of a child's going wrong by putting the smallest possible number of temptations in his way.

MODEL QUESTIONS

Multiple Choice Questions

1. **In which poisoning we avoid gastric lavage or use lavage cautiously?**
   (a) Tablets (b) Cosmetics
   (c) Kerosene (d) All of these
2. **The drug used as antidotes for opiods analgesics poisoning.**
   (a) Diazepam (b) Pantoprazole
   (c) Naloxone (d) Flumazenil
3. **Otitis media is the infection of ......**
   (a) Middle ear (b) Outer ear
   (c) Nose (d) All of these
4. **The portal of entry of measles virus are......**
   (a) Respiratory tract (b) GI tract
   (c) Ear (d) Genital tract
5. **Poliomyelitis caused by ....**
   (a) Enterovirus (b) DNA virus
   (c) Both (a) and (b) (d) None of these
6. **Which one of the following is complication of mumps?**
   (a) Sterility in male (b) Oophoritis
   (c) DM (d) All of these
7. **The *aedes* mosquito caused ....**
   (a) Dengue (b) Malaria
   (c) Both (a) and (b) (d) Polio
8. **Corynebacterium diphtheriae caused ....**
   (a) Tetanus (b) TB
   (c) Diphtheria (d) All of these
9. **Schick test is done for ....**
   (a) Diphtheria (b) TB
   (c) Mumps (d) Measles
10. **Whooping cough also known as ....**
    (a) Cough and cold (b) Pneumonia
    (c) Both a and b (d) Pertussis
11. **Whooping cough transmission is mainly from...**
    (a) Droplet infection (b) Coughing
    (c) Direct contact (d) All of these
12. **The 1st dose of DPT vaccine should be started at..........**
    (a) 4 weeks (b) 6 weeks
    (c) 10 weeks (d) 12 weeks
13. **Miliary tuberculosis is ....**
    (a) Miliary TB (b) Primary TB
    (c) Secondary TB (d) All of these

14. Mantoux test done for the detection of .... disease.
(a) TB (b) Cholera
(c) Typhoid (d) Diphtheria

15. Hansen disease is also known as
(a) Typhoid (b) Pertussis
(c) Leprosy (d) Hernia

16. The sudden outburst or violent display of anger in toddler children called.......
(a) Pica (b) Breath holding
(c) Temper tantrum (d) Thumb sucking

17. Tics are sudden ....movement
(a) Voluntary (b) Only hand movement
(c) Both a and b (d) Involuntary

True or False

1. Schick test is done in typhoid.
2. Pica eating is one type of behavioral disorders.
3. Measles is not a congenital disease.
4. Encopresis is the involuntary discharge of urine.
5. Amenorrhea is the pain during menses.
6. Temper tantrum is the behavioral disorder in adolescent age.
7. Helminthic infestation is the worm infestation.
8. Accidental injury is sudden occurrence.

Fill in the Blanks

1. Causative organism of the TB.............
2. The complication of mumps is.............
3. ....vaccine given for measles.
4. Otitis media is the infection in which area of ear........
5. Breast enlargement in male the condition known as ....
6. Write one organism cause STDs................
7. Temper tantrum mainly occurs in ....age group.

Short Answer Questions 1 × 5 = 5

(a) Poisoning
(b) Temper tantrum
(c) Otitis media
(d) Obesity
(e) Poliomyelitis

Long Answer Questions 1 × 15 = 15

1. (a) Define diarrhea.
   (b) What are the causative factor responsible for diarrhea?
   (c) Explain the management of diarrhea according to plan A, B and C.
2. (a) Define communicable disease.
   (b) List down the communicable disease.
   (c) Explain any one communicable disease and its management.

ANSWER KEY

Multiple Choice Questions

1. (c)	2. (c)	3. (a)	4. (a)	5. (a)	6. (d)	7. (a)
8. (c)	9. (a)	10. (d)	11. (d)	12. (b)	13. (c)	14. (a)
15. (c)	16. (c)	17. (b)				

True or False

1. False	2. True	3. False	4. False	5. False	6. False	7. True
8. True						

Fill in the Blanks

1. *Mycobacterium tuberculosis*
2. Diabetic mellitus, male-sterility
3. MMR
4. Middle
5. Gynecomastia
6. HIV
7. Toddler (1–3 years)

Chapter 6

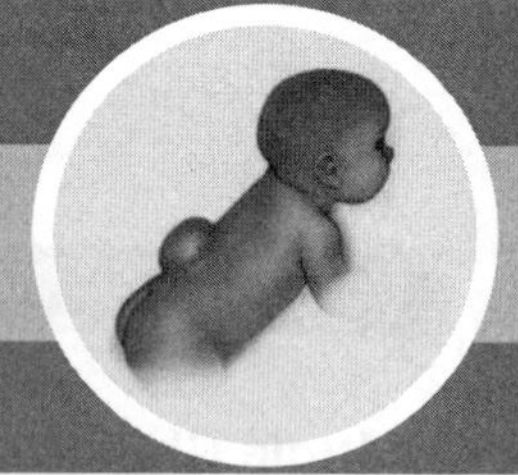

Child with Congenital Disorders

- **Malformations of Central Nervous System (CNS)**
  - Cranial Deformities
  - Spina Bifida (or) Meningocele and Myelomeningocele
  - Hydrocephalus
  - Cerebral Palsy
- **Skeletal Defects**
  - Cleft Lip and Cleft Palate
- **Gastrointestinal Tract Defects**
  - Tracheoesophageal Fistula and Esophageal Atresia
  - Anorectal Malformations
  - Hernia (Umbilical or Inguinal) in Children
  - Congenital Diaphragmatic Hernia (CDH)
  - Pyloric Stenosis
  - Congenital Hypertrophic Pyloric Stenosis (HPS)
- **Defects of Genitourinary Tract**
  - Hypospadiasis and Epispadiasis
  - Epispadias
  - Bladder Exstrophy
  - Phimosis and Paraphimosis
  - Cryptorchidism (Undescended Testes)
  - Polycystic Kidney Disease (PKD)
- **Sexual Abnormalities**
  - Ambiguous Genitalia
- **Defects of Cardiovascular System**
  - Congenital Heart Defects
  - Cyanotic Heart Diseases
  - Transposition of Great Arteries/Vessels (TGA)

- Total Anomalous Pulmonary Venous Connection (TAPVC)
- Truncus Arteriosus
- Hypoplastic Left Heart Syndrome
- Eisenmenger Syndrome or Complex
- Acyanotic Heart Diseases

• **Atrial Septal Defect (ASD)**
• **Patent Ductus Arteriosus (PDA)**
• **Pulmonary Hypertension**
• **Atrioventricular Canal Defect (AV Canal or AVC)**
• **Coarctation of the Aorta (CoA)**
  - Pulmonary Stenosis
• **Aortic Stenosis**
• **Congenital Mitral Stenosis (MS)**
• **Orthopedic Abnormalities**
  - Congenital Talipes Equinovarus (Club Foot)
  - Congenital Dislocation of Hips
• **Chromosomal Abnormalities**
  - Down Syndrome
  - Turner's Syndrome

MALFORMATIONS OF CENTRAL NERVOUS SYSTEM (CNS)

CRANIAL DEFORMITIES

Introduction

The medical term for positional skull deformities is occipital plagiocephaly. The formal definition of occipital plagiocephaly is 'oblique head.' When viewed from above, the head has a parallelogram appearance caused by constant pressure to the back of one side of baby's head. Occipital plagiocephaly also results from prolonged positioning on the back of the head, causing it to flatten unevenly across the back, thus resulting in an altered head shape. The cranial asymmetry may be present at birth or may develop during the first few months of life. Over the past several years, pediatricians have seen an increase in the number of children with cranial asymmetry, particularly unilateral flattening of the occiput.

Definition

Plagiocephaly is derived from the Greek words meaning 'oblique head.' The condition can result from either premature closure of the lambdoidal suture (synostotic plagiocephaly) or positional head deformity (nonsynostotic plagiocephaly).

Types

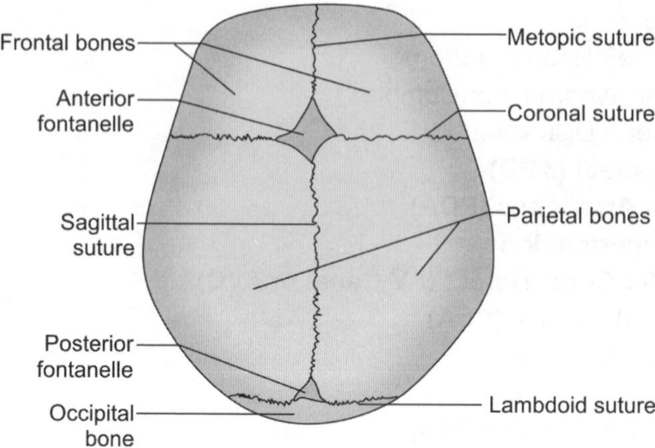

Fig. 6.1: Normal skull of the newborn

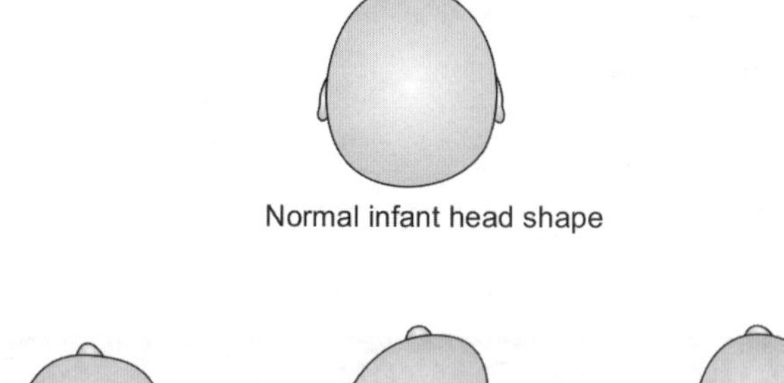

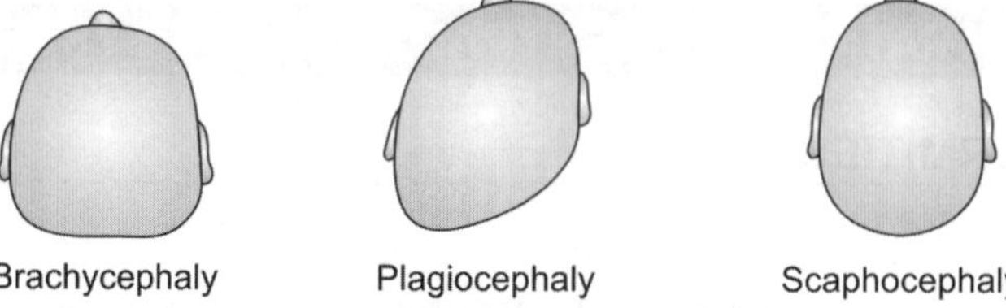

Fig. 6.2: Types of cranial deformities

Risk Factors

- Premature birth
- Hypotonic muscle disorders
- Congenital torticollis, and intrauterine constraint (such as in multiple gestation or oligohydramnios).

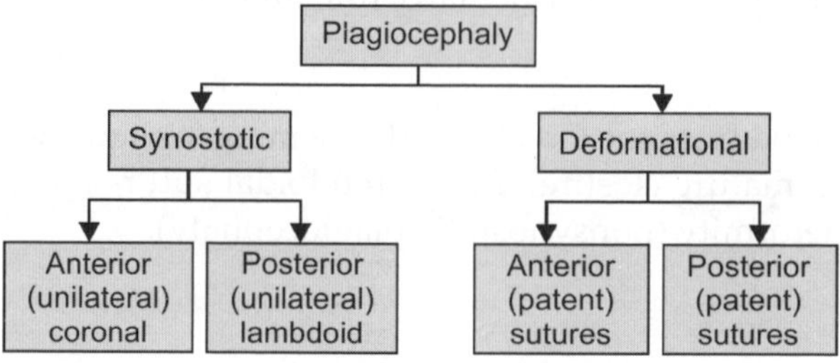

Causes

- Genetic problems
- Congenital anomalies
- Breech positioning
- Multiple fetuses
- An inadequate amount of amniotic fluid
- Difficult or prolonged delivery.

Signs and Symptoms

- High pressure on the brain (increased ICP)
- Headaches
- Untreated children may develop learning disabilities
- Vision problems
- Poor brain development
- Developmental delays.

Table 6.1: Identification of positional head deformity (PHD) and synostotic plagiocephaly

Examination	Signs of PHD or Synostosis
Palpate lambdoidal suture	Palpable ridge suggests synostosis
Check ear position	Ear on flattened side more posterior than the other ear suggests synostosis
	Ear on flattened side more anterior than the other ear suggests PHD
Assess facial symmetry	Forehead protruding on the side of the flattening suggests PHD
Observe unilateral 'bald spot'	A unilateral bald spot suggests PHD. Physician should palpate occiput for flattening
Inspect by aerial view	'Parallelogram-shaped' head suggests PHD

Diagnostic Evaluation

- History collection
- Physical examination
- X-ray
- CT/MRI scan.

Management

- Management of deformational plagiocephaly involves preventive counseling of parents, mechanical adjustments, and exercises.
- Parental compliance with the management plan is pivotal in lessening the likelihood and severity of skull deformity.
- Skull molding helmets are an option for patients with severe deformity or skull shape that is refractory to therapeutic physical adjustments and position changes.
- Surgery is rarely necessary but may be indicated in severe refractory cases of deformational plagiocephaly or in patients with craniosynostosis.

Mechanical Adjustments and Exercises

- The parent should be made aware of the condition and the mechanical adjustments that can be instituted. In general, most infants improve if the appropriate measures are conducted for a 2- to 3-month period.
- These include positioning the infant so that the rounded side of the head is placed dependent against the mattress. Additionally, the position of the crib in the room may be changed to require the child to look away from the flattened side to see the parents and others in his or her room.
- The pediatrician should continue to encourage supervised 'tummy time' on firm surfaces when the infant is awake and being observed.
- Torticollis perpetuates the position of the head on the flattened side and can add to a greater facial deformity. Therefore, if torticollis is present, neck motion exercises should be taught to the parents as part of management. Neck exercises should be done with each diaper change.
- There are three repetitions per exercise, and it is estimated to take approximately two additional minutes per diaper change. One hand is placed on the child's upper chest, and the other hand rotates the child's head gently so that the chin touches the shoulder.
- This is held for approximately 10 seconds. The head is then rotated toward the opposite side and held for the same count.
- This will stretch out the sternocleidomastoid. Next, the head is tilted so that the infant's ear touches his or her shoulder. Again, the position is held for a count of 10 and repeated for the opposite side.
- This second exercise stretches the trapezius muscle. Additionally, the parents may be taught the rotating chair or stool technique to enhance neck motion in the infant.

Skull-Molding Helmets

- The head-molding devices in infants to reshape a typically shaped skull into a different but desired skull form. Conversely, skull-molding helmets can be used to correct atypical skull shapes, and similar devices are now proposed for this purpose.
- The best response for helmets occurs in the age range of 4 to 12 months because of the greater malleability of the young infant skull bone and the normalizing effect of the rapid growth of the brain.
- There is less modification of the cranial configuration when used after 12 months of age. The use of helmets and other related devices seems to be beneficial primarily when there has been a lack of response to mechanical adjustments and exercises.

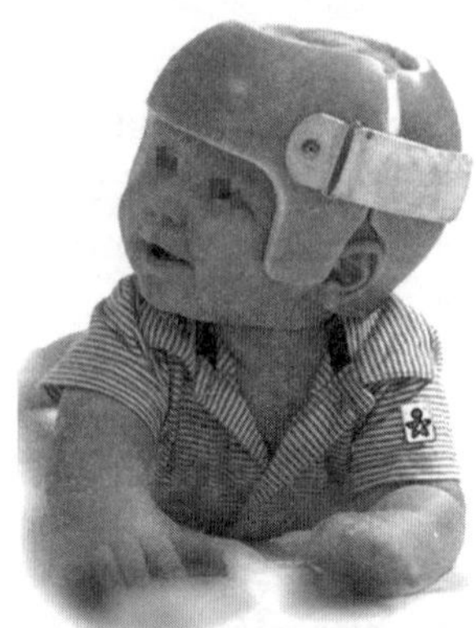

Fig. 6.3: Child with skull-molding helmet

- In most situations, an improvement to repositioning and neck exercise is seen over a 2- to 3-month period if these measures are instituted as soon as the condition is recognized.
- Because use of skull-molding helmets incurs significant cost, further studies are needed to identify outcomes with and without them.

Preventive Measures

- To prevent the head deformity, the parents should be counseled during the newborn period (by 2 to 4 weeks of age) when the skull is maximally deformable.
- Parents should be instructed to lay the infant down to sleep in the supine position, alternating positions (i.e. left and right occiputs). When awake and being observed, the infant should spend time in the prone position.
- The infant should spend minimal time in car seats (when not a passenger in a vehicle) or other seating that maintains supine positioning.
- Once deformational plagiocephaly has developed, these same preventive strategies may be used to minimize progression.
- Additionally, it is important to monitor head shape closely until there is confidence that improvement will continue, usually when the infant is old enough to sit, crawl, and spend less time on his or her back, and until any associated torticollis is completely corrected.

Surgical Management

Management of deformational skull deformities can include surgery. Surgery is almost always indicated for craniosynostosis and it has been used in rare instances for deformational plagiocephaly without synostosis when the deformities are severe and resistant to nonsurgical measures.

Standard Craniosynostosis Surgery

Strip sagittal craniectomy: This technique is used for children who are not candidates for endoscopic procedures. An incision is made over the top of the head from ear to ear and the scalp is moved forward. A strip of bone encasing the fused suture approximately two inches wide is removed from behind the 'soft spot' to the back of the head. The child will spend the first night in the intensive care unit and moved to a regular room the next morning. Children are discharged on the third or fourth day if they are feeding well.

Frontal-orbital advancement (FOA): This procedure is recommended for older infants with severe metopic synostosis or coronal synostosis. An incision is made over the top of the scalp from ear to ear. The bone of the skull is removed from above the eyes to behind the forehead. The bone is reformed and then replaced.

Children spend the first night in the intensive care unit. If the blood counts are stable, the child is moved to a regular room the following day. Their eyes will become swollen over the first 12 to 24 hours and may be swollen shut for two to three days. As soon as the eyes are open, the blood counts are stable, there is no fever and the child is eating well they may go home. The length of hospital stay is usually five to seven days.

Frontal-occipital reversal (FOR): This procedure is advised for children 6 months of age or older who have fusion of the sagittal suture or have multiple sutures that are fused. An incision is made over the top of the scalp from ear to ear. The scalp is drawn back and the skull bone is removed from above the eyes to the back of the head. The bone is divided into several pieces, which are reshaped and then replaced over the crown of the head. Tiny plates and screws are used to fix the bones into proper position. These children spend the first night in the intensive care unit. Significant swelling is expected around the face and eyes, which lasts for several days.

Nursing Management

- Monitor for postoperative complication
- Provide for family education: Support parents by providing them with information on the complex decision-making process
- Assess coping skills
- Parental knowledge deficit.

SPINA BIFIDA (OR) MENINGOCELE AND MYELOMENINGOCELE

Introduction

The term spina bifida comes from Latin and literally means 'split' or 'open' spine. This defect happens at the end of the first month of pregnancy, when a baby's spine and spinal cord (a bundle of nerves that runs down the center of the spine) are developing. Spina bifida is the most common permanently disabling birth defect, that the spinal bones protect the spinal cord has not formed completely while a baby is developing in the mother's uterus. This happens very early in pregnancy. Spina bifida can happen anywhere along a baby's back between the head and the hips. It occurs most often in the lumbar spine.

Children with spina bifida may have health problems because of the condition. They may be paralyzed (not able to move their legs) or have decreased movement of their legs, changes or loss of feeling in their legs. They may have problems with their bladder and bowel function.

Definition

Spina bifida is part of congenital defects called as neural tube defects. The neural tube is the embryonic structure that eventually develops into the baby's brain and spinal cord and the tissues that enclose them. Normally, the neural tube forms early in the pregnancy and closes by the 28th day after conception. In babies with spina bifida, a portion of the neural tube fails to develop or close properly, causing defects in the spinal cord and in the bones of the spine.

Spina bifida occurs in various forms of severity. When treatment for spina bifida is necessary, it is done surgically, although such treatment does not always completely resolve the problem.

Incidence

About 1 baby in every 2,500 babies has some form of spina bifida.

Types of Spina Bifida

There are 4 main types of spina bifida: Spina bifida occulta, meningocele, and myelomeningocele. 'Meningo' refers to the lining of the spinal cord. 'Myelo' refers to the spinal cord itself. 'Cele' means bulging out.

Spina Bifida

The neural tube does not fully close during fetal development, spina bifida can result. In spina bifida occulta, some vertebral arches are missing, but the spinal cord and meninges usually do not protrude through. There may be a dimple or patch of hair. In meningocele, the meninges that surround the spinal cord protrude through the gap in the vertebral canal. Myelomeningocele also has a fluid filled sac which protrudes, but the sac also contains some spinal cord and spinal nerves.

Spina Bifida Occulta

Spina bifida occulta occurs when the outer part of the vertebrae (the bones of the spine) have not completely joined, leaving an opening. In this type of spina bifida, the spinal cord and its coverings (the meninges) are not damaged and they do not protrude or bulge through the opening. There may be a dimple, tuft of hair, birthmark, or fatty bulge at the site of the defect. This type of spina bifida is not detected before birth.

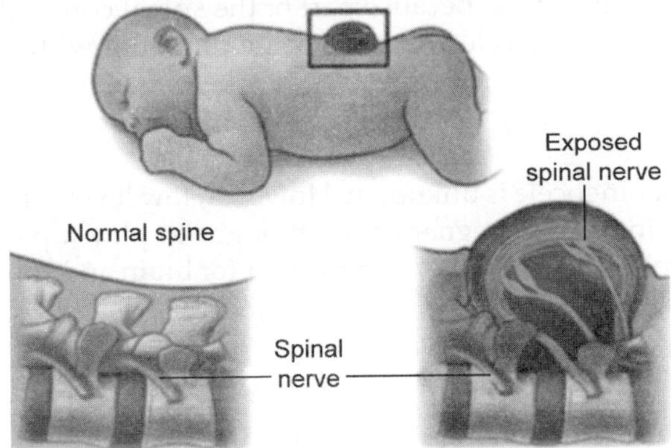

Fig. 6.4: Anatomical difference between normal and spina bifida spine

Meningocele

A meningocele (meh-NING-go-seal) occurs when the outer part of the vertebrae have not completely closed, leaving an opening. The spinal cord itself may not be affected, but its coverings (the meninges) are damaged and pushed through the opening. With a meningocele, the spinal cord stays inside the back where it belongs. This means that most children with a meningocele will have normal movement and normal feeling in their legs and feet.

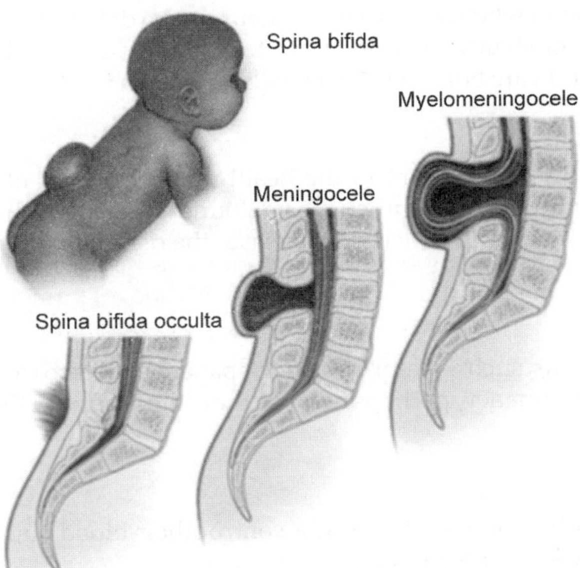

Fig. 6.5: Types of spina bifida

Myelomeningocele

A myelomeningocele (MY-ell-oh-meh-NING-go-seal) occurs when the outer part of the vertebrae have not completely closed, creating an abnormal opening. With a myelomeningocele, both the covering of the spinal cord (the meninges) and the spinal cord itself are pushed out the opening. Usually they protrude into a covered, fluid-filled sac that has a very thin membrane and can easily split, exposing its delicate contents. This is the most serious form of spina bifida. Because part of the spinal cord bulges into the sac, most children with a myelomeningocele will have some difficulty with movement and feeling in their legs and feet.

Causes

The cause of myelomeningocele is unknown. However, low levels of folic acid in a woman's body before and during early pregnancy are thought to play a part in this type of birth defect. The vitamin folic acid (or folate) is important for brain and spinal cord development.

Risk Factors

Race

Spina bifida is more common among Whites and Hispanics.

Sex

Girls are affected more often.

Family History of Neural Tube Defects

Couples who have had one child with a neural tube defect have a slightly higher chance of having another baby with the same defect. That risk increases if two previous children have been affected by the condition.

In addition, a woman who was born with a neural tube defect, or who has a close relative with one, has a greater chance of giving birth to a child with spina bifida. However, most babies with spina bifida are born to parents with no known family history of the condition.

Folic Acid Deficiency

Folic acid (vitamin B_9) is important to the healthy development of a baby. Folate is the natural form of vitamin B_9. The synthetic form, found in supplements and fortified foods, is called folic acid. A Folic acid deficiency increases the risk of spina bifida and other neural tube defects.

Some Medications

Antiseizure medications, such as valproic acid (Depakene), seem to cause neural tube defects when taken during pregnancy, perhaps because they interfere with the body's ability to use folate and folic acid.

Diabetes

Pregnant women with diabetes who do not control their blood sugar well have a higher risk of having a baby with spina bifida.

Obesity

Prepregnancy obesity is associated with an increased risk of neural tube birth defects, including spina bifida.

Increased Body Temperature

Some evidence suggests that increased body temperature (hyperthermia) in the early weeks of pregnancy may increase the risk of spina bifida. Elevating your core body temperature, due to fever or the use of saunas or hot tubs, has been associated with increased risk of spina bifida.

Signs and Symptoms

A newborn may have a sac sticking out of the mid to lower back.

Symptoms include:

- Loss of bladder or bowel control
- Partial or complete lack of sensation
- Partial or complete paralysis of the legs
- Weakness of the hips, legs/feet of a newborn baby.

Other signs symptoms may include:

- Abnormal feet or legs, such as clubfoot
- Build up of fluid inside the skull (hydrocephalus).

Clinical Features

Table 6.2: Clinical features of meningocele vs myelomeningocele

Meningocele	Myelomeningocele
• Urinary frequency, urgency and incontinence	• Development of hydrocephalous characterized by macrocephaly, headache, vomiting, urinary incontinence
• Urinary retention	• Spastic weakness of all four limbs
• Constipation and diarrhea	• An abnormally small sized head
• An allergy to latex	• Uncoordinated muscle movements
• Scoliosis	• Delayed developmental milestones
• Hydrocephalus (in 90% of cases)	• Vision problems
• Difficulty in walking	• Mental and growth retardation
• Poor coordination in walking	• Seizures
• Paralysis of lower limbs	
• Numbness of lower limbs	
• Pain and heaviness in lower limbs	
• Loss of sensation in perianal and genital area	

Diagnostic Evaluation

Spina Bifida can be diagnosed on physical examination of the lower back of a baby just after birth. In doubtful conditions, the following investigations can be carried out to diagnose myelomeningocele:

- *X-rays:* Spine
- *MRI:* Spine

Prenatal diagnosis by following screening tests, though these are nonspecific:
- Serum alpha-fetoprotein levels
- Quadruple/triple screen
- Ultrasonography
- Amniocentesis.

Maternal Serum Alpha-Fetoprotein (MSAFP) Test

A common test used to check for myelomeningocele is the maternal serum alpha-fetoprotein (MSAFP) test. To perform this test, your doctor draws a blood sample and sends it to a laboratory, where it is tested for alpha-fetoprotein (AFP) a protein that is produced by the baby.

It is normal for a small amount of AFP to cross the placenta and enter the mothers bloodstream, but abnormally high levels of AFP suggest that the baby has a neural tube defect, most commonly spina bifida or anencephaly, a condition characterized by an underdeveloped brain and an incomplete skull.

Some spina bifida cases do not produce a high level of AFP. On the other hand, when a high level of AFP is found, a neural tube defect is present only a small percentage of the time.

Varying levels of AFP can be caused by other factors including a miscalculation in fetal age or multiple babies so your doctor may order a follow-up blood test for confirmation. If the results are still high, you will need further evaluation, including an ultrasound examination.

Other Blood Tests

Along with MSAFP test with two or three other blood tests, which may detect other hormones, such as human chorionic gonadotropin (hCG), inhibin A and estriol.

Depending on the number of tests, the combination is called a triple screen or quadruple screen (quad screen). These tests are commonly done with the MSAFP test, but their objective is to screen for trisomy 21 (Down syndrome), not neural tube defects.

Ultrasound

Most of the obstetricians rely on ultrasonography to screen for spina bifida. If blood tests indicate high AFP levels, your doctor will suggest an ultrasound exam to help determine why. The most common ultrasound exams bounce high-frequency sound waves off tissues in your body to form black-and-white images on a video monitor.

The information these images provide can help establish whether there is more than one baby and can help confirm gestational age, two factors that can affect AFP levels. An advanced ultrasound can also detect signs of spina bifida, such as an open spine or particular features in your baby's brain that indicate spina bifida.

In expert hands, ultrasound today is quite effective in detecting spina bifida and assessing its severity. Ultrasound is safe for both mother and baby.

Amniocentesis

If a blood test shows high levels of AFP in your blood but the ultrasound is normal, your doctor may offer amniocentesis. During amniocentesis, your doctor uses a needle to remove a sample of fluid from the amniotic sac that surrounds the baby.

An analysis indicates the level of AFP present in the amniotic fluid. A small amount of AFP is normally found in amniotic fluid.

However, when an open neural tube defect is present, the amniotic fluid contains an elevated amount of AFP because the skin surrounding the baby's spine is gone and AFP leaks into the amniotic sac.

Management

Surgical Management

Meningocele involves surgery to put the meninges back in place and close the opening in the vertebrae. Myelomeningocele also requires surgery, usually within 24 to 48 hours after birth. Performing the surgery early can help minimize risk of infection that is associated with the exposed nerves and may also help protect the spinal cord from additional trauma.

During the procedure, a neurosurgeon places the spinal cord and exposed tissue inside the baby's body and covers them with muscle and skin. Sometimes a shunt to control hydrocephalus in the baby's brain is placed during the operation on the spinal cord.

Children who also have *hydrocephalus* may need a ventriculoperitoneal shunt placed.

- In a ventriculostomy, a small opening is made in the bottom of the third ventricle (one of four ventricles in the brain) to allow fluid to exit the brain.
- In a shunt procedure, a thin tube is placed within the brain to drain extra fluid down to the belly, where the body can absorb it.

Two types of prenatal repair can be performed. These include:

1. Open prenatal fetal surgery
2. Minimal invasive surgery.

Ongoing Care

Treatment does not end with the initial surgery, though. In babies with myelomeningocele, irreparable nerve damage has already occurred and ongoing care from a multidisciplinary team of surgeons, physicians and therapists is usually needed. Babies with myelomeningocele may need further operations for a variety of complications.

Paralysis and bladder and bowel problems often remain, and treatment for these conditions typically begins soon after birth. Babies with myelomeningocele may also start exercises that will prepare their legs for walking with braces or crutches when they are older.

Many have a tethered spinal cord, a condition in which the spinal cord is bound to the scar of the closure and is less able to properly grow in length as the child grows. This progressive 'tethering' can cause loss of muscle function to the legs, bowel or bladder. Surgery can limit the degree of disability and may also restore some function.

Complications of Spina Bifida

- Traumatic birth and difficult delivery of the baby
- Frequent urinary tract infections
- Fluid buildup on the brain (hydrocephalus)
- Loss of bowel or bladder control
- Low blood oxygen level in the baby

- Brain infection (meningitis)
- Permanent weakness or paralysis of legs.

Preventive Measures

- Folic acid supplements may help reduce the risk of neural tube defects such as myelomeningocele. It is recommended that any woman considering becoming pregnant take 0.4 mg of folic acid a day. Pregnant women need 1 mg per day.
- It is important to remember that folic acid deficiencies must be corrected before becoming pregnant, because the defects develop very early.
- Prospective mothers may be screened to determine the amount of folic acid in their blood.

Nursing Management

- Newborn child has a condition such as spina bifida can naturally cause you to feel grief, anger, frustration, fear and sadness.
- There is good reason to hope, however, because most people with spina bifida live active, productive and full lives especially with encouragement and support from loved ones.
- Even with severe spina bifida, most children can walk for at least short distances, usually with the assistance of braces, canes or crutches, although they may require wheelchairs for longer distances.
- Using these devices can help a child compensate for his or her condition and gain more independence.
- Many children with spina bifida have normal intelligence, but they may need early educational intervention for learning problems. They may also need extra help from teachers and counselors to adapt to school.
- A physical disability like spina bifida can also cause emotional and social problems.
- Children with spina bifida need encouragement to participate in activities with their peers and to lead independent lives, within their physical limitations and capabilities.
- It may be helpful to remember that these children have never known what is accepted as normal function and often adapt to their condition in remarkable ways.

HYDROCEPHALUS

Introduction

Hydrocephalus can be defined broadly as a disturbance of formation, flow, or absorption of cerebrospinal fluid (CSF) that leads to an increase in volume occupied by this fluid in the CNS. This condition also could be termed a hydrodynamic disorder of CSF. Conditions such as cerebral atrophy and focal destructive lesions also lead to an abnormal increase of CSF in CNS. In these situations, loss of cerebral tissue leaves a vacant space that is filled passively with CSF. Such conditions are not the result of a hydrodynamic disorder and therefore are not classified as hydrocephalus. An older misnomer used to describe these conditions was hydrocephalus.

Normal pressure hydrocephalus (NPH) describes a condition that rarely occurs in patients younger than 60 years. Enlarged ventricles and normal CSF pressure at lumbar puncture

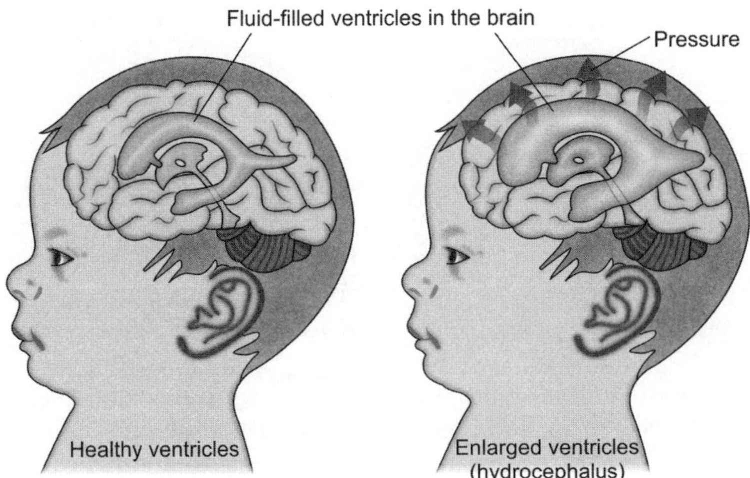

Fig. 6.6: Normal and hydrocephalus child

(LP) in the absence of Papilledema led to the term NPH. However, intermittent intracranial hypertension has been noted during monitoring of patients in whom NPH is suspected, usually at night. The classic Hakim triad of symptoms includes gait apraxia, incontinence, and dementia. Headache is not a typical symptom in NPH.

Benign external hydrocephalus is a self-limiting absorption deficiency of infancy and early childhood with raised intracranial pressure (ICP) and enlarged subarachnoid spaces. The ventricles usually are not enlarged significantly, and resolution within 1 year is the rule.

Definition

Hydrocephalus defined as disturbance of formation, flow, or absorption of cerebrospinal fluid (CSF) that leads to an increase in volume occupied by this fluid in the CNS. This condition also could be termed a hydrodynamic disorder of CSF.

Types/Classification

Major Classification

- Communicating hydrocephalus
- Noncommunicating hydrocephalus.

Minor Classification

- Acute hydrocephalus
- Subacute hydrocephalus
- Chronic hydrocephalus.

Communicating Hydrocephalus

- It occurs when full communication occurs between the ventricles and subarachnoid space. It is caused by overproduction of CSF (rarely), defective absorption of CSF (most often), or venous drainage insufficiency (occasionally).
- Communicating hydrocephalus with surrounding 'atrophy' and increased periventricular and deep white matter signal on fluid-attenuated inversion recovery (FLAIR) sequences.

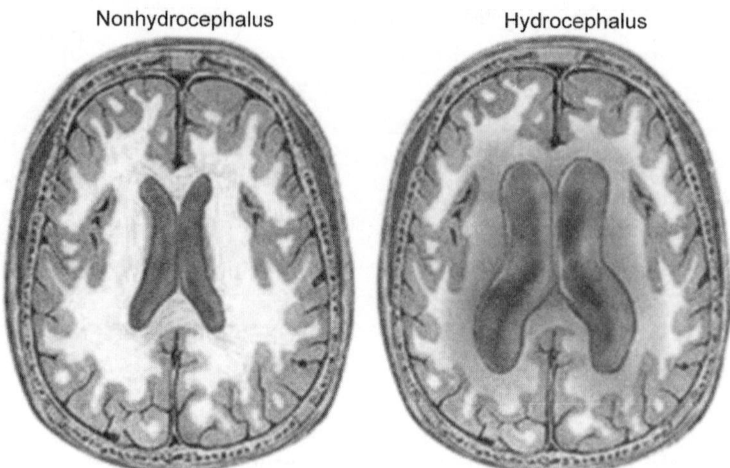

Fig. 6.7: Major types of hydrocephalus

- Note that apical cuts (lower row) do not show enlargement of the sulci, as is expected in generalized atrophy.
- Pathological evaluation of this brain demonstrated hydrocephalus with no microvascular pathology corresponding with the signal abnormality (which likely reflects transependymal exudate) and normal brain weight (indicating that the sulci enlargement was due to increased subarachnoid cerebrospinal fluid [CSF] conveying a pseudoatrophic brain pattern).

Noncommunicating Hydrocephalus

- It occurs when CSF flow is obstructed within the ventricular system or in its outlets to the arachnoid space, resulting in impairment of the CSF from the ventricular to the subarachnoid space.
- The most common form of noncommunicating hydrocephalus is obstructive and is caused by intraventricular or extraventricular mass-occupying lesions that disrupt the ventricular anatomy.
- Congenital hydrocephalus applies to the ventriculomegaly that develops in the fetal and infancy periods, often associated with macrocephaly.
- The most common causes of congenital hydrocephalus are obstruction of the cerebral aqueduct flow, Arnold-Chiari malformation or Dandy-Walker malformation.
- These patients may stabilize in later years due to compensatory mechanisms but may decompensate, especially following minor head injuries.
- During this decompensation, determining the extent to which any new neurological deficits may be due to the new acute event, compared with hydrocephalus that may have gone unnoticed for many years, is difficult.

Incidence

International

Incidence of acquired hydrocephalus is unknown. About 100,000 shunts are implanted each year in the developed countries, but little information is available for other countries.

- In untreated hydrocephalus, death may occur by tonsillar herniation secondary to raised ICP with compression of the brain stem and subsequent respiratory arrest.
- Shunt dependence occurs in 75% of all cases of treated hydrocephalus and in 50% of children with communicating hydrocephalus.
- Children are hospitalized for scheduled shunt revisions or for treatment of shunt complications or shunt failure.
- Poor development of cognitive function in infants and children, or loss of cognitive function in adults, can complicate untreated hydrocephalus.
- It may persist after treatment. Visual loss can complicate untreated hydrocephalus and may persist after treatment.

Sings and Symptoms

Symptoms in Infants

- Poor feeding
- Irritability
- Reduced activity
- Vomiting.

Symptoms in Children

- Slowing of mental capacity.
- Headaches (initially in the morning) that are more significant than in infants because of skull rigidity.
- Neck pain suggesting tonsillar herniation.
- Vomiting, more significant in the morning.
- *Blurred vision:* This is a consequence of papilledema and later of optic atrophy.
- *Double vision:* This is related to unilateral or bilateral sixth nerve palsy.
- Stunted growth and sexual maturation from third ventricle dilatation: This can lead to obesity and to precocious puberty or delayed onset of puberty.
- Difficulty in walking secondary to spasticity: This affects the lower limbs preferentially because the periventricular pyramidal tract is stretched by the hydrocephalus.
- Drowsiness.

Symptoms in Adolescent/Adults

- *Cognitive deterioration:* This can be confused with other types of dementia in the elderly.
- *Headaches:* These are more prominent in the morning because cerebrospinal fluid (CSF) is reabsorbed less efficiently in the recumbent position. This can be relieved by sitting up. As the condition progresses, headaches become severe and continuous. Headache is rarely if ever present in normal pressure hydrocephalus (NPH).
- *Neck pain:* If present, neck pain may indicate protrusion of cerebellar tonsils into the foramen magnum.
- Nausea that is not exacerbated by head movements.
- *Vomiting:* Sometimes explosive, vomiting is more significant in the morning.

- *Blurred vision (and episodes of 'graying out'):* These may suggest serious optic nerve compromise, which should be treated as an emergency.
- Double vision (horizontal diplopia) from sixth nerve palsy.
- Difficulty in walking.
- Drowsiness.
- *Incontinence (urinary first, fecal later if condition remains untreated):* This indicates significant destruction of frontal lobes and advanced disease.

Symptoms of NPH

- Gait disturbance is usually the first symptom and may precede other symptoms by months or years. Magnetic gait is used to emphasize the tendency of the feet to remain 'stuck to the floor' despite patients' best efforts to move them.
- Dementia should be a late finding in pure (shunt-responsive) NPH. It presents as an impairment of recent memory or as a 'slowing of thinking.' Spontaneity and initiative are decreased. The degree can vary from patient to patient.
- Urinary incontinence may present as urgency, frequency, or a diminished awareness of the need to urinate.
- Other symptoms that can occur include personality changes and Parkinsonism. Seizures are extremely rare and should prompt consideration for an alternative diagnosis.

Causes

Congenital Causes in Infants and Children

- *Brainstem malformation causing stenosis of the aqueduct of Sylvius:* This is responsible for 10% of all cases of hydrocephalus in newborns.
- *Dandy-Walker malformation:* This affects 2–4% of newborns with hydrocephalus.
- Arnold-Chiari malformation type 1 and type 2.
- Agenesis of the foramen of Monro.
- Congenital toxoplasmosis.
- *Bickers-Adams syndrome:* This is an X-linked hydrocephalus accounting for 7% of cases in males. It is characterized by stenosis of the aqueduct of Sylvius, severe mental retardation, and in 50% by an adduction-flexion deformity of the thumb.

Acquired Causes in Infants and Children

- *Mass lesions:* Mass lesions account for 20% of all cases of hydrocephalus in children. These are usually tumors (e.g. medulloblastoma, astrocytoma), but cysts, abscesses, or hematoma also can be the cause.
- *Hemorrhage:* Intraventricular hemorrhage can be related to prematurity, head injury, or rupture of a vascular malformation.
- *Infections:* Meningitis (especially bacterial) and, in some geographic areas, cysticercosis can cause hydrocephalus.
- *Increased venous sinus pressure:* This can be related to achondroplasia, some craniostenoses, or venous thrombosis.
- *Iatrogenic:* Hypervitaminosis A, by increasing secretion of CSF or by increasing permeability of the blood-brain barrier, can lead to hydrocephalus. As a caveat,

hypervitaminosis A is a more common cause of idiopathic intracranial hypertension, a disorder with increased CSF pressure but small rather than large ventricles.
- Idiopathic.

Causes of Hydrocephalus in Adolescent/Adults

- Subarachnoid hemorrhage (SAH) causes one third of these cases by blocking the arachnoid villi and limiting reabsorption of CSF. However, communication between ventricles and subarachnoid space is preserved.
- Idiopathic hydrocephalus represents one third of cases of adult hydrocephalus.
- Head injury, through the same mechanism as SAH, can result in hydrocephalus.
- Tumors can cause blockage anywhere along the CSF pathways. The most frequent tumors associated with hydrocephalus are ependymoma, subependymal giant cell astrocytoma, choroid plexus papilloma, craniopharyngioma, pituitary adenoma, hypothalamic or optic nerve glioma, hamartoma, and metastatic tumors.
- Prior posterior fossa surgery may cause hydrocephalus by blocking normal pathways of CSF flow.
- Congenital aqueductal stenosis causes hydrocephalus but may not be symptomatic until adulthood. Special care should be taken when attributing new neurological deficits to congenital hydrocephalus, as its treatment by shunting may not correct these deficits.
- Meningitis, especially bacterial, may cause hydrocephalus in adults.
- All causes of hydrocephalus described in infants and children are present in adults who have had congenital or childhood-acquired hydrocephalus.

Causes of NPH

(Most cases are idiopathic and are probably related to a deficiency of arachnoid granulations.)
- SAH
- Head trauma
- Meningitis.

Pathophysiology

Normal CSF production is 0.20–0.35 mL/min; most CSF is produced by the choroid plexus, which is located within the ventricular system, mainly the lateral and fourth ventricles. The capacity of the lateral and third ventricles in a healthy person is 20 mL. Total volume of CSF in an adult is 120 mL. Normal route of CSF from production to clearance is the following: From the choroid plexus, the CSF flows to the lateral ventricle, then to the interventricular foramen of Monro, the third ventricle, the cerebral aqueduct of Sylvius, the fourth ventricle, the two lateral foramina of Luschka and 1 medial foramen of Magendie, the subarachnoid space, the arachnoid granulations, the dural sinus, and finally into the venous drainage.

ICP rises if production of CSF exceeds absorption. This occurs if CSF is overproduced, resistance to CSF flow is increased, or venous sinus pressure is increased. CSF production falls as ICP rises. Compensation may occur through transventricular absorption of CSF and also by absorption along nerve root sleeves. Temporal and frontal horns dilate first, often asymmetrically. This may result in elevation of the corpus callosum, stretching or perforation of the septum pellucidum, thinning of the cerebral mantle, or enlargement of the third ventricle downward into the pituitary fossa (which may cause pituitary dysfunction).

The mechanism of NPH has not been elucidated completely. Current theories include increased resistance to flow of CSF within the ventricular system or subarachnoid villi; intermittently elevated CSF pressure, usually at night; and ventricular enlargement caused by an initial rise in CSF pressure; the enlargement is maintained despite normal pressure because of the Laplace law. Although pressure is normal, the enlarged ventricular area reflects increased force on the ventricular wall.

Diagnostic Evaluation

Laboratory Studies

- No specific blood tests are recommended in the workup for hydrocephalus.
- Genetic testing and counseling might be recommended when X-linked hydrocephalus is suspected.
- Evaluate cerebrospinal fluid (CSF) in posthemorrhagic and postmeningitic hydrocephalus for protein concentration and to exclude residual infection.

Imaging Studies

- CT can assess the size of ventricles and other structures.
- MRI can evaluate for Chiari malformation or cerebellar or periaqueductal tumors. It affords better imaging of the posterior fossa than CT. MRI can differentiate normal pressure hydrocephalus (NPH) from cerebral atrophy although the distinctions may be challenging. Flow voids in the third ventricle and transependymal fluid exudates are helpful. However, numerous suitable patients have a brain pattern suggestive of atrophy and small vessel ischemic disease that may ultimately be NPH. Guidelines for imaging studies in suspected NPH have been established.
- CT/MRI criteria for acute hydrocephalus include the following:
  - Size of both temporal horns is greater than 2 mm, clearly visible. In the absence of hydrocephalus, the temporal horns should be barely visible.
  - Ratio of the largest width of the frontal horns to maximal biparietal diameter (i.e. Evans ratio) is greater than 30% in hydrocephalus.
  - Transependymal exudate is translated on images as periventricular hypoattenuation (CT) or hyperintensity (MRI T2-weighted and fluid-attenuated inversion recovery [FLAIR] sequences).
  - Ballooning of frontal horns of lateral ventricles and third ventricle (i.e. 'Mickey mouse' ventricles) may indicate aqueductal obstruction.
  - Upward bowing of the corpus callosum on sagittal MRI suggests acute hydrocephalus.
- CT/MRI criteria for chronic hydrocephalus include the following:
  - Temporal horns may be less prominent than in acute hydrocephalus.
  - Third ventricle may herniate into the sella turcica.
  - Sella turcica may be eroded.
  - Macrocrania (i.e. occipitofrontal circumference > 98th percentile) may be present.
  - Corpus callosum may be atrophied (best appreciated on sagittal MRI). In this case, parenchymal atrophy and ex-vacuo (rather than true) hydrocephalus from a neurodegenerative disease should be considered.

- Ultrasonography through the anterior fontanelle in infants is useful for evaluating subependymal and intraventricular hemorrhage and in following infants for possible development of progressive hydrocephalus.
- Radionuclide cisternography can be done in NPH to evaluate the prognosis with regard to possible shunting. If a late scan (48–72 hour) shows persistence of ventricular activity with a ventricular to total intracranial activity (V/T ratio) greater than 32%, the patient is more likely to benefit from shunting. Because of its poor sensitivity in predicting shunt response when the V/T ratio is less than 32%, this test is no longer commonly used.
- Skull radiographs may depict erosion of sella turcica, or 'beaten copper cranium' (called by some authors 'beaten silver cranium'). The latter can also be seen in craniosynostosis.
- MRI cine is an MRI technique to measure CSF stroke volume (SV) in the cerebral aqueduct. Cine phase-contrast MRI measurements of SV in the cerebral aqueduct does not appear to be useful in predicting response to shunting.
- Diffusion tensor imaging (DTI) is a novel imaging technique that detects differences in fractional anisotropy (FA) and mean diffusivity (MD) of the brain parenchyma surrounding the ventricles. Impairment of FA and MD through DTI allows the recognition of microstructural changes in periventricular white matter region that may be too subtle on conventional MRI.

Other Tests

- After shunt insertion, confirm correct positioning of installed hardware with a plain radiograph
- EEG if seizure occurs
- Lumbar puncture (LP).

Management

Medical Management

Medical treatment in hydrocephalus is used to delay surgical intervention. It may be tried in premature infants with posthemorrhagic hydrocephalus (in the absence of acute hydrocephalus). Normal CSF absorption may resume spontaneously during this interim period. Medical treatment is not effective in long-term treatment of chronic hydrocephalus. It may induce metabolic consequences and thus should be used only as a temporizing measure.

Medications Affect CSF Dynamics by the Following Mechanisms

Decreasing CSF secretion by the choroid plexus—Acetazolamide and furosemide—Increasing CSF reabsorption—Isosorbide (effectiveness is questionable).

Medication

- *Acetazolamide (ACZ) and Furosemide (FUR):* Treat posthemorrhagic hydrocephalus in neonates. Both are diuretics that also appear to decrease secretion of CSF at the level of the choroid plexus. ACZ can be used alone or in conjunction with FUR. The combination enhances efficacy of ACZ in decreasing CSF secretion by the choroid plexus. If ACZ is used alone, it appears to lower risk of nephrocalcinosis significantly. Medication as treatment for hydrocephalus is controversial. It should be used only as a temporary measure for posthemorrhagic hydrocephalus in neonates.

- *Carbonic anhydrase inhibitors:* These agents inhibit an enzyme found in many tissues of the body that catalyzes a reversible reaction in which carbon dioxide becomes hydrated and carbonic acid dehydrated. These changes may result in a decrease in CSF production by the choroid plexus.
- *Acetazolamide (Diamox):* Noncompetitive reversible inhibitor of enzyme carbonic anhydrase, which catalyzes the reaction between water and carbon dioxide, resulting in protons and carbonate. This contributes to decreasing CSF secretion by choroid plexus. Pediatric, 25 mg/kg/d PO tid; not to exceed 100 mg/kg/d.
- *Loop diuretics:* These agents increase excretion of water by interfering with the chloride-binding cotransport system, which results from inhibition of reabsorption of sodium and chloride in the ascending loop of Henle and distal renal tubule.
- *Furosemide (Lasix):* Mechanisms proposed for lowering ICP include lowering cerebral sodium uptake, affecting water transport into astroglial cells by inhibiting cellular membrane cation-chloride pump, and decreasing CSF production by inhibiting carbonic anhydrase. Pediatric: 1 mg/kg/d IV.

Surgical Management

Surgical treatment is the preferred therapeutic option. Repeat lumbar punctures (LPs) can be performed for cases of hydrocephalus after intraventricular hemorrhage, since this condition can resolve spontaneously. If reabsorption does not resume when the protein content of cerebrospinal fluid (CSF) is less than 100 mg/dL, spontaneous resorption is unlikely to occur. LPs can be performed only in cases of communicating hydrocephalus.

Alternatives to Shunting Include the Following

Choroid plexectomy or choroid plexus coagulation may be effective. Opening of a stenosed aqueduct has a higher morbidity rate and a lower success rate than shunting, except in the case of tumors. However, lately cerebral aqueductoplasty has gained popularity as an effective treatment for membranous and short-segment stenosis of the sylvian aqueduct. It can be performed through a coronal approach or endoscopically through suboccipital foramen magnum trans-fourth ventricle approach. In these cases, tumor removal cures the hydrocephalus in 80%. Endoscopic fenestration of the floor of the third ventricle establishes an alternative route for CSF toward the subarachnoid space. It is contraindicated in communicating hydrocephalus.

Shunts eventually are performed in most patients. Only about 25% of patients with hydrocephalus are treated successfully without shunt placement. The principle of shunting is to establish a communication between the CSF (ventricular or lumbar) and a drainage cavity (peritoneum, right atrium, pleura). Remember that shunts are not perfect and that all alternatives to shunting should be considered first. A ventriculoperitoneal (VP) shunt is used most commonly. The lateral ventricle is the usual proximal location. The advantage of this shunt is that the need to lengthen the catheter with growth may be obviated by using a long peritoneal catheter. A ventriculoatrial (VA) shunt also is called a 'vascular shunt.' It shunts the cerebral ventricles through the jugular vein and superior vena cava into the right cardiac atrium. It is used when the patient has abdominal abnormalities (e.g. peritonitis, morbid obesity, or after extensive abdominal surgery). This shunt requires repeated lengthening in a growing child. A lumboperitoneal shunt is used only for communicating hydrocephalus, CSF fistula, or pseudotumor cerebri.

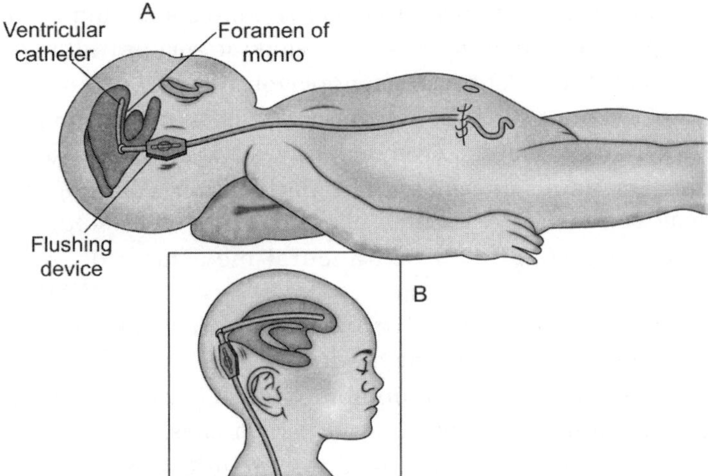

Fig. 6.8: Child with ventriculoperitoneal (VP) shunt

A Torkildsen shunt is used rarely. It shunts the ventricle to cisternal space and is effective only in acquired obstructive hydrocephalus. A ventriculopleural shunt is considered second line. It is used if other shunt types are contraindicated. Rapid-onset hydrocephalus with increased intracranial pressure (ICP) is an emergency.

Types of Shunts

- Ventricular tap in infants
- Open ventricular drainage in children and adults
- LP in posthemorrhagic and postmeningitis hydrocephalus
- VP or VA shunt.

Complications

Related to Progression of Hydrocephalus

- Visual changes
  - Occlusion of posterior cerebral arteries secondary to downward transtentorial herniation
  - Chronic papilledema injuring the optic disc
  - Dilatation of the third ventricle with compression of optic chiasm.
- Cognitive dysfunction
- Incontinence
- Gait changes.

Related to Medical Treatment

- Electrolyte imbalance
- Metabolic acidosis.

Related to Surgical Treatment

- Signs and symptoms of increased intracranial pressure (ICP) can be a consequence of undershunting or shunt obstruction or disconnection.

- Subdural hematoma or hygroma is secondary to overshunting. Headache and focal neurological signs are common.
- Treat seizures with antiepileptic drugs.
- Shunt infection occasionally can be asymptomatic. In neonates, it manifests as alteration of feeding, irritability, vomiting, fever, lethargy, somnolence, and a bulging fontanelle.
- Older children and adults present with headache, fever, vomiting, and meningismus. With ventriculoperitoneal (VP) shunts, abdominal pain may occur.
- Shunts can act as a conduit for extraneural metastases of certain tumors (e.g. medulloblastoma).
- Hardware erosion through the skin occurs in premature infants with enlarged heads and thin skin who lie on 1 side of the head.
- VP shunt complications include peritonitis, inguinal hernia, perforation of abdominal organs, intestinal obstruction, volvulus, and CSF ascites.
- Ventriculoatrial (VA) shunt complications include septicemia, shunt embolus, endocarditis, and pulmonary hypertension.
- Lumboperitoneal shunt complications include radiculopathy and arachnoiditis.

Nursing Management

- Child with shunt-dependent hydrocephalus should be admitted for consideration of shunt revision, if shunt malfunction or infection is suspected.
- In children, shunt revisions are scheduled according to growth rate.
- Child on acetazolamide (ACZ) or furosemide (FUR) should be followed for possible electrolyte imbalance and metabolic acidosis. Clinical signs that should prompt attention are lethargy, tachypnea, or diarrhea.
- Child with shunts should be re-evaluated periodically, including assessment of distal shunt length in growing children.
- The first follow-up examination usually is scheduled 3 months after surgery, and CT scan or MRI of the head should be done at that time.
- Follow-up is performed every 6–12 months in the first 2 years of life. In children aged 2 years and older, follow-up is performed every 2 years.
- Medications include acetazolamide and furosemide. These are helpful for temporizing the hydrocephalus until compensation occurs. If compensation does not occur, then shunting is indicated.
- Medications should not be used in patients with functional shunts.
- Medication is not effective in long-term treatment of chronic hydrocephalus, and it may induce metabolic consequences.
- If seizures occur, antiepileptic drugs are recommended.

Prognosis

- Long-term outcome is related directly to the cause of hydrocephalus.
- Up to 50% of patients with large intraventricular hemorrhage develop permanent hydrocephalus requiring shunt.

- Following removal of a posterior fossa tumor in children, 20% develop permanent hydrocephalus requiring a shunt. The overall prognosis is related to type, location, and extent of surgical resection of the tumor.
- Satisfactory control was reported for medical treatment in 50% of hydrocephalic patients younger than 1 year who had stable vital signs, normal renal function, and no symptoms of elevated ICP.

Parental Education

- Knowledge of the signs and symptoms of shunt malfunction or infection and the necessity for emergent medical evaluation in these instances is mandatory in patients, family members, and caregivers.
- The patient, family, and caregivers should know that periodic re-evaluation is necessary.
- Pumping the shunt is contraindicated in most cases.
- Patients with vascular shunts, and some patients with other types of shunts, should receive prophylactic antibiotics before dental procedures or instrumentation of the bladder.

CEREBRAL PALSY

Introduction

Cerebral palsy (CP) describes a group of permanent disorders of the development of movement and posture, causing activity limitation, that are attributed to nonprogressive disturbances that occurred in the developing fetal or infant brain. The motor disorders of cerebral palsy are often accompanied by disturbances of sensation, perception, cognition, communication, and behavior, by epilepsy, and by secondary musculoskeletal problems. There are many types and subtypes of CP, none of them have a known cure. Usually, medical intervention is limited to the treatment and prevention of complications arising from CP's effects.

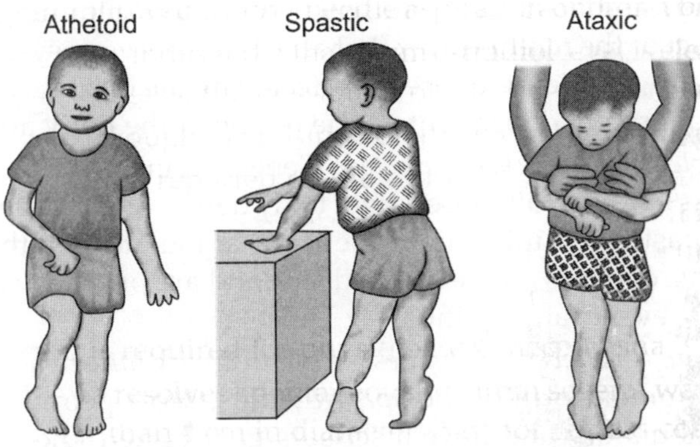

Fig. 6.9: Cerebral palsy child

History

Cerebral palsy formerly known as 'Cerebral Paralysis,' was first identified by English surgeon William Little in 1860. Little raised the possibility of asphyxia during birth as a chief cause of the disorder. It was not until 1897 that Sigmund Freud, then a neurologist, suggested that a difficult birth was not the cause but rather only a symptom of other effects on fetal development. Research conducted during the 1980s by the National Institute of Neurological Disorders and Stroke (NINDS) suggested that only a small number of cases of CP are caused by lack of oxygen during birth.

Incidence

In the industrialized world, the incidence of cerebral palsy is about 2 per 1000 live births. The incidence is higher in males than in females; the Surveillance of Cerebral Palsy in Europe (SCPE) reports a M:F ratio of 1.33:1. Variances in reported rates of incidence across different geographical areas in industrialized countries are thought to be caused primarily by discrepancies in the criteria used for inclusion and exclusion. When such discrepancies are taken into account in comparing two or more registers of patients with cerebral palsy (for example, the extent to which children with mild cerebral palsy are included), the incidence rates converge toward the average rate of 2:1000.

Classification

CP is divided into five major classifications to describe different movement impairments. These classifications also reflect the areas of the brain that are damaged. The five major classifications are:

1. Spastic cerebral palsy: Causes stiffness and movement difficulties
2. Athetoid cerebral palsy: Leads to involuntary and uncontrolled movements
3. Ataxic cerebral palsy: Causes a disturbed sense of balance and depth perception
4. Hypotonic cerebral palsy
5. Hypertonic cerebral palsy.

1. *Spastic cerebral palsy:* The most common form of cerebral palsy is spastic diplegia. Spastic cerebral palsy is by far the most common type, occurring in 70% to 80% of all cases. Spastic CP accompanies one of the other types in 30% of all cases. Child with this type is hypertonic and has a neuromuscular condition stemming from damage to the corticospinal tract or the motor cortex that affects the nervous system's ability to receive gamma amino butyric acid in the area(s) affected by the disability. Spastic CP is further classified by topography dependent on the region of the body affected; these include:
   - *Spastic hemiplegia (one side being affected):* Generally, injury to muscle-nerves controlled by the brain's left side will cause a right body deficit, and vice versa. Typically, people that have spastic hemiplegia are the most ambulatory, although they generally have dynamic equinus on the affected side and are primarily prescribed ankle-foot orthoses to prevent said equinus.
   - *Spastic diplegia (the lower extremities are affected with little to no upper-body spasticity):* The most common form of the spastic forms. Most people with spastic diplegia are fully ambulatory and have a scissors gait. Flexed knees and hips to varying degrees are common. Hip problems, dislocations, and in three-quarters of spastic diplegics, also strabismus (crossed eyes), can be present as well. In addition, these individuals are often nearsighted. The intelligence of a person with spastic diplegia is unaffected by the condition.
   - *Spastic quadriplegia (all four limbs affected equally):* People with spastic quadriplegia are the least likely to be able to walk, or if they can, to want to walk, because their muscles

are too tight and it is too much effort to do so. Some children with quadriplegia also have hemiparetic tremors, an uncontrollable shaking that affects the limbs on one side of the body and impairs normal movement.

- Other medical terms such as monoplegia, paraplegia, triplegia, and pentaplegia may also be used to refer to specific manifestations of the spasticity.

2. *Ataxic cerebral palsy:* Ataxia CP is a type symptoms can be caused by damage to the cerebellum. The forms of ataxia are less common types of cerebral palsy, occurring in at most 10% of all cases. Some of these individuals have hypotonia and tremors. Motor skills such as writing, typing, or using scissors might be affected, as well as balance, especially while walking. It is common for individuals to have difficulty with visual and/or auditory processing.

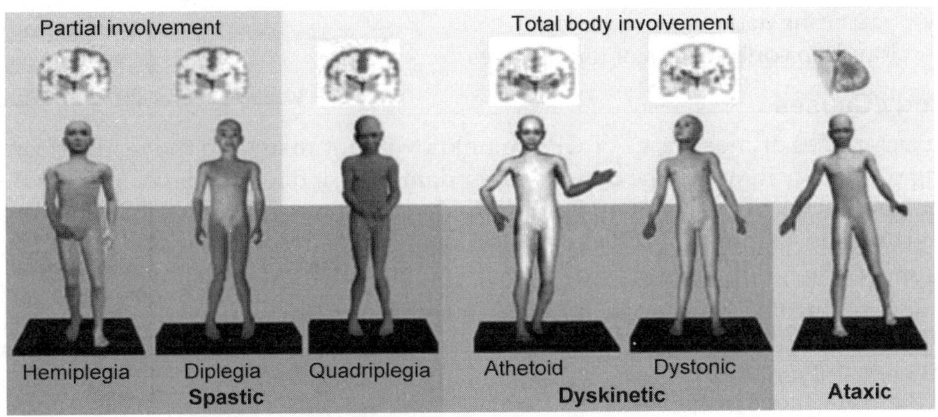

Fig. 6.10: Types of cerebral palsy

3. *Athetoid/Dyskinetic:* Athetoid or dyskinetic is mixed muscle tone of child with athetoid CP have trouble holding themselves in an upright, steady position for sitting or walking, and often show involuntary motions. For some people with athetoid CP, it takes a lot of work and concentration to get their hand to a certain spot (like scratching their nose or reaching for a cup). Because of their mixed tone and trouble keeping a position, they may not be able to hold onto objects (such as a toothbrush or pencil). About one quarter of all people with CP have athetoid CP. The damage occurs to the extrapyramidal motor system and/or pyramidal tract and to the basal ganglia. It occurs in 10 to 20% of all cases. In newborn infants, high bilirubin levels in the blood, if left untreated, can lead to brain damage in certain areas (kernicterus). This may also lead to athetoid cerebral palsy.
4. *Hypotonic cerebral palsy:* Hypotonic cerebral palsy is a form of the disorder marked by floppy (overly relaxed) muscles; hypotonic CP is rarer than the spastic forms of the disorder. Hypotonic cerebral palsy have noticeably 'floppy' muscles and no control of their head. The arms and legs hang down like a 'rag doll.' Joints may be lax. Reflexes may be poor, and walking is usually difficult. The condition causes posture problems and may cause breathing and swallowing difficulties. Speech may also be difficult, although intelligence is usually unaffected.

Hypotonia means less muscle tone. It can be caused by several factors: Cerebral palsy, muscular dystrophy, Down's syndrome, myotonic dystrophy, Tay-Sachs disease, and Prader-Willi syndrome. Hypotonic cerebral palsy is hypotonia which is caused by brain damage or brain malformation; it is generally congenital (present at birth).

5. *Hypertonic cerebral palsy:* The word hypertonic comes from hypertonia. It refers to the rigidity, stiffness and heightened tension in the person's muscles. While a physician usually will not make a diagnosis for months after a child's birth, common signs that this form of cerebral palsy is affecting your child include:
   - Uncomfortable movements
   - Awkward movements
   - Muscle resistance when your child tries to move
   - Spastic movements
   - Muscle spasms
   - Poor balance
   - Scissoring actions with the legs
   - Random contractions of the muscles

Etiology/Causes

The exact causes of most cases of CP are unknown, but many are the result of problems during pregnancy in which the brain is either damaged or does not develop normally. This can be due to infections, maternal health problems, or something else that interferes with normal brain development. Problems during labor and delivery can cause CP in some cases.

- Common in multiple births
- Other causes include toxins, severe jaundice, lead poisoning
- Physical brain injury
- Shaken baby syndrome
- CP is not genetic or hereditary.

Signs and Symptoms

All types of cerebral palsy are characterized by abnormal muscle tone (i.e. slouching over while sitting), reflexes, or motor development and coordination. There can be joint and bone deformities and contractures (permanently fixed, tight muscles and joints).

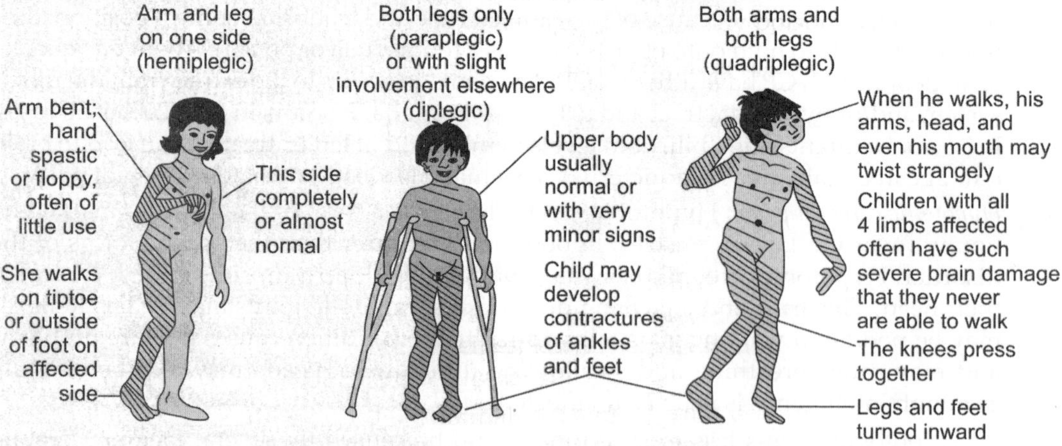

Fig. 6.11: Signs and symptoms of cerebral palsy

The classical symptoms are spasticity:

- Muscles spasms
- Involuntary movements (e.g. Facial gestures)
- Unsteady gait
- Problems with balance
- Decreased muscle mass
- Scissor walking
- Toe walking

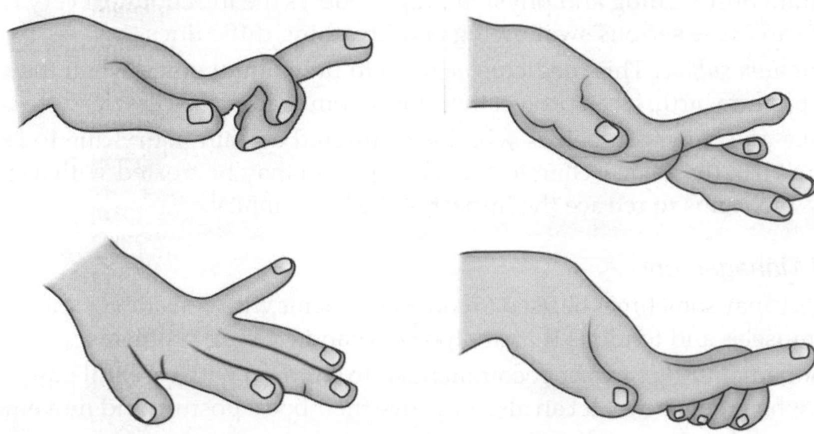

Fig. 6.12: Symptoms of cerebral palsy

- Motor dysfunction
- Babies born with severe CP often have an irregular posture
- Child bodies may be either very floppy or very stiff
- Birth defects, such as spinal curvature, a small jawbone, or a small head sometimes occur along with CP. Symptoms may appear or change as a child gets older
- Secondary condition can include seizures, epilepsy, apraxia, dysarthria or other communication disorders, eating problems, sensory impairments, mental retardation, learning disabilities, and behavioral disorders
- Speech and language disorders are common in people with CP.

Diagnostic Evaluation

- History collection
- Physical examination
- CT and MRI scan.

Management

A cerebral palsy is a lifelong disability. There are many interventions to reduce its impact on the body and the individual's quality of life. An intervention is a service that aims to improve the condition of cerebral palsy and the day-to-day experience of the person living with it.

Medical Management

The medications are taken orally (e.g. diazepam) and others are injected or delivered through surgically implanted pumps (e.g. Baclofen). Many children with cerebral palsy benefit from Botulinum toxin type A injections into muscles affected by spasticity. This intervention is used from about two years of age and is most effective when used in conjunction with therapy.

- *Botulinum toxin:* Cerebral palsy child has muscle stiffness affecting a specific muscle or group of muscles, injections of a medication called Botulinum toxin can be recommended. The effects of botulinum toxin injections normally last between three and six months, but repeat injections can be given. The treatment is most effective when a program of stretching and physiotherapy follows the injections. In very rare cases, this drug can cause serious swallowing and breathing difficulties.
- *Magnesium sulfate:* This medicine is given to pregnant women when they are at risk of very preterm birth. It can protect the babies from brain injury that leads to cerebral palsy.
- *Cooling cap:* Newborn babies who have suffered a brain injury due to lack of oxygen before birth (hypoxic ischemic encephalopathy) may be treated with a special cooling cap which aims to reduce the impact of the brain injury.

Surgical Management

- Surgery may sometimes be used to correct problems with bones and joints, by lengthening any muscles and tendons that are too short and causing problems.
- Orthopedic surgery can be recommended to children with cerebral palsy causing them pain when they move. It can also improve their body posture and movement as well as their confidence and self-esteem.
- Selective Dorsal Rhizotomy (SDR) is a neurosurgical procedure that is used in a small percentage of children with cerebral palsy to permanently reduce spasticity in their legs.

Physiotherapy and Occupational Therapy

The four main goals of physiotherapy are:

- To prevent the weakening of muscles that is not normally practiced by child with cerebral palsy.
- To prevent muscles shortening and losing their normal range of movement (known as a contracture)
- Physiotherapists and occupational therapists focus on encouraging a person's day-to-day movement skills such as sitting, walking, playing, dressing and toileting.
- They will use a range of specialist interventions such as movement training and equipment, e.g. walking frames, wheelchairs, supportive seating, footwear and orthotics.

Conclusion

The primary care of the child with Cerebral Palsy can be challenging to treat. Providing the support needed by these children and their families can be incredibly rewarding. Knowing the common problems seen in these families along with treatment options can help the practitioner optimize the function of the child and support the family in caring for their child.

SKELETAL DEFECTS

CLEFT LIP AND CLEFT PALATE

Introduction

Cleft lip and cleft palate are openings or splits in the upper lip, the roof of the mouth (palate) or both. Cleft lip and cleft palate result when facial structures that are developing in an unborn baby do not close completely.

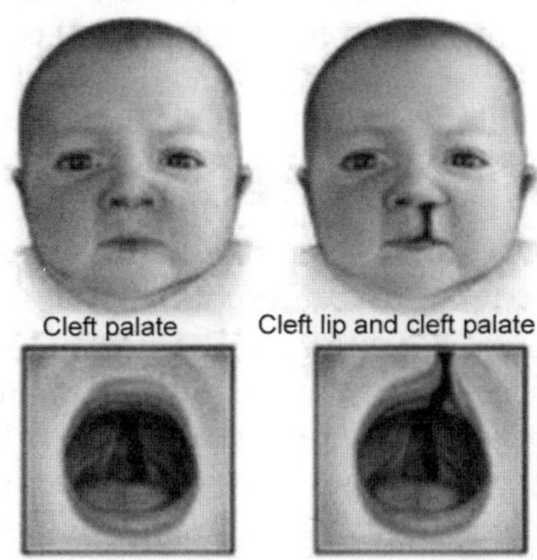

Fig. 6.13: Child with cleft lip and cleft palate

The cleft lip and cleft palate which can also occur together as cleft lip and palate are variations of a type of clefting congenital deformity caused by abnormal facial development during gestation periods. A cleft is a fissure or opening a gap. It is the nonfusion of the body's natural structures that form before birth. Approximately 1 in 700 children born have a cleft lip and/or a cleft palate.

Cleft lip and palate can also affect other parts of the face, such as the eyes, ears, nose, cheeks, and forehead. A cleft lip or palate can be successfully treated with surgery, especially so if conducted soon after birth or in early childhood.

History

Hippocrates (400 BC) and Galen (150 AD) mention cleft lip, but not cleft palate in their writings. For centuries, perforations of the palate were considered to be secondary to syphilis, and cleft palate was not recognized as a congenital disorder until 1556, by Fanco. The first successful closure of a soft palate defect was reported in 1764 by LeMonnier, a French dentist. The first closure of the hard palate was performed in 1834 by Dieffenbach. In the 1930s, Kilner and Wardill independently developed the 'pushback' procedure.

Definition of Cleft Lip

The cleft does not affect the palate structure of the mouth it is referred to as cleft lip. Cleft lip is formed in the top of the lip as either a small gap or an indentation in the lip (partial or incomplete cleft) or it continues into the nose (complete cleft). Lip cleft can occur as a one sided (unilateral) or two sided (bilateral). It is due to the failure of fusion of the maxillary and medial nasal processes (formation of the primary palate).

Definition of Cleft Palate

Cleft palate is a condition in which the two plates of the skull that form the hard palate (roof of the mouth) are not completely joined. The soft palate is in these cases cleft as well. In most of the cases cleft lip is also present. Palate cleft can occur as complete (soft and hard palate, possibly including a gap in the jaw) or incomplete (a 'hole' in the roof of the mouth, usually as a cleft soft palate). When cleft palate occurs, the uvula is usually split. It occurs due to the failure of fusion of the lateral palatine processes, the nasal septum or the median palatine processes (formation of the secondary palate). The hole in the roof of the mouth caused by a cleft connects the mouth directly to the nasal cavity.

Classification/Types

- Clefts of the lip are incomplete or complete. Incomplete means only a portion of the lip is involved, and may mean anything from a muscular diastasis only, to a large cleft with only a small band of tissue connecting the two sides. A complete cleft lip involves the entire thickness of the lip. Cleft lips are unilateral or bilateral.
- The primary palate is anterior to the incisive foramen, and the secondary palate is posterior to the foramen. Clefts of the palate are unilateral if on one side the palatal process of the maxilla is fused with the nasal septum. A bilateral cleft is not attached to the nasal septum, and the septum is visible through the cleft. A complete palatal cleft involves the primary and secondary palate; an incomplete cleft involves the secondary palate only.

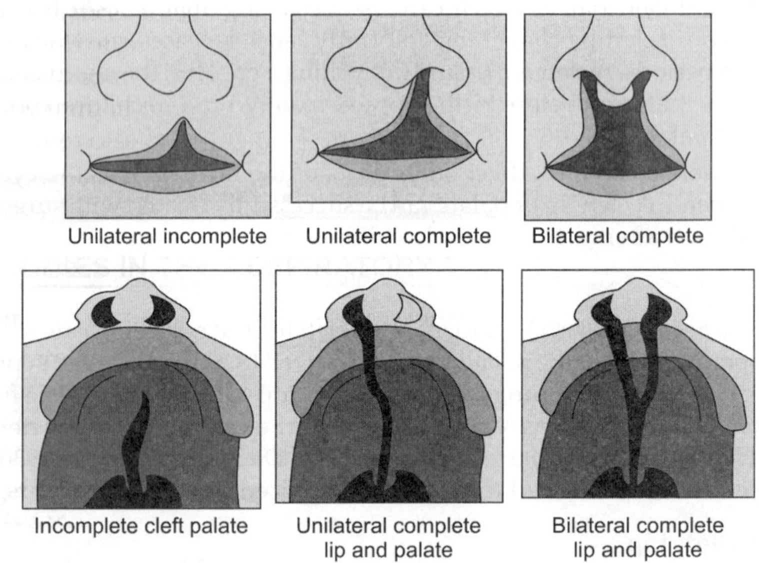

Fig. 6.14: Classification of cleft lip and cleft palate

Causes

- Its Common congenital anomalies, and caused by the interaction between genetic and environmental factors. In those instances, genetic factors create susceptibility for

clefts. When environmental factors (i.e. triggers) interact with a genetically susceptible genotype, a cleft develops during an early stage of development.
- The proportion of environmental and genetic factors varies with the sex of the individual affected with cleft. In cleft lip and cleft palate, it also varies with the severity and the unilaterality or bilaterality of the cleft anomaly; the highest proportion of genetic factors are in the subgroup of females with a bilateral cleft, and the smallest proportion is in the subgroup of males with a unilateral cleft.
- This process is very vulnerable to multiple toxic substances, environmental pollutants, and nutritional imbalance. The biologic mechanisms of mutual recognition of the two cabinets, and the way they are glued together, are quite complex and obscure despite intensive scientific research.

Other Causes

- Seasonal causes (such as pesticide exposure)
- Poor maternal diet and vitamin intake
- Anticonvulsant drugs
- Alcohol and cigarette smoking
- Nitrate compounds, organic solvents, parental exposure to lead
- Illegal drugs (cocaine, crack cocaine, heroin, etc.)
- Current research continues to investigate the extent to which folic acid can reduce the incidence of clefting.

Signs and Symptoms

- Difficulty with feedings
- Difficulty swallowing with potential for liquids or foods to come out the nose
- Nasal speaking voice
- Chronic ear infections.

Diagnostic Evaluation

- Complete history collection
- Head to foot physical examination
- Recent advances in prenatal diagnosis have allowed obstetricians to diagnose facial clefts *in utero*.
- USG, CT and MRI scan.

Management

Neonatal Care

When a neonate with a cleft is born, a pediatrician has three major concerns:

1. Risk of aspiration because of communication between oral and nasal cavities
2. Airway obstruction (in addition to sequelae of aspiration, especially in Robin sequence in which the cleft palate [CP] is combined with micrognathia and the tongue has a normal size)
3. Difficulties with feeding of a child with a cleft and nasal regurgitation.

These three factors are influenced by the presence of other major or minor anomalies that may, in association with a cleft, represent 1 of 300 known cleft syndromes. Therefore, a neonate with an orofacial cleft should be seen by a medical geneticist as soon as possible. As with any other medical condition, each case is different. A child with a severe cleft may do very well, whereas a child with a much less severe condition may experience many problems. An individual approach is necessary; however, several major rules apply to every neonate born with a cleft.

Common Treatment Protocol

- *Newborn:* Diagnostic examination, general counseling of parents, feeding instructions, palatal obturator (if necessary); genetic evaluation and specification of diagnosis; empiric risk of recurrence of cleft calculated; recommendation of a protocol for the prevention of a cleft recurrence in the family.
- *Age 3 months:* Repair of cleft lip (and placement of ventilation tubes).
- *Age 6 months:* Pre-surgical orthodontics, if necessary; first speech evaluation.
- *Age 9 months:* Speech therapy begins.
- *Age 9–12 months:* Repair of cleft palate (placement of ventilation tubes if not done at the time of cleft lip repair).
- *Age 1–7 years:* Orthodontic treatment.
- *Age 7–8 years:* Alveolar bone graft.
- *Older than 8 years:* Orthodontic treatment continues.

Other surgical procedures can be performed in patients with severe clefts as necessary.

In view of these complications, the reconstructive surgeon is faced with timing the cleft repair so that hearing and speech are optimized, but effects on midface growth are minimized. Cleft lip repair is usually planned at approximately ten weeks of age, if the baby weighs ten pounds, and the hemoglobin is ten grams. Cleft palate repair is usually scheduled at approximately six to 12 months of age.

Surgical Management

The closure of the cleft lip is the first major procedure that tremendously changes children's future development and ability to thrive. Variations occur in timing of the first lip surgery; however, the most usual time occurs at approximately age 3 months. Pediatricians used to strictly follow a rule of 'three 10s' as a necessary requirement for identifying the child's status as suitable for surgery (i.e. 10 lb, 10 mg/L of hemoglobin, and age 10 weeks). Although pediatricians are presently much more flexible, and some surgeons may well justify a neonatal lip closure, considering the rule of three 10s is still very useful.

Anatomical differences predispose children with cleft lip and palate and with isolated cleft palate to ear infections. Therefore, ventilation tubes are placed to ventilate the middle ear and prevent hearing loss secondary to otitis media with effusion. In multidisciplinary teams with significant participation of an otolaryngologist, the tubes are placed at the initial surgery and at the second surgery routinely.

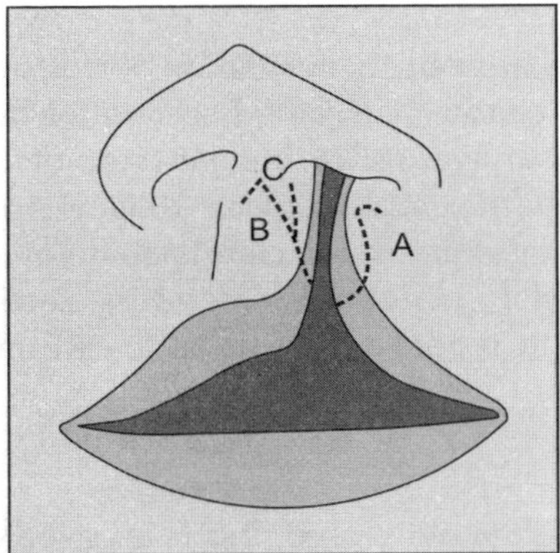

The dotted lines indicate incisions

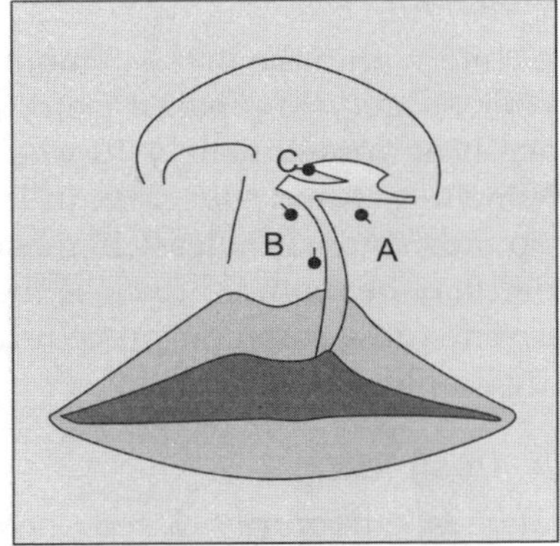

Movement of the flaps; flap A is moved between B and C. C is rotated slightly while B is pushed down

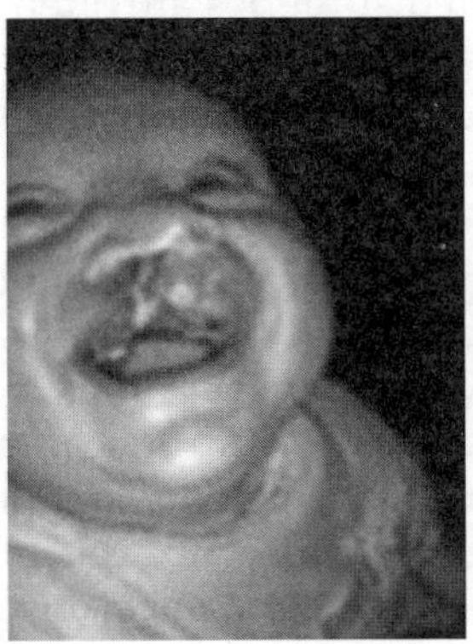

Preoperation

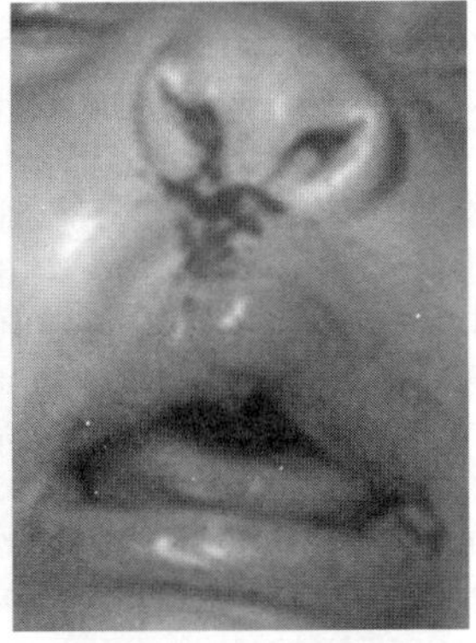

Postoperation, the lip is swollen from surgery and will get a more natural look within a couple of weeks

Fig. 6.15: Surgical closure of the cleft lip

The hearing is tested after the first placement when ears are clear with tubes. If no cleft surgery is planned early, placing the tubes by age 6 months and monitoring hearing with repeated testing is recommended. Complications include eardrum perforation and otorrhea, particularly in patients with open secondary palates in which closure is planned for later. For preventive reasons, ear tubes are usually placed when the child is still under general anesthesia for cleft repair.

Detailed surgical treatment is described elsewhere (see surgical articles Craniofacial, Bilateral Cleft Lip Repair, Craniofacial, Bilateral Cleft Nasal Repair, Craniofacial, Unilateral Cleft Nasal Repair, Craniofacial, Unilateral Cleft Lip Repair). Pediatricians may find it useful to inform parents of the kinds of procedures with a child with cleft may undergo.

Cleft Lip Treatment

To treat the child within the first 2–3 months after birth, surgery is performed to close the cleft lip. While surgery to repair a cleft lip can be performed soon after birth, the often preferred age is at approximately 10 weeks of age, following the 'rule of 10s' coined by surgeons Wilhelmesen and Musgrave in 1969 (the child is at least 10 weeks of age; weights at least 10 pounds, and has at least 10 g hemoglobin). If the cleft is bilateral and extensive, two surgeries may be required to close the cleft, one side first, and the second side a few weeks later. The most common procedure to repair a cleft lip is the Millard procedure pioneered by Ralph Millard.

Cleft Palate Treatment

The cleft palate is temporarily closed, the cleft is not closed, but it is covered by a palatal obturator (a prosthetic device made to fit the roof of the mouth covering the gap). Cleft palate can also be corrected by surgery, usually performed between 6 and 12 months.

Approximately 20–25% only requires one palatal surgery to achieve a competent velopharyngeal valve capable of producing normal, nonhypernasal speech. However, combinations of surgical methods and repeated surgeries are often necessary as the child grows. One of the new innovations of cleft lip and cleft palate repair is the Latham appliance. The Latham is surgically inserted by use of pins during the child's 4th or 5th month.

Speech and Hearing Treatments

A tympanostomy tube is often inserted into the eardrum to aerate the middle ear. This is often beneficial for the hearing ability of the child. Speech problems are usually treated by a speech-language pathologist. In some cases pharyngeal flap surgery or augmentation pharyngoplasty is performed to reduce the escape of nasal airflow in speech sounds requiring oral air pressure, to improve the pronunciation of those sounds, and reduce nasality in those parts of speech that are not normally nasalized. The speech-language pathologist may also be called on to correct incorrect speaking habits that the child developed before the cleft was corrected surgically.

Complications

The Children with cleft lip with or without cleft palate face a variety of challenges, depending on the type and severity of the cleft.

- *Difficulty feeding:* The most immediate concerns after birth is feeding. While most babies with cleft lip can breastfeed, a cleft palate may make sucking difficult.
- *Ear infections and hearing loss:* Most of the child with cleft palate is especially at risk of developing middle ear fluid and hearing loss.
- *Dental problems:* If the cleft extends through the upper gum, tooth development may be affected.
- *Speech difficulties:* Because the palate is used in forming sounds, the development of normal speech can be affected by a cleft palate. Speech may sound too nasal.
- *Challenges of coping with a medical condition:* Children with clefts may face social, emotional and behavioral problems due to differences in appearance and the stress of intensive medical care.

Nursing Management

Breastfeeding an Infant with a Cleft

- The infant mother typically does not experience feeding problems beyond learning how to 'latch on' to the nipple at the beginning of the feeding. Infants with cleft palate must squeeze the milk out of the nipple by compressing the nipple between the tongue and whatever portion of the palate that remains.

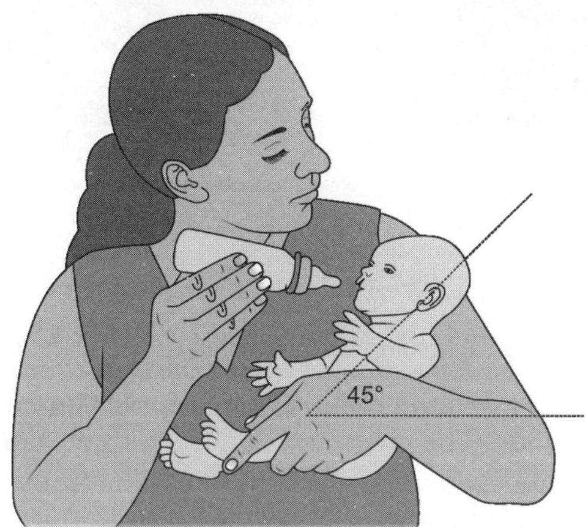

Fig. 6.16: Feeding a baby with cleft palate or cleft lip

- Massaging the breast and applying hot packs on the breast 20 minutes before nursing usually helps.
- The mother should apply pressure to the areola with her fingers to help the engorged nipple protrude. She should hold the infant in a semi-upright, straddle, or football position. She should support the breast by holding it between her thumb and middle finger, making sure that the infant's lower lip is turned out and the tongue is under the nipple.
- If the infant cannot hold onto the nipple any more, the mother can collect the remaining milk using an electrical or manual breast pump or by squeezing the breast with both hands and can finish the feeding with collected milk in a bottle.
- The mother should increase her fluid intake (drink lots of water).

Feeding Breast Milk with a Bottle

- Particularly for infants with bilateral cleft lip and palate, breastfeeding is not possible.
- The mother can use a breast pump (an electric pump ensures the highest level of success). Then, she can feed the baby with a bottle.

Feeding Milk Formula with a Bottle

- The most appropriate milk formula should be selected by a pediatrician or feeding specialist.
- Various nipples and bottles are made specifically for infants with clefts. The goal is to find a nipple and bottle that make feeding easy for the infant and still allow ample opportunity to suck.
- A soft nipple is generally better than a hard nipple (some can be softened by boiling).

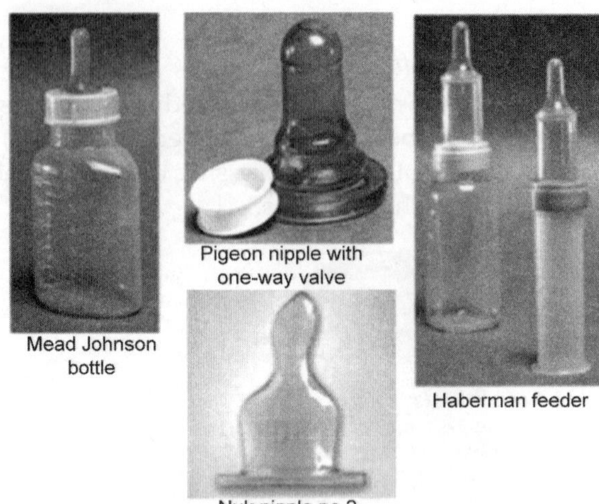

Fig. 6.17: Special feeding bottle for cleft lip and cleft palate child

- Use a crosscut nipple to prevent choking. Any nipple can be crosscut manually using a single-edged razor blade. The crosscut is on the tongue side.
- The bottle should be squeezed and released, not continually squeezed.
- The nipple is angled to a side of the mouth, away from the cleft.

GASTROINTESTINAL TRACT DEFECTS

TRACHEOESOPHAGEAL FISTULA AND ESOPHAGEAL ATRESIA

Introduction

As a fetus is growing and developing in its mother's uterus before birth, different organ systems are developing and maturing. The trachea and the esophagus begin developing as one single tube. At about four to eight weeks after conception, a wall forms between the fetus' esophagus and trachea to separate them into two distinct tubes. If this wall does not form properly, TE fistula and/or esophageal atresia can occur.

- *Esophagus:* Tube that connects the mouth to the stomach
- *Trachea:* 'Windpipe'
- *Atresia:* Absence of a normal opening
- *Congenital:* Found at birth.

Definition

Tracheoesophageal Fistula

Tracheoesophageal fistula is an abnormal connection in one or more places between the esophagus (the tube that leads from the throat to the stomach) and the trachea (the tube that leads from the throat to the windpipe and lungs). Normally, the esophagus and the trachea are two separate tubes that are not connected. Tracheoesophageal fistula is also known as TE fistula or simply TEF. TE fistula is a birth defect, which is an abnormality that occurs as a fetus is forming in the mother's uterus.

A baby with a TE fistula swallows the liquid can pass through the abnormal connection between the esophagus and the trachea. When this happens, liquid gets into the baby's lungs. This can cause pneumonia and other problems.

Fistula

Abnormal passage from a body organ to the body surface or between two internal body organs.

- Congenital esophageal atresia (EA) represents a failure of the esophagus to develop as a continuous passage. It ends as a blind pouch.
- Tracheoesophageal fistula (TEF) represents an abnormal opening between the trachea and esophagus.
- EA and TEF can occur separately or together.
- EA and TEF are diagnosed in the ICU at birth and treated immediately.

Esophageal Atresia

TE fistula often occurs with another birth defect known as esophageal atresia. The esophagus is a tube that leads from the throat to the stomach. With esophageal atresia, the esophagus does not form properly while the fetus is developing before birth resulting in two segments.

One part that connects to the throat and other part that connects to the stomach. The two segments do not connect to each other. Since the esophagus is in two segments, liquid that a baby swallows cannot pass normally through the esophagus and reach the stomach. Liquid that a baby swallows can pass through the connection between the esophagus and the trachea and go into the lungs. This can cause pneumonia and other problems.

Types

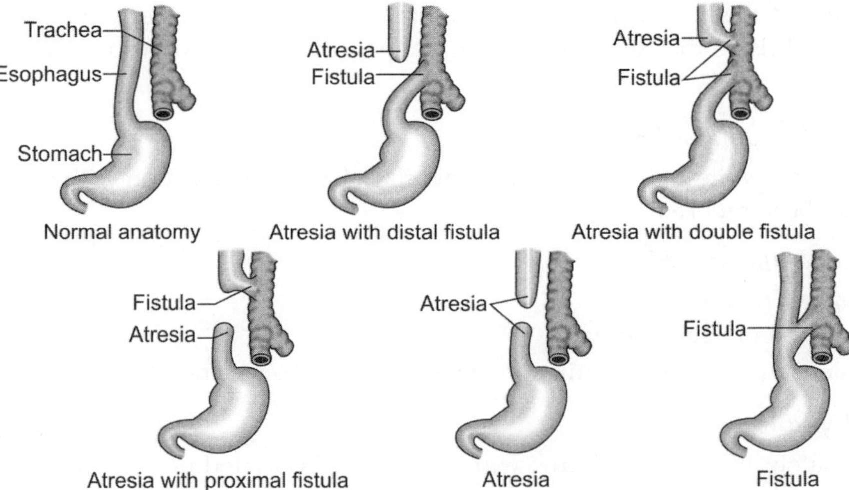

Fig. 6.18: Tracheoesophageal fistula

Introduction

A tracheoesophageal fistula (TEF) is a congenital or acquired communication between the trachea and esophagus. TEFs often lead to severe and fatal pulmonary complications.

Incidence

TEFs are a common congenital anomaly with an incidence of 1 case in 2000–4000 live births. Acquired TEFs are quite rare and incidence rates have not been well documented.

Anatomic characteristics	Percent of cases
Esophageal atresia with distal TEF	87
Isolated esophageal atresia without TEF	8
Isolated TEF	4
Esophageal atresia with proximal TEF	1
Esophageal atresia with proximal and distal TEF	1

Mortality/Morbidity

- Surgical and preoperative management of congenital TEFs have improved significantly. Survival rates of 100% can be achieved in infants who do not have severe associated congenital anomalies.
- Patients may develop morbidities following TEF repair, including tracheomalacia, esophageal dysmotility, gastroesophageal reflux, and dysphagia. Additionally, patients may develop pulmonary problems from recurrent aspiration.
- Child with acquired TEFs have high mortality and morbidity rates because of critical illnesses and comorbidities.
- Congenital TEFs are primarily observed in neonates and during the first year of life.
- Adults rarely present with congenital TEFs that were undiagnosed during their early years of life.
- Acquired TEFs may occur in individuals of any age, and elderly individuals are at increased risk if they become ventilator dependent because of respiratory failure.

Causes

Causes of Congenital TEF

Although no definite cause exists for congenital TEFs, an association with trisomy 18, 21, and 13 has been reported.

Causes of Acquired TEFs

- Iatrogenic injury
- Blunt chest or neck trauma
- Prolonged mechanical ventilation via endotracheal or tracheostomy tube.

Pathophysiology

Approximately 17–70% of children with TEFs have associated developmental anomalies. These anomalies include Down syndrome, duodenal atresia, and cardiovascular defects. The following congenital anomalies have been reported with variable frequency:

- Cardiac anomalies include ventricular septal defect, patent ductus arteriosus, tetralogy of Fallot, atrial septal defect, and right-sided aortic arch.
- Genitourinary anomalies include renal agenesis or dysphagia, horseshoe kidney, polycystic kidney, ureteral and urethral malformations, and hypospadias.

- Gastrointestinal anomalies include imperforate anus, duodenal atresia, malrotation, intestinal malformation, Meckel diverticulum, and annular pancreas.
- Musculoskeletal anomalies include hemivertebrae, radial dysphagia or amelia, polydactyly, syndactyly, rib malformation, scoliosis, and lower limb defect.

Clinical Manifestation

- Esophageal atresia in the fetus should be considered as a cause of maternal polyhydramnios.
- Absence of stomach gas on prenatal ultrasound is another indication of esophageal atresia.
- Neonates with esophageal atresia usually develop copious, fine white frothy bubbles of mucus in the mouth and nose. Secretions recur despite suctioning.
- Infants may develop rattling respiration and episodes of coughing and choking in association with cyanosis.
- Symptoms worsen during feeding in the presence of a TEF.
- The symptoms induced by malignant TEFs are cough, aspiration, and fever.
- The average duration of symptoms from onset to diagnosis is approximately 12 days.

Diagnostic Evaluation

- Detail history collection
- Perform a careful physical examination to document/exclude other associated developmental anomalies
- In the presence of a TEF, abdominal distention may occur secondary to collection of air in the stomach.

Prenatal Diagnosis of Congenital TEFs

- Prenatal ultrasound may reveal polyhydramnios
- Absence of fluid-filled stomach
- Small abdomen
- Lower-than-expected fetal weight
- A distended esophageal pouch.

Postnatal Diagnosis of Congenital TEFs

- Plain chest radiographs may reveal tracheal compression and deviation.
- Absence of a gastric bubble indicates esophageal atresia without a TEF or esophageal atresia with a proximal TEF.
- Chest radiography leads to the diagnosis of TEF in most cases of congenital TEF.
  - Aspiration pneumonia in the posterior segments of the upper lobes may occur secondary to aspiration of the contents from the esophageal pouch or stomach. Recurrent or massive aspiration may lead to acute lung injury in some patients. (Infiltrates occur diffusely in these patients).
  - Insertion of a nasogastric tube may show coiling in the mediastinum of patients who have concomitant esophageal atresia. This finding is diagnostic of TEFs associated with esophageal atresia.

- Contrast studies are seldom required to confirm the diagnosis. These studies have the risk of aspiration pneumonitis and pulmonary injury, and they add minimal information to the diagnostic workup. If the contrast study is performed, 1–2 mL of barium is instilled through an 8 F catheter placed into the esophagus. Chest radiographs are taken in the lateral decubitus position as well as the anteroposterior position to detect spilling of the contrast into the trachea.
- Use of multidetector-row CT scans have made 3-dimensional (3D) displays of many organs and structures a popular clinical examination tool, as the quality of images has markedly improved. Presence of TEF was correctly diagnosed with multidetector-row CT esophagography.

The VACTERL Association

V = Vertebral, problems with the bones in the spine

A = Imperforate anus, a problem with the way a baby's anus or rectum has formed

C = Cardiac, problems with the heart

TE = Tracheoesophageal fistula and esophageal atresia

R = Renal (kidney) problems

L = Limb, problems with the bones in the arms.

Diagnostic Procedures

Flexible esophagoscopy or flexible bronchoscopy may be useful in the diagnosis of acquired TEFs. Either or both of these procedures may be required to evaluate the anatomy of these structures and to exclude an unsuspecting mucosal lesion. The role of endoscopic procedures is especially important in localizing the acquired nonmalignant or malignant TEF.

Management

Surgical Repair is Required for TEF

In healthy infants without pulmonary complications, primary repair is performed within the first few days of life. Repair is delayed in patients with low birth weight, pneumonia, or other major anomalies. Initially, treat child conservatively with parenteral nutrition, gastrostomy, and upper pouch suction until they are considered to be low risk.

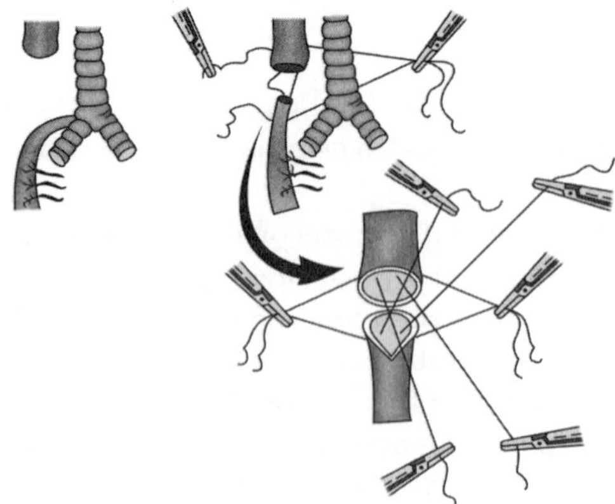

Fig. 6.19: Surgical repair of child with TEF

Preoperatively a cuffed endotracheal tube is placed distal to the fistula site in order to prevent reflux of gastric contents into the lungs. The ongoing mechanical ventilation following tracheal reconstruction is associated with recurrence of TEFs or restenosis.

- A conservative approach is therefore used until the patient is weaned from the mechanical ventilator. A tracheostomy tube is placed distally to the TEF if possible.
- The head of the bed is elevated, and oral secretions are frequently suctioned. A gastrostomy tube is placed to minimize gastroesophageal reflux, and a Jejunostomy feeding tube is placed for nutritional purposes.
- If soilage of the respiratory tract continues, esophageal diversion procedures may be required. Since acquired TEFs do not close spontaneously, surgical repair is planned if the patient is stable enough. Critically ill child are managed conservatively until stable enough for a major surgical procedure.

Treatment of malignant TEFs must be individualized, and the treatment should be instituted promptly. The therapy is generally palliative. Palliation consists of relief of obstruction and diversion of contamination from the respiratory tract. The procedures offered include esophageal exclusion or bypass, resection, direct closure, or endoprosthesis. Supportive therapy is recommended for patients who present late in the course of the fistula and already have pulmonary sepsis. The supportive measures include nasogastric drainage, tracheostomy, gastrostomy, and intravenous hydration and antibiotics.

Burt reported that bypass therapy and radiation therapy were the only treatments that significantly prolonged survival compared to supportive care. With radiation therapy, TEFs initially heal but usually recur, leading to respiratory tract contamination. Esophageal bypass with gastric, colonic, or Jejunal interposition would have significantly improved survival rates but has a high risk of immediate mortality.

Surgical Management

Congenital TEFs

In the preoperative phase, risk of aspiration should be reduced. Continuous suctioning of the blind esophageal pouch with an 8 F catheter may decrease the risk of aspiration. The infant's head should be elevated, and he or she should be hydrated and provided energy intake (caloric intake) via intravenous dextrose solution.

If the patient develops acute respiratory failure, endotracheal intubation and mechanical ventilation are performed. Administer broad-spectrum antibiotics for patients who may have developed lower respiratory tract infection. For patients known to have pneumonia or other pulmonary problems, a gastrostomy for gastric decompression may be required to prevent further reflux of gastric contents into the trachea. The use of proton pump inhibitors may be helpful.

Operative Repair

Timing of operation and choice of surgical approach in congenital TEFs are crucial. Make decisions based on the size and condition of the infant. Most infants are recommended to undergo primary care; however, a staged repair several weeks following birth is recommended for infants who are premature and have severe respiratory distress syndrome.

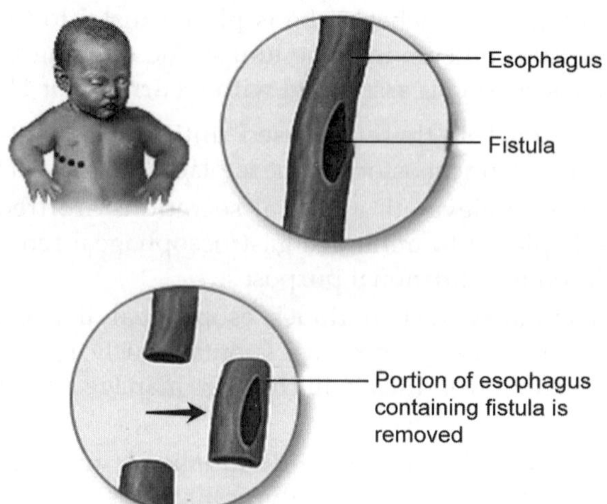

Fig. 6.20: Surgical repair of TEF

The presence of other severe comorbidities, such as aspiration pneumonia, congenital cardiac disease, or other life-threatening conditions, should also delay the primary repair. Tracheostomy is required only if planning a staged repair. Infants who have severe respiratory distress syndrome may require the use of a Fogarty balloon catheter to obliterate the TEF while awaiting surgery.

The repair is performed via right Thoracotomy in the left lateral decubitus position, and the head of table is elevated to avoid gastric reflux. A posterolateral thoracotomy incision is made through the fourth intercostal space, and a retro pleural exposure is obtained. During the dissection, the azygos vein is divided and the vagus nerve is identified. The distal esophagus is identified and dissected distal to the TEF.

The fistula is divided and closure is performed with stay sutures. Dissection is carefully performed to avoid interruption of blood supply or the branches coming off the vagus nerve. Tracheal suture line may be covered with a flap of mediastinal pleura. Prior to esophageal anastomosis, the proximal pouch of the trachea is mobilized.

If a fistula lies between the esophageal pouch and trachea, it is divided and closed. The esophageal anastomosis is performed in 1–2 layers and is covered with mediastinal pleura. A nasogastric feeding tube is placed through the esophagus into the stomach prior to the chest closure, and a chest tube is placed in the retropleural space. Postoperatively, the infant is ventilated as needed, nasogastric or gastrostomy feedings are resumed, and a contrast swallow radiographic examination is performed on the seventh postoperative day. If no leak is detected, oral feedings are resumed. Approximately 3 weeks later, the esophagus is dilated up to a 24 F size in order to prevent future esophageal stenosis.

The most common complications of surgery are pneumonia and atelectasis leading to respiratory failure in postoperative period. A leak at the anastomotic site and pneumothorax are other complications. Most patients who develop an anastomotic leak also develop strictures, which may be dilated later. Rarely, a recurrent TEF may develop. The management of recurrent TEFs usually requires repeat surgical repair. Some patients develop periodic apneic spells that are likely secondary to gastroesophageal reflux and associated laryngospasm.

Repair of esophageal atresia and tracheoesophageal fistula has traditionally been performed via thoracotomy. Recent attempts at thoracoscopic repair have shown that such repair is feasible but technically challenging. However, more data are needed for further evaluation of this approach, particularly in long-gap defects that require more extensive dissection and difficult anastomosis.

Esophageal Endoprosthesis

Placement of an esophageal endoprosthesis has been used to palliate patients with malignant TEFs. A variety of stents are currently available; these include plastic stents (e.g. Medoc, Atkinson, Celestin) and self-expanding metallic stents. Some authors have proposed the esophageal stents as the first line of therapy for malignant strictures associated with a TEF.

The placement of an endoprosthesis may be complicated by an inability to see the endoprosthesis well, enlargement of the TEF, and ongoing contamination of the respiratory tract. Other complications associated with esophageal stents include migration, obstruction, ulceration, esophageal necrosis, and delayed perforation. Insertion of plastic stents requires aggressive dilatation.

- Patients should be seen by a gastroenterologist or pulmonologist for diagnostic workup.
- Consultation with a thoracic surgeon is required for definitive surgical repair.
- Any patient who is ill must be cared for in the intensive care unit, so that the staff can monitor the patient's respiratory system and ensure adequate nutrition.

Nursing Management

- Transfer infants and children with TEF to a pediatric center experienced with surgical repair of TEF.
- The center should be experienced with providing support of critically ill pediatric patients.
- Adults who develop acquired TEF must be transferred to a facility with thoracic surgery support and other adequate support services.
- Child on prolonged ventilatory support is at risk of developing a TEF. The incidence of TEFs has decreased markedly following the introduction of endotracheal tube cuffs of high volume and low pressure.
- In critically ill patients cuff pressure of 30–40 mm Hg may decrease capillary perfusion and result in tissue ischemia. Cuff pressures should be maintained below 25 mm Hg, even at the expense of a small leak.
- Optimal nutrition and use of flexible, small-caliber nasogastric feeding tubes may be of further help.

Complications

Congenital and acquired TEFs are associated with multiple complications, including recurrent pneumonia, acute lung injury, acute respiratory distress syndrome, lung abscess, poor nutrition, bronchiectasis from recurrent aspiration, respiratory failure, and death.

In patients with esophageal atresia and a TEF, abnormal esophageal motility is always present because of abnormal development and innervations of esophagus. Long-term follow-up studies have reported complications of esophagitis, Barrett esophagus, and hiatal hernia.

The major postoperative complications are tracheal stenosis and recurrent fistula. Tracheal stenosis occurs in patients who have extensive injury to the posterior tracheal wall. Surgical repair of tracheal stenosis may be performed at a later date. Recurrent fistulas develop in patients who require continued postoperative intubation. This generally occurs from breakdown of the repair, and the risk of infection spreading into the soft tissue planes, neck, and mediastinum is high.

Gastroesophageal reflux disease may later occur in half of patients who had repair for esophageal atresia and TEFs during the neonatal period. Treatment for reflux is antisecretory therapy. Rare complications of reflux are Barrett esophagus and esophageal carcinoma.

Prognosis

The survival rate in healthy infants who undergo surgical repair for a congenital TEF may be 100%. In groups of infants who have comorbidities or who are not fit enough for early repair, the survival rate is 80–95%. In a series of 118 children, overall survival was more than 90%.

ANORECTAL MALFORMATIONS

Introduction

Anorectal malformations comprise a wide spectrum of diseases, which can affect boys and girls, and involve the distal anus and rectum as well as the urinary and genital tracts. They occur in approximately 1 in 5000 live births. Defects range from the very minor and easily treated with an excellent functional prognosis, to those that are complex, difficult to manage, are often associated with other anomalies, and have a poor functional prognosis.

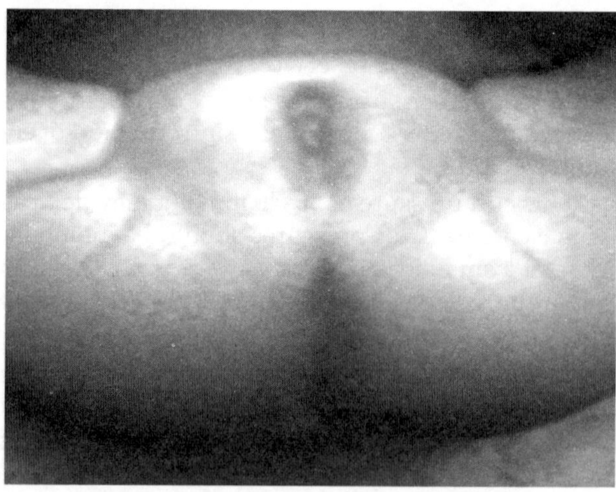

Fig. 6.21: Child with anorectal malformations

Definition

Anorectal malformations comprise a wide spectrum of diseases, which can affect boys and girls, and involve the distal anus and rectum as well as the urinary and genital tracts. Defects range from the very minor and easily treated with an excellent functional prognosis, to those that are complex, difficult to manage, are often associated with other anomalies, and have a poor functional prognosis.

Incidence

Anorectal malformations are congenital anomalies that occur in approximately 1 in 5000 live births.

History of Diseases

Imperforate anus has been a well-known condition since antiquity. For many centuries, physicians, as well as individuals who practiced medicine, created an orifice in the perineum of children with imperforate anus. Those that survived most likely suffered from a type of defect that would now be recognized as 'low'.

Those with a 'high' defect did not survive that treatment. Amussat, in 1835 was the first individual who sutured the rectal wall to the skin edges, which could be considered the first anoplasty. During the first 60 years of the 20th century, surgeons performed a perineal operation without a colostomy for the so-called low malformations. High imperforate anus was usually treated with a colostomy performed in the newborn period, followed by an abdominoperineal pull-through some time later in life, but surgeons lacked objective anatomic guidelines. Unfortunately this left many patients incontinent and was not an appropriate solution to the spectrum of malformations.

The surgical approach to repairing these defects changed dramatically in 1980 with the introduction of the posterior sagittal approach, which allowed surgeons to view the anatomy of these defects clearly, to repair them under direct vision, and to learn about the complex anatomic arrangement of the junction of rectum and genitourinary tract. It has become the predominant surgical method for anorectal anomalies. In cases when the rectum or the vagina are very high and an abdominal approach as well is needed, laparoscopy can be used in combination with the posterior sagittal approach.

Classification

The traditional classification such as:

- High
- Intermediate
- Low defects render the results dubious.

The classification presented here attempts to group together defects that have common diagnostic, therapeutic and prognostic features.

The posterior approach and direct visualization of the anatomy have allowed us to learn about important features. For instance, rectovaginal fistula are almost nonexistent, in retrospect it seems that most of the previously reported 'rectovaginal fistula' cases were misdiagnosed cloacas.

This assertion is supported by the authors' experience of cloaca reoperations where it has been found that most patients who were originally operated on by a surgeon who classified the defect as a 'rectovaginal fistula' had only the rectal component of the cloaca repaired and had been left with a persistent urogenital sinus.

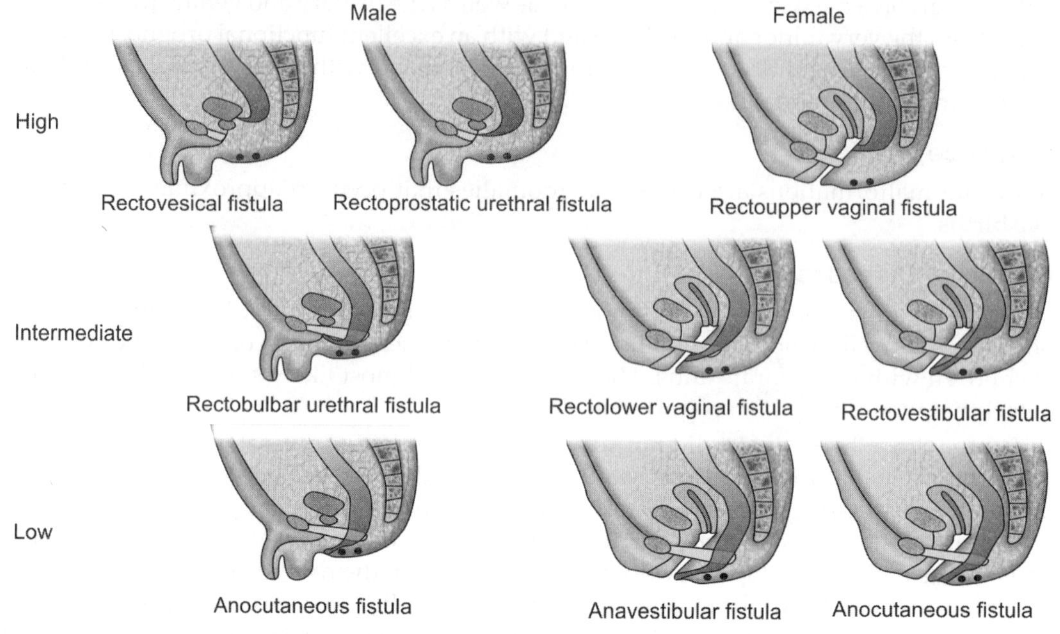

Fig. 6.22: Classification of anorectal malformation

Etiology

Anorectal malformations (ARM) represent a spectrum of abnormalities ranging from mild anal anomalies to complex cloacal malformations. The etiology of such malformations remains unclear and is likely multifactorial.

- There are however reasons to believe there is a genetic componenet. As early as the 1950s, it was recognized that there was an increased risk for a sibling of a patient with ARM to be born with a malformation, as much as 1 in 100, compared with the incidence of about 1 in 5000 in the general population.
- Since that time there have been reports of families with two or more affected members and associations of ARMs with multisystem syndromes.
- In particular, mutations in specific genes encoding transcription factors have been described in patients having such as:
  - Townes-Brocks syndrome
  - Currarino syndrome
  - Pallister-Hall syndrome, each of which have autosomal dominant modes of inheritance.
- In addition, it has been found that there is not only an increased incidence of ARM in patient with trisomy 21 (Down syndrome), but that 95% of patients with trisomy 21 and ARM have imperforate anus without fistula, compared with only 5% of all patients with ARM.

- Based on this evidence, it is likely that the mutation of a variety of different genes can result in ARM, or that the etiology of ARM is multigenic.

Diagnostic Evaluation

- History collection
- Physical examination
- X-ray.

The radiologic evaluation of a newborn with imperforate anus includes an abdominal ultrasound to evaluate for urologic anomalies. In the case of persistent cloaca a distended vagina (hydrocolpos) can be identified. Plain radiographs of the spine can show spinal anomalies such as spina bifida and spinal hemivertebrae.

A spinal ultrasound in the newborn period and up to age 3 months (at which time the sacrum becomes ossified) can look for evidence of a tethered spinal cord and other spinal anomalies. A cross table lateral radiograph can help show the air column in the distal rectum in the small percentage of patients for whom clinical evidence does not delineate in 16–24 hours the likely anorectal anomaly.

Management

- The early management of a newborn infant born with an anorectal anomaly is crucial and two important questions must be answered during the first 24 to 48 hours of life.
- Babies born with persistent cloaca, the surgeon must also determine whether a dilated vagina is present and if it should be drained, as well as determining whether urinary diversion will be required. These maneuvers are intended to prevent sepsis or metabolic acidosis.
- The decision to perform an anoplasty in the newborn period or to delay the repair and to perform a colostomy is based on the infant's physical examination, the appearance of the perineum, and any changes that occur over the first 24 hours of life.
- After the baby is born, an intravenous line is placed for fluids and antibiotics.
- A nasogastric tube is inserted to keep the stomach decompressed to avoid the risk of vomiting and aspiration. Meconium is usually not seen at the perineum in a baby with a rectoperineal fistula until at least 16–24 hours.
- Therefore, the decision of whether to perform a colostomy or an anoplasty must wait for these 16–24 hours while the surgeon observes for clinical evidence of the baby's anorectal anomaly.

Clinical inspection of the buttocks is important. A flat 'bottom' or flat perineum, as evidenced by the lack of a midline gluteal fold and the absence of an anal dimple indicates that the patient has very poor muscles in the perineum. These findings are associated with a high malformation and therefore a colostomy should be performed. Perineal signs found in patients with low malformations include the presence of meconium at the perineum, a 'bucket-handle' malformation (a prominent skin tag located at the anal dimple below which an instrument can be passed), and an anal membrane (through which one can see meconium).

Male Newborns

- In 80–90% of male newborns, clinical evaluation and urinalysis will provide enough information for the surgeon to decide whether the baby requires a colostomy.

- Male newborns with rectoperineal fistula do not need a colostomy. They can undergo a posterior sagital anoplasty whereas male babies with evidence of a rectourinary tract communication should undergo fecal diversion with a colostomy.
- If none of the clinical signs to determine the location of the anorectal anomaly becomes evident by 24 hours, a cross-table lateral film with the baby in prone position, with the pelvis elevated, and with a radio-opaque marker placed on the perineum is performed.
- This X-ray on rare occasion may show the column of air in the distal rectum to be within 1 cm of the perineum, and if this is the case, the baby can be treated like those with a rectoperineal fistula, and a newborn perineal operation can be performed. If the air column is greater than 1 cm from the perineum, a colostomy is indicated.
- A definitive repair in the newborn period avoids a colostomy but there is considerable risk to the urinary tract with this practice because the surgeon does not know the precise anorectal defect. The only way to definitively determine the patient's anorectal defect is to perform a distal colostogram, which of course requires the presence of a colostomy. Without this information an operation in the newborn period is essentially a blind perineal exploration.
- The surgeon may not be able to find the rectum and may find and damage other, unexpected, structures, such as the posterior urethra, seminal vesicles, vas deferens, and ectopic ureters during the search for the rectum. Finally, without fecal diversion, there is the risk of dehiscence and infection.
- These complications may compromise the ultimate functional prognosis.

Female Newborns

- Managing the female newborns are less complicated. In 90% of patients, a meticulous perineal inspection will demonstrate the anorectal defect. Waiting 16–24 hours for enough abdominal distension to demonstrate the presence of a rectoperineal fistula or rectovestibular fistula applies to females as well.
- The most common anomaly in females is a rectovestibular fistula. Perineal inspection shows a normal urethra, normal vagina, and another orifice, which is the rectal fistula in the vestibule.

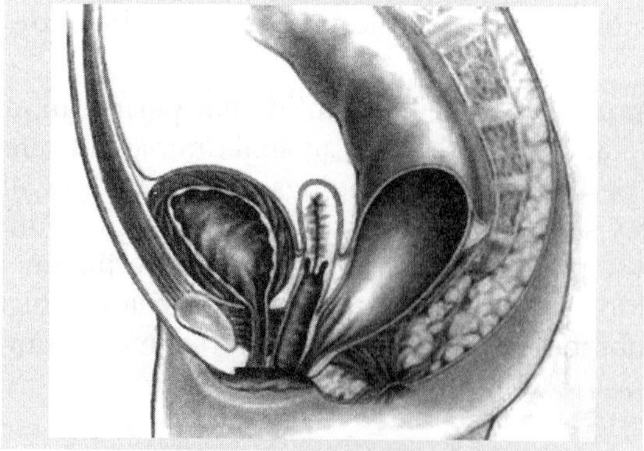

Fig. 6.23: Rectovestibular fistula in females

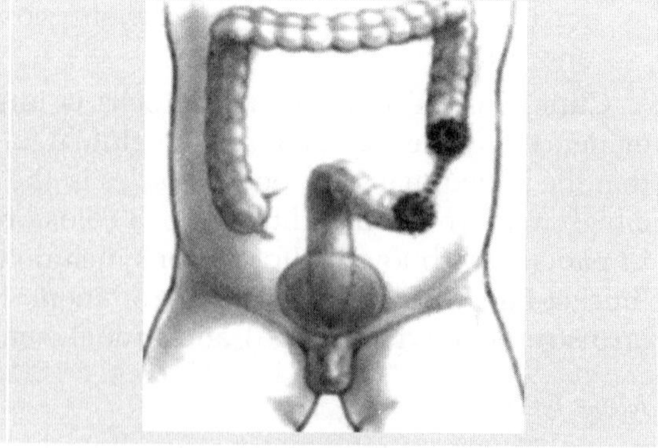

Fig. 6.24: Rectoperineal fistula in male child

- The safest option for a surgeon without extensive experience in anorectal anomalies when faced with a baby with clinical evidence of a rectovestibular fistula is to perform a diverting colostomy.
- Colostomy prior to the main repair avoids the complications of infection and dehiscence. Definitive repair of this anomaly in the newborn period should be reserved for surgeons with significant experience repairing these defects.
- This anomaly has an excellent prognosis and therefore complications that could affect future continence must be avoided.

Surgical Management

As discussed previously, the surgeon must decide in the newborn period whether the child requires fecal diversion with a colostomy, or can undergo a primary repair procedure.

Colostomy

The preferred colostomy is a descending colostomy, i.e. made from the descending portion of the colon located in the lower-left quadrant of the abdomen, with separated stomas. The proximal stoma is connected to the upper gastrointestinal tract and drains stool. The distal stoma, also called a mucous fistula, is connected to the rectum and will drain small amounts of mucus material.

The advantages of this type of colostomy are many:

- It defunctionalizes only a small portion of distal colon
- In cases of large rectourinary fistulae in which the patient passes urine into the bowel, the urine comes out easily through the mucous fistula, avoiding problems of hyperchloremic acidosis due to urine absorption. Urinary tract infections are also avoided
- It is relatively easy to wash and clean the part of the colon distal to the colostomy
- Distal colostograms are easy to perform
- The sigmoid loop is kept distal to the colostomy which provides enough length to reach the perineum during the definitive pull-through procedure
- The separated stomas prevent spillage of stool from proximal to distal bowel, which avoids impacted distal stool and urinary tract infections
- There is a low incidence of prolapse with this technique. Proximal stoma prolapse in a normally rotated colon should not happen with this technique because the colon is well fixed to the retroperitoneum just before the colostomy rises to the skin level.

The distal stoma may prolapse because it is in a mobile portion of the colon. To avoid this, the distal stoma must be made intentionally small, as it will be used only for irrigations and radiologic studies. When performing the colostomy in the newborn, the distal bowel should be irrigated to remove all of the meconium. This prevents formation of a megasigmoid, which may be responsible for the future development of constipation.

Colostomy Procedures

- If the colostomy is placed too distal, it will interfere with the pull-through.
- During attempts to perform a transverse colostomy, cases of inadvertent sigmoid colostomy placed in the right upper quadrant have occurred. Anchoring of the sigmoid in the right upper quadrant would interfere with the pull-through procedure.

- A loop colostomy does not completely divert the stool and allows for distal stool impaction and urinary tract infections.
- Transverse colostomies produce megarectum

Posterior Sagittal Approach

Anorectal Repair

The repair of an anorectal malformation requires a meticulous and delicate technique and a surgeon with experience in the management of these defects. The posterior sagittal approach is an ideal method of defining and repairing anorectal anomalies. If the baby growing well, the repair can be performed at 1–2 months of age.

Ninety percent of male patients can be approached with a posterior sagittal approach alone, while 10% require an abdominal component (with laparotomy or laparoscopically) to mobilize a very high rectum. All female malformations, with the exception of about 30% of cloacas can be repaired with this approach. In 30% of cloacas, the rectum or vagina is so high as to require an abdominal approach as well.

Rectobladder Neck Fistula

In the rare case of a true supralevator malformation (rectobladder neck fistula), the operation involves both a posterior sagittal incision and an abdominal component, which can be done with laparoscopy or laparotomy.

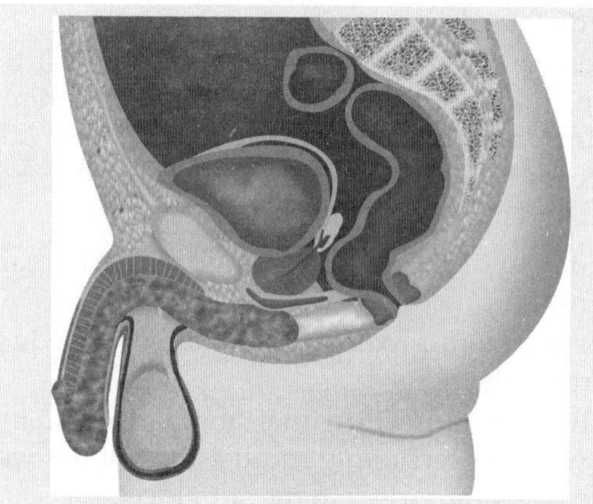

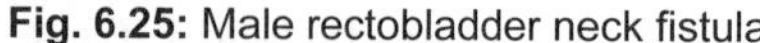

Fig. 6.25: Male rectobladder neck fistula

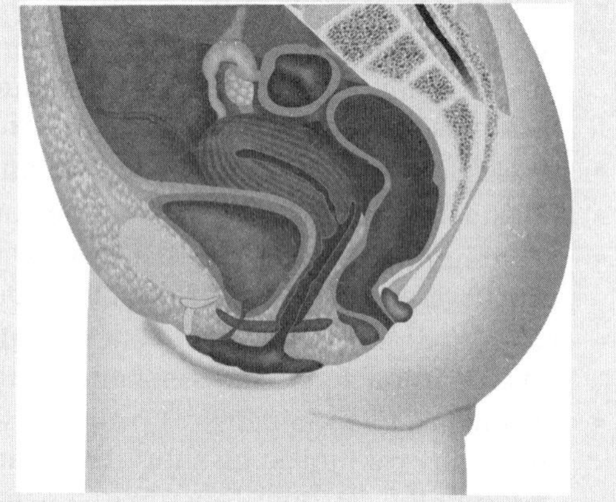

Fig. 6.26: Female rectobladder neck fistula

Imperforate Anus without Fistula

In patients with imperforate anus without fistula, the same meticulous dissection is required to separate the distal rectum from the urinary tract as in patient with rectourinary fistulae because the rectum and urethra still share a common wall.

Rectovestibular Fistula

In cases of rectovestibular fistula, the posterior sagittal incision can be shorter than in male patients with rectourethral fistulae. Often the entire levator mechanism needs not be divided and only the external sphincter, muscle complex, and part of the lower portion of the levator mechanism need to be divided. The rectum and posterior vagina share a common wall, and it is this separation that is the most difficult part of the operation. Once the rectum is completely mobilized, a perineal body is constructed, and the rectum is placed within the limits of the sphincter mechanism.

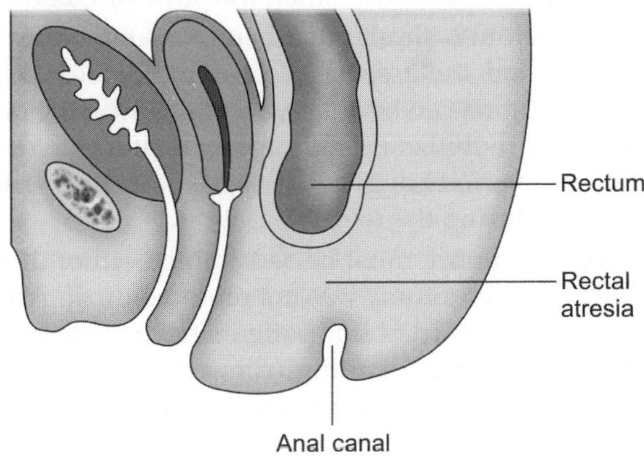

Fig. 6.27: Female rectal atresia

Rectal Atresia

A very rare malformation, rectal atresia, occurs in 1% of cases. The anal canal is normal and externally the anus appear normal. However, there is a blockage 1–2 cm from the anal skin, usually found when the nurse tries to pass a thermometer. These babies should undergo colostomy at birth, and then their definitive repair involves a posterior sagittal approach and an end-to-end anastomosis between the upper rectal pouch and the anal canal.

Persistent Cloacas

The repair of persistent cloacas represents a serious technical challenge that should be performed in specialized centers by pediatric surgeons dedicated to the care of these complicated patients. This malformation represents a wide spectrum of defects by itself. The defect involves fusion of the rectum, vagina, and urethra together to form a common channel.

The length of this common channel can range from 1 to 10 cm. The rectum and vagina share a common wall and the vagina and urinary tract likewise have a common wall. The goals of surgical treatment are to achieve bowel control, urinary control, and normal sexual function. Sometimes all three goals are achieved, sometimes only two, often *Persistent cloaca* only one, and occasionally none.

Prognostic factors include the quality of the sacrum, the quality of the muscles, and the length of the common channel. We have arbitrarily defined two groups of patients.

The repair of patients with a common channel less than three cm is reproducible and is feasible for most pediatric surgeons. For patients with a common channel greater than three cm, the repair should be performed at a specialized center by a surgeon with experience managing the urologic anomalies and able to performing complex vaginal reconstructions.

If the common channel is less than 3 cm, the posterior sagittal approach without an abdominal approach can be used to repair the defect.

For patients with a common channel greater than three cm, a laparotomy is usually required. Often the vagina and urinary tract must be separated trying to gain length, and the urethra must then be reconstructed. The surgeon must be prepared to open the bladder and to reimplant the ureters if necessary. Complex vaginal mobilizations are often required and frequenly a vaginal replacement with small intestine or colon is necessary.

The pullthrough of the rectum is similar to other anorectal malformations. It is the repair of the vagina, the urethra, and the associated urologic defects that represents the main surgical challenge. A large vagina can be an advantage during the definitive repair because the surgeon can more easily mobilize it and has more alternatives for the vaginal repair. About 50% of patients have various degrees of vaginal or uterine septation. These can be totally or partially repaired during the main operation.

The precise gynecologic anatomy must be ascertained either during the main repair or during colostomy closure (if a laparotomy was not required during the main repair). We have learned that approximately one third of our patients have obstructed Mullerian structures which can lead to severe problems resulting from retrograde menstruation. Predictions of future problems such as amenorrhea in cases of atretic uteri, or hydrometrocolpos and retrograde menses can be made in the newborn period. Presentations of pelvic pain or amenorrhea as teenagers should prompt the assumption of anomalous gynecologic structures.

Laparoscopically Assisted Anorectal Approach

The laparoscopically-assisted anorectal approach consists in mobilizing and bringing the rectum through the pelvic floor sphincter muscles through a minimal posterior incision. Perianal dissection towards the laparoscopic light source favors accurate placement of a trocar to pull the rectum through the external sphincter muscle complex. Laparoscopically-assisted anorectal repair can either be performed in the newborn period without a colostomy or in a stage-approach. This new technique, described by KE Georgeson et al. needs further long-term evaluation in terms of fecal continence.

Anterior Sagittal Approach

Anterior sagittal approach, involving anterior perineal dissection (from the base of the scrotum to the posterior part of the anoderm), is used by some surgeons, with the aim of preserving the internal anal sphincter. But it should be noticed that this approach might damage the vesical nerve plexus when the rectourethral-fistula is dissected up to its junction with the urethra. Furthermore, an internal sphincter saving technique has been devised when performing the posterior sagittal approach.

Postoperative Management

Anoplasty

The posterior sagittal incision is relatively painless. In patients with a rectourethral fistula, the Foley's catheter stays in place for about 5–7 days, and occasionally longer. At two weeks postoperatively, anal calibration is performed, followed by a program of anal dilatations. The anus must be dilated twice daily and every week the size of the dilator is increased. The final size to be reached depends on the age of the patient. Once the desired size is reached, the colostomy can be closed. Dilatations are a vital part of the postoperative management to avoid a stricture at the anoplasty. After colostomy closure, severe diaper rash is common because the perineal skin has never before been exposed to stool.

Complication

Constipation

The most frequent functional disorder encountered after treatment for imperforate anus in which the rectum has been preserved is constipation.

It is also the most important problem to avoid after definitive repair for female patients with rectovestibular or rectoperineal fistula and for male patients with rectobulbarurethral fistula, imperforate anus without fistula, and rectoperineal fistula. Failure to avoid constipation can result in megarectum and megasigmoid, and can lead to fecal impaction and overflow incontinence. The origin of the problem of constipation is unknown. It was originally thought that the perirectal dissection caused a degree of denervation that resulted in constipation. However, on careful review of the largest series of these patients, it became clear that those with the most benign defects and thus the least amount of perirectal dissection had the worst constipation.

Continence

Less frequently than constipation, some patients may experience soiling. While in a patient with a good prognosis, this may be overflow incontinence, it may also represent true fecal incontinence in cases of very high imperforate anus or poor muscles and an abnormal sacrum. A contrast enema is helpful in differentiating these two groups of patients. Patients with real incontinence require a bowel management program, which involves cleaning of the child's colon once a day by the use of a suppository, an enema or a colonic irrigation.

Giving the enema after the main meal of the day allows a more efficient cleansing of the bowel by taking advantage of the gastrocolic reflex. Antegrade enema procedures, whereby enema is introduced in a conduit via appendicocecostomy, has been devised to help the patient clean its bowel. The artificial bowel sphincter and electrically stimulated gracilis neosphincter are two relatively new techniques that have been used for the treatment of patients with severe refractory fecal incontinence.

The child shows signs that he is 'feeling' while having a bowel movement as he pushes. On the other end of the spectrum, a child who suffers from fecal incontinence passes stool constantly without any evidence of pushing or feeling. A child with a normal bowel movement pattern is trainable, whereas a child with the second pattern will likely need a bowel management program. For that child, one should not expect him to achieve voluntary bowel control.

Prognosis

When evaluating the results of the treatment of anorectal defects, we feel that one cannot group patients according to the traditional nomenclature into 'high,' 'intermediate,' and 'low' defects, as malformations classified in a same group can have different treatments and different prognoses. For instance, rectoprostatic fistula and bladderneck fistula, both considered as 'high' defects are actually very different. We believe that an anatomic classification would have more clinical value. The functional results of the repair of anorectal anomalies seem to have significantly improved since the advent of the posterior sagittal approach. However, the results of this approach are difficult to compare with those of other methods because terminology and classification are not consistent.

HERNIA (UMBILICAL OR INGUINAL) IN CHILDREN

Introduction

A hernia occurs when a section of intestine protrudes through a weakness in the abdominal muscles. A soft bulge is seen underneath the skin where the hernia has occurred. A hernia that occurs in the groin area is called an inguinal hernia.

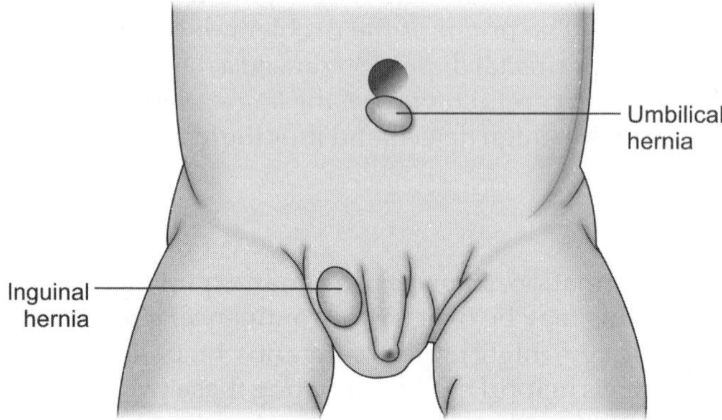

Fig. 6.28: Child with inguinal hernia

Inguinal hernia is the most common surgical problem of childhood. It results from a small sac that comes through the inguinal ring that is normally open during fetal life and closes around the time of birth. For reasons we do not understand, it does not close in some infants. This sac then makes a pathway for abdominal organs to come through the inguinal ring into the groin. In boys, the organ is usually a loop of bowel and, in girls, it may be bowel or an ovary. In boys and girls, the hernia first appears as a bulge in the groin, and may appear and disappear, or may be present all the time. It will usually 'pop out' when the child cries or strains. If only fluid comes through the inguinal ring into the sac, the problem is called a hydrocele.

Definition

A hernia is a bulge created by an organ or tissue. The bulge pushes through a weakness in the area of the body that normally contains it. The most common place that a hernia occurs is in the abdomen.

Types of hernias in children are:

- An *umbilical hernia* occurs when a part of the intestine sticks through the abdominal wall through the navel.
- An *inguinal hernia* occurs when part of the intestine pushes through the abdominal wall in or around the groin. Inguinal hernias occur in up to 5 out of 100 babies.

Umbilical Hernia

The soft bulge this creates is an umbilical hernia. It is most obvious when the baby cries, coughs, or strains. Umbilical hernias are more common in females, those of African heritage, and low birth weight babies. These hernias range in size from less than ½ inch (2 centimeters) to more than 2 inches (6 centimeters).

In most instances an umbilical hernia causes no discomfort. Usually, a doctor can easily push it back in. An infant's umbilical hernia (unlike an adult's) rarely obstructs or strangulates. In fact, most umbilical hernias, even the larger ones, tend to close up on their own by age two. That is why the doctor usually advises waiting and watching this kind of hernia in an infant rather than operating.

Inguinal Hernia

In infants, an inguinal hernia is most often caused by a protrusion of a loop or portion of intestine or a fold of membrane from the abdomen—or in girls, from an ovary or fallopian tube — through an opening into the groin (the area where the abdomen meets the top of the thigh). The opening is caused by the presence of a fold of the peritoneal membrane, which produces a sac. Within this sac, the loop of bowel can protrude.

The hernia is apparent as a bulge in the groin area, especially when the child cries, coughs, or stands. Sometimes, in male child are the inguinal hernia extends beyond the groin into the scrotum (the sac that holds the testicles). In girls, it can extend to one of the outer labia (the larger lips of tissue around the vaginal opening). In these cases, an enlargement or swelling can be seen that extends from the groin into the scrotum or labium.

More common on the right side, inguinal hernias occur far more often in boys than girls child and are most common in preemies, baby boys with undescended testicles, and kids with cystic fibrosis. Kids with a family history of hernias are also at risk.

Causes of Hernia

Most common causes are between 12 to 14 weeks of fetal development, the testicles or ovaries form in the abdomen near the kidneys. They gradually move down into the lower part of the abdomen as the baby continues to develop. As they move down, a portion of the peritoneum (a thin layer of tissue that lines the inside of the abdomen) that attaches to the testicle is drawn with it into the scrotum, forming a pouch or sac.

Common Causes

- Increased pressure within the abdomen
- A pre-existing weak spot in the abdominal wall
- A combination of increased pressure within the abdomen and a pre-existing weak spot in the abdominal wall.
- Straining during bowel movements or urination
- Heavy lifting
- Fluid in the abdomen (Ascites)
- Pregnancy
- Excess weight
- Chronic coughing or sneezing.

Umbilical Hernia

The navel has very little muscle beneath the skin. It is a weak area. When a baby cries or pushes out his belly, the pressure sometimes pushes part of an organ or tissue through the navel.

Inguinal Hernia

Male children are more likely to have this type of hernia. The inguinal canal is the passage through which the testes descend into the scrotum. Normally, this canal closes shortly after birth. If it does not close completely, it leaves a hole through which a loop of the intestine can pass into the groin or scrotum. This creates a bulge under the skin. This is an inguinal hernia.

Risk factors for an inguinal hernia include:

- *Being male:* Male children are likely to develop an inguinal hernia. Also, the vast majority of newborns and children who develop inguinal hernias are boys.
- *Family history:* Inguinal hernia increases if you have a close relative, such as a parent or sibling, who has the condition.
- *Certain medical conditions:* People who have cystic fibrosis, a life-threatening condition that causes severe lung damage and often a chronic cough, are more likely to develop an inguinal hernia.
- *Chronic cough:* A chronic cough, such as from smoking, increases your risk of inguinal hernia.
- *Chronic constipation:* Straining during bowel movements is a common cause of inguinal hernias.
- *Excess weight:* Being moderately to severely overweight puts extra pressure on your abdomen.
- *Pregnancy:* This can both weaken the abdominal muscles and cause increased pressure inside your abdomen.
- *Premature birth:* Infants who are born early are more likely to have inguinal hernias.
- *History of hernias:* Previously if child had one inguinal hernia, it is much more likely to develop another usually on the opposite side.

Signs and Symptoms of Hernia

Umbilical Hernia

An umbilical hernia usually appears a few weeks after birth. It usually occurs after the umbilical cord has fallen off. In general, it goes away before 2 years of age without treatment.

- A soft swelling around the navel
- The swelling may appear later in the day
- The swelling gets bigger if your child coughs, cries, sneezes, or stiffens his abdominal muscles.

Inguinal Hernia

- A soft swelling above the groin or in the scrotum
- The swelling may appear later in the day
- The swelling gets bigger if your child cries, coughs, sneezes, or stiffens his abdominal muscles.

Diagnostic Evaluation

A physical exam is usually all that is needed to diagnose an inguinal hernia.

- History collection
- Physical examination
- Abdominal X-ray
- CT scan
- Ultrasound scan
- MRI scan.

Surgical Management

- Herniorrhaphy
- Laparoscopy

Techniques

Open Repair

This involves making an incision just below the belt line and dissecting down to the hole in the muscle layer. This hernia is closed with stitches. The deeper tissues and skin are then sewn together with dissolvable sutures that are hidden under the skin so that there are no stitches to be removed. In teenagers, it is sometimes necessary to use a patch to help repair the hernia.

Open Repair with Laparoscopic Exploration

This is the same as the open repair except that before closing the hernia hole, a small camera (about 3 mm in diameter) is passed into the abdomen to examine the opposite groin from the inside. The surgeon will recommend this laparoscopic exploration in certain circumstances to rule out a potential hernia on the opposite side. If a hernia is detected, a matching incision is made on the opposite side to allow repair of the second hernia.

Laparoscopic Repair

In this approach the hernia is closed using laparoscopic techniques. A 3-mm or 5-mm camera is inserted through the belly button and additional instruments are introduced through needle holes to perform the hernia closure. There a number of different laparoscopic hernia repair techniques in children (eversion technique, intracorporeal suturing technique, single stitch technique) that a surgeon can use depending upon the particular patient.

Complications

If a loop of intestine or another organ or tissue becomes trapped in its hole, its blood supply can become blocked. This is called a strangulated hernia. When this occurs, the area becomes discolored and painful. Your child may vomit. If this happens, take your child to the doctor immediately, or go to the nearest Emergency Department right away.

Complications of an inguinal hernia include:

- *Pressure on surrounding tissues:* Most inguinal hernias enlarge over time if they are not repaired surgically. Large hernias can put pressure on surrounding tissues. In men, large hernias may extend into the scrotum, causing pain and swelling.

- *Incarcerated hernia:* If the omentum or a loop of intestine becomes trapped in the weak point in the abdominal wall, it can obstruct the bowel, leading to severe pain, nausea, vomiting, and the inability to have a bowel movement or pass gas.
- *Strangulation:* An incarcerated hernia may cut off blood flow to part of your intestine. This condition is called strangulation, and it can lead to the death of the affected bowel tissue. A strangulated hernia is life-threatening and requires immediate surgery.

CONGENITAL DIAPHRAGMATIC HERNIA (CDH)

Introduction

The topic of congenital diaphragmatic hernia (CDH) has frequently appeared in the medical literature since its first description in the early 18th century. Initial theories about the pathophysiology of this condition centered on the presence of the herniated viscera within the chest and the need for its prompt removal.

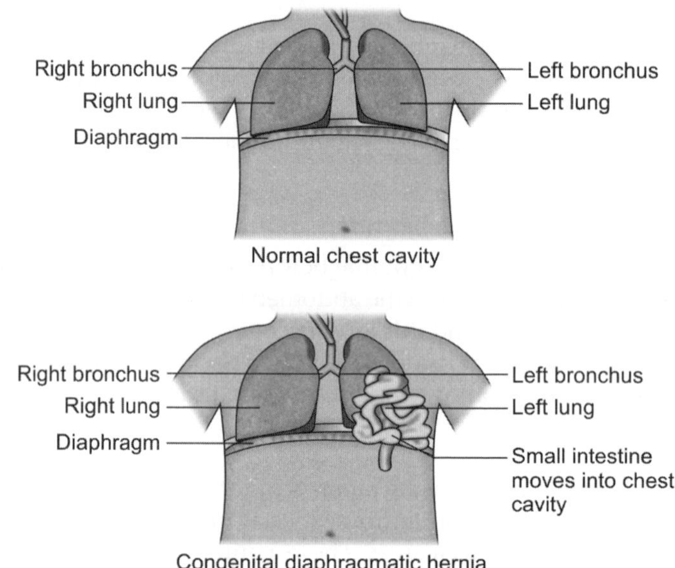

Fig. 6.29: Anatomical difference between normal and diaphragmatic herniation chest cavity

In 1946, Gross reported the first successful repair of a neonatal diaphragmatic hernia in the first 24 hours of life. The medical literature for the next decade addressed congenital diaphragmatic hernia as a surgical problem and discussed various technical aspects of surgical repair, including techniques required to close large defects. In the 1960s, however, Areechon and Reid observed that the high mortality rate of congenital diaphragmatic hernia was related to the degree of pulmonary hypoplasia at birth.

Over the past 20 years, pulmonary hypertension and pulmonary hypoplasia have been recognized as the two cornerstones of the pathophysiology of congenital diaphragmatic hernia. In recent years, evidence suggests that cardiac maldevelopment may further complicate the pathophysiology of congenital diaphragmatic hernia.

Definition

Congenital diaphragmatic hernia (CDH) defined as congenital malformation (birth defect) of the diaphragm. A hole in the diaphragm allows abdominal organs to move into the chest, which prevents the lungs from developing normally, resulting in pulmonary hypoplasia.

CDH is a life-threatening pathology in infants, and a major cause of death due to two complications:

- Pulmonary hypoplasia and pulmonary hypertension. Experts disagree on the relative importance of these two conditions:
  - Hypoplasia
  - Hypertension
- Newborns with CDH often have severe respiratory distress which can be life-threatening unless treated appropriately.

Incidence

Congenital diaphragmatic hernia occurs in one of every 2000–3000 live births and accounts for 8% of all major congenital anomalies. The risk of recurrence of isolated (i.e. nonsyndromic) congenital diaphragmatic hernia in future siblings is approximately 2%. Familial congenital diaphragmatic hernia is rare (< 2% of all cases), and both autosomal recessive and autosomal dominant patterns of inheritance have been reported. Congenital diaphragmatic hernia is a recognized finding in Cornelia de Lange syndrome and also occurs as a prominent feature of Fryns syndrome, an autosomal recessive disorder with variable features, including diaphragmatic hernia, cleft lip or palate, and distal digital hypoplasia.

Types of Congenital Diaphragmatic Hernia

- A Bochdalek hernia is a hole in the back of the diaphragm. Ninety percent of CDHs are this type
- A Morgagni hernia involves a hole in the front of the diaphragm
- Diaphragm eventration.

The diagnosis of congenital diaphragmatic eventration is used when there is abnormal displacement (i.e. elevation) of part or all of an otherwise intact diaphragm into the chest cavity. This rare type of CDH occurs because in the region of eventration the diaphragm is thinner, allowing the abdominal viscera to protrude upwards. This thinning is thought to occur because of incomplete muscularization of the diaphragm, and can be found unilaterally or bilaterally. Minor forms of diaphragm eventration are asymptomatic, however in severe cases infants will present with respiratory distress similar to Bochdalek hernia.

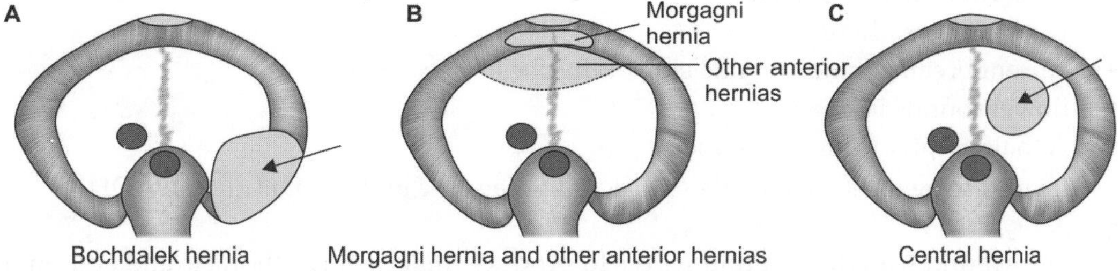

Fig. 6.30: Types of congenital hernia

Etiology (Causes)

- The diaphragm initially develops as a septum between the heart and liver, progresses posterolaterally, and closes at the left Bochdalek foramen at approximately 8–10 weeks' gestation.
- Congenital diaphragmatic hernias are idiopathic; their cause is unknown. However, chromosomal abnormalities have been implicated in about 30 percent of cases.

Signs and Symptoms

This condition can often be diagnosed before birth and fetal intervention can sometimes help, depending on the severity of the condition. Infants born with diaphragmatic hernia experience respiratory failure due to both pulmonary hypertension and pulmonary hypoplasia. The first condition is a restriction of blood flow through the lungs thought to be caused by defects in the lung. Pulmonary hypoplasia or decreased lung volume is directly related to the abdominal organs presence in the chest cavity which causes the lungs to be severely undersized, especially on the side of the hernia.

Symptoms may include the following:

- Difficulty in breathing
- Tachypnea
- Tachycardia
- Cyanosis (blue color of the skin due to low oxygen levels)
- Abnormal chest development, with one side being larger than the other
- Abdomen that appears caved in (concave).

Pathophysiology

Congenital diaphragmatic hernia is characterized by a variable degree of pulmonary hypoplasia associated with a decrease in cross-sectional area of the pulmonary vasculature and dysfunction of the surfactant system. The lungs have a small alveolar capillary membrane for gas exchange, which may be further decreased by surfactant dysfunction. In addition to parenchymal disease, increased muscularization of the intra-acinar pulmonary arteries appears to occur. In very severe cases, left ventricular hypoplasia is observed. Pulmonary capillary blood flow is decreased because of the small cross-sectional area of the pulmonary vascular bed, and flow may be further decreased by abnormal pulmonary vasoconstriction.

Diagnostic Evaluation

Physical Examination

- Abnormal chest movements
- Difficulty breathing
- Absent breath sounds on one side of the chest
- Bowel sounds in chest
- A 'half empty' feeling abdomen

The following tests are usually sufficient to diagnose both a CDH and an ADH:

- X-ray
- Ultrasound scan (uses sound waves to produce images of the thoracic and abdominal cavities and their contents)

- CT scan (allows for direct viewing of the abdominal organs)
- Arterial blood gases (takes blood directly from an artery and tests for levels of oxygen, carbon dioxide, and acidity, or pH level).

Chromosome Studies

Obtain chromosome studies because of the frequent association with chromosomal anomalies. In rare cases (e.g. Pallister–Killian syndrome), chromosomal disorders that can be diagnosed only based on skin biopsy findings may be present. If dysmorphic features are observed upon examination, a consultation with a geneticist is often helpful in evaluating the infant and ensuring that chromosome studies include appropriate deletion analysis.

Serum Electrolytes

As with all critically ill neonates, monitor levels of serum electrolytes, ionized calcium, and glucose initially and frequently. Maintaining glucose levels in the reference range and maintaining calcium homeostasis are particularly important.

Other Tests

Pulse Oximetry

Continuous pulse oximetry is valuable in the diagnosis and management of PPHN. Place oximeter probes at preductal (right-hand) and postductal (either foot) sites to assess for a right-to-left shunt at the ductus arteriosus level.

Histological Findings

- Both lungs appear abnormal, although histological changes are more severe on the affected side. Bronchi are less numerous, and the overall number of alveoli is reduced.
- In addition, the lungs appear to be less mature with fewer mature alveoli.
- Pulmonary vascular abnormalities occur in addition to parenchymal abnormalities, characterized by both a reduction in the cross-sectional area of the pulmonary vascular bed and an abnormal increase in muscularization of pulmonary arteries and arterioles.

Differential Diagnoses

- Cystic adenomatoid malformation
- Disorders of the thoracic cavity and pleura
- Pneumothorax
- Pulmonary hypertension
- Persistent newborn.

Management

Medical Management

Because of associated persistent pulmonary hypertension of the newborn (PPHN) and pulmonary hypoplasia, medical therapy in patients with congenital diaphragmatic hernia (CDH) is directed toward optimizing oxygenation while avoiding barotrauma.

Medical therapy in congenital diaphragmatic hernia (CDH) is directed toward stabilizing blood pressure and circulating volume, pulmonary distress, and hypoxemia.

Vasoactive Agents

Judicious use of vasoactive agents may increase cardiac output without affecting systemic or pulmonary vascular resistance.

Dopamine (Intropin)

Dopamine increases blood pressure primarily via stimulation of alpha-adrenergic receptors; however, its mechanism of action in newborn infants remains controversial because of developmental differences in endogenous norepinephrine stores and expression and function of alpha-adrenergic receptors. Dosage must be individualized.

Pediatric dose: 2–20 mcg/kg/min IV continuous infusion Phenytoin, alpha- and beta-adrenergic blockers, general anesthesia, and MAOIs increase and prolong effects of dopamine.

Dobutamine (Dobutrex)

Increases blood pressure primarily via stimulation of beta1-adrenergic receptors. It appears to have a more prominent effect on cardiac output than on blood pressure.

Pediatric dose: 2–25 mcg/kg/min IV continuous infusion, Beta-adrenergic blockers antagonize effects of dobutamine; general anesthetics may increase toxicity.

Fentanyl (Duragesic, Sublimaze)

Synthetic opioid that is 75–200 times more potent than morphine. It is highly lipophilic and protein-bound. Prolonged exposure leads to accumulation in fat and delays the weaning process. Used alone, fentanyl causes minor cardiovascular compromise, although the addition of benzodiazepines or other sedatives may result in decreased cardiac output and blood pressure.

Pediatric dose: Intermittent: 1–5 mcg/kg IV q2h by slow bolus. Continuous infusion: 1–10 mcg/kg/min IV, Phenothiazines may antagonize analgesic effects of opiate agonists; tricyclic antidepressants may potentiate adverse effects of fentanyl when both drugs are used concurrently.

Pulmonary Vasodilation Agents

Nitric oxide is an important mediator of vascular tone that was recently approved as a therapeutic modality for infants with PPHN. It is delivered as an inhaled gas. At least two multicenter studies did not show that inhaled nitric oxide decreases mortality or the need for extracorporeal support in infants with CDH; however, it may be useful in stabilizing an infant while evaluating or transferring for ECMO.

Mechanical Ventilation

A diaphragmatic hernia is a life-threatening illness. Most affected babies are unable to breathe well enough on their own because their lungs are underdeveloped and/or prevented from expanding by the abdominal organs in the chest area. Most babies will need to be placed on a breathing machine called a mechanical ventilator to help their breathing. In addition, a suction catheter is placed into the baby's stomach, from the nose or mouth, in order to remove any fluid or air that fills-up the stomach in order to prevent further pressure on the lungs.

Extra Corporeal Membrane Oxygenation (ECMO)

Some infants with severe breathing problems may need to be placed on a temporary heart/lung bypass machine called ECMO. ECMO does the job that the heart and lungs would be doing: putting oxygen in the bloodstream and pumping blood to the body. ECMO may be used temporarily while a baby's condition stabilizes and improves.

Surgical Management

Fetal Surgery

Theoretically, fetal surgery for congenital diaphragmatic hernia provides an elegant solution to the difficult problem of congenital diaphragmatic hernia. Unfortunately, this is far from reality. Harrison et al reported the first human fetal surgery for congenital diaphragmatic hernia in 1990. However, a randomized trial published in 1998 showed that in utero repair did not improve survival compared with standard therapy.

Subsequent trials of fetal intervention focused on occluding the fetal trachea. The fetal lung secretes fluid by active ion transport through gestation, and this lung fluid provides a template for lung growth. Occlusion of the fetal trachea traps this fluid and stimulates lung growth, either by retention of growth factors within the lung or stimulation of local growth factors by the gentle distension provided by the fluid. Unfortunately, a randomized trial in humans found that fetal tracheal occlusion did not improve outcome compared with standard treatment. Currently, fetal intervention is not indicated in congenital diaphragmatic hernia.

Postnatal Surgical Care

Until recently, specialists believed that reduction of the herniated viscera and closure of the diaphragmatic defect should be emergently performed following birth. However, a delayed surgical approach that enables preoperative stabilization decreases morbidity and mortality.

This change in protocol is due to the recent understanding that the medical problems of pulmonary hypoplasia and PPHN are largely responsible for the outcome of congenital diaphragmatic hernia and that the severity of these pathophysiologies is largely predetermined in utero. Herniated viscera in the chest does not appear to exacerbate the pathophysiology as long as bowel decompression with a nasogastric tube is continuous.

Several reports indicate that circulatory stability, respiratory mechanics, and gas exchange deteriorate after surgical repair. The ideal time to repair a congenital diaphragmatic hernia is unknown. Some suggest that repair 24 hours after stabilization is ideal, but delays of up to 7–10 days are typically well tolerated, and many surgeons now adopt this approach. Some surgeons prefer to operate on these neonates when normal pulmonary artery pressure is maintained for at least 24–48 hours based on echocardiography.

Chest Tube Placement

Chest tube drainage is necessary when a tension pneumothorax is present; however, whether routine chest drainage has a role is controversial. Some clinicians report improved survival when chest drainage is not used. Others think that balanced intrathoracic drainage, in which a closed gated pressure system is used to maintain intrathoracic pressure within the normal physiologic range, may minimize risk of pulmonary injury.

Lung Transplantation

Transplantation of a single lung has been reported in one case. Lung transplantation may allow the remaining hypoplastic lung to grow and to recover from injury while still allowing adequate oxygenation and ventilation. However, this approach has not been widely used because of the substantial problems associated with donor lung availability and immunosuppression.

Nursing Management

Pulmonary care in congenital diaphragmatic hernia (CDH) severely affected infants have chronic lung disease. These infants may require prolonged therapy with supplemental oxygen and diuretics, an approach similar to that for bronchopulmonary dysplasia. The use of steroids, particularly high doses for prolonged periods, is controversial and may hinder appropriate lung and brain development.

Late pulmonary hypertension has been successfully treated with low-dose inhaled nitric oxide. This therapy can be delivered via nasal cannula following extubation. In this setting, the delivered dose is diluted because of entrainment of room air. In a recent report, the median duration of treatment using inhaled nitric oxide delivered via nasal cannula was 17 days.

Neurologic Evaluation

Following recovery, a neurologist or developmental pediatrician should perform an examination that includes an evaluation for CNS injury using head CT scanning.

The incidence of hearing loss appears to be particularly high in patients with congenital diaphragmatic hernia (approximately 40% of infants). An automated hearing test should be performed prior to discharge.

Gastroesophageal Reflux

- The incidence of significant gastroesophageal reflux is very high in patients who survive congenital diaphragmatic hernia, and studies document an incidence of 45–85%.
- The need for a diaphragmatic patch may be a significant predictor of gastroesophageal reflux. Severe reflux may result in chronic aspiration and is, therefore, aggressively treated.
- Although most infants can be medically treated with H2 blockers or proton pump inhibitors in combination with a motility agent such as metoclopramide, surgical intervention is sometimes required.

Home Management

Growth Assessment

Failure to thrive is common, and, in some studies, more than 50% of patients are below the 25th percentile for height and weight during the first year of life. In one study, one third of infants required gastrostomy tube placement to improve caloric intake.

The need for supplemental oxygen at the time of discharge is a significant predictor for subsequent growth failure. Possible causes include increased caloric requirements due to chronic lung disease, oral aversion after prolonged intubation, poor oral feeding due to neurologic delays, and gastroesophageal reflux.

Prognosis

- *Pulmonary recovery:* Overall reported survival varies among institutions. Remember that a single institution's results may look better than those provided by population-based studies because of case-selection biases. When all resources, including ECMO, are provided, reported survival rates range from 40–90%. The ELSO registry reports the ECMO survival rate at 52%.

- *Long-term morbidity:* As noted, survivors are at risk for significant long-term morbidity, including chronic lung disease, growth failure, gastroesophageal reflux, hearing loss, and neurodevelopmental delay. The risk appears to be highest in infants with severe lung disease (need for supplemental oxygen), need for patch closure of the diaphragm, and need for gastrostomy tube feeding.

PYLORIC STENOSIS

Introduction

Pyloric stenosis, also known as infantile hypertrophic pyloric stenosis (IHPS), is the most common cause of intestinal obstruction in infancy. According to Pandya and Heiss, current recommendations include ultrasonography for diagnosis, preoperative corrections of electrolytes, and use of minimally invasive treatment techniques.

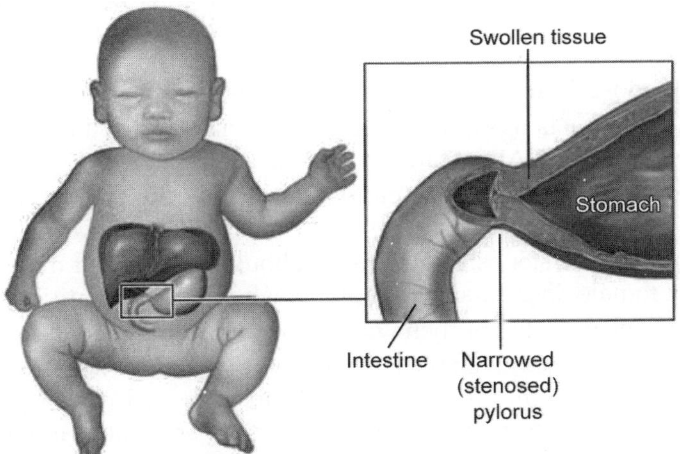

Fig. 6.31: Child with pyloric stenosis

Pyloric stenosis, a condition that may affect the gastrointestinal tract during infancy, it can cause your baby to vomit forcefully and often may cause other problems such as dehydration and salt and fluid imbalances. Immediate treatment for pyloric stenosis is extremely important.

Also called *infantile hypertrophic pyloric stenosis,* pyloric stenosis is a form of *gastric outlet obstruction,* which means a blockage from the stomach to the intestines.

Definition

Pyloric stenosis is the narrowing of the lower portion of the stomach (pylorus) that leads into the small intestine. The muscles in this part of the stomach thicken, narrowing the opening of the pylorus and preventing food from moving from the stomach to the intestine.

Pyloric stenosis is a narrowing of the pylorus, the lower part of the stomach through which food and other stomach contents pass to enter the small intestine. When an infant has pyloric stenosis, the muscles in the pylorus have become enlarged and cause narrowing within the pyloric channel to the point where food is prevented from emptying out of the stomach.

Pyloric stenosis can lead to forceful vomiting, dehydration and weight loss. Babies with pyloric stenosis may seem to be hungry all the time.

Incidence

This problem typically occurs in infants between 2 and 8 weeks of age and affects one out of every 500 to 1,000 live births.

Causes

It is believed that babies who develop pyloric stenosis are not born with it, but that the progressive thickening of the pylorus occurs after birth. A baby will start to show symptoms when the pylorus is so thickened that the stomach can no longer empty properly.

The causes of pyloric stenosis are unknown, but genetic and environmental factors might play a role. Pyloric stenosis usually is not present at birth and probably develops afterward.

Risk Factors

- *Sex:* Pyloric stenosis is more common in boys, especially firstborn children than in girls.
- *Race:* Pyloric stenosis is more common in Caucasians of northern European ancestry, less common in African-Americans and rare in Asians.
- *Premature birth:* Pyloric stenosis is more common in babies born prematurely than in full-term babies.
- *Family history:* Pyloric stenosis develops in about 20 percent of male descendants and 10 percent of female descendants of mothers who had the condition.
- *Smoking during pregnancy:* This behavior can nearly double the risk of pyloric stenosis.
- *Early antibiotic use:* Babies given certain antibiotics in the first weeks of life erythromycin to treat whooping cough, for example have an increased risk of pyloric stenosis. In addition, babies born to mothers who took certain antibiotics in late pregnancy also may have an increased risk of pyloric stenosis.

Signs and Symptoms

Signs of pyloric stenosis usually appear within three to five weeks after birth. Pyloric stenosis is rare in babies older than age 3 months.

Vomiting after feeding: The baby may vomit forcefully, ejecting breast milk or formula up to several feet away (projectile vomiting). Vomiting might be mild at first and gradually become more severe as the pylorus opening narrows. The vomit may sometimes contain blood.

Persistent hunger: Babies who have pyloric stenosis often want to eat soon after vomiting.

Stomach contractions: She may notice wave-like contractions (peristalsis) that ripple across your baby's upper abdomen soon after feeding, but before vomiting. This is caused by stomach muscles trying to force food through the narrowed pylorus.

Changes in bowel movements: Since pyloric stenosis prevents food from reaching the intestines, babies with this condition might be constipated.

Weight problems: Pyloric stenosis can keep a child from gaining weight, and sometimes can cause weight loss.

Other symptoms appear several weeks after birth and may include:

- Abdominal pain
- Burping
- Constant hunger
- Dehydration (gets worse as vomiting gets worse)
- Failure to gain weight or weight loss
- Wave-like motion of the abdomen shortly after feeding and just before vomiting occurs.

Diagnostic Evaluation

History collection and physical examination generally reveals a firm mass, the size of an olive, in the mid-abdomen.

These procedures include:

- *Blood tests:* This test done to evaluate the dehydration and mineral imbalances.
- *Abdominal ultrasound:* This is the gold standard for diagnosing pyloric stenosis. This is an imaging technique that uses high frequency sound waves and a computer to create images of blood vessels, tissues, and organs. It is used to determine the thickness and length of the pyloric muscle.
- *Barium swallow/upper GI series:* This test examines the organs comprising the upper part of the digestive system, which are the esophagus, stomach, and duodenum (the first section of the small intestine). Dense, chalky fluid called barium, which is used to coat the inside of organs so they will show up on an X-ray, is swallowed. X-rays are then taken to evaluate the digestive organs. This test will also demonstrate a delayed emptying of the stomach content as well as the narrowing of the pylorus.

Management

Medical Management

Pyloric stenosis is treated in two stages:

1. Fluids are given intravenously to treat dehydration
2. Restore the body's normal minerals.

Surgical Management

Pyloromyotomy

A surgical procedure called *pyloromyotomy,* which involves cutting through the thickened muscles of the pylorus, is performed to relieve the blockage that results from pyloric stenosis. The pylorus is examined through a very small incision, and the muscles that are overgrown and thickened are spread and relaxed.

The surgery can also be performed through *laparoscopy*. This is a technique that uses a tiny scope placed in an incision in the belly button allowing the doctor to see the area of the pylorus. With the help of other small instruments placed in nearby incisions, the surgery is completed.

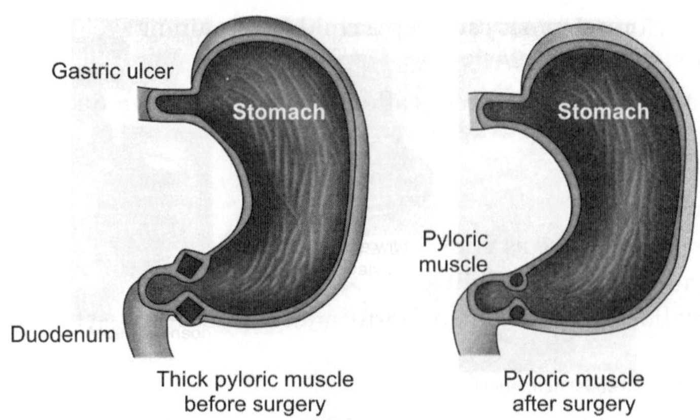

Fig. 6.32: Comparative image of before and after the pyloromyotomy surgery

Most babies are able to return to normal feedings fairly quickly, usually 3 to 4 hours after the surgery. Because of swelling at the surgery site, the baby may still vomit small amounts for a day or so after surgery. As long as there are no complications, most babies who have undergone pyloromyotomy can return to a normal feeding schedule and be sent home within 24 to 48 hours of the surgery.

If you are breastfeeding, you may be concerned about being able to continue feeding while your baby is hospitalized. The hospital should be able to provide you with a breast pump and assist you in its use so that you can continue to express milk until your baby can once again feed regularly.

After a successful pyloromyotomy, your infant will not need to follow any special feeding schedules. Your doctor will probably want to examine your child at a follow-up appointment to make sure the surgical site is healing properly and that your baby is feeding well and maintaining or gaining weight.

Pyloric stenosis should not recur after a complete pyloromyotomy. If your baby continues to display symptoms weeks after the surgery, it may suggest another medical problem, such as inflammation of the stomach (gastritis) or GERD or it could indicate that the initial pyloromyotomy was incomplete.

Role of Nurse after the Surgery

Pain

While in the operating room, your baby will receive a pain medication that is injected into the incision. This should allow him/her to feel and appear comfortable for about six to eight hours after surgery. If necessary, acetaminophen (medication such as Tylenol) may also be given to help ease discomfort.

Feedings

Within two hours after surgery, small amounts of milk or liquids are given. Over a 24- to 48-hour period, feedings are gradually increased. As soon as your baby can tolerate normal feedings (usually one to two days after surgery), he/she will be discharged from the hospital. After discharge, it is strongly recommended to do no more than 3 ounces every three hours for the next three days.

Vomiting

Although a baby often vomits for 24 to 48 hours after surgery, this usually disappears without any further treatment. Occasionally, however, vomiting may persist for four to five days.

Incision

The surgical incision should be kept clean and dry, and no tub baths should be given for one week after surgery. Steri-strips (bandage-like tape) that are placed over the incision should be left in place and then removed according to the instructions of your pediatric surgeon. They are generally left in place for seven to 10 days.

Prognosis

In this condition basically surgery will relieves all the symptoms. As soon as several hours after surgery, the infant can start small amount of frequent feedings.

CONGENITAL HYPERTROPHIC PYLORIC STENOSIS (HPS)

Definition

The congenital hypertrophic pyloric stenosis (HPS) is defined as functional gastric outlet obstruction which results in hypertrophy and hyperplasia of muscular layers of the pylorus. In infants periods this condition is most common and cause of gastric outlet obstruction and the most common surgical cause of vomiting.

Causes

- Congenital hypertrophic pyloric stenosis is more common in boys and manifested at 3–8 weeks of life.
- Its diagnosis can easily be made by ultrasonography and depends on visualization of thickened pyloric muscle layer (> 3 mm) and elongated pyloric canal (> 15 mm).

Signs and Symptoms

- Typical presentation is onset of initially nonbloody and nonbilious vomiting at 4–8 weeks of age.

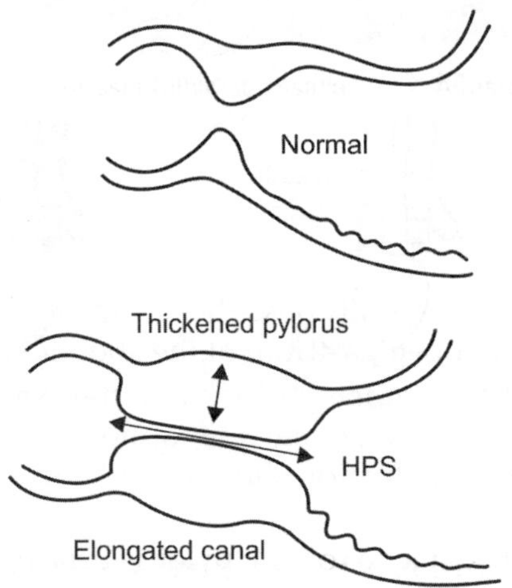

Fig. 6.33: Difference between normal and HPS

- Infrequent and projectile vomiting ensues
- Slight hematemesis of either bright-red flecks or a coffee-ground appearance is sometimes observed
- Dehydration
  - Poor weight gain and malnutrition
- Metabolic alterations and lethargy.

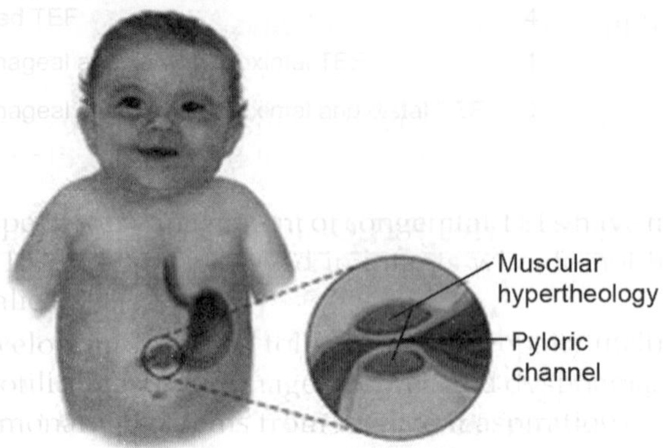

Fig. 6.34: Shape of congenital HPS

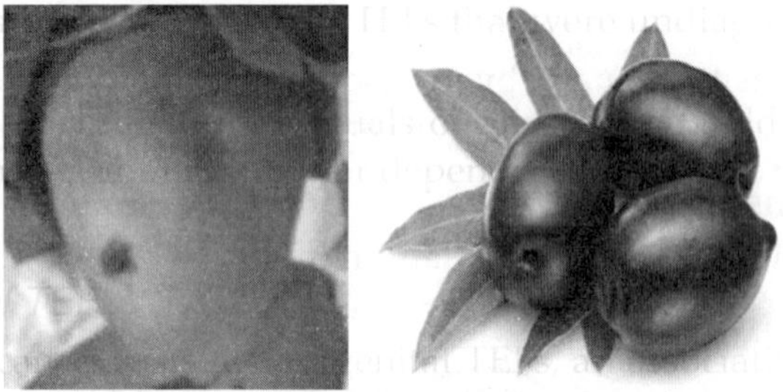

Fig. 6.35: Comparison of olive to congenital HPS

Diagnostic Evaluation

- History collection
- Physical examination
  - An enlarged pylorus, classically described as an 'olive shape' can be palpated in the right upper quadrant or epigastrium of the abdomen in 60–80% of infants.
  - The infant should be in supine position and the examiner on the child's left side, gently palpate the liver edge near the xiphoid process, then displace the liver superiorly; downward palpation should reveal the pyloric olive just on or to the right of the midline.
  - To be assure yourself, able to roll the pylorus beneath the examining finger.
  - The tumor (mass) is best felt after vomiting or during, or at the end of the feeding.

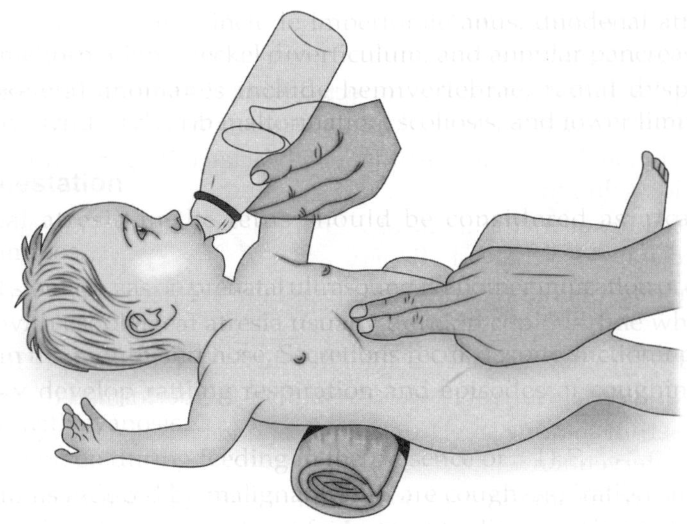

- Ultrasonography
  - Basically in this condition muscle wall thickness 3 mm or greater and pyloric channel length 14 mm or greater are considered abnormal in infants younger than 30 days.
- Barium meal upper GI study
  - This method is more effective when ultrasonography is not diagnostic properly
  - It should be demonstrate an elongated pylorus with antral indentation from the hypertrophied muscle
  - It may show the 'double track' sign when thin tracks of barium are compressed between thickened pyloric mucosa or the 'shoulder' sign when barium collects in the dilated prepyloric antrum
  - After upper GI barium meal study, irrigating and removing any residual barium from the stomach is advisable to avoid aspiration.
- Endoscopy.

Management

Surgical Management

- In this condition Ramstedt pyloromyotomy is the standard procedure
- The usual approach is via a right upper quadrant transverse incision that splits the rectus muscle and fascia
- Laparoscopic pyloromyotomy may also be used
- Endoscopic pyloromyotomy is a simple procedure and can be performed as an outpatient procedure
- Endoscopic balloon dilatation of hypertrophic pyloric stenosis after failed pyloromyotomy can be used
- A supraumbilical curvilinear approach has gained popularity with good cosmetic results.

Preoperative Nursing Management

- Assess the general condition of the child
- The infants can have their fluid status corrected within 24 hours and severely dehydrated children sometimes require several days for correction
- Administer an initial fluid bolus of 10 ml/kg with lactated Ringer solution or 0.45 isotonic sodium chloride solution
- Continue IV therapy at an initial rate of 1.25–2 times the normal maintenance rate until adequate fluid status is achieved
- Adequate amounts of both chloride and potassium are necessary to correct metabolic alkalosis
- Unless renal insufficiency is a concern, initially add 2–4 mEq of KCl per 100 mL of IV fluid
- Urine output and serial electrolyte determinations are performed during resuscitation
- Correction of serum chloride level to 90 mEq/L or greater is usually adequate to proceed with surgical intervention
- Before induction of anesthesia, aspirate the infant's stomach with a large-caliber suction tube to remove any residual gastric fluid or barium; saline irrigation is occasionally necessary to remove a large quantity of barium.

Postoperative Nursing Management

- Provide comfortable postoperative bed to the child
- She should be continue the IV fluid therapy until the infant is able to tolerate enteral feedings
- In most instances, feedings can begin within 8 hours following surgery
- Graded feedings can usually be initiated every 3 hours, starting with pedialyte and progressing to full-strength formula
- Schedules that advance the volume of feeds more quickly or those that begin with ad lib feeds are associated with more frequent episodes of vomiting but do not increase morbidity and actually may decrease the time to hospital discharge
- Addition of an H2 receptor blocker sometimes can be beneficial
- Treat persistent vomiting expectantly because it usually resolves within 1–2 days
- Avoid the temptation to repeat ultrasonography or upper GI barium study; these invariably demonstrate a deformed pylorus, and results are difficult to interpret.

Complications

- Severe electrolyte disturbance (hypokalemic and hypochloremic metabolic alkalosis).
- Operative complications include mucosal perforation, continued postoperative bleeding (very rare), and persistent vomiting due to incomplete pyloromyotomy (rare).
- Foveolar cell hyperplasia (FCH) has been reported as a rare cause of persistent gastric outlet obstruction in patients with IHPS. An extended pyloromyotomy is required to manage this.

Prognosis

- In this condition prognosis status is excellent unless diagnosis is delayed and prolonged severe dehydration occurs.
- Mortality rate is very rare in this condition after the surgery (pyloromyotomy).

DEFECTS OF GENITOURINARY TRACT

HYPOSPADIASIS AND EPISPADIASIS

Hypospadiasis

Introduction

Hypospadias (hi-poe-SPAY-dee-us) is a condition in which the opening of the urethra is on the underside of the penis, instead of at the tip. It is one of the most common birth defects among boys, hypospadias is caused by the incomplete development of the urethra, the canal that carries urine from the bladder out of the body and also serves as the passageway for semen. The defect results in a urethra that opens on the underside of the penis. In the most serious cases, boys cannot urinate normally unless they are treated.

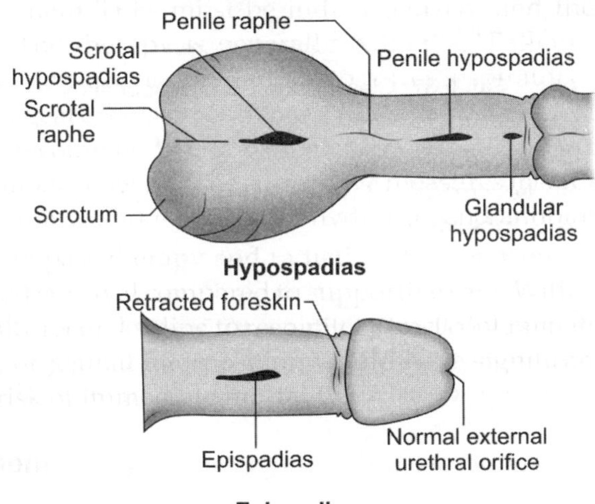

Fig. 6.36: Child with hypospadias

There is a family tendency towards hypospadias, with an increased rate noted in boys whose father or brothers have hypospadias. Other than inherited cases, the cause is usually unknown.

Hypospadias occurs in about one in 100 to 1 in 200 boys. There are different degrees of hypospadias, some minor and others more severe. Surgical correction of hypospadias involves straightening of any chordee and then extension of the urinary tube (urethra) out to the tip of the penis (the glans).

Definition

Hypospadias is defined as abnormal opening on the ventral aspect (Lower surface of the penile shaft) of the penis. It is common congenital malformation of male children.

Classification of Hypospadias

The types of hypospadias according to their anatomic location, but one must always determine whether or not there is associated chordee.

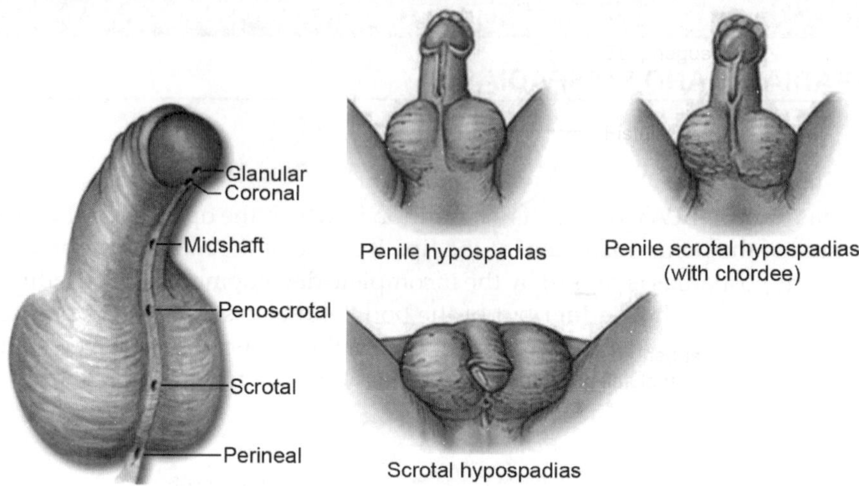

Fig. 6.37: Classification of hypospadias

Causes

The exact reason this defect occurs is unknown. Hypospadias is present at birth (congenital). Sometimes hypospadias is inherited.

Risk Factors

The cause of hypospadias is unknown, both environmental and genetic factors have been associated with the condition, including:

- *Family history:* This condition is more common in infants with a family history of hypospadias.
- *Maternal age over 40:* An increased risk of hypospadias in infant males born to women of an advanced age.
- *Exposure to smoking and chemicals:* There is some speculation about an association between a mother's exposure to pesticides and hypospadias, but further studies are needed to confirm this.

Signs and Symptoms

- Opening of the urethra below the tip on the bottom side of the penis
- Abnormal appearance of the glans penis (the tip of penis)
- Incomplete foreskin in which the foreskin extends only around the top of the penis
- Curvature of the penis during an erection (called chordee)
- Buried penis
- Abnormal position of scrotum with respect to penis.

Problems resulting from hypospadias include deviation of the urinary stream, cosmetic and psychological considerations and potential adverse effects on sexual functioning.

Diagnostic Evaluation

Hypospadias is typically diagnosed during a newborn examination. The opening of the urethra is below the tip of the penis. The penis may be curved and the foreskin not completely formed around the entire tip of the penis. Occasionally, a specific type of hypospadias, known as mega-meatus intact prepuce variant of hypospadias is not noted until a circumcision has been performed.

- History collection
- Physical examination
- Ultrasound scan
- X-ray

Management

Hypospadias is treated with surgery to correct the placement of the urethral opening, usually during the first year of life. There are different types of surgery.

- To create a straight penis by repairing any curvature (orthoplasty)
- To create a urethra with its meatus at the tip of the penis (urethroplasty)
- To reform the glans into a more natural conical configuration (glansplasty)
- To achieve cosmetically acceptable penile skin coverage.

The goal of surgical correction is to reconstruct a straight penis with a urethral opening as close to the tip of the penis as possible. This will result in a properly directed urinary stream, straightened penis upon erection and an appearance similar to a circumcised penis.

The surgery is performed under general anesthesia and often your child will be admitted and discharged from the hospital on the same day. About half of the cases involve the more complicated hypospadias repairs, which require a catheter to be left in the bladder to drain the urine for seven to 10 days.

Postoperative Instructions for Hypospadias Repaired Child

Catheter Care

- Sometime the child may be discharged with a catheter. If the child wears a diaper, the catheter will drain into his diaper.
- The child is older; the catheter will drain into a bag on his leg. Urine may leak around the tube or spurt through the tube.
- This is common and is not a problem, as long as most of the urine drains through the tube. Excessive leaking might indicate the tube is blocked.
- The tube may cause bladder spasms while the child is sleeping. He may arch his back, bring his knees up to his chest and urine may squirt through or around the tube. Spasms are not harmful, but may be uncomfortable.
- A spot or two of blood on the diaper is normal. Do not apply powder or ointments to the genital area. The child has loose bowel movements and soils his surgical dressing clean. It gently with soapy water and a washcloth away from his penis.
- Children who do not have a catheter may complain of discomfort or cry while urinating through the repaired area for one or two days.

Medications

- An antibiotic upon discharge from the hospital. Continue to give the antibiotic for several days after the removal of the catheter.
- Tylenol with or without codeine, may be given for discomfort.

- Encourage your child to drink lots of fluids.
- Most children will be given a nerve block during surgery to reduce pain. This block will wear off in four to six hours.
- The children experience more discomfort than usual for 15 to 20 minutes when the block wears off. To help prevent this, give Tylenol or Tylenol with codeine about three-and-a-half to four hours after the surgery, even if your child is comfortable.

Wound Dressings

- The child will go to home with a 'dressing' or covering consisting of a clear plastic over gauze, or plain gauze taped around his penis. It may become soiled and loose from urine and stool.
- Do not remove the soiled dressing unless there is stool underneath the plastic dressing, in contact with the gauze. If the dressing is covered with stool, clean with soapy water, wiping toward the rectum and away from child's penis.
- Remove the dressing two days after your son's surgery. This can be done easily in the bath. If the child has a urethral catheter be mindful of the tube.
- Expect some swelling and discoloration of the penis after the surgery, which will resolve in time. Some oozing from the penis resulting in spotting on the dressings, diaper or underpants is normal.

Child Bathing

- Sponge-bathe the child until the dressing is removed.
- Provide tub baths when the dressing falls off or two days after the surgery, whichever occurs first.
- The child can take a tub bath even while the catheter is in. When you resume regular bathing, use tepid water without soap.
- Do not scrub the area and do not directly wash the penis; just allow the water to soak the area. Gently pat the area dry with a clean towel.

Diet Management

The child can resume a normal diet at home. Encourage fluids for example, ice pops, juice, soup to keep the child urine clean. Some children may have nausea or vomiting from the anesthesia, but most will be fine. Gradually child appetite will return to normal and he can have any food he likes.

Nursing Management

Encourage child to drink more fluids that will be help to urinate. A follow-up visit should be scheduled for four weeks after the tube is removed.

The nurse should manage the child following problems:

- Temperature greater than 101 °F
- Excessive bleeding (some spotting or blood stains on the dressing is normal)
- Extreme irritability
- Excessive pain
- Increasing redness of the penis
- Disinterest in eating and drinking (particularly after 24 hours)

- Continuous vomiting
- Change in urination
- Difficulty urinating (pushing when he urinates).

EPISPADIAS

Introduction

Congenital malformations of the male genitalia include a wide range of clinical conditions such as hypospadias, epispadias (in females, bifid clitoris) with bladder exstrophy, and hidden penis. Epispadias is an uncommon congenital malformation of the penis and is often part of the condition termed epispadias-exstrophy of the bladder.

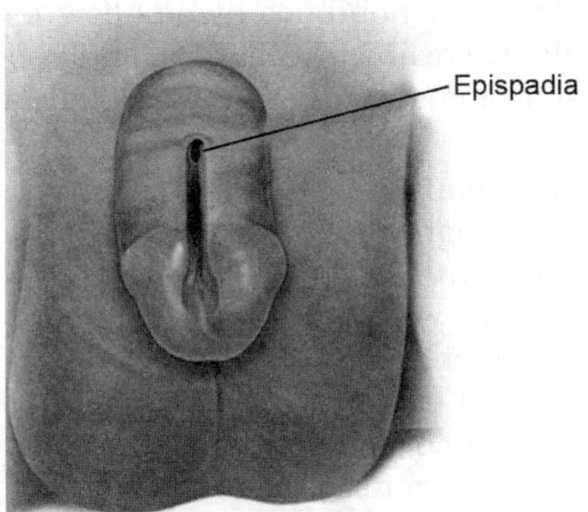

An *epispadias* is a rare type of malformation of the penis in which the urethra ends in an opening on the upper aspect (the dorsum) of the penis. It can also develop in females when the urethra develops too far anteriorly. It occurs in around one in 120,000 male and one in 500,000 female births.

Definition

An *epispadias* is a rare type of malformation of the penis in which the urethra ends in an opening on the upper aspect (the dorsum) of the penis. Epispadias is a rare congenital (present from birth) defect located at the opening of the urethra. In this condition, the urethra does not develop into a full tube and the urine exits the body from an abnormal location.

Causes

- Epispadias is an uncommon and partial form of a spectrum of failures of abdominal and pelvic fusion in the first months of embryogenesis known as the exstrophy-epispadias complex.
- Epispadias is inherent in all cases of exstrophy. It can also, much less frequently, appear in isolation as the least severe form of the complex spectrum.
- It occurs as a result of defective migration of the genital tubercle primordii to the cloacal membrane, and so malformation of the genital tubercle, at about the 5th week of gestation.

- They are not thought to involve androgens nor to be primarily genetic, although there is some increased genetic frequency. The leading theory is that of a virus during pregnancy, manifesting as a moderate to serious common cold
  - The causes of epispadias are unknown at this time. It may be related to improper development of the pubic bone.
  - In boys with epispadias, the urethra generally opens on the top or side of the penis rather than the tip. However, it is possible for the urethra to be open along the entire length of the penis.
  - In girls, the opening is usually between the clitoris and the labia, but may be in the belly area. Epispadias can be associated with bladder exstrophy, an uncommon birth defect in which the bladder is inside out, and sticks through the abdominal wall. However, epispadias can also occur with other defects.
  - Epispadias occurs in 1 in 117,000 newborn boys and 1 in 484,000 newborn girls. The condition is usually diagnosed at birth or shortly thereafter.

Types of Epispadias

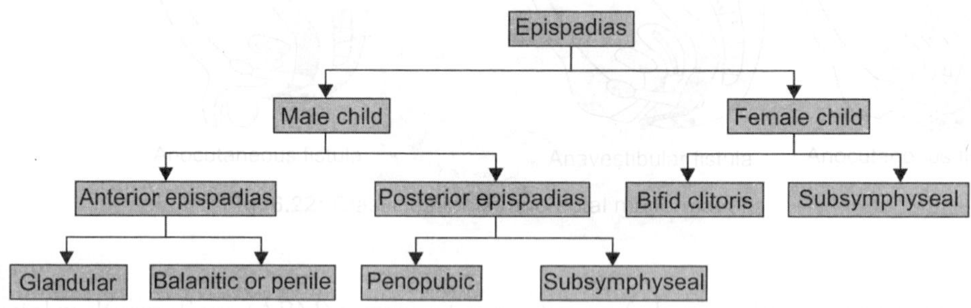

Signs and Symptoms

In Male Children

- Abnormal opening from the joint between the pubic bones to the area above the tip of the penis
- Backward flow of urine into the kidney (reflux nephropathy)
- Short, widened penis with an abnormal curvature
- Urinary tract infections
- Widened pubic bone.

In Female Children

- Abnormal clitoris and labia
- Abnormal opening from the bladder neck to the area above the normal urethral opening
- Backward flow of urine into the kidney (reflux nephropathy)
- Widened pubic bone
- Urinary incontinence
- Urinary tract infections.

Pathophysiology

In male children epispadias causes impotentia coeundi, which results from the dorsal curvature of the penile shaft, and Impotentia generandi, which results from the incomplete urethra. Also reported are frequent ascending infections to the prostate or bladder and kidneys and psychological problems related to the deformity. If epispadias is distal to the bladder neck, urinary continence may not be present.

Diagnostic Evaluation

Laboratory Studies

Obtain a complete blood cell count.

Imaging Studies

- Obtain a chest radiograph if indicated based on examination findings or the patient's history.
- Radiologic (e.g. intravenous pyelogram)
- Ultrasound evaluations of the urogenital system (e.g. kidneys, ureters, bladder; urethra, genitalia) are usually necessary to evaluate the extent of the defect.

Other Tests

Obtain an ECG for operating room guidelines.

Diagnostic Tests

- Blood test to check electrolyte levels
- Intravenous pyelogram (IVP), a special X-ray of the kidneys, bladder, and ureters
- MRI and CT scans, depending on the condition
- Pelvic X-ray
- Ultrasound of the urogenital system.

Management

The main treatment for isolated epispadias is a comprehensive surgical repair of the genito-urinary area usually during the first 7 years of life, including reconstruction of the urethra, closure of the penile shaft and mobilization of the corpora.

The most popular and successful technique is known as the *modified Cantwell-Ransley* approach. In recent decades however increasing success has been achieved with the *complete penile disassembly* technique despite its association with greater and more serious risk of damage.

Medical Management

There is no any specific medical intervention for epispadias.

Surgical Management

Most of the repair techniques are based on multistaged reconstruction procedures used in hypospadias correction. The first stage addresses correction of the eventually stenotic meatus, the second stage addresses elimination of the dorsal chordee and penile straightening, and the third stage addresses the urethroplasty. Together with the progress in surgical treatment of hypospadias, one-stage procedures have also been used to correct epispadias.

The goals of surgical procedures such as:

- Correction of the curvature
- Reconstruction of the missing portion of urethra
- Restoration of the normal aspect of the external genitalia
- Reconstruction of the anterior wall of the bladder when necessary.

Surgery differs according to the complexity of the malformation.

Epispadias is treated with the same technique as hypospadias located in the same anatomic position, with the exception that the repair is reversed and the epispadias reconstruction is on the dorsal surface.

Continence is a difficult goal in exstrophy-epispadias complex repair. Presumably, all anatomic components involved in the exstrophy-epispadias abnormality are present but are displaced laterally and anteriorly. A staged approach has often been used for the management of the exstrophy-epispadias complex. The Cantwell-Ransley repair and the Young procedure have also been used.

Postoperative Details

Arm and leg restraints may be necessary. The dressings remain in place for 4 days if no problems occur. Remove the diverting urinary catheter after 8 to 10 days. Discharge the patient after removal of the urinary diversion and when spontaneous voiding occurs without difficulty.

Repair of Hypospadias and Chordee

The children have surgery to correct hypospadias at about six to nine months of age. Although we try and correct most children with one operation, about 10% will require a second surgical procedure to manage complications. If that is necessary, the second operation is delayed for one year. By performing the first operation early in life, both operations can be completed before the child is finished toilet training.

The operations performed to correct the hypospadias vary according to the degree of abnormality. The extra foreskin is sometimes needed to construct a new urethra. When the operation is completed, the extra skin is removed so the child will look circumcised. To protect the newly constructed urethra (neourethra) the urine is usually diverted with a stent (a silastic tube through the neourethra). We also leave a plastic dressing on the penis, which can be removed by the parent at home.

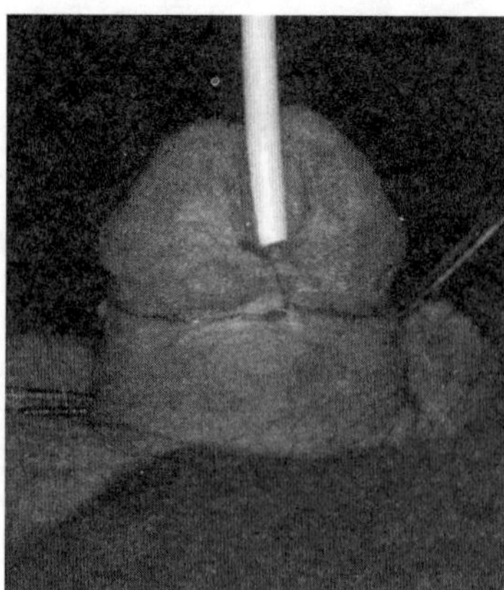

Fig. 6.38: Distal penile epispadias

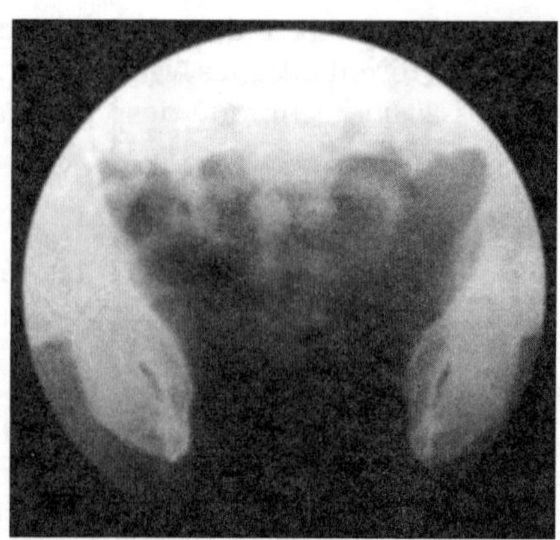

Fig. 6.39: Wide diastasis of the pubic bone and external displacement of the hips in epispadias

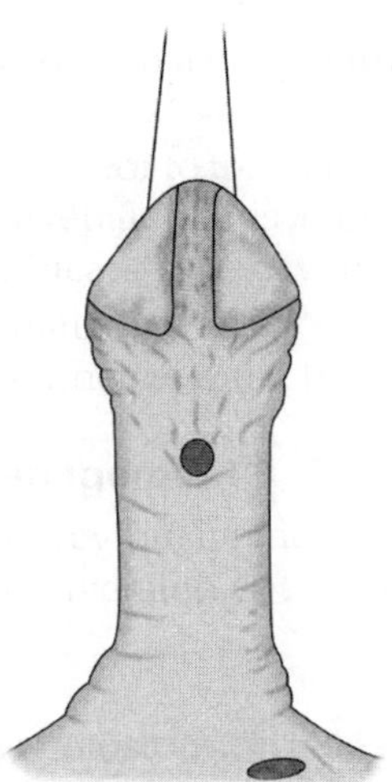

Fig. 6.40: Distal epispadias. Outlining of local flaps from the glans to reconstruct the distal urethra

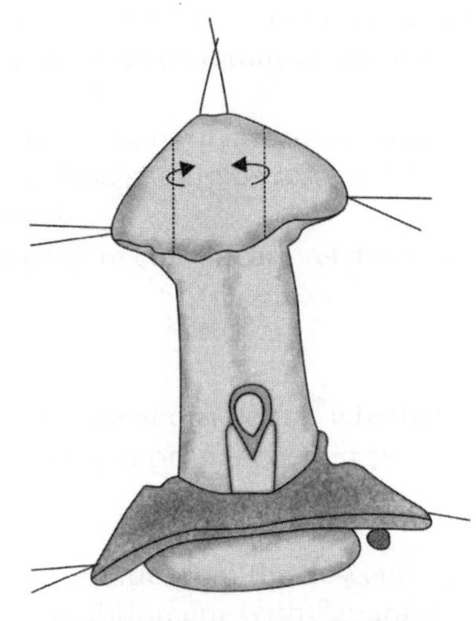

Fig. 6.41: Reconstruction of distal penile urethra using local flaps (arrows)

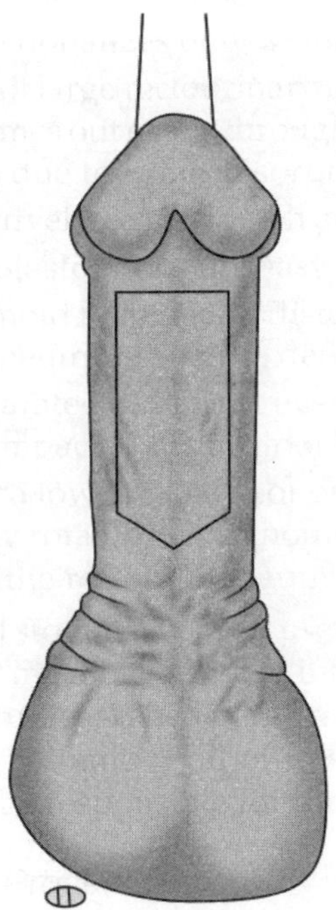

Fig. 6.42: Vertical island flap drawn on the ventral aspect of the penis

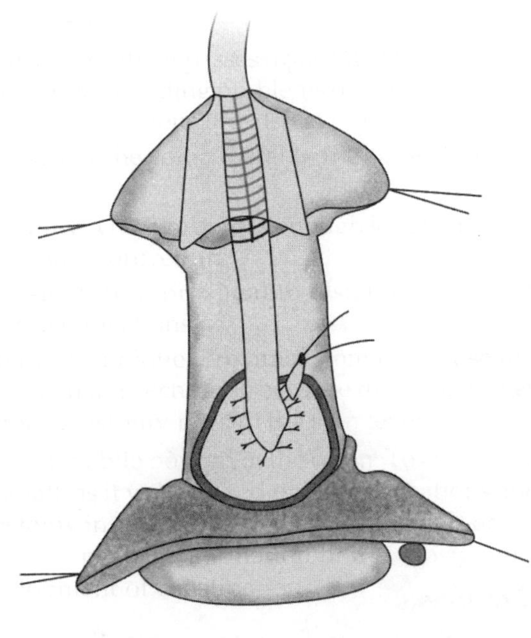

Fig. 6.43: Island flap transferred dorsally and anastomosed to the urethra

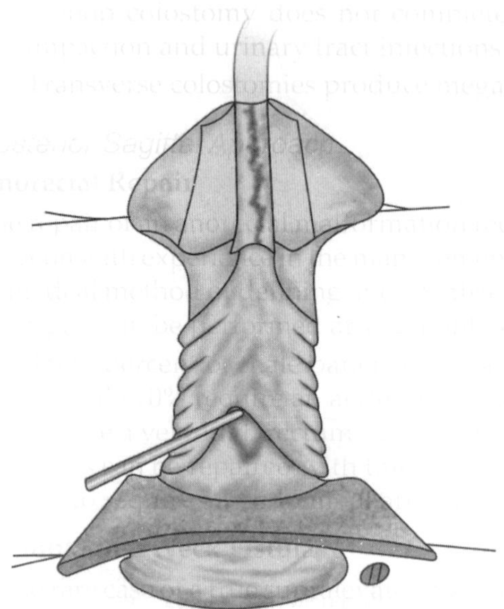
Fig. 6.44: Island flap sutured into a tube to reconstruct the missing portion of the urethra

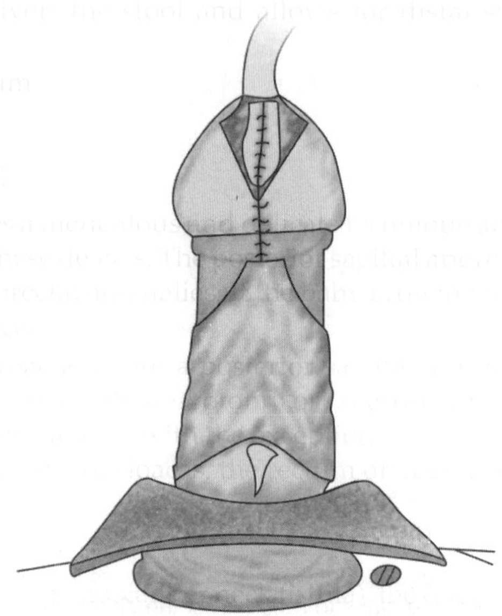
Fig. 6.45: Urethral reconstruction is completed

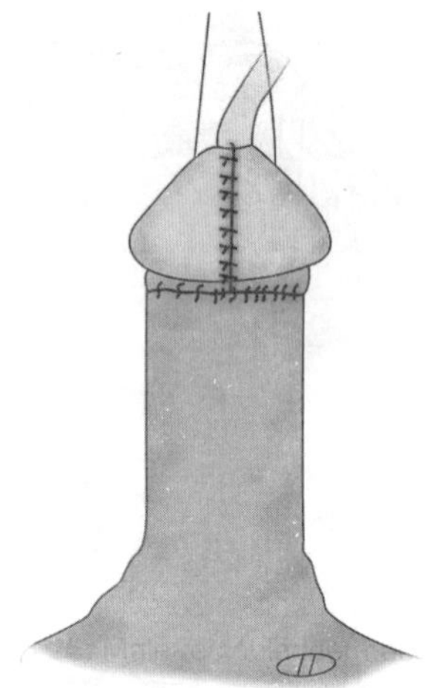
Fig. 6.46: Drawing of the final appearance at the end of the operation

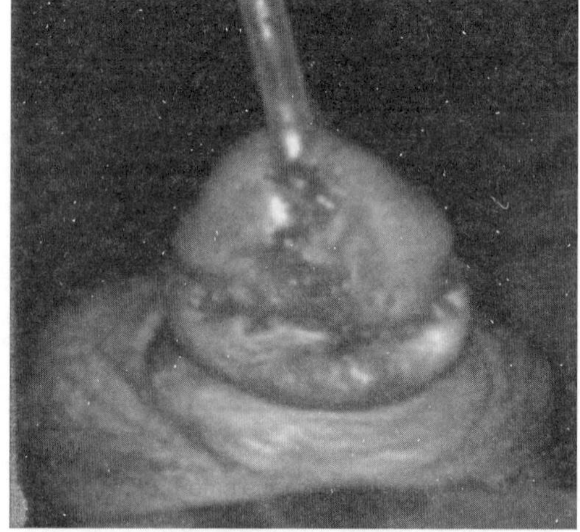
Fig. 6.47: Image of the final appearance at the end of the healing process

Prognosis

In terms of overall success rates, the incidence of fistulas or stenosis, and the mean hospitalization time, functional results obtained with one-stage epispadias correction have proved to be superior to those obtained with multistage procedures; the prognosis is good. For one-stage reconstruction, the use of a well-nourished and innervated flap with a long and pliable pedicle is necessary to achieve the high success rate reported in the literature.

Surgical repair generally results in both continence (ability to control the flow of urine) and a good cosmetic outcome. Successful reconstruction of epispadias improves the body image and enables the patient to perform sexually.

- Even with successful surgery, child may have long-term problems with incontinence
- Depression and psychosocial complications
- Sexual dysfunction.

Complications

- Early complications include bleeding, infection
- Wound separation, flap necrosis, and edema
- Urethrocutaneous fistula with urinary leakage from the new urethra and urethral stricture occur in approximately 10–19% of all epispadias repairs.

Nursing Management

- She should be monitor child with a urine flow rate study at 3 weeks and at 3 and 12 months postoperatively.
- If a mild urethral stenosis is noticed, dilate the urethra with probes of increasing sizes and repeat the flow rate study after 3 weeks.
- Question child parents about persistence of the curvature 3 weeks postoperatively.
- Long-term follow-up care is necessary at least through puberty to exclude late failure due to hypertrophic urethral scarring or undetected chronic inflammation.

BLADDER EXSTROPHY

Introduction

The bladder exstrophy and epispadias complex comprises a spectrum of congenital abnormalities that includes classic bladder exstrophy, epispadias, cloacal exstrophy, and

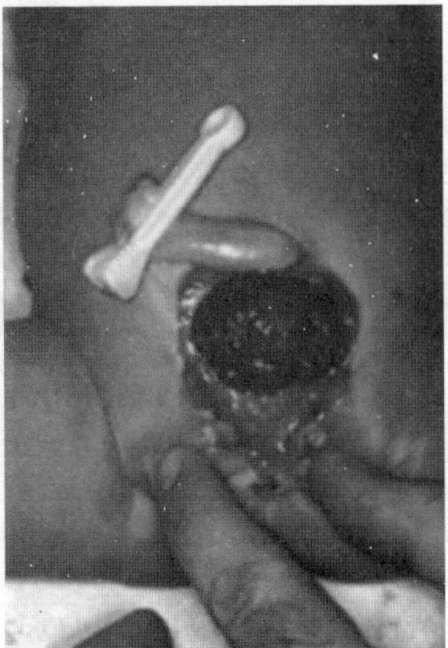

Fig. 6.48: Open bladder plate and urethra with bifid clitoris in female patient with classic bladder exstrophy. Note low-set umbilicus and interiorly displaced anus

several variants. Each of these anomalies is thought to result from the same embryologic defect. Separation of the primitive cloaca into the urogenital sinus and hindgut occurs during the first trimester at approximately the same time as maturation of the anterior abdominal wall.

Failure of mesenchyme to migrate between the ectodermal and endodermal layers of the lower abdominal wall leads to instability of the cloacal membrane. Premature rupture of the membrane before its caudal translocation leads to this complex of infraumbilical anomalies. Rupture of the cloacal membrane after complete separation of the genitourinary and GI tracts results in classic bladder exstrophy.

Classification

The cloacal exstrophy must be distinguished from the condition of persistent cloaca or cloacal malformation. The latter terms refer to the most extreme form of anorectal malformation in female infants. This complex anomaly involves incomplete separation of the urinary tract, genital tract and hindgut. No abdominal wall defect is present in persistent cloaca.

Classification of Bladder Exstrophy (See figures A to M)

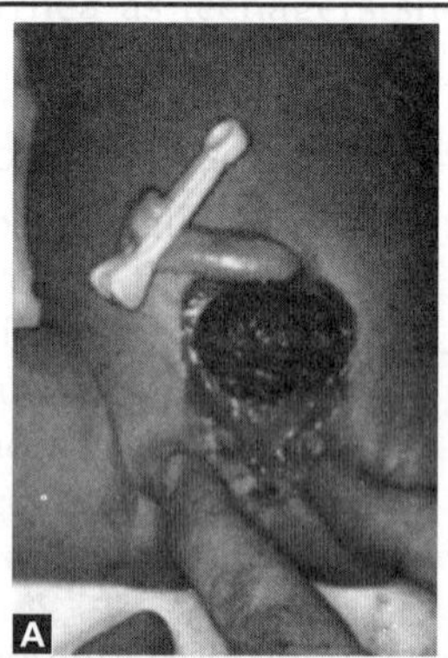 A	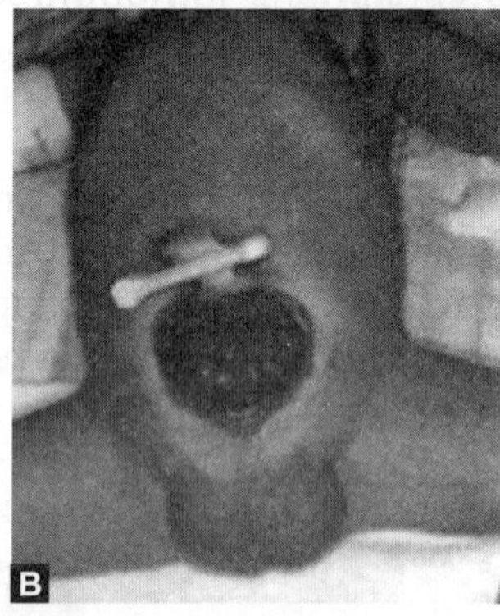 B
Open bladder plate and urethra with bifid clitoris in female patient with classic bladder exstrophy. Note low-set umbilicus and anteriorly displaced anus.	Male with classic bladder exstrophy. Note low-set umbilicus and short, broad, upturned phallus. Distance between phallus and scrotum is abnormal.
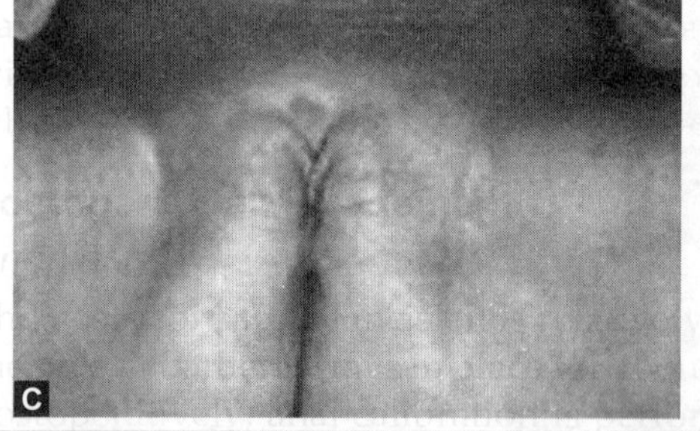 C	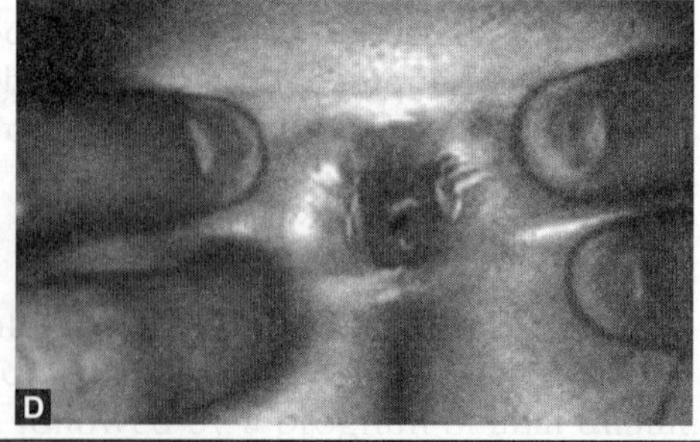 D
External view in female patient with epispadias. Labia are separated anteriorly.	Female child with epispadias with labia retracted. The clitoris is bifid, and the urethra is open dorsally.

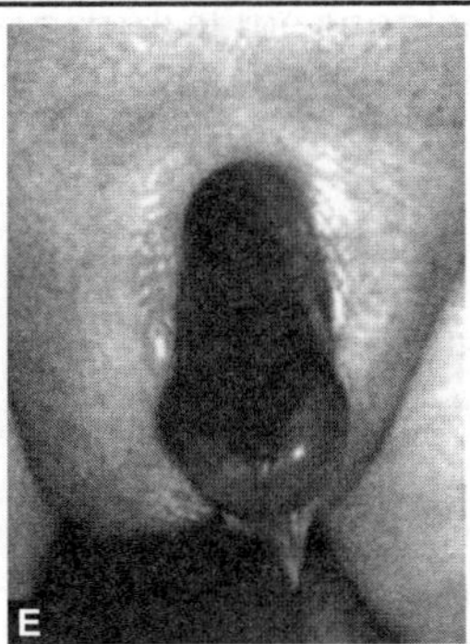	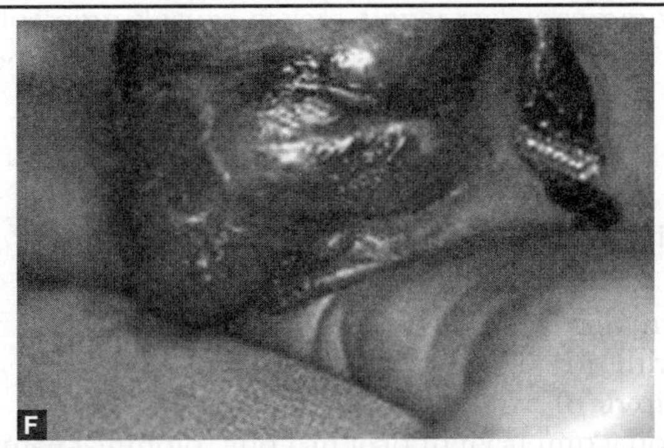
Penopubic epispadias in male child. Typical spade like configuration of glans penis with incomplete foreskin, dorsal urethral plate, and open bladder neck.	46, XY newborn with cloacal exstrophy. A very large omphalocele is present, and the hemibladders flank the exstrophic cecal plate. The phallus is small and bifid, with the hemiglans and hemiscrotum located just distal to the bladder.
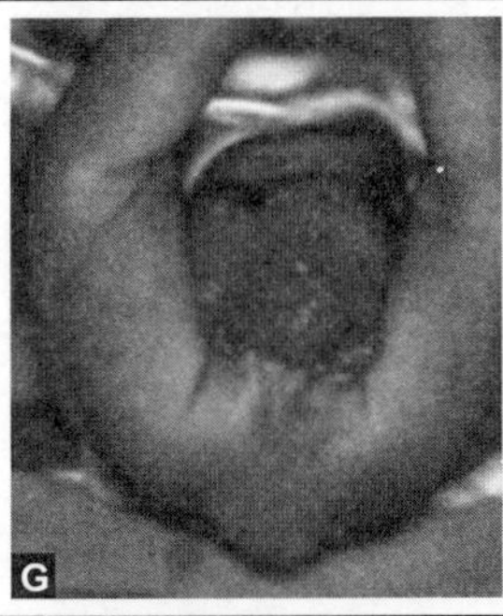	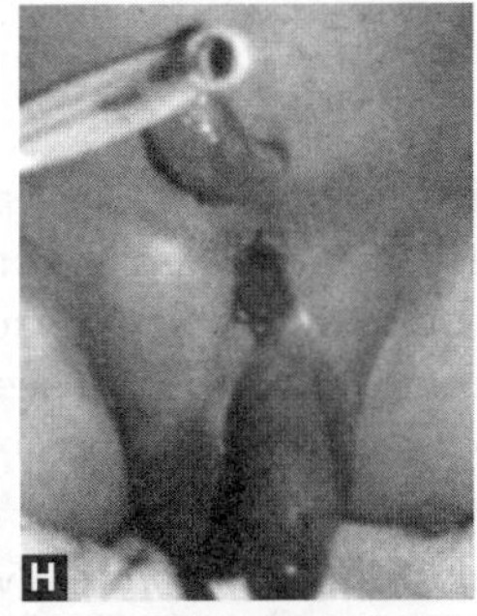
Lipomeningocele in the same newborn shown in Image F, a 46, XY newborn with cloacal exstrophy.	Superior vesical fissure variant of exstrophy. Genitalia are normal. Patent urachus is considered in the differential diagnosis, although the opening is well below the umbilicus. Rectus abdominis and pubic abnormalities are found in the exstrophic variant but not with patent urachus.
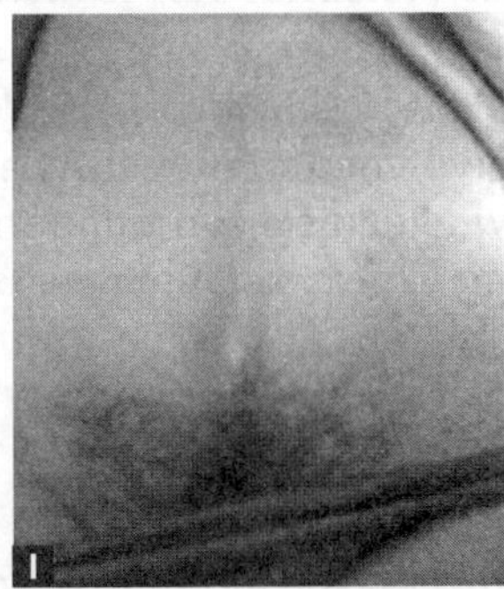	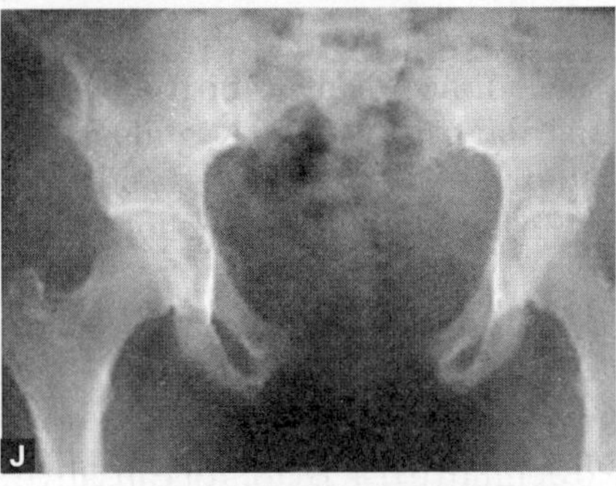
Female with covered exstrophy. The umbilicus is very low, the pubic bones are widely separated, and the rectus muscles are divergent. The bladder is intact, but the patient has undergone bladder neck reconstruction to achieve urinary continence. The external genitalia are normal.	Typical appearance of pelvis in patient with exstrophy-epispadias complex with wide separation of pubic symphysis.

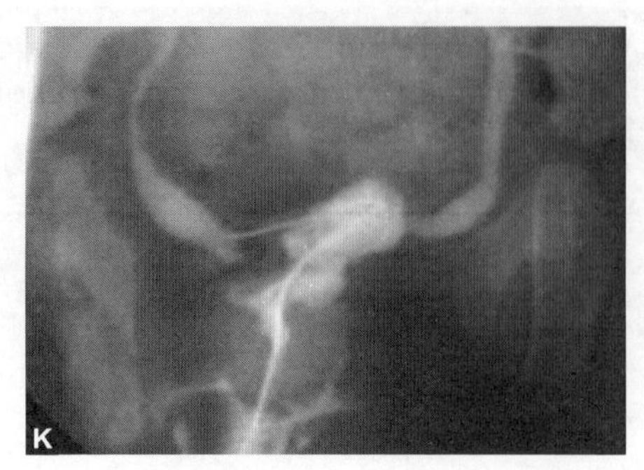

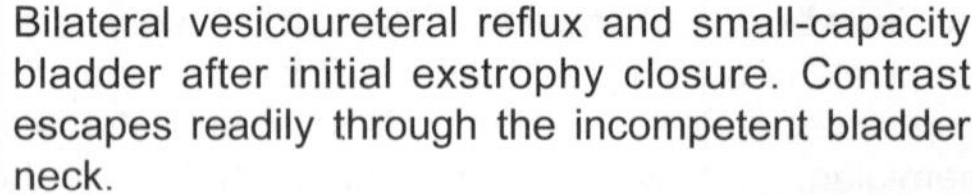
Bilateral vesicoureteral reflux and small-capacity bladder after initial exstrophy closure. Contrast escapes readily through the incompetent bladder neck.

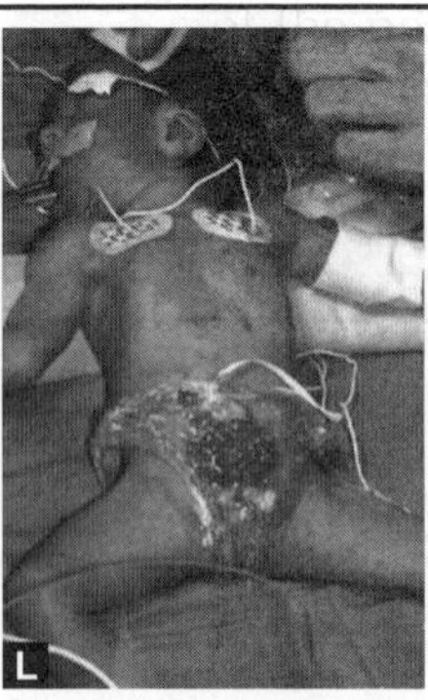

Use of plastic wraps to protect the delicate bladder mucosa in a newborn with bladder exstrophy.

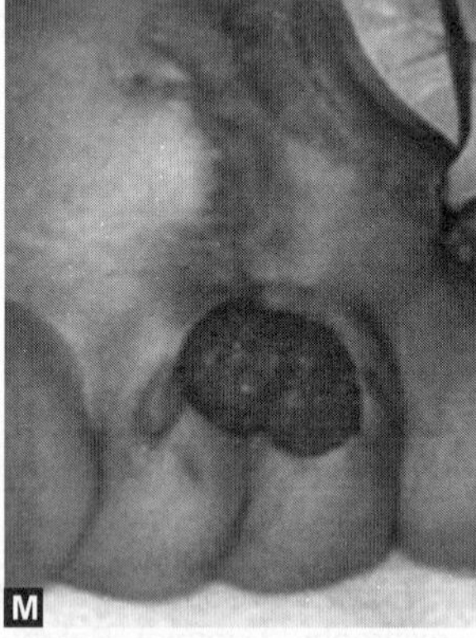

Subtotal prolapse of bladder wall through patulous bladder neck after bladder closure in female with cloacal exstrophy. The bladder mucosa appears healthy, and urine is draining freely.

Incidence

Prevalence of classic bladder exstrophy is 3.3 per 100,000 births; male epispadias occurs one in 117,000 births, female epispadias one in 484,000 births, and cloacal exstrophy one in 200,000–400,000 births.

- For classic bladder exstrophy, the male-to-female ratio is 2.3:1 and as high as 6:1 in some series.
- Because this is a congenital abnormality, newborns are affected.

Causes

- No definitive risk factors or causative agents are known. Based on the known embryologic principles of cloacal development any inciting event would occur early in pregnancy.
- Offspring of patients with exstrophy-epispadias complex have a one in 70 risk (500 times that of the general population) of being affected. Nevertheless, familial occurrence is uncommon in large series.

- Exstrophy has been reported in twins. Concordance rates show strong evidence of genetic effects, but less than 100% concordance among identical twins suggests some role for environmental effect on development of exstrophy-epispadias.
- A higher incidence of bladder exstrophy is observed in infants of younger mothers and in those with relatively high parity.
- Maternal tobacco exposure is associated with more severe defects (cloacal vs classic exstrophy).
- Growing evidence suggests an increased incidence of cloacal exstrophy and bladder exstrophy-epispadias in vitro fertilization (IVF) pregnancies.
- Heredity of cloacal exstrophy has not been established because no offspring have been reported.

Signs and Symptoms

Antenatal ultrasonography findings suggestive of exstrophy-epispadias complex include the following:

- Repeated failure to visualize the bladder on ultrasonography
- Lower abdominal wall mass
- Low-set umbilical cord
- Abnormal genitalia
- Increased pelvic diameter.

Pathophysiology

The true cause of bladder exstrophy has not been elucidated. In classic bladder exstrophy, the lower urinary tract, genitalia, and musculoskeletal system are affected. Cloacal exstrophy is a much more severe abnormality, with significant involvement of the GI tract and CNS. In epispadias, only the urethra and external genitalia are involved.

Diagnostic Evaluation

Physical Examination

- *Classic bladder exstrophy or epispadias:* Patients typically appear as term infants.
- *Cloacal exstrophy:* Patients are often preterm. They may have respiratory embarrassment requiring mechanical ventilation.
- Abdomen
  - *Classic bladder exstrophy:* The bladder is open on the lower abdomen, with mucosa fully exposed through a triangular fascial defect. The abdominal wall appears long because of a low-set umbilicus on the upper edge of the bladder plate. The distance between the umbilicus and anus is foreshortened. Rectus muscles diverge distally, attaching to the widely separated pubic bones. Indirect inguinal hernias are frequent (> 80% of males, > 10% of females) due to wide inguinal rings and the lack of an oblique inguinal canal.
  - *Epispadias:* The pubic symphysis is generally widened. The rectus muscles are divergent distally.
  - *Cloacal exstrophy:* Nearly all patients have an associated omphalocele. The bladder is open and separated into two halves, flanking the exposed interior of the cecum.

Openings to the remainder of the hindgut and to one or two appendices are evident within the cecal plate. Terminal ileum may prolapse as a 'trunk' of bowel onto the cecal plate.

- *Exstrophy variants:* The pubic symphysis is widely separated, and rectus muscles diverge distally. The umbilicus is low or elongated. A small superior bladder opening or a patch of isolated bladder mucosa may be present. The intact bladder may be externally covered by only a thin membrane. Isolated ectopic bowel segments have been reported. Patent urachus is a differential diagnosis for the superior vesical fissure variant of exstrophy-epispadias. However, patent urachus lacks the typical musculoskeletal abnormalities of exstrophy and is open at the umbilicus. Superior vesical fissure is infraumbilical.

- *Genitalia* (When describing the anatomy of the penis, the terms 'dorsal' and 'ventral' refer to a normal phallus in the erect state. The dorsal surface is in continuity with the abdominal wall, and the ventral surface is in continuity with the scrotum.)
  - *Classic bladder exstrophy (male):* The phallus is short and broad with upward curvature (dorsal chordee). The glans lies open and flat like a spade, and the dorsal component of the foreskin is absent. The urethral plate extends the length of the phallus without a roof. The bladder plate and urethral plate are in continuity, with the verumontanum and ejaculatory ducts visible within the prostatic urethral plate. The anus is anteriorly displaced with a normal sphincter mechanism.
  - *Epispadias (male):* The phallus is short and broad with upward curvature (dorsal chordee). The glans lies open and flat like a spade, and the dorsal component of the foreskin is absent. The urethral meatus is located on the dorsal penile shaft, anywhere between the penopubic angle and the proximal margin of the glans.
  - *Classic bladder exstrophy (female):* The clitoris is uniformly bifid with divergent labia superiorly. The open urethral plate is in continuity with the bladder plate. The vagina is anteriorly displaced. The anus is anteriorly displaced with a normal sphincter mechanism.
  - *Epispadias (female):* The clitoris is most often bifid with divergent labia superiorly. The dorsal aspect of the urethra is open distally. The urethra and bladder neck are patulous and may allow visualization of bladder. Bladder mucosa may prolapse through the bladder neck.
  - *Cloacal exstrophy:* The penis is generally quite small and bifid, with a hemiglans located just caudal to each hemibladder. Infrequently, the phallus may be intact in the midline. In females, the clitoris is bifid and 2 vaginas are present. The anus is absent.
  - *Exstrophy variants:* Genitalia generally are intact, though epispadias can occur.
- Musculoskeletal
  - *Classic bladder exstrophy:* The pubic symphysis is widely separated. Divergent rectus muscles remain attached to the pubis. External rotation of the innominate bones results in a waddling gait in ambulatory patients but does not appear to result in orthopedic problems later in life.
  - *Cloacal exstrophy:* Examination is the same as for bladder exstrophy. As many as 65% of patients have a clubfoot or major deformity of a lower extremity. As many as 80% of patients have vertebral anomalies.

- *Exstrophy variants:* In these split-symphysis variants of exstrophy, the pubic symphysis is widely separated, and the rectus muscles are divergent.
- Neurologic
  - In cloacal exstrophy, as many as 95% of patients have myelodysplasia
  - Which may include myelomeningocele, lipomeningocele, meningocele, or other forms of occult dysraphism. These patients are at risk of neurologic deterioration, and they should be observed closely. Early neurosurgical consultation is appropriate if a radiographic abnormality of the spinal cord or canal is observed.

Laboratory Studies

The following studies are indicated in exstrophy and epispadias:

- Information about baseline renal function is important before complex reconstruction of the urinary tract.
- Losses from the terminal ileum short-gut physiology can result in significant electrolyte abnormalities in patients with cloacal exstrophy.

Imaging Studies

- **Renal ultrasonography**
  - Baseline examination of the kidneys is recommended for all patients with exstrophy because increased bladder pressure after bladder closure can lead to hydronephrosis and upper urinary tract deterioration.
  - Congenital upper urinary tract anomalies are uncommon with classic exstrophy and epispadias but are present in approximately one third of patients with cloacal exstrophy (e.g. ectopic pelvic kidney, renal agenesis, hydronephrosis).
- **Spinal ultrasonography or radiography**
  - Myelodysplasia should be excluded in newborns with cloacal exstrophy. This can be accomplished through ultrasonography early in life.
  - MRI is recommended in cloacal exstrophy to help identify occult abnormalities that may predispose to symptomatic spinal cord tethering.
- **Voiding cystourethrography**
  - Bilateral vesicoureteral reflux is present in nearly all patients with classic bladder exstrophy.
  - This study is performed in early childhood to assess bladder capacity in preparation for reconstructive continence surgery.
  - Evaluation of the bladder neck and proximal urethra is recommended in patients with epispadias in order to plan surgical management.

Histological Findings

- Histological studies are not routinely performed. However, clinical investigations have revealed an increased ratio of extracellular matrix to muscle within the bladder wall. In particular, the amount of type III collagen is increased.
- This ratio seems to approach a more normal range (i.e. relative increase in muscle) after successful bladder closure. Exstrophied bladders also have fewer myelinated nerve fibers than unaffected bladders.

Management

Medical Management

- In neonates with exstrophy and epispadias, initiate general supportive care appropriate for the overall condition and associated anomalies.
- Institute parenteral nutrition early for patients with cloacal exstrophy.
- Place clean plastic wrap over the bladder plate. Avoid moistened or impregnated gauze, which is irritating to the delicate bladder mucosa. Mist tents may be used to protect exposed tissue.
- Start antibiotic therapy after delivery and continue through the early postoperative period.
  - Daily prophylactic antibiotic therapy may be continued in the weeks after bladder closure. Surgeon's philosophies on this matter vary.
  - Infections may be related to poor emptying and are to be prevented in light of the high incidence of vesicoureteral reflux. Institute latex precautions due to high incidence of latex sensitization in patients with exstrophy-epispadias complex.

Medication

Antibiotics are given to prevent urinary tract infections in patients with exstrophy and epispadias.

Broad-spectrum Antibiotics

These agents are used for prevention of perioperative tissue infection due to preoperative colonization of urinary tract or multiple indwelling catheters.

1. *Ampicillin (Marcillin, Omnipen, Polycillin):* Bactericidal activity against susceptible organisms. Started at birth in classic bladder exstrophy or cloacal exstrophy and continued through early postoperative period.

   Pediatric: 50 mg/kg IV q6h Probenecid and disulfiram elevate levels; allopurinol decreases effects and has additive.
2. *Gentamicin (Garamycin):* Aminoglycoside antibiotic for gram-negative coverage. Started at birth in classic bladder exstrophy or cloacal exstrophy and continued through early postoperative period.

   Pediatric: 2 mg/kg IV q8h, Coadministration with other aminoglycosides, cephalosporins, penicillins, or amphotericin B may increase nephrotoxicity; aminoglycosides enhance effects of neuromuscular blocking agents and thus prolonged respiratory depression may occur. Coadministration with loop diuretics may increase auditory toxicity of aminoglycosides; possible irreversible hearing loss of varying degrees may occur (monitor regularly), Documented hypersensitivity; renal insufficiency.
3. *Prophylactic Antibiotics:* These agents are used for prevention of urinary tract infection in light of vesicoureteral reflux and possible inefficient bladder emptying.

   Amoxicillin (Trimox, Amoxil, Biomox): First-line choice for prophylaxis in newborns. Interferes with synthesis of cell wall mucopeptides during active multiplication, resulting in bactericidal activity against susceptible bacteria. Used as prophylaxis in certain PO, GI, or genitourinary procedures.

   Pediatric: 20 mg/kg PO qhs. Risk of rash increased by allopurinol. Documented hypersensitivity.

Surgical Management

Reconstruction of exstrophy-epispadias complex remains one of the greatest challenges facing the pediatric urologist. Many modifications in surgical procedures have improved the outcome for these patients, but the optimal approach remains uncertain. Longitudinal prospective assessment of both surgical approaches (staged procedure versus total reconstruction) is critical to optimize functional and cosmetic outcomes.

Goals of therapy include provision of urinary continence with preservation of renal function and reconstruction of functional and cosmetically acceptable genitalia. Creation of a neoumbilicus is also important to many of these patients.

Surgical techniques include the following:

- Staged functional closure for classic bladder exstrophy (i.e. modern staged repair of exstrophy [MSRE])
  - Traditional approach comprises a series of operations.
  - Initial bladder closure is completed within 72 hours of birth. If delayed, pelvic osteotomies are required to facilitate successful closure of the abdominal wall and to allow the bladder to lie within a closed and supportive pelvic ring.
  - Epispadias repair with urethroplasty at age 12–18 months allows enough increase in bladder outlet resistance to improve the bladder capacity.
  - Bladder neck reconstruction at age 4 years (typically a modified Young-Dees-Leadbetter repair) allows continence and correction of vesicoureteral reflux. Multiple modifications have been proposed. The procedure is delayed until bladder capacity is adequate; better results are reported with a capacity greater than 85 mL.
- Complete primary repair for classic bladder exstrophy (CPRE)
  - This is a relatively newer approach to exstrophy closure.
  - Primary bladder closure, urethroplasty, and genital reconstruction are performed in a single stage in newborns. This procedure involves complete penile disassembly in males and mobilization of the urogenital complex in females. Hypospadias is a common outcome in males and requires subsequent reconstruction.
  - The goal is early bladder cycling. A subset of patients have achieved continence without bladder neck reconstruction.
- Urinary diversion for classic bladder exstrophy
  - This procedure was the original surgical treatment of choice.
  - Diversion may be performed in a patient with an extremely small bladder plate not suitable for functional closure.
  - In Europe, early diversion has been widely used, with success for most exstrophy patients.
- Closure for cloacal exstrophy
  - Treatment of myelodysplasia and GI anomalies has priority over management of urinary and genital anomalies.
  - Closure can be staged or performed in one stage, depending on the overall condition of the child and the severity of the abdominal wall defect. A large omphalocele may limit the success of closing the abdomen and the bladder in one stage.
  - First stage involves separation of the GI and genitourinary tracts, closure of the colon, creation of a colostomy, and closure of the omphalocele. The bladder plates are brought together in the midline.

  - The hindgut should be incorporated into the GI tract to maximize absorptive surface area, since virtually all of these patients have some element of short-gut syndrome. Ileostomy should be avoided because of the high incidence of recurrent hospitalizations for dehydration and severe electrolyte abnormalities. A decision for rectal pull-through versus permanent colostomy is based on surgeon preference and projected potential for social fecal continence.
  - Subsequent bladder closure is as in classic bladder exstrophy. The principles of complete primary repair have been applied at this point as well. Consideration may be given to continent diversion as the second stage, based on poor potential for volitional voiding and continence. Because of more severe pubic diastasis, pelvic osteotomies are required. Staged osteotomies with gradual closure of the pelvis may be needed in severe cases.
- Gender reassignment
  - Historically, all males with cloacal exstrophy underwent early gender conversion because of inadequate male genitalia.
  - Testicular histology is normal despite frequent cryptorchidism.
  - Evidence suggesting that testosterone in utero has a significant impact on the developing brain has led to a change in surgical philosophy, as has anecdotal evidence suggesting that raising a 46, XY cloacal exstrophy patient as female can result in significant gender dysphoria. Cloacal exstrophy is now included as a subset of disorders of sex development. Multidisciplinary evaluation and both early and long-term counseling should be offered.

Complications

- In the treatment of complex congenital anomalies, the distinction between technical complications and problems inherent to the anomaly is not always obvious.
- Failure of closure may occur.
  - If the bladder plate is adequate, reclosure with pelvic osteotomies is recommended. In this instance, bladder closure and epispadias repair are performed in one stage.
  - Urinary diversion is the alternative therapy.
- A vesicocutaneous fistula or urethrocutaneous fistula may form after primary closure or urethral reconstruction. If spontaneous closure does not occur, surgical repair is required.
- Loss of the hemiglans or corporal body has been reported as a result of complete primary repair.
- Minor orthopedic complications may occur after osteotomy or immobilization.
- Upper urinary tract deterioration is a potential complication. Causes include excessive outlet resistance and high pressure in a small-capacity reservoir and persistent vesicoureteral reflux.
- Abnormal bladder function may result in poor emptying. Clinical problems related to poor emptying include recurrent febrile infections, epididymitis, bladder stones, acute urinary retention, and rupture of the native bladder.
- Bladder prolapse is a potential complication.
  - Posterior bladder wall may prolapse through the patulous bladder neck after primary closure.

  - Recurrent prolapse, congestion, ischemia of bladder mucosa, or failure of ureteral drainage warrants early surgical correction.
- Complications of short-gut syndrome are as follows:
  - Paucity of hindgut and, in many cases, limited small intestine can result in electrolyte abnormalities in patients with cloacal exstrophy.
  - Dehydration is particularly a concern during an acute GI illness with diarrhea.
  - Nutritional supplementation may be required.

Prognosis

Even with successful surgery, patients may have long-term problems:
- Incontinence
- Urinary reflux
- Repeated urinary tract infections
- Bladder adenocarcinoma
- Colonic adenocarcinoma
- Sexual dysfunction
- Pain
- Uterine prolapsed

Nursing Management

- After surgery, patients with exstrophy remain in the hospital in modified Bryant traction (legs adducted and pelvis slightly elevated) for 3 weeks after bladder closure. Alternative techniques of immobilization may be used based on osteotomies or institutional protocol.
- Bladder and kidneys are drained fully with multiple catheters during the first few weeks after closure.
- Nutritional support is mandatory for patients with cloacal exstrophy. Patients with classic bladder exstrophy may also have early difficulties feeding because of the body position in traction.
- Remaining urinary drainage catheters are removed as part of outpatient follow-up care. Prophylactic antibiotics are continued.
- Lifelong follow-up care with a urologist is important to monitor for urinary tract infections, deterioration in bladder function, or damage to the kidneys and to direct appropriate surgical or medical therapy.
- Patients with cloacal exstrophy require long-term follow-up care with a neurosurgeon, orthopedic surgeon, and general surgeon.
- Counseling for school-age children may be offered preemptively or as concerns arise.
- Maintain oral antibiotic prophylaxis as described in Medication.

Patient Education

- Because of the potential long-term implications of exstrophy, patient education is critical. Exstrophy support groups are established at several major medical centers.

Diet

- Some young patients with cloacal exstrophy are seriously affected by short-gut syndrome and may depend on long-term supplemental parenteral nutrition for growth and development.

Activity

- Patient is kept in modified Bryant traction for 3 weeks after exstrophy closure. Alternatively, spica casts, lower extremity wraps, and external pelvic fixators are used based upon performance of osteotomies and institutional protocol.
- In childhood, patient may have a waddling gait because of abnormal pelvic rotation, but activity is unrestricted and no long-term orthopedic sequelae occur.

PHIMOSIS AND PARAPHIMOSIS

Introduction

Phimosis is a constriction of the opening of the foreskin so that it cannot be drawn back over the tip of the penis. This condition is a normal occurrence in the newborn boy, but over time, the skin that adheres to the tip of the penis can be retracted as the foreskin loosens. By age 17, 99% of males will be able to completely retract their foreskin.

Paraphimosis occurs when the foreskin is retracted behind the corona (or crown) of the penis and cannot be returned to the unretracted position. This can cause entrapment of the penis, impairing the drainage of blood, and may be serious.

Definition

Phimosis defines an inability to retract the foreskin after it was previously retractible or after puberty, usually secondary to distal scarring of the foreskin. *Paraphimosis* is the entrapment of a retracted foreskin behind the coronal sulcus.

Types

- Physiologic phimosis is the normal condition in which children are born with a tight foreskin and separation occurs during late childhood and early adolescence.
- Pathologic phimosis occurs due to infection, inflammation, or scarring and is usually found in uncircumcised adult men.

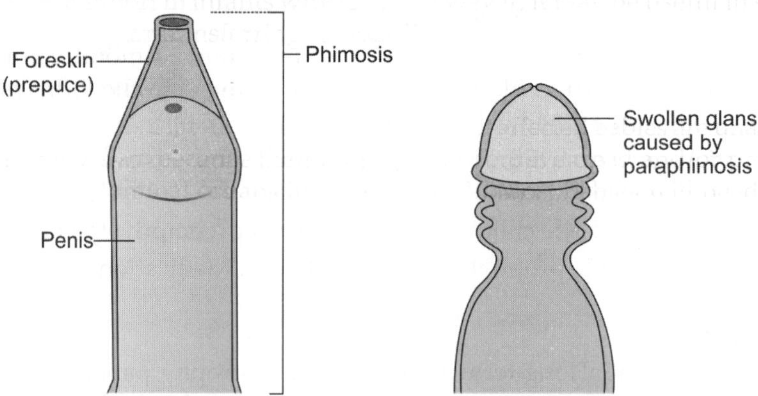

Fig. 6.49: Classification of phimosis vs paraphimosis

Signs and Symptoms

The inability of the foreskin to retract can lead to difficulty cleaning of the area which can cause balanitis.

Other symptoms phimosis include:

- Bulging of the foreskin during urination, (like a balloon inflating)
- Inability to completely retract the foreskin by age 3 years
- Difficulty urinating
- Painful urination
- Painful erection
- Urinary tract infections.

Symptoms of Paraphimosis

- Swelling of the tip of the penis as the foreskin is retracted or pulled back
- Pain
- Inability to pull the foreskin back over the tip of the penis
- Discoloration, either dark red or bluish color of the tip of the penis.

Diagnostic Evaluation

- History collection
- Physical examination.

Management

- *Phimosis:* Treatment may involve application of a steroid cream to the foreskin three to four times per day for about one month to loosen the adhesive ring. Each time the cream is applied, it should be done while using gentle, steady pressure to retract the foreskin for one minute. If the cream does not work and the child continues to have adverse phimosis symptoms, a circumcision may be recommended.

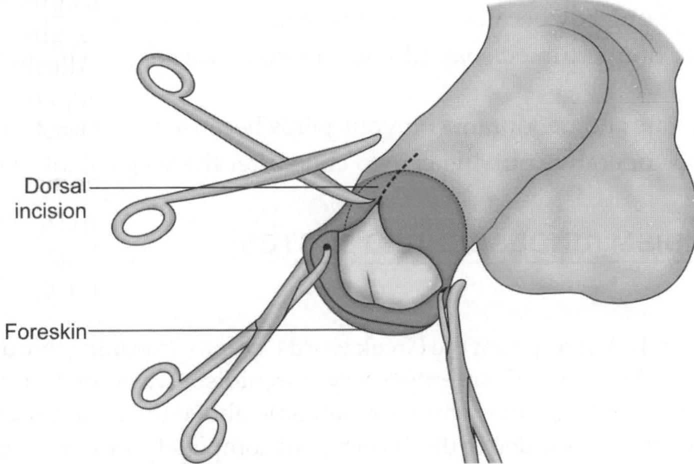

Fig. 6.50: Surgical procedures (circumcision)

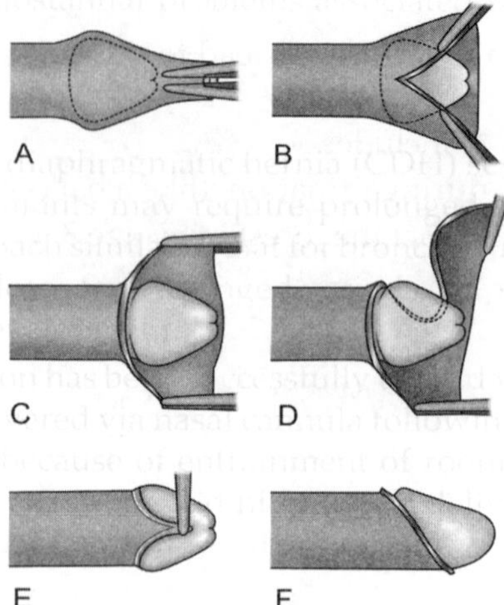

Fig. 6.51: Steps in surgical management of phimosis

- *Paraphimosis:* Treatment may involve lubricating the foreskin and tip of the penis and then gently squeezing the tip of the penis while pulling the foreskin forward. A bandage may also be wrapped from the tip of the penis towards the base to try to reduce the swelling. If this is ineffective, a small incision to relieve the tension may be performed. In some cases, an emergency circumcision may be recommended.
- *Circumcision:* Surgical removal of all or part of the foreskin.

Nursing Management

- Gently wash the child penis with warm water each day while providing a bath or showering
- Gently pull back the penis foreskin and wash underneath; do not pull back the foreskin of a baby or young boy because it could be painful and cause harm
- Use a mild or nonperfumed soap (if you choose to use soap) to reduce the risk of skin irritation
- Avoid using talc and deodorants on your penis because they may cause irritation
- Providing postoperative nursing care to child after the surgical intervention.

CRYPTORCHIDISM (UNDESCENDED TESTES)

Introduction

The cryptorchidism is derived from the Greek words 'crypto' (meaning 'hidden') and 'orchid' (meaning 'testicle'). During the last century, cryptorchidism was sometimes restricted to the subset of undescended testes that were not palpable above the scrotum or in the inguinal canal those that were truly hidden in the abdomen or completely absent. In recent decades the distinction is no longer made in most contexts, and the two terms are used interchangeably. Cryptorchism is an older variant of the same term.

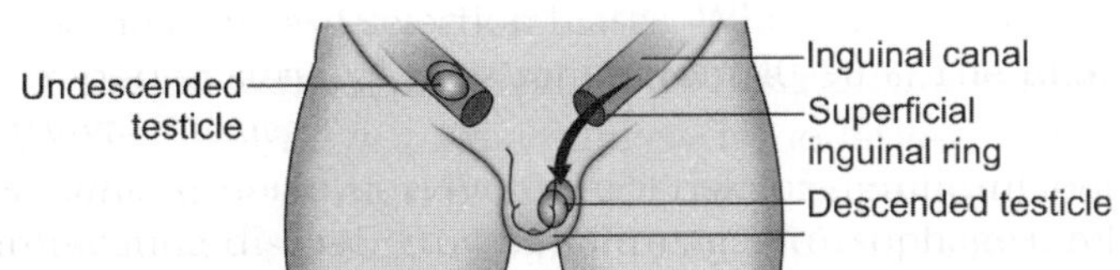

Fig. 6.52: Diagram of undescended testicle

Definition

Cryptorchidism is defined as the absence of one or both testes from the scrotum. This usually represents failure of the testis to move, or 'descend,' during fetal development from an abdominal position, through the inguinal canal, into the ipsilateral scrotum.

Types

A testis absent from the normal scrotal position can be:

- Found anywhere along the 'path of descent' from high in the posterior (retroperitoneal) abdomen, just below the kidney, to the inguinal ring

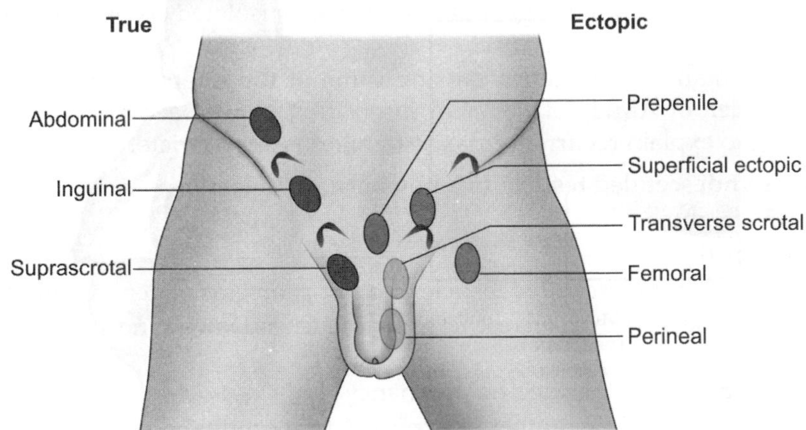

Fig. 6.53: Types of cryptorchidism

- Found in the inguinal canal
- Ectopic, that is, found to have 'wandered' from that path, usually outside the inguinal canal and sometimes even under the skin of the thigh, the perineum, the opposite scrotum, and femoral canal
- Found to be undeveloped (hypoplastic) or severely abnormal (dysgenetic)
- Found to have vanished (also see anorchia).

Causes and Risk Factors

In most full-term infant boys with cryptorchidism but no other genital abnormalities, a cause cannot be found, making this a common, sporadic, unexplained (idiopathic) birth defect.

Causes

- Severely premature infants can be born before descent of testes.
- There is a strong association of cryptorchidism with low birthweight due to either prematurity or intrauterine growth retardation. In these infants, there is usually no evidence of hormonal malfunction. Inguinal hernias associated with low birthweight are common.
- A contributing role of environmental chemicals endocrine disruptors that interfere with normal fetal hormone balance has been proposed and is rarely possible to implicate a specific chemical exposure for an individual child.
- Rare iatrogenic cases have also been reported, in which a hernia repair or other surgery in the inguinal area resulted in trapping of a testis above the scrotum.
- Environmental risk factors may include exposure to regular alcohol consumption during pregnancy (5 or more drinks per week, associated with a three time increase in cryptorchidism, when compared to nondrinking mothers), exposure to pesticides, gestational diabetes, being a twin, and being born to pregnant women who drink caffeine (at least three drinks per day).
- A small percentage of cases of isolated cryptorchidism are familial. It has been reported that about 4% of fathers and 6–10% of brothers of affected boys have also had cryptorchidism. Few specific genes associated with isolated cryptorchidism have been identified.
- In contrast, many of the genes causing some of the intersex conditions associated with androgen or AMH deficiency or insensitivity have been identified, and genetic counseling to explain recurrence risk to families is appropriate.

Risk factor of undescended testicle in a newborn includes:

- Low birth weight
- Premature birth
- Family history of undescended testicle or other problems of genital development
- Conditions of the fetus that can restrict growth, such as Down syndrome or an abdominal wall defect
- Alcohol use by the mother during pregnancy
- Cigarette smoking by the mother or exposure to secondhand smoke
- Obesity in the mother
- Diabetes in the mother type 1 diabetes, type 2 diabetes or gestational diabetes
- Parents' exposure to some pesticides.

Pathophysiology

Potential explanations for the pathophysiology of cryptorchidism have been proposed, including gubernacular abnormalities, reduced intra-abdominal pressures, intrinsic testicular and/or epididymal abnormalities, and endocrine abnormalities, as well as anatomic anomalies (e.g. fibrous bands within the inguinal canal or abnormal arrangement of the cremasteric muscle fibers). The gubernaculum testis is a structure that attaches the lower portion of the tunica vaginalis to base of the scrotum. The gubernaculum is thought to aid in testicular descent by widening the inguinal canal and guiding the testis down to the scrotum. Therefore, anomalies in this attachment may contribute to cryptorchidism.

Diagnostic Evaluation

Physical Examination

A general physical examination that emphasizes the signs of syndromic features may reveal an underlying reason for cryptorchidism, The genitalia should be examined for evidence of hypospadias or ambiguity. Concurrence of hypospadias and undescended testis is commonly associated with states of intersexuality, especially mixed gonadal dysgenesis and true hermaphroditism.

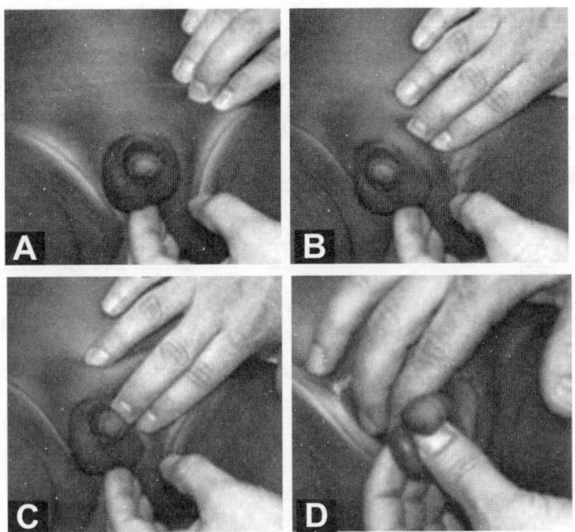

Fig. 6.54: Examination of the groin for an undescended testicle is often enhanced with the use of lubrication. (A) The examining hand is swept along the inguinal canal, starting at the superiolateral extent of the inguinal canal. If the testicle is present, it will either 'pop' under the examiner's fingers (B,C), or be manipulated into the scrotum, where it will be palpated by the opposite hand (D).

Evaluation of the Bilateral Nonpalpable Testis

A phenotypically male newborn with bilateral nonpalpable testicles should be considered to be a genetic female with congenital adrenal hyperplasia until proved otherwise. Congenital adrenal hyperplasia may rarely present with a normal male phenotype and is a life-threatening condition. Ultrasound examination of the pelvic structures, karyotyping and measurements of serum electrolytes, testosterone, Müllerian-inhibiting hormone, and adrenal hormones and metabolites (17 hydroxyprogesterone) should be considered in the initial evaluation. An older child with bilateral nonpalpable testicles should be evaluated hormonally for testicular absence.

Serum studies should include testosterone:

- Luteinizing hormone (LH)
- Follicle-stimulating hormone (FSH) and Müllerian-inhibiting substance (MIS).
- Elevations in LH and FSH, as well as the absence of detectable MIS, suggest testicular absence. Measurements of thyroid hormone and cortisol levels should be considered because hypogonadism may occur with pituitary aplasia.

- A stimulation test using intramuscular human chorionic gonadotropin (hCG) can be administered to check for evidence of testosterone production.
- Radiologic evaluation of the nonpalpable testicle is not warranted. None of the commonly applied studies, such as ultrasonography, computed tomography or magnetic resonance imaging, is sensitive enough to detect the majority of intra-abdominal testes, and none is specific enough to exclude an intra-abdominal testis.
- Whether or not a testicle is located by the radiologic study, surgical exploration is required.
- Ultrasound examination may be advisable in the infant with bilateral nonpalpable testes to look for gonads and to exclude the presence of a uterus, which would suggest a state of intersexuality. Ultrasound examination may also be helpful in the overweight child to detect inguinal testicles that are difficult to palpate.

Management of Cryptorchidism

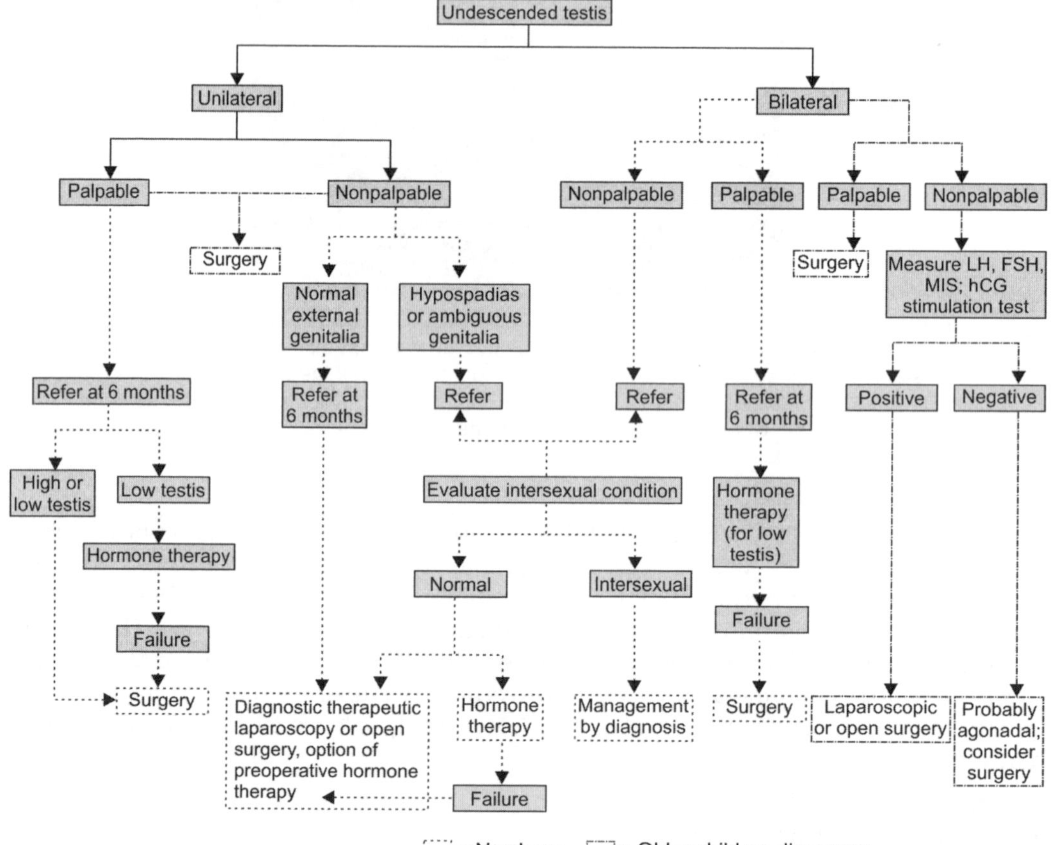

Fig. 6.55: Management of the infant with cryptorchidism, including suggested times for referral to a pediatric urologist. Older children should be referred on discovery of an undescended testicle. (LH = luteinizing hormone; FSH = follicle-stimulating hormone; MIS = Müllerian inhibiting substance; hCG = human chorionic gonadotropin)

Surgical Management of the Nonpalpable Testis

The primary management of cryptorchidism is surgery, called orchiopexy. It is usually performed in infancy, if inguinal testes have not descended after 4–6 months, often by a pediatric urologist or pediatric surgeon, but in many communities still by a general urologist or surgeon.

Surgery becomes more complicated if the blood supply is not ample and elastic enough to be stretched into the scrotum. In these cases, the supply may be divided, some vessels sacrificed with expectation of adequate collateral circulation. In the worst case, the testis must be 'auto-transplanted' into the scrotum, with all connecting blood vessels cut and reconnected ('anastomosed').

The testis is in the abdomen, the first stage of surgery is exploration to locate it, assess its viability, and determine the safest way to maintain or establish the blood supply. Multi-stage surgeries, or auto-transplantation and anastomosis, are more often necessary in these situations. Just as often, intra-abdominal exploration discovers that the testis is nonexistent ('vanished'), or dysplastic and not salvageable.

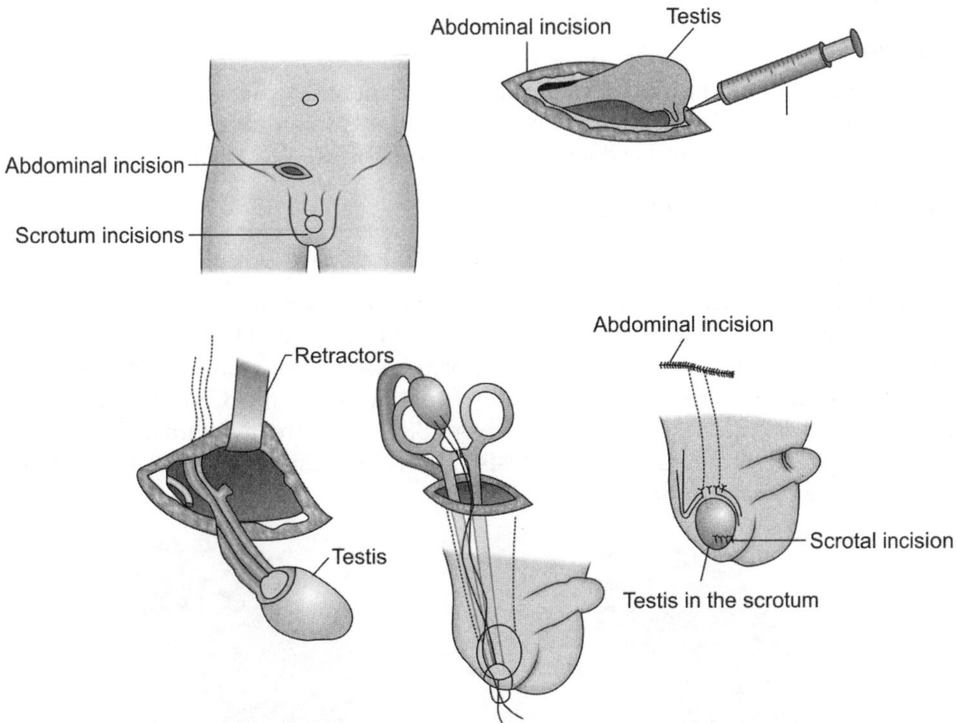

Fig. 6.56: Surgical (orchiopexy) management of undescended testicles

The two initial surgical approaches to the nonpalpable testis are the open inguinal and diagnostic laparoscopic techniques. In the open inguinal approach, the groin is explored. If cord structures or testicular remnants are found, they are removed, and the procedure is terminated. If the groin exploration is negative, the incision is extended, and the peritoneum is entered in a search for an intra-abdominal testis.

The second surgical approach to the nonpalpable testis is laparoscopic. Diagnostic laparoscopy, which is a safe procedure in experienced hands, is performed initially. Using a laparoscope placed through the umbilicus, the inguinal rings are examined, and the status of the processes vaginalis (patent or nonpatent), wolffian structures and testicular vessels can be easily identified. The presence of blind-ending spermatic vessels confirms an absent testis, allowing termination of the procedure without a groin incision. If vessels and vas deferens exit the internal ring, the groin can be explored. If an intra-abdominal testis is identified, the physician can then choose the best surgical approach.

Complications

Complications related to the surgical correction following:
- Testicular atrophy (5%)
- Injury to vas deferens (1–2%)
- Reascent of the testicle or abnormal anatomic position (< 10%)
- Epididymoorchitis
- Hydrocele.

Prognosis

Most cases get better on their own, without any treatment. Medical or surgical correction of the condition is usually successful. About 5% of patients with undescended testicles do not have testicles that can be found at the time of surgery. This is called a vanished or absent testis.

POLYCYSTIC KIDNEY DISEASE (PKD)

Introduction

Polycystic kidney disease is a genetic disorder that causes numerous cysts to grow in the kidneys. A kidney cyst is an abnormal sac filled with fluid. PKD cysts can greatly enlarge the kidneys while replacing much of their normal structure, resulting in chronic kidney disease (CKD), which causes reduced kidney function over time. CKD may lead to kidney failure, described as end-stage kidney disease or ESRD when treated with a kidney transplant or blood-filtering treatments called dialysis. The two main types of PKD are autosomal dominant PKD and autosomal recessive PKD.

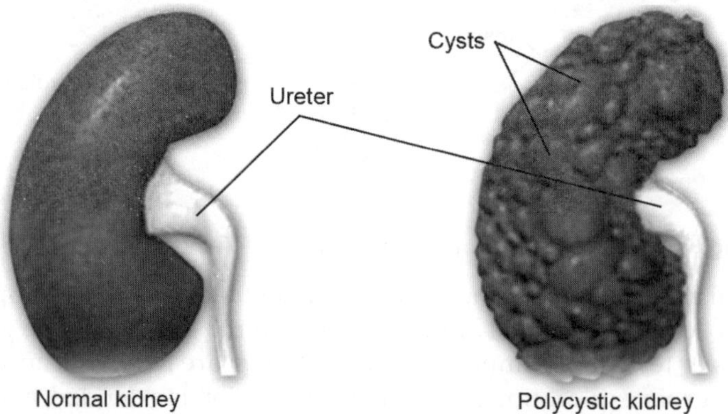

Fig. 6.57: Anatomical view of normal and polycystic kidney

Definition

Polycystic kidney disease (PKD) defined as an inherited genetic disorder in which clusters of cysts develop primarily within kidneys. Cysts are noncancerous round sacs containing water-like fluid. A common complication of polycystic kidney disease is high blood pressure. Kidney failure is another common problem for people with polycystic kidney disease.

Causes/Types

There are two types of polycystic kidney diseases:

- Autosomal dominant PKD
- Autosomal recessive PKD

Abnormal genes cause polycystic kidney disease, and the genetic defects mean the disease runs in families. A genetic mutation can be the cause of polycystic kidney disease.

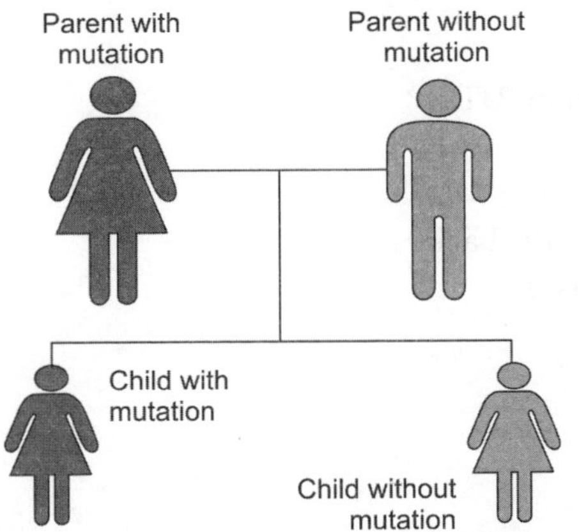

Fig. 6.58: Autosomal dominant polycystic kidney disease

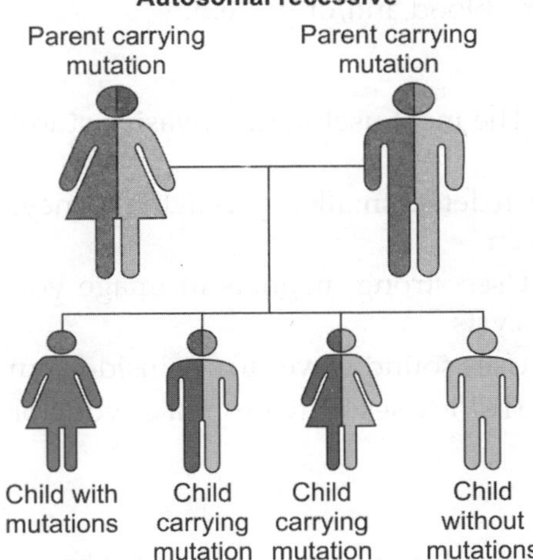

Fig. 6.59: Autosomal recessive polycystic kidney disease

- *Autosomal dominant polycystic kidney disease (ADPKD):* Signs and symptoms of ADPKD often develop between the ages of 30 and 40. In the past this type was called adult polycystic kidney disease, but children can develop the disorder.
- *Autosomal recessive polycystic kidney disease (ARPKD):* This type is far less common than is ADPKD. The signs and symptoms often appear shortly after birth. Sometimes, symptoms do not appear until later in childhood or during adolescence.

Both types of parents must have abnormal genes to pass on this form of the disease. If both parents carry a gene for this disorder, each child has a 25 percent chance of getting the disease.

Signs and Symptoms

The main symptoms of PKD include:

- Pain or tenderness in the abdomen
- Blood in the urine
- Frequent urination
- Pain in the sides
- Urinary tract infection (UTI)
- Kidney stones.

Other symptoms include:

- Pain or heaviness in the back
- Skin that bruises easily
- Pale skin color
- Fatigue
- Joint pain
- Nail abnormalities.

Diagnostic Evaluation

- A complete blood count (CBC) looking for anemia or signs of infection
- A urinalysis looking for blood and/or protein.

Imaging Study Includes

- *Abdominal ultrasound:* The most useful, noninvasive study using sound waves to look for cysts
- *Abdominal CT scan:* It can detect smaller cysts in the kidney; uses X-rays to build a cross-section of your abdomen
- *Abdominal MRI scan:* Uses strong magnets to image your body to visualize kidney structure and look for cysts
- *Abdominal ultrasound:* Uses sound waves to see inside your body
- *Intravenous pyelogram (IVP):* Uses a dye to make your blood vessels show up more clearly on an X-ray.

Genetic Testing

The health care provider may refer a person suspected of having autosomal dominant PKD to a geneticist. Genetic testing can show whether a person's cells carry a gene mutation that causes autosomal dominant PKD. A health care provider may also use genetic testing results to determine whether someone with a family history of PKD is likely to develop the disorder in the future. Prenatal testing can diagnose autosomal recessive PKD in unborn children.

Two factors limit the usefulness of genetic testing for PKD:

1. Detection of a mutated gene cannot predict the onset of symptoms or how serious the disorder will be.
2. Even if a health care provider finds a mutated gene, no specific cure for the disorder exists.

Management

The goal of PKD treatment is to manage symptoms. Especially controlling high blood pressure is the most important part of treatment.

Treatment may include:

- Pain medication
- Blood pressure medication
- Antibiotics (to treat UTI)
- A low-sodium (salt) diet
- Diuretics (to help remove excess fluid)
- Surgery (to drain cysts and help relieve discomfort).

Complication

Autosomal dominant PKD	Autosomal recessive PKD
• Pain	• Death due to breathing problems
• High blood pressure	• Kidney failure
• Kidney failure	• Liver scarring
• Urinary tract infections (UTIs)	• High blood pressure
• Kidney stones	• UTIs
• Liver cysts	
• Pancreatic cysts	
• Abnormal heart valves	
• Diverticula	
• Brain aneurysms	

SEXUAL ABNORMALITIES

AMBIGUOUS GENITALIA

Introduction

Ambiguous genitalia is a rare condition in which an infant's external genitals do not appear to be clearly either male or female. In a baby with ambiguous genitalia, the genitals may not be well-formed or the baby may have characteristics of both sexes. The external sex organs may not match the internal sex organs or genetic sex. It is referred to as a disorder of sexual development.

Definition

Ambiguous genitalia defined as (otherwise known as atypical genitalia) birth defect of the sex organs that make it unclear whether an affected newborn is a girl or boy. This condition occurs approximately once in every 4,500 births. The baby seems to have a mixture of both female and male parts. For example, they may have both a vulva and testicles.

Classification

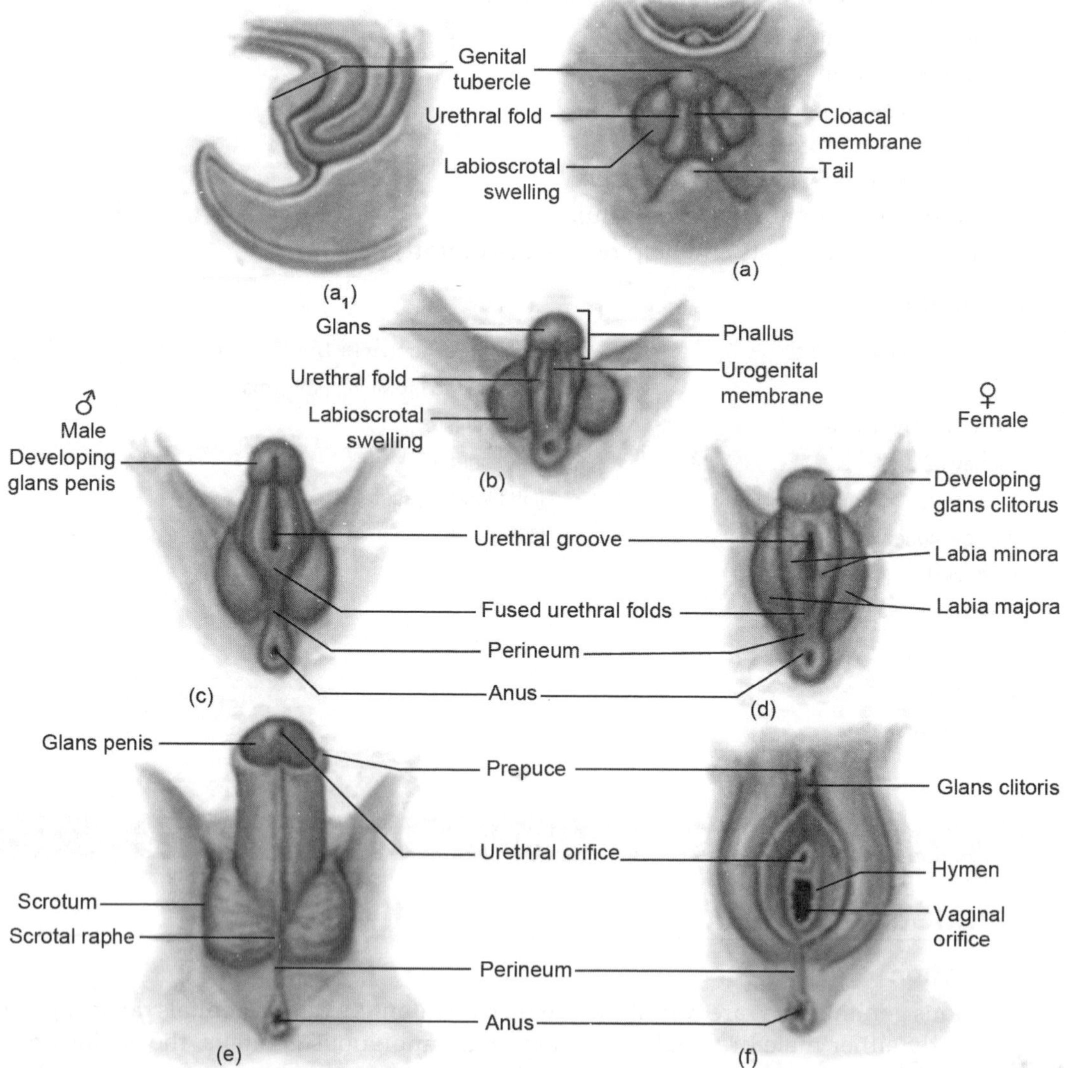

Fig. 6.60: Classification of ambiguous genitalia of male and female child

Causes

There are a number of different causes of ambiguous genitalia, with the most common described below. The cause, in many cases, is not known and the disorder appears to occur by chance. A disruption of the steps that determine sex can result in a mismatch between the appearance of the external genitals and the internal sex organs or the genetic sex (XX or XY).

- A lack or deficiency of male hormones in a genetic male fetus can cause ambiguous genitalia, while exposure to male hormones during development results in ambiguous genitalia in a genetic female.
- Mutations in certain genes can influence fetal sex development and cause ambiguous genitalia.
- Chromosomal abnormalities, such as a missing sex chromosome or an extra one, also can cause ambiguous genitalia.
- In some cases, the cause of ambiguous genitalia may not be determined.

Causes in Genetic Females

- *Congenital adrenal hyperplasia:* Certain forms of this genetic condition cause the adrenal glands to make excess male hormones (androgens).
- *Prenatal exposure to male hormones:* Certain drugs that contain male hormones or that stimulate production of the male hormones in a pregnant woman can cause developing female genitals to become more masculine. A developing baby also may be exposed to excess male hormones if the mother has a disease or condition that causes hormone imbalance.
- *Tumors*: A tumor in the mother can produce male hormones.

Causes in Genetic Males

- *Impaired testicle development:* This may be due to genetic abnormalities or unknown causes.
- *Androgen insensitivity syndrome*: In this condition, developing genital tissues do not respond normally to male hormones made by the testes.
- *Abnormalities with testes or testosterone:* Various abnormalities can interfere with the testes' activity. This may include structural problems with the testes, problems with production of the male hormone testosterone or problems with cellular receptors that respond to testosterone.
- *5a-reductase deficiency*: This enzyme defect impairs normal male hormone production.

Risk Factors

- Unexplained deaths in early infancy
- Infertility absent menstrual periods or excess facial hair in females
- Genital abnormalities
- Abnormal physical development during puberty
- Congenital adrenal hyperplasia.

Signs and Symptoms

Female (with two X chromosomes) may have:

- An enlarged clitoris, which may resemble a small penis
- Closed labia, or labia that include folds and resemble a scrotum
- Lumps that feel like testes in the fused labia.

Male (with one X and one Y chromosome) may have:

- A condition in which the narrow tube that carries urine (urethra)
- Does not fully extend to the tip of the penis (hypospadias)
- An abnormally small penis with the urethral opening closer to the scrotum
- The absence of one or both testicles in what appears to be the scrotum
- Undescended testicles and an empty scrotum that has the appearance of a labia with or without a micropenis.

Diagnostic Evaluation

- Complete medical history
- Physical examination
- A pelvic ultrasound (to check for the presence of female reproductive organs)
- A genitourethrogram to look at the urethra and vagina if present
- A chromosomal analysis (to help determine genetic sex: 46, XX or 46, XY)
- Fertility potential of a female pseudohermaphrodite
- Size and potential for growth of a penis present in a male pseudohermaphrodite
- Ability of an internal reproductive organ to produce appropriate sex hormones for the gender 'assigned' to the child
- Risk of future health conditions (i.e. cancer) that may develop in the original reproductive organs later in life.

Management

- Treatment for ambiguous genitalia depends of the type of the disorder but will usually include corrective surgery to remove or create reproductive organs appropriate for the gender of the child.
- *Parental counseling:* Successful sex assignment and identity for the child depends largely on the attitude of the parents. It is important that both the mother and father are fully informed about their child's condition. Support groups may provide help in this area.
- *Surgery:* Surgical gender assignment depends heavily on what genital structures the surgeons have to work with. The majority of babies with ambiguous genitalia have been brought up as girls. A few operations may be needed, usually begun in the child's first year. Further surgery might be required during adolescence. Some intersex support groups feel that surgery is not always the answer, particularly when the gender of the child is not clear. Others suggest that surgery should wait until the child is old enough to decide for themselves. However most medical professionals advocate early surgical and hormonal intervention for the sake of clearly establishing the child's gender and sense of belonging in society.
- *Counseling for the child:* The child needs to be informed and talked to about their diagnosis in a very careful way.
- *Hormone therapy:* During their teenage years, the child may need hormone supplementation therapy to help bring on puberty. A child with CAH will need to have daily hormone therapy.

Complication

- *Infertility:* Whether people with ambiguous genitalia can have children depends on the specific diagnosis. For example, genetic females with congenital adrenal hyperplasia usually can get pregnant if they so choose.
- *Increased risk of certain cancers:* Some disorders of sex development are associated with an increased risk of certain types of cancer.

DEFECTS OF CARDIOVASCULAR SYSTEM

CONGENITAL HEART DEFECTS

Introduction

Congenital heart defects have been divided into two categories. *Acyanotic defects and Cyanotic defects.* In clinical practice this system is problematic because children with acyanotic defects may develop cyanosis. Also, more often, those with cyanotic defects may appear pink and have more clinical signs of congestive heart failure (CHF).

A more useful classification system is based on hemodynamic characteristics (blood flow patterns within the heart). These blood flow patterns are such as:

- Increased pulmonary blood flow
- Decreased pulmonary blood flow
- Obstruction to blood flow out of the heart
- Mixed blood flow, in which saturated and desaturated blood mix within the heart or great arteries. As a comparison, both classification systems are outlined.

Incidence

The overall incidence of congenital heart diseases is about 8–10 percent per 1000 live births.

Defect	Percentage
• VSD	• 25–30%
• PDA	• 10%
• ASD	• 10%
• Coarctation of aorta	• 6%
• TOF	• 5–9%

Etiology

Hereditary Factors

- CHD affects 8–12 of every 1000 neonates
- Associated factor for CHD include
- Fetal or Maternal infection during the first trimester (Rubella)
- Chromosomal abnormality (Trisomy 21, 18, 13)
- Maternal diabetes
- Teratogenic effects of drugs and alcohol.

Syndromes that include CHD

- Marfan's syndrome: Mitral value prolapse
- Turner's syndrome: Aortic value stenosis, COA

- William's syndrome: Dysplastic pulmonary value
- Down syndrome: Trisomy

Classification of Congenital Cardiac Defects

Congenital heart diseases			
Cyanotic heart diseases (R to L shunt)		**A cyanotic heart diseases (L to R shunt)**	
Decreased pulmonary blood flow	**Mixed blood flow**	**Increased pulmonary blood flow**	**Obstructive heart diseases**
• Tetralogy of Fallot (TOF)	• Trans position of great arteries	• VSD (ventricular Septal defect)	• Coarctation of aorta (COA)
- Ventricular septal defect	• Total anomalous of pulmonary venous connection (TAPVC)	• ASD (Atrial Septal defect)	• Pulmonary stenosis (PS)
- Pulmonic stenosis	• Truncus arteriosus	• PDA (patent ductus arteriosus)	• Aortic stenosis (AS)
- Overriding aorta	• Hypoplastic left heart syndrome	• Pulmonary hypertension (PH)	• Congenital mitral stenosis
- Right ventricular hypertrophy	• Eisenmenger syndrome or complex	• Atrial ventricular canal (AVC)	• Hypoxemia
• Tricuspid atresia (TA)			

CYANOTIC HEART DISEASES

Tetralogy of Fallot (TOF)

Definition

Tetralogy of Fallot (TOF) is a complex of anatomic abnormalities arising from the maldevelopment of the right ventricular infundibulum. Tetralogy of Fallot (TOF) is a cardiac anomaly that refers to a combination of four related heart defects that commonly occur together.

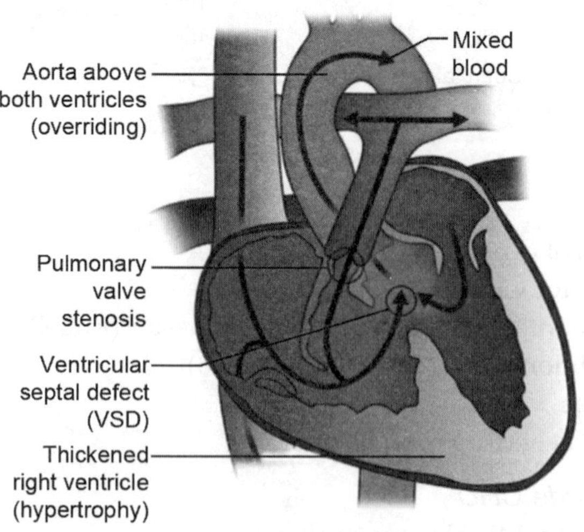

Fig. 6.61: Anatomic findings in tetralogy of Fallot

The four defects are:

1. *Ventricular Septal Defect (VSD)*
2. *Overriding of aorta:* The aortic valve is enlarged and appears to arise from both the left and right ventricles instead of the left ventricle as in normal hearts.
3. *Pulmonary value stenosis*: Narrowing of the pulmonary valve and outflow tract or area below the valve that creates an obstruction (blockage) of blood flow from the right ventricle to the pulmonary artery.
4. *Right ventricular hypertrophy:* Thickening of the muscular walls of the right ventricle, which occurs because the right ventricle is pumping at high pressure.

Causes

- The exact cause of tetralogy of Fallot is unknown
- Tetralogy of Fallot occurs during Fetal growth, when the baby's heart is developing
- While factors such as poor maternal nutrition
- Viral illness or genetic disorders might increase the risk of this condition.

Risk factors include:

- A viral illness during pregnancy, such as rubella (German measles)
- Alcoholism during pregnancy
- Poor nutrition during pregnancy
- A mother older than age 40 years
- A parent who has tetralogy of Fallot
- The presence of Down syndrome.

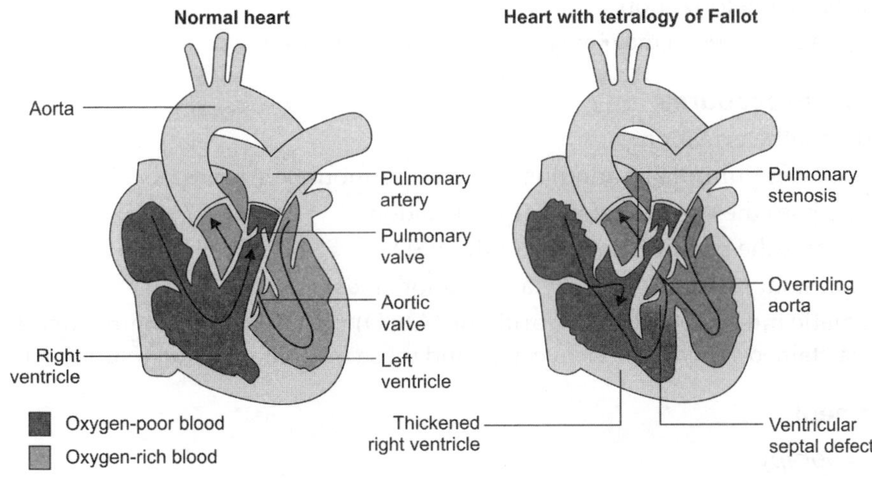

Fig. 6.62: Comparison of normal and TOF heart

Signs and Symptoms

Tetralogy of Fallot is most often diagnosed in the first few weeks of life due to either a loud murmur or cyanosis. Babies with tetralogy of Fallot usually have a patent ductus arteriosus at birth that provides additional blood flow to the lungs, so severe cyanosis is rare early after birth.

- A bluish coloration of the skin caused by blood low in oxygen (cyanosis)
- Shortness of breath and rapid breathing, especially during feeding or exercise
- Loss of consciousness (fainting)
- Clubbing of fingers and toes: An abnormal, rounded shape of the nail bed
- Poor weight gain
- Tiring easily during play or exercise
- Irritability
- Prolonged crying
- A heart murmur.

Diagnostic Evaluation

- History collection
- Physical examination (Pulse, blood pressure, temperature and number of breaths a baby takes a minute)
- Listening with a stethoscope for changes in heart sounds
- An oxygen saturation monitor to see how much oxygen is getting into the blood
- A chest X-ray to see the size and position of the heart
- An ECG (electrocardiogram) to check the electrical activity
- An ultrasound scan (echocardiogram) to see how the blood moves through the heart
- Checks for chemical balance in blood and urine
- A cardiac catheterization
- MRI (magnetic resonance imaging) test may be needed.

Diagnostic Procedures

- Cardiac catheterization
  - Assesses pulmonary annulus size and pulmonary arteries
  - Assesses the severity of RVOT obstruction
  - Locates the position and size of the VSD
  - Rules out possible coronary artery anomalies.
- Automatic internal cardiac defibrillator (AICD) placement: Recommended in patients with sustained ventricular tachycardia and those resuscitated after a sudden death event.

Management

Oxygen Therapy

- Once tetralogy of Fallot is diagnosed, the immediate management focuses on determining whether the child's oxygen levels are in a safe range.
- If oxygen levels are critically low soon after birth, a prostaglandin infusion is usually initiated to keep the ductus arteriosus open which will provide additional pulmonary blood flow and increase the child's oxygen level.

Medication

The goals of tetralogy of Fallot (TOF) therapy are to reduce the ventilatory drive, decrease systemic venous return, and increase peripheral venous return.

- *Analgesics:* These agents reduce ventilatory drive. Pain control ensures patient comfort and promotes pulmonary toilet. Most analgesics have sedating properties, which are beneficial for patients who are having hypercyanotic episodes.
- *Morphine sulfate:* Narcotic analgesia because of its reliable and predictable effects, safety profile, and ease of reversibility with naloxone. Administered IV, may be dosed in number of ways and commonly titrated until desired effect obtained.
  Pediatric dose: 0.05–0.2 mg/kg dose IV prn; not to exceed 15 mg/dose
- *Phenylephrine (non-synephrine):* Strong postsynaptic alpha-receptor stimulant with little beta-adrenergic activity; produces vasoconstriction of arterioles, increasing peripheral venous return.
  Pediatric dose: 5–20 mcg/kg/dose IV bolus q10–15 min prn, 0.1–0.5 mcg/kg/min IV infusion

Surgical Management

- These infants will usually require surgical intervention in the neonatal period. Infants with normal oxygen levels or only mild cyanosis are usually able to go home in the first week of life.
- Complete repair is usually done electively when children are about 6 months of age, as long as the oxygen levels remain adequate. Progressive or sudden decreases in oxygen saturation may prompt earlier corrective repair.
- Surgical correction of the defect is always necessary. Occasionally, the child will require a surgical palliative procedure prior to the final correction.
- Corrective repair of tetralogy of Fallot involves closure of the ventricular septal defect with a *synthetic dacron patch* so that the blood can flow normally from the left ventricle to the aorta.
- The narrowing of the pulmonary valve and right ventricular outflow tract is then augmented (enlarged) by a combination of cutting away (resecting) obstructive muscle tissue in the right ventricle and by enlarging the outflow pathway with a patch.
- The coronary arteries will branch across the right ventricular outflow tract where the patch would normally be placed. In these babies, an incision in this area to place the patch would damage the coronary artery, so this cannot safely be done.
- When this occurs, a hole is made in the front surface of the right ventricle (avoiding the coronary artery) and a conduit (tube) is sewn from the right ventricle to the bifurcation of the pulmonary arteries to provide unobstructed blood flow from the right ventricle to the lungs.

Palliative Surgery in Tetralogy of Fallot (TOF)

- Blalock-Taussig shunt
- Potts procedure
- Waterston shunt.

Definitive Surgery in Tetralogy of Fallot

Total surgical correction with patch closure of the ventricular septal defect (VSD) and relief of the ventricular outflow obstruction is preferred. The image below shows an example of typical postoperative ECG findings.

Complications

Complications of tetralogy of Fallot include the following:

- Erythrocytosis
- Brain abscess
- Acute gouty arthritis
- Infective endocarditis
- Cerebrovascular thrombosis
- Delayed puberty
- Postoperative complications.

Congestive heart failure (right or left, residual outflow obstruction, VSD, and/or pulmonic regurgitation atrial flutter, ventricular arrhythmias, right bundle-branch block, or left anterior hemiblock—arrhythmias were identified in up to 38.9% of patients with symptoms suggestive of rhythm disturbances, infective bacterial endocarditis.

TRANSPOSITION OF GREAT ARTERIES/VESSELS (TGA)

Introduction

Transposition of the great arteries is a serious but rare heart defect present at birth (congenital), in which the two main arteries leaving the heart are reversed (transposed). Transposition of the great arteries changes the way blood circulates through the body, leaving a shortage of oxygen in blood flowing from the heart to the rest of the body. Without an adequate supply of oxygen-rich blood, the body cannot function properly and your child faces serious complications or death without treatment. Transposition of the great arteries is usually detected within the first hours to weeks of life.

Definition

Transposition of the great arteries (TGA) is the most common cyanotic congenital heart lesion that presents in neonates. The hallmark of transposition of the great arteries is ventriculo arterial discordance, in which the aorta arises from the morphologic right ventricle and the pulmonary artery arises from the morphologic left ventricle.

Transposition of the great vessels is a heart defect that occurs from birth (congenital).

The two major vessels that carry blood away from the heart:

1. The aorta
2. The pulmonary artery.

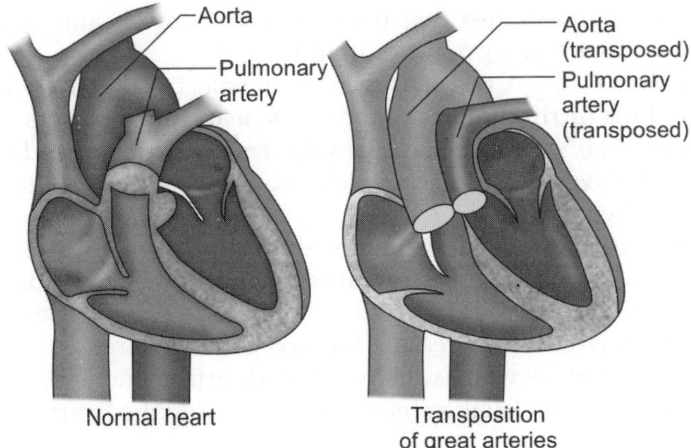

Fig. 6.63: Difference between normal and TGA heart

Causes

- Etiology for transposition of the great arteries is unknown and is presumed to be multifactorial.
- Embryology likely involves abnormal persistence of the subaortic conus with resorption or underdevelopment of the subpulmonary conus (infundibulum).
- This abnormality aligns the aorta anterior and superior with the right ventricle during development.

Risk Factors

- A history of German measles (rubella) or another viral illness in the mother during pregnancy
- A family history of transposition of the great arteries or another congenital heart defect
- Poor nutrition during pregnancy
- Drinking alcohol during pregnancy
- A mother older than age 40
- A mother who has poorly controlled diabetes
- Down syndrome in the baby.

Signs and Symptoms

- Clubbing of the fingers or toes
- Poor feeding
- Blue color of the skin (cyanosis)
- Shortness of breath
- Lack of appetite
- Poor weight gain.

Diagnostic Evaluation

- Detail history collection from the parents
- Physical examination

- Pulse oximetry (to check blood oxygen level)
- *Chest X-ray:* A diagnostic test that uses invisible X-ray beams to produce images of internal tissues, bones, and organs onto film.
- *Electrocardiogram (ECG):* A test that records the electrical activity of the heart, shows abnormal rhythms (arrhythmias), and detects heart muscle stress.
- *Echocardiogram (echo):* A procedure that evaluates the structure and function of the heart by using sound waves recorded on an electronic sensor to produce a moving picture of the heart and heart valves.
- *Cardiac catheterization:* A cardiac catheterization is an invasive procedure that gives very detailed information about the structures inside the heart. Under sedation, a small, thin, flexible tube (catheter) is inserted into a blood vessel in the groin, and guided to the inside of the heart. Blood pressure and oxygen measurements are taken in the four chambers of the heart, as well as the pulmonary artery and aorta. Contrast dye is also injected to more clearly visualize the structures inside the heart.

Complication

- *Lack of oxygen to tissues:* The child tissues will receive too little oxygen, (hypoxia). Unless there is some mixing of oxygen-rich blood and oxygen-poor blood within child body, he or she will not be able to survive.
- *Heart failure:* Heart failure a condition in which the heart cannot pump enough blood to meet the bodys needs may develop over time because the right ventricle is pumping under higher pressure than usual. This added stress may make the muscle of the right ventricle stiff or weak.
- *Lung damage:* The lack of oxygenated blood causes damage to the lungs, making breathing difficult.

Surgery is required for all babies with transposition of the great arteries early in life, usually within the first week. Complications of surgery to correct transposition of the great arteries may occur later in life, including:

- Narrowing of the arteries that supply blood to the heart (coronary arteries)
- Heart rhythm abnormalities (arrhythmias)
- Heart muscle weakness or stiffness leading to heart failure
- Leaky heart valves.

Management

Medication

- *Medication:* The medication prostaglandin E1 (alprostadil) helps keep the connection between the aorta and pulmonary artery open (ductus arteriosus), increasing blood flow and improving mixing of oxygen-poor and oxygen-rich blood until surgery can be performed.
- *Atrial septostomy:* This procedure usually done using cardiac catheterization rather than surgery enlarges a natural connection between the hearts upper chambers (atria). It allows for the oxygen-rich and oxygen-poor blood to mix and results in improved oxygen delivery to your baby's body.

Surgical Management

- *Arterial switch operation:* This is the surgery that surgeons most often use to fix transposition of the great arteries. This is usually perform this surgery within the first month of life. During an arterial switch operation, the pulmonary artery and the aorta are moved to their normal positions. The pulmonary artery is connected to the right ventricle, and the aorta is connected to the left ventricle. The coronary arteries also are reattached to the aorta.

- *Atrial switch operation:* In this surgery, the surgeon makes a tunnel (baffle) between the heart's two upper chambers (atria). This diverts the oxygen-poor blood to the left ventricle and the pulmonary artery and the oxygen-rich blood to the right ventricle and the aorta. With this procedure, the right ventricle must pump blood to the entire body, instead of just to the lungs as it would do in a normal heart. Possible complications of the atrial switch operation include irregular heartbeats, baffle obstructions or leaks, and heart failure due to problems with right ventricle function.
- *Rastelli's operation*
- *Beffe's operation*

TOTAL ANOMALOUS PULMONARY VENOUS CONNECTION (TAPVC)

Definition

Total anomalous pulmonary venous connection (TAPVC) consists of an abnormality of blood flow in which all 4 pulmonary veins drain into systemic veins or the right atrium with or without pulmonary venous obstruction. Systemic and pulmonary venous blood mix in the right atrium. An Atrial defect or foramen ovale (part of the complex) is important in left ventricular output both in fetal and in newborn circulation.

Total anomalous pulmonary venous connection (TAPVC), defined as total anomalous pulmonary venous return (TAPVR), is a cyanotic congenital defect in which all four pulmonary veins fail to make their normal connection to the left atrium. This results in drainage of all pulmonary venous return into the systemic venous circulation.

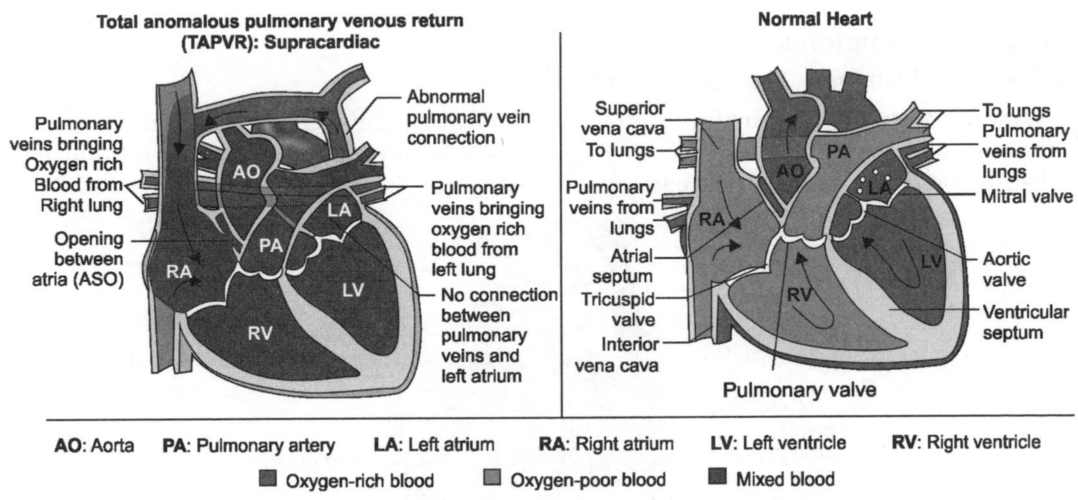

Fig. 6.64: Comparison of normal heart and TAPVC heart

Incidence

The incidence of total anomalous pulmonary venous connection (TAPVC) ranges from 0.6 to 1.2 per 10,000 live births. Among the children born with congenital heart disease (CHD). The incidence of TAPVC ranges between 0.7 and 1.5 percent. It is the fifth most common cause of cyanotic CHD.

Types

Supracardiac Total Anomalous Pulmonary Venous Return

The pulmonary veins drain to the right atrium via the superior vena cava. In this type of TAPVR, the pulmonary veins first come together behind the heart and then drain upwards to an abnormal 'vertical vein.' This vertical vein joins the innominate vein which connects to the right superior vena cava and drains to the right atrium.

Cardiac Total Anomalous Pulmonary Venous Return

The pulmonary veins come together behind the heart and then drain to the right atrium through the coronary sinus. The coronary sinus is the vein that normally returns blood from the heart muscle itself back to the right atrium after its oxygen has been depleted. The coronary sinus drains directly into the right atrium.

Infracardiac Total Anomalous Pulmonary Venous Return

The pulmonary veins drain to the right atrium via the hepatic (liver) veins and inferior vena cava. In this type, the pulmonary veins join together behind the heart and then typically drain downwards, connecting to the liver's portal vein system. They then drain through the vascular bed of the liver and enter the right atrium from the hepatic veins.

Causes

- The cause of total anomalous pulmonary venous return (TAPVR) is unknown
- Genetic problems
- Hereditary.

Signs and Symptoms

Child with Pulmonary Vein Obstruction

Pulmonary venous obstruction occurs in virtually all children with subdiaphragmatic drainage and in approximately 50% of patients with supracardiac drainage. Child with obstruction develop symptoms early, usually at age 24–36 hours.

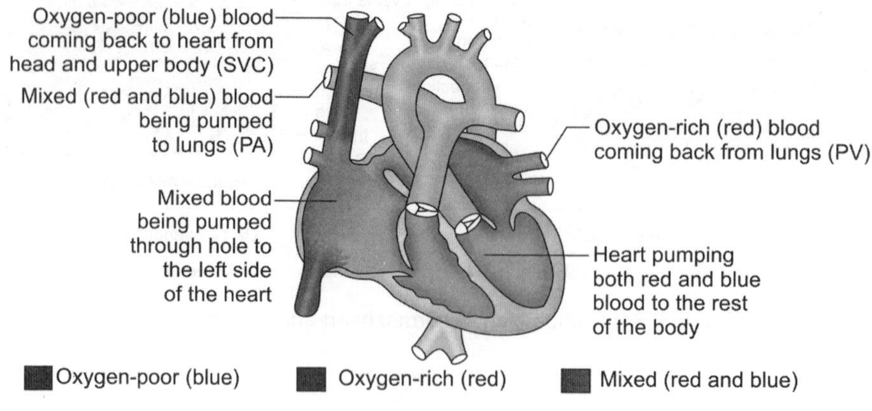

- Tachypnea
- Tachycardia and cyanosis.
- Pulmonary hypertension progress with decreasing pulmonary blood flow and worsening cyanosis.
- The pulmonary component of the second heart sound is increased.
- A murmur usually is not present.
- Peripheral pulses are usually normal after birth but may decrease as heart failure progresses.
- Liver enlargement commonly occurs.

Child without Pulmonary Venous Obstruction

Child with unobstructed pulmonary venous flow present with symptoms more similar to a very large atrial septal defect.

- Mild failure to thrive
- Pulmonary outflow murmur with or without a tricuspid diastolic murmur
- Cyanosis infrequently occurs in the first year of life
- Pulmonary hypertension
- Tachypnea
- Pulmonary venous congestion.

Other Symptoms

Newborns

- Tachypnea
- Cyanosis
- Signs of pulmonary venous congestion
- Mitral stenosis
- Hypoplastic left heart syndrome
- Coarctation or interrupted aortic arch
- Transposition of the great vessels
- Persistent fetal circulation.

Infants (Age Usually > 6 weeks)

- Large ventricular septal defect
- Common arteriovenous canal
- Truncus arteriosus
- Single ventricle.

Children Older than one Year

- Large atrial septal defect
- Common atrium partial anomalous pulmonary venous connection.

Diagnostic Evaluation

- Cardiac catheterization can confirm the diagnosis by showing that the blood vessels are abnormally attached

- ECG shows enlargement of the ventricles (ventricular hypertrophy)
- Echocardiogram may show that the pulmonary vessels are attached
- MRI of the heart can show the connections between the pulmonary vessels
- X-ray of the chest shows a normal to small heart with fluid in the lungs.

Other Tests

- ECG reveals significant right ventricular hypertrophy in most of these patients, usually with a qR pattern in the right chest leads by age 5–7 days. Right atrial enlargement rarely occurs in these younger patients.

Diagnostic Procedures

- In some child with multiple sites of pulmonary venous connection, cardiac catheterization serves to better define sites of pulmonary venous obstruction, when other associated cardiac defects are present (i.e. pulmonary atresia), and to directly measure foramen ovale size when surgery is delayed.

Management

Total anomalous pulmonary venous return is a defect which requires surgical correction. The timing of the surgical repair varies depending on the type of total anomalous pulmonary venous return present as well as the condition of the child.

Surgical repair is used as treatment for total anomalous pulmonary venous connection whenever it best serves the individual patient. Stabilizing the child prior to surgery as much as possible from a cardiovascular and metabolic standpoint is important. In a newborn with obstructive total anomalous pulmonary venous connection, stabilization often involves mechanical ventilation, correction of acidosis, inotropic support, and administration of prostaglandin E_1 for patency of patent ductus arteriosus and, in child with total anomalous pulmonary venous connection type III, for patency of the ductus venous.

Nitric oxide may be useful as a pulmonary dilator postoperatively in patients experiencing episodic pulmonary hypertension that is affecting cardiac output. Reports indicate that magnesium sulfate is a useful pulmonary vasodilator in these patients. Extracorporeal membrane oxygenation (ECMO) may be life saving in some patients. If transesophageal echocardiography is used intraoperatively in infants with pulmonary vein obstruction, waiting for probe insertion until after chest is opened may be safer.

Interventional Cardiac Catheterization

A cardiac catheterization procedure can be used as a diagnostic procedure, as well as initial treatment procedure for some heart defects. A cardiac catheterization procedure will usually be done to evaluate the defect(s) and the amount of blood that is mixing. As part of the cardiac catheterization, a procedure called balloon atrial septostomy may be done to improve mixing of oxygen-rich (red) and oxygen-poor (blue) blood:

- A special catheter with a balloon in the tip is used to create an opening in the atrial septum (wall between the left and right atria)
- The catheter is guided through the foramen ovale
- The balloon is inflated
- The catheter is quickly pulled back through the hole, into the right atrium, enlarging the hole, allowing blood to mix between the atria

- An IV medication called prostaglandin E1 may be given to keep the ductus arteriosus from closing.

Complications

- Breathing difficulties
- Heart failure
- Irregular, fast heart rhythms (arrhythmias)
- Lung infections
- Pulmonary hypertension.

Prognosis

- Most of the children survive surgery without late cardiovascular problem manifestations.
- An increased incidence of neurodevelopment difficulties has been reported, with fine motor function, visual-motor integration, and attention difficulties noted.

TRUNCUS ARTERIOSUS

Introduction

Truncus arteriosus (TA) is an uncommon congenital cardiovascular anomaly that is characterized by a single arterial trunk arising from the normally formed ventricles by means of a single semilunar valve (i.e. truncal valve).

There is usually also a large hole between the two ventricles (ventricular septal defect). As a result, the blue (without oxygen) and red (oxygen-rich) blood mix.

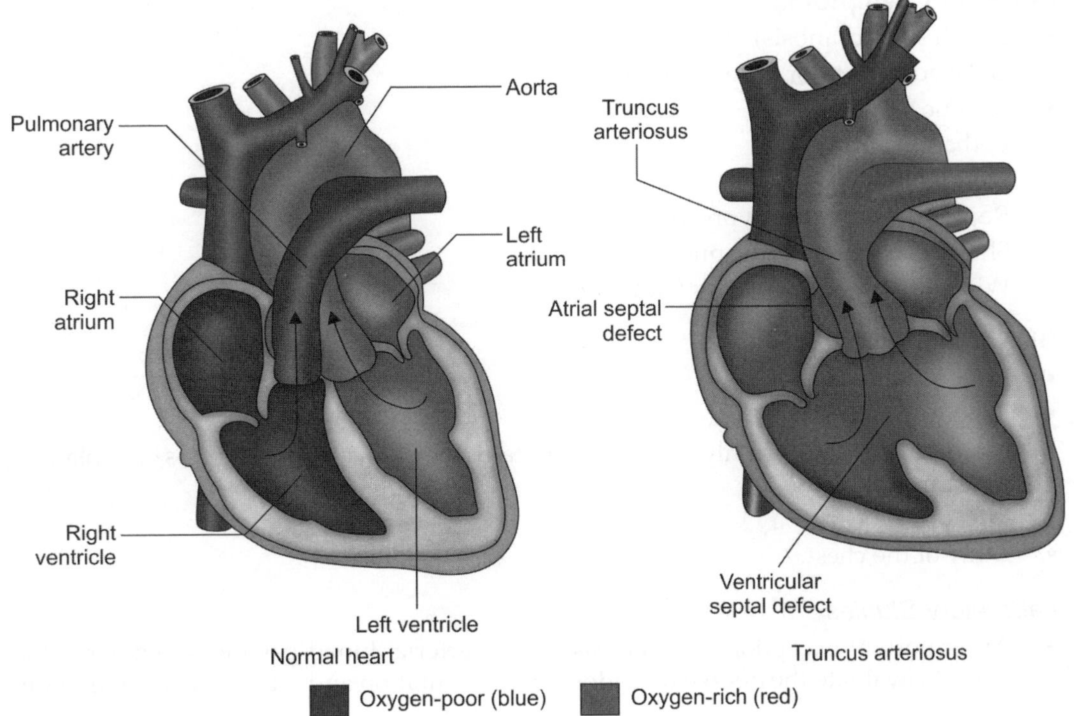

Definition

Truncus arteriosus defined as its rare congenital heart defect that is present at birth. A single blood vessel (truncus arteriosus) comes out of the right and left ventricles, instead of the normal two vessels (pulmonary artery and aorta). As a result of truncus arteriosus, less oxygenated blood enter to the lungs and oxygen-rich blood that go to the rest of the body are mixed together. This creates severe circulatory problems. If left untreated, truncus arteriosus can be fatal.

Causes

It is a congenital heart disease the causes of truncus arteriosus are unknown.

Pathophysiology

Pathophysiology of truncus arteriosus is typified by cyanosis and systemic ventricular volume overload. Outflow from both ventricles is directed into the common arterial trunk. Pulmonary blood flow is derived from this combined ventricular output and its magnitude depends on the ratio of resistances to flow in the pulmonary and systemic vascular beds.

Because of the mixing (although not complete) of left and right ventricular output that occurs primarily during systole and at the level of the common arterial trunk, subnormal systemic arterial oxygen saturation is common. Similarly, because the systemic and pulmonary circulations are essentially in parallel, pulmonary blood flow typically is at least 3-fold higher than systemic blood flow with pulmonary over circulation and increased myocardial works that result in increased resting oxygen demand and decreased metabolic reserve.

Signs and Symptoms

- Bluish skin (cyanosis)
- Delayed growth or growth failure
- Fatigue
- Lethargy
- Poor feeding
- Rapid breathing (tachypnea)
- Shortness of breath (dyspnea)
- Widening of the finger tips (clubbing).

Diagnostic Evaluation

- ECG
- Echocardiogram
- Heart catheterization (only needed in rare cases to help with the diagnosis or in planning a treatment strategy)
- MRI of the heart
- X-ray of the chest.

Laboratory Studies

- An important exception in some cases is an arterial blood gas measurement, which helps to evaluate the degree of acidosis on presentation and may aid in differentiating cardiac disease from primary pulmonary pathology when performed before and after administration of 100% inspired oxygen (hyperoxia test).

- Measurement of serum electrolytes, including total and ionized calcium, is important in patients with truncus arteriosus, given the common association with DiGeorge syndrome, which frequently may include hypoparathyroidism and hypocalcemia.

Imaging Studies

Chest Radiography

- Upon presentation, obtain a chest radiograph in most patients with truncus arteriosus.
- Cardiomegaly and increased pulmonary vascular markings are typically present, and fullness in the region of the truncal root may possibly be discerned. In patients with a right aortic arch, this radiographic finding in association with increased pulmonary vascular markings suggests truncus arteriosus.

Echocardiography

- Echocardiography with cross-sectional and doppler flow analysis is sufficient to confirm diagnosis of truncus arteriosus and fully characterize the various anatomic features in most patients. A full complement of echocardiographic views is necessary to ensure complete and accurate definition of the anatomy and potential associated anomalies.

MRI

- MRI is rarely necessary in patients with truncus arteriosus.
- MRI modality provides excellent imaging for characterizing anatomy, and may be especially useful in reconstructing complex pulmonary arterial anatomy in older patients with truncus arteriosus.

Other Tests

Electrocardiography (ECG)

- Electrocardiographic (ECG) findings in young infants with truncus arteriosus do not distinguish this lesion from others on the differential diagnosis.
- A normal sinus rhythm, normal intervals, and either a normal QRS axis or minimal right-axis deviation are generally observed. Biventricular hypertrophy is a characteristic finding.

Procedures

Cardiac Catheterization

- Standard angiographic images from the truncal root can aid in the assessment of coronary arterial anatomy, if echocardiography is inadequate, and in the assessment of regurgitation through the truncal valve.
- Cardiac catheterization is generally not required prior to repair in neonates and infants with truncus arteriosus.
- Catheterization is an important tool for evaluating some of the most common anatomic problems in patients with repaired truncus arteriosus, such as obstruction of the surgical reconstructed right ventricular outflow tract, branch pulmonary arterial stenosis, truncal valve regurgitation, and, in patients repaired later in life, pulmonary vascular obstructive disease.

Transcatheter Balloon Dilation

- Treatment of pulmonary outflow tract or pulmonary arterial obstruction with transcatheter balloon dilation or stenting is an effective therapy for these problems in many children.

Management

Medical Management

- Medications to control congestive heart failure such as diuretics are often begun.
- Some of the neonates with truncus arteriosus display some evidence of congestive heart failure; they are usually treated with digitalis and diuretic medicines.
- Intravenous prostaglandin is often administered in patients with truncus arteriosus upon presentation because the differential diagnosis includes numerous anomalies with duct-dependent systemic or pulmonary blood flow. However, it is beneficial only in patients with associated interruption of the aortic arch or aortic coarctation.
- Other preoperative medications are not generally indicated although specific circumstances may dictate after load reducing agents, inotropic medications, or antiarrhythmics.
- Full-term and premature newborns with truncus arteriosus may be at increased risk for necrotizing enterocolitis, either preoperatively or postoperatively, and appropriate evaluation should be undertaken in any newborn exhibiting signs or symptoms of necrotizing enterocolitis.

Surgical Management

Surgical correction is typically carried out in the first few weeks of life after the infant is maximally stabilized. The surgical repair of truncus arteriosus requires the use of heart-lung bypass machine support.

Indications

- Truncus arteriosus invariably requires operative repair
- Symptoms typically develop in the early neonatal period
- Indicating that complete repair is required at this point.

It involves three major components:

1. Separating the pulmonary arteries from the main truncus (the truncus will remain as the first part of the aorta)
2. Closure of the ventricular septal defect using a patch
3. Creating a connection between the right ventricle and the pulmonary arteries using a conduit, usually a homograft pulmonary artery.

Nursing Management

- Administer routine postoperative care, initially in the cardiac intensive care unit, following correction of truncus arteriosus.
- Support patients with mechanical ventilation, inotropic medications, and sedation as necessary.
- Restore fluid balance with diuretic therapy and continue tube thoracostomy until pleural and pericardial effusions have resolved.

- Focus remainder of inpatient stay on providing sufficient enteral nutrition, parental education, and elucidation of the maintenance pharmacologic regimen (if any) that is adopted.
- Postoperative care after repair of truncus arteriosus requires attention to issues that are common to patients with complex congenital heart disease (e.g. support of cardiac output) and prevention or management of arrhythmias and end-organ dysfunction.
- Management issues include maintenance of intravascular volume and ventricular filling, inotropic support, and acid-base and electrolyte homeostasis.
- Management with extended periods of anesthesia, including neuromuscular blockade and continuous fentanyl infusion, often is helpful. Ventilatory strategies aimed at minimizing pulmonary vascular resistance also may be effective. In refractory cases, inhaled nitric oxide or extracorporeal membrane oxygenation may be indicated.
- Maintain close follow-up care in young children after repair of truncus arteriosus.
- Infants are often discharged on cardiac medications and may usually be weaned over the following months.
- Frequently a mild degree of regurgitation occurs through the right ventricle-to-pulmonary arterial conduit but, in most cases does not pose a significant load on the heart.
- In most patients, conduit regurgitation and obstruction becomes an important issue after early repair; however, reintervention usually is not required for a year or more.
- Truncus valve regurgitation, which may progress even if it was not severe before repair, may become an important cause of persistent failure to thrive, and repair or replacement of the valve may be indicated.
- In patients with associated interruption of the aortic arch, pay particular attention to potential recurrent arch obstruction and compression of the bronchi, both of which may manifest within weeks or months of the initial repair.
- Routine clinical and echocardiographic follow-up care is sufficient to monitor most patients.
- Cardiac catheterization may be performed for the purpose of balloon dilation, stenting, or both of the pulmonary arteries or pulmonary outflow conduit, for evaluation of the pulmonary vascular bed in patients who are older and have evidence of pulmonary hypertension, or for other diagnostic indications according to the preference of the physicians.

HYPOPLASTIC LEFT HEART SYNDROME

Introduction

The term hypoplastic left heart syndrome (HLHS), initially proposed by Noonan and Nadas, describes a spectrum of cardiac abnormalities characterized by marked hypoplasia of the left ventricle and ascending aorta. This is the same disorder characterized as hypoplasia of the aortic tract complex by Lev. The aortic and mitral valves are atretic, hypoplastic, or stenotic.

A patent foramen ovale or an atrial septal defect is usually present. The ventricular septum is usually intact. A large patent ductus arteriosus supplies blood to the systemic circulation. Systemic arterial desaturation may be present because of complete mixing of pulmonary and systemic venous blood in the right atrium. Coarctation of the aorta is also commonly present.

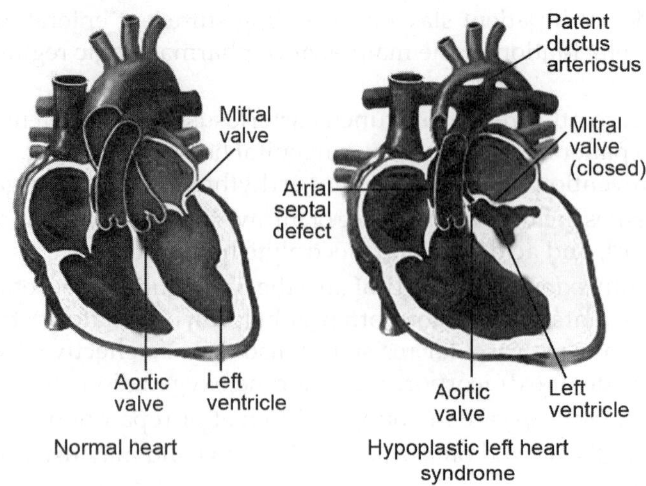

Fig. 6.65: Anatomical view of normal and PDA heart

Definition

Hypoplastic left heart syndrome is defined as a complex and rare heart defect present at birth (congenital). In this condition the child left side of the heart is critically underdeveloped.

Incidence

Incidence of hypoplastic left heart syndrome is 0.16–0.36 per 1000 live births. It comprises 1.2–1.5% of all congenital heart defects. Hypoplastic left heart syndrome accounts for 7–9% of all congenital heart disease diagnosed in the first year of life. Before surgical treatment was available, hypoplastic left heart syndrome was responsible for 25% of cardiac deaths in the neonatal period.

Causes

- The exact cause of hypoplastic left heart syndrome is unknown.
- Genetic causes with autosomal recessive inheritance have been reported, hypoplastic left heart syndrome is generally postulated to follow multifactorial mode of inheritance.

Pathophysiology

The oxygenated blood from the placenta is returned to the inferior vena cava and is not shunted preferentially across the patent foramen ovale into the left atrium; instead, it mixes with the superior vena caval blood in the right atrium. The pulmonary veins drain into the left atrium, and the pulmonary venous blood gets shunted across the atrial septum into the right atrium because of mitral valve obstruction. The vena caval and pulmonary venous blood along with the coronary sinus flow enters the right ventricle and the pulmonary artery.

Because of widely patent ductus arteriosus and high pulmonary vascular resistance in the fetus, a small portion of the blood from the right heart enters the lungs. Most of the blood is directed into the aorta via the ductus. Once in the aorta, the blood gets distributed into the brachiocephalic vessels, ascending aorta, and descending aorta. The quantitative distribution into these different vascular beds depends on their relative vascular resistances. The ascending aortic blood flows in a reverse direction and supplies the coronary arteries.

Postnatal Circulation

The newborn infant with hypoplastic left heart syndrome has a complex cardiovascular physiology. Fully saturated pulmonary venous blood returning to the left atrium cannot flow into the left ventricle because of atresia, hypoplasia, or stenosis of the mitral valve. Therefore, pulmonary venous blood must cross the atrial septum. In most babies, a patent foramen ovale is present and is small and partially obstructive. This blood mixes with desaturated systemic venous blood in the right atrium. The right ventricle then must pump this mixed blood to both the pulmonary and the systemic circulations that are connected in parallel, rather than in series, by the ductus arteriosus. Blood exiting the right ventricle may flow (1) to the lungs via the branch pulmonary arteries or (2) to the body via the ductus arteriosus. The amount of blood that flows into each circulation is based on the resistance in each circuit.

The postnatal circulation in hypoplastic left heart syndrome depends on three major factors:

1. Adequacy of interatrial communication
2. Patency of the ductus arteriosus
3. Level of pulmonary vascular resistance.

Signs and Symptoms

The clinical features of hypoplastic left heart syndrome (HLHS) largely depend on the patency of the ductus arteriosus, the level of pulmonary vascular resistance, and the size of the interatrial communication. As the ductus arteriosus begins to close normally over the first 24–48 hours of life, symptoms of cyanosis, tachypnea, respiratory distress, pallor, lethargy, metabolic acidosis, and oliguria develop. Without intervention to reopen the ductus arteriosus, death rapidly ensues.

- Grayish-blue skin color
- Rapid, difficult breathing
- Poor feeding
- Cold hands and feet
- Being unusually drowsy or inactive.

Signs of shock include:

- Cool, clammy skin that may be pale or gray
- A weak and rapid pulse
- Abnormal breathing that may be either slow and shallow or very rapid
- Dilated pupils
- Lackluster eyes that seem to stare.

Diagnostic Evaluation

- Routine ultrasound exam during the second trimester of pregnancy.
- CBC count
  - Measure hemoglobin levels, because severe neonatal anemia can cause high-output congestive heart failure (CHF) and cardiogenic shock.

- The hemoglobin level is usually normal in hypoplastic left heart syndrome.
- Obtain a total WBC count with differential. Sepsis can cause symptoms of shock.
- The WBC count is typically normal.

- Electrolytes
  - Electrolyte abnormalities may be present in infants with poor oral intake secondary to CHF.
  - Use carbon dioxide and bicarbonate to assess acid-base status.
  - Electrolyte levels are usually normal. The carbon dioxide level may be low if a metabolic acidosis is present.
  - The carbon dioxide level may be high if respiratory failure sets in.
- BUN/creatinine
  - Infants with critical illness and significantly reduced systemic perfusion may show evidence of renal failure.
  - The creatinine level may be transiently elevated.
- Liver function tests
  - Infants with critical illness and significantly reduced systemic perfusion and CHF may show evidence of hepatocellular damage.
  - Aspartate aminotransferase (AST) and alanine aminotransferase (ALT) levels may be transiently elevated.
- ABG and lactic acid
  - Assessing acid-base status is paramount, especially to rule out metabolic acidosis. Most infants have some evidence of metabolic acidosis, which should be immediately corrected.
  - This is usually secondary to decreased systemic perfusion. Appropriate intervention to augment systemic flow should be promptly undertaken.
  - Elevated levels of serum lactic acid generally precede a fall in pH, as acidosis develops.
  - Assessment of PaO_2 and $PaCO_2$ is important for respiratory management and manipulation of pulmonary vascular resistance by mechanical ventilation and the addition of supplemental inhaled nitrogen. The PaO_2 is optimally 30–45 mm Hg, and the $PaCO_2$ is ideally 45–50 mm Hg.
- Karyotype
  - Chromosomal analysis is indicated for infants with dysmorphic features.
  - Nearly 25% of infants have chromosomal abnormalities.

Other Tests

Electrocardiography

- Electrocardiography typically reveals sinus tachycardia, right-axis deviation
- Right atrial enlargement, and right ventricular hypertrophy with a QR configuration in the right precordial leads.
- A paucity of left ventricular forces is noted in the left precordial leads.
- ST-T wave changes suggestive of myocardial ischemia may be present in some patients.

Management

The approach to the treatment of neonates with hypoplastic left heart syndrome (HLHS). Supportive care, multistage surgical intervention (i.e. Norwood, Glenn, and Fontan procedures) and cardiac transplantation are available options. A thorough explanation of each of these options, including their advantages and disadvantages, should be provided to the parents. Occasionally, some anatomic features favor one choice over the others. In the presence of severe tricuspid or pulmonary valve anomalies, the multistage surgical approach is not likely to be beneficial; cardiac transplantation is the only surgical choice. In most cases, the choice of treatment is based on the parents' preference. While such a decision is being made, the infant should be stabilized. If supportive care is chosen by the parents, they need strong emotional support because the condition is fatal without active treatment.

Medical Management

Successful preoperative management depends on providing adequate systemic blood flow while limiting pulmonary overcirculation.

- Open the ductus arteriosus
  - Blood flow to the systemic circulation (coronary arteries, brain, liver, kidneys) depends on flow through the ductus arteriosus. If a diagnosis of hypoplastic left heart syndrome is suspected, start prostaglandin E_1 infusion immediately to establish ductal patency and ensure adequate systemic perfusion.
  - If the diagnosis is made prenatally or when the infant is relatively asymptomatic, a smaller dose of prostaglandin E_1 may be sufficient to keep the ductus arteriosus patent while limiting its side effects.
  - A larger dose of prostaglandin E_1 is often required to reopen the ductus arteriosus if an infant has cardiovascular collapse and shock due to ductal closure.
  - Ideally, prostaglandin E_1 is administered centrally via an umbilical venous catheter.
- Correct metabolic acidosis
  - Metabolic acidosis indicates inadequate cardiac output to meet the metabolic demands of the body. Acidosis adversely affects the myocardium.
  - Correction of metabolic acidosis with sodium bicarbonate infusion is essential in early management. This therapy is futile if the ductus arteriosus remains constricted.
- Manipulate pulmonary vascular resistance
  - The pulmonary vascular resistance of a newborn is slightly less than the systemic vascular resistance and begins to fall soon after birth. In the patient with hypoplastic left heart syndrome, decreased pulmonary vascular resistance causes increased pulmonary blood flow and an undesirable obligatory decrease in systemic blood flow. Increased alveolar oxygen decreases pulmonary vascular resistance, leading to increased pulmonary blood flow. Therefore, oxygen should not be administered unless pulmonary parenchymal disease or pulmonary edema, causing severe hypoxemia, is present. The oxygen should be discontinued once these abnormalities resolve.
  - Consequently, most infants should remain in room air with acceptable oxygen saturation (pulse oximeter) in the low 70s. An exceptional circumstance is the infant with severe hypoxemia caused by pulmonary venous hypertension.

- Achieving a slightly higher $PaCO_2$, in the range of 45–50 mm Hg, can increase pulmonary vascular resistance. This can be accomplished by intubation, sedation, mechanical hypoventilation, or the addition of nitrogen or carbon dioxide (FIO_2 of 15–19%) to the infant's inspired gas via the endotracheal tube or hood.
- Intubation is not preferred. However, intubation and ventilation along with measures to balance pulmonary and systemic flows may improve tricuspid regurgitation.
- Serial blood gas analysis is necessary. Initially, an umbilical arterial catheter is useful to obtain frequent blood samples.
- Although administration of subambient inspired oxygen to balance systemic and pulmonary blood flows is an attractive concept and should be applied during stabilization of the neonate, it should not be pursued for long periods because severe pulmonary hypertension may complicate the postoperative course. However, this does not seem to adversely affect the pulmonary vasculature on long-term follow-up.

- Inotropes
  - Inotropic support is indicated only in severely ill neonates with concurrent sepsis or profound cardiogenic shock and acidosis.
  - The administration of inotropes can adversely affect the balance between pulmonary and systemic vascular resistance.
  - If needed, wean from inotropic support as soon as the infant is clinically stable.
- Diuretics
  - Consider diuretics to manage pulmonary overcirculation before surgery.
  - Agents commonly used include furosemide and spironolactone.
- Antibiotics
  - Antibiotics are indicated if the infant is at risk for antepartum infection.
  - Discontinue antibiotics after obtaining negative blood cultures.

Surgical Management

- Sinha and associates, Caylor and colleagues and Dotty and associates proposed various palliative operations; however, survival was not feasible until Norwood and associates demonstrated that a multistage operative approach could be used to treat hypoplastic left heart syndrome.
- After Fontan and Kreutzer's initial description of the physiologically corrective operation for tricuspid atresia corrective surgery was widely adapted to treat this entity. The concept was extended to treat other cardiac defects with a functionally single ventricle, including hypoplastic left heart syndrome.
- The originally described Fontan operation consisted of the following:
  - Superior vena cava-to-right pulmonary artery end-to-end anastomosis (Glenn procedure),
  - Anastomosis of the proximal end of the divided right pulmonary artery to the right atrium directly or by means of an aortic homograft,
  - Closure of the atrial septal defect,
  - Insertion of a pulmonary valve homograft into the inferior vena caval orifice, and
  - Ligation of the main pulmonary artery, thus completely bypassing the right ventricle.

- Kreutzer performed anastomosis of the right atrial appendage and pulmonary artery directly or via a pulmonary homograft and closed the atrial septal defect. A Glenn procedure was not performed, and a prosthetic valve was not inserted into the inferior vena cava. Fontan's concept was to use the right atrium as a pumping chamber therefore; he inserted prosthetic valves into the inferior vena cava and right atrial–pulmonary artery junction. Kreutzer's view was that the right atrium may not function as a pump and that the left ventricle functions as a suction pump in the system.

Numerous modifications to the aforementioned procedures were undertaken by these and other workers in the field (see Tricuspid Atresia). Currently, staged total cavopulmonary connection is the procedure of choice. The goal of surgical reconstruction of hypoplastic left heart syndrome is to eventually separate the pulmonary and systemic circulations by achieving a Fontan circulation. The right ventricle remains the systemic ventricle while blood passively flows to the lungs. This ultimate reconstruction is accomplished in the following 3 stages.

Norwood Procedure (Stage I)

This procedure is usually performed during the first weeks of life, after the infant has been stabilized in the neonatal intensive care unit (ICU). The goals of the procedure are: (1) To establish reliable systemic circulation without the ductus arteriosus, and (2) To provide enough pulmonary blood flow for adequate oxygenation, while simultaneously protecting the pulmonary vascular bed in preparation for stages II and III.

The Norwood procedure includes: (1) Performing an atrial septectomy to provide unrestricted blood flow across the atrial septum, (2) Ligating the ductus arteriosus, (3) Creating an anastomosis between the main pulmonary artery and the aorta to provide systemic blood flow, (4) Eliminating coarctation of the aorta, and (5) Placing an aorta-to-pulmonary artery shunt (usually a modified Blalock-Taussig shunt) to provide pulmonary circulation. More recently, connecting a Gore-Tex graft from the right ventricular outflow tract to the pulmonary artery (i.e. Sano operation) has been advocated instead of conventional modified Blalock-Taussig shunt. Some surgeons have shown better results with the Sano procedure than with the conventional Norwood approach.

Upon hospital discharge, most infants remain on digoxin to augment cardiac function, on diuretics to help manage right ventricular volume overload, and on aspirin to prevent thrombosis of the shunt. If tricuspid regurgitation is present, use afterload reduction with captopril. Oxygen saturation is typically 70–80% in room air.

Bidirectional Glenn Procedure (Stage II)

This procedure is performed approximately 6 months after the Norwood procedure. Before surgery, perform a cardiac catheterization to assess right ventricular function, pulmonary artery anatomy, and pulmonary vascular resistance. If results are favorable, schedule elective surgery.

The bidirectional Glenn procedure includes creating an anastomosis between the superior vena cava and the right pulmonary artery, end-to-side so that venous return from the upper body can flow directly into both lungs. In the hemi-Fontan, the superior vena cava-right atrial junction is closed with a patch that is removed during the next stage. Blood from the inferior vena cava continues to drain into the right atrium. The aorta-to-pulmonary artery shunt that was placed at stage I is ligated.

When both right and left superior vena cava are present, bilateral bidirectional Glenn shunts should be performed, especially if the bridging innominate vein is absent or small. At the time of bidirectional Glenn, repair of pulmonary artery narrowing, if present, should be undertaken. Issues related to tricuspid valve regurgitation, restrictive atrial septum and any other abnormalities should also be addressed. At discharge, infants usually remain on digoxin, diuretics, aspirin, and captopril for the reasons mentioned above.

Fontan Procedure (Stage III)

The Fontan procedure is performed approximately 12 months after the bidirectional Glenn procedure. Again, catheterization is necessary to ensure that the child is a candidate for surgery. Completion of the Fontan procedure includes directing blood flow from the inferior vena cava to the pulmonary arteries either via a lateral tunnel procedure or via an extracardiac conduit. Extracardiac conduit diversion of inferior vena caval blood into the right pulmonary artery is currently preferred by most surgeons. To address the growth issue related to extracardiac Fontan, some surgeons use autologous pericardial roll grafts. At the conclusion of the procedure, systemic venous blood returns to the lungs passively without passing through a ventricle.

Choussat et al. criteria have been modified by many cardiologists and surgeons. Patients violating these criteria are at a higher risk for poor prognosis following Fontan operation than patients within the limits set by Choussat. In this high-risk group, the concept of leaving a small atrial septal defect open to facilitate decompression of the right atrium has been advanced. Laks et al advocated closure of the atrial defect by constricting the preplaced suture in the postoperative period whereas Bridges et al used a transcatheter closure technique. Although the fenestrated Fontan was initially conceived for high-risk patients, it has since been used in patients with modest or even low risk. Rare reports of cerebrovascular or other systemic arterial embolic events following the fenestrated Fontan procedure tend to contraindicate its use in non-high-risk patients. Some studies suggest routine fenestration is unnecessary.

At discharge, most children remain on digoxin, diuretics, aspirin, and captopril if necessary. In an uncomplicated case, most of these medications can be weaned over 6 months following the Fontan operation. Some cardiologists advocate using aspirin indefinitely. Routine use of more aggressive anticoagulation with Coumadin is debated.

Heart transplantation is another surgical option. The infant must remain on prostaglandin E1 infusion to keep the ductus arteriosus patent while waiting for a donor heart to become available. Approximately 20% of infants listed for heart transplantation die while waiting for a suitable donor organ. After successful cardiac transplantation, infants require multiple medications for modulation of the immune system and prevention of graft rejection. Perform frequent outpatient surveillance to identify rejection early and prevent lasting damage to the transplanted heart. Periodic endomyocardial biopsy usually is performed for more precise monitoring.

Emerging Therapies Include the Following

Catheter-assisted Fontan

Following Norwood procedure, second stage cavopulmonary connection is currently recommended for achieving Fontan circulation. Konert et al. proposed a staged surgical-catheter approach they initially perform a modified hemi-Fontan procedure that is later completed by transcatheter methodology. This reduces the total number of operations required.

The modified hemi-Fontan procedure involves the usual bidirectional Glenn procedure. The lower end of the divided superior vena cava is anastomosed to the undersurface of the right pulmonary artery. The superior vena cava is then banded around a 16-gauge catheter with 6–0 Prolene slightly above the cavoatrial junction. A lateral tunnel with a Gore-Tex baffle is created, diverting the inferior vena caval blood toward the superior vena cava. The Gore-Tex baffle is then fenestrated with three to five 5-mm holes. Thus, the first stage achieves a physiologic bidirectional Glenn procedure.

At the time of the second stage (the transcatheter stage), the superior vena caval constriction is balloon dilated, and fenestrations are closed with devices or by placement of covered stent. These procedures have been performed in a limited number of patients, and preliminary data suggest that the usual post-Fontan operation complications, such as pleural effusion and ascites, have not occurred with this approach. Additional experience is reported however, scrutiny of results of larger experience and longer-term follow-up and ready availability of covered stents are necessary for routine application of this innovative approach.

Sano's Modification of the Norwood Procedure

Because of high mortality that Sano and his associates observed with the conventional Norwood procedure, they performed right ventricular outflow-to-pulmonary artery Gore-Tex graft anastomosis to provide for the pulmonary blood flow instead of conventional modified aortopulmonary shunt. Significant improvement was demonstrated in both immediate and late mortality with this modification. Currently, an ongoing multi-institutional study is comparing the results of these 2 types of stage I palliation of hypoplastic left heart syndrome.

Other hybrid approaches: Again, because of high mortality following stage I Norwood reconstruction, several groups have performed bilateral banding of the branch pulmonary arteries via median sternotomy and implant stent in the ductus arteriosus. Maintaining ductal patency with long-term prostaglandin infusion instead of ductal stenting is advocated by some. At the time of the second stage, aortic arch reconstruction, atrial septectomy, and bidirectional Glenn shunt are performed. This is followed by Fontan conversion. Although reduction of early mortality is theoretically feasible, larger experience with this approach than is currently available is necessary prior to general adaptation of this method of management of hypoplastic left heart syndrome.

Prevention by fetal intervention: Fetal echocardiography studies have shown development of hypoplastic left heart syndrome in fetuses initially found to have severe/critical aortic stenosis. Some data suggest that fetal intervention to relieve aortic valve stenosis (by balloon aortic valvuloplasty) may promote normal development of the left ventricle. Further research into this type of approach is needed.

Complications

- Preoperative complications include acidosis, congestive heart failure (CHF), renal failure, liver failure, necrotizing enterocolitis, sepsis, and death.
- Postoperative complications include acidosis, CHF, renal failure, liver failure, necrotizing enterocolitis, sepsis, pericardial or pleural effusion, phrenic or recurrent laryngeal nerve

damage, stroke, coarctation of the aorta, and death. Early graft rejection and opportunist infection may occur after cardiac transplantation.

- Major complications following the Norwood procedure include aortic arch obstruction at the site of surgical anastomosis and progressive cyanosis caused by limited blood flow through the shunt. An inadequate atrial communication contributes to progressive cyanosis.
- Major complications following the bidirectional Glenn/hemi-Fontan procedure include transient superior vena cava syndrome and persistent pleural or pericardial effusion. The development of systemic venous to pulmonary venous collateral vessels is possible.
- Major complications following the Fontan procedure include persistent pleural or pericardial effusion. Neurodevelopmental abnormalities are reported and may be inherent in some patients with hypoplastic left heart syndrome.
- Arrhythmias, obstructed venous pathways, and protein-losing enteropathy are some of the other complications observed following the Fontan operation.

Nursing Management

- Initial preoperative management and postoperative care of hypoplastic left heart syndrome (HLHS) take place in the neonatal, pediatric, or cardiac ICUs.
- When postoperative patients are clinically stable, transfer them to the general cardiac unit for adjusting oral medications, addressing feeding issues, and completing discharge teaching.
- Involve a pediatric cardiologist during any noncardiac hospital admission of a patient who is status post (S/P) Norwood procedure. This is because of the complex cardiovascular physiology in infants after this surgery.
- Hospitalization and inpatient care may be required for cardiac catheterizations, catheter interventions and surgical procedures and for treatment of intercurrent infections as well as for management of postsurgical complications, including those after Fontan operation.
- Schedule outpatient follow-up care 2 weeks after discharge in the typical postoperative patient.
- Schedule those who are S/P cardiac transplantation earlier for necessary laboratory studies.
- Earlier follow-up care is also necessary if a pericardial effusion is discovered on the discharge echocardiogram.
- Periodic follow-up visits after stage I, II, and III operations are mandatory. Individualize outpatient follow-up care based on the needs of each patient.

Diet

Adequate nutrition is important before and after surgery. Many infants require nasogastric feeding with increased-calorie breast milk or formula after the Norwood procedure. However, normal oral feeding is re-established with time. Adequate oral iron intake prevents development of iron deficiency anemia. After completion of the Fontan operation, specific dietary restrictions are not necessary unless protein-losing enteropathy develops. In such cases, a medium-chain triglyceride diet may be helpful.

Activity

- Specific activity restrictions are not imposed on children after completion of the Fontan operation. In general, encourage children to participate in activities that they are able to tolerate. Children who underwent a Fontan procedure may not be able to tolerate highly competitive sports.
- Studies have shown that these children may have impaired exercise performance when compared to age-matched peers. Perform an exercise stress test when the child is old enough.
- Neurodevelopmental abnormalities occur often in patients with hypoplastic left heart syndrome.

Parental Education

- *General:* At the outset, appropriately warn the parents and other caregivers that hypoplastic left heart syndrome is a complex heart defect that requires multiple hospitalizations, surgeries, catheter interventions and long-term follow-up.
- Medication
  - Educate parents regarding the doses and side effects of their child's cardiac medications.
  - Discuss interactions with other medications with the family and the infant's general pediatrician.
- Feeding
  - Many infants require nasogastric tube feeding after discharge from the hospital. Parents must become comfortable with placement of the nasogastric feeding tube.
  - Frequently, increased-calorie formula is required for adequate growth. Provide the formula recipe or a source for purchasing it to the caregiver.

Conclusion

The newborn with hypoplastic left heart syndrome (HLHS) dies rapidly if untreated. Surgical techniques, both reconstruction and heart transplantation, offer an opportunity to preserve the newborn's life. Survival rates given above represent the best results and reflect only survival, not quality of life. Mortality rates in many centers exceed those mentioned. Incidence of neurodevelopmental abnormalities in hypoplastic left heart syndrome appears to exceed that of other single-ventricle conditions.

Hypoplastic left heart syndrome affects family structure. For example, reproductive studies indicate that the incidence of subsequent pregnancy is significantly lower in mothers of a living patient with hypoplastic left heart syndrome than in mothers after death of an infant with hypoplastic left heart syndrome. For these reasons, most pediatric cardiologists continue to offer no treatment as an acceptable option to parents of a newborn with hypoplastic left heart syndrome. It is incumbent on physicians caring for a newborn with hypoplastic left heart syndrome to clearly communicate all of this information to the parents. An ethically appropriate consent for surgery requires this. Allowing an affected infant to die without surgical intervention is a difficult decision but is still chosen by some families and should not be discouraged.

Ethical issues related to transplantation compared with multistage reconstructive surgery were recently reviewed. Although the decision regarding this choice must be made in the best interest of the infant with hypoplastic left heart syndrome, considerations such as interests of the family members and society-at-large may have to be taken into account.

EISENMENGER SYNDROME OR COMPLEX

Introduction

Eisenmenger syndrome was initially described in 1897, when Victor Eisenmenger reported on a patient with symptoms of dyspnea and cyanosis from infancy who subsequently developed heart failure and succumbed to massive hemoptysis.

Eisenmenger syndrome occurs when the increased pressure of the blood flow in the lung becomes so great that the direction of blood flow through the shunt reverses. Oxygen-poor (blue) blood from the right side of the heart flows into the left ventricle and is pumped to your body so you do not receive enough oxygen to all your organs and tissues.

Definition

A heart defect that causes a hole (shunt) to develop between two chambers of heart is the most common cause of Eisenmenger syndrome. This hole causes blood to circulate abnormally in heart and lungs. Increased blood flow returns to lungs instead of going to the rest of body. The blood vessels in lung arteries become stiff and narrow, increasing the pressure in lungs' arteries. This permanently damages the blood vessels in lungs.

Incidence

- The frequency of pulmonary hypertension and the subsequent development of reversed shunting vary depending on the specific heart defect and operative interventions.
- Approximately 50% of infants with a large, nonrestrictive VSD or patent ductus arteriosus (PDA) develop pulmonary hypertension by early childhood.

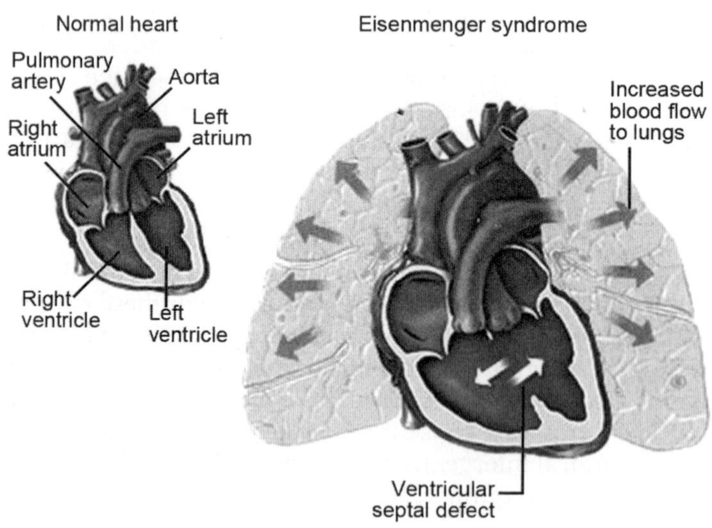

Fig. 6.66: Comparison of normal and Eisenmenger heart

- Forty percent of patients with VSD or PDA and transposition of the great arteries develop pulmonary hypertension within the first year of life.
- The natural history of a large secundum Atrial Septal Defect (ASD) differs in that the 10% of cases that progress to pulmonary hypertension do so more slowly and usually not until after the third decade of life.
- All children with persistent truncus arteriosus and unrestricted pulmonary blood flow, and almost all patients with common atrioventricular canal, develop severe pulmonary hypertension by the second year of life.
- The frequency of pulmonary hypertension in surgically created systemic-to-pulmonary shunts varies depending on size and anatomy.
- Ten percent of those with a *Blalock-Taussig anastomosis* (subclavian artery to pulmonary artery) develop pulmonary hypertension compared to 30% of those with a Waterston (ascending aorta to pulmonary artery) or a Potts (descending aorta to pulmonary artery) shunt.

Causes

Eisenmenger syndrome, the cause of their condition is due to a hole (shunt) between the main blood vessels or chambers of heart. This shunt is a heart defect you are born with (congenital). Heart defects that can cause Eisenmenger syndrome include:

- *Ventricular septal defect:* This shunt in the wall of tissue that divides the right and left sides of heart's main pumping chambers (ventricles) is the most common cause of Eisenmenger syndrome.
- *Atrial septal defect:* An atrial septal defect is a shunt in the wall of tissue that divides the right and left sides of the upper chambers of heart (atria).
- *Patent ductus arteriosus:* This heart defect is an opening between the pulmonary artery that carries oxygen-poor blood to the lungs and the artery that carries oxygen-rich blood to the rest of body (aorta).
- *Atrioventricular canal defect:* In this heart defect, there is a large hole in the center of the heart where the walls between the upper chambers (atria) and lower chambers (ventricles) meet. Some of the valves in heart also may not function properly.

Signs and Symptoms

General Signs and Symptoms

- Bluish or grayish skin color (cyanosis)
- Large, rounded fingernails or toenails (clubbing)
- Easily tiring and shortness of breath with activity
- Shortness of breath while at rest
- Chest pain or tightness
- Skipped or racing heartbeats (palpitations)
- Fainting (syncope)
- Coughing up blood (hemoptysis)
- Dizziness
- Numbness or tingling in the fingers or toes

- Headaches
- Abdominal swelling.

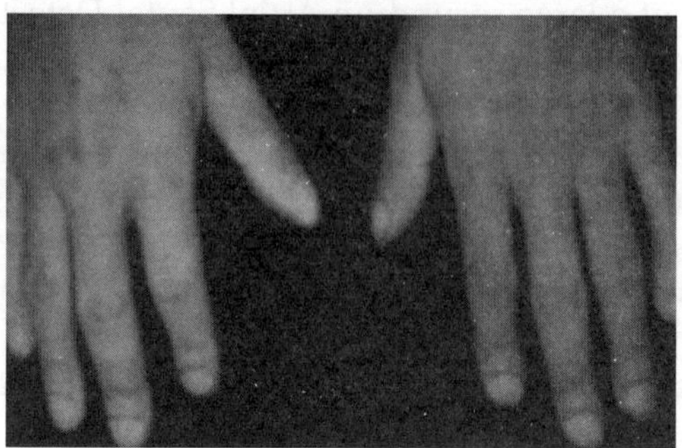

Clubbing and cyanosis in Eisenmenger
Clubbing and cyanosis of the fingers in patient with Eisenmenger syndrome due to an atrial septal defect.

Specific Signs and Symptoms

Symptoms related specifically to pulmonary hypertension result from the inability to increase pulmonary blood flow in response to physiological stress. Other symptoms are caused by the variety of multisystem complications associated with cyanotic congenital heart disease.

Pulmonary hypertension	**Heart failure**
• Breathlessness	• Exertional dyspnea
• Fatigue	• Orthopnea
• Lethargy	• Paroxysmal nocturnal dyspnea
• Severely reduced exercise tolerance with a prolonged recovery phase	• Edema
• Presyncope	• Ascites
• Syncope	• Anorexia
Erythrocytosis	• Nausea
• Myalgias	**Bleeding tendency**
• Muscle weakness	• Mild mucocutaneous bleeding
• Anorexia	• Epistaxis
• Fatigue	• Menorrhagia
• Lassitude	• Pulmonary hemorrhage
• Paresthesias of the digits and lips	**Vasodilation**
• Tinnitus	• Presyncope
• Blurred or double vision	• Syncope
• Scotomata (visual migraine)	**Cholelithiasis**
• Headache	• Right upper quadrant pain
• Dizziness	• Biliary colic
• Decreased alertness	• Fever

Contd...

Contd...

Pulmonary hypertension	Heart failure
Nephrolithiasis	• Pale stools
• Renal colic	• Jaundice
• Secondary gout	• Paradoxical embolus can cause symptoms of localized vascular insufficiency end-organ ischemia.
• Joint pain and swelling	• Hypertrophic osteoarthropathy can cause long bone pain and tenderness.
	• Retinal complications include episodes of transient visual loss and spontaneous hyphemas (completely block vision)

Diagnostic Evaluation

Physical Examination Findings of Cardiovascular

- Central cyanosis (differential cyanosis in the case of a PDA)
- Clubbing
- Jugular venous pulse wave may be A-wave dominant, and, in the presence of a significant tricuspid regurgitation, the V-wave may be prominent; central venous pressure may be elevated.
- Precordial palpation reveals a right ventricular heave and, frequently, a palpable S_2.
- Loud P_2
- High-pitched early diastolic murmur of pulmonic insufficiency
- Right-sided fourth heart sound
- Pulmonary ejection click
- Single S_2
- As the pulmonary vascular resistance progressively rises, the holosystolic murmur of nonrestrictive VSD shortens and softens, first becoming early systolic in timing, before disappearing entirely as the shunt is reversed.
- The continuous murmur of a PDA disappears when Eisenmenger physiology develops; a short systolic murmur may remain audible.

Laboratory Studies

- Complete blood count
  - Erythrocytosis increases hematocrit and hemoglobin concentration
  - Phlebotomy-related iron deficiency decreases the mean corpuscular volume and mean corpuscular hemoglobin concentration.
- Red cell mass is increased with erythrocytosis
- Bleeding time is prolonged by platelet dysfunction
- Biochemical profile
  - Increased conjugated bilirubin
  - Increased uric acid
  - Urea and creatinine sometimes elevated

- Erythrocytic hypoglycemia is an artifactually low blood glucose level caused by increased in vitro glycolysis in the setting of increased red cell mass.
- Iron studies
  - Reduced serum ferritin due to phlebotomy-related iron store reduction
  - Increased total iron binding capacity.
- Urine biochemical analysis reveals proteinuria
- Arterial blood gases
  - Reduced resting $PaCO_2$ due to resting tachypnea and reduced PaO_2 due to right-to-left shunting
  - Mixed respiratory and metabolic acidosis.

Imaging Studies

Chest Radiograph

- Right ventricular and right atrial enlargement
- Features of pulmonary hypertension, including dilated main pulmonary artery, increased hilar vascular markings, and pruned peripheral vessels.

Transthoracic Echocardiogram

- The structural cardiac defect responsible for the shunt can be defined by the two-dimensional imaging
- The location of cardiac shunt can usually be demonstrated by color doppler
- The pressure gradient across the defect can be estimated
- Estimated pulmonary artery systolic and diastolic pressures
- Left and right ventricular size and function: A study by Salehian et al reported that left ventricular dysfunction (defined as LVEF < 50%), right ventricular hypertrophy, and signs and symptoms of heart failure predict mortality in patients with Eisenmenger syndrome
- Identification of surgical systemic-to-pulmonary shunts
- The addition of supine bicycle ergometry can demonstrate increased right-to-left shunting with exercise.

Other Tests

- Electrocardiogram
  - Almost always abnormal results and includes signs of right heart hypertrophy in addition to abnormalities associated with the underlying defect
  - Frontal plane QRS right axis deviation
  - Tall monophasic R wave in V_1, deep S wave in V_6, ± ST and T wave abnormalities
  - P pulmonale.

Histological Findings

In severe pulmonary vascular disease, histological analysis reveals abnormal extension of muscle into small peripheral arteries, severe medial smooth muscle hypertrophy of existing muscular arteries, plexiform lesions and increased intercellular material, and a reduction in the overall concentration and size of arteries.

Management

Medical Management

- Fluid balance and climate control
  - Avoid sudden fluid shifts or dehydration, which may increase right-to-left shunting.
  - Avoid very hot or humid conditions, which may exacerbate vasodilation, causing syncope and increased right-to-left shunting.
- Oxygen therapy
  - The use of oxygen supplementation is controversial.
  - Oxygen therapy has been shown to have no impact on exercise capacity and survival in adult patients with Eisenmenger syndrome.
  - Some patients might benefit from nocturnal supplementation, although it is most useful as a bridge to heart-lung transplant.
- Pulmonary vasodilator therapy
- *Anticoagulation:* Silversides et al reported that the incidence of proximal pulmonary artery thrombus in this patient population was 21%. This study raised the issue of anticoagulation in Eisenmenger patients. These patients are at increased risk of bleeding; hence, the use of anticoagulation is still not routinely recommended.
- Contraception, pregnancy and genetic counseling
  - Avoid pregnancy. Tubal ligation is strongly recommended in women with Eisenmenger syndrome.
  - If patients refuse tubal ligation, hormone therapy (controlled release levonorgestrel or norethindrone and ethinyl estradiol preparations) is preferred over intrauterine devices, which can cause significant menorrhagia and potentially increase the risk of endocarditis.
  - The fetal mortality rate is approximately 25%, and the maternal mortality rate exceeds 50%.
  - Therapeutic abortion is recommended for women in the early stages of pregnancy.
  - The risk of congenital heart defects in offspring is approximately 10% and sometimes higher, depending on the primary natural cardiac defect.
  - Fetal echocardiography is recommended for pregnant patients or siblings.

Medication

The medical treatment of Eisenmenger syndrome is directed toward improvement of symptoms related to heart failure and pulmonary hypertension and preventing and managing complications related to cyanotic congenital heart disease.

Diuretics

These agents are useful to remove fluid and reduce preload and afterload in the treatment of heart failure.

Furosemide (Lasix)

Increases excretion of water by interfering with chloride-binding cotransport system, which in turn results inhibits sodium and chloride reabsorption in the ascending loop of Henle and distal renal tubule. Dose must be individualized to patient. Depending on response, administer at increments of 20–40 mg, no sooner than 6–8 h after the previous dose, until desired diuresis occurs. When treating infants, titrate with 1 mg/kg per dose increments until a satisfactory effect is achieved.

Digoxin (Lanoxin, Lanoxicaps)

Cardiac glycoside with direct inotropic effects in addition to indirect effects on the cardiovascular system. Acts directly on cardiac muscle, increasing myocardial systolic contractions. Its indirect actions result in increased carotid sinus nerve activity and enhanced sympathetic withdrawal for any given increase in mean arterial pressure.

Epoprostenol (Flolan)

Strong vasodilator of all vascular beds. May decrease thrombogenesis and platelet clumping in the lungs by inhibiting platelet aggregation. Continuous chronic infusion should be administered through a central venous catheter.

Surgical Management

Procedures

Cardiac catheterization can be of value, after collecting clinical and noninvasive data, to confirm and/or demonstrate the following:

- Severity of pulmonary arterial hypertension
- Conduit patency and pressure gradient
- Coexisting coronary artery anomalies (rare)
- Degree of shunting
- Heart-lung transplantation
  - Heart-lung transplantation is the procedure of choice if repair of the underlying cardiac defect is not possible.
  - It was performed successfully for the first time in 1981. Since then, the outcome has improved due to better immunosuppressive therapy, new antiviral agents, and improved patient selection.
  - Reported actuarial survival rates are 68% at 1 year, 43% at 5 years, and 23% at 10 years.
  - The main complications are infection, rejection, and obliterative bronchiolitis.
- Bilateral lung transplantation
  - Repair of the underlying cardiac defect is required, but it is considered the preferable procedure if the cardiac defect is simple.
  - Bilateral lung transplantation is better than single-lung transplantation in terms of mortality, New York Heart Association functional class, cardiac output, and postoperative pulmonary edema.
- Corrective surgery
  - Repair of the primary defect is contraindicated in the context of established severe pulmonary arterial hypertension. However, corrective surgery may be possible in certain cases if a significant degree of left-to-right shunting remains and if responsiveness of the pulmonary circulation to vasodilator therapy can be demonstrated.

- Limitations include a transient dynamic right ventricular outflow tract obstruction, and exact indications for this approach have not yet been defined.

Nursing Management

- Transfer patient to a specialized cardiology unit
- Monitor patient in an intensive care unit
- Patient should follow-up at a specialized cardiology clinic within 2 weeks of discharge, and every 3 months when stable.

Diet

- Patients with right-sided congestive heart failure should avoid excessive sodium intake.
- Sodium restriction must be balanced with the need to maintain intravascular volume.

Activity

- Intense athletic activities carry the risk of sudden death
- Patients should not participate in competitive sports
- In certain patients, an exercise prescription can be individualized based on exercise testing that documents a level of activity that meets the following three criteria:
    1. Oxygen saturations remain greater than 80%
    2. No symptomatic arrhythmias occur
    3. No evidence of symptomatic ventricular dysfunction is present.

Prevention Measures

- Educate patients regarding infective endocarditis risk reduction
- Avoid situations that exacerbate vasodilation
- Avoid abrupt, strenuous, or isometric exercise
- Restrict activities that may result in further oxygen desaturation, symptomatic arrhythmias, or right ventricular dysfunction
- Stop steady-state exercise at onset of symptoms.

Prognosis

- Survival is limited by complications and deteriorating ventricular function
- Sudden death always is a threat.

ACYANOTIC HEART DISEASES

Introduction

The congenital heart defects that do not normally interfere with the amount of oxygen or blood that reaches the tissues of the body are called acyanotic heart defects. A bluish tint of the skin is not common in babies with acyanotic heart defects, although it may occur. If a bluish tint occurs, it often is during activities when the baby needs more oxygen, such as when crying and feeding.

Types of Acyanotic Heart Diseases

Acyanotic heart diseases (left to right shunt)	
Increased pulmonary blood flow	**Obstructive heart diseases**
• VSD (Ventricular septal defect)	• Coarctation of aorta (CoA)
• ASD (Atrial septal defect)	• Pulmonary stenosis (PS)
• PDA (Patent ductus arteriosus)	• Aortic stenosis (AS)
• Pulmonary hypertension (PH)	• Congenital mitral stenosis
• Atrial ventricular canal (AVC)	• Hypoxemia

Ventricular Septal Defect (VSD)

Introduction

A ventricular septal defect (VSD), a hole in the heart, is a common heart defect that is present at birth (congenital). The hole occurs in the wall that separates the heart's lower chambers (septum) and allows blood to pass from the left to the right side of the heart. The oxygen-rich blood then gets pumped back to the lungs instead of out to the body, causing the heart to work harder. A small ventricular septal defect may cause no problems, and many small VSDs close on their own. Larger VSDs need surgical repair early in life to prevent complications.

The ventricular septum is made up of different types of tissue, with one part composed of mainly muscle and another part made of thinner, fibrous tissue. The location and size of the hole within the septum will determine in part the consequences of the ventricular septal defect.

Definition

Ventricular septal defect defined as one or more holes in the wall that separates the right and left ventricles of the heart. Ventricular septal defect is one of the most common congenital (present from birth) heart defects.

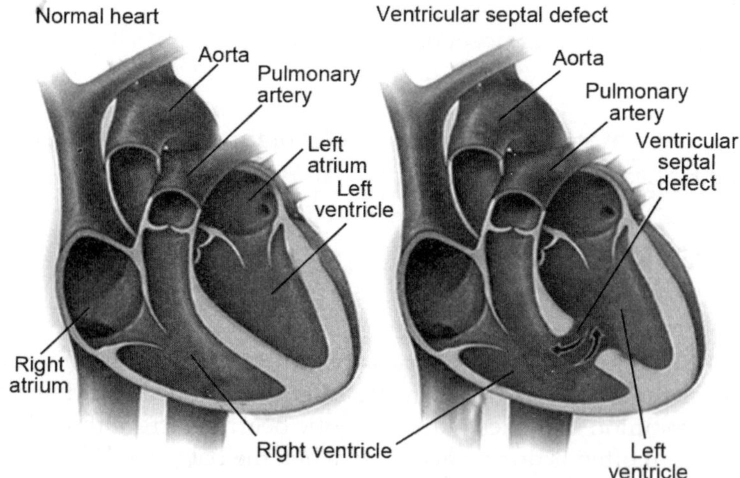

Fig. 6.67: Anatomical difference of normal and VSD heart

A ventricular septal defect (VSD) is a defect in the septum between the right and left ventricle. The septum is a wall that separates the heart's left and right sides. Septal defects are sometimes called a 'hole' in the heart. It is the most common congenital heart defect in the newborn; it is less common in older children and adults because some VSDs close on their own. —*American Heart Association*

Causes

- The exact cause is not known
- Genetics and environmental factors probably play a role. Ventricular reptal defects can occur alone or with other congenital heart defects
- During fetal development, a ventricular septal defect occurs when the muscular wall separating the heart into left and right sides (septum) fails to form fully between the lower chambers of the heart (ventricles)
- Ventricular septal defect is one of the most common congenital heart defects. The baby may have no symptoms, and the hole can eventually close as the wall continues to grow after birth. If the hole is large, too much blood will be pumped to the lungs, leading to heart failure.

Types of VSD

- *Type 1:* Subarterial/Supracristal/Infundibular
  - Found in 5–7% of patients, more in Asians, related to the pulmonary valve
- *Type 2:* Perimembranous/Paramembranous
  - Most common variety found in 70%
- *Type 3:* Inlet/AV canal type
  - Commonly associated with atrioventricular septal defect, found in about 5%
- *Type 4:* Muscular
  - Located in the muscular septum, found in 20%. Can be subclassified again based on the location into anterior, apical, posterior and mid.

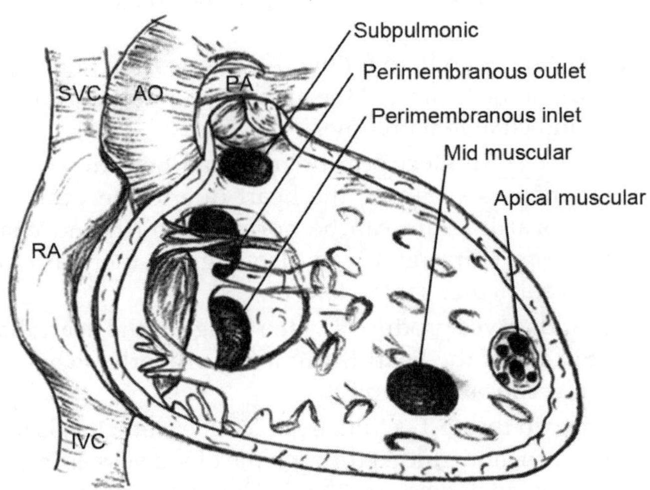

Fig. 6.68: Types of VSD

Abbreviation: SVC: Superior vena cava; AO: Aorta; RA: Right atrium; IVC: Inferior vena cava

Signs and Symptoms

Ventricular septal defects have a very characteristic murmur, to the point where a cardiologist may be able to pinpoint the location and estimate the size of a ventricular septal defect just by how it sounds.

Symptoms

- Poor eating, failure to thrive
- Fast breathing or breathlessness
- Easy tiring.

The most common symptoms include:

- Shortness of breath
- Fast breathing
- Hard breathing
- Paleness
- Failure to gain weight
- Fast heart rate
- Sweating while feeding
- Frequent respiratory infections.

Diagnostic Evaluation

Most ventricular septal defects can be diagnosed on physical exam, due to their characteristic murmur. The murmur can change with time either due to the hole closing, or in the case of large ventricular septal defects, due to more blood flow across the hole.

The heart can sometimes be seen or felt to be beating hard because of the extra work it is performing. Babies can be continuously breathing fast or hard and have a fast heart rate. Listening with a stethoscope usually reveals a heart murmur (the sound of the blood crossing the hole). The loudness of the murmur is related to the size of the defect and amount of blood crossing the defect.

- *Chest X-ray:* A chest X-ray can help follow the progression of congestive heart failure by looking at the size of the heart and the amount of blood flow to the lungs. This may be normal at birth and change with time.
- *Electrocardiogram (ECG):* An electrocardiogram can help determine the sizes of the chambers to see if there is strain on the heart due to the ventricular septal defect. However, the electrocardiogram can be normal at birth and change with time as congestive heart failure worsens. It can also suggest there are other heart defects associated with the ventricular septal defect.
- *Echocardiogram:* Sound waves produce a video image of the heart that can help doctors see if there is a VSD and if the heart is pumping properly. Echocardiography can be used on a fetus (fetal echocardiography).
- *Cardiac catheterization:* In this test, a thin, flexible tube (catheter) is inserted into a blood vessel at the groin or arm and guided through the blood vessels into the heart. Through catheterization, doctors can diagnose congenital heart defects and determine the function of the heart valves and chambers.

- *Pulse oximetry:* A small clip on the fingertip measures the amount of oxygen in the blood.
- *MRI of the heart*: Used to find out how much blood is getting to the lungs.

Management

The defect is small, no treatment is usually needed. However, the baby should be closely monitored by a health care provider to make sure that the hole eventually closes properly and signs of heart failure do not occur. Babies with a large VSD who have symptoms related to heart failure may need medicine to control the symptoms and surgery to close the hole. Medications may include digitalis (digoxin) and diuretics. If symptoms continue despite medication, surgery to close the defect with a Gore-tex patch is needed. Some VSDs can be closed with a special device during a cardiac catheterization, although this is infrequently done. Surgery for a VSD with no symptoms is controversial. This should be carefully discussed with your health care provider.

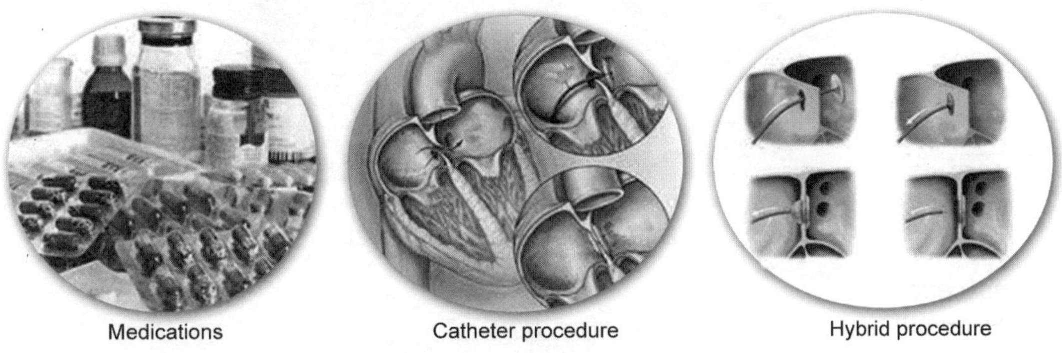

Fig. 6.69: Treatment of VSD

Medical Management

Medications for ventricular septal defect may include those to:

- *Increase the strength of the heart's contractions:* Examples include digoxin (Lanoxin).
- *Decrease the amount of fluid in circulation and in the lungs:* Doing so reduces the volume of blood that must be pumped. These medications, called diuretics, include furosemide (Lasix).
- *Keep the heartbeat regular:* Examples include beta blockers (Lopressor, Inderal LA, others) and digoxin (Lanoxin, Lanoxin Pediatric).

Surgical Management

Surgical treatment for ventricular septal defects involves plugging or patching the abnormal opening between the ventricles, using one of these procedures:

- *Surgical repair:* This procedure of choice in most cases usually involves open-heart surgery under general anesthesia. The surgery requires a heart-lung machine and an incision in the chest. The doctor uses a patch or stitches to close the hole.
- *Catheter procedure:* Closing a VSD during catheterization does not require opening the chest. Rather, the doctor inserts a thin tube (catheter) into a blood vessel in the groin and guides it to the heart. The doctor then uses a specially sized mesh device to close the hole.

- *Hybrid procedure:* A hybrid procedure uses surgical and catheter-based techniques. Access to the heart is usually through a small incision, and the procedure may be performed without stopping the heart and using the heart-lung machine. A device closes the VSD via a catheter placed through the incision. Recovery from this procedure is quicker than with standard surgery.

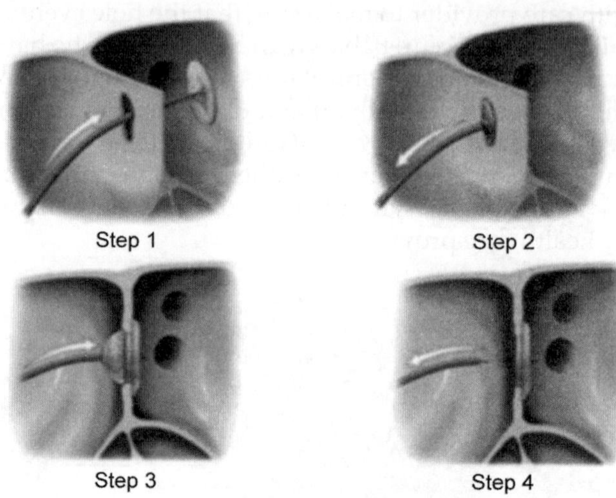

Fig. 6.70: Hybrid procedure for VSD

Complications

- Heart failure
- Infective endocarditis (bacterial infection of the heart)
- Aortic insufficiency (leaking of the valve that separates the left ventricle from the aorta)
- Damage to the electrical conduction system of the heart during surgery (causing arrhythmias)
- Delayed growth and development (failure to thrive in infancy)
- Pulmonary hypertension (high blood pressure in the lungs) leading to failure of the right side of the heart.

Most often, this condition is diagnosed during routine examination of an infant. Call your infant's health care provider if the baby seems to be having difficulty breathing, or if the baby seems to have an unusual number of respiratory infections.

Prevention

Except for the case of heart attack associated VSD, this condition is always present at birth. Drinking alcohol and using the antiseizure medicines depakote and dilantin during pregnancy have been associated with increased incidence of VSDs. Other than avoiding these things during pregnancy, there is no known way to prevent a VSD.

Prognosis

Many small defects will close on their own. For those defects that do not spontaneously close, the outcome is good with surgical repair. Complications may result if a large defect is not treated.

ATRIAL SEPTAL DEFECT (ASD)

Introduction

This defect allows oxygen-rich blood to leak into the oxygen-poor blood chambers in the heart. ASD is a defect in the septum between the heart's two upper chambers (atria). The condition is present from birth (congenital). Small atrial septal defects may close on their own during infancy or early childhood. Large and long-standing atrial septal defects can damage your heart and lungs. Small defects may never cause a problem and may be found incidentally. An adult who has had an undetected atrial septal defect for decades may have a shortened life span from heart failure or high blood pressure that affects the arteries in the lungs (pulmonary hypertension).

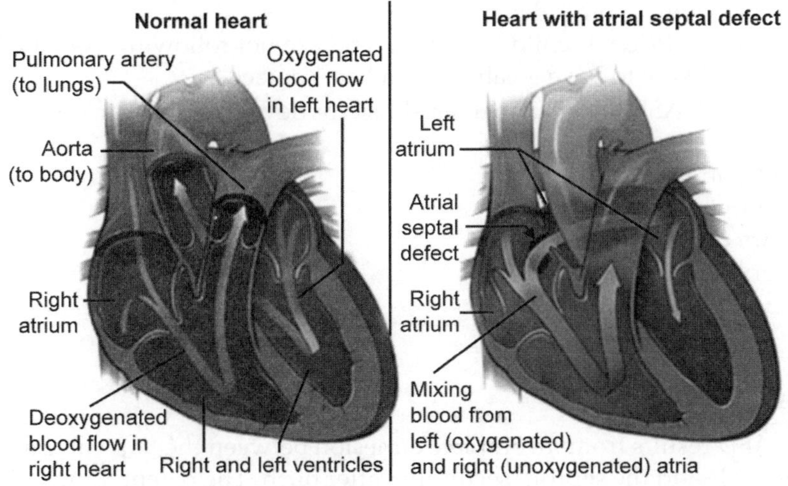

Fig. 6.71: Anatomical difference between normal and ASD heart

Definition

An atrial septal defect (ASD) is defined as a shunt in the wall between the two upper chambers of your heart (atria). Small atrial septal defects may close on their own during infancy or early childhood.

Incidence

Isolated secundum atrial septal defects account for approximately 7% of congenital cardiac defects. Congenital heart defects of significance occur in approximately 8 per 1000 live births. Therefore, 5–6 cases of secundum atrial septal defect occur per 10,000 live births. This number refers only to defects that are large enough to come to clinical attention. Many small defects that remain undetected occur in addition to numerous cases of patent foramen ovale, as mentioned above.

Causes

- Genetics and environmental factors
- Down syndrome
- Ebstein's anomaly

- Fetal alcohol syndrome
- Holt–Oram syndrome
- Lutembacher's syndrome.

Risk Factors

- *Rubella infection:* Becoming infected with rubella (German measles) during the first few months of pregnancy can increase the risk of fetal heart defects.
- *Drug, tobacco or alcohol use, or exposure to certain substances:* Use of certain medications, tobacco, alcohol or drugs, such as cocaine, during pregnancy can harm the developing fetus.
- *Diabetes or lupus:* If child have diabetes or lupus, you may be more likely to have a baby with a heart defect.
- *Obesity:* Being extremely overweight (obese) may play a role in increasing the risk of having a baby with a birth defect.
- *Phenylketonuria (PKU):* If child have PKU and are not following your PKU meal plan, may be more likely to have a baby with a heart defect.

Individuals with ASD are at an increased risk for developing a number of complications including:

- Atrial fibrillation (in adults)
- Heart failure
- Pulmonary overcirculation
- Pulmonary hypertension
- Stroke.

Types

Ostium Secundum ASD

This type of ASD results from incomplete adhesion between the flap valve associated with the foramen ovale and the septum secundum after birth. The patent foramen ovale usually

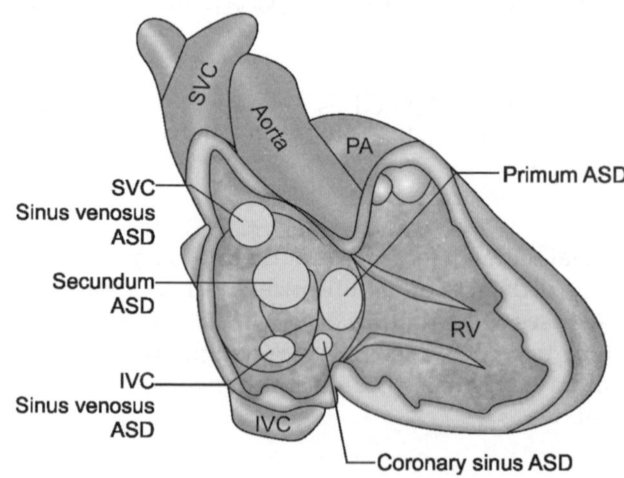

Fig. 6.72: Types of ASD
Abbreviation: SVC: Superior vena cava; ASD: Atrial septal defect; PA-Pulmonary artery; RV-Right ventricle: IVC: Inferior vena cava

results from abnormal resorption of the septum primum during the formation of the foramen secundum. Resorption in abnormal locations causes a fenestrated or netlike septum primum. Excessive resorption of the septum primum results in a short septum primum that does not close the foramen ovale. An abnormally large foramen ovale can occur as a result of defective development of the septum secundum. The normal septum primum does not close this type of abnormal foramen ovale at birth. A combination of excessive resorption of the septum primum and a large foramen ovale produces a large ostium secundum ASD.

Ostium Primum ASD

These defects are caused by incomplete fusion of septum primum with the endocardial cushion. The defect lies immediately adjacent to the atrioventricular (AV) valves, either of which may be deformed and incompetent. In most cases, only the anterior or septal leaflet of the mitral valve is displaced, and it is commonly cleft. The tricuspid valve is usually not involved.

Sinus Venosus ASD

Abnormal fusion between the embryologic sinus venosus and the atrium causes these defects. In most cases, the defect lies superior in the atrial septum near the entry of superior vena cava. Often there is associated anomalous drainage of the right superior pulmonary vein. The relatively uncommon inferior type is associated with partial anomalous drainage of the right inferior pulmonary vein. Anomalous drainage can be into the right atrium, the superior vena cava, or the inferior vena cava.

Coronary Sinus ASD

Coronary sinus defect is characterized by unroofed coronary sinus and persistent left superior vena cava that drains into the left atrium. A dilated coronary sinus often suggests this defect. This can result is desaturation due to right-to-left shunt into the left atrium. The diagnosis can be made by injecting contrast agent into left upper extremity; coronary sinus opacification precedes right atrial opacification.

Pathophysiology

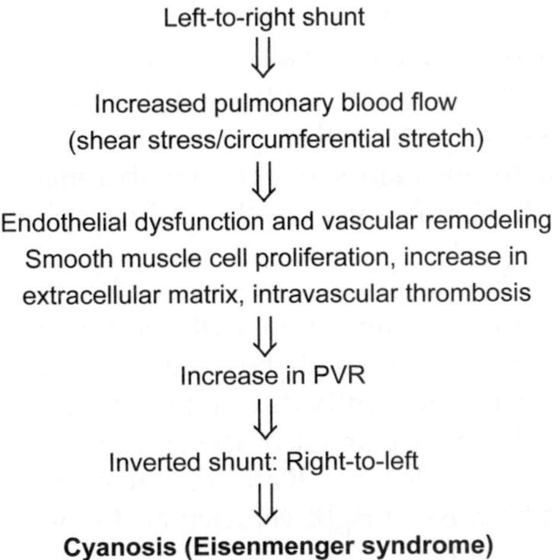

Signs and Symptoms

The child with ostium secundum atrial septal defects rarely has symptoms resulting directly from the defect. Decreased exercise tolerance in relation to peers may occur in older children and young adults. Some reports suggest that children with secundum atrial septal defects are smaller than other children; if so, this is an association. A cause-and-effect relationship has not been established.

Symptoms that may occur can include:

- Difficulty breathing (dyspnea)
- Frequent respiratory infections in children
- Shortness of breath with activity
- Fatigue
- Swelling of legs, feet or abdomen
- Heart palpitations or skipped beats
- Frequent lung infections
- Stroke
- Heart murmur, a whooshing sound that can be heard through a stethoscope.

Diagnostic Evaluation

Laboratory Studies

There is no specific laboratory blood tests are necessary in the evaluation of patients with an ostium secundum atrial septal defect. A small degree of right-to-left shunt may occur with a large atrial septal defect. This may be detected by observing a mild decrease in cutaneous oxygen saturation to 93–95%. Although this may increase hemoglobin and hematocrit minimally, it is insufficient to cause clinical cyanosis.

Imaging Studies

- Routine chest radiography is not essential in the evaluation of a child with a suspected secundum atrial septal defect. They demonstrate increased pulmonary arterial vascularity with a prominent pulmonic trunk, right atrial enlargement, no evidence of left atrial enlargement, and right ventricular dilation.
- Echocardiography is essential in the evaluation of a child with a suspected atrial septal defect. The right atrium and right ventricle are dilated; paradoxical motion of the ventricular septum is usually present.
- MRI is not indicated in the evaluation of a child with a suspected secundum atrial septal defect and does not add significantly to echocardiography findings.

Other Tests

An ECG demonstrates sinus rhythm, often with evidence of right atrial enlargement manifested by tall, peaked P waves (usually best seen in leads II and V_2) and prolongation of the PR interval. The QRS axis is slightly directed to the right (+ 100°), and the precordial leads reveal right ventricular enlargement of the so-called volume overload type that is characterized by an rSR′ pattern in leads V_3 R and V_1 with normal T waves. The QRS duration may be mildly prolonged because of right ventricular dilation. This mimics the finding in right ventricular conduction delay.

A significant proportion (20–40%) of children with secundum atrial septal defect may not have abnormal ECG findings. Uncommonly, a patient with a secundum atrial septal defect may demonstrate a superior QRS axis with right ventricular enlargement, mimicking findings observed in the ECG of a patient with an ostium primum atrial septal defect (Atrial Septal Defect, Ostium Primum).

Management

Medical Management

Small-to-moderate-sized ostium secundum atrial septal defects diagnosed in the infant demonstrate significant likelihood of either spontaneous closure or reduction in size to the point that medical intervention no longer is indicated. Such patients should be followed until age 3 to 4 years before considering either device use or surgical closure.

Medication

Drug therapy is not currently a component of the standard of care for this condition. No specific medications are indicated for patients with a secundum atrial septal defect. Bacterial endocarditis prophylaxis is required for the first 6 months following device closure or surgical closure with a patch. Preoperatively, antibiotic prophylaxis is not required in an isolated ostium secundum atrial septal defect. For information regarding antibiotics used for endocarditis prophylaxis, see Antibiotic Prophylactic Regimens for Endocarditis.

Surgical Management

Minimally invasive cardiac surgery techniques allow closure without the use of blood or blood products in appropriately sized patients.

- The skin incision is short because complete vertical division of the sternum is not necessary.
- If the defect is moderate in size and oval in shape, direct suture closure may be appropriate. Larger or rounder defects require patch closure. The patch can be fashioned from the patient's pericardium or made from Dacron.
- Results of surgery are excellent; a 100% closure rate should be achieved. Risk of mortality does not exceed that of general anesthesia.
- Inpatient hospital stay now averages 2–3 days. Perform postoperative echocardiography to confirm closure.
- Postoperative care includes bacterial endocarditis precautions for 6 months if a patch was placed.

Open-heart Surgery

This type of surgery is done under general anesthesia and requires the use of a heart-lung machine. Through an incision in the chest, surgeons use patches to close the hole. This procedure is the preferred treatment for certain types of atrial septal defects (primum, sinus venosus and coronary sinus), and these types of atrial defects can only be repaired through open-heart surgery.

Cardiac Catheterization

- Transcatheter device closure of secundum atrial septal defect now represents a standard of care for this abnormality. Experience at centers throughout the world is extensive; the success rate has been high, and the risk of complications has been low. Indication for closure in the pediatric age range is a shunt of sufficient size to be clinically apparent. The reason for closure is to prevent development of complications (e.g. atrial dysrhythmia, right heart dysfunction) that may appear in the adult. Small defects in children that are detectable only by echocardiography do not require closure.

- In adult patients who experience a suspected thrombotic stroke and who manifest a patent foramen ovale (15–20% of all adults demonstrate a patent foramen ovale on echocardiography), concern arises that the stroke may have been caused by a paradoxical embolus. In these patients, device closure of the communication is often recommended and accomplished. Studies remain controversial regarding the appropriateness of this treatment.
- Transcatheter device occlusion of a secundum atrial septal defect should be accomplished only by physicians properly trained and experienced in the procedure. Proper sizing of the defect and anatomic evaluation to assure reliable seating of the device is essential.
- The device is placed in the atrial septum via a catheter introduced into a femoral vein. Most operators advise monitoring the procedure with transesophageal echocardiography. Multiple studies indicate a high degree of success, with complete closure rates only slightly less than those obtained by surgery.
- Studies comparing device closure with surgery establish that hospital stay is shorter in patients undergoing device closure. Total costs of the 2 techniques do not significantly differ, apparently because of the cost of the device.
- Complications of device occlusion include hemorrhage, vascular disruption, pain, nausea and vomiting, and arterial or venous obstruction from thrombosis or spasm. Other complications include rupture of blood vessel, tachyarrhythmias, bradyarrhythmias, and vascular occlusion. Embolization of the device during placement rarely occurs but can result in emergency surgery for removal. The most common complication is incomplete closure of the defect.

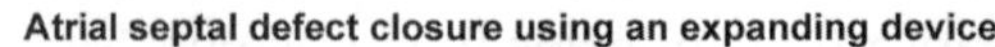

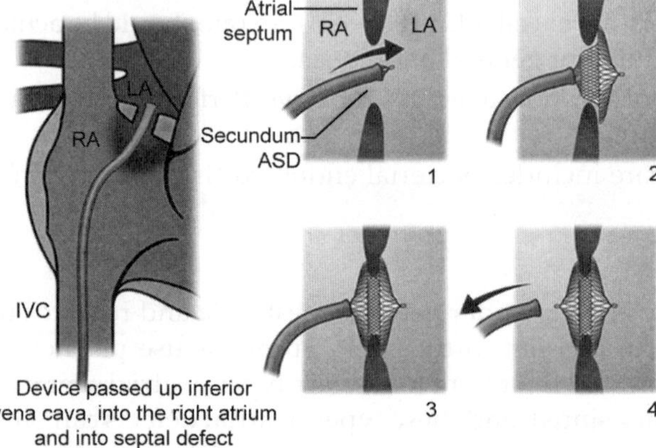

Fig. 6.73: Atrial septal defect closure procedures
Abbreviation: RA: Right atrium; LA: Left atrium; IVC: Inferior vena cava; ASD: Atrial septal defect

Complications

- Surgical damage to the sinoatrial node occurs rarely when experienced individuals accomplish closure. Short and long-term postoperative rhythm disturbances can occur, however, particularly when closure of a large defect is delayed beyond early childhood (i.e. > 8 y).
- Late complications of device closure can include rhythm disturbance, perforation of the heart, fracture of the supporting structures of the device, and residual shunts. Long-term late complications remain unknown.

Nursing Management

- No further inpatient care is required in patients with ostium secundum atrial septal defect.
- If the immediate postoperative echocardiography confirms complete closure, a follow-up visit one year following closure is adequate to evaluate possible long-term complications (rare).
- Patients who undergo closure of a large defect late in childhood (when > 8 y) should be advised to continue infrequent cardiology evaluations with electrocardiographic studies approximately every 5 years to monitor for the possible occurrence of a dysrhythmia.
- Patients who undergo device closure of a secundum atrial septal defect should continue cardiology evaluations until long-term published studies establish the absence of late complications.
- No medications are required, except bacterial endocarditis prophylaxis for 6 months following either device or patch closure.
- Evaluation and treatment should be carried out at a center specializing in congenital heart disease.

Activity

No activity restrictions are required except for a few weeks following either device closure or heart surgery.

Parental Education

- No patient restrictions are indicated. Families and patients should have some familiarity with symptoms of cardiac dysrhythmias.
- Genetic counseling is advised for all patients and their families, especially if other family members are affected.
- When a child with a secundum atrial septal defect reaches maturity education regarding the significance of the defect is advisable.

Prognosis

The surgical mortality rate should be less than 0.1%. If defects are closed in children younger than 8 years, the prognosis is excellent, with rare short-term or long-term cardiac abnormalities. Patients with incomplete closure or closure at older age remain at risk for development of cardiac rhythm disturbances. Whether closure of a secundum atrial septal defect in a person older than 40 years alters the patient's risk of either cardiac disability or limitation of life remains controversial.

PATENT DUCTUS ARTERIOSUS (PDA)

Introduction

Patent ductus arteriosus (PDA) is one of the more common congenital heart defects. Depending on the size of the patent ductus arteriosus, the gestational age of the neonate and the pulmonary vascular resistance, a premature neonate may develop life-threatening pulmonary over circulation in the first few days of life. During antenatal period the fetus's blood does not need to go to the lungs to get oxygenated. The ductus arteriosus is a hole that allows the blood to skip the circulation to the lungs. However, when the baby is born, the blood must receive oxygen in the lungs and this hole is supposed to close. If the ductus arteriosus is still open (or patent) the blood may skip this necessary step of circulation. The open hole is called the patent ductus arteriosus.

Definition

Patent ductus arteriosus (PDA) is defined as a persistent opening between two major blood vessels leading from the heart. The opening, called the ductus arteriosus is a normal part of a fetal heart circulatory system before birth that usually closes shortly after birth. If it remains open after birth also called a patent ductus arteriosus.

The ductus arteriosus is a fetal blood vessel that closes soon after birth. In a PDA, the vessel does not close and remains 'patent' (open), resulting in irregular transmission of blood between the aorta and the pulmonary artery. PDA is common in newborns with persistent respiratory problems such as hypoxia and has a high occurrence in premature newborns.

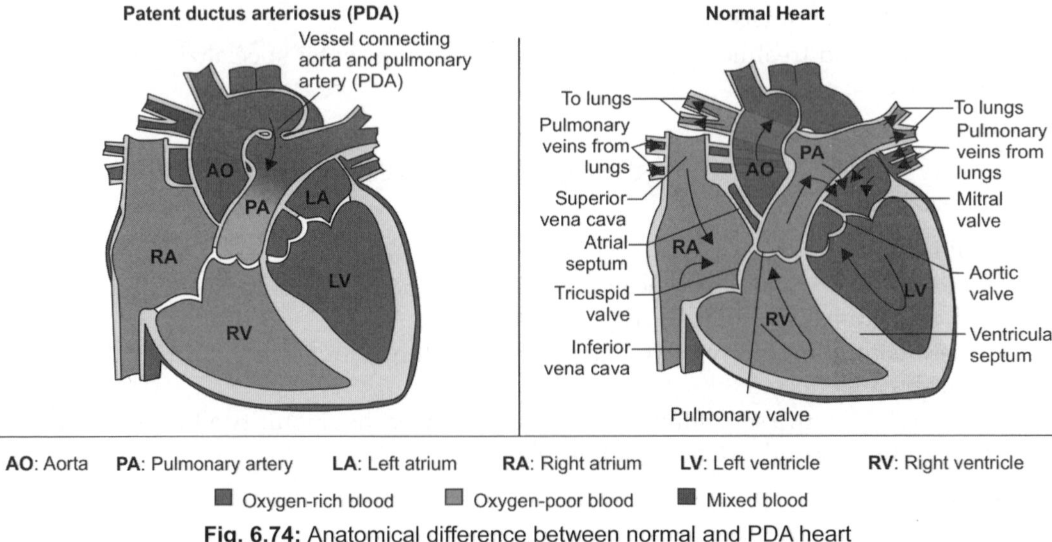

Fig. 6.74: Anatomical difference between normal and PDA heart

Incident

The estimated incidence in children born at term is between 0.02% and 0.006% of live births. This incidence is increased in children who are born prematurely, children with a history of perinatal asphyxia, and, possibly, children born at high altitude. Perinatal asphyxia usually only delays the closure of the ductus, and, over time, the ductus typically closes without specific therapy. The female-to-male ratio is 2:1 if not associated with other risk factors. In patients in whom the patent ductus arteriosus is associated with a specific teratogenic exposure, such as congenital rubella, the incidence is equal between the sexes.

The ductus arteriosus is always patent in the fetus if the cardiovascular system is otherwise normal. Normally, the ductus arteriosus closes functionally in the first 10–18 hours of life. Prematurity, perinatal distress, and hypoxia delay closure of the ductus arteriosus; however, most children who are found to have a ductus arteriosus have no history of precedent risk factors.

Causes

- Preterm birth
- Congenital rubella syndrome
- Chromosomal abnormalities (e.g. Down syndrome)
- Genetic conditions such as Loeys-Dietz syndrome (would also present with other heart defects)
- Genetic cause has not been determined
- Implicated teratogens include congenital rubella (associated with patent ductus arteriosus and pulmonary artery branch stenosis)
- Fetal alcohol syndrome, maternal amphetamine use and maternal phenytoin use.

Pathophysiology

A patent ductus arteriosus produces a left-to-right shunt. In other words, it allows blood to go from the systemic circulation to the pulmonary circulation. Therefore, pulmonary blood flow is excessive (see the image below).

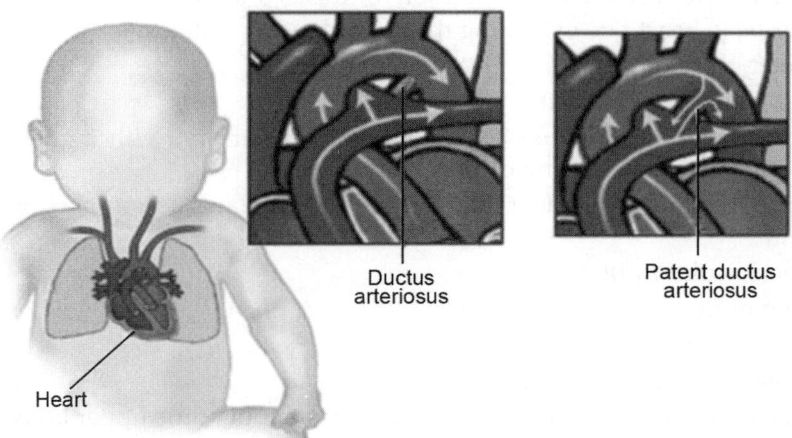

Fig. 6.75: Schematic diagram of left-to-right shunt of blood flow from descending aorta via patent ductus arteriosus (PDA) to main pulmonary artery

The magnitude of the excess pulmonary blood flow depends on relatively few factors. The larger the internal diameter of the narrowest portion of the ductus arteriosus, the larger the left-to-right shunt. If the ductus arteriosus is restrictive, then the length of the narrowed area also affects the magnitude of the shunt. A longer ductus is associated with a smaller shunt. Finally, the magnitude of the left-to-right shunt is partially controlled by the relationship of the pulmonary vascular resistance to the systemic vascular resistance.

If the systemic vascular resistance is high and/or the pulmonary vascular resistance is low, the flow through the ductus arteriosus is potentially large. Beginning at the ductus arteriosus, the course of blood flow in a typical patent ductus arteriosus with pulmonary overcirculation is as follows: patent ductus arteriosus, pulmonary arteries, pulmonary capillaries, pulmonary veins, left atrium, left ventricle, aorta, patent ductus arteriosus.

Therefore, a large left-to-right shunt through a patent ductus arteriosus results in left atrial and left ventricular enlargement. Additionally, the pulmonary veins and the ascending aorta can be dilated with a sufficiently large patent ductus arteriosus. Also, if little or no restriction is present at the level of the patent ductus arteriosus, pulmonary hypertension results.

The ductus arteriosus is normally patent during fetal life. This patency is promoted by continual production of prostaglandin E_2 (PGE2) by the ductus. Prostaglandin antagonism such as maternal use of nonsteroidal anti-inflammatory medications can cause fetal closure of the ductus arteriosus. This can be associated with severe fetal cardiovascular compromise.

Normal functional closure of the ductus arteriosus occurs by about 15 hours of life in healthy infants born at term. This occurs by abrupt contraction of the muscular wall of the ductus arteriosus, which is associated with increases in the partial pressure of oxygen (PO_2) coincident with the first breath.

Signs and Symptoms

The typical child with a patent ductus arteriosus (PDA) is asymptomatic. A history of premature birth, perinatal distress, or perinatal hypoxia may be present. Babies that have a more severe clinical course of hyaline membrane disease may have a higher prevalence of patent ductus arteriosus. The exact reason for this is unclear.

- Tachycardia (a heart rate exceeding the normal resting rate)
- Respiratory problems
- Dyspnea (shortness of breath)
- Heart murmur (usually from aorta to pulmonary artery, with higher flow during systole and lower flow during diastole)
- Cardiomegaly (enlarged heart, reflecting ventricular dilation and blood volume overload)
- Left subclavicular thrill
- Bounding pulse
- Widened pulse pressure
- Poor growth and development
- Cyanosis, i.e. Cyanosis of the lower extremities but not of the upper body.

Diagnostic Evaluation

Chest Radiography

Significantly left-to-right shunt through the patent ductus arteriosus is present, the pulmonary arteries, pulmonary veins, left atrium, and left ventricle are enlarged. Also the ascending aorta may be prominent. The chest radiographic findings are normal until the magnitude of the ratio of pulmonary to systemic circulation (QP/QS) exceeds 2:1. With marked pulmonary overcirculation, pulmonary edema may occur. In elderly individuals, the patent ductus arteriosus may calcify and may be visible on a standard radiograph.

Doppler Echocardiography

The echocardiographic findings are typically diagnostic. Relying on alternative imaging techniques to make the diagnosis of patent ductus arteriosus is unusual. By two-dimensional echocardiography, the patent ductus arteriosus can be seen most easily in the parasternal short axis view and from the suprasternal notch. The classic patent ductus arteriosus connects the junction of the main pulmonary artery and the left pulmonary artery with the aorta just below and opposite the left subclavian artery.

Other Tests

A small patent ductus arteriosus, the ECG findings are typically normal. Left ventricular hypertrophy may be present with a larger patent ductus arteriosus. This is typically seen as tall R waves in the lateral precordial leads (V6). In the neonate, especially the premature neonate with a large patent ductus arteriosus, T-wave inversion and ST segment depression may be present, suggesting ischemia or a supply-demand mismatch. This is thought to be related to increased myocardial work due to the left-to-right shunt and pulmonary overcirculation in the face of low aortic and coronary diastolic blood pressure due to the runoff of blood from the aorta into the pulmonary arteries.

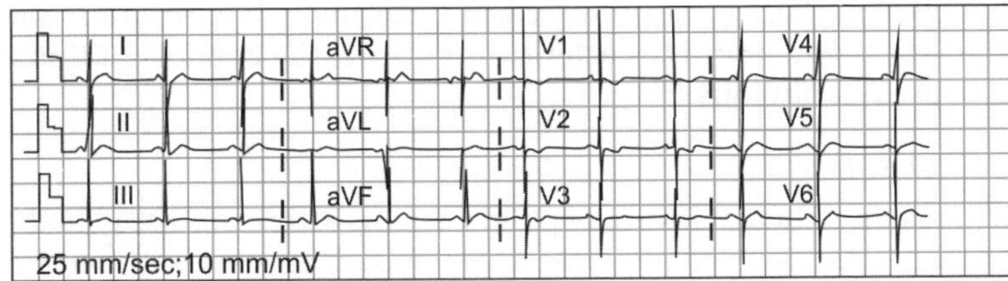

Management

Medications

In a premature baby, nonsteroidal anti-inflammatory drugs (NSAIDs) such as ibuprofen (Advil, Infant's Motrin, others) or indomethacin (Indocin) might be used to help close a PDA. NSAIDs block the hormone like chemicals in the body that keep the PDA open. NSAIDs would not close a PDA in full-term babies, children or adults.

Catheter Procedures

Premature babies are too small for catheter procedures. However, if the child does not have PDA-related health problems, the doctor will be recommend to waiting until the baby is older to do a catheter procedure to correct the PDA. Catheter procedures can also be used to treat full-term babies, children and adults.

In a catheter procedure, a thin tube (catheter) is inserted into a blood vessel in the groin and threaded up to the heart. Through the catheter, a plug or coil is inserted to close the ductus arteriosus. If the procedure is done on an outpatient basis, your child probably would not stay overnight in the hospital. Complications from catheter procedures include bleeding, infection, or movement of the plug or coil from where it was placed in the heart.

Surgical Management

Open Heart Surgery

The medications are not effective and child's condition is severe or causing complications, open-heart surgery might be recommended. A surgeon makes a small cut between child's ribs to reach the child's heart and repair the open duct using stitches or clips.

After the surgery child will remain in the hospital for several days for observation. It usually takes a few weeks for a child to fully recover from open-heart surgery. Open-heart surgery might also be recommended for adults who have a PDA that is causing health problems. Possible risks include hoarseness, bleeding, infection and a paralyzed diaphragm.

Surgical ligation or surgical ligation and division remain the standard treatment of large patent ductus arteriosus that require treatment in infancy. This is a particularly successful procedure in the hands of an experienced pediatric cardiovascular surgeon. The techniques are reviewed in Patent Ductus Arterious: Surgical Perspective.

When performed by an experienced pediatric cardiac surgeon, patent ductus arteriosus ligation is a low-risk procedure with excellent results. This is true even in the smallest premature babies. The risks include hemorrhage, vessel damage, ligation of the wrong vessel (left pulmonary artery or aorta), recurrent laryngeal nerve or phrenic nerve damage, or infection.

While indomethacin therapy is preferred in most intensive care nurseries as the first-line approach to effect patent ductus arteriosus closure, the benefits of this approach over surgical ligation are not obvious.

Nursing Management

The patients who have catheter closure of patent ductus arteriosus are usually sent home on the day of the procedure. Even patients who have standard surgery with a thoracotomy rarely are hospitalized for longer than 2 or 3 days. The appropriate care and length of hospitalization of premature neonates with a patent ductus arteriosus are primarily determined based on abnormalities of other organ systems. However, babies who have effective closure of patent ductus arteriosus appear to have shorter hospital stays than babies whose patent ductus arteriosus remains a problem.

Nursing Diagnosis for Patent Ductus Arteriosus (PDA)

- Decreased cardiac output related to malformations of the heart.
- Impaired gas exchange related to pulmonary congestion.
- Activity intolerance related to imbalance between oxygen consumption by the body and oxygen supply to the cells.
- Delayed growth and development related to an inadequate supply of oxygen and nutrients to the tissues.
- Imbalanced nutrition less than body related to fatigue at mealtime and increased caloric needs.
- Risk for infection related to decreased health status.

Nursing Interventions for Patent Ductus Arteriosus (PDA)

Maintain Adequate Cardiac Output

- Observation of the quality and strength of heart rate, peripheral pulses, skin color and warmth
- Enforce the degree of cyanosis (circumoral, mucous membranes, clubbing)
- Monitor signs of CHF (restlessness, tachycardia, tachypnea, spasms, fatigue, periorbital edema, oliguria, and hepatomegaly)
- Collaboration of drugs in accordance with the order, using toxicity hazard prevention techniques
- Provide treatment to reduce afterload
- Give diuretics as indicated.

Reduce the Increase in Pulmonary Vascular Resistance

- Monitor the quality and rhythm of breathing
- Adjust the position of the child with Fowler position
- Avoid children from an infected person
- Give adequate rest
- Provide optimal nutrition
- Give oxygen if indicated.

Maintaining Adequate Levels of Activity

- Allow the child to rest frequently, and avoid disturbances during sleep
- Encourage to engage in play and light activity
- Help child to choose activities appropriate to the age, condition and abilities
- Avoid the ambient temperature is too hot or too cold
- Avoid the things that cause fear/anxiety in children.

Provide Support for the Growth and Development

- Assess the level of development of the child
- Give the stimulation of growth and development, play activities, gaming, watching TV, puzzles, drawing, and others according to the condition and age of the child
- Involve the family in order to continue to provide stimulation during care.

Maintaining Growth in Weight and Height Appropriate

- Provide a balanced diet, high nutrients for adequate growth
- Monitor height and weight, documented in the form of graphs to determine the trend of growing children
- Measure weight every day with the same weight and the same time
- Record intake and output correctly
- Provide food with small portions but often to avoid fatigue during meals
- Children who receive diuretics are usually very thirsty, and therefore not restricted fluid.

Children will not Show Signs of Infection
- Avoid contact with infected individuals
- Give adequate rest
- Provide optimal nutritional needs.

Complications
- Endocarditis
- Congestive heart failure
- Pulmonary vascular obstructive disease
- Aortic rupture.

Prognosis
The patent ductus arteriosus closure, patients experience no further symptoms and have no further cardiac sequelae. Premature infants who had a significant patent ductus arteriosus are more likely to develop bronchopulmonary dysplasia.

PULMONARY HYPERTENSION

DEFINITION
Pulmonary hypertension is high blood pressure in the arteries to lungs. It is a serious condition for which there are treatments but no cure. The blood vessels that carry oxygen-poor blood from your heart to your lungs become hard and narrow. Idiopathic pulmonary artery hypertension (IPAH), previously referred to as primary pulmonary hypertension (PPH), is a relatively recently described entity with an unclear etiology. A new classification scheme has been defined, based on the World Health Organization conference on pulmonary hypertension in 2003.

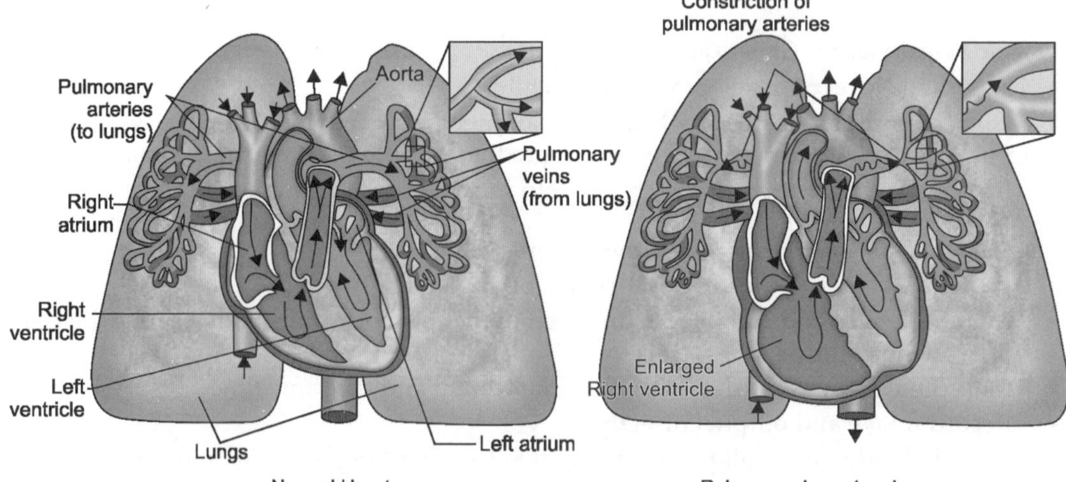

Fig. 6.76: Anatomical difference between normal lungs and pulmonary hypertension

Types

The classification system includes the following:

Pulmonary Artery Hypertension (Group 1)

- Idiopathic pulmonary hypertension
- Familial
- Pulmonary hypertension associated with the following:
  - Collagen vascular disease
  - Congenital heart disease with left-to-right shunt
  - Portal hypertension
  - Human immunodeficiency virus (HIV) infection
  - Drugs (Anorexigens or other toxins)
  - Thyroid disorders
  - Other entities (Gaucher disease, hereditary hemorrhagic telangiectasia, hemoglobinopathies)
- Persistent pulmonary hypertension of the newborn
- Pulmonary veno-occlusive disease.

Pulmonary Hypertension with Left Heart Disease (Group 2)

- Left atrial or left ventricular disease
- Left-sided valvular disease.

Pulmonary Hypertension Associated with Respiratory Disorders and/or Hypoxemia (Group 3)

- Chronic obstructive lung disease
- Interstitial lung disease
- Sleep-disordered breathing
- Alveolar hypoventilation
- Chronic exposure to high altitude
- Neonatal lung disease
- Alveolar-capillary dysplasia
- Other.

Pulmonary Hypertension Due to Chronic Thrombotic/Embolic Disease (Group 4)

- Thrombotic obstruction of proximal pulmonary arteries
- Obstruction of distal pulmonary arteries
  - Pulmonary embolism (thrombus, tumor, parasites)
  - *In situ* thrombosis.

Incidence

The age of vasodilator therapy, most children died within 1–2 years of diagnosis whereas adults had a median survival of 2–3 years. Survival has improved, although morbidity and mortality remain significant. Morbidity and mortality rates vary and depend on the age, the degree of pulmonary hypertension, and the response to vasodilator therapy. Death as a result of both acute and chronic right heart failure and its associated arrhythmias may occur. Additionally, patients can be affected by the complications associated with low output. In 2009, the United Kingdom Pulmonary Hypertension Service for Children reported survival rates of 85.6% at 1 year, 79.9% at 3 years, and 71.9% at 5 years. Finally, the morbidity associated with chronic vasodilator therapy and frequent intravenous line infections in patients on long-term continuous intravenous prostacyclin as well as long-term anticoagulation are well known.

Causes

- The exact pathogenesis and pathophysiology of idiopathic pulmonary artery hypertension are unclear. The mechanism that is most widely accepted is that of pulmonary vasoconstriction. Many studies suggest that individuals who are predisposed may be exposed to certain stimuli that initiate the characteristic vascular lesions.
- Various triggers, such as high altitude, hypoxemia, drugs, toxins, sympathetic tone, and autoimmune disorders, can cause pulmonary vasoconstriction in susceptible individuals.
- Other studies also invoke an imbalance of vasoactive mediators favoring vasoconstriction as important in the pathophysiology of idiopathic pulmonary artery hypertension. Factors such as thromboxane, arachidonate metabolites, and prostacyclin and other endothelial factors have been invoked.
- In addition, coagulation abnormalities may occur, supported by the finding of microthrombi in the pulmonary vascular bed, noted at the time of lung biopsy, autopsy, or in explanted lungs at the time of lung transplantation. Whether this is a primary or secondary finding is unknown.

Clinical Manifestation

Infants and children with idiopathic pulmonary artery hypertension (IAH):

- Poor appetite
- Poor growth
- Nausea
- Vomiting
- Lethargy
- Sweating
- Tachypnea
- Tachycardia.

Physical Examination Findings

The physical examination findings are typical of the findings of pulmonary hypertension.

- Typically, the pulmonic component of the second heart sound is accentuated.
- A right ventricular heave with or without chest wall distortion may be noted as a result of right ventricular hypertrophy and/or dysfunction.
- Tricuspid regurgitation is common.
- Clinical signs of right heart failure, such as hepatomegaly, peripheral edema, and acrocyanosis, are rare in infants but can be observed in older children and adults.

Diagnostic Evaluation

Flow chart: Diagnostic evaluation

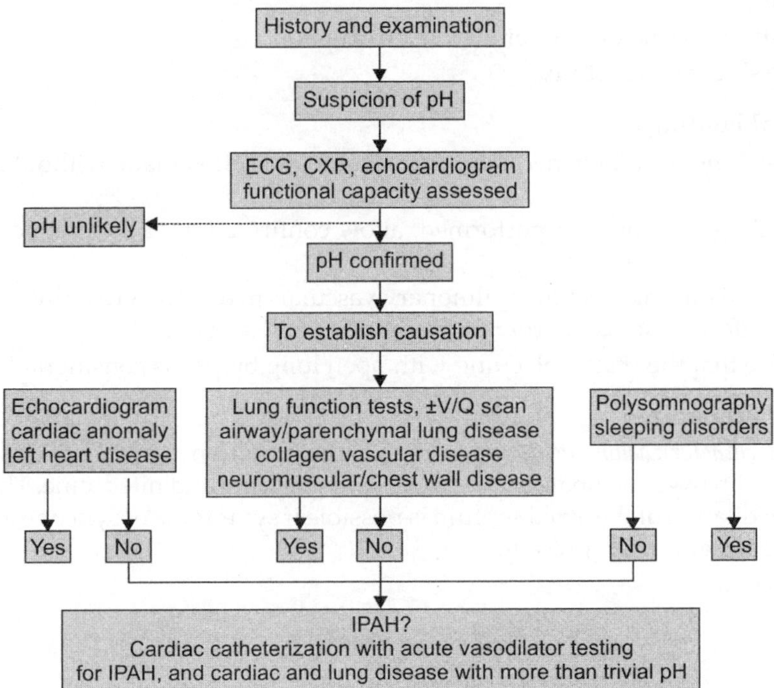

Laboratory Studies

The following studies are indicated in idiopathic pulmonary artery hypertension (IPAH):

- CBC count with differential
- Liver function tests
- Coagulation studies
  - Coagulation profile
  - Bleeding time
  - Platelet aggregation studies.

Imaging Studies

- Chest radiography
- ECG
- Two-dimensional echocardiography
- Ventilation-perfusion imaging to rule out pulmonary thromboembolic disease
- MRI to assess airways and branch pulmonary arteries
- Radionuclide angiography to assess right ventricular function
- Evaluation for lung transplantation.

Other Tests

- Pulmonary function tests, including lung volumes, diffusion capacity, and bronchodilator response
- Sleep study to rule out upper airway obstruction
- Progressive exercise study.

Histological Findings

Lung biopsy is not routinely necessary; the diagnosis is often made without this diagnostic procedure.

- The findings at biopsy, if performed, allow confirmation of the diagnosis as well as a determination of severity.
- The typical findings include pulmonary vascular medial hypertrophy, intimal fibrosis, and plexiform lesions in order of progression and severity.
- Be aware that the risk of bleeding with open lung biopsy is considerable.

Diagnostic Procedures

- *Cardiac catheterization:* Perform cardiac catheterization with acute vasodilator drug testing with oxygen, inhaled nitric oxide, prostacyclin, and nifedipine. The Trans-septal balloon dilation of the atrial septum is possible if symptoms of syncope associated with right heart failure are present.
- Lung biopsy

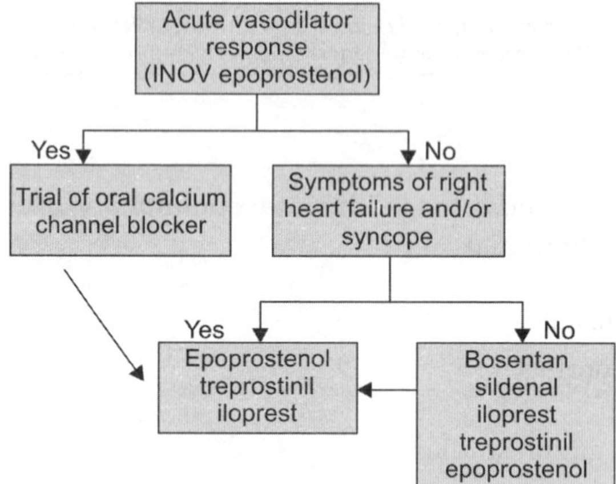

Arrow depict potential change in therapy of clinical response is poor or incomplete

Fig. 6.77: Algorithm for treatment of pediatric pulmonary artery hypertension

Medical Management

General medical measures and the care of the pediatrician for this group of children are very important.

- Annual influenza vaccination is important. Also consider immunization with palivizumab in infants and young children with idiopathic pulmonary artery hypertension (IPAH).

- In addition, treat respiratory illnesses aggressively in order to minimize or prevent increases in pulmonary bed reactivity from ventilation-perfusion mismatching and/or hypoxia.
- Fevers should be aggressively treated to reduce the metabolic demands.
- Any infectious illness can potentiate pulmonary hypertensive crises requiring maximization of vasodilator therapy.
- Supplemental oxygen
  - Note that a current recommendation suggests performing a sleep study as part of the diagnostic workup for patients with IPAH to rule out sleep apnea and/or upper airway obstruction as the underlying cause for pulmonary hypertension.
  - Oxygen is certainly well known as a pulmonary vasodilator. Some authors recommend that supplemental oxygen be available at all times for emergency use and in the presence of an intercurrent pulmonary infection that might potentially result in systemic desaturation, even if treated in the outpatient setting.
  - Additionally, some children demonstrate desaturation with sleep secondary to hypoventilation. This group of patients may also benefit from nocturnal supplemental oxygen therapy.

Medication

Treatment for idiopathic pulmonary artery hypertension (IPAH) has significantly improved over the past 20 years. Therapy now offers children with idiopathic pulmonary artery hypertension hope for a much better prognosis and a relatively reasonable quality of life.

Anticoagulant Agents

Adult studies have suggested that long-term anticoagulation with warfarin to achieve an international normalized ratio (INR) of 2.5–3 decreases the morbidity and mortality rates associated with idiopathic pulmonary artery hypertension. This is based on the pathologic finding of microthrombi in the pulmonary vasculature. Whether this is a primary or secondary finding is not known. The major precautions relate to bleeding risks.

Surgical Management

Child with severe pulmonary hypertension resulting in recurrent syncope or right-to-left intracardiac shunting have a poor prognosis. The former group does not have an intra-atrial communication.

Syncopal spells are often exercise related and are a result of systemic vasodilation with the concomitant inability to augment cardiac output because of idiopathic pulmonary artery hypertension and right heart dysfunction. This group of patients may benefit from palliation with blade atrial septostomy or balloon dilation of the atrial septum.

This procedure can be performed in the cardiac catheterization laboratory. Although the arterial oxygen saturation decreases, cardiac output and oxygen delivery increases with successful decompression of the atrial septum. The procedure is not without risk but is a very good palliative bridge for the symptomatic patient with idiopathic pulmonary artery hypertension. Open lung biopsy is occasionally performed for diagnostic purposes. Risks are associated with this intervention in this population of patients, including bleeding as well as the risks of anesthesia.

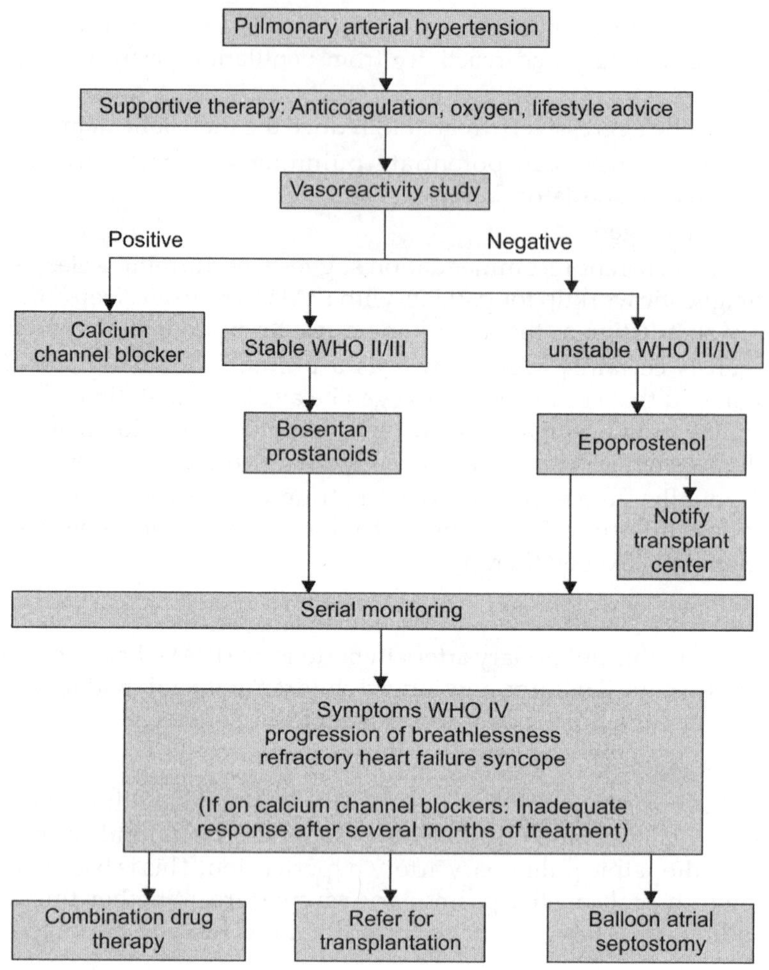

Nursing Management

Diet Management

- No specific diet is recommended other than one that prevents constipation
- Valsalva maneuvers can reduce venous return to an already dysfunctional right ventricular with resultant syncope.

Activity

- Many children with idiopathic pulmonary artery hypertension are activity restricted and not allowed to participate in competitive athletics.
- In some instances, children may be allowed to participate in activities. This is more likely the case in a child with a pop-off lesion who has no adverse cardiopulmonary effects at exercise testing. This decision must only be made by a specialist familiar with pulmonary hypertension in children and only after a complete evaluation, including a progressive exercise test.

ATRIOVENTRICULAR CANAL DEFECT (AV CANAL OR AVC)

DEFINITION

Atrioventricular canal is a congenital (present at birth) heart defect. Other terms used to describe this defect are endocardial cushion defect and atrioventricular septal defect (AVSD). As the fetus is growing, something occurs to affect heart development during the first 8 weeks of pregnancy and certain areas of the heart do not form properly. AV canal is a complex heart problem that involves several abnormalities of structures inside the heart.

Types

- *Atrial septal defect*: An opening in the atrial septum or dividing wall between the two upper chambers of the heart known as the right and left atria.

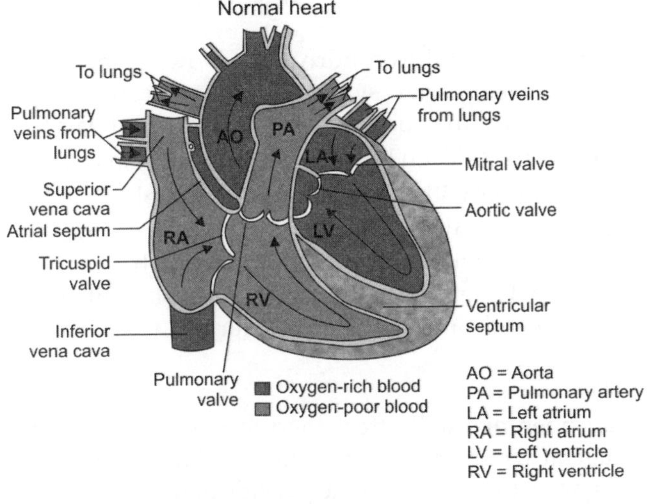

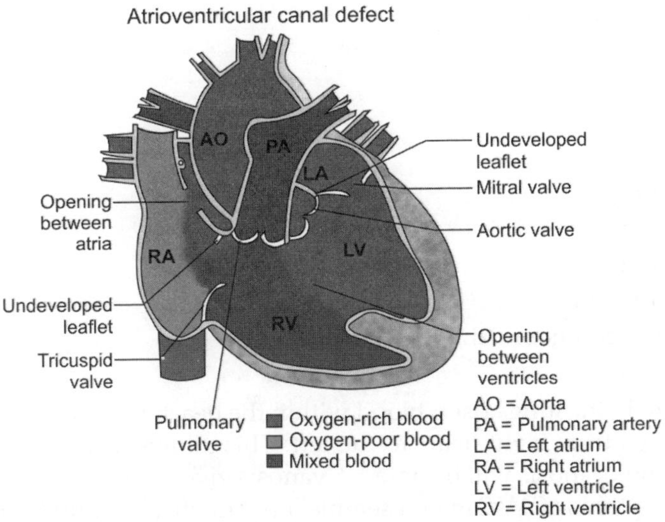

Fig. 6.78: Difference between normal heart and AVSD heart

- *Ventricular septal defect*: An opening in the ventricular septum or dividing wall between the two lower chambers of the heart known as the right and left ventricles.
- *Improperly formed mitral and/or tricuspid valves:* The valves that separate the upper heart chambers (atria) from the lower heart chambers (ventricles) are improperly formed.

Causes

The heart is forming during the first 8 weeks of fetal development. It begins as a hollow tube, then partitions within the tube develop that eventually become the septa (or walls) dividing the right side of the heart from the left. Atrial and ventricular septal defects occur when the partitioning process does not occur completely, leaving openings in the atrial and ventricular septum. The valves that separate the upper and lower heart chambers are being formed in the latter portion of this eight-week period and for some reason, they do not develop properly either. There may be genetic influences on the development of atrioventricular canal.

- CHD is present in half of children born with Down syndrome, and 45 percent of these cases have AV canal; Down syndrome is caused by the presence of three #21 chromosomes in the cells of the body, rather than the usual pair (two) of chromosomes.
- Similarly one-third of all children born with AV canal also have Down syndrome.
- Fourteen percent of mothers with an AV canal defect give birth to a child with the disease.
- Other chromosome abnormalities (in addition to Down syndrome) are linked to the development of atrioventricular canal. Maternal age can have an effect on the prevalence of AV canal, which may be related to the increased probability of a woman giving birth to a child with Down syndrome as she gets older.

Signs and Symptoms

The size of the septal openings will affect the type of symptoms noted, the severity of symptoms, and the age at which they first occur. The larger the openings, the greater the amount of blood that passes through from the left side of the heart to the right and overloads the right heart and the lungs.

- Fatigue
- Sweating
- Pale skin
- Cool skin
- Rapid breathing
- Heavy breathing
- Rapid heart rate
- Congested breathing
- Disinterest in feeding, or tiring while feeding
- Poor weight gain.

As the pressure in the lungs rises, blood within the heart will eventually 'shunt' through the septal openings from right heart to the left. This allows oxygen-poor (blue) blood to reach the body, and cyanosis will be noted. Cyanosis gives a blue color to the lips, nailbeds, and skin. The symptoms of AVC may resemble other medical conditions or heart problems.

Diagnostic Evaluation

A heart murmur is simply a noise caused by the turbulence of blood flowing through the opening from the left side of the heart to the right. Symptoms your child exhibits will also help with the diagnosis. The location within the chest that the murmur is heard best, as well as the loudness and quality of the murmur (harsh, blowing, etc.)

- *Chest X-ray*: A diagnostic test which uses invisible electromagnetic energy beams to produce images of internal tissues, bones and organs onto film.
- *Electrocardiogram (ECG or EKG)*: A test that records the electrical activity of the heart, shows abnormal rhythms (Arrhythmias or Dysrhythmia), and detects heart muscle stress.
- *Echocardiogram (echo):* A procedure that evaluates the structure and function of the heart by using sound waves recorded on an electronic sensor that produce a moving picture of the heart and heart valves. An echo can show the pattern of blood flow through the septal openings and determine how large the openings are as well as how much blood is passing through them.
- *Cardiac catheterization:* A cardiac catheterization is an invasive procedure that gives very detailed information about the structures inside the heart. Under sedation, a small, thin, flexible tube (catheter) is inserted into a blood vessel in the groin, and guided to the inside of the heart. Blood pressure and oxygen measurements are taken in the four chambers of the heart, as well as the pulmonary artery and aorta. Contrast dye is also injected to more clearly visualize the structures inside the heart.

Management

Medical Management

Most of the children will eventually need to take medications to help the heart and lungs work better, due to strain from the extra blood passing through the septal defects. Medications that may be prescribed include the following:

- *Digoxin*: Helps strengthen the heart muscle, enabling it to pump more efficiently.
- *Diuretics:* The body's water balance can be affected when the heart is not working as well as it could. These medications help the kidneys remove excess fluid from the body.
- *ACE (Angiotensin-converting enzyme) inhibitors:* Dilate the blood vessels, making it easier for the heart to pump blood forward into the body.

Surgical Management

The goal is to repair the septal openings and repair the valves before the lungs become damaged from too much blood flow and pressure. The operative methods used to repair atrioventricular canal have improved greatly in the past decade, and the operation has a high likelihood of success. Most children undergo surgery by the age of 6 months. Children with Down syndrome may develop lung problems earlier than other children, and may need to have surgical repair at an earlier age.

The operation is performed under general anesthesia. The atrial and ventricular septal defects are often closed with a pericardial patch made from the membrane that covers the outside surface of the heart, or a patch made from synthetic material. The valve repair technique will differ according to the abnormality and the surgeon's preferences.

Nursing Management

Adequate Nutrition

Infants may become tired when feeding, and may not be able to eat enough to gain weight. Options that can be used to ensure your baby will have adequate nutrition include:

High-Calorie Formula or Breast Milk

Special nutritional supplements may be added to formula or pumped breast milk that increase the number of calories in each ounce, thereby allowing your baby to drink less and still consume enough calories to grow properly.

Supplemental Tube Feedings

Feedings given through a small, flexible tube that passes through the nose, down the esophagus, and into the stomach, can either supplement or take the place of bottle feedings. Infants who can drink part of their bottle, but not all, may be fed the remainder through the feeding tube. Infants who are too tired to bottle feed may receive their formula or breast milk through the feeding tube alone.

Infection Control

Children with certain heart defects are at risk for developing an infection of the inner surfaces of the heart known as bacterial endocarditis. A common procedure that puts your child at risk for this infection is a routine dental check-up and teeth cleaning. Other procedures may also increase the risk of the heart infection occurring. However, giving children with heart defects an antibiotic by mouth before these procedures can help prevent bacterial endocarditis. It is important that you inform all medical personnel that your child has an atrioventricular canal defect, so they may determine if the antibiotics are necessary before a procedure.

- Coarctation of aorta (COA)
- Aortic stenosis (AS)
- Pulmonary stenosis (PS)
- Congenital mitral stenosis
- Hypoxemia.

COARCTATION OF THE AORTA (COA)

INTRODUCTION

Coarctation of the aorta (CoA) is a relatively common defect that accounts for 5–8% of all congenital heart defects. Coarctation of the aorta may occur as an isolated defect or in association with various other lesions, most commonly bicuspid aortic valve and ventricular septal defect (VSD). The diagnosis of coarctation of the aorta may be missed unless an index of suspicion is maintained, and diagnosis is often delayed until the patient develops congestive heart failure (CHF), which is common in infants, or hypertension, which is common in older children. This article discusses the pathology, pathophysiology, clinical features, noninvasive and invasive evaluation, and therapy in patients with coarctation of the aorta.

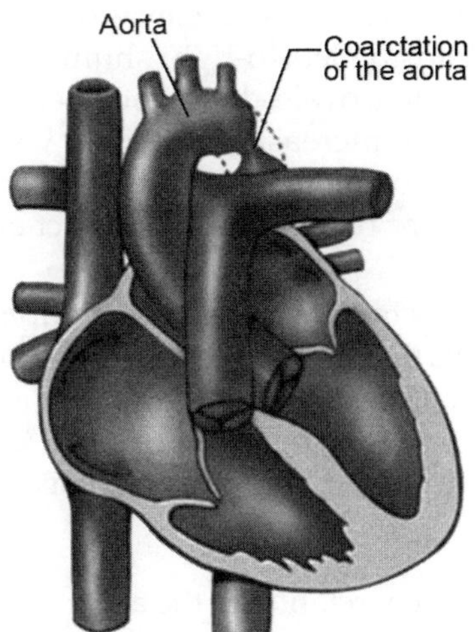

Incidence

Past autopsy studies suggest that the mortality rate in patients in whom coarctation of the aorta is not surgically repaired is 90% by age 50 years, with a mean age of 35 years. In the current era, coarctation of the aorta mortality is often determined by patient age, patient size, and associated major cardiovascular anomalies. Associated problems that may contribute to death or morbidity include hypertension, intracranial hemorrhage, aortic rupture or dissection, endocarditis, and CHF.

The male-to-female ratio is 2:1, although this ratio is not valid in abdominal coarctation of the aorta, in which this rare lesion predominantly affects females. The ratio of abdominal-to-thoracic coarctation is approximately 1:1000. The male preponderance observed in older patients is not seen in infants with coarctation of the aorta.

Causes

Coarctation of the aorta manifests when the ductus closes starting at the pulmonary end, with gradual involution of ductal tissue toward the aorta.

Similar to most forms of congenital heart disease (CHD), the etiology of coarctation of the aorta may be explained by multifactorial inheritance hypothesis. The prevalence of coarctation of the aorta in genetic abnormalities such as Turner syndrome (45, X), is as high as 15–20%. Familial patterns of inheritance of coarctation have been reported, as well as for other left heart obstructive lesions. An increase in seasonal occurrence of coarctation of the aorta is reported in September and November.

Pathophysiology

Coarctation of the aorta imposes significant after load on the left ventricle (LV), which results in increased wall stress and compensatory ventricular hypertrophy. The afterload may be imposed acutely, as occurs following closure of the ductus arteriosus in neonates with severe coarctation. These infants may rapidly develop CHF and shock. Rapid constriction of the ductus arteriosus, producing sudden severe aortic obstruction, seems to be the most likely explanation. As the ductus (aortic end) constricts, the left ventricular afterload rapidly increases, with a resultant increase in left ventricular pressures (systolic and diastolic). This causes elevation of the left atrial pressure, which may open the foramen ovale, causing left-to-right shunt and dilatation of the right atrium and right ventricle. If the foramen ovale does not open, pulmonary venous pressures and pulmonary artery pressures increase, and right ventricular dilatation develops. Cardiomegaly revealed by chest roentgenography and right ventricular hypertrophy seen on ECG and echocardiography are related to the indirect effects of rapid development of severe aortic obstruction.

LV afterload may also gradually increase, allowing children with less severe coarctation to develop arterial collateral vessels that partially bypass the aortic obstruction. These children may be asymptomatic until hypertension is detected or another complication develops. The mechanism for development of hypertension is not clearly understood; mechanical obstruction and renin-angiotensin-mediated humoral mechanisms have been postulated.

Clinical Manifestation

The presentation of patients with coarctation of the aorta (CoA) varies but may be discussed relative to the patients who present early, often with congestive heart failure (CHF) and the patients who present later, most often with hypertension.

Early Presentation

The presence of associated defects and aortic arch anomalies, the extent of patency of the ductus arteriosus, the rapidity of the process of closure of the ductus arteriosus, and the level of pulmonary vascular resistance determine the timing of clinical presentation and the severity of symptoms. Young child may present in the first few weeks of life with poor feeding, tachypnea, and lethargy and progress to overt CHF and shock. These patients may have appeared well prior to hospital discharge, and deterioration coincides with closure of the patent ductus arteriosus. Presentation may be abrupt and acute with ductal closure. Development of symptoms is often accelerated by the presence of associated major cardiac anomalies, such as ventricular septal defect (VSD). Symptoms may be subtle at first and child may make repeated trips to the physician before finally presenting in extremis.

Late Presentation

Children often present after the neonatal period with hypertension or a murmur. These patients often have not developed overt CHF because of the presence of arterial collateral vessels. Diagnosis is often made after hypertension is noted as an incidental finding during evaluation of other problems, such as trauma or more routine illness. Other presenting symptoms may include headaches, chest pain, fatigue, or even life-threatening intracranial hemorrhage. True claudication is rare, although an occasional child may experience pain or weakness in the legs. Many patients are asymptomatic except for the incidentally noted hypertension. Frequently, coarctation of the aorta is not recognized by the primary care physician. Palpation of femoral pulses and measurement of blood pressure during routine examination is necessary to avoid a delay in the diagnosis.

Diagnostic Evaluation

Laboratory Studies

- Laboratory studies in neonatal patients who present in shock include the following:
  - Septic workup includes blood, urine, and cerebral spinal fluid (CSF) cultures.
  - Electrolyte levels, BUN, creatinine, and glucose concentrations should be tested.

  - Measure arterial blood gases and serum lactate levels.
- Laboratory studies in older patients who present with hypertension include urinalysis, electrolyte levels, BUN, creatinine, and glucose concentrations.

Imaging Studies

Chest Radiography

- Radiography in patients with early onset of coarctation of the aorta may reveal cardiomegaly, pulmonary edema, and other signs of congestive heart failure (CHF).
- Radiography in patients with late onset of coarctation of the aorta may reveal cardiomegaly. An inverted '3' sign of the barium-filled esophagus or a '3' sign on a highly penetrated chest radiograph (frontal view) may be visualized. Rib notching secondary to collateral vessels may also be seen.

Echocardiography

Echocardiography delineates intracardiac anatomy and allows assessment of associated significant intracardiac anomalies. The suprasternal notch two-dimensional echocardiographic view allows evaluation of the aortic arch to assess the transverse aortic arch, isthmus, and severity of coarctation. Doppler echocardiography is used to measure the gradient at the site of coarctation and to identify the pattern of diastolic runoff typically seen in patients with severe obstruction.

MRI and CT

MRI and CT are useful in older or postoperative patients to assess residual arch obstruction, arch hypoplasia, or formation of aneurysms. Ultrafast CT scanning is preferable if multiple surgical clips or a stent is present in the area of coarctation.

Histological Findings

- Coarctation of the aorta results from marked ridgelike thickening of the media of the aortic wall opposite the insertion of the patent ductus arteriosus or ligamentum arteriosum.
- Intima in this area may be thin initially but may thicken over time.
- This ridge or shelf becomes an obstruction when the patent ductus involutes and when ductal tissue in the wall of the aorta involutes.

Medical Management

Early Presentation of Coarctation of the Aorta (CoA)

- Treatment in patients with congestive heart failure (CHF) includes the use of diuretics and inotropic drugs.
- Prostaglandin E1 (0.05–0.15 mcg/kg/min) is infused intravenously to open the ductus arteriosus.
- Ventilatory assistance is provided to patients with markedly increased work of breathing.
- Infusion of inotropic drugs (dopamine, dobutamine, epinephrine) is useful when ventricular dysfunction is present, especially with hypotension.
- A Foley catheter is inserted to monitor renal perfusion and urine output.
- ABGs are tested to monitor acidosis.

- An umbilical artery catheter may be placed in neonates to assess the response to prostaglandin infusion with regard to improving lower-body blood flow.
- Patients stabilized by the above interventions are better candidates for surgical or catheter intervention.
- In the presence of associated defects, the significance of coarctation on the clinical course of the patient should be assessed with echo-Doppler and/or catheterization and angiographic studies. If the coarctation has a significantly adverse effect on the physiology of the associated defects, and consequently the clinical status, the coarctation should be initially relieved with surgery or balloon angioplasty and the patient reassessed with regard to need for intervention for the associated defects. Based on the authors' experience and that of others, the aortic obstruction is usually a major contributing factor for the symptomatology, and relief of the obstruction may postpone or avert the need for additional surgical intervention for the associated cardiac defects.

Late Presentation of Coarctation of the Aorta

Treatment of Hypertension

- Preoperative hypertension can be effectively treated using beta-blockers. The goal should be to reduce upper extremity hypertension, but remember that vigorous attempts to achieve normal upper extremity blood pressure (BP) may result in inadequate lower-body perfusion. Beta-blocker therapy prior to surgery may reduce the severity of postoperative hypertension, although most patients with preoperative hypertension require at least transient postoperative therapy. Remember that relieving the aortic obstruction promptly rather that attempting to treat hypertension with antihypertensive medications is better.
- Postoperative hypertension can be treated short-term with vasodilators, such as sodium nitroprusside, and intravenous beta-blockers, such as esmolol. When longer-term antihypertensive therapy is required, beta-blockers may be continued, and if no residual arch obstruction exists, ACE inhibitors or angiotensin II antagonists (pediatric dosing not established for angiotensin II antagonists) may be added if hypertension persists despite beta-blocker therapy.
- Guidelines regarding beta-adrenergic receptor blockers have been established.
- A recent study concluded that data is not sufficient to discourage or recommend the use of beta-blockers in children with CHF.
  - Evaluate associated abnormalities, such as aortic stenosis, subaortic stenosis, or mitral valve disease.
  - Evaluate adequacy of collateral blood vessels to assess the safety of surgical intervention.

Surgical Management

Significant hypertension or congestive heart failure (CHF) is an indication for intervention. Surgical relief of the aortic obstruction and catheter interventional techniques (balloon angioplasty and stents) are available alternatives. Symptomatic neonates and infants should undergo urgent intervention soon after the infant is stabilized. Asymptomatic infants, children, adolescents, and adults should undergo the procedure electively. If neither hypertension nor heart failure is present, elective surgical or balloon therapy in children aged 2–5 years is suggested. Waiting beyond age 5 years for surgery or balloon therapy to relieve aortic obstruction is not advisable because of the evidence of residual hypertension if intervention is performed after age 5 years.

Since the introduction of surgical correction by Crafoord and Nylin (1945) and by Gross and Hufnagel (1945) in the early 1940s, surgical therapy has been the preferred treatment for aortic coarctation. Various surgical techniques have been used to treat patients with coarctation of the aorta, namely, resection and end-to-end anastomosis, patch aortoplasty, left subclavian flap aortoplasty, and tubular bypass grafts. The techniques are occasionally combined or modified to fit the individual patient's anatomy.

For instance, a reverse left subclavian flap aortoplasty may be used, turning the left subclavian artery as a patch back toward the left carotid artery to enlarge an area of transverse arch hypoplasia. In addition, an extended end-to-end repair may be used, in which the segment of descending aorta is beveled and brought up to the underside of the transverse arch to enlarge areas of transverse arch hypoplasia. The exact technique used varies depending on the patient's age at presentation, size, associated abnormalities, and arch anatomy. A surgical approach from a median sternotomy, rather than the classic left lateral thoracotomy, is used commonly in complex arch repairs.

Balloon Angioplasty

Gruntzig's technique of balloon angioplasty was adopted by Sos et al (1979), Singer et al (1982), and Sperling et al (1983) for enlargement of coarcted aortic segments in a postmortem specimen, postsurgical recoarctation, and native coarctation, respectively. Other cardiologists then used this technique to treat native coarctation of the aorta. Numerous investigators reported their experiences with balloon angioplasty of native aortic coarctations. However, the use of balloon angioplasty for treatment of native aortic coarctation is controversial. This section describes the technique and the results of balloon angioplasty.

Complications

Vessel disruption, displacement of stent, stent fracture, and aneurysms are rare but do occur. Balloon rupture that results in inadequate stent expansion and stent migration has been reported but may be prevented by avoiding curvature of the balloon or stent assembly, the use of newer stents with less injurious ends, and the use of BIB catheters. Because of the large size of the sheath required, loss of pulse and bleeding from a puncture site may occur. Use of vascular closure devices may help circumvent this problem. Rare complications included myocardial infarction and retroperitoneal hemorrhage.

Coarctation of the aorta is a lifelong disease with complications that may not be evident until many years following an initial and apparently successful repair.

- Recurrent coarctation
- Aortic aneurysm
- Hypertension
- Cerebral aneurysms
- Paralysis
- Cardiomyopathy
- Valvar aortic stenosis.

Nursing Management

- Focus postoperative recovery of patients with coarctation of the aorta (CoA) on control of blood pressure (BP), slow advancement of diet, manipulation of antihypertensive medications, progressive ambulation, and pulmonary therapy to improve left lung atelectasis (common after left thoracotomy).
- Hospitalization and inpatient care may be required for cardiac catheterizations, catheter interventions, and surgical procedures for treatment of recoarctation or other complications.
- Focus early outpatient follow-up care on wound healing, resolution of lung atelectasis, and adjustment of antihypertensive medications.
- Assess postoperative BP response to exercise prior to discontinuation of antihypertensive therapy.
- Many patients may be weaned from antihypertensive therapy over months or years following repair of coarctation. Other patients may require some form of ongoing antihypertensive therapy.
- Search for late complications of coarctation repair, including recurrent coarctation and aneurysm formation.
- Child should receive antibiotic prophylaxis before undergoing any bacteremia-producing surgery or procedures, especially in view of reported incidence of bacterial endocarditis during follow-up.
- Educate patients with coarctation of the aorta and their families regarding the need for lifelong follow-up care to detect recurrent coarctation or late complications.
- Educate patients regarding a healthy lifestyle by instructing them to avoid smoking and obesity, get plenty of aerobic exercise, control BP appropriately, and reduce other factors that influence cardiovascular disease.

Diet Management

- Persistent hypertension has been shown to increase the incidence of coronary artery disease (CAD) therefore, periodically examine patients who have undergone coarctation of the aorta repair for hypertension and recommend a healthy low-fat, and perhaps, low-salt diet.
- Measure cholesterol levels and intervene pharmacologically in older patients as indicated, with a total cholesterol goal of less than 200 g/dL.
- Patients with persistent hypertension may require varying degrees of salt restriction.
- Emphasize dietary counseling and avoidance of obesity and smoking.

Activity

- Child with coarctation of the aorta and hypertension who are awaiting surgical repair should limit heavy isometric exercises to a degree commensurate with the degree of hypertension.
- Generally, the duration of hypertension after coarctation of the aorta repair is related in part to the duration of hypertension prior to diagnosis and repair of coarctation. Patients who undergo repair of coarctation in infancy usually remain normotensive in the absence of significant residual arch obstruction and require no specific activity

restrictions or limitations. With growth, coarctation may recur, and some patients may be normotensive at rest but have significant upper extremity hypertension provoked by exercise. Such patients who desire to participate in competitive athletics should undergo exercise stress testing prior to clearance.

- Child who undergo repair later in life and who have had a significant period of preoperative hypertension are at particular risk for sustained postoperative hypertension, which may be permanent. Restrict heavy isometric exercise and other activities in these patients, commensurate with the degree of hypertension and BP control. Use exercise testing to assess BP response to exercise as a means of delineating reasonable exercise limitations.

PULMONARY STENOSIS

Introduction

Diseases of the pulmonary valve are most often congenital, and only rarely do acquired disorders such as carcinoid and rheumatic fever affect the pulmonary valve. The pulmonary valve may be stenotic or atretic, or the leaflets of the valve may be absent. Pulmonary stenosis may be valvar, supravalvar, or subvalvar (i.e. double-chambered right ventricle); it may also be in the branch pulmonary arteries. These lesions are collectively associated with obstruction of the right ventricular outflow tract. In this article, only valvar pulmonary stenosis is reviewed.

A stenotic pulmonary valve may occur without associated congenital abnormalities, although it is most often associated with other structural abnormalities of the heart. To distinguish the former from the latter, terms such as pulmonary stenosis with a normal aortic root or pulmonary stenosis with an intact ventricular septum have been used. However, the term isolated pulmonary valve stenosis is preferred. The term isolated may be used even when a patent foramen ovale or a small atrial septal defect is present. The term congenital need not be used because most are congenital.

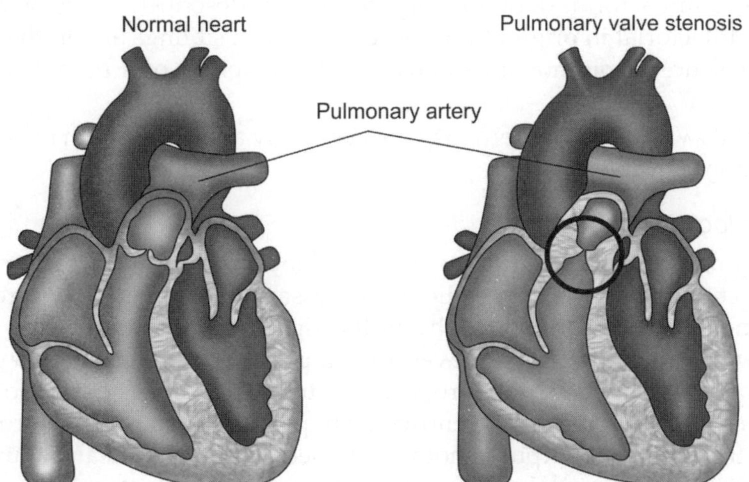

Fig. 6.79: Anatomical difference between normal heart and pulmonary valve stenosis heart

Incidence

The severity of the valvar dysplasia determines its related morbidity and mortality. Mild-to-moderate valvar pulmonary stenosis is extremely well tolerated. Severe pulmonary stenosis can be associated with decreased pulmonary flow, right ventricular hypertrophy, early congestive heart failure (CHF) with critical obstructions, and cyanosis. The morbidity formerly associated with surgery is lessened with balloon pulmonary valvuloplasty.

The male-to-female ratio is 1:1.

Causes

- Pulmonary valve stenosis is primarily due to maldevelopment of the pulmonary valve tissue and the distal portion of the bulbus cordis, which is characterized by fusion of leaflet commissures, resulting in a thickened and domed appearance of the valve.

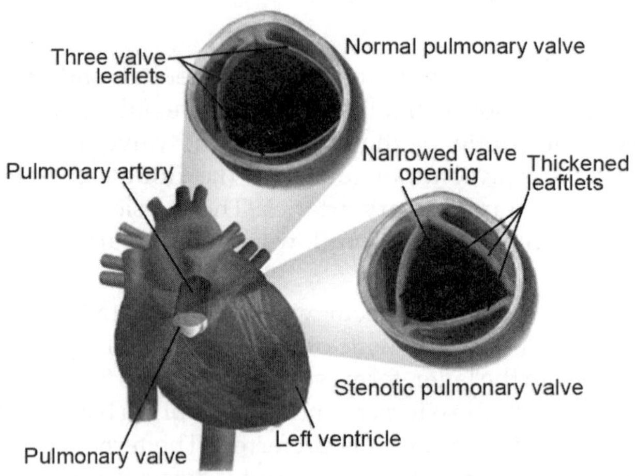

Fig. 6.80: An example of pulmonary stenosis

- Although familial forms of pulmonary stenosis are described, it is generally considered to be multifactorial in origin. Rates of recurrence in siblings are on the order of 2–3%. The prevalence of pulmonary stenosis in the offspring of a parent with pulmonary stenosis is 3.6%.
- Aberrant flow patterns in utero may also be partly associated with maldevelopment of the pulmonary valve.

Pathophysiology

Clinically significant narrowing of a valve or a blood vessel increases pressure proximal to the obstruction. This pressure gradient is necessary to maintain flow across the stenotic site. In pulmonic stenosis, hypertrophy of the right ventricle ensues and maintains this forward flow. The magnitude of right ventricular pressure and the pressure gradient across the pulmonary valve are generally proportional to the degree of obstruction. Under usual circumstances, proportional right ventricular hypertrophy maintains normal pulmonary blood flow. If the normal output is not maintained, right-sided heart failure ensues. This occurs in neonates with critical pulmonary stenosis and in patients with severe obstruction that occurs in childhood or adulthood.

Changes in the geometry of the left ventricle and decreased left ventricular function can also occur. The changes are proportional to the degree of right ventricular hypertrophy; however, they revert to normal after obstruction of the right ventricular outflow tract is relieved.

With increasing right ventricular hypertrophy, right ventricular compliance decreases with a resultant increase in end-diastolic pressure and with prominent a waves in the right atrium. As right atrial pressure rises, a right-to-left shunt may occur if the foramen ovale is patent or if an atrial septal defect is present; this change results in systemic arterial desaturation and clinically discernible cyanosis. This shunting may occur even without measurable elevation of right atrial pressure and is attributable to decreased right ventricular compliance. Such a right-to-left shunt can also occur in patients with an underdeveloped (hypoplastic) right ventricle.

Clinical Manifestation

- Most children with pulmonic stenosis, particularly those with trivial and mild pulmonary stenosis, present with asymptomatic cardiac murmurs that are detected during routine examination.
- Child with moderate or severe pulmonary stenosis may have mild exertional dyspnea. Adults may be asymptomatic irrespective of the severity of their obstruction.
- Child with severe or critical obstruction may present with signs of systemic venous congestion, which are usually interpreted as signs of congestive heart failure (CHF). The signs are due to severe right ventricular dysfunction or to cyanosis secondary to a right-to-left shunt across a patent foramen ovale or an atrial septal defect.
- Lightheadedness, syncope and chest pain that resembles angina pectoris are rare but even in patients with severe obstruction.

Diagnostic Evaluation

Laboratory Studies

- Laboratory evaluation is usually not helpful in pulmonary valve stenosis.
- Hemoglobin and hematocrit measurements in patients with cyanosis may be helpful in that they are increased in patients with right-to-left shunt.
- Oximetry provides information of potential right-to-left shunting in borderline cyanotic lesions but does not help in identifying the cause of the shunt (pulmonary, interatrial, interventricular, great arterial).
- Although ABG analysis is usually not needed, one notable exception is the hyperoxia test in the newborn with cyanosis of undetermined origin.
- The fraction of inspired oxygen (FIO_2) of 1 (100% oxygen) generally does not increase the partial pressure of oxygen to more than 100 mm Hg in patients with a cyanotic congenital heart defect (right-to-left intracardiac shunt).

Imaging Studies

Chest radiography: Chest radiographs reveal a prominent main pulmonary artery segment, but the size of the heart is usually normal.

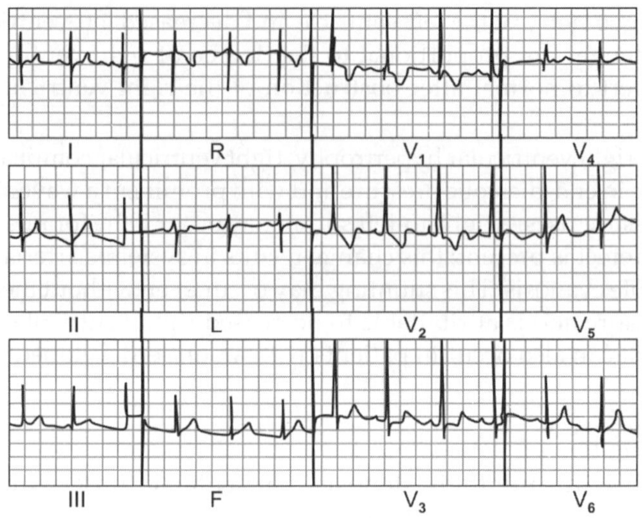

Other Tests

ECG

- ECG findings are usually normal in mild pulmonary stenosis.
- Right-axis deviation and right ventricular hypertrophy occur in moderate and severe valvar pulmonary stenosis.
- The degree of right ventricular hypertrophy is well correlated with the severity of pulmonary stenosis.
- Right atrial hypertrophy and right ventricular hypertrophy with strain pattern are observed when pulmonary stenosis is severe.
- A superior QRS axis (left-axis deviation) is seen with dysplastic pulmonary valves and Noonan syndrome.

Staging

- The severity of pulmonary valve obstruction may be categorized (staged) as follows, based on peak-to-peak catheter-measured pulmonary valvar gradient:
  - *Trivial:* Gradient of less than 25 mm Hg
  - *Mild:* Gradient of 25–49 mm Hg
  - *Moderate:* Gradient of 50–79 mm Hg
  - *Severe:* Gradient of more than 80 mm Hg.

Medical Management

Prehospital care in patients with pulmonary valve stenosis:

- Collect essential information about vital signs, including the patient's pulse, respiratory rate, work of breathing, and blood pressure (BP) in the upper and lower extremities. Note the presence or absence of cyanosis.
- Associated congenital cardiac anomalies should be anticipated until proven otherwise.

- If the patient has a known large left-to-right shunt, such as patent ductus arteriosus (PDA) or ventricular septal defect (VSD), and if the patient is in respiratory distress, diuresis should be attempted. Diuresis is effective in reducing the cyanosis secondary to pulmonary edema, which is unusual in patients with isolated pulmonary valve stenosis.
- Use of oxygen may reduce pulmonary artery pressure in patients with a reactive pulmonary vasculature, increasing pulmonary blood flow, which is also unusual in patients with isolated pulmonary valve stenosis.
- Administer oxygen to any patient with cyanosis and respiratory distress. However, cyanosis-related intracardiac right-to-left shunting does not resolve hypoxemia.

Surgical Management

Balloon Pulmonary Valvuloplasty

Complications

- *Hypercontractile residual obstructing muscular hypertrophy in the infundibulum:* This complication is associated with surgical or balloon valvuloplasty for severe pulmonary stenosis.
- *Infundibular obstruction:* This phenomenon, which occurs after valvar stenosis repair by means of surgery or valvuloplasty, has led to the designation of a suicide right ventricle. Beta-blockers and volume replacement are used to treat this condition, which occurs more frequently in relatively old patients with long-standing pulmonary stenosis.
- Late atrial arrhythmias
- Persistent repolarization abnormalities.

Prognosis

- Mild valvar pulmonary stenosis usually does not progress, but moderate-to-severe disease does tend to progress.
- After the stenosis is relieved by means of balloon valvuloplasty, 8–10% patients require repeat intervention. The condition does not recur in the remaining patients, and right ventricular hypertrophy regresses.
- Pulmonary valve regurgitation may need reintervention and further long-term studies are required to assess the impact of this issue on long-term outcome.
- The outcome after balloon or surgical valvulotomy is generally excellent. The probability of survival is similar to that of the general population, and the vast majority of patients are asymptomatic.

Nursing Management

- The neonate with critical pulmonary valve stenosis requires special consideration.
  - Patients with critical pulmonary stenosis may present with near-pulmonary atresia (cyanotic lesion) with a small and often inadequate right ventricle. These patients survive because of a patent ductus arteriosus (PDA).
  - Although balloon pulmonary valvuloplasty produces good results, nearly 25% patients require reintervention to address related complications, restenosis, and associated defects.
- Child with associated severe infundibular or supravalvar pulmonary stenosis require surgical intervention.

- Definitive repair may not be possible if the right ventricle is hypoplastic or if single ventricular palliation (e.g. the Fontan procedure or a variation of this) is needed. The modified Fontan procedure currently used is staged cavopulmonary connection.
- Clinical, ECG, and Doppler echocardiographic evaluation are recommended at 1 month, 6 months, and 12 months after balloon pulmonary valvuloplasty and yearly thereafter.
- Patients with trivial and mild pulmonary stenosis do not need intervention to relieve the pulmonary valve obstruction. However, they should be clinically followed-up at periodic intervals (e.g. on a yearly basis).
- Routine well-child care, including immunizations, as per the primary physician, is suggested.
- Physical activity should be normal.
- Most patients with pulmonary stenosis are given prophylaxis for subacute bacterial endocarditis (SBE).
- Opinions differ about the need for SBE prophylaxis in patients with valvar pulmonary stenosis because of the extremely low incidence of pulmonary valve endocarditis in this relatively large subpopulation. The author recommends SBE prophylaxis for all patients with valvar pulmonary stenosis.

Parental Education

- Reassure parents of children with mild valvar pulmonary stenosis that this condition is not related to or associated with coronary artery disease, dysrhythmia, or sudden death.
- Insurability may become a factor in obtaining further care. Patients are no more at risk for disastrous health consequences than is the usual population.
- Provided the patient is asymptomatic and acyanotic and provided that initial Doppler echocardiograms show only mild valvar pulmonary stenosis, yearly screening examination and ECG are prudent follow-up care.
- If evaluations performed a few years after the initial evaluation reveal no clinically significant change, the patient may be followed-up once every 3–5 years.
- For excellent patient education resources, visit eMedicine's Heart Center. Also, see eMedicine's patient education article Tetralogy of Fallot.

AORTIC STENOSIS

INTRODUCTION

Aortic stenosis (AS) is the narrowing of the exit of the left ventricle of the heart such that problems result. It may occur at the aortic valve as well as above and below this level. Congenital heart disease occurs in 8 of 1000 live births. Aortic valve stenosis results from minor to severe degrees of aortic valve maldevelopment. This stenosis causes mild to severe obstruction of left ventricular outflow that may be associated with other left heart obstructive lesions or extracardiac malformations, including genetic disorders. This article focuses on presentation, clinical features, and therapeutic options associated with aortic valve stenosis. Bicuspid aortic valves without stenosis or insufficiency in adult patients can be associated with progressive pathologic enlargement of the aortic root of uncertain etiology, which infrequently leads to surgical aortic root replacement.

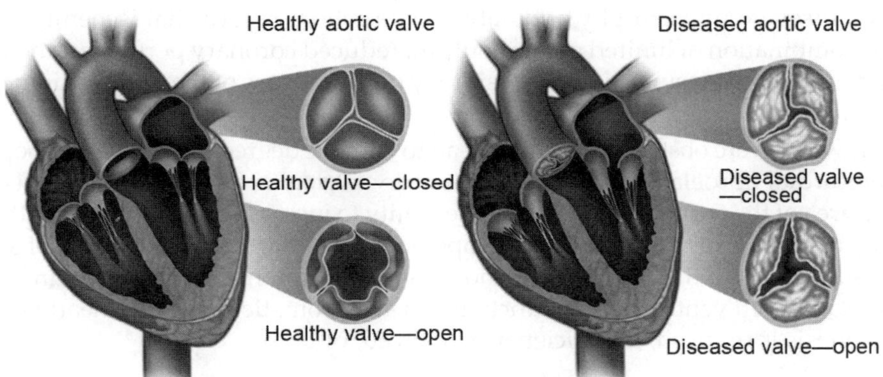

Fig. 6.81: Anatomical difference between normal heart and aortic stenosis

Definition

The aorta is the main artery that carries blood out of the heart to the rest of the body. Blood flows out of the heart and into the aorta through the aortic valve. In aortic stenosis mean narrowing of the aortic valve. This decreases blood flow from the heart. This obstructs blood flow from heart into aorta and onward to the rest of child body.

Incidence

Mortality is higher in patients presenting with severe or critical aortic valve stenosis during the first year of life, specifically in the neonatal period. Mortality is in part influenced by associated congenital cardiac anomalies, which occur in as many as 20% of patients. These include patent ductus arteriosus, coarctation of aorta, ventricular septal defect, mitral valve abnormalities, and left ventricular hypoplasia. Undetected, severe aortic valve stenosis is a known cause of sudden death and accounts for approximately 1% of all causes of sudden death in young people.

Causes

- Causes of aortic valve stenosis are multifactorial, although studies suggest a higher rate of recurrence of left ventricular outflow tract obstructive lesions than other forms of congenital heart disease
- Other forms of left heart obstructive disease may occur repeatedly within families (e.g. Hypoplastic left heart syndrome in a child whose older sibling had coarctation of the aorta).
- A definite genetic defect for aortic valve stenosis has not been identified, but the presence of a bicuspid aortic valve has been documented in multiple family members and is a common congenital heart defect in patients with Turner syndrome (monosomy X).

Pathophysiology

Pure aortic valve stenosis results in compensatory ventricular hypertrophy proportional to the degree of obstruction. Mild degrees of obstruction are usually well tolerated, with minimal hypertrophy and normal left ventricular function. As stenosis progresses, often in association with periods of rapid somatic growth, hypertrophy increases and reduces wall stress. With severe hypertrophy and valvar obstruction, myocardial ischemia may result from the combination of limited cardiac output, reduced coronary perfusion, and increased myocardial oxygen consumption. Fibrosis may occur in areas of the myocardium damaged by ischemia.

Infants with severe obstruction in utero lead to variable degrees of left heart hypoplasia and endomyocardial fibroelastosis, causing reduced ventricular function. A small, fixed cross-sectional area of the aortic valve can limit the ability to increase cardiac output with exercise. This may result in exercise-induced syncope or sudden death. Development of significant aortic insufficiency in the absence of stenosis is less common and may result in ventricular dilation. Rarely, left ventricular dysfunction and symptomatic congestive heart failure occur unless stenosis is reduced, insufficiency is relieved, or both.

Clinical Manifestation

- *Chest discomfort:* The chest pain may get worse with activity and reach into the arm, neck, or jaw. The chest may also feel tight or squeezed.
- Cough with blood
- Breathing problems when exercising
- Becoming easily tired
- Feeling the heart beat (palpitations)
- Fainting, weakness, or dizziness with activity.

In infants and children:

- Becoming easily tired with exertion (in mild cases)
- Failure to gain weight
- Poor feeding
- Serious breathing problems that develop within days or weeks of birth (in severe cases)
- Children with mild or moderate aortic stenosis may get worse as they get older.

Diagnostic Evaluation

The following may be indicated in patients with aortic valve stenosis:

- History collection and physical examination.
- The evaluation for sepsis in infants presenting with shock includes blood, urine, and cerebrospinal fluid (CSF) cultures.
- Pulse oximeter assessment is performed both preductally (typically in the right arm) and postductally (typically in a lower extremity).
- Oxygen saturation may be lower in the legs (postductal circulation) because of right-to-left shunting at the level of the ductus arteriosus.
- *Electrocardiogram (ECG):* Impulses are recorded as waves displayed on a monitor or printed on paper. An ECG can provide clues about whether the left ventricle is thickened or enlarged, a problem which can occur with aortic valve stenosis.
- *Chest X-ray:* An X-ray image of child chest allows checking the size and shape of your heart to determine whether the left ventricle is enlarged a possible indicator of aortic valve stenosis.
- *Cardiac catheterization:* Which helps your arteries become visible on an X-ray (coronary angiogram). This test helps show any blockages in arteries to child heart that can

coexist with aortic valve stenosis that may need surgical treatment along with aortic valve stenosis.

- *Exercise tests:* In exercise tests child allow to do the exercise to increase heart rate and check heart work harder. If child have severe aortic valve stenosis but are not experiencing symptoms, doctor may order exercise tests to evaluate how your heart responds to exertion (exercise) and to measure child tolerance for activity.
- *Computerized tomography (CT) scans:* A CT scan uses a series of X-rays to create detailed images of child heart and heart valves. Doctors may use this test to measure the size of aorta and look at child aortic valve more closely.
- *Magnetic resonance imaging (MRI):* An MRI uses powerful magnets and radio waves to create detailed images of heart and heart valves. Doctors may inject a dye into your blood vessels to highlight the heart and blood vessels in images (magnetic resonance angiography). Doctors may use this test to measure the size of aorta.

Medical Management

Medicines are used to treat symptoms of heart failure or abnormal heart rhythms (most commonly atrial fibrillation). These include diuretics (water pills), nitrates and beta-blockers. High blood pressure should also be treated. Medications can reduce symptoms of aortic valve stenosis. However, the only way to eliminate aortic valve stenosis is surgery to repair or replace the valve and open-up the passageway.

Surgical Management

Transcatheter balloon dilation in the 1980s were encouraging although morbidity related to aortic valve insufficiency and femoral artery compromises were considered limitations of the procedure. With the advent of improved catheter technology, percutaneous balloon valvuloplasty has become the procedure of choice in most centers for severe congenital aortic valve stenosis and can be safely performed with virtually no mortality and minimal morbidity.

Balloon Valvuloplasty

- A balloon valvuloplasty is an option. Balloon valvuloplasty uses a soft, thin tube (catheter) tipped with a balloon. A guides the catheter through a blood vessel in the groin to heart and into narrowed aortic valve. Once in position a balloon at the tip of the catheter is inflated.
- The balloon pushes open the aortic valve and stretches the valve opening, improving blood flow. The balloon is then deflated and the catheter with the balloon is guided back out of child body.
- Balloon valvuloplasty may relieve aortic valve stenosis and its symptoms especially in infants and children. However, in adults, the valve tends to narrow again even after initial success.

Aortic Valve Replacement

- This is the primary surgical treatment for severe aortic valve stenosis. The surgeon removes the narrowed aortic valve and replaces it with a mechanical valve or a tissue valve. This procedure is generally performed during open-heart surgery.

- Mechanical valves, made from metal, are durable, but they carry the risk of blood clots forming on or near the valve.
- If child receive a mechanical valve need to provide an anticoagulant medication, such as warfarin (Coumadin), for life to prevent blood clots.
- *Tissue valves:* This may come from a pig, cow or human deceased donor, often eventually narrow over the years and need to be replaced. Another type of tissue valve replacement that uses your own pulmonary valve (autograft) is sometimes possible but less likely in an older person. Doctor can discuss the risks and benefits of each type of heart valve with parents. Aortic valve replacement can relieve aortic valve stenosis and its symptoms.

Transcatheter Aortic Valve Replacement (TAVR)

- Aortic valve replacement, the most common treatment for aortic valve stenosis, has traditionally been performed with open-heart surgery.
- A less invasive approach—transcatheter aortic valve replacement—involves replacing the aortic valve with a prosthetic valve via the femoral artery in leg (transfemoral) or the left ventricular apex of heart (transapical).
- In TAVR insert a catheter with a balloon at the tip in an artery in your leg or in a small incision in chest and guide it to heart and into aortic valve.
- A balloon at the tip of the catheter, which has a folded valve around it, is then inflated. This pushes open the aortic valve and stretches the valve opening and expands the folded valve into the aortic valve.
- In some cases, a valve can be inserted via a catheter into a tissue replacement valve that needs to be replaced (valve-in-valve procedure).
- TAVR is usually reserved for individuals with severe aortic valve stenosis who are at increased risk of complications from aortic valve surgery. This procedure can relieve severe aortic valve stenosis and its symptoms in those who are at increased risk of complications from aortic valve surgery. TAVR has a higher risk of stroke and vascular complications than aortic valve replacement surgery. The technique is relatively new and is evolving quickly, and there are newer valves and indications occurring frequently. TAVR is sometimes referred to as transcatheter aortic valve implantation (TAVI).

Surgical Valvuloplasty

- In rare cases, surgical repair may be a more effective option than balloon valvuloplasty.
- Such as in infants born with an aortic valve in which the leaflets of the valve are fused together.
- Using traditional surgical tools, a cardiac surgeon operates on the valve and separates these leaflets to reduce stenosis and improve blood flow.

The Ross Procedure

- This procedures (pulmonary autograft) or autotransplantation of a pulmonary valve to the aortic position is favored by some surgeons because of the potential for growth of the pulmonary autograft valve through childhood.
- Such growth has been documented, as has adequate performance of a pulmonary valve in the aortic position. Problems with this procedure in children include development of early stenosis or insufficiency of a pulmonary homograft placed in the pulmonary position.

- This can necessitate multiple interventional catheterizations or surgical reoperations during childhood to alleviate the obstruction or insufficiency of the homograft.
- Significant enlargement of the neoaortic root, especially within the sinuses, may occur, and aortic insufficiency occasionally develops.
- This procedure does avoid the need for anticoagulation and serious sport restrictions, especially in active, injury-prone children.

Complications

- Congestive heart failure
- Myocardial injury and fibrosis
- Syncope
- Endocarditis
- Calcific aortic stenosis
- Progressive aortic insufficiency
- Systemic embolization
- Arrhythmias
- Sudden death.

Prognosis

The prognosis for patients with congenital aortic valve stenosis depends on the valve anatomy and its response to intervention. The severity of the disorder is widely varies, ranging from no symptoms in children with only a bicuspid aortic valve and minimal stenosis to critical illness in neonates who face the prospect of serial interventions. The main goal is to preserve the native aortic valve and ventricular function for as long as possible until aortic valve replacement is necessary.

Nursing Management

- Manage congestive heart failure in child with aortic valve stenosis
- Monitor for arrhythmias and initiate antiarrhythmics therapy as needed
- Monitor postprocedural or postsurgical recovery
- Provide patient education
- Manage congestive heart failure
- Provide physical rehabilitation
- Perform exercise stress testing to determine response to therapy or activity restrictions
- Provide patient education
- Use subacute bacterial endocarditis (SBE) prophylaxis for indicated procedures
- Prescribe other medicines as indicated for treatment of specific conditions such as congestive heart failure and arrhythmias.

Diet

Dietary restrictions are necessary.

Activity

- Activity limitations depend on the degree of severity of aortic valve stenosis and, in older children, the results noted on exercise stress testing.

- Strenuous isometric sports should be avoided; specific recommendations regarding sports participation have been published by the American Heart Association.

Parental Education

- Education is indicated for affected families regarding signs of progressive aortic stenosis, congestive heart failure, and low cardiac output. Education regarding good dental care and avoidance of risk factors for endocarditis is imperative. Other goals of parent education include setting reasonable goals for exercise participation that allow for a healthy lifestyle but downplaying long-term goals for competitive athletics at a high level until complete relief of aortic valve disease is accomplished by aortic valve repair or replacement.
- Similarly, emphasize that treatment of aortic valve disease is a lifelong process and is best introduced early and reinforced often to ensure that patients with aortic valve stenosis continue to receive ongoing follow-up care as they make the transition from an adolescent lifestyle at home to the independent lifestyle of young adulthood.

Special Concerns

- The choice of an aortic valve for aortic valve replacement may be more complicated in female patients contemplating pregnancy.
- The choice of a mechanical valve, a bioprosthetic valve, or a Ross procedure should be reviewed at length for all patients, particularly those contemplating valve replacement.
- Teratogenic effects of warfarin, management issues of anticoagulation during pregnancy, and need for reoperation, as well as durability of various valve options, should be reviewed at length.

CONGENITAL MITRAL STENOSIS (MS)

INTRODUCTION

The mitral valve is a one-way valve in the left side of the heart that allows blood to fill its 'pump,' the left ventricle. When a child has mitral valve stenosis (also known simply as 'mitral stenosis'), her mitral valve cannot open fully creating a problematic blockage.

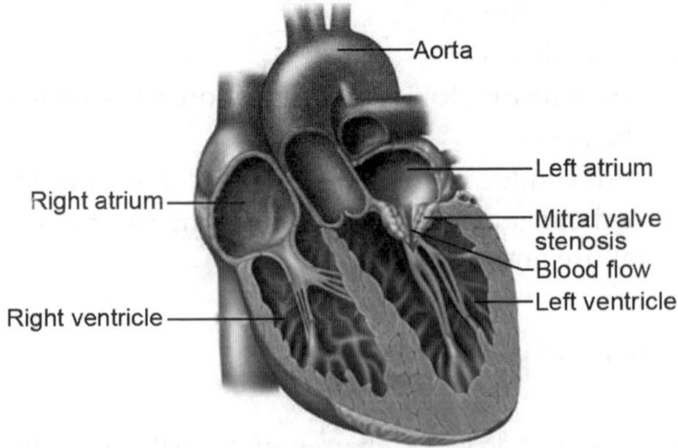

Fig. 6.82: Anatomy of normal heart with valves

Causes

- Mitral valve stenosis is typically caused by rheumatic fever. This is usually a childhood disease, and it results from the body's immune response to an infection with the streptococcal bacteria. It is a serious complication of strep throat or scarlet fever.
- Birth defect such as:
  - A narrowed mitral valve
  - A damaged or malformed mitral valve.

Rare causes for mitral valve stenosis include:

- Tumors
- Blood clots
- Radiation treatments
- Calcium buildup on valves
- Congenital heart defects.

Signs and Symptoms of Mitral Valve Stenosis

Most of the children with mitral valve stenosis show no outward signs, since they are in the mild to moderate stages of the condition and their symptoms have not yet progressed to a more serious level. The only identifiable symptoms in most cases are rapid breathing, slow growth/weight gain or a soft heart murmur.

- Rapid or labored breathing
- Frequent coughing or wheezing
- Slow growth/weight gain
- Feeding difficulties
- Fatigue
- Frequent respiratory infections
- Irregular heartbeats or heart palpitations
- Chest pain
- Swelling in ankles and/or feet
- Respiratory infections
- Plum-colored cheeks.

Pathophysiology

MS obstructs blood flow into the LV, elevating left atrial pressure in proportion to severity of the stenosis. This, in turn, restricts pulmonary venous return to the left atrium, elevating pulmonary vascular and, consequently, right heart pressures. Elevated hydrostatic pressure in the pulmonary capillaries forces fluid into the alveoli and interstitial space, producing pulmonary congestion. Congested bronchial veins may encroach on small bronchioles, with subsequent increase in airway resistance.

As a compensatory mechanism, pulmonary vasoconstriction occurs. The right ventricle (RV) pressure increases, resulting in RV hypertrophy. Elevated pulmonary pressure can progress to fixed pulmonary arterial hypertension from medial hypertrophy and intimal thickening of the pulmonary arterioles. The RV eventually fails, and pulmonary blood flow decreases, decreasing systemic blood flow. If the reduction in cardiac output is critical, end organ failure with renal and/or hepatic insufficiency, shock, and metabolic acidosis can occur. RV failure results in systemic venous congestion with development of hepatomegaly, ascites, and pedal edema.

Hemodynamic changes in severe congenital mitral valve stenosis (MS). MS causes an obstruction (in diastole) to blood flow from the left atrium (LA) to the left ventricle (LV). Increased LA pressures are transmitted retrograde to pulmonary veins and pulmonary capillaries, resulting in capillary leak with subsequent development of pulmonary edema. To overcome pulmonary edema, the arterioles constrict, increasing pulmonary pressures. With time, capillaries develop intimal thickening, causing fixed (permanent) pulmonary hypertension. The right ventricle (RV) hypertrophies to generate enough pressure to overcome the increased afterload. Eventually, the RV fails, which manifests as hepatomegaly and/or ascites, edema of the extremities, and cardiomegaly on radiography.

Diagnostic Evaluation

Imaging Studies

Chest Radiography

- Left atrial dilation
- Posteroanterior (PA) dilation secondary to high pulmonary vascular pressure and resistance
- Pulmonary venous congestion
- Right ventricular enlargement.

Echocardiography

- Echocardiography is the most important diagnostic tool to evaluate patients with mitral stenosis (MS). This noninvasive imaging modality provides excellent anatomic and hemodynamic assessment of MS.

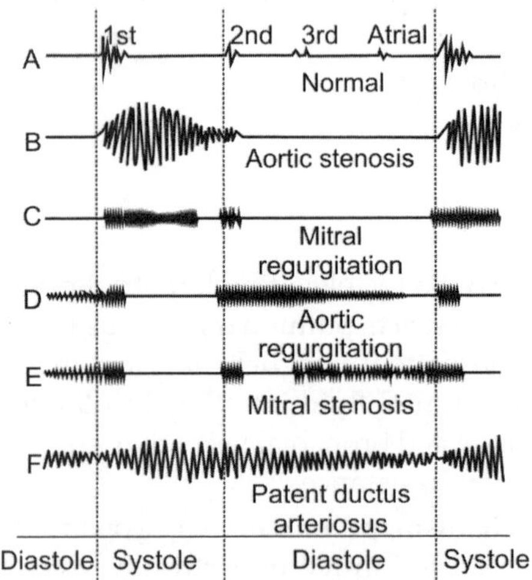

Phonocardiograms from normal and abnormal heart sounds

Cardiac Catheterization

- This may be used to obtain direct intracardiac pressure measurements, the mitral valve gradient, pulmonary vascular resistance, and systemic cardiac output.
- The diagnosis and hemodynamic assessment of most patients with MS is performed noninvasively with echocardiography. However, cardiac catheterization is used only when echocardiography does not provide complete information or if the patient undergoes mitral balloon valvuloplasty.

Other Tests

- Electrocardiography findings may be normal in patients with mild MS. Hemodynamically significant stenosis results in ECG findings of left atrial or biatrial enlargement and RV enlargement in proportion to severity of the obstruction.
- MRI is used infrequently; however, experience with this imaging modality in MS is more limited than with echocardiography.

Management

Asymptomatic patients with mild mitral stenosis (MS) require no significant therapy. They should undergo yearly follow-up care with physical examination, chest radiography, and ECG with echocardiography as indicated by this assessment. These patients may remain stable for decades before MS progresses and the patient requires surgical intervention.

- More significant stenosis producing mild symptoms can be managed with diuretics alone. Direct careful attention to proper diet and to early intervention for pulmonary disease.
- For the patient with congestive heart failure, administer loop diuretics plus potassium-sparing diuretics. Digoxin may improve right ventricular function in the setting of pulmonary hypertension.
- Address cardiac rhythm abnormalities with appropriate medications.
- Patients with chronic uncontrolled atrial tachyarrhythmias should be on anticoagulant therapy.

Medication

Medical therapy is used to avoid or decrease pulmonary congestion as well as to treat atrial tachyarrhythmias. These require medical therapy to prevent thromboembolic complications, anticoagulants (blood thinners)

- Diuretics (to reduce fluid buildup through increased urine output)
- Antiarrhythmics (medications to treat abnormal heart rhythms)
- Beta-blockers (medications to slow your heart rate).

Loop Diuretics

By promoting renal excretion of water and electrolytes, loop diuretics decrease pulmonary congestion. Pulmonary congestion results from back-flow to the lungs caused by obstruction across a narrowed mitral valve orifice.

Furosemide

Furosemide acts by inhibiting absorption of the electrolytes sodium and chloride in the proximal and distal tubules and in the loop of Henle, thereby promoting excretion of salt (sodium chloride) and water. It acts as a diuretic and as an antihypertensive.

Surgical Management

Therefore balloon dilation of congenital MS, although performed in some centers, is not always successful. According to a recent study, younger patients and those who develop significant mitral regurgitation after balloon-dilation have a worse outcome. However, because the 5-year survival is still relatively poor in those with severe congenital MS, regardless of treatment modality, the optimal therapeutic strategy remains unclear. Surgical options depend on specific mitral valve pathology.

Mitral Valve Repair

- Commissurotomy consists of an incision of fused mitral valve commissures and shaving of thickened mitral valve leaflets. Open surgical commissurotomy is preferable.
- Divide fused chordae tendineae and papillary muscles to relieve subvalvular stenosis.
- Resect any supravalvular tissue contributing to the MS.

Mitral Valve Replacement with Mechanical Valve or Bioprosthesis

- This is reserved for patients with severe MS in whom mitral valve repair is not possible. In older children for whom warfarin (Coumadin) therapy may be contraindicated, mitral valve replacement can be performed using a bioprosthesis, although the durability of tissue valves is less than mechanical prosthesis.
- The risk of warfarin therapy should be weighed against the disadvantage of progressive bioprosthetic valve deterioration resulting in the certain need for reoperation.
- Mitral valve replacement is best avoided in infants and small children because of frequent size mismatch between the smallest mechanical valves and the hypoplastic mitral valve annulus. In addition, somatic growth in children leads to the need for subsequent mitral prosthesis replacements.
- Warfarin therapy is also more difficult to administer and to monitor in children. A less-than-perfect mitral valve repair is frequently preferable to mitral valve replacement in this group of patients.
- Complications after mitral valve replacement include the risks of anticoagulation, valve thrombosis, valve dehiscence, infective endocarditis, valve malfunction, and embolic events.
- However, in complex anatomy, replacement is the only solution to achieve an acceptable result. The Ross II operation, which uses a pulmonary autograft, is a difficult technique that may be useful in the youngest patient group when prosthetic devices cannot be used. This technique is still under clinical evaluation.

Prevention

- Antibiotics for endocarditis prophylaxis are required for patients with certain cardiac conditions, such as mitral stenosis, before performing procedures that may cause bacteremia. For more information, see Antibiotic Prophylactic Regimens for Endocarditis.
- Avoid excessive salt intake, which increases fluid retention and may worsen symptoms.
  - Avoid excessive heat, excessive use of diuretics, and dehydration, which may decrease LV output by reducing preload.
  - Patients taking anticoagulants should avoid contact sports because of risks of cerebral, splenic, renal, or other internal organ bleeding. Pregnant women should avoid warfarin because of its teratogenic effects and risk of miscarriage.

Complications

- If MS is left untreated, the following complications may arise:
  - Pulmonary edema
  - Right heart failure with progression to congestive heart failure
  - Renal insufficiency (due to congestive heart failure)
  - Progression to pulmonary hypertension
  - Atrial arrhythmias: Atrial arrhythmias such as fibrillation or flutter occur more frequently in patients with chronic left atrial enlargement. Initiation and perpetuation of these arrhythmias has been attributed to a vertical line of conduction delay that runs between the pulmonary veins.
  - Thrombus formation in the dilated left atrium (due to stasis of blood)
  - Embolization of left atrial thrombus, stroke
  - Dysphagia from compression of esophagus by the enlarged left atrium.
- Complications of medical treatment
  - Diuretics may provoke dehydration (decreased preload) with subsequent compromise in cardiac output that may precipitate prerenal renal failure.
  - Warfarin may cause bleeding, such as intracranial hemorrhage and GI bleeding.
- Complications of surgery
  - Mitral commissurotomy may cause significant postoperative mitral regurgitation, which may necessitate subsequent mitral valve replacement.
  - The risks of mitral valve replacement include those associated with anticoagulation, valve thrombosis, valve dehiscence, infective endocarditis, valve malfunction, and embolic events.

Prognosis

- Untreated newborns with severe MS have a grim prognosis. Surgical intervention is ideally avoided for as long as possible. Mechanical mitral valve replacement in a small infant or child is a high-risk procedure and carries a guarded prognosis.
- Operative results and long-term outcome are widely variable and highly depends on the abnormalities that are present.
- Mitral valve replacement entails a less than 5% mortality risk in young, healthy patients without other significant cardiac abnormalities.

Nursing Managements

- Critically ill patients or patients unable to take oral medication may receive intravenous medications. Admission to the ICU and endotracheal intubation may be required because of ineffective breathing caused by pulmonary edema.
- Monitor the patient's anticoagulation therapy to prevent thrombus formation and to decrease the risk of embolization in case of a mechanical mitral valve. Remember that embolization is to the systemic circulation because these emboli come from the left atrium and many emboli reach the brain.
- Regular visits to the pediatrician and/or generalist to monitor general health status, depending on the severity of the mitral stenosis (MS).
- Regular visits to the pediatric cardiologist to monitor hemodynamic status, antiarrhythmic drug levels, and anticoagulation.

- *Serial echocardiography to monitor anatomic and hemodynamic progression of the MS:* The frequency varies according to the patient's general health status and according to the cardiologist's criteria.
- *Stress Doppler hemodynamics using a supine bicycle or treadmill:* Hemodynamics may be measured using transthoracic echocardiographic Doppler. This noninvasive test has replaced the traditional exercise stress test in the catheterization laboratory.

Diet Managements

- Restrict salt and avoid excessive fluids. Maintain proper nutrition. Caloric supplementation may be necessary in the symptomatic infant.

Activity

- Patients should avoid strenuous exercise because an increased heart rate decreases diastolic filling time. If atrial flutter and atrial fibrillation are present and atrial kick is lost, a further decrease in LV stroke volume occurs. This may result in syncope from decreased cerebral perfusion.

Parental Education

- Counsel the patient and families regarding the appearance and worsening of symptoms.
- Prior to any invasive or surgical application, advise the patient regarding subacute bacterial endocarditis prophylaxis.
- Monitor prothrombin time (PT) and international normalized ratio (INR) if the patient is on anticoagulation medication.
- Advise pregnant mothers to avoid taking warfarin, avoid strenuous activity and excessive salt intake, and have their blood pressure frequently monitored.
- For excellent patient education resources, visit eMedicine's Heart Center.

Special Concerns

- Asymptomatic or minimally symptomatic patients may only require close observation, but severely symptomatic patients may require urgent surgical intervention.
- Pregnant women who require anticoagulation because of a prosthetic mitral valve should receive heparin, which does not cross the placental barrier. They should not receive warfarin because of its teratogenic effects and fetal wastage.
- Pregnant women with underlying heart disease require antibiotic prophylaxis with ampicillin and gentamicin or with amoxicillin if they undergo potentially bacteremic procedures.
- Of note, cesarean delivery or uncomplicated abdominal delivery are not indications for antibiotic prophylaxis.

ORTHOPEDIC ABNORMALITIES

CONGENITAL TALIPES EQUINOVARUS (CLUB FOOT)

Introduction

Talipes equinovarus (Club foot) is a deformity of the foot and ankle that a child can be born with this problem. It is not clear exactly what causes talipes. In most of the cases it is diagnosed by the typical appearance of a baby's foot after they are born. The Ponseti method is now a widely used treatment for talipes. This treatment gives good results for most children and so major surgery is not usually needed to correct the foot deformity.

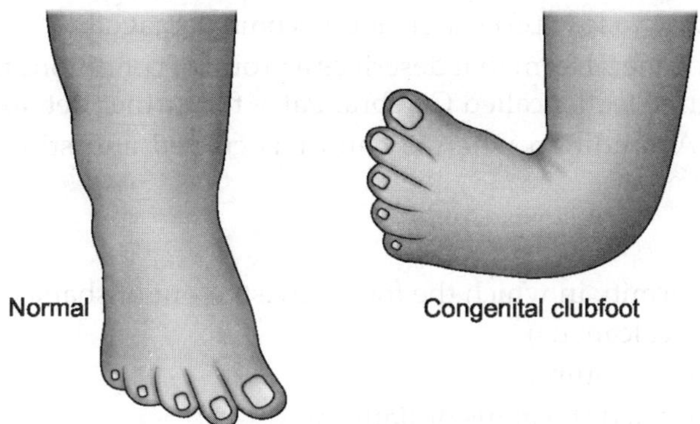

Fig. 6.83: Anatomical difference between normal and club foot

Definition

Clubfoot or Talipes Equinovarus is a congenital anomaly in which the foot is plantar flexed at the ankle and subtalar joints, the hind foot is inverted, and the midfoot and forefoot are adducted and inverted.

A deformity of the foot and ankle called club foot, in which the foot is twisted and relatively fixed in an abnormal position. Talipes refers to deformities that involve the foot and ankle, where as refers only to deformities of the foot. Kinds of talipes include talipes calcaneo-valgus, talipes calcaneo-varus, and talipes equinovarus.

Incidence

According to the National Institutes of Health (NIH), USA, approximately 1 in every 1,000 babies is born with club foot. Males are twice as likely to have the condition as females. According to the National Health Service (NHS), UK, if one child is born with club foot there is a 1 in 30 chance that his/her younger sibling will also be affected.

Causes

It is not clear exactly why talipes develops. It is thought that there may possibly be some genetic factors involved. There is about a 3–4 in 100 chances that a brother or sister born after them will also have talipes equinovarus. Babies born to a parent who has talipes also have an increased risk of being born with the problem themselves. If both parents have talipes, this risk is higher. Talipes may also have something to do with the position of the baby's foot when the baby is in the womb.

This foot abnormality can be multi-factorial in nature, meaning there could be several different predisposing factors.

- *Extrinsic:* This type is usually mild and supple. The cause can be due to intrauterine compression (large baby, abnormally shaped or small uterus, or abnormal intrauterine fluid levels).
- *Intrinsic:* This type is commonly more severe, rigid and the calf muscle is smaller. The foot may be smaller and there can be a bone deformity of the talus.

Clubfoot present at birth can point to further health problems because clubfoot can be linked with other conditions such as:
- *Spina bifida:* A condition where the bones of the spine do not form properly, causing the nerves of the spine to lose protection and become damaged.
- *Cerebral palsy:* A general term that describes a group of conditions that cause movement problems. Separate leaflet called Cerebral Palsy for further details.
- *Arthrogryposis:* A condition where a child has curved and stiff joints and abnormal muscle development.

Types

It is a congenital deformity in which the foot is twisted out of shape or position.
- Indorsiflexion (t. calcaneus)
- In plantar flexion (t. equinus)
- Abducted and everted (t. valgus or flatfoot)
- Abducted and inverted (t. varus)
- Various combinations (t. calcaneovalgus, t. calcaneovarus, t. equinovalgus, or t. equinovarus).

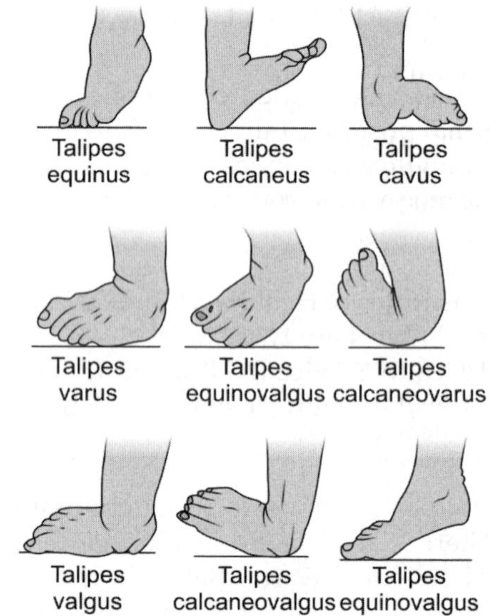

Fig. 6.84: Types of congenital talipes equinovarus

Signs and Symptoms

- Usually clubfoot is painless in a children
- Discomfort and become a noticeable disability
- The foot will remain twisted out of shape and the affected leg may be shorter and smaller than the other
- Poor child growth and development
- Body image disturbance

- The calf muscles are generally underdeveloped
- Stiff, rigid, foot of varying degrees.

Diagnostic Evaluation

- History collection
- Physical examination
- Ultrasound scanning during pregnancy
- X-rays.

Management

There have been some changes to the treatment for talipes over recent years. Major surgery was often a common treatment used. However, the results of medical research studies have shown that other treatments without major surgery, particularly a treatment known as the Ponseti method, seem to give good long-term results for most children. The Ponseti method is now the preferred treatment by most orthopedic surgeons throughout the world. Although the Ponseti method is usually preferred, there are other treatment methods available. One example is the French functional method. The French functional method involves daily manipulation as well as immobilization with adhesive bandages and pads.

The Ponseti Method

The specialist gently manipulates (holds, stretches and moves) the child's foot with their hands into a position in which the foot deformity is put right (corrected) as much as possible. This is not painful or uncomfortable for the child. Once in this position, a plaster cast is put on to hold the child's foot in position. This plaster cast usually goes from the child's toes to their groin area.

The aim is to correct the bend in the foot. Then a plaster cast is applied from the patient's toes to their thigh to hold the foot in correct position. Each session is generally done once a week. The manipulation and casting are done very gently and the child should experience no pain. At each session the plaster cast is changed, and each time the foot is corrected a tiny bit more. The whole process may be done 4 to 10 times (4 to 10 new casts used).

Surgical Management

The physician will decide whether a minor operation on the Achilles tendon (to release it) is needed. When the foot is eventually corrected, the patient has to wear special boots attached to a brace to hold the foot (feet) in the best position. For two to three months the boots are worn 23 hours a day; eventually they are just worn at night and during daytime naps—until the patient is about four years old. For the Ponseti method to be effective it has to be done very early on and parents have to make sure the boots are worn according to instructions. If instructions are not followed strictly, the foot may go back to the way it was, and treatment has to start again.

- Soft tissue surgery that releases the tight tissues around the joints and results in lengthening of tendons so the foot can assume a more corrected position.
- Bony procedures such as 'breaking bone' and resetting the bone to correct deformities, or fusing joints together to stabilize joints to enable the bones to grow solidly together.
- Tendon transfers to move the tendons to a different position, so they can move the foot into a corrected position.

The French Functional Method

It consists of daily stretching, exercise, massage, and immobilization of the foot with non-elastic tape to slowly move the foot to the correct position. These therapy sessions are performed primarily by a physical therapist for the first three months, when most of the improvement occurs, but parents receive training during this time in order to perform some of the treatments at home. The taping and splinting continues until the child is two years old.

Denis-Browne Bar and Shoes

A child's foot will continue to grow, change and shape for several years. Once the casting is completed, the child will be transitioned into a set of special shoes to keep the foot in correct alignment. This next step in the treatment process is the longest and most important. The special pair of shoes with a bar attached at the bottom will be made for the baby. These are called Denis-Browne Shoes and Bar and they are fit at an orthotist office. The bar, not the shoes, is the main workhorse of this treatment and must be used at all times.

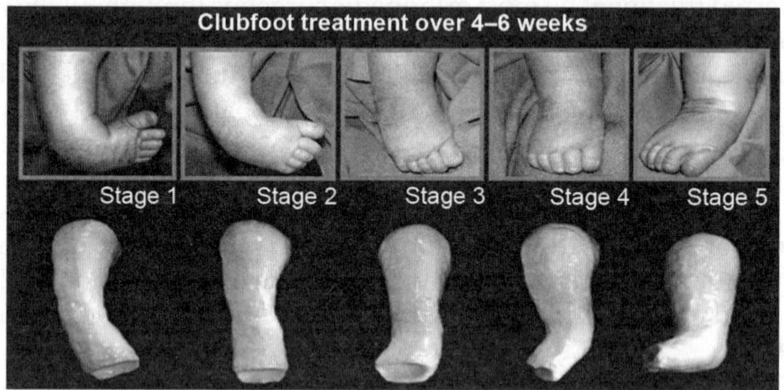

Fig. 6.85: The Ponseti method of clubfoot management

Nursing Management

It is important to keep regular follow-up appointments after the casts are completed. The orthopedist may be able to notice subtle changes in the child's foot alignment or flexibility that would suggest the correction is not being maintained with the bar and shoes. If caught early, this alignment can be corrected with some short term cast application.

Cast Care and Daily Concerns

It is important to check the baby's toes every hour or so during the first day of casting with each cast change. This is to insure the circulation is good. After the first day, the toes should be checked about every 12 hours. Lightly pinching the toes should cause them to turn pale and then return to pink within a few seconds. The foot is not properly aligned in the cast, the correction will be lost. (This tip will be useful with the Denis-Browne shoes as well. If you cannot see all the toes at the edge of the shoes, the foot may not be seated all the way into the shoe and the correction will not be maintained.)

- The cast should become very wet where it falls apart, or if the cast literally falls off just from kicking.
- The baby seems to be crying more than usual and seems to be in pain, and if the toes are not maintaining a warm and pink appearance.

- The child has had a surgical procedure, and the child should develop a temperature over 101 °F through the night, treat the elevated temperature and contact the orthopedic center the next morning.
- If she has questions at any time the staff nurses will be happy to assist parents and child.

CONGENITAL DISLOCATION OF HIPS

Introduction

The hip is a 'ball-and-socket' joint. In a normal hip, the ball at the upper end of the thighbone (femur) fits firmly into the socket, which is part of the large pelvis bone. In babies and children with developmental dysplasia (dislocation) of the hip (DDH), the hip joint has not formed normally. The ball is loose in the socket and may be easy to dislocate.

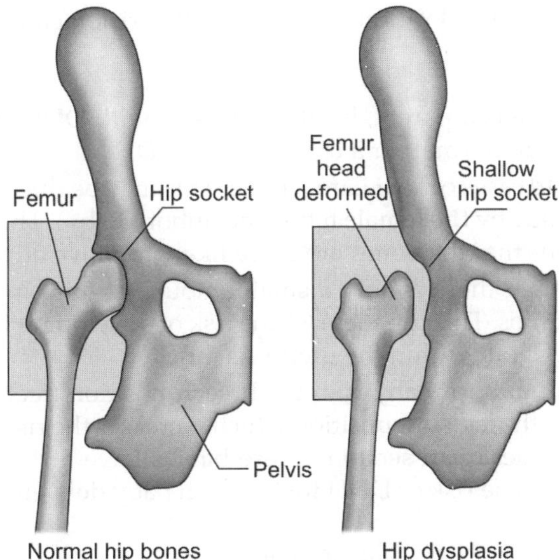

Definition

Congenital hip dislocation (CHD) occurs when a child is born with an unstable hip due to abnormal formation of the hip joint during their early stages of fetal development.

Types

The degree of hip looseness, or instability, varies among children with DDH.

- *Subluxatable:* In mild cases of DDH, the head of the femur is simply loose in the socket. During a physical examination, the bone can be moved within the socket, but it will not dislocate.
- *Low dislocation:* In the most severe cases of DDH, the head of the femur is completely out of the socket.
- *High dislocation:* In these cases, the head of the femur lies within the acetabulum, but can easily be pushed out of the socket during a physical examination.

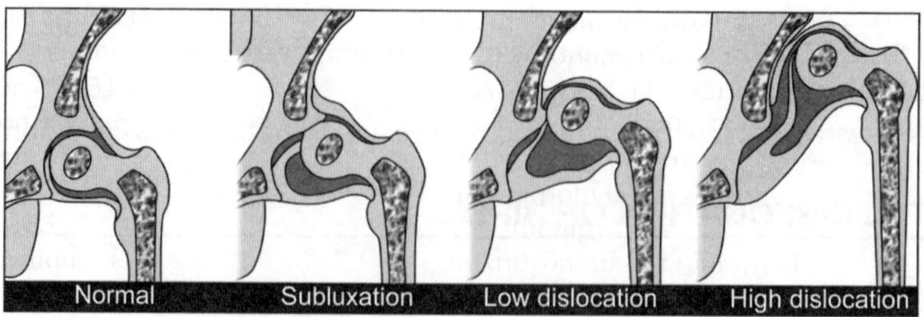

Fig. 6.86: Types of hip dislocation

Causes

The exact cause is not clear. There are factors that are known to contribute to the chance of a baby being born with DDH. Only 1 in 75 babies with a risk factor have a dislocated hip.

Risk Factors Include

- *Family history:* If there is a parent, brother or sister with DDH then this makes it five times more likely than normal for a child to have DDH.
- *Gender:* About 8 in 10 cases of DDH are female. This may be due to estrogen (the female hormone) that is made by the female fetus (the unborn baby). This makes the ligaments stretchier and means that the bones are more likely to move out of position.
- *Pregnancy conditions:* If there is only a small amount of fluid in the womb (uterus) is called oligohydramnios. This can increase the risk of developing DDH because the baby is not able to move about within the uterus as much.
- *Breech position:* If an unborn baby is in the breech position (feet down position in the uterus), this can put the legs in a position which increases the risk of DDH. Most breech babies are born by caesarean section. These babies have a risk of DDH seven times higher than normal. (The risk of DDH for a breech baby delivered vaginally is 17 times higher than normal.)
- *Firstborn baby:* About 6 in 10 cases of DDH occur in firstborn children. This may be because the uterus is tighter and less elastic than in future pregnancies so that the baby has less room to move.
- *Other abnormalities:* If the baby has cerebral palsy, spinal cord problems or other nerve and muscle disorders, this increases the risk of developing DDH. DDH is also more common in premature babies or babies born weighing more than 5 kg.

Signs and Symptoms

Symptoms that may occur in a newborn can include:

- Leg with hip problem may appear to turn out more
- Reduced movement on the side of the body with the dislocation
- Shorter leg on the side with the hip dislocation
- Uneven skin folds of thigh or buttocks
- After 3 months of age, the affected leg may turn outward or be shorter than the other leg.

Once the child begins walking symptoms can include:
- Waddling or limping while walking
- One shorter leg, so the child walks on their toes on one side and not the other side
- The child's lower back is rounded inward.

Diagnostic Evaluation
- History collection
- Physical examination
- Ultrasound scan
- X-ray

The screening for CHD occurs at birth and throughout the first year of your child's life. The most common screening method is a physical exam. The child's doctor will gently maneuver the child's hip and legs while listening for clicking or clunking sounds that may indicate a dislocation.

This exam consists of two tests:
- *Ortolani test:* The pediatrician will apply upward force while they move your child's hip away from the child's body. Movement away from the body is called abduction.
- *Barlow test:* The pediatrician will apply downward force while they move the child's hip across child's body. Movement toward the body is called adduction.

These tests are only accurate before the child is 3 months old. In older babies and children, findings that indicate CHD include limping, limited abduction, and a difference in leg lengths if they have a single affected hip.

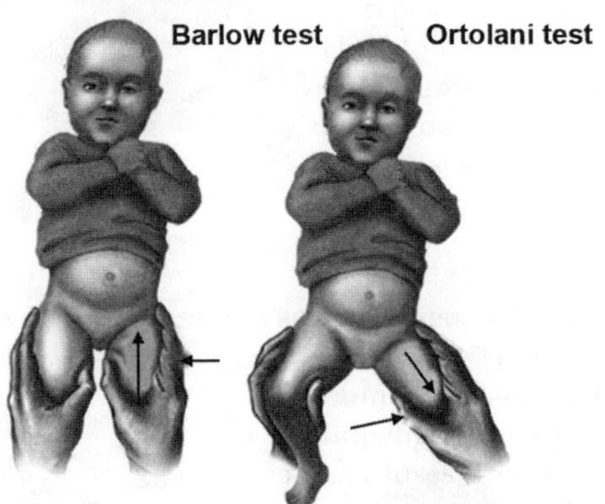

Fig. 6.87: Screening test for assessment of hip dislocation

Management
- Treatment is needed because if the head of the femur is left in an abnormal position then the hip joint develops abnormally. The earlier treatment is started after birth, the greater the likely success of treatment and the lower rate of long-term complications.
- The goal of treatment is to relocate the head of the femur into the acetabulum. This then allows the structures of the rapidly developing hip joint (femur, acetabulum, supporting ligaments, etc) to become established normally.

- The treatment goal can be achieved through a variety of methods, depending on the age of your child. The success rate of simple nonsurgical treatments reduces significantly after 7 weeks of age.

Pavlik Harness

This is a device that is used to hold the hips in the correct position. It is often the first treatment used in children under 6 months old. It usually needs to be worn for at least six weeks full-time and six weeks part-time in young babies. Older babies may need to wear it for longer. During this time, ultrasound scans are usually done to check that the hip is in the correct position. This harness keeps the legs bent and turned outwards, but allows certain movements. It does not allow child to straighten their legs or turn them inwards. The harness is adjusted as the child grows and as the hip stabilises.

- Mild DDH (subluxation) harness works in more than 9 in 10 children if used at this young age.
- In severe DDH (dislocation), the harness is effective in about 8 in 10 children.
- The main possible complication of the harness is called avascular necrosis.

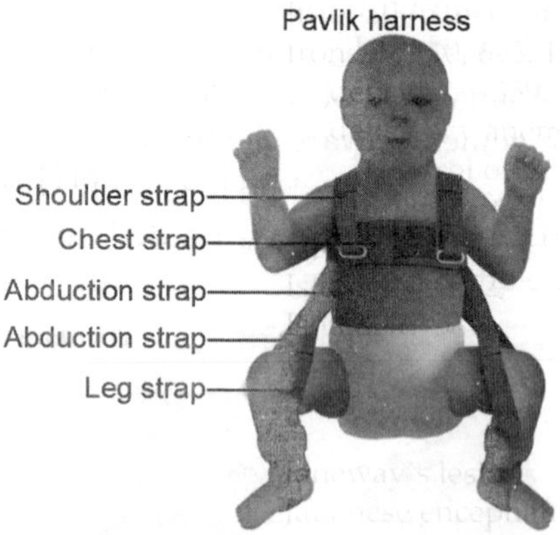

Closed Reduction and Hip Spica

This method is used in children over 6 months of age, or if the Pavlik harness is not effective. This involves your child being given an anesthetic. While they are anesthetized, the doctor

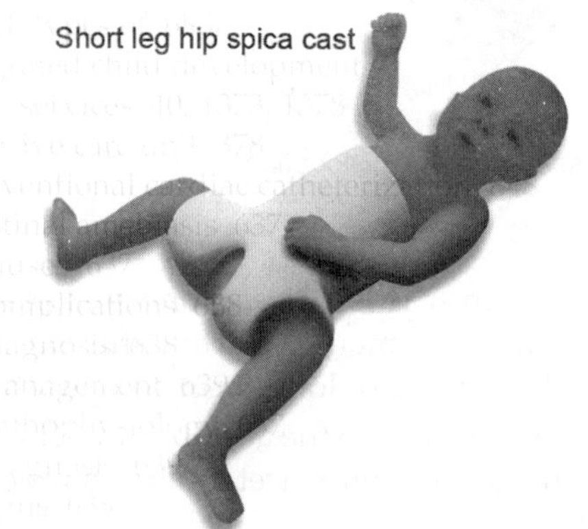

Fig. 6.88: Short leg hip spica cast

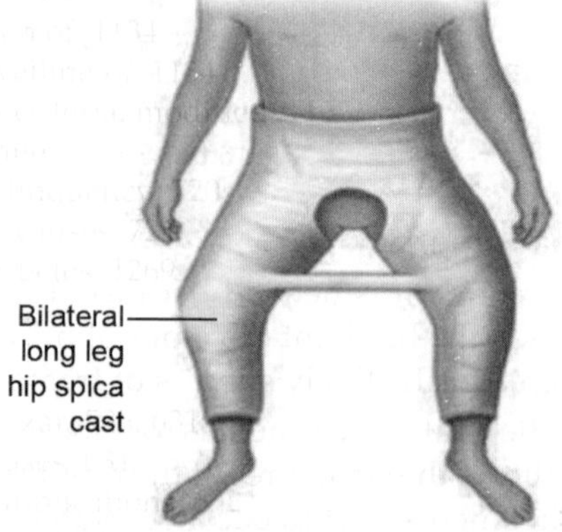

Fig. 6.89: Bilateral long leg spica cast

positions the hip the correct way and then applies a special cast or plaster to keep the hip in the right position. The position of the hip is confirmed as correct by an MRI or CT scan done after the procedure. This cast is kept on for at least 12 weeks.

Surgical Management

Open Reduction

The child is much older when DDH is diagnosed, then an operation is needed. The operation involves loosening the tendons around the hip and removing anything that is stopping the hip from moving freely. Once the bones are in a good position, the joint is strengthened.

- *Six months to two years:* If a closed reduction procedure is not successful in putting the thighbone is proper position, open surgery is necessary. In this procedure, an incision is made at the baby's hip that allows the surgeon to clearly see the bones and soft tissues.

  The thighbone will be shortened in order to properly fit the bone into the socket. X-rays are taken during the operation to confirm that the bones are in position. Afterwards, the child is placed in a spica cast to maintain the proper hip position.
- *Older than two years:* In some children, the looseness worsens as the child grows and becomes more active. Open surgery is typically necessary to realign the hip. A spica cast is usually applied to maintain the hip in the socket.

Nursing Management

- Pain relief
- Protect operated joint from further injury
- RICE therapy (rest, ice, compression, elevation)
- Immobilization
- Family support
- Making sure that the family understand the rehabilitation program
- Demonstrating the adaptation required for patients in cast
- Making sure that the family understand how to check for suture line infections and if there are drainage or bad odor from the cast, the importance of reporting them immediately.

CHROMOSOMAL ABNORMALITIES

DOWN SYNDROME

Introduction

Down's syndrome otherwise called as Down syndrome, it is a genetic condition that typically causes some level of learning disability and characteristic physical features. Genes carry the codes responsible for all of our inherited traits and are grouped along rod-like structures called chromosomes. Typically, the nucleus of each cell contains 23 pairs of chromosomes, half of which are inherited from each parent. Down syndrome occurs when an individual has a full or partial extra copy of chromosome 21. A few of the common physical traits of Down syndrome are low muscle tone, small stature, an upward slant to the eyes, and a single deep crease across the center of the palm-although each person with Down syndrome is a unique individual.

Definition

Down syndrome is defined as it is a genetic disorder caused when abnormal cell division results in extra genetic material from chromosome trisomy 21. This genetic disorder which varies in severity causes lifelong intellectual disability and developmental delays and in some people it causes health problems.

Causes

At the time of conception a fetus inherits genetic information from its parents in the form of 46 chromosomes: Twenty three from the mother and twenty three from the father. In most cases of Down syndrome, a child gets an extra chromosome 21 for a total of 47 chromosomes instead of 46. It is this extra genetic material that causes the physical features and developmental delays associated with Down syndrome.

- Exact causes still unknown
- Genetic causes (trisomy 21 defect).

Advancing Maternal Age

A woman's chances of giving birth to a child with Down syndrome increase with age because older eggs have a greater risk of improper chromosome division. A woman who has more risk of getting Down syndrome baby:

- 20 years of age has a risk of one in 1,500
- 30 years of age has a risk of one in 800
- 35 years of age has a risk of one in 270
- 40 years of age has a risk of one in 100
- 45 years of age has a risk of one in 50 or greater.

Types of Down's Syndrome

There are three forms of Down's syndrome, although the effects of each type are usually very similar.

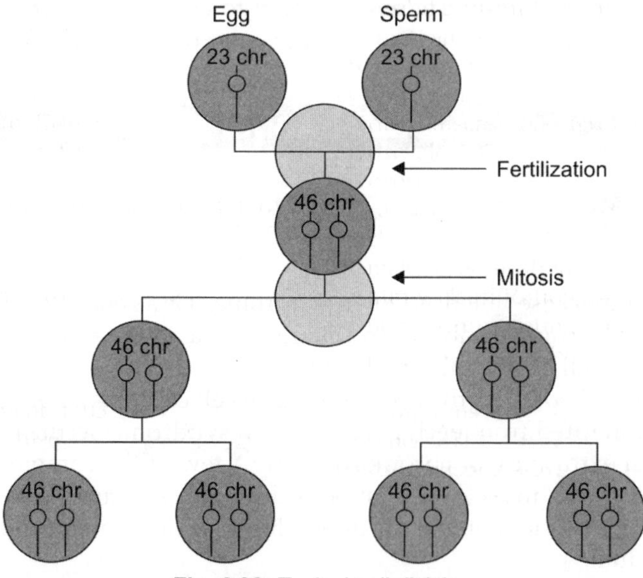

Fig. 6.90: Typical cell division

- *Trisomy 21* is the most common type, affecting around 94% of people with Down's syndrome. It is where every cell in the body has an extra copy of chromosome 21.
- *Translocation* is where an extra piece of chromosome 21 attaches itself to another chromosome. It affects around 4% of people with Down's syndrome. In this situation, there are only 46 chromosomes in each cell but one of them has extra material attached, so the total amount of genetic material in the cell is similar to that seen in a trisomy.
- *Mosaicism* is the least common type, affecting around 2% of people with Down's syndrome. Only some of the cells have an extra copy of chromosome 21, which can mean people with mosaic Down's syndrome experience less delay with some aspects of their development.

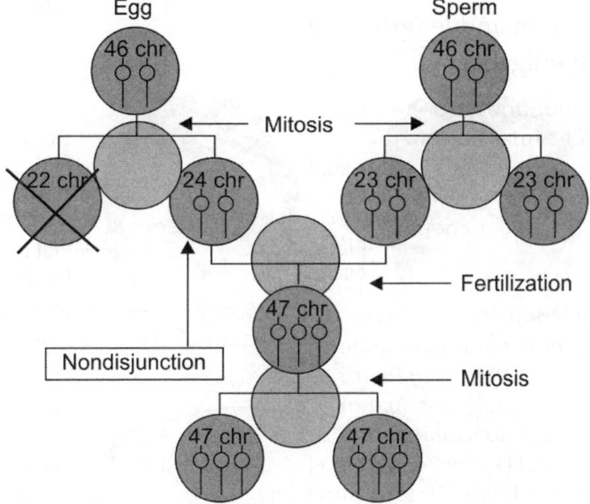

Fig. 6.91: Trisomy 21 cell division

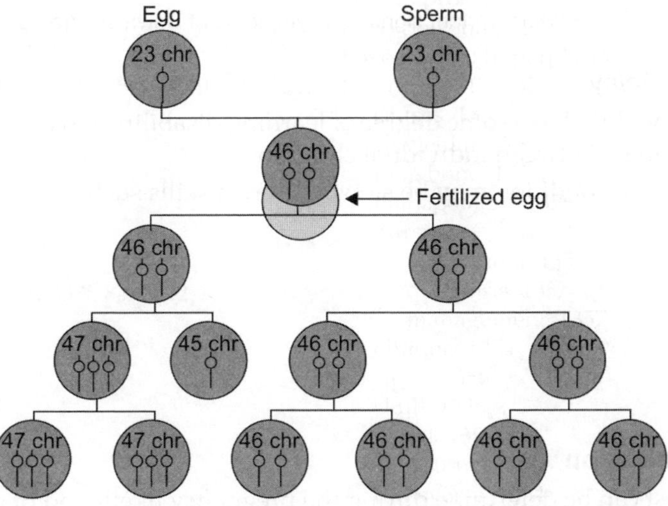

Fig. 6.92: Mosaic cell division

Signs and Symptoms

Physical appearance
- A flat back of the head
- Eyes that slant upwards and outwards
- A small nose and flat nasal bridge
- A small mouth with a protruding tongue
- Low muscle tone (called *Hypotonia*)
- A big space between the first and second toe (sandal gap)
- Broad hands with short fingers
- Their palm may have only one crease across it (single transverse palmar crease)
- Below-average weight and length at birth
- Below-average intelligence.

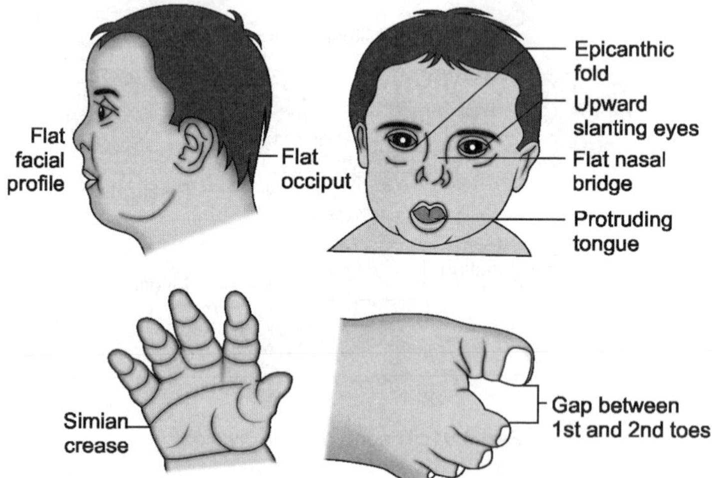

Fig. 6.93: Important signs and symptoms of Down syndrome

Developmental Delay

Down's syndrome child have some degree of learning disability and delayed development, but this varies widely between individual children.

Children with the condition may be slower to learn skills such as:
- Talking
- Reading
- Writing
- Standing
- Sitting
- Walking

Diagnostic Evaluation

The screening test can be determine during the pregnancy likelihood of a baby being born with Down's syndrome, but in many cases the condition is only diagnosed after birth.

The screening tests are:

- A blood test plus nuchal translucency ultrasound scan (nuchal translucency is a collection of fluid at the back of the baby's neck): This is called the combined test, and is offered between 11 and 14 weeks of pregnancy.
- A blood test that can be offered between 14 and 20 weeks of pregnancy if you are too far along to have the combined test: This blood test is less accurate than the combined test.
- *Cell-free fetal DNA analysis:* The cell-free fetal DNA test checks for fetal DNA circulating in the mother's blood. This test is usually recommended for women who have a higher risk of having a baby with Down syndrome or in response to risk detected by one of the previous tests. The mother's blood can be tested during pregnancy after 10 weeks gestation.
- *A genetic ultrasound:* A detailed ultrasound is often performed at 18 to 20 weeks in conjunction with the blood tests, and it checks the fetus for some of the physical traits abnormalities associated with Down syndrome.

There are three main tests used to diagnose a baby with Down's syndrome while it is still in the womb:

- *Chorionic villus sampling (CVS):* A sample of the placenta (an organ attached to the lining of your womb during pregnancy) is removed with a needle or tube for examination; this is usually done from week 11 of pregnancy.
- *Amniocentesis:* A sample of amniotic fluid (the fluid that surrounds the fetus in the womb) is removed with a needle for examination; this is usually carried out from week 15 of pregnancy.
- *Cordocentesis:* In this test, also known as percutaneous umbilical blood sampling or PUBS, fetal blood is taken from a vein in the umbilical cord and examined for chromosomal defects. Physician can perform this test between 18 and 22 weeks of pregnancy. This test carries a significantly greater risk of miscarriage than does amniocentesis or CVS, so it is only offered when results of other tests are unclear and the desired information cannot be obtained any other way.

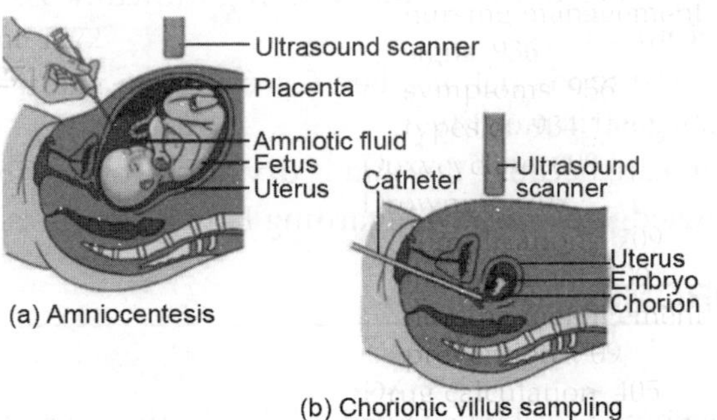

Fig. 6.94: Amniocentesis and chorionic villus sampling

Management

An early treatment for infants and children with Down syndrome can make a major difference in realizing their potential abilities and promote their quality of life.

An early intervention program can include:

- *Speech and language therapy:* To help the child with any problems in communicating or feeding
- *Physiotherapy:* To help the child with any muscle weakness or movement difficulties
- Individual home teaching programmes
- *Family counseling:* This therapy involves regular sessions with a qualified counselor who has experience working with families who have children with Down syndrome
- Coping and support the child in all aspect.

Preventive Measures

There is no way to prevent Down syndrome. If the parents are at high risk of having a child with Down syndrome or already have one child with Down syndrome, you should inform them to consult a genetic counselor before becoming pregnant. A genetic counselor can help you understand your chances of having a child with Down syndrome. He or she can also explain the prenatal tests that are available and help explain the pros and cons of testing.

Nursing Management

- Assess for associated Down syndrome problems.
- Administer medications which prescribed by the physician for associated problems.
- Implement a plan of care that is the same as for mental retardation. Include planning and intervention strategies for associated problems and features.
- Encourage genetic counseling to parents.
- Explain hypertonicity and joint hyperextensibility to parents, and that the child's resultant lack of clinging is physiologic and not a sign of detachment.
- Prevent respiratory infections by clearing the nose with a bulb syringe, using a cool mist vaporizer, performing chest physiotherapy when needed, providing good handwashing and avoiding exposure to infection.
- When feeding infants and young children, use a small, straight-handled spoon to push food to the side and back of the mouth. Feeding difficulties occur due to a protruding tongue and hypotonia.
- Encourage fluids and foods rich in fiber. Constipation results from decreased muscle tone, which affects gastric motility.
- Provide good skin care because the skin is dry and prone to infection.
- Improve the knowledge of parents regarding Down syndrome condition.

TURNER'S SYNDROME

Introduction

Turner's syndrome is named for Henry Turner who, in 1938, was one of the first doctors to report on the disorder in the medical literature. Turner syndrome is one of the most common chromosomal disorders and likely the most common genetic disorder of females.

Turner syndrome otherwise called as:

- 45, X syndrome
- Monosomy X

- Ullrich-Turner syndrome
- Bonnevie-Ullrich syndrome

The disorder is characterized by partial or complete loss (monosomy) of one of the X chromosomes. Affected females can potentially develop a wide variety of symptoms, affecting many different organ systems. Common symptoms include short stature and premature ovarian failure, which can result in the failure to attain puberty.

Most of the girls and women with Turner syndrome have normal intelligence. Developmental delays, nonverbal learning disabilities, and behavioral problems are possible, although these characteristics vary among affected individuals.

Definition

Turner syndrome is a rare chromosomal disorder that affects females. The disorder is characterized by partial or complete loss (monosomy) of one of the X chromosomes. Turner syndrome is highly variable and can differ dramatically from one person to another.

Incidence

Turner syndrome is a genetic disorder that affects about 1 in every 2,500 baby girls and only affects females. But it is much more common among pregnancies that do not survive to term (miscarriages and stillbirths).

Types

- *Classic Turner syndrome:* Where one of the X chromosomes is completely missing
- *Mosaic Turner syndrome:* Most cells one X chromosome is complete and the other is partially missing or abnormal in some way, but in some cells there may be just one X chromosome or rarely, two complete X chromosomes.

Causes

A girl with Turner syndrome only has one normal X sex chromosome, rather than the usual two (XX). Turner syndrome is caused by partial or complete loss (monosomy) of one of the X chromosomes in the child. Chromosomes are found in the nucleus of all body cells. They carry the genetic characteristics of each individual. Pairs of human chromosomes are numbered from 1 through 22, with an unequal 23rd pair that normally consists of one X and one Y chromosome for males and two X chromosomes for females. Thus, females with a normal chromosome make-up (karyotype) have 46 chromosomes, including two X chromosomes (46,XX karyotype); they receive one chromosome from the mother and one from the father in each of the 23 pairs.

The genetic alterations of Turner syndrome may be one of the following:

- *Monosomy or X-chromosome:* The complete absence of an X chromosome generally occurs because of an error in the father's sperm or in the mother's egg. This results in every cell in the body having only one X chromosome.
- *Mosaicism:* In most of the child an error occurs in cell division during early stages of fetal development. This results in some cells in the body having two complete copies of the X chromosome. Other cells have only one copy of the X chromosome, or they have one complete and one altered copy.

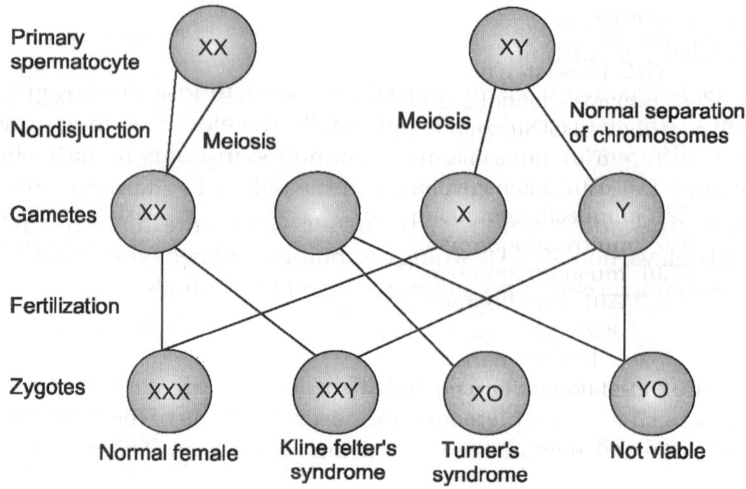

Fig. 6.95: Genetic structure of Turner's syndrome

- *Y-chromosome material:* In a very few percentage of Turner syndrome cases, some cells have one copy of the X chromosome and other cells have one copy of the X chromosome and some Y chromosome material. These individuals develop biologically as girls, but the presence of Y chromosome material increases the risk of developing a type of cancer called gonadoblastoma.

Signs and Symptoms

In this condition most of girls with Turner syndrome will grow-up to be shorter than average, with underdeveloped ovaries.

Antenatal Periods

Prenatal ultrasound of a baby with Turner syndrome may show:

- Thick neck tissue
- Swelling of the neck (cystic hygroma)
- Being a small baby
- Heart conditions
- Kidney abnormalities.

At Birth/During Infancy Periods

Signs of Turner syndrome at birth or during infancy may include:

- Wide or weblike neck
- Receding or small lower jaw
- High, narrow roof of the mouth (palate)
- Low-set ears
- Low hairline at the back of the head
- Broad chest with widely spaced nipples
- Short fingers and toes

- Arms that turn outward at the elbows
- Fingernails and toenails that are narrow and turned upward
- Swelling of the hands and feet, especially at birth
- Slightly smaller than average height at birth
- Delayed growth.

In Older Girls/Teens Age Women

Signs and symptoms in older girls, teenagers and young women that may indicate Turner syndrome include:

- No growth spurts at expected times in childhood
- Short stature with an adult height of about 8 inches (20 centimeters)
- Learning disabilities
- Difficulty in social situations, such as problems understanding other people's emotions or reactions
- Failure to begin sexual changes expected during puberty
- Sexual development that 'stalls' during teenage years
- Early end to menstrual cycles not due to pregnancy.

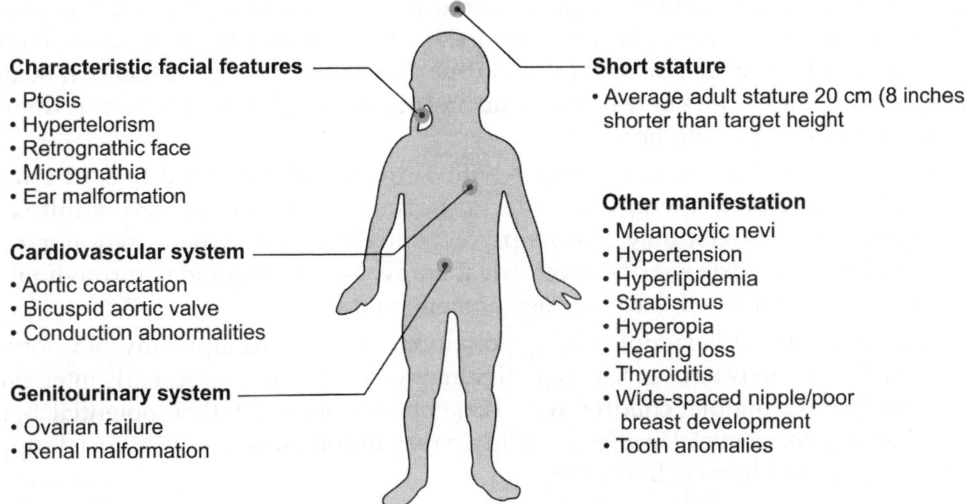

Fig. 6.96: Illustrated signs and symptoms of Turner's syndrome

Diagnostic Evaluation

A diagnosis of Turner's syndrome is based upon identification of characteristic symptoms, a detailed patient history, a thorough clinical evaluation, and a variety of specialized tests. Turner syndrome should be suspected in girls with growth deficiency or short stature of unknown cause.

- History collection
- Physical examination
- Ultrasound scan
- Chorionic villus sampling
- Amniocentesis

Karyotyping

Karyotyping is a test that involves analyzing the 23 pairs of chromosomes (strands of genes present in all human cells). It is often used where Turner syndrome is suspected. The test can either be carried out while the baby is inside the womb by taking a sample of amniotic fluid (amniocentesis) or after birth by taking a sample of the baby's blood.

Management

The treatment of Turner syndrome is directed toward the specific symptoms that are apparent in each individual. Treatment may require the coordinated efforts of a team of specialists. Genetic counseling may be of benefit for affected individuals and their families.

There is no cure for Turner syndrome, but therapies have been developed that can improve physical development. With proper medical care, females with Turner syndrome should be able to lead full, productive lives. The primary therapies for affected individuals are growth hormone therapy and estrogen therapy.

- *Growth hormone:* Growth hormone therapy is recommended for most girls with Turner syndrome. The goal is to increase height as much as possible at appropriate times during childhood and teen years. Growth hormone treatment is usually given several times a week as injections of somatropin (Humatrope, Genotropin, Saizen, others). If height is very short, some doctors may recommend an androgen called oxandrolone (Oxandrin) in addition to the growth hormone.
- *Estrogen therapy:* The most of the girls with Turner syndrome need to start estrogen and related hormone therapy in order to begin puberty and achieve adult sexual development. Estrogen may also help your daughter grow when used along with growth hormone. Estrogen replacement therapy usually continues throughout life, until a woman reaches the average age of menopause.

Additional treatment is symptomatic and supportive. For exmaple, thyroid hormone replacement therapy may be used to treat individuals with thyroid disease. Early intervention is important in ensuring that children with Turner syndrome reach their potential. Special services that may be beneficial to affected children may include special psychosocial support, speech therapy, and other such services.

Nursing Management

Turner syndrome cannot be cured because it is a genetic condition. However, growth hormone started early and estrogen replacement treatment in adolescence can help girls with the disorder grow to a normal height and achieve normal sexual development. Early diagnosis of Turner syndrome is important because growth hormone treatment should be started in childhood.

Estrogen replacement therapy is not started until the girl is twelve to fifteen years old as it will slow down her growth in height if given earlier. Girls with Turner syndrome should continue to receive estrogen until they reach the normal age of menopause in order to prevent osteoporosis.

Child with Turner syndrome require careful monitoring throughout life for such possible complications as recurrent ear infections and possible hearing loss; kidney or thyroid disorders; heart problems; diabetes; and high blood pressure. They should have annual blood tests as part of routine physical checkups.

In addition, they should watch their weight carefully because obesity increases their already high risk of diabetes. Although women with Turner syndrome are infertile because their ovaries do not develop normally, they can become pregnant with the help of assisted reproductive techniques. They should, however, consult a heart specialist before considering pregnancy because of the risk of aortic rupture or other heart complications.

The most girl children with Turner syndrome have normal intelligence, and many are intellectually gifted. Those who have difficulty with mathematics or related areas of study may need special tutoring in those fields. In general, however, TS should not interfere with children ability to complete schooling and be successful in a wide variety of occupations. Several studies have shown that many women with Turner syndrome have higher-than-average educational achievements.

Prognosis

The prognosis of Turner syndrome depends partly on whether the patient has monosomy X, a damaged second X chromosome or mosaic Turner syndrome. In general, patients with monosomy X have a greater chance of developing heart or kidney problems than those with other forms of Turner syndrome and require more careful monitoring of their health. Most patients have an overall good prognosis with a slightly shorter than average life expectancy.

MODEL QUESTIONS

Multiple Choice Questions

1. **Boot shaped heart is seen in ....**
   (a) TOF (b) Aortic stenosis
   (c) Coarctation of aorta (d) PDA
2. **Acyanotic heart defect includes all except**
   (a) VSD (b) TOF
   (c) ASD (d) None of these
3. **Cyanotic heart disease includes all except**
   (a) TOF (b) Tricuspid atresia
   (c) Truncus arteriosus (d) ASD
4. **Aortic septal defect is an abnormal opening between ....**
   (a) Wall separating right and left atrium
   (b) Wall separating left atrium and ventricles

(c) Wall separating right atrium and ventricles
(d) Wall separating right atrium and left ventricle

5. **........... is the normal pathway in the fetal circulation system.**
(a) PDA
(b) VSD
(c) ASD
(d) TOF

6. **............ is an autoimmune disease caused by B-hemolytic *Streptococcus*.**
(a) TOF
(b) RHD
(c) ASD
(d) VSD

7. **TEF stands for ....**
(a) Tracheoesophageal atresia
(b) Total esophageal atresia
(c) Tracheoesophageal fistula
(d) None of these

8. **Omphalocele is the herniation of the ....**
(a) Genital organ
(b) Respiratory organ
(c) Cardiac organ
(d) Abdominal organ

9. **Rule of ten is used for ....**
(a) Cleft lip
(b) TEF
(c) CHD
(d) None of these

10. **Abnormal communication between trachea and esophagus is known as..........**
(a) Pyloric stenosis
(b) Hirschsprung disease
(c) Esophagitis
(d) TEF

11. **Herniation of abdominal organs into the umbilical cord is known as ....**
(a) Fistula
(b) Ascitis
(c) Omphalocele
(d) PDA

12. **Wilms tumor is tumor of ....**
(a) Lung
(b) Brain
(c) Kidney
(d) Intestine

13. **Manifestation of Wilms tumor include ....**
(a) A firm abdominal mass
(b) Abdominal pain
(c) Hematuria
(c) All of these

14. **Features of nephrotic syndrome are ....**
(a) Edema
(b) Hypoalbuminemia
(c) Proteinuria
(d) All of these

15. **Management of nephrotic syndrome are except ....**
(a) Low sodium and high protein diet
(b) High sodium and low protein diet
(c) Complete bed rest
(d) Care of edematous skin

16. **Thalasemia is a ....**
(a) Cardiac disorder
(b) Hemolytic anemia
(c) Respiratory problem
(d) Endocrinal disorder

17. **Hemophilia is a ....**
   (a) Cardiac disorder
   (b) Blood coagulation disorder
   (c) Respiratory disorder
   (d) Endocrine disorder

18. **Regurgitation and non-bilious vomiting is a clinical features of ....**
   (a) Hirschprung's disease
   (b) Congenital hernia
   (c) Necrotizing enteocolitis
   (d) Pyloric stenosis

19. **Narrowing and obstruction of the lower portion of stomach is termed as ....**
   (a) Duodenal stenosis
   (b) Cardiac stenosis
   (c) Fundal stenosis
   (d) Pyloric stenosis

True or False

(a) Cleft lip is more common in females than males.
(b) Cleft palate is more common in females in compare to males.
(c) During the surgical treatment of cleft lip and palate, closure of cleft lip is done first and then palate.
(d) Type–III TEF is the most common type of tracheoesophageal fistula.
(e) Rectourinary fistula is diagnosed by observing presence of meconium in urine.
(f) An approximate 50% of ASD are due to persistent of ostium secundum.
(g) Ventricular septal defect (VSD) are found about 25% of all congenital heart defect.
(h) Pulmonary stenosis is a severe form of pulmonary atresia.
(i) Teratology of fallot (TOF) is a common congenital defect having four defects.
(j) School age children are less susceptible for rheumatic fever.
(k) In hypospadia, surgical correction is generally performed as 6 years of age.
(l) Nephrotic syndrome can be present in any age but ususually between 1 and 7 years.
(m) In pseudocryptorchidism condition, testis are localizing in the abdomen and inguinal canal which affects to poor spermatogenesis.

Fill in the Blanks

(a) Congenital malformation are also called as ....
(b) In.................... urethral opening is situated on the ventral side of penis.
(c) In .... the urethral opening is present on the dorsal side of penis.
(d) Type V TEF is also known as ....
(e) .... leads to obstruction to the outflow of blood from left ventricle.
(f) In.................. the renal tissue is full of multiple small cysts.
(g) Cleft lip is also known as ....
(h) Cleft palate is also known as ....
(i) The procedure for cleft lip repair is called ....
(j) Fredet-Ramstedt procedure is done as corrective surgery for ....
(k) Inward bending of foot is called ....

Short Answer Questions

(a) Club foot
(b) Congenital hypothyroidism
(c) Spina Bifida
(d) Rheumatic heart disease
(e) Enlist congenital disorder

Long Answer Questions

1 × 15 = 15

1. (a) What is rheumatic heart disease?
   (b) Discuss the clinical presentation and management of rheumatic heart disease.
2 (a) Define tetralogy of fallot.
   (b) Enlist the defects occurring in TOF.
   (c) Describe the clinical features and diagnosis of tetralogy of fallot.
   (d) Discuss the management of TOF.
3. Define club foot. What are its types and clinical features? Describe management of talipes equinovarus.
4. Enlist the various congenital disorders of genitourinary system and describes exstrophy of bladder in details.
5. (a) Classify congenital cardiac defects.
   (b) Enlist the various disorders in each category.
   (c) Discuss the nursing management of children undergoing cardiac surgery.

ANSWER KEY

Multiple Choice Questions

1. (a)	2. (b)	3. (d)	4. (a)	5. (a)	6. (b)	7. (c)
8. (a)	9. (a)	10. (d)	11. (c)	12. (c)	13. (c)	14. (a)
15. (a)	16. (b)	17. (b)	18. (d)	19. (b)		

True or False

(a) False	(b) True	(c) True	(d) True	(e) True	(f) False	(g) True
(h) False	(i) True	(j) False	(k) False	(l) True	(m) False	

Fill in the Blanks

(a) Congenital anomalies/birth defects
(b) Hypospadias
(c) Epispadias
(d) H type
(e) Aortic stenosis
(f) Polycystic kidneys
(g) Palatoschisis
(h) Cheiloschisis
(i) Millard procedure
(j) Hypertrophied pyloric stenosis
(k) Club foot

Chapter 7

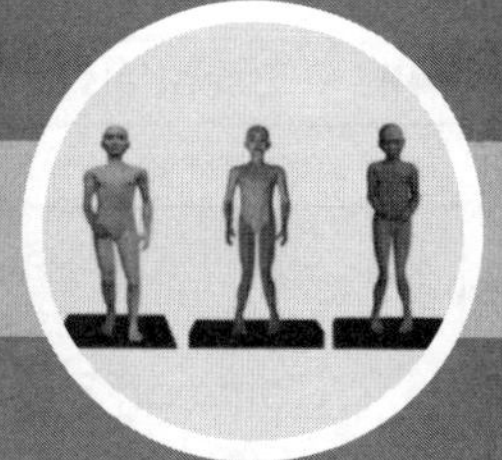

Children with Various Disorders and Diseases

Definition, Etiology, Signs and Symptoms, Complications, Prevention, Medical, Surgical and Nursing Management of Child with:

- **Renal System**
  - Nephrotic Syndrome
  - Glomerulonephritis
  - Renal Failure
  - Acute Renal Failure (ARF)
  - Chronic Renal Failure (CRF)
- **Respiratory System**
  - Child with URI and LRI
  - Upper Respiratory Tract Infection
  - Child with Rhinitis
  - Rhinosinusitis
  - Sinusitis
  - Common Cold
  - Acute Pharyngitis
  - Epiglottitis
  - Laryngitis (Croup)
  - Tonsillitis
  - Epistaxis
  - Lower Respiratory Tract Infections
  - Bronchitis
  - Acute Bronchitis
  - Chronic Bronchitis
  - Bronchiolitis
  - Pneumonia
  - Child with Asthma
  - Status Asthmaticus

- Cystic Fibrosis
- Lung Abscess
- Common Respiratory Disorders in Neonates, Infants and Young Children
- Apnea of Prematurity
- Bacterial Tracheitis (Pseudomembranous Croup)
- Bronchopulmonary Dysplasia (BPD)
- Croup (Laryngotracheobronchitis)
- Meconium Aspiration Syndrome
- Persistent Pulmonary Hypertension of the Newborn
- Pulmonary Air-leak Syndromes
- Respiratory Distress Syndrome (Hyaline Membrane Disease)
- Transient Tachypnea of the Newborn (Neonatal Wet Lung Syndrome)

• **Gastrointestinal (GI) System**
- Intestinal (Bowel) Obstruction
- Small Bowel Obstruction (SBO)
- Hirschsprung's Disease (HD)
- Malabsorption Syndromes
- Inflammatory Conditions: Ulcerative Colitis/Inflammatory Bowel Disease
- Child with Appendicitis
- Meckel's Diverticulum (Ulcerative Colitis)
- Worm Infestation

• **Cardiovascular System (CVS)**
- Rheumatic Fever
- Congestive Heart Failure (CHF)
- Infective Endocarditis
- Myocarditis
- Pericarditis

• **Hematological System: Child with Blood Disorders**
- Child with Anemia
- Iron Deficiency Anemia
- Megaloblastic Anemia
- Sickle Cell Anemia
- Aplastic Anemia
- Thalassemia
- Hemophilia in Children
- Polycythemia
- Thrombocytopenia or Idiopathic Thrombocytopenia Purpura (ITP)
- Disseminated Intravascular Coagulation (DIC)
- Child with Purpura
- Childhood Leukemia

- **Neurological System**
  - Meningitis
  - Encephalitis
  - Convulsive Disorders
  - Epilepsy
  - Febrile Seizures
  - Craniocerebral Trauma
  - Head Trauma (Injury)
- **Endocrine System**
  - Endocrine Disorders
  - Pituitary Disorders
  - Pituitary Tumors
- **Growth Hormone Deficiency in Children**
  - Hypopituitarism
  - Hyperpituitarism
  - Diabetes Insipidus
  - Diabetes Mellitus (IDDM and NIDDM)
  - Hyperthyroidism (Graves' Disease)
  - Hypothyroidism
  - Phenylketonuria (PKU)
  - Galactosemia
  - Adrenal Disorders
- **Developmental Problem**
  - Child with Disabilities (or) Handicapped Children
  - Learning Disability
  - Mental Retardation
  - Dyslexia
  - Hearing and Vision Impairment
  - Vision Impairment
- **Other Condition**
  - Fluid and Electrolyte Imbalance
  - Child with Burns
- **Problems with Locomotion**
  - Poliomyelitis
  - Osteomyelitis
  - Kyphosis, Lordosis and Scoliosis (or) Spine Curvature Disorders
  - Kyphosis
  - Lordosis
  - Scoliosis
  - Fractures
  - Pre and Post Operative Care of Children Undergoing Surgery

RENAL SYSTEM

NEPHROTIC SYNDROME

Introduction

Nephrotic syndrome is a set of signs or symptoms that may point to kidney problems. The kidneys are two bean-shaped organs found in the lower back. They clean the blood by filtering out excess water and salt and waste products from food. Nephrotic syndrome is a condition that is often caused by any of a group of diseases that damage the kidneys' filtering system. The structure of the glomeruli prevents most of protein from getting filtered through into the urine. There are three main symptoms of nephrotic syndrome associated with protein leaking into the urine:

1. Hypoalbuminemia (low level of albumin in the blood)
2. Edema (swelling)
3. Hyperlipidemia

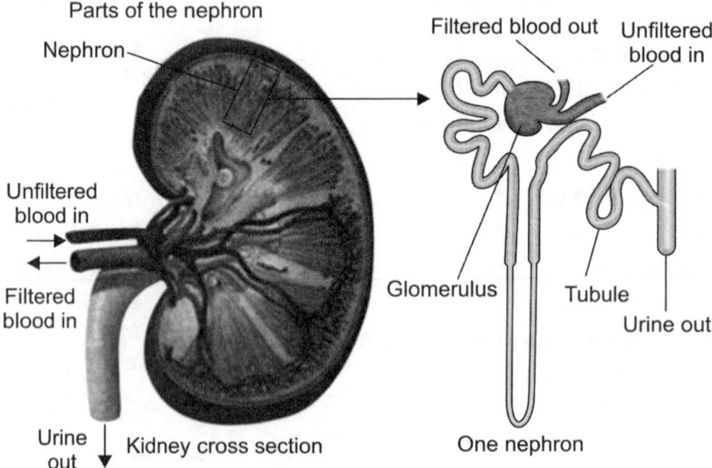

Fig. 7.1: Anatomy of kidney and nephron

Definition

Nephrotic syndrome is defined as group of kidney disease with proteinuria, hypoalbuminemia and edema. Nephrotic range proteinuria is 3 grams per day or more. On a single, 'spot' urine collection, it is 2 grams of protein per gram of urine creatinine.

Types

- Congenital nephrotic syndrome
- Idiopathic or primary nephrotic syndrome
- Secondary nephrotic syndrome

Congenital Nephrotic Syndrome

- It is rare but serious and fatal problem usually associated with other congenital abnormalities of kidney.

- It is inherited as autosomal recessive disease.
- ` Severe renal insufficiency and urinary infections along with this condition result is poor prognosis.

Idiopathic or Primary Nephrotic Syndrome

- Subgroup of this type
  - Minimal change nephrotic syndrome (85%)
  - Proliferative nephrotic syndrome (5%)
  - Focal sclerosis nephrotic syndrome (10%)
- It is the most common type (about 90%) and regarded as autoimmune phenomenon as it responds to immunosuppressive therapy.

Secondary Nephrotic Syndrome

- It occurs in children about 10% of all cases. This condition may occur due to some form of chronic glomerulonephritis or due to diabetes mellitus, systemic lupus erythematosis (SLE), malaria, malignant hypertension, hepatitis 'B', infective endocarditis, drug toxicity, lymphomas and syphilis.

Causes

Primary causes of nephrotic syndrome include:

- Minimal-change nephropathy
- Focal glomerulosclerosis
- Membranous nephropathy
- Hereditary nephropathies

Secondary causes include:

- Diabetes mellitus
- Lupus erythematosus
- Amyloidosis and paraproteinemias
- Viral infections (e.g. hepatitis B, hepatitis C, human immunodeficiency virus [HIV])
- Preeclampsia

Most of these diseases tend to occur more often in certain age groups:

- Less than 1 year old
  - Congenital nephrosis
- Less than 15 years old
  - Focal segmental glomerulosclerosis (FSGS)
- Age 15 to 40 years
  - Focal segmental glomerulosclerosis (FSGS)
  - Other causes
- Over age 40 years
  - Membranous GN
  - Diabetic nephropathy
- Above 60 years
  - Amyloidosis may account for up to 20 percent of cases.

Risk Factors

- Medical conditions:
  - Diabetes
  - Lupus
  - Amyloidosis
  - Minimal change disease and other kidney diseases.
- *Certain medications:* Most common medications that can cause nephrotic syndrome include nonsteroidal anti-inflammatory drugs (NSAIDs) and drugs used to fight infections.
- *Certain infections:* The infection that increases the risk of nephrotic syndrome includes HIV, hepatitis B, hepatitis C and malaria.

Signs and Symptoms

A child with nephrotic syndrome has these signs:

- High levels of protein in the urine, a condition called proteinuria
- Low levels of albumin in the blood
- Swelling resulting from build-up of salt and water
- Less frequent urination
- Weight gain from excess water.

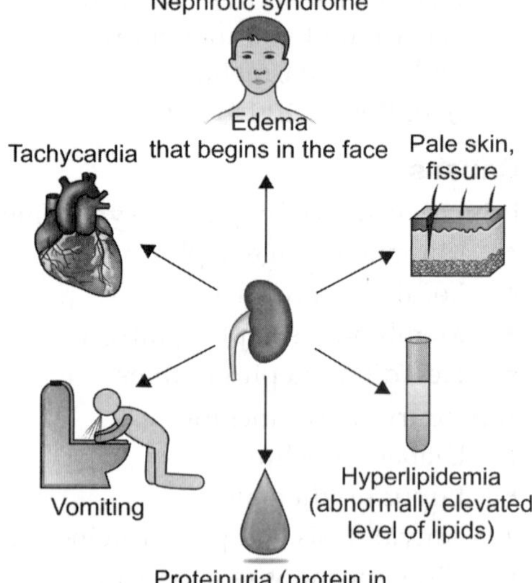

Fig. 7.2: Signs and symptoms of nephrotic syndrome

Diagnostic Evaluation

- Blood analysis
- Urinalysis
- Kidney biopsy

Blood Analysis

The blood analysis shows that high cholesterol levels and low albumin. Blood urea nitrogen (BUN) and creatinine may or may not be elevated. If BUN and creatinine are elevated the patient has renal failure and the prognosis is worse.

Urinalysis

Evaluation of the urine by a simple urine dipstick in the office can give preliminary information on the amount of protein in the urine. However, this test is a qualitative test. In order to determine the actual amount of protein in the urine, a 24-hour quantitative test must be done, which indicates levels of protein and creatinine in the urine. A comparison of protein to creatinine based on a single sample is used to determine 24-hour protein loss. This is helpful for quicker results or when the patient cannot collect urine over 24 hours.

Kidney Biopsy

A kidney biopsy procedure may be used to determine the underlying cause and extent of disease with the exception of the following cases:

- **Children** with Nephrotic Syndromens most often have minimal change disease and respond well to a short course of steroids. A biopsy should only be considered if they do not show a favorable response to the steroids within 6–8 weeks.
- **Adult child** with a history of diabetes who have tested negative to other disorders such as myeloma, infections and collagen vascular diseases. It is presumed the cause of the proteinuria is diabetic nephropathy and a kidney biopsy is not necessary. If the duration of diabetes has been short or the severity of the NS is profound, a kidney biopsy is considered.
- **Elderly child**, child who are not expected to live long, or those for whom immunosuppressive drug therapy is not advisable are typically not candidates for a biopsy.

Pathophysiology

The main functional units of the kidneys, where the blood filtering happens, are tiny organs called nephrons. Each kidney has about a million nephrons and each nephron has one **glomerulus** (singular of glomeruli) a ball of tiny blood vessels, or capillaries. The glomerulus is the nephron's filter. This is where the process of removing waste products and fluids from the blood begins.

When the glomeruli stop filtering the urine properly, they allow too much protein to leave the blood. Protein helps hold fluids in the blood, so when there is less protein in the blood, the fluids can move to other parts of the body and cause a type of swelling (edema) in the face, belly, hands, arms and other extremities. When this happens, it is called nephrotic syndrome.

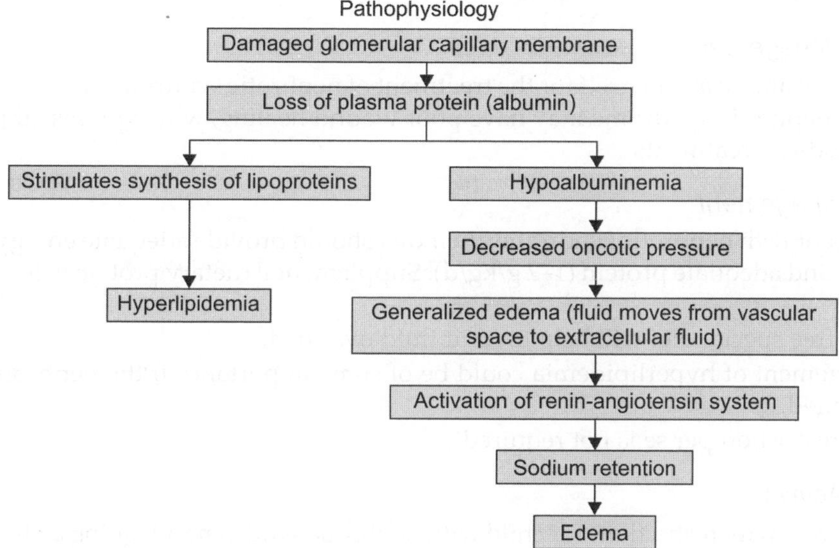

Fig. 7.3: Pathophysiology of nephrotic syndrome

Management

Medical Management

There is no cure for nephrotic syndrome, but there are treatments that can help you manage symptoms and prevent more kidney damage.

- *Blood pressure medications:* The drugs angiotensin-converting enzyme inhibitors reduce blood pressure and also reduce the amount of protein released in urine. Medications in this category include benazepril (Lotensin), captopril (Capoten) and enalapril (Vasotec). Another group of drugs that works in a similar way is called angiotensin II receptor blockers and includes losartan (Cozaar) and valsartan (Diovan).
- *Antidiuretic:* Diuretics will be needed; furosemide (1 mg/kg/d) and spironolactone (2 mg/kg/d) will help when fluid retention is severe, provided no signs of renal failure or volume contraction are evident. Achieving a satisfactory diuresis is difficult when the patient's serum albumin level is less than 1.5 g/dL. Albumin at 1 g/kg may be given, followed by intravenous furosemide.
- *Cholesterol-reducing medications:* Medications called statins can help lower cholesterol levels. However, it's currently unclear whether or not cholesterol-lowering medications can specifically improve the outcomes of people with nephrotic syndrome, such as avoiding heart attacks or decreasing the risk of early death. Statins include atorvastatin (Lipitor), fluvastatin (Lescol), lovastatin (Altoprev, Mevacor), pravastatin (Pravachol), rosuvastatin (Crestor) and simvastatin (Zocor).
- *Blood thinners:* Medications called anticoagulants help decrease your blood's ability to clot and reduce your risk of developing blood clots. Anticoagulants include heparin or warfarin (Coumadin).
- *Immune system-suppressing medications:* Medications to control the immune system, such as corticosteroids, may decrease the inflammation that accompanies certain kidney disorders, such as minimal change disease.

Surgical Management

Surgery is not applicable in itself for the treatment of nephrotic syndrome. It is possible that child with nephrotic syndrome may have poor wound healing, which places emphasis on optimal medical treatments.

Dietary Management

- The client with nephrotic syndrome, their diet should provide adequate energy (caloric) intake and adequate protein (1–2 g/kg/d). Supplemental dietary protein is of no proven value.
- A salt free special diet will help to limit fluid overload.
- Management of hyperlipidemia could be of some importance if the nephrotic state is prolonged.
- Fluid restriction per se is not required.

Physical Activity

There are no activity restrictions for child with nephrotic syndrome. Ongoing activity, rather than bed rest, will reduce the risk of blood clots.

Complications

Infection is a major concern in nephrotic syndrome; children have an increased susceptibility to infection with *Streptococcus pneumoniae, Haemophilus influenzae, Escherichia coli* and other gram-negative organisms. Varicella infection is also common. The most common infectious complications are bacterial sepsis, cellulitis, pneumonia and peritonitis. Proposed explanations for these complications include decreased immunoglobulin levels, edema fluid acting as a culture medium, protein deficiency, decreased bactericidal activity of the leukocytes, immunosuppressive therapy, decreased perfusion of the spleen caused by hypovolemia and urinary loss of a complement factor (properdin factor B) that opsonizes certain bacteria.

The occurrence of hyperlipidemia may be considered a typical feature of the nephrotic syndrome, rather than a mere complication. It is related to the hypoproteinemia and low serum oncotic pressure of nephrotic syndrome, which then leads to reactive hepatic protein synthesis, including of lipoproteins. Some of the elevated serum lipoproteins are filtered at the glomerulus, leading to lipiduria and the classical findings of oval fat bodies and fatty casts in the urine sediment.

Nursing Management

- Continuous monitoring of fluid retention or exudation is an important nursing function.
- Strict intake and output records are essential but may be difficult to obtain from very young children.
- Other methods of monitoring progress include urine examination for albumin, daily weight and measurement of abdominal girth.
- Vital signs are monitored to detect any early signs of complications such as shock or an infective process
- Continuous support of the child and family is one of the major nursing considerations
- Bed rest is required during the stage of edema
- Diet should be low in sodium and high in proteins
- The fluid intake requirement is calculated according to the output and weight of the child
- Dyspnea due to as cites can be relieved by sitting position and abdominal paracentesis to relieve upward pressure on the diaphragm
- Proteins may be given 1 gm/kg/day of body weight according to serum protein levels and tolerance of the child adequate calories should be supplied.

Parental Advice

- Explain the parents about the follow-up and a risk of relapse
- Emphasize on the high protein diet. Demonstrate urine test for albumin
- The maintenance dose should be explained which may be done over 8 to 12 months period
- They should be explained about the continuation of the treatment according to the doctor's prescription.

GLOMERULONEPHRITIS

Introduction

Glomerulonephritis (GN) otherwise called as **glomerular nephritis**, most of the renal diseases are characterized by inflammation either of the glomeruli or the small blood vessels in the kidneys. Nephritis is an older term used to clinically denote a child with hypertension,

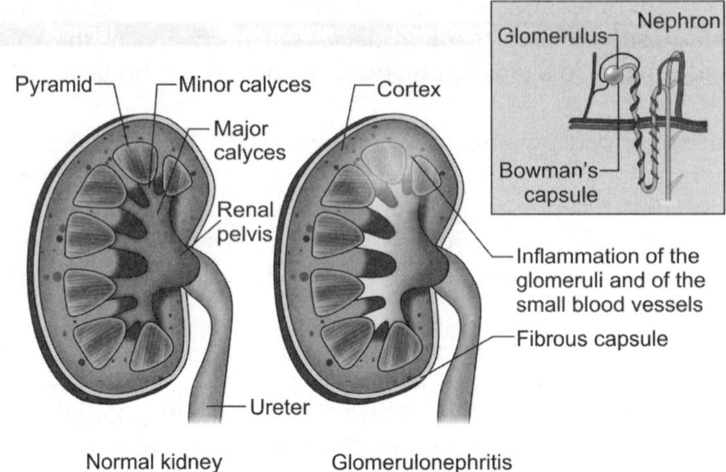

Fig. 7.4: Acute and chronic glomerulonephritis

decreased renal function, hematuria and edema. Technically term nephritis suggests a non-infectious inflammatory process that involves the nephron.

Acute glomerulonephritis comprises a specific set of renal diseases in which an immunologic mechanism triggers inflammation and proliferation of glomerular tissue that can result in damage to the basement membrane or capillary endothelium.

In chronic glomerulonephritis, scarring of the glomeruli impedes the filtering process, trapping waste products in the blood while allowing red blood cells or proteins to escape into the urine, eventually producing the characteristic signs of high blood pressure and swelling in the legs and ankles.

Diseases that produce GN are usually classified as:

- *Primary*: Diseases in which the kidney is the primarily affected organ.
- *Secondary*: Systemic disorders that involve the kidneys in addition to other organs, such as systemic lupus erythematosus.

Definition

Glomerulonephritis is a group of diseases that injure the part of the kidney that filters blood (called glomeruli). Other terms are nephritis and nephrotic syndrome. When the kidney is injured, it cannot get rid of wastes and extra fluid in the body. If the illness continues, the kidneys may stop working completely, resulting in kidney failure.

Acute glomerulonephritis is defined as the sudden onset of hematuria, proteinuria and red blood cell (RBC) casts. This clinical picture is often accompanied by hypertension, edema, azotemia (i.e. decreased glomerular filtration rate [GFR] and renal salt and water retention. Acute GN can be due to a primary renal disease or to a systemic disease.

Chronic glomerulonephritis is defined as a kidney disorder caused by slow, cumulative damage and scarring of the tiny blood filters in the kidneys. These filters, known as glomeruli, remove waste products from the blood.

Types

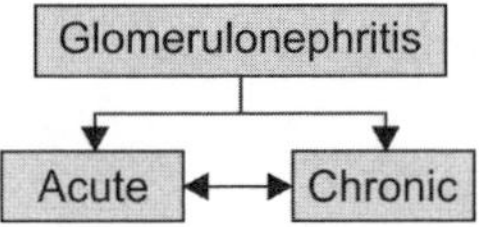

Causes

Acute Glomerulonephritis

Acute GN can be a response to an infection such as strep throat or an abscessed tooth. It may be due to problems with child immune system overreacting to the infection.

Common causes in children and adolescents include:

- Hemolytic uremic syndrome
- Henoch-Schönlein purpura
- IgA nephropathy
- Poststreptococcal glomerulonephritis

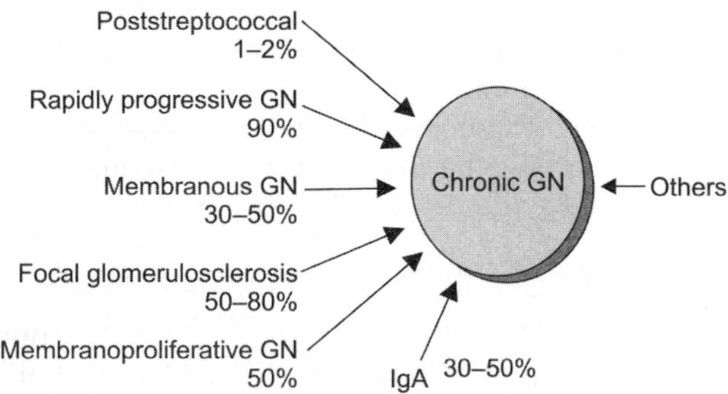

Fig. 7.5: Causes of chronic GN

Chronic Glomerulonephritis

The chronic form of GN can develop over several years with no or very few symptoms. This can cause irreversible damage to child kidneys and ultimately lead to complete kidney failure. A genetic disease can sometimes cause chronic GN. Hereditary nephritis occurs in young men with poor vision and poor hearing.

Immune diseases may also cause chronic GN. A history of cancer may also put you at risk. Having the acute form of GN may make you more likely to develop the chronic form later on. Exposure to some hydrocarbon solvents may increase the risk of chronic GN. Chronic GN does not always have a clear cause. Twenty-five percent of people with the condition have no history of kidney disease.

Symptoms of Glomerulonephritis

Acute Glomerulonephritis

Early symptoms of acute GN include:
- Puffiness in the face (edema)
- Urinating less often
- Blood in urine (dark, rust-colored urine)
- Extra fluid in your lungs, causing coughing
- High blood pressure.

Chronic Glomerulonephritis

The chronic form of glomerulonephritis can creep up without any symptoms. There may be slow development of symptoms similar to the acute form.
- Blood or excess protein in urine, which may be microscopic and show up in urine tests
- High blood pressure
- Swelling in ankles and face (edema)
- Frequent nighttime urination
- Bubbly or foamy urine (from excess protein)
- Abdominal pain
- Frequent nosebleeds.

Pathophysiology

Reduction in nephron mass from the initial injury reduces the GFR. This reduction leads to hypertrophy and hyperfiltration of the remaining nephrons and to the initiation of intraglomerular hypertension. These changes occur in order to increase the GFR of the remaining nephrons, thus minimizing the functional consequences of nephron loss. The changes, however, are ultimately detrimental because they lead to glomerulosclerosis and further nephron loss.

A substantial decline in the GFR may lead to only slight increases in serum creatinine levels. Azotemia (i.e. a rise in blood urea nitrogen [BUN] and serum creatinine levels) is apparent when the GFR decreases to less than 60–70 mL/min. In addition to a rise in BUN and creatinine levels, the substantial reduction in the GFR results in the following:
- Decreased production of erythropoietin, thus resulting in anemia.
- Decreased production of vitamin D, resulting in hypocalcemia, secondary hyperparathyroidism, hyperphosphatemia and renal osteodystrophy.
- Reduction in acid, potassium, salt and water excretion, resulting in acidosis, hyperkalemia, hypertension and edema.
- Platelet dysfunction, leading to increased bleeding tendencies.

Accumulation of toxic waste products (uremic toxins) affects virtually all organ systems. Azotemia occurring with the signs and symptoms listed above is known as uremia. Uremia occurs at a GFR of approximately 10 mL/min. Some of these toxins (e.g. BUN, creatinine, phenols and guanidines) have been identified, but none has been found to be responsible for all the symptoms.

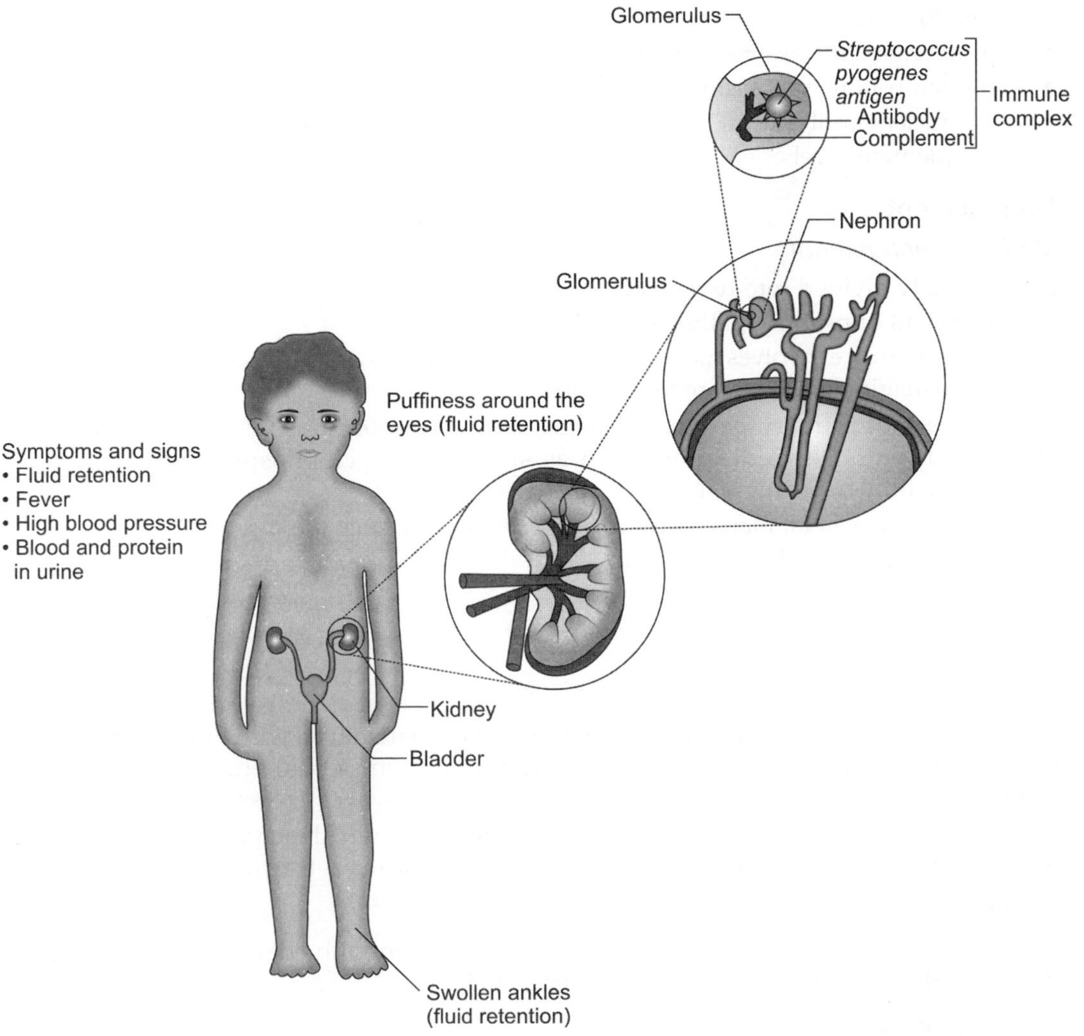

Fig. 7.6: Pathophysiology

Diagnostic Evaluation

Urine Tests

- Creatinine clearance
- Total protein in the urine
- Urine concentration
- Urine specific gravity
- Urine red blood cells (RBCs)
- Urine osmolality

Blood Tests

- Red blood cell levels in the blood
- Abnormal albumin levels
- Abnormal blood urea nitrogen
- High creatinine levels.

Immunology Testing

- Antiglomerular basement membrane antibodies
- Antineutrophil cytoplasmic antibodies
- Antinuclear antibodies
- Complement levels.

Management

Medical Management

GN is usually divided into two major components:

1. Treatment of primary pathology and supportive care.
2. Supportive care involves managing hypertension and fluid and electrolyte abnormalities and managing decreased renal function.

Treatment of primary pathology ranges from postinfectious GN, to treatment with immunosuppressive medication, such as steroids or cyclophosphamide in lupus or tubulointerstitial nephritis (TIN).

Hypertension can be managed with antihypertensive such as:

- Calcium channel–blocking agents
- Ace inhibitors
- Angiotensin receptor–blocking agents
- Peripheral vasodilators
- Diuretics.

The most common fluid abnormality is hypovolemia managed with fluid restriction and diuretics or dialysis if renal function is too poor to respond to diuretics. Hyponatremia is usually dilutional and responds at least partially to removal of excess fluid.

Hypocalcemia may respond to oral or intravenous calcium, depending on severity. Mild metabolic acidosis may be present but rarely requires primary treatment.

Diuretic Agents

These agents are used to remove excess fluid in children with edema secondary to renal disease and as an adjunct to manage hypertension.

Furosemide (Lasix)

A loop diuretic. Often effective in removing fluid even when GFR is reduced secondary to nephritis. Increases excretion of water by interfering with chloride-binding cotransport system, which, in turn, inhibits sodium and chloride reabsorption in ascending loop of Henle and distal renal tubule.

Adult

20–80 mg/d PO/IV/IM; titrate up to 600 mg/d for severe edematous states.

Pediatric

1–2 mg/kg PO/IV up to 6 mg/kg/d.

Nursing Management

- Provide best rest during the acute phase.
- Perform passive range of motion exercises for the patient on bed rest.

- Allow the patient to resume normal activities gradually as symptoms subside.
- Consult the dietician about a diet high in calories and low in protein, sodium, potassium and fluids.
- Protect the debilitated patient against secondary infection by providing good nutrition and hygienic technique and preventing contact with infected people.
- Check the patient's vital signs and electrolyte values.
- Monitor intake and output and daily weight.
- Report peripheral edema or the formation of ascites.
- Explain to the patient taking diuretics that he may experience orthostatic hypotension and dizziness when he changes positions quickly.
- Provide emotional support for the patient and his family.
- If the patient is scheduled for dialysis, explain the procedure fully.

Nursing Diagnosis for Glomerulonephritis

- Ineffective tissue perfusion related to water retention and hypernatremia
- Risk for imbalanced fluid volume related to oliguria
- Risk for imbalanced nutrition less than body requirements related to anorexia.
- Activity intolerance related to fatigue.
- Risk for disturbed sleep pattern related to immobilization and edema.

Diet Management

In children with acute renal failure secondary to GN who have lost the ability to excrete a water load, fluid restriction may prevent fluid overload. TIN usually produces non-oliguric acute renal failure (ARF). Fluid restriction of 300 mL/m^2/d plus losses may allow management of acute renal failure for 2–3 days without dialysis. In child with hypertension, sodium restriction to recommended daily allowances (RDA) of 2–4 mEq/kg/d may aid in management. In children with renal failure, potassium restriction is justified to prevent hyperkalemia. A short-term high-carbohydrate diet may prevent catabolism of body protein as an energy source. Calcium supplementation is useful to maintain normal serum calcium.

Complications

- Primary complications associated with hypertension
  - Seizure
  - Encephalopathy
  - Stroke
  - End-organ damage.
- Primary complications associated with kidney failure
  - Fluid overload
  - Electrolyte abnormality
  - Uremic symptoms
  - Anemia
  - Abnormal bone mineralization
  - Sexual dysfunction
  - Poor growth

- Anorexia
- Endocrine abnormalities.

Prognosis

The overall prognosis for survival in children with all forms of nephritis is good.

RENAL FAILURE

Introduction

Renal failure is the inability of the kidneys to excrete waste material, concentrate urine and conserve electrolytes. It can occur suddenly (acute renal failure) in response to inadequate profusion, kidney disease or urinary react obstruction, or it can develop slowly (chronic renal failure) as a result of long standing kidney disease or an anomaly.

Definition

Renal failure is defined as temporary or permanent damage of the kidneys that results in loss of normal kidney function. There are two different types of renal failure, acute and chronic. The causes, symptoms, treatments and outcomes of acute and chronic are different.

Types

There are three types of renal failure:

- Acute renal failure (ARF).
- Chronic renal failure (CRF) progresses slowly over at least 3 months and can lead to permanent renal failure.
- ESRD (End Stage Renal Failure).

Table 7.1: Types of renal failure

Kidney failure	
Acute renal failure (ARF)	A sudden loss of kidney function caused by an illness an injury, or a toxin that stresses the kidneys (kidney function may recover)
Chronic renal failure (CRF)	A long and usually slow process where the kidneys lose their ability to function
End-stage renal failure (ESRD)	When the kidneys have completely and permanently shut down

Table 7.2: Difference between acute and chronic renal failure

Acute renal failure (ARF)	Chronic renal failure (CRF)
Decreased blood flow to the kidneys for a period of time. This may occur from blood loss, surgery, or shock.	A prolonged urinary tract obstruction or blockage.
An obstruction or blockage along the urinary tract.	Alport syndrome, an inherited disorder that causes deafness, progressive kidney damage and eye defects.
Hemolytic uremic syndrome, usually caused by an *E. coli* infection, kidney failure develops as a result of obstruction to the small functional structures and vessels inside the kidney.	Nephrotic syndrome. A condition that has several different causes. Nephrotic syndrome is characterized by protein in the urine, low protein in the blood, high cholesterol levels and tissue swelling.
Taking certain medications that may cause toxicity to the kidneys.	Polycystic kidney disease. A genetic disorder characterized by the growth of numerous cysts filled with fluid in the kidneys.

Contd...

Contd...

Glomerulonephritis, a type of kidney disease that involves glomeruli. During glomerulonephritis, the glomeruli become inflamed and harm the kidney's ability to filter urine.	Cystinosis an inherited disorder in which the amino acid cystine (a common protein-building compound) collects within specific cellular bodies of the kidney, known as lysosomes.
Any condition that may impair the flow of oxygen and blood to the kidneys, such as cardiac arrest.	

ACUTE RENAL FAILURE (ARF)

Definition

Acute renal failure (ARF) is defined as an acute decline in renal function characterized by an increase in blood urea nitrogen (BUN) and serum creatinine values, often accompanied by hyperkalemia, metabolic acidosis and hypertension. Significant morbidity and mortality can accompany ARF. Child who have ARF, recover their renal function either partially or completely or they develop end-stage renal disease.

Causes

- Glomerulonephritis and hemolytic uremic syndrome
- Poor renal perfusion
- Urinary tract obstruction
- Acute renal injury.

Types

ARF is divided into three forms:

1. Pre-renal failure (most common)
2. Post-renal failure
3. Intrinsic renal failure.

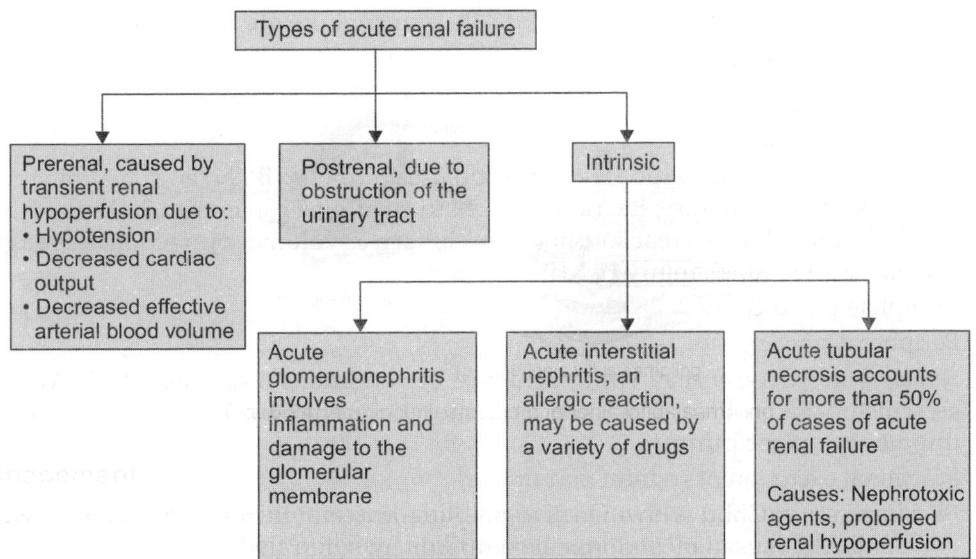

Fig. 7.7: Types of ARF

Signs and Symptoms

- Hemorrhage
- Fever and rash
- Bloody diarrhea
- Severe vomiting
- Abdominal pain
- No urine output or high urine output
- History of recent infection
- History of taking certain medications
- History of trauma
- Swelling of the tissues
- Inflammation of the eye
- Detectable abdominal mass
- Exposure to heavy metals or toxic solvents.

Pathophysiology

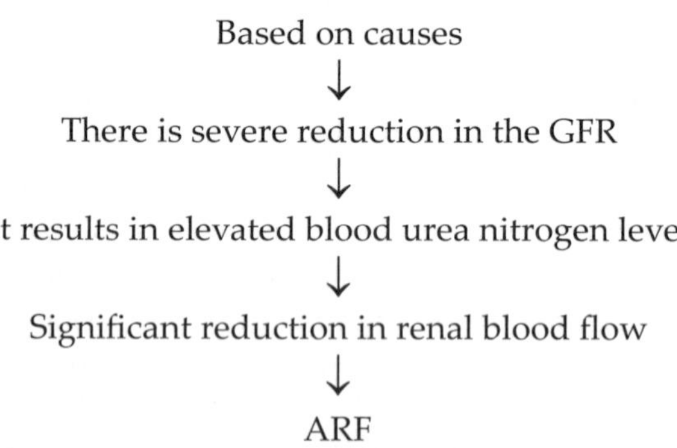

Diagnostic Evalution

- History collection
- Physical examination
- *Renal function test*: Increased levels of blood urea nitrogen (BUN) and creatinine are the hallmarks of renal failure; the ratio of BUN to creatinine can exceed 20:1 in conditions that favor the enhanced reabsorption of urea, such as volume contraction (this suggests prerenal acute kidney injury [AKI])
- Complete blood count
- Peripheral smear
- *Serologic tests*: These may show evidence of conditions associated with AKI, such as schistocytes in disorders such as hemolytic-uremic syndrome and thrombotic thrombocytopenic purpura
- Fractional excretion of sodium and urea
- *Bladder pressure*: Child with a bladder pressure above 25 mm Hg should be suspected of having AKI caused by abdominal compartment syndrome

- *Ultrasonography*: Renal ultrasonography is useful for evaluating existing renal disease and obstruction of the urinary collecting system
- *Renal biopsy*: Can be useful in identifying intrarenal causes of AKI.

Management

Initially a Foley catheter is inserted to rule out urine retention to collect available urine for analysis.

- Monitor results of diuretic administration
- The catheter may or may not be removed during oliguric phase
- The amount of exogenous water provided should not exceed the amount needed to maintain zero water balance
- When the output begins to increase either spontaneously or in response to diuretic therapy the intake of fluid, potassium and sodium must be monitored and adequate replacement provided to prevent depletion and its consequences.

Complications

- Hyperkalemia is the most immediate threat to the life of the child with ARF.
- Hypertension is a frequent and serious complication of ARF and to detect it early blood pressure measurements are made every 4 to 6 hrs.
- Anemia is frequently associated with ARF but transfusion is not recommended unless the hemoglobin drops below 68/dL.
- Seizures occur rather often when renal failure progresses to uremic and are leached to hypertension, hyponatremia and hyperkalemia
- Cardiac failure with pulmonary edema is almost always associated with hyper volume.

Prognosis

- The prognosis of ARF depends largely on the nature and severity of the causative factor or participating event and the promptness and competence of management.

CHRONIC RENAL FAILURE (CRF)

Introduction

The kidneys are able to maintain the chemical composition of fluids within normal limits until more than 50% of functional renal capacity is destroyed by disease or injury. Chronic renal insufficiency or failure begins when the diseased kidneys can no longer maintain the normal chemical structure of body fluids under normal conditions.

The term chronic renal insufficiency was used to characterize child who had progressive decline in renal function, defined as a glomerular filtration rate (GFR) of less than 75 mL/min per 1.73 m^2 body surface area. Chronic kidney disease (CKD) is the new term defined by the National Kidney Foundation Kidney Disease and Outcome Quality Initiative (KDOQI) Group to classify any patient who has kidney damage lasting for at least 3 months with or without a decreased GFR or any patient who has a GFR of less than 60 mL/min per 1.73 m^2 lasting for 3 months with or without kidney damage.

Definition

Chronic kidney disease (CKD) refers to a state of irreversible kidney damage and/or reduction of kidney function, which can be progressive. The accepted term in the pediatric nephrology community, replacing the clinical terms of chronic renal failure (CRF) and chronic renal insufficiency (CRI), which describe kidney dysfunction of varying degrees from severe to mild in nature.

Causes

- Congenital renal and urinary tract malformation
- Recurrent urinary tract infection (UTI)
- Chronic pyelonephritis
- Glomerulonephritis
- Anaphylactic purpura and lupus erythematosus
- Obstruction to kidneys that can prevent blood from getting to them
- Reflux from bladder back up into kidneys that can cause chronic infection
- Dysplastic kidneys.

Stages

- *Stage 1*: Kidney damage with a normal or increased GFR (> 90 mL/min per 1.73 m^2)
- *Stage 2*: Mild reduction in the GFR (60 to 89 mL/min per 1.73 m^2)

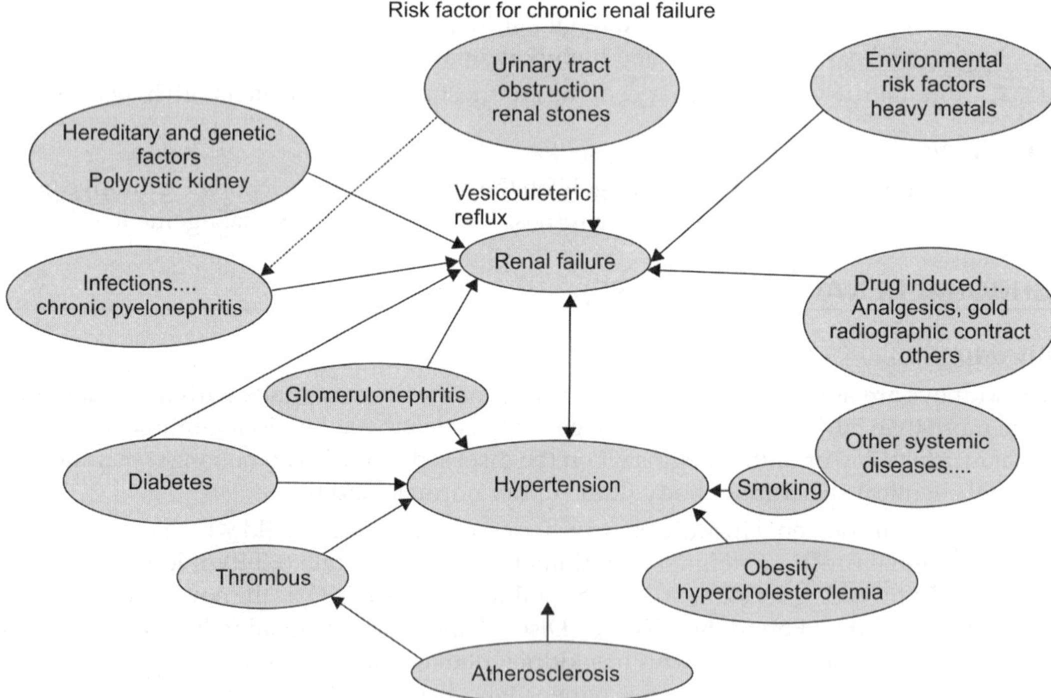

Fig. 7.8: Risk factors of CRF

- *Stage 3*: Moderate reduction in the GFR (30 to 59 mL/min per 1.73 m^2)
- *Stage 4*: Severe reduction in the GFR (15 to 29 mL/min per 1.73 m^2)
- *Stage 5*: Kidney failure (GFR $<$ 15 mL/min per 1.73 m^2 or dialysis)

Pathophysiology

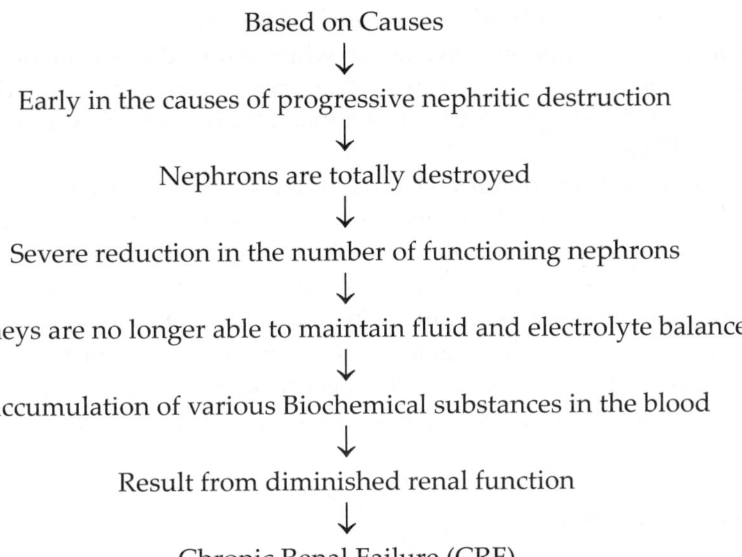

Signs and Symptoms

A CRF is challenging to diagnose early because in its earliest stages, it often does not cause visible symptoms. When symptoms do appear, they are often nonspecific and do not necessarily indicate a problem with child's kidneys.

- Fatigue
- Problems concentrating
- Trouble sleeping, restless leg syndrome
- Generally feeling unwell
- Fever
- Loss of appetite.

Collection of symptoms and signs centered around four major components:

1. Protein in urine
2. Low levels of protein in the blood since it is being lost in the urine
3. Swelling in the body (edema), particularly around the ankles and eyes. This happens because the proteins that hold water inside the child's blood vessels are lost in the urine, so water seeps into the body's tissues.
4. High cholesterol to compensate for the low levels of protein, the body makes fat in the form of cholesterol.

Diagnostic Evaluation

- History collection
- Physical Examination
- *Kidney biopsy:* A small sample of tissue is taken from through a needle and sent to a lab for analysis. The biopsy may indicate focal segmental glomerulosclerosis (FSGS) or the presence of another acquired disease, such as lupus.
- *Kidney ultrasound:* A non-invasive test in which a transducer is passed over the kidney producing a picture of the organ on a video screen. The test is used to determine the size and shape of the kidney and to detect a mass, kidney stone, cyst or other obstruction or abnormalities.
- *Nuclear medicine study:* A non-invasive, painless tests that can reveal important information about child's health. Nuclear medicine uses short-lived radiopharmaceuticals and specialized cameras to create images of the human body.
- *Kidney function tests:* There are two main ways to test child's kidney functioning: By measuring her creatinine level and glomerular filtration rate (GFR).
- *Creatinine* is a waste product that the body makes in a constant amount (depending on muscle mass) each day. Creatinine level is checked through a simple blood test.
- *Glomerular filtration rate test:* It is a measure of how efficiently kidneys are able to filter blood.
- *Other blood tests* may be used to check cholesterol level and for the level of a blood protein called albumin.

Table 7.3: Normal ranges for lab values commonly affected by CRF

Lab	Normal range	Effect in CRF
Bun	8–25 mg/dl	Elevated
Creatinine	0.6–1.2 mg/dl	Elevated
Potassium	3.5–5 mEq/L	Elevated
Sodium	135–145	Decreased
Bicarbonate	22–26	Decreased
pH	7.35–7.45	Decreased

Management

- Promote maximum renal function
- Maintain body fluid and electrolyte balance
- Treat systemic complications
- Diet regulation is the most effective means short of dialysis for reducing the quantity of material is that require renal excretion.
- Diet in renal failure is to provide sufficient calories and protein for growth white liming the excretory demands made on kidney, to minimize metabolic bone disease (Osteodystrophy).
- Sodium and water are not usually limited unless there is evidence of edema or hypertension and potassium is not usually restricted.

- Dietary phosphorus is controlled to prevent or correct the calcium/phosphorus imbalance by the reduction of protein and milk intake.
- Serum calcium levels are increased from the calcium carbonate, vitamin and therapy is begun to increase calcium absorption.
- Metabolic acidosis is alleviated through administration of alkalizing agents such as sodium bicarbonate or combination of Ne and K citrate.

Growth failure in one major consequence of CRF (chronic Renal failure), especially in the preadolescent. These children grow purely both before and after the initiation of hemodialysis.

- Dental care is especially important in these children.
- Anemia in children with CRF is related to decreased production of erythrism protein.
- Recombinant human erythrism protein is being offered to these children as thrice weekly or weekly subcutaneous injections and is replacing the need for frequent blood transfusions.
- Hypertension of advanced renal disease may be managed initially by cautious use of a low sodium diet, fluid restriction.
  - *Antihypertensive (blood pressure pills):* There are various types of medicines that help reduce blood pressure and because they work in different ways, sometimes two or more types may be used together to lower blood pressure.
  - *Red blood cell stimulating agents (e.g. erythropoietin):* These medications, given by a needle, stimulate the bone marrow to produce red blood cells and so prevent anemia.
  - *Phosphate binders (e.g. calcium carbonate):* These medications are taken with meals to prevent phosphate from being absorbed from the digestive tract into the body (they 'bind' phosphate in the intestines and it is passed out in the stool).
  - *Vitamin D:* A special 'activated' form of Vitamin D that helps keep bones healthy.
  - *'Kidney' multivitamin pills:* A special combination of vitamins those are suitable for people living with kidney disease.

Dialysis

The kidneys remove waste products and extra water from the blood. If the kidneys fail before, transplantation is possible, child may need some form of dialysis to do this job. Each type of dialysis will affect family's lifestyle.

Hemodialysis

Hemodialysis filters the blood, removing harmful wastes and extra salts and fluids. A few ounces of blood at a time are pumped through a dialysis machine, where the blood is cleaned before it is returned to the body. Our nurses have special training to help your child with hemodialysis.

Types

- Continuous venovenous hemofiltration (CVVH)
- Continuous venovenous hemodialysis (CWHD)
- Continuous venovenous hemodiafiltration (CVVHDF)

These continuous renal replacement therapies are used in antiretroviral therapy (ART), severe fluid overload in born of peritoneal metabolism.

Procedures

- In hemodialysis a child's blood is sent through a filter to remove harmful wastes, extra salt and extra water. Hemodialysis helps control blood pressure and keeps the proper balance of potassium, sodium, calcium and bicarbonate. Hemodialysis uses a special filter called a dialyzer.
  - During treatment, blood travels from the child's body through tubes into the dialyzer, which filters out wastes and extra water. Then the cleaned blood flows through another set of tubes back into the child's body.
  - The dialyzer is connected to a machine that monitors blood flow and disposes of the wastes. Hemodialysis usually takes place in a clinic three times a week, but it may be required more often in smaller children.
  - Each treatment lasts from 3 to 4 hours. Some clinics offer home hemodialysis, which allows more flexibility in scheduling but requires the caregiver to take weeks of training. During treatment, the child can do homework, read, write, sleep, talk, or watch TV.
  - If she chooses hemodialysis, the doctor will need to create an access to the bloodstream (vascular access) several months before the first treatment. The child may be able to complete the procedure for the vascular access in one day or may need to stay overnight in the hospital.

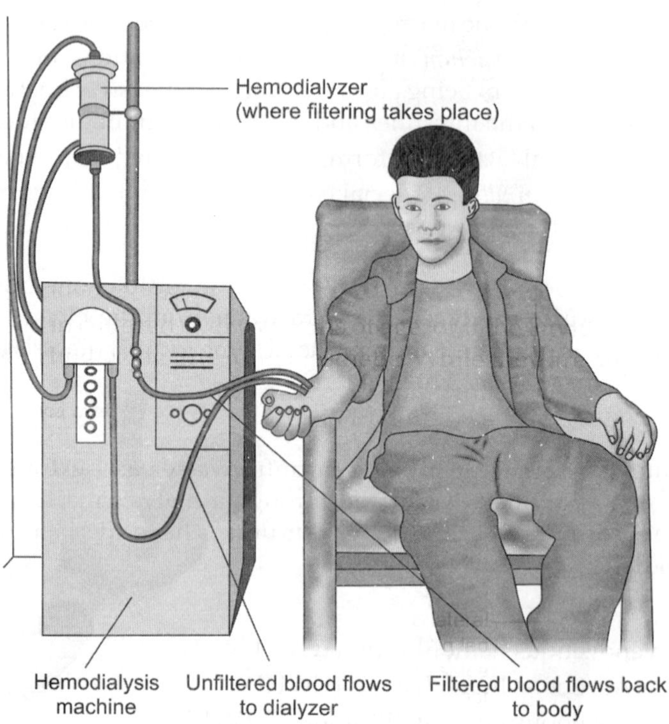

Fig. 7.9: Hemodialysis

When a child starts hemodialysis, problems can be caused by rapid changes in the body's water and chemical balance during treatment.

- Muscle cramps and a sudden drop in blood pressure are two common side effects. Low blood pressure, called hypotension, can make a child feel weak, dizzy, or nauseated.
- Most children need a few months to adjust to hemodialysis. Side effects can often be treated quickly and easily, so you should always report them to your doctor and dialysis staff.
- She can avoid many side effects by making sure your child gets a proper diet, limits liquid intake and takes all medicines as directed.

Peritoneal Dialysis

The abdominal cavity acts as a semipermeable membrane through which water and solutes of small molecular size move by osmosis and diffusion according to their respective concentrations on either side of the membrane.

There are two types of peritoneal dialysis:

1. Continuous ambulatory peritoneal dialysis
2. Continuous cycling peritoneal dialysis.

Vascular Access

A venous fistula is an access in which a vein and artery are connected surgically. The prefunded sites are the radial artery and forearm vein that produces dilation and thickening of the vessels of the forearm to provide easy access for repeated vein puncture.

Arteriovenous graft by anastomosing artery and vein with a synthetic prosthetic graft for circulatory access. For external vascular access devices percutaneous catheters are inserted in

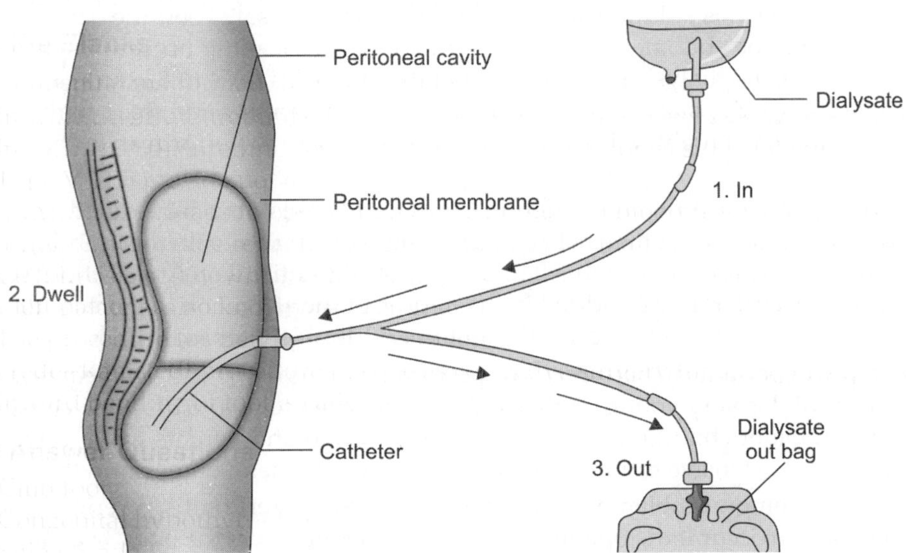

Fig. 7.10: Peritoneal dialysis

femoral subclavian or internal jugular veins even in very small children. A more permanent form of external access is available via a central catheter inserted surgical into the meal jugular vein. This catheter has a dual lumen which allows a large volume of blood flow with minimum recalculation. This procedure is usually performed three times per week for 4 to 6 hours, depending on the size of the child.

Procedures

Peritoneal dialysis uses the lining of child's abdomen, called the peritoneal membrane, to filter blood. A mixture of minerals and sugar dissolved in water, called dialysis solution, is inserted into child's abdomen through a soft tube.

The sugar, called dextrose, draws wastes, chemicals and extra water from the tiny blood vessels in the peritoneal membrane into the dialysis solution. After some time, the used solution—now loaded with the wastes and extra fluid that the kidneys would have filtered out—is drained from child's abdomen through the tube. The period that dialysis solution is in the abdomen is called the dwell time. The abdomen is filled again with fresh dialysis solution and the cycle repeats. The process of emptying and refilling the abdomen is called an exchange and takes about 30 to 40 minutes.

Before the first treatment, a surgeon will place a small, soft tube called a catheter into child's abdomen. The catheter tends to work better if the insertion site has time—usually from 10 days to 3 weeks—to heal. The catheter stays there to help transport dialysis solution to and from the abdomen and is removed only after a successful transplant is in place.

Peritoneal dialysis can be done with or without a cycling machine.

- *Continuous ambulatory peritoneal dialysis (CAPD):* CAPD requires no machine and can be done in any clean, well-lit place. With CAPD, child's blood is always being cleaned. The dialysis solution passes from a plastic bag through the catheter and into the abdomen, where it stays for several hours with the catheter sealed. After the dwell time, the child drains the dialysis solution into a drain bag for disposal. Then the same catheter is used to refill the abdomen with fresh solution so the cleaning process can begin again. With CAPD, the dialysis solution stays in the abdomen for 4 to 6 hours or more. Most people change the dialysis solution at least four times a day and sleep with solution in their abdomen at night. With CAPD, it is not necessary to perform an exchange during the night.
- *Continuous cycling peritoneal dialysis (CCPD):* CCPD uses a machine called a cycler to fill and empty child's abdomen many times at night during sleep. In the morning, the child begins one exchange with a dwell time that lasts the entire day. An additional exchange without the cycler may be added in the middle of the afternoon to increase the amount of waste removed and to reduce the amount of fluid left behind.

Both types of peritoneal dialysis can be performed in the home without help from a nurse or doctor. If child is very young, pediatric nurse will need to help with the exchanges or set up the cycler. Older children can do it themselves. Child and parents will receive detailed instructions and extensive training so you feel confident when you perform the exchanges.

The most common problem with peritoneal dialysis is peritonitis, a serious abdominal infection that can occur if the opening where the catheter enters the body becomes infected or if contamination occurs as the catheter is connected or disconnected from the bags. Peritonitis requires antibiotic treatment prescribed by child's nephrologist.

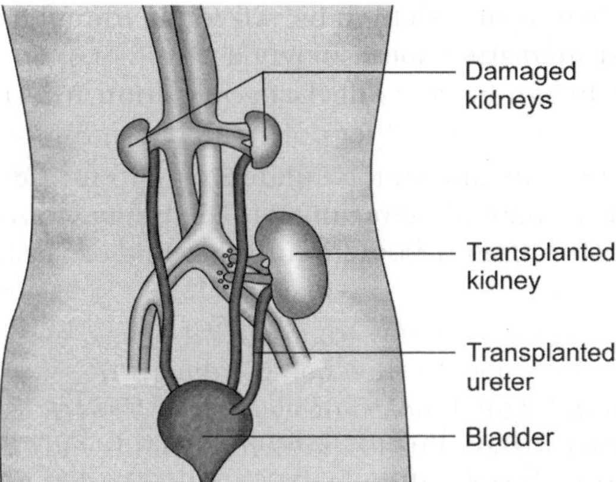

Fig. 7.11: Renal (kidney) transplantation

Renal Transplantation

Renal transplantation is surgery to place a healthy kidney from someone who has just died or a living donor, usually a family member, into a person's body to take over the job of the failing kidney. Once kidneys fail because of chronic kidney disease (CKD), function cannot be restored, so transplantation is the closest thing to a cure. Children with a transplant will need to take medications everyday to prevent their body from rejecting the new kidney and get regular checkups to make sure the new kidney is accepted and functioning properly.

To receive a donor kidney, a child first undergoes a thorough medical evaluation at a transplant center. Kidney transplantation is surgery to place a healthy kidney from someone who has just died or a living donor, usually a family member, into a person's body to take over the job of the failing kidney.

Deceased Donor Kidneys

If the medical evaluation shows that the child does not have a condition that would prevent a successful transplant, the transplant coordinator places the child on a waiting list.

Transplant coordinators register those needing a deceased donor organ with the United Network for Organ Sharing (UNOS), which maintains a centralized computer network linking all regional organ procurement organizations (OPOs) and transplant centers. A child can be registered with multiple transplant centers; most centers require a separate medical evaluation.

The length of time a child has to wait for a transplant depends on many things; however, it is determined primarily by how good the match is between the child and the donor.

A child's place on the list depends on the following:

- *Tissue typing:* A blood test that checks six antigens, or proteins, that make each person different. Tissue typing lets the transplant surgeon know how many antigens the donor shares with the recipient.
- Blood type.
- Length of time on the waiting list.
- Age of child waiting.

- Blood antibody levels, which show how active the immune system is at the current time, a factor than can increase the risk of rejection.
- The immune system normally protects people from infection by identifying and destroying bacteria, viruses and other potentially harmful foreign substances.

When a kidney becomes available, the OPO reports to UNOS and a central computer generates a ranked list of compatible recipients. The transplant center keeps each child's updated contact and health status information, so the child can be found immediately when a kidney becomes available.

Living Donor Kidneys

About half of the kidneys transplanted into children are from living donors, often a parent, family member, or family friend. Potential donors need to be tested for matching factors and to make sure that donating a kidney will not endanger their health.

A kidney from a living donor often has advantages over a kidney from a deceased donor because:

- A kidney from a parent is more likely to be a better tissue match than a kidney from someone who is not related to the child.
- Living donation allows for greater preparation; for example, the operation can be scheduled in advance.
- The kidney does not have to be transported from one site to another, so it may be in better condition.

Nursing Management

Dialysis is the process of separating colloids and crystalline sustained in solution by the difference in their rate of diffusion through a semipermeable membrane.

Nursing Care Plans for Child with ARF or AKI

Nursing Priorities

- Reestablish or maintain fluid and electrolyte balance.
- Prevent complications.
- Provide emotional support for client and significant other (SO).
- Provide information about disease process, prognosis and treatment needs.

Nursing Diagnosis

1. Excess fluid volume related to compromised regulatory mechanism.
2. Risk for decreased cardiac output (RF may include: Fluid overload, fluid shifts, fluid deficit).
3. Risk for imbalanced nutrition: Less than body requirements.
4. Risk for infection.
5. Deficient knowledge.

1. Excess Fluid Volume

Nursing Diagnosis

- Excess fluid volume

As evidenced by:

- Intake greater than output, oliguria; changes in urine specific gravity
- Venous distension; blood pressure (BP)/central venous pressure (CVP) changes
- Generalized tissue edema, weight gain
- Changes in mental status, restlessness
- Decreased Hb/hematocrit (Hct), altered electrolytes; pulmonary congestion on X-ray.

Desired Outcomes

- Display appropriate urinary output with specific gravity/laboratory studies near normal; stable weight, vital signs within patient's normal range; and absence of edema.

Nursing interventions	Rationale
Accurately record intake and output (I & O) noting to include 'hidden' fluids such as IV antibiotic additives, liquid medications, frozen treats, ice chips. Religiously measure gastrointestinal losses and estimate insensible losses (sweating), including wound drainage, nasogastric outputs and diarrhea.	Decrease in output (to less than 400 mL per 24 hours) may indicate acute failure, especially in high-risk child. Accurate monitoring of I & O is necessary for determining renal function and fluid replacement needs and reducing risk of fluid overload. Do note that hypovolemia usually occurs in anuric phase of ARF and may mask the symptoms.
Monitor urine specific gravity.	Measures the kidney's ability to concentrate urine. In intrarenal failure, specific gravity is usually equal to or less than 1.010, indicating loss of ability to concentrate the urine.
Weigh daily at same time of day, on same scale, with same equipment and clothing.	Daily body weight is best monitor of fluid status. A weight gain of more than 0.5 kg/day suggests fluid retention.
Assess skin, face, dependent areas for edema. Evaluate degree of edema (on scale of +1–+4).	Edema occurs primarily in dependent tissues of the body, (hands, feet, Lumbosacral area). Patient can gain up to 10 lb (4.5 kg) of fluid before pitting edema is detected. Periorbital edema may be a presenting sign of this fluid shift because these fragile tissues are easily distended by even minimal fluid accumulation.
Monitor heart rate (HR), BP and JVD/CVP.	Tachycardia and hypertension can occur because of: (1) failure of the kidneys to excrete urine, (2) excess fluid resuscitation during efforts to treat hypovolemia and/or hypotension or convert oliguric phase of renal failure, (3) changes in the renin-angiotensin system. Invasive monitoring may be needed for assessing intravascular volume, especially in child with poor cardiac function.
Auscultate lung and heart sounds.	Fluid overload may lead to pulmonary edema and HF evidenced by development of adventitious breath sounds, extra heart sounds.
Assess level of consciousness. Investigate changes in mentation, presence of restlessness.	May reflect fluid shifts, accumulation of toxins, acidosis, electrolyte imbalances, or developing hypoxia.
Scatter desired beverages throughout the 24-hour period and give various offering (hot, cold, frozen).	Helps avoid periods without fluids, minimizes boredom of limited choices and reduces sense of deprivation and thirst.
Correct any reversible cause of ARF: Replace blood loss, maximize cardiac output, discontinue nephrotoxic drug, relieve obstruction via surgery.	Kidneys may be able to return to normal functioning, preventing or limiting residual effects.

Contd...

Contd...

Nursing interventions	Rationale
Use appropriate safety measures (raising side rails and restraints.	Patient with central nervous system (CNS) involvement may be dizzy and/or confused.
Administer medication as indicated:	
Diuretics: Furosemide (Lasix), bumetanide (Bumex), torsemide (Demadex), mannitol (Osmitrol).	Given early in oliguric phase of ARF in an effort to convert to non-oliguric phase, flush the tubular lumen of debris, reduce hyperkalemia and promote adequate urine volume.
Antihypertensives: Clonidine (Catapres), methyldopa (Aldomet), prazosin (Minipress).	May be given to treat hypertension by counteracting effects of decreased renal blood flow and/or circulating volume overload.
Calcium channel blockers	Given early in nephrotoxic acute tubular necrosis (ATN) to reduce influx of calcium into kidney cells, thereby helping to maintain cell integrity and improve GFR.
Prostaglandins	Vasodilatory effect may improve circulating volume and reestablish renal blood flow to aid in clearing nephrotoxic agents from nephrons.
Insert indwelling catheter, as indicated.	Catheterization excludes lower tract obstruction and provides means of accurate monitoring of urine output during acute phase; however, indwelling catheterization may be contraindicated because of increased risk of infection.
Prepare for dialysis as indicated: Hemodialysis, peritoneal dialysis, or continuous renal replacement therapy (CRRT).	Done to correct volume overload, electrolyte and acid-base imbalances and to remove toxins. The type of dialysis chosen for ARF depends on the degree of hemodynamic compromise and patient's ability to withstand the procedure.
During peritoneal dialysis, position the patient carefully: Elevate the head of the bed.	Doing so would reduce the pressure on the diaphragm and can aid in respiration.
Watch out for complications such as peritonitis, atelectasis, hypokalemia, pneumonia and/or shock.	These complications are common for child undergoing peritoneal dialysis.

2. Risk for Decreased Cardiac Output

Nursing Diagnosis

- Risk for decreased cardiac output

Risk factors may include

- Fluid overload (kidney dysfunction/failure, overzealous fluid replacement)
- Fluid shifts, fluid deficit (excessive losses)
- Electrolyte imbalance (potassium, calcium), severe acidosis
- Uremic effects on cardiac muscle/oxygenation.

Desired Outcomes

Maintain cardiac output as evidenced by BP and HR/rhythm within patient's normal limits; peripheral pulses strong and equal with adequate capillary refill time.

Nursing interventions	Rationale
Monitor BP and HR	Fluid volume excess, combined with hypertension (common in renal failure) and effects of uremia, increases cardiac workload and can lead to cardiac failure. In ARF, cardiac failure is usually reversible.
Observe ECG or telemetry for changes in rhythm.	Changes in electromechanical function may become evident in response to progressing renal failure and accumulation of toxins and electrolyte imbalance. Peaked T wave, wide QRS, prolonged PR interval is usually associated with **hyperkalemia**. Flat T wave, peaked P wave and appearance of the U waves usually indicate **hypokalemia**. Prolonged QT interval may reflect **calcium deficit**.
Auscultate heart sounds.	Development of S_3/S_4 is indicative of failure. Pericardial friction rub may be only manifestation of uremic pericarditis, requiring prompt intervention and possibly acute dialysis.
Assess color of skin, mucous membranes and nail beds. Note capillary refill time.	Pallor may reflect vasoconstriction or anemia. Cyanosis is a late sign and is related to pulmonary congestion and/or cardiac failure.
Note occurrence of slow pulse, hypotension, flushing, nausea and vomiting and depressed level of consciousness.	Use of drugs (like antacids) containing magnesium can result in hypermagnesemia, potentiating the neuromuscular dysfunction and risk of a respiratory or cardiac arrest. Use aluminum-hydroxide-based antacid.
Monitor for GI bleeding by guaiac testing all stools for blood.	Gastrointestinal bleeding is a known complication of renal failure; however, its pathogenesis remains uncertain. Some have attributed gastrointestinal bleeding to the effects of uremia on the gastrointestinal mucosa; others have suggested that uremia may affect platelet adhesiveness, which may explain the prolonged gastrointestinal bleeding seen in child with renal failure. In addition, the role of heparinization and the widespread use of antiplatelet agents in child on dialysis have been implicated in the etiology of gastrointestinal bleeding.
Investigate reports of muscle cramps, numbness of fingers, with muscle twitching, hyper-reflexia.	Neuromuscular indicators of hypocalcemia, which can also affect cardiac contractility and function.
Maintain bed rest or encourage adequate rest and provide assistance with care and desired activities.	Reduces oxygen consumption and cardiac workload.
Administer medications as indicated:	
Inotropic agents: Digoxin (Lanoxin)	May be used to improve cardiac output by increasing myocardial contractility and stroke volume. Dosage depends on renal function and potassium balance to obtain therapeutic effect without toxicity.
Calcium gluconate	Serum calcium is often low but usually does not require specific treatment in ARF. Calcium gluconate may be given to treat hypocalcemia and to offset the effects of hyperkalemia by modifying cardiac irritability.
Aluminum hydroxide gels (Amphojel, Basaljel)	Increased phosphate levels may occur as a result of failure of glomerular filtration and require use of phosphate-binding antacids to limit phosphate absorption from the GI tract.
Glucose and/or insulin solution	Temporary measure to lower serum potassium by driving potassium into cells when cardiac rhythm is endangered.

Contd...

Contd...

Nursing interventions	Rationale
Sodium bicarbonate or sodium citrate	May be used to correct acidosis or hyperkalemia (by increasing serum pH) if patient is severely acidotic and not suffering from fluid overload.
Sodium polystyrene sulfonate (Kayexalate) with or without sorbitol.	Exchange resin trades sodium for potassium in the GI tract to lower serum potassium level. Sorbitol may be included to cause osmotic diarrhea to help excrete potassium.
Prepare for/assist with dialysis as necessary.	May be indicated for persistent dysrhythmias, progressive Heart failure (HF) unresponsive to other therapies.

Nursing Care Plans for Child with CRF or CKD

Nursing Priorities

- Maintain homeostasis.
- Prevent complications.
- Provide information about disease process/prognosis and treatment needs.
- Support adjustment to lifestyle changes.

Discharge Goals

- Fluid/electrolyte balance stabilized.
- Complications prevented/minimized.
- Disease process/prognosis and therapeutic regimen understood.
- Dealing realistically with situation; initiating necessary lifestyle changes.
- Plan in place to meet needs after discharge.

Risk for Decreased Cardiac Output

- Fluid imbalances affecting circulating volume, myocardial workload and systemic vascular resistance (SVR)
- Alterations in rate, rhythm, cardiac conduction (electrolyte imbalances, hypoxia)
- Accumulation of toxins (urea), soft-tissue calcification (deposition of calcium phosphate).

Desired Outcomes

- Maintain cardiac output as evidenced by BP and heart rate within patient's normal range; peripheral pulses strong and equal with prompt capillary refill time.

Nursing interventions	Rationale
Auscultate heart and lung sounds. Evaluate presence of peripheral edema, vascular congestion and reports of dyspnea.	S_3 and S_4 heart sounds with muffled tones, tachycardia, irregular heart rate, tachypnea, dyspnea, crackles, wheezes, edema and jugular distension suggest HF.
Assess presence and degree of hypertension: monitor BP; note postural changes (sitting, lying, standing).	Significant hypertension can occur because of disturbances in the renin-angiotensin-aldosterone system (caused by renal dysfunction). Although hypertension is common, orthostatic hypotension may occur because of intravascular fluid deficit, response to effects of antihypertensive medications, or uremic pericardial tamponade.

Contd...

Contd...

Nursing interventions	Rationale
Investigate reports of chest pain, noting location, radiation, severity (0–10 scale) and whether or not it is intensified by deep inspiration and supine position.	Although hypertension and chronic HF may cause MI, approximately half of CRF child on dialysis develop pericarditis, potentiating risk of pericardial effusion or tamponade.
Evaluate heart sounds (note friction rub), BP, peripheral pulses, capillary refill, vascular congestion, temperature and sensorium or mentation.	Presence of sudden hypotension, paradoxic pulse, narrow pulse pressure, diminished or absent peripheral pulses, marked jugular distension, pallor and a rapid mental deterioration indicate tamponade, which is a medical emergency.
Assess activity level, response to activity.	Weakness can be attributed to HF and anemia.

Risk for Ineffective Protection

- Abnormal blood profile (suppressed erythropoietin production/secretion; decreased RBC production and survival; altered clotting factors; increased capillary fragility).

Desired Outcomes

- Experience no signs/symptoms of bleeding/hemorrhage.
- Maintain/demonstrate improvement in laboratory values.

Nursing interventions	Rationale
Note reports of increasing fatigue, weakness. Observe for tachycardia, pallor of ski and mucous membranes, dyspnea and chest pain. Plan patient activities to avoid fatigue.	May reflect effects of anemia and cardiac response necessary to keep cells oxygenated.
Monitor level of consciousness and behavior.	Anemia may cause cerebral hypoxia manifested by changes in mentation, orientation and behavioral responses.
Evaluate response to activity, ability to perform tasks. Assist as needed and develop schedule for rest.	Anemia decreases tissue oxygenation and increases fatigue, which may require intervention, changes in activity and rest.
Limit vascular sampling, combine laboratory tests when possible.	Recurrent or excessive blood sampling can worsen anemia.
Observe for oozing from venipuncture sites, bleeding, ecchymotic areas following slight trauma, petechiae; joint swelling or mucous membrane involvement (bleeding gums, recurrent epistaxis, hematemesis, melena and hazy or red urine.	Bleeding can occur easily because of capillary fragility and altered clotting functions and may worsen anemia.
Hematest GI secretions and stool for blood.	Mucosal changes and altered platelet function due to uremia may result in gastric mucosal erosion and GI hemorrhage.
Provide soft toothbrush, electric razor; use smallest needle possible and apply prolonged pressure following injections or vascular punctures.	Reduces risk of bleeding and hematoma formation.
Administer medications as indicated:	
Erythropoietin preparations (Epogen, EPO, Procrit);	Corrects many of the symptoms of CRF resulting from anemia by stimulating the production and maintenance of RBCs, thus decreasing the need for transfusion.

Contd...

Contd...

Nursing interventions	Rationale
Iron preparations: Folic acid (Folvite), cyanocobalamin (Rubesol-1000).	Useful in managing symptomatic anemia related to nutritional or dialysis-induced deficits. Note: Iron should not be given with phosphate binders because they may decrease iron absorption.
Cimetidine (Tagamet), ranitidine (Zantac); antacids;	May be given prophylactically to reduce or neutralize gastric acid and thereby reduce the risk of GI hemorrhage.
Hemostatics or fibrinolysis inhibitors such as aminocaproic acid (Amicar)	Inhibits bleeding that does not subside spontaneously or respond to usual treatment.
Stool softeners (Colace); bulk laxative (Metamucil).	Straining to pass hard-formed stool increases likelihood of mucosal and rectal bleeding.

Disturbed Thought Process

- *Physiological changes:* Accumulation of toxins (e.g. urea, ammonia), metabolic acidosis, hypoxia; electrolyte imbalances, calcifications in the brain
- Disorientation to person, place, time
- Memory deficit; altered attention span, decreased ability to grasp ideas
- Impaired ability to make decisions, problem-solve
- *Changes in sensorium:* Somnolence, stupor, coma
- *Changes in behavior:* Irritability, withdrawal, depression, psychosis.

Desired Outcomes

- Regain/maintain optimal level of mentation.
- Identify ways to compensate for cognitive impairment/memory deficits.

Nursing interventions	Rationale
Assess extent of impairment in thinking ability, memory and orientation. Note attention span.	Uremic syndrome's effect can begin with minor confusion, irritability and progress to altered personality or inability to assimilate information and participate in care. Awareness of changes provides opportunity for evaluation and intervention.
Ascertain from SO patient's usual level of mentation.	Provides comparison to evaluate progression and resolution of impairment.
Provide SO with information about patient's status.	Some improvement in mentation may be expected with restoration of more normal levels of BUN, electrolytes and serum pH.
Provide quiet or calm environment and judicious use of television, radio and visitation.	Minimizes environmental stimuli to reduce sensory overload and confusion while preventing sensory deprivation.
Reorient to surroundings, person and so forth. Provide calendars, clocks, outside window.	Provides clues to aid in recognition of reality.
Present reality concisely, briefly and do not challenge illogical thinking.	Confrontation potentiates defensive reactions and may lead to patient mistrust and heightened denial of reality.
Communicate information and instructions in simple, short sentences. Ask direct, yes or no questions. Repeat explanations as necessary.	May aid in reducing confusion and increases possibility that communications will be understood and remembered.

Contd...

Contd...

Nursing interventions	Rationale
Establish a regular schedule for expected activities.	Aids in maintaining reality orientation and may reduce fear and confusion.
Promote adequate rest and undisturbed periods for sleep.	Sleep deprivation may further impair cognitive abilities.
Monitor laboratory studies such as BUN and Cr, serum electrolytes, glucose level and ABGs (PO_2, pH).	Correction of elevations or imbalances can have profound effects on cognition or mentation.
Provide supplemental O_2 as indicated.	Correction of hypoxia alone can improve cognition.
Avoid use of barbiturates and opiates.	Drugs normally detoxified in the kidneys will have increased half-life and cumulative effects, worsening confusion.
Prepare for dialysis.	Marked deterioration of thought processes may indicate worsening of azotemia and general condition, requiring prompt intervention to regain homeostasis.

RESPIRATORY SYSTEM

CHILD WITH URI AND LRI

Introduction

The human respiratory system is a series of organs responsible for taking in oxygen and expelling carbon dioxide. The primary organs of the respiratory system are lungs, which carry out this exchange of gases as we breathe.

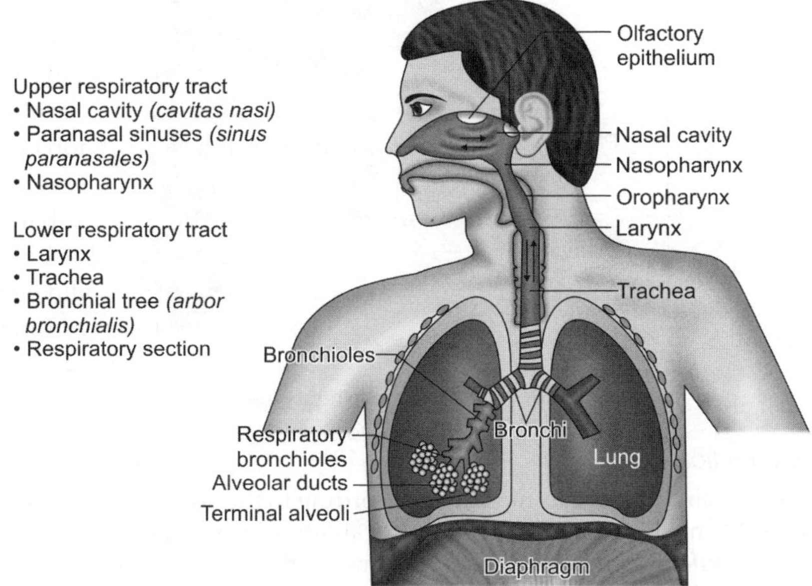

Fig. 7.12: Anatomical view of upper and lower respiratory tract

Red blood cells collect the oxygen from the lungs and carry it to the parts of the body where it is needed, according to the American Lung Association. During the process, the red blood cells collect the carbon dioxide and transport it back to the lungs, where it leaves the body when we exhale. The human body needs oxygen to sustain itself. A decrease in oxygen is known as hypoxia and a complete lack of oxygen is known as anoxia.

In humans, the average rate of breathing is dependent upon age. A newborn's normal breathing rate is about 40 times each minute and may slow to 20 to 40 times per minute when the baby is sleeping. For adults, the average resting respiratory rate for adults is 12 to 16 breaths per minute. Physical exertion also has an effect on respiratory rate and healthy adults can average 45 breaths per minute during strenuous exercise.

- *The upper respiratory tract* includes the mouth, nose, sinus, throat, larynx (voice box) and trachea (windpipe). Upper respiratory infections are often referred to as 'colds.'
- *The lower respiratory tract* includes the bronchial tubes and the lungs. Bronchitis and pneumonia are infections of the lower respiratory *tract*.

UPPER RESPIRATORY TRACT INFECTION

Introduction

Upper respiratory tract infections, (URI or URTI), are the illnesses caused by an acute infection which involves the upper respiratory tract: Nose, sinuses, pharynx or larynx.

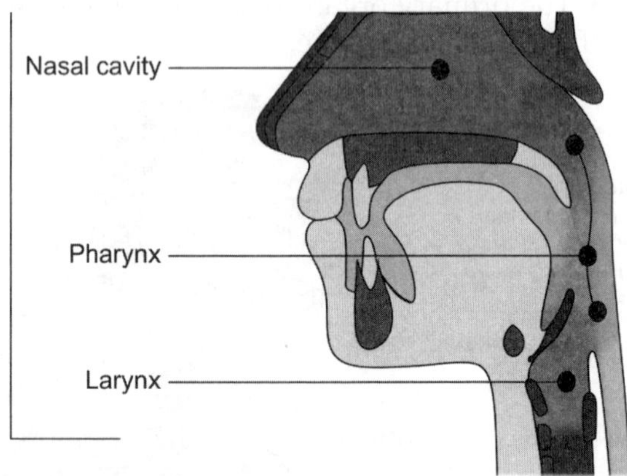

Fig. 7.13: Upper respiratory tract

Respiratory Infection

Infection of the respiratory tract is described according to the anatomic area of involvement. URI represents the most common acute illness evaluated. URI range from the common cold, typically a mild self-limited, catarrhal syndrome of the nasopharynx to life threatening illnesses, such as epiglottis.

Definitions

Upper respiratory tract infection (URI) is defined as nonspecific term used to describe acute infections involving the nose, paranasal sinuses, pharynx, larynx, trachea and bronchi. The prototype is the illness known as the common cold, pharyngitis, sinusitis and tracheobronchitis.

Common URI terms are defined as follows:

- *Rhinitis*: Inflammation of the nasal mucosa
- *Rhinosinusitis or sinusitis*: Inflammation of the nares and paranasal sinuses, including frontal, ethmoid, maxillary and sphenoid
- *Nasopharyngitis (rhinopharyngitis or the common cold)*: Inflammation of the nares, pharynx, hypopharynx, uvula and tonsils
- *Pharyngitis*: Inflammation of the pharynx, hypopharynx, uvula and tonsils
- *Epiglottitis (supraglottitis):* Inflammation of the superior portion of the larynx and supraglottic area
- *Laryngitis:* Inflammation of the larynx
- *Laryngotracheitis:* Inflammation of the larynx, trachea and subglottic area
- *Tracheitis:* Inflammation of the trachea and subglottic area.

Causes

Upper respiratory tract infection (URTI) or 'the common cold' is a symptom complex usually caused by several families of virus; these are the rhinovirus, coronavirus, parainfluenza, respiratory syncytial virus (RSV), adenovirus, human metapneumovirus and influenza. Occasionally the enterovirus is implicated in summer.

The most common virus is called the rhinovirus. Up to 15% of acute pharyngitis cases may be caused by bacteria, commonly Group A streptococcus in Streptococcal pharyngitis ('Strep Throat'). Influenza (the flu) is a more severe systemic illness which typically involves the upper respiratory tract.

Mode of Transmission

Transmission is via respiratory droplets or by virus-contaminated hands. Upper respiratory tract (nose, throat, sinuses) mucosa inflammation causes increased secretions, rhinorrhea and results in sneezing and coughing facilitating the spread.

Signs and Symptoms

Acute upper respiratory tract infections include rhinitis, pharyngitis/tonsillitis and laryngitis often referred to as a common cold and their complications: Sinusitis, ear infection and sometimes bronchitis (though bronchi are generally classified as part of the lower respiratory tract.)

Symptoms of URI's commonly include cough, sore throat, runny nose, nasal congestion, headache, low grade fever, facial pressure and sneezing. Onset of the symptoms usually begins 1–3 days after the exposure to a microbial pathogen.

The illness usually lasts 7–10 days. Group-A beta hemolytic streptococcal pharyngitis/ tonsillitis (strep throat) typically presents with a sudden onset of sore throat, pain with swallowing and fever. Strep throat does not usually cause runny nose, voice changes or cough. Pain and pressure of the ear caused by a middle ear infection (otitis media) and the reddening of the eye caused by viral conjunctivitis are often associated with upper respiratory infections.

Table 7.4: Comparison of URI symptom with major causes

Symptoms	Allergy	URI	Influenza
Itchy, watery eyes	Common	Rare (conjunctivitis may occur with adenovirus)	Soreness behind eyes, sometimes conjunctivitis
Nasal discharge	Common	Common	Common
Nasal congestion	Common	Common	Sometimes
Sneezing	Very common	Very common	Sometimes
Sore throat	Sometimes (postnasal drip)	Very common	Sometimes
Cough	Sometimes	Common (mild to moderate, hacking)	Common (dry cough, can be severe)
Headache	Uncommon	Rare	Common
Fever	Never	Rare in adults, possible in children	Very common (100–102 °F [or higher in young children], lasting 3–4 days; may have chills)
Malaise	Sometimes	Sometimes	Very common
Fatigue, weakness	Sometimes	Sometimes	Very common, can last for weeks, extreme exhaustion early in course
Myalgias	Never	Slight	Very common, often severe

Management

According to a Cochrane review single oral dose of nasal decongestant in the common cold is modestly effective for the short-term relief of congestion in adults; however, 'there is insufficient data on the use of [Decongestants] in children.' Therefore decongestants are not recommended for use in children under 12 years of age with the common cold. Oral decongestants are, also, contraindicated in child with hypertension, coronary artery disease and history of bleeding strokes.

The use of Vitamin C in the inhibition and treatment of upper respiratory infections has been suggested since the initial isolation of vitamin C in the 1930s. Some evidence exists to indicate that it could be justified in persons exposed to brief periods of severe physical exercise and/or cold environments. There is no evidence to support the age-old advice to rest when you are sick with an upper respiratory illness. In fact, moderate exercise in sedentary subjects with a URI has been shown to have no effect on the overall severity and duration of the illness. Based on these findings, it was concluded that previously sedentary people who have acquired a URI and who have initiated an exercise program may continue to exercise. Increasing fluid intake or 'drinking plenty of fluids' during a cold is not supported by medical evidence, according to a literature review published in the British Medical Journal.

CHILD WITH RHINITIS

Introduction

Rhinitis commonly known as a stuffy nose is the medical term describing irritation and inflammation of some internal areas of the nose. The primary symptom of rhinitis is nasal dripping. It is caused by chronic or acute inflammation of the mucous membrane of the nose due to viruses, bacteria or irritants. Rhinitis has also been found to adversely affect more than just the nose, throat and eyes. It has been associated with sleeping problems, ear conditions and even learning problems. Rhinitis is caused by an increase in histamine. This increase is most often caused by airborne allergens. These allergens may affect an individual's nose, throat, or eyes and cause an increase in fluid production within these areas.

Definition

The inflammation results in the generating of excessive amounts of mucus, commonly producing the aforementioned runny nose, as well as nasal congestion and postnasal drip.

Types

Rhinitis is categorized into three types:

1. Infective rhinitis includes acute and chronic bacterial infections.
2. Nonallergic (vasomotor) rhinitis includes autonomic, hormonal, drug-induced, atrophic and gustatory rhinitis, as well as rhinitis medicamentosa.
3. Allergic rhinitis, the reaction triggered by pollen, mold, animal dander, dust and other similar inhaled allergens.

Signs and Symptoms

Pediatric allergic rhinitis includes the following:

- Rhinorrhea, nasal congestion, postnasal drainage
- Pale nasal turbinates, with or without clear nasal discharge
- Repetitive sneezing
- Itching of the palate, nose, ears or eyes
- Snoring
- Frequent sore throats
- Constant clearing of the throat, cough
- Headaches.

Nonallergic Rhinitis

Nonallergic rhinitis refers to runny nose that is not due to allergy. Nonallergic rhinitis can be classified as either:

- Noninflammatory rhinitis.
- Inflammatory rhinitis.

Noninflammatory or nonallergic rhinitis that is sometimes confused with allergy is called vasomotor rhinitis in which certain nonallergic triggers such as smells, fumes, smoke, dusts and temperature changes, cause rhinitis.

There is still much to be learned about this entity, but it is thought that these nonallergic triggers cause dilation of the blood vessels in the lining of the nose, which results in swelling and drainage.

Vasomotor rhinitis can coexist with allergic rhinitis and this is called 'mixed rhinitis.' Vasomotor rhinitis appears to be significantly more common in women than men, leading some researchers to believe hormones to play a role. In general, age of onset occurs after 20 years of age, in contrast to allergic rhinitis which can be developed at any age. Individuals suffering from vasomotor rhinitis typically experience symptoms year-round, though symptoms may exacerbate in the spring and autumn when rapid weather changes are more common.

Allergic Rhinitis

Allergic rhinitis is the most common childhood ailment caused by allergies. Symptoms include a runny and itchy nose, sneezing, postnasal drip and nasal congestion (blockage). A child with allergies may also have itchy, watery, red eyes and chronic ear problems. Even though it is commonly known as 'hay fever,' allergic rhinitis is not triggered by hay and does not cause fever.

Management

The management of rhinitis depends on the underlying cause.

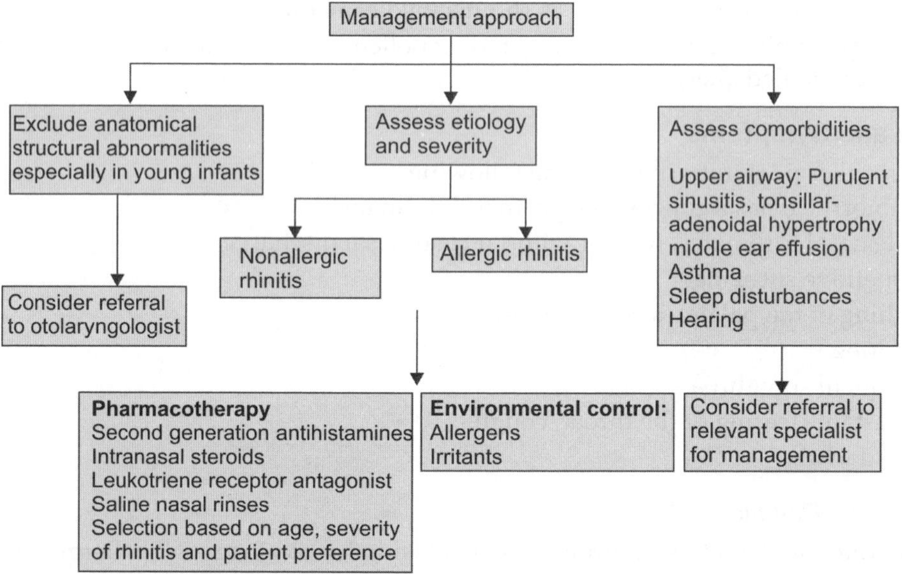

Fig. 7.14: Management process of rhinitis

RHINOSINUSITIS

Introduction

Rhinosinusitis is a very common disease worldwide population. It is a common disease in children but may be under diagnosed. Several reasons may account to the disease being missed in children. The symptoms in children are limited and can be very similar to the common cold or allergic symptoms. Cough and nasal discharge may be the only symptoms present in children.

A high index of suspicion is necessary to make the diagnosis of rhinosinusitis in these children. The majority of those children are treated medically. Only a few numbers will require surgical intervention when medical treatment fails. Complications of rhinosinusitis, even though rare, can carry a high morbidity and mortality rate.

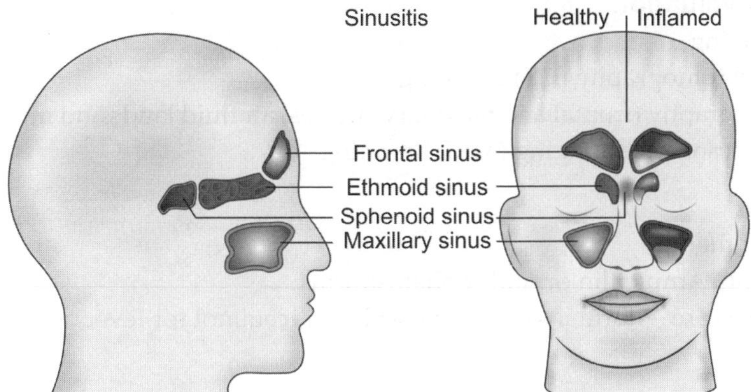

Fig. 7.15: Comparison of child with normal and inflamed sinus

Definition

Inflammation of the nares and paranasal sinus including frontal, ethmoid, maxillary and sphenoid.

Incidence

Sinusitis is common in persons with Viral URTS (Upper airway tracts), 80% child with uncomplicated viral upper respiratory tract infections, 2% of children with bacterial rhinosinusitis.

Causes

Acute Viral or Bacterial Rhinosinusitis

The presentation of rhinosinusitis is often similar to that of nasopharyngitis because many viral upper respiratory infection directly involve the paranasal sinuses. Symptoms may have a biphasic pattern wherein cold like symptoms initially improve but then coarsen. Acute bacterial rhinosinusitis is not common in child whose symptoms have lasted fever more than 7 days, unilateral and localizing symptoms raise the suspicion for sinus involvement.

Clinical Manifestation

- Nasal discharge
- Secondary to nasal inflammation
- Facial or dental pressure or pain
- Maxillary sinus inflammation may manifest as pain in the upper teeth on the affected sides.

- Halitosis—foul breath
- Cough—upper airway cough syndrome
- Fever
- Fatigue or malaise
- Periorbital swelling
- Sinus cavity opacification on transillumination.

Diagnostic Evaluation

- Sinus imaging
- Computed tomography (CT) scanning
- Plain radiography (frontal and maxillary sinuses) air fluid lauds and muwsal thickening
- Magnetic resonance imaging (MRI) scanning.

Management

- Antibiotic therapy
- Amoxicillin, Ampicillin or oral cephalosporins
- Supportive care—normal saline in nostrils paracetamol for fever and pain relief.

SINUSITIS

Introduction

The sinuses are cavities, or air-filled pockets, near the nasal passage. Such as nasal passage, the sinuses are lined with mucous membranes.

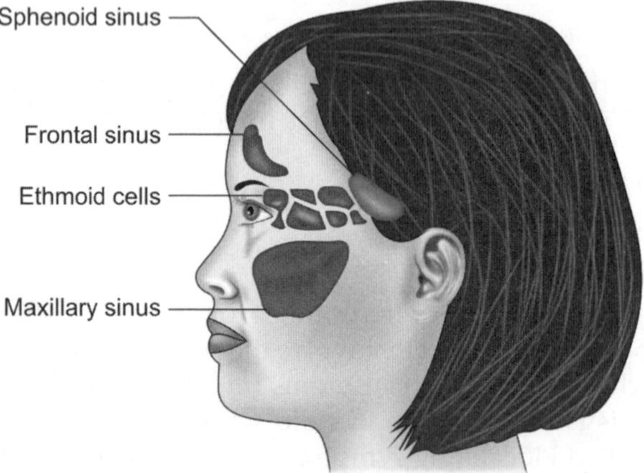

Fig. 7.16: Anatomical review of sinuses

There are four different types of sinuses:

1. *Sphenoid sinus*: Located deep in the face, behind the nose. This sinus does not develop until adolescence.
2. *Frontal sinus*: Located inside the face, in the area of the forehead. This sinus does not develop until around 7 years of age.

3. *Ethmoid sinus*: Located inside the face, around the area of the bridge of the nose. This sinus is present at birth and continues to grow.
4. *Maxillary sinus*: Located inside the face, around the area of the cheeks. This sinus is also present at birth and continues to grow.

Definition

Sinusitis is defined as an inflammation of the paranasal sinuses, which may be due to infection, allergy or autoimmune issues. Most cases are due to a viral infection and resolve over the course of 10 days. It is a common condition with more than 24 million cases occurring in the United States annually.

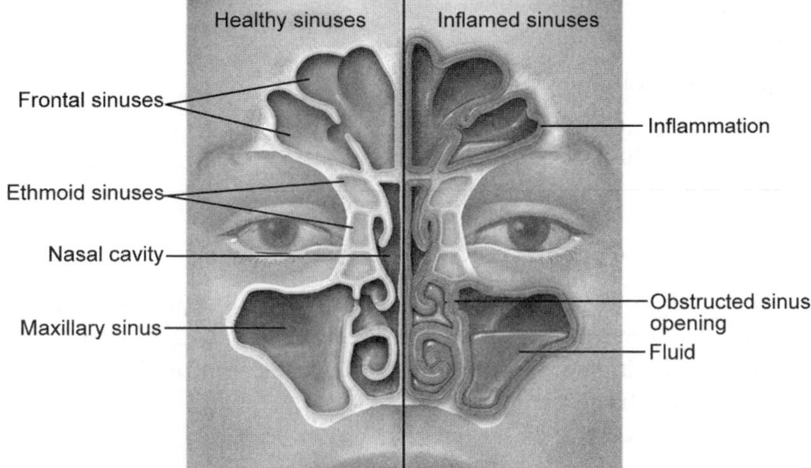

Fig. 7.17: Anatomical difference between normal and inflamed sinus

Classification

A sinusitis is an infection of the sinuses near the nose. These infections usually occur after a cold or after an allergic inflammation.

There are four types of sinusitis:

1. *Acute sinusitis*: Symptoms of this type of infection last less than four weeks and get better with the appropriate treatment.
2. *Subacute sinusitis*: This type of infection does not get better with treatment initially and symptoms last four to eight weeks.
3. *Chronic sinusitis*: This type of infection happens with repeated acute infections or with previous infections that were inadequately treated. These symptoms last eight weeks or longer.
4. *Recurrent sinusitis*: Three or more episodes of acute sinusitis a year.

Causes and Risk Factors

The URI causes inflammation of the nasal passages that can block the opening of the paranasal sinuses and result in a sinus infection. Allergies can also lead to sinusitis because of the swelling of the nasal tissue and increased production of mucus.

The most common bacteria that cause sinusitis include the following:

- *Streptococcus pneumonia*
- *Haemophilus influenzae*
- *Moraxella catarrhalis*

There are other possible conditions that can block the normal flow of secretions out of the sinuses and can lead to sinusitis including the following:

- Abnormalities in the structure of the nose
- Enlarged adenoids
- Diving and swimming
- Infections from a tooth
- Trauma to the nose
- Foreign objects stuck in the nose
- Cleft palate
- Gastroesophageal reflux disease (GERD)
- Secondhand smoke

Incubation Period

Sinusitis can be acute (going on less than four weeks), subacute (4–8 weeks) or chronic (going on for 8 weeks or more). All three types of sinusitis have similar symptoms and are thus often difficult to distinguish. Acute sinusitis is very common. Roughly ninety percent of adults have had sinusitis at some point in their life.

Location

There are several paired paranasal sinuses, including the frontal, ethmoid, maxillary and sphenoid sinuses. The ethmoid sinuses is further subdivided into anterior and posterior ethmoid sinuses, the division of which is defined as the basal lamella of the middle turbinate. In addition to the severity of disease, discussed below, sinusitis can be classified by the sinus cavity which it affects:

- *Maxillary sinusitis*: It cause pain or pressure in the maxillary (cheek) area (e.g. toothache, headache)
- *Frontal sinusitis*: It cause pain or pressure in the frontal sinus cavity (located behind/above eyes), headache
- *Ethmoid sinusitis*: It cause pain or pressure pain between/behind the eyes and headaches
- *Sphenoid sinusitis*: It cause pain or pressure behind the eyes, but often refers to the vertex, or top of the head.

Recent theories of sinusitis indicate that it often occurs as part of a spectrum of diseases that affect the respiratory tract (i.e. the 'one airway' theory) and is often linked to asthma. All forms of sinusitis may either result in, or be a part of, a generalized inflammation of the airway, so other airway symptoms, such as cough, may be associated with it.

Pathophysiology

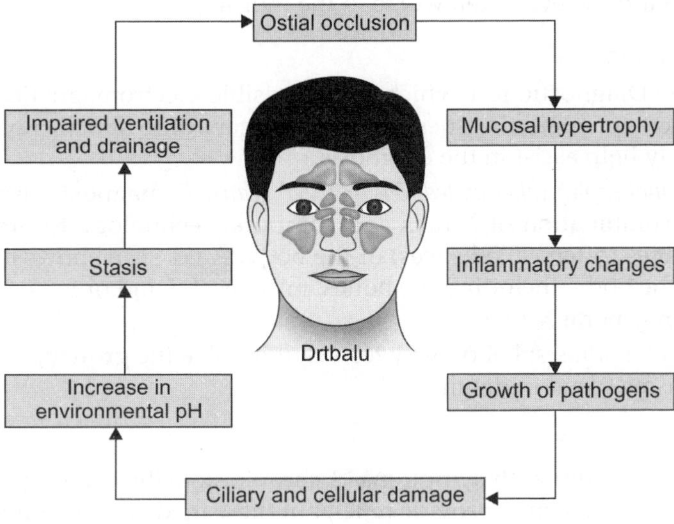

Fig. 7.18: Pathophysiology of sinusitis

Signs and Symptoms

Younger Children (Birth to 5 Years)

- Runny nose
  - Lasts longer than 7 to 10 days
  - Discharge is usually thick green or yellow, but can be clear
- Nighttime cough
- Occasional daytime cough
- Swelling around the eyes
- Usually no headaches younger than 5 years of age.

Older Children and Adults (6 to 18 Years)

In older child and teens, the most common sinusitis symptoms are a cough that does not improve after the first 7 days of cold symptoms, fever, worsening congestion, foul breath, dental pain, ear pain, or tenderness in the face. Sometimes, teens who have sinusitis also develop upset stomachs, nausea, headaches and pain behind the eyes.

- Runny nose or cold symptoms lasting longer than seven to 10 days
- Drip in the throat from the nose
- Headaches
- Facial discomfort
- Bad breath
- Cough
- Mild to severe fever

- Sore throat
- Swelling around the eye, often worse in the morning

Diagnostic Evaluation

- *Sinus X-rays*: Diagnostic test which uses invisible electromagnetic energy beams to produce images of internal tissues, bones and organs onto film. (X-rays are not typically used, but may help assist in the diagnosis.)
- *Computed tomography (also called CT or CAT scan)*: A diagnostic imaging procedure that uses a combination of X-rays and computer technology to produce horizontal, or axial, images (often called slices) of the body. A CT scan shows detailed images of any part of the body, including the bones, muscles, fat and organs. CT scans are more detailed than general X-rays.
- *Cultures from the sinuses*: Laboratory tests that involve the growing of bacteria or other microorganisms to aid in diagnosis.

Management

Nasal irrigation may help with symptoms of chronic sinusitis. Decongestant nasal sprays containing oxymetazoline may provide relief, but these medications should not be used for more than the recommended period. Longer use may cause rebound sinusitis.

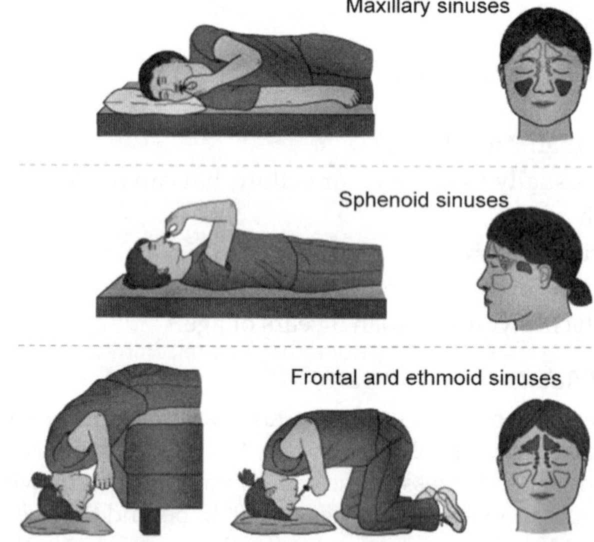

Fig. 7.19: Medication position for different types of sinusitis

Antibiotic Therapy

- The vast majority of cases of sinusitis is caused by viruses and will therefore resolve without antibiotics. However, if symptoms do not resolve within 7 days, amoxicillin is a reasonable antibiotic to use first for treatment with amoxicillin/clavulanate (Augmentin) is being indicated when the patient's symptoms do not improve on amoxicillin alone.
- Fluoroquinolones and some of the newer macrolide antibiotics such as clarithromycin and doxycycline are used in child who is allergic to penicillin.

- Antibiotics are usually ineffective and overall may be no more effective than placebos, as one study found 60 to 90% of people do not experience resolution of symptoms using antibiotics. Thus, antibiotics may not improve the long-term clinical outcomes of sinusitis.
- Though a short-course (3–7 days) of antibiotics seems to be effective for child who present without severe disease or any complicating factors.

Corticosteroids

Acute sinusitis, intranasal corticosteroids have not been found to be better than placebo either alone or in combination with antibiotics. However for cases confirmed by radiology or nasal endoscopy treatment with corticosteroids alone or in combination with antibiotics is supported.

Surgical Management

Chronic or recurring sinusitis, referral to an otolaryngologist specialist may be indicated and treatment options may include nasal surgery. However, for most child the surgical approach is not superior to appropriate drug treatment. Surgery should only be considered for those child who do not experience sufficient relief from optimal medication.

A relatively recent advance in the treatment of sinusitis is a type of surgery called functional endoscopic sinus surgery. This surgery removes anatomical and pathological obstructions associated with sinusitis in order to restore normal clearance of the sinuses. This replaces prior open techniques requiring facial or oral incisions and refocuses the technique to the natural openings of the sinuses instead of promoting drainage by gravity, the idea upon which the Caldwell-Luc surgery was based.

A number of surgical approaches can be used to access the sinuses and these have generally shifted from external/extranasal approaches to intranasal endoscopic ones. The benefit of the Functional Endoscopic Sinus Surgery is its ability to allow for a more targeted approach to the affected sinuses, reducing tissue disruption and minimizing postoperative complications. Another recently developed treatment is balloon sinuplasty. This method, similar to balloon angioplasty used to 'unclog' arteries of the heart, utilizes balloons in an attempt to expand the openings of the sinuses in a less invasive manner. The utility of this treatment for sinus disease is still under debate but appears promising.

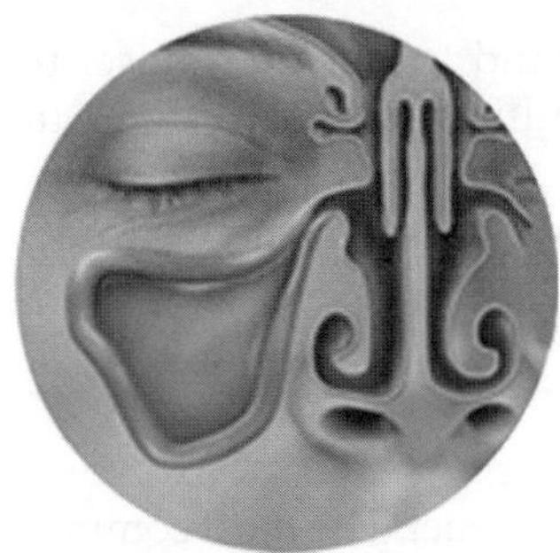

Blocked sinus pathway

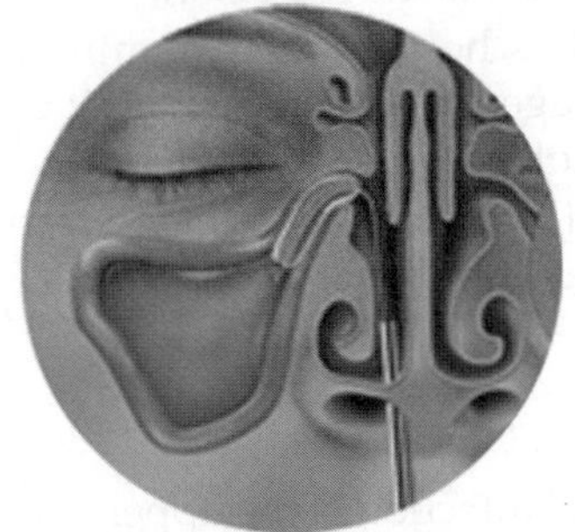

Balloon inflated

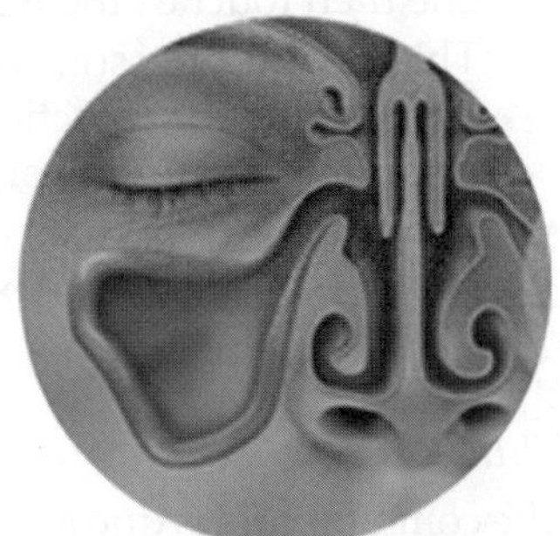

Drainage restored

Fig. 7.20: Balloon sinuplasty

Persistent symptoms and disease in child who have failed medical and the functional endoscopic approach's, older techniques can be used to address the inflammation of the maxillary sinus, such as the Caldwell-Luc radical antrostomy. This surgery involves an incision in the upper gum, opening in the anterior wall of the antrum, removal of the entire diseased maxillary sinus mucosa and drainage is allowed into inferior or middle meatus by creating a large window in the lateral nasal wall.

Complications

The close proximity of the brain to the sinuses makes the most dangerous complication of sinusitis, particularly involving the frontal and sphenoid sinuses, infection of the brain by the invasion of anaerobic bacteria through the bones or blood vessels. Abscesses, meningitis and other life-threatening conditions may result. In extreme cases the patient may experience mild personality changes, headache, altered consciousness, visual problems and, finally seizures, coma and possibly death.

COMMON COLD

Definition

Common colds are caused by viruses, which are extremely small infectious organisms (much smaller than bacteria). A sneeze or a cough may directly transfer a virus from one person to another. The common cold is the most frequent infectious disease in humans with on average two to four infections a year in individual adults and up to 6–12 in individual children. Common symptoms include a sore throat, runny nose and fever. There is no cure; however, symptoms usually resolve spontaneously in 7 to 10 days, with some symptoms possibly lasting for up to three weeks.

Incidence

The common cold accounts for approximately 22 million missed days of school and 20 million absences from work, including time away from work caring for ill children.

Mode of Transmission

- Droplet infection: A child or adult infected with the virus will, in coughing, sneezing, or touching her nose, transfer some of the virus particles onto her hand.
- She then touches the hand of a healthy person.
- This healthy person touches her newly contaminated hand to her own nose, thus introducing the infectious agent to a place where it can multiply and grow in the nose or throat. Symptoms of a cold soon develop.
- The cycle then repeats itself, with the virus being transferred from this newly infected child or adult to the next susceptible one and others.

Cause

Viruses

The common cold is due to a viral infection of the upper respiratory tract. The most commonly implicated virus is a

- Rhinovirus (30–50%)
- A type of picornavirus with 99 known serotypes

- Others include: Corona-virus (10–15%)
- Influenza (5–15%)
- Human para-influenza viruses
- Human respiratory syncytial virus
- Adenoviruses
- Enteroviruses and metapneumovirus.

Risk Factors

- Spending time in an enclosed area with an infected person or in close contact with an infected person. Common colds are droplet-borne infections, which means that they are primarily transmitted through breathing in tiny particles that the infected person emits when he or she coughs, sneezes, or exhales.
- Frequently touching eyes, nose, or mouth with contaminated fingers. This behavior somewhat increases the likelihood of transferring viruses from the surface of the hands, where they are harmless, into the upper respiratory tract, where they can infect the tissues.
- A history of smoking extends the duration of illness by about three days.
- Getting fewer than seven hours of sleep per night has been associated with a risk three times higher of developing an infection when exposed to a rhinovirus, compared to those who sleep more than eight hours per night.
- Low blood vitamin D levels are associated with an increased risk of getting a common cold. Whether this relation is causal has yet to be determined.
- Common colds are seasonal, occurring more frequently during winter outside of tropical zones. This is believed to be partly due to a change in behaviors such as increased time spent indoors, which puts infected people in close proximity to other people, rather than to exposure to cold temperatures.
- Low humidity increases viral transmission rates. One theory is that dry air causes evaporation of water, thus allowing small viral droplets to disperse farther and stay in the air longer.

Signs and Symptoms

- Fever of 100.4 °F (38 °C) in newborns up to 12 weeks
- Cough, sore throat and runny nose.
- Nasal congestion
- Conjunctivitis (pink eye)
- Muscle aches, fatigue, headaches, shivering
- Loss of appetite.

Pathophysiology

The common cold virus is transmitted mainly from contact with the saliva or nasal secretions of an infected child, either directly by coughs or sneezes, or by touching a contaminated surface and then touching the nose or eyes.

Influenza can be distinguished by its sudden onset of fever and cough.

The common cold is self-limiting, and the host's immune system effectively deals with the infection. Within a few days, the body's immune response begins producing specific antibodies that can prevent the virus from infecting cells.

The cell-mediated immune response, leukocytes destroy the virus through phagocytosis and destroy infected cells to prevent further viral replication.

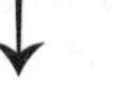

In healthy children immunocompetent individuals, the common cold resolves in seven days on average.

Management

Treatments that help alleviate symptoms include:

- Analgesics/antipyretics such as ibuprofen and acetaminophen/paracetamol.
- Getting plenty of rest
- Advise the child to drink sufficient fluids to maintain hydration
- Gargling with warm salt water are reasonable conservative measures.
- Evidence for encouraging the active intake of fluids in acute respiratory infections is lacking as is the use of heated humidified air.
- Saline nasal drops may help alleviate nasal congestion.

Antibiotics and Antiviral

Antibiotics are not effective against the viruses that cause the common cold and due to their side effects cause overall harm. There are no approved antiviral drugs for the common cold even though some preliminary research has shown benefit.

Common Cold Complications

- *Ear infection*: In this 5 and 19 percent of children with a cold develop a bacterial or viral ear infection. If a child develops a fever (temperature higher than 100.4 °F or 38 °C) after the first three days of cold symptoms, an ear infection may be to blame.
- *Asthma*: Colds can cause wheezing in children who have not wheezed before, or worsening of asthma in children who have a history of this condition.
- *Sinusitis*: Children who have nasal congestion that does not improve over the course of 10 days may have a bacterial sinus infection.
- *Pneumonia*: Children who develop a fever after the first three days of cold symptoms may have bacterial pneumonia, especially if the child also has a cough and is breathing rapidly.

Preventive Measures

The best prevention is staying away from people who are infected, because the overwhelming majority of infections are acquired by inhaling virus-laden air that an infected person has coughed, sneezed, or breathed out. Additionally, experts frequently recommend thorough and regular washing of the hands, especially in health care environments, as this reduces the likelihood of transmission through the less common route of direct contact.

- Handwashing is an essential and highly effective way to prevent the spread of infection. Hands should be wet with water and plain soap and rubbed together for 15 to 30 seconds. It is not necessary to use antibacterial hand soap. Teach children to wash their hands before and after eating and after coughing or sneezing.
- Alcohol-based hand rubs are a good alternative for disinfecting hands if a sink is not available. Hand rubs should be spread over the entire surface of hands, fingers and wrists until dry and may be used several times. These rubs can be used repeatedly without skin irritation or loss of effectiveness.
- It may be difficult or impossible to completely avoid people who are ill, although parents should try to limit direct contact.
- Most children with colds need not be excluded from day care or school. It is likely that they spread the virus before they developed cold symptoms.
- Advise the mother to using a household cleaner that kills viruses, such as phenol/ alcohol (sample brand name: Lysol), may help to reduce viral transmission.

ACUTE PHARYNGITIS

Definition

Pharyngitis is an inflammation of the throat or pharynx. In most cases it is painful and the initial infection can extend for a lengthy time period. It is the most common cause of a sore throat. Like many types of inflammation, pharyngitis can be acute—characterized by a rapid onset and typically a relatively short course or chronic. Pharyngitis can result in very large tonsils which cause trouble swallowing and breathing.

Incidence

Acute cases are caused by viral infections (40–80%), with the remainder caused by bacterial infections, fungal infections or irritants such as pollutants or chemical substances. Treatment of viral causes are mainly symptomatic while bacterial or fungal causes may be amenable to antibiotics and anti-fungal respectively.

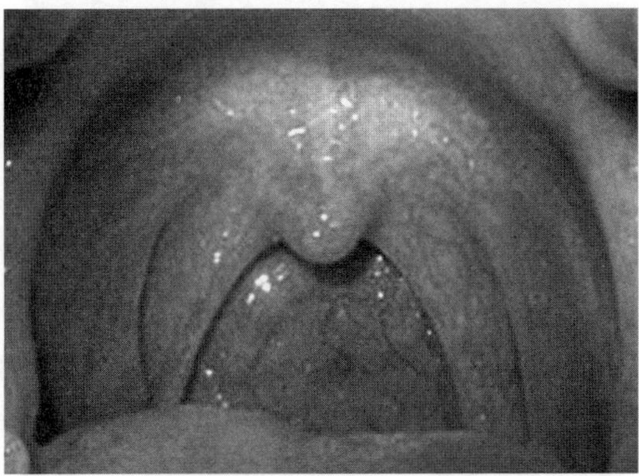

Fig. 7.21: Acute pharyngitis

Cause

Acute pharyngitis is one of the upper respiratory tract infectious diseases.

The majority of cases are due to an infectious organism acquired from close contact with an infected individual.

- Group-A Streptococcus (GAS) causes 37% of cases of acute pharyngitis in children older than 5 years.
- Other bacterial causes of pharyngitis are Group *C. Streptococcus* (5% of total cases).
- *C. pneumoniae* (1%).
- *M. pneumoniae* (1%) and anaerobic species (1%).
- Coronavirus and adenovirus account for the 30% of the total cases.
- Epstein barr virus for 1%, influenza and parainfluenza virus for about 4%.

Types

Viral Pharyngitis

- *Adenovirus*: The most common of the viral causes. Typically the degree of neck lymph node enlargement is modest and the throat often does not appear red, although it is very painful.
- *Orthomyxoviridae which cause influenza*: Present with rapid onset high temperature, headache and generalized ache. A sore throat may be associated.
- *Infectious mononucleosis ('glandular fever') caused by the Epstein-Barr virus*. This may cause significant lymph gland swelling and an exudative tonsillitis with marked redness and swelling of the throat. The heterophile test can be used if this is suspected.
- Herpes simplex virus can cause multiple mouth ulcers.
- Measles
- *Common cold:* Rhinovirus, coronavirus, respiratory syncytial virus, parainfluenza virus can cause infection of the throat, ear and lungs causing standard cold-like symptoms and often extreme pain.
- Primary HIV.

Bacterial Pharyngitis

A number of different bacteria can infect the human throat. The most common is:

- Group A streptococcus
- Corynebacterium diphtheriae
- Neisseria gonorrhea
- Chlamydophila pneumonia
- Mycoplasma pneumonia.

Streptococcal Pharyngitis

Streptococcal pharyngitis or strep throat is caused by group A beta-hemolytic streptococcus (GABHS). It is the most common bacterial cause of cases of pharyngitis (15–30%). Common symptoms include fever, sore throat and large lymph nodes. It is a contagious infection, spread by close contact with an infected individual. A definitive diagnosis is made based on the results of a throat culture. Antibiotics are useful to both prevent complications and speed recovery.

Corynebacterium Diphtheria

Diphtheria is a potentially life threatening upper respiratory infection caused by *Corynebacterium diphtheriae* which has been largely eradicated in developed nations since the introduction of childhood vaccination programs, but is still reported in the Third World and increasingly in some areas in Eastern Europe. Antibiotics are effective in the early stages, but recovery is generally slow.

Diagnostic Evaluation

It is hard to differentiate a viral and a bacterial cause of a sore throat based on symptoms alone. Thus often a throat swab is done to rule out a bacterial cause.

- History collection
- Physical examination
- Throat culture
- Blood tests.

Management

The majority of time treatment is symptomatic. Specific treatments are effective for bacterial, fungal and herpes simplex infections.

Medications

- Analgesics such as NSAIDs and acetaminophen can help reduce the pain associated with a sore throat.
- Steroids (such as dexamethasone) have been found to be useful for severe pharyngitis.
- Viscous lidocaine relieves pain by numbing the mucus membranes of the throat.
- Antibiotics are useful if a group a streptococcus is the cause of the sore throat. For viral infections, antibiotics have no effect.

Alternative Treatments Used for the Common Cold

Alternative medicines are promoted and used for the treatment of sore throats. They are however poorly supported by evidence and up-to-date, an evidence-based peer-reviewed resource, recommends that they not be used to treat pharyngitis.

To prevent pharyngitis

- Avoid sharing food, drinks and eating utensils
- Avoid individuals who are sick
- Wash your hands often, especially before eating and after coughing or sneezing
- Use alcohol-based hand sanitizers when soap and water are not available
- Avoid smoking and inhaling secondhand smoke.

EPIGLOTTITIS

Introduction

Epiglottitis is characterized by inflamed tissue in epiglottis. It is a potentially life-threatening illness. The epiglottis is at the base of the tongue. It is made up of mostly cartilage. It helps prevent food from entering to windpipe. The tissue that makes up the epiglottis can swell and block your airway.

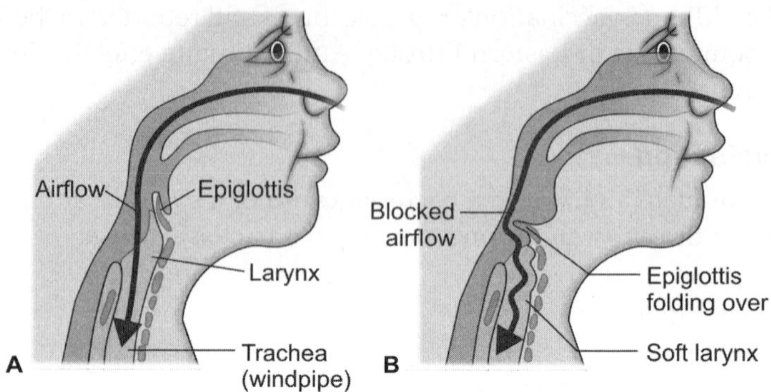

Fig. 7.22: (A) Normal epiglottis; (B) Epiglottitis

Definition

Epiglottitis is inflammation of the epiglottis—it is a rapidly progressive bacterial infection of the epiglottis and surrounding tissues that may lead to sudden respiratory obstruction and death. Symptoms include severe sore throat, Dysphagia, high fever, drooling and inspiratory stridor.

Epiglottitis is a rapid-onset bacterial infection that results in sudden inflammation of the epiglottis and the tissues around the epiglottis. It can lead to blockage of the upper airway and death.

Cause

Epiglottitis is usually caused by an infection with Haemophilus influenzae type B (Hib) bacteria. Epiglottitis can either be bacterial or viral in origin. The following causes the occurrence of this condition:

- H. influenzae type B
- Pneumococci
- Streptococci
- Staphylococci
- Echovirus
- Respiratory syncytial virus

Risk Factors

Age

Children younger than 2 months of age are at a higher risk for developing Epiglottitis. This is because these children have not yet received a Hib vaccine. Children ranging from 3–7 years of age who live in countries not offering vaccines or where the vaccine is hard to come by are at increased risk. Children whose parents purposely refrain from vaccinating with the Hib vaccine are also at increased risk for epiglottitis.

Sex

Males are more likely to develop epiglottitis than females. The reason for this is unclear.

Environment

If your children live with a large number of people, the child more likely to catch the germs of others and develop an infection. Likewise, heavily populated environments such as schools or day care centers may increase your child's exposure to bacteria, fungi and viruses. The risk of getting epiglottitis is increased in those environments.

Immune System

A weakened immune system can make it more difficult for your body to fight germs. Poor immune function makes it easier for epiglottitis to develop.

Injury

Physical injury, such as a direct blow to the throat, can cause epiglottitis. So can burns from drinking very hot or caustic liquids.

- Swallow a chemical
- Swallow a foreign object
- Smoke drugs, such as crack cocaine.

Signs and Symptoms Common in Children

- A high degree temperature (fever) of 38 °C (100.4 °F) or above
- A severe sore throat
- Difficulty in swallowing
- Difficulty breathing, which may improve when leaning forwards
- Breathing that sounds abnormal and high-pitched (stridor)
- Irritability and restlessness
- Muffled or hoarse voice
- Drooling

Diagnostic Evaluation

- *History collection and Physical examination.*
- *Throat examination*: The fiber-optic-lighted tube (laryngoscopy) can be used to identify the problem. A local anesthetic can be used to relieve pain and discomfort.
- *Chest or neck X-ray*: The danger of sudden breathing problems, X-ray may reveal what looks like a thumbprint in the neck, an indication of an enlarged epiglottis.
- *Throat culture and blood tests*: An epiglottis is wiped with a cotton swab and the tissue sample is checked for Hib. Blood cultures are usually taken because bacteremia.

Management

Epiglottitis requires urgent endotracheal intubation to protect the airway. Given in the initial stages to reduce symptoms, but this will not treat the underlying cause. It should also be noted that if stridor becomes quieter, obstruction is likely to follow and thus intubation should be expedited even further. In addition, child should be given antibiotic such as second- or third generation cephalosporins (either alone or in combination with penicillin or ampicillin for streptococcal coverage).

- Adequate airway ensured.
- Endotracheal intubation.
- Antibiotics (e.g. ceftriaxone).
- IV steroids can reduce swelling around the windpipe.
- IV fluids are used in order to address dehydration.

In children with epiglottitis, the airway must be secured immediately, preferably by nasotracheal intubation. Securing the airway can be quite difficult and should, if possible, be done by experienced personnel in the operating room.

An endotracheal tube is usually required until the patient has been stabilized for 24 to 48 hours (usual total intubation time is < 60 hours). Alternatively, a tracheotomy is done. If respiratory arrest occurs before an airway is established, bag-mask ventilation may be a life-saving temporary measure. For emergency care of children with epiglottitis, each institution should have a protocol that involves critical care, otolaryngology, anesthesia and pediatrics.

A β-lactamase–resistant antibiotic, such as ceftriaxone 50 to 75 mg/kg IV once/day (maximum 2 g), should be used empirically, pending culture and sensitivity test results. Epiglottitis caused by *H. influenzae* type B can be effectively prevented with the *H. influenzae* type B *(HiB)* conjugate vaccine.

Nursing Management

- Administer the moist air to reduce the epiglottal inflammation.
- Provide the oxygen if cyanosis is present.
- Should administer the antibiotic therapy such as a second-generation cephalosporin as per doctors order.
- The antibiotic such as Cefuroxime may be prescribed to the patient for a full 7 to 10 days. After the antibiotic therapy the epiglottal inflammation recedes rapidly.
- To maintain hydration in child with epiglottitis, intravenous fluid therapy is needed since these children cannot swallow.
- It is important that the nurse should prepare a tracheostomy or entracheal intubation set at the bedside. Children with epiglottitis may need a prophylactic tracheostomy or necessitate endotracheal intubation to prevent total airway obstruction.
- Never attempt to visualize the epiglottis directly with a tongue depressor because the gagging procedure causes complete obstruction of the glottis and results to respiratory failure.
- Throat culture should NOT be done UNLESS a means of providing an artificial airway such as a tracheostomy or endotracheal intubation is readily available.

Nursing Diagnosis and Intervention

Nursing Diagnosis

Ineffective breathing patterns associated with upper airway edema.

Intervention

- Assess the signs and symptoms of respiratory disorders of children, including dyspnea, tachypnea, cyanosis, saliva and wheezing.
- Prepare emergency means of intubation and tracheostomy child's bed side at all times.
- Avoid direct stimulation of the airway by pressing the tongue, culture swabs, suction catheter, or laryngoscope.
- Let the child in a position comfortable as possible from the horizontal position (head higher above the bed). Monitor continuously run private child's skin color, respiratory status and heart rate to ensure free airway.

Nursing Diagnosis

Risk reduction in fluid volume associated with decreased fluid intake.

Intervention

- Do not give children fluids by mouth prior to intubation.
- Provide and monitor fluid IV as directed.
- Monitor children carefully in relation to fluid intake and output.
- Assess for signs of dehydration in children, including poor skin turgor, dry mucous membranes and hollow crown and eyeballs.

LARYNGITIS (CROUP)

Introduction

Laryngitis is inflammation of the vocal cords located in the larynx or voice box. The larynx is the voice box that allows us to speak, shout, whisper and sing. The larynx consists of a cartilage skeleton that houses the vocal cords, which are covered by a mucus lining. Muscles inside the larynx adjust the position, shape and tension of the vocal cords, allowing the voice to make different sounds like whispering, singing and shouting. The larynx is located at the junction of the mouth and trachea (where air enters the lungs). There is a flap-like covering called the epiglottis.

Definition

Laryngitis is defined as inflammation of the voice box or larynx, which results in voice changes, for example, hoarseness or complete loss of the voice (Dysphonia) because of irritation to the vocal folds (vocal cords).Croup is defined as an infection of the throat and vocal cords (larynx). It is caused by several viruses. When children younger than 5 years of age have the infection, it is called croup. In older children, it is called laryngitis.

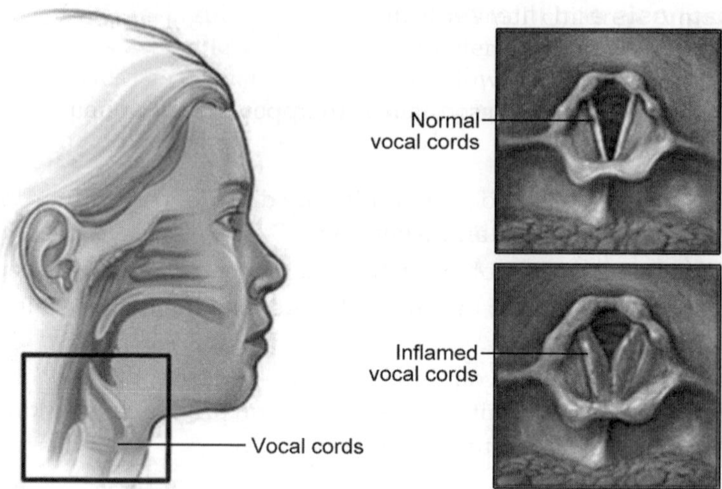

Fig. 7.23: Normal and inflamed vocal cords

Types

Laryngitis is categorized as acute if it lasts less than a few days. Otherwise it is categorized as chronic and may last over 3 weeks.

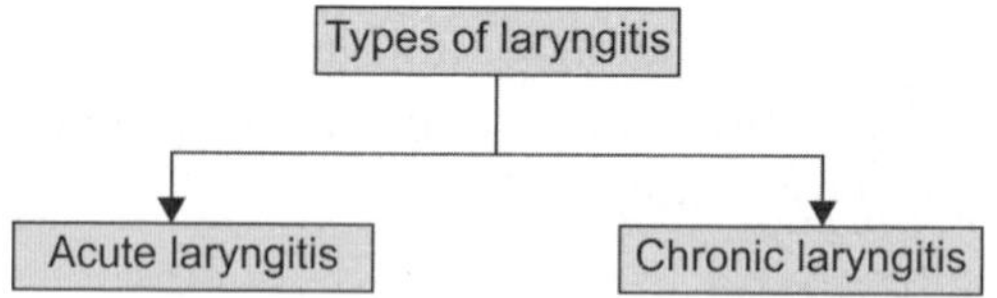

Acute Laryngitis

Acute laryngitis is a temporary condition caused by an underlying infection or overuse. Treating the underlying condition will cause the laryngitis to go away.

Chronic Laryngitis

Chronic laryngitis results from long-term exposure to irritants. This type of laryngitis tends to be more severe and have effects that last longer.

Causes

Acute laryngitis includes:

- Viral infections
- Straining vocal cords by talking or yelling more than normal sound
- Bacterial infections (rare).

Chronic laryngitis includes:

- Frequent exposure to harmful chemicals or allergens
- GERD Reflux (gastroesophageal reflux disease)
- Frequent sinus infections

- Smoking or secondary smokers (adolescents and adults)
- Voice abuse
- Low-grade yeast infections caused by frequent use of an asthma inhale
- excessive coughing or alcohol consumption
- Allergies.

Signs and Symptoms

Croup

In infants and small children, certain symptoms indicate a form of bacterial laryngitis called croup. Croup, which is inflammation of the throat, can lead to the development of epiglottitis.

- Dysphagia (Trouble in swallowing)
- Dyspnea (Problems in breathing)
- Excessive salivation
- Noisy or high-pitched sounds while breathing (during inspiration)
- A fever over 103 °F
- A barking cough.

Laryngitis

- Weakened voice
- Loss of voice (Dysphonia)
- Hoarse, dry throat
- Constant tickling or minor throat irritation
- Dry cough.

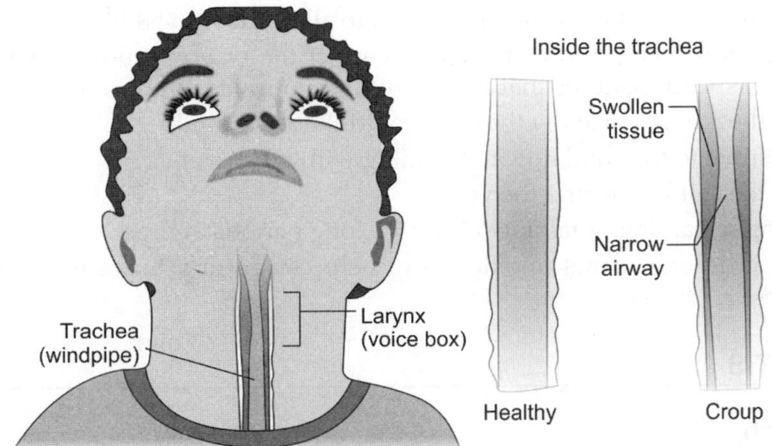

Fig. 7.24: Healthy trachea and croup

Diagnostic Evaluation

- History collection
- Physical examination

- Laryngoscopy
- Biopsy.

Management

Antibiotics are only administered if any secondary infection is suspected; otherwise they are of limited use. Sometimes oral steroids are given to reduce the inflammation and swelling.
- Antibiotics
- Corticosteroids.

Preventive Measures

- Do not smoke and avoid secondhand smoke.
- Avoid the alcohol and caffeine.
- *Drink plenty of water*: Fluids help keep the mucus in throat thin and easy to clear.
- *Avoid eating spicy foods*: Spicy foods can cause stomach acid to move into the throat or esophagus, it causing heartburn or gastroesophageal reflux disease (GERD).
- *Advise the parents to include whole grains*: Fruits and vegetables in diet. These foods contain vitamins A, E and C and help keep the mucus membranes that line the throat healthy.
- *Avoid clearing your throat*: This does more harm than good, because it causes an abnormal vibration of your vocal cords and can increase swelling. Clearing throat also it cause throat to secrete more mucus and feel more irritated, making you want to clear throat again.
- Avoid upper respiratory infections. Wash your hands often and avoid contact with people who have upper respiratory infections such as colds.

Nursing Management

- Provide the humidifier or inhaling steam to alleviate dryness
- Getting vocal therapy to analyze and correct the way you use your voice and any abnormal speech patterns that place stress on your vocal cords and voice box
- Advise the parents to allow the child to drink lots of fluids
- Demonstrate to the child how to Gargling with salt water
- Advise the child to resting the voice
- Avoiding screaming or talking loudly for long periods of time
- Avoiding decongestants (medicines to help clear stuffy noses by drying out nasal passages).

TONSILLITIS

Introduction

Tonsillitis is inflammation of the tonsils. It is usually caused by a viral infection or less commonly a bacterial infection.

Tonsillitis is an inflammation of the tonsils, the almond-shaped lymph nodes that hang down at both sides of the back of the throat and it is very common in children. The tonsils filter out germs in the throat, but when a virus or bacteria is too strong, it can cause the tonsils to swell. Difficulty swallowing and refusal to eat are typically the first signs of tonsillitis.

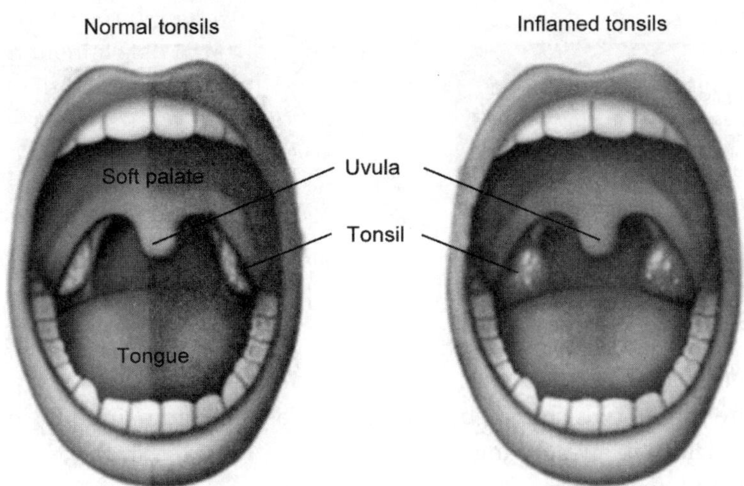

Fig. 7.25: Normal tonsils and inflamed tonsils

Definition

Tonsillitis is defined as an inflammation of the tonsils and characterized by sore throat and fever. It is most common in children aged 3 to 7 years.

Types

There are 2 main types of tonsillitis:

1. Acute tonsillitis
2. Chronic tonsillitis.

Acute tonsillitis can either be bacterial or viral in origin. Subacute tonsillitis is caused by the *bacterium Actinomyces*. Chronic tonsillitis can last for long periods of time if not treated and is mostly caused by bacterial infection and will show pus on the tonsils.

Causes

Common causes of tonsillitis:

- *Group-A streptococcus*: Which are common bacteria that cause throat infections in 1 in 5 people, including adults. Many people have no symptoms but they can still transmit the bacteria. Group A streptococcus can also cause strep throat. It is also capable under some circumstances of causing more serious illness, such as rheumatic fever.
- *Various respiratory viruses*: Flu viruses, account for most cases of tonsillitis. These infections can be sometimes milder than bacterial infections, but it is often difficult to tell the difference between a viral and bacterial infection.
- *Infectious mononucleosis*: It caused by the Epstein-Barr virus, can also produce symptoms of tonsillitis, especially in children.

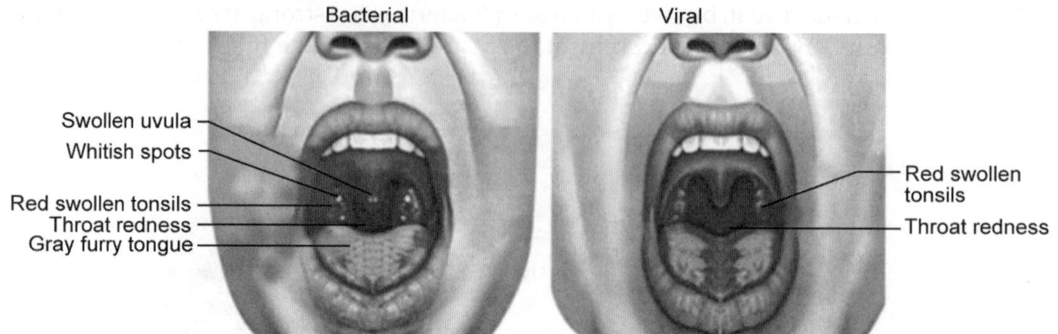

Fig. 7.26: Difference between bacterial and viral infective tonsils

Signs and Symptoms

Acute Tonsillitis

- Severe sore throat, (which may be experienced as referred pain to the ears).
- Painful/difficulty in swallowing.
- Coughing and headache.
- Myalgia (muscle aches).
- Fever and chills.
- Tonsillitis is characterized by signs of red, swollen tonsils which may have a purulent exudative coating of white patches (i.e. Pus).
- Swelling of the eyes, face and neck may occur.

Chronic Tonsillitis is a Persistent Infection in the Tonsils

- Difficulty swallowing
- Ear pain
- Fever and chills
- Headache
- Sore throat-lasts longer than 48 hours and may be severe
- Tenderness of the jaw and throat
- Voice changes, loss of voice.

Diagnostic Evaluation

The health care provider will look in the mouth and throat for swollen tonsils. The tonsils are usually reddened and may have white spots on them. The lymph nodes in the jaw and neck may be swollen and tender to the touch.

Tests that may be done include:

- Detailed history collection
- Physical examination
- Rapid strep test
- Throat swab culture

Pathophysiology

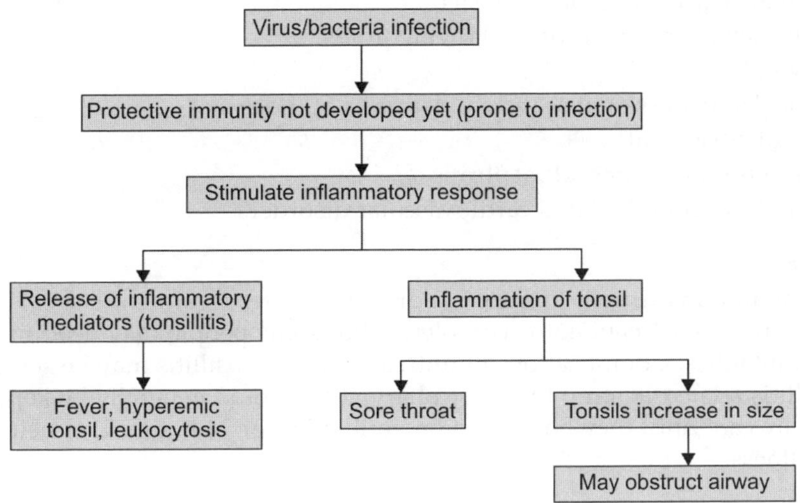

Fig. 7.27: Pathophysiology of tonsillitis

Management

Medical Management

Treatments of tonsillitis consist of pain management medications and lozenges. If the tonsillitis is caused by bacteria, then antibiotics are prescribed, with penicillin being most commonly used. Erythromycin and clarithromycin are used for child allergic to penicillin.

In many cases of tonsillitis, the pain caused by the inflamed tonsils warrants the prescription of topical anesthetics for temporary relief. Viscous lidocaine solutions are often prescribed for this purpose and anesthetic throat lozenges containing benzocaine, lignocaine, benzydamine and flubiprofen are widely available without prescription.

- Ibuprofen or other analgesics such as aspirin or paracetamol can help to decrease the edema and inflammation, which will ease the pain and allow the patient to swallow liquids sooner.
- Tonsillitis is caused by a virus; the length of illness depends on which virus is involved. Usually, a complete recovery is made within one week; however, some rare infections may last for up to two weeks.
- Chronic cases may indicate tonsillectomy (surgical removal of tonsils) as a choice for treatment. Additionally,
- Gargling with a solution of warm water and salt may reduce pain and swelling.

Surgical Management

- *Tonsillectomy*: Surgical removal of the tonsils (partial or full)
- *Adenoidectomy*: Surgical removal of the adenoids who have hypertrophied adenoids that obstruct nasal breathing.

Complications

- Blocked airway from swollen tonsils
- Dehydration from difficulty swallowing fluids
- Kidney failure
- Peritonsillar abscess or abscess in other parts of the throat
- Pharyngitis-bacterial
- Poststreptococcal glomerulonephritis
- Rheumatic fever and related cardiovascular disorders.

Prognosis

Tonsillitis symptoms usually improve 2 or 3 days after treatment starts. The infection usually is cured after treatment is completed, but some people may need more than one course of antibiotics. Complications of untreated strep tonsillitis may be severe. Children with tonsillitis related to strep throat or pharyngitis should generally be kept home from school or day care until they have been on antibiotics for 24 hours. This helps reduce the spread of illness.

Nursing Management

- Providing comfort and minimizing activities or interventions that precipitate bleeding
- Soft liquid diet
- Cool mist vaporizer keeps the mucus membrane moist during periods of month breathing
- Warm salt water gargles
- Analgesic/antipyretic drugs Acetaminophen
- Opioid and nonpaid tablets

Nursing Diagnoses

- Ineffective breathing pattern related to inflammatory process
- Ineffective airway clearance related to increased secretions.

EPISTAXIS

Introduction

Epistaxis is common in children. Epistaxis otherwise called as nose bleeding and its rare condition in children. Frequent minor nosebleeds can be both bothersome and alarming

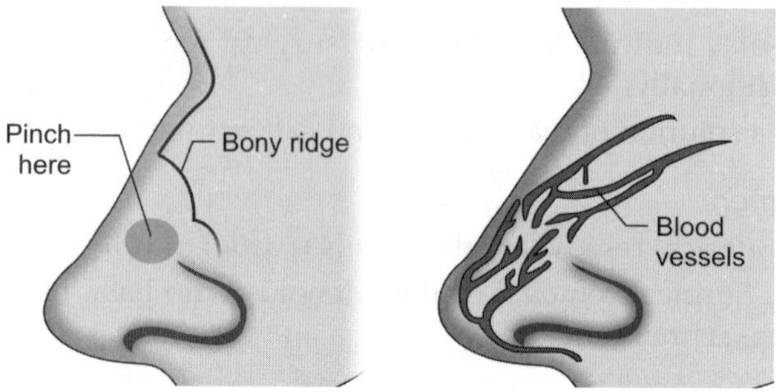

Anatomical review of nose

for parents and children. Most epistaxis in children is minor and is easily managed with direct compression of the nasal for 5 to 10 minutes. Children with refractory epistaxis or underlying local or systemic factors (e.g. nasal tumor or bleeding disorder) that predispose to epistaxis require an individualized approach to management and specialty consultation.

Definition

Epistaxis is defined as acute hemorrhage from the nostril, nasal cavity, or nasopharynx and Epistaxis in children is usually from Little's area of nose. The bleeding is usually venous, is of brief duration and is often recurrent. The two most important factors in childhood epistaxis are: Minor trauma—from nose picking, rubbing, sneezing, coughing or straining.

Causes

- Local trauma (i.e. nose picking) is the most common cause, followed by facial trauma, foreign bodies, nasal or sinus infections and prolonged inhalation of dry air.
- A disturbance of normal nasal airflow, as occurs in a deviated nasal septum, may also be a cause of epistaxis.
- Iatrogenic causes include nasogastric and nasotracheal intubation.
- Topical nasal drugs such as antihistamines and corticosteroids, especially when applied directly to the nasal septum instead of the lateral walls, may cause mild epistaxis.
- Children usually present with epistaxis due to local irritation or recent upper respiratory infection (URI).
- Vascular abnormalities that contribute to epistaxis may include the following:
  - Sclerotic vessels
  - Hereditary hemorrhagic telangiectasia
  - Arteriovenous malformation
  - Neoplasm
  - Aneurysms
  - Septal perforation, deviation
  - Endometriosis.

Signs and Symptoms

Bleeding usually occurs from only one nostril. If the bleeding is heavy enough, the blood can fill up the affected nostril and overflow into the nasopharynx (the area inside the nose where the two nostrils converge), causing simultaneous bleeding from the other nostril as well. Blood can also drip into the back of the throat or down into the stomach, causing a person to spit up or even vomit blood.

Signs of excessive blood loss include:

- Dizziness
- Weakness
- Confusion
- Fainting.

Pathophysiology

Epistaxis is classified on the basis of the primary bleeding site as anterior or posterior. Hemorrhage is most commonly anterior, originating from the nasal septum. A common source of anterior epistaxis is the Kiesselbach plexus, an anastomotic network of vessels on the anterior portion of the nasal septum, also referred to as Little's area. It receives blood supply from both the internal and external carotid arteries. Anterior bleeding may also originate anterior to the inferior turbinate. Posterior hemorrhage originates from branches of the sphenopalatine artery in the posterior nasal cavity or nasopharynx.

Diagnostic Evaluation

- Routine laboratory studies are rarely indicated or helpful for nosebleeds but are recommended in the presence of major bleeding or if a coagulopathy is suspected.
  - Obtain a hematocrit count and type and cross if a history of persistent heavy bleeding is present.
  - Obtain a complete blood count (CBC) if a history of recurrent epistaxis, a platelet disorder, or neoplasia is present.
  - The bleeding time is an excellent screening test if suspicion of a bleeding disorder is present.
  - Obtain the international normalized ratio (INR)/prothrombin time (PT) if the patient is taking warfarin or if liver disease is suspected.

Imaging Studies

- Sinus films are rarely indicated for a nosebleed.
- CT scanning and/or nasopharyngoscopy may be performed if a tumor is the suspected cause of bleeding.
- Angiography is rarely indicated.

Management

Emergency Care

- As always, first address the patient's airway, breathing and circulation (ABCs). Rarely, severe epistaxis may necessitate endotracheal intubation.
- Stable child should be instructed to grasp and pinch their entire nose, maintaining continuous pressure for at least 10 minutes. Make sure to compress the soft nose tissues against the nasal septum. Pinching the hard, incompressible nasal bones will not aide hemorrhage control.
- Gowns, gloves and protective eyewear should be worn. Adequate light is best provided by a headlamp with an adjustable narrow beam. Child should be positioned comfortably in a seated position, holding a basin under their chin.
- Child with significant hemorrhage should receive an IV line and crystalloid infusion, as well as continuous cardiac monitoring and pulse oximetry. Child frequently presents with an elevated blood pressure; however, a significant reduction can usually be obtained with analgesia and mild sedation alone. Specific antihypertensive therapy is rarely required and should be avoided in the setting of significant hemorrhage.

- Insert pledgets soaked with an anesthetic-vasoconstrictor solution into the nasal cavity to anesthetize and shrink nasal mucosa. Soak pledgets in 4% topical cocaine solution or a solution of 4% lidocaine and topical epinephrine (1:10,000) and place them into the nasal cavity. Allow them to remain in place for 10–15 minutes.
- If a bleeding point is easily identified, gentle chemical cautery may be performed after the application of adequate topical anesthesia. The tip of a silver nitrate stick is rolled over mucosa until a grey eschar forms. To avoid septal necrosis or perforation, only one side of the septum should be cauterized at a time. To be effective, cautery should be performed after bleeding is controlled. Thermal cautery using an electric cautery device is reserved for more aggressive bleeding under local or general anesthesia.
- If attempts to control hemorrhage with pressure or cautery fail, the nose should be packed. Options include traditional nasal packing, a prefabricated nasal sponge, an epistaxis balloon, or absorbable materials.

The proper technique for placement of a gauze pack is as follows:

- Grasp the gauze ribbon, about 6 inches from its end, with bayonet forceps. Place it in the nasal cavity as far back as possible, ensuring that the free end protrudes from the nose. On the first pass, the gauze is pressed onto the floor of nasopharynx with closed bayonets.
- Next, grasp the ribbon about 4–5 inches from the nasal alae and reposition the nasal speculum so that the lower blade holds the ribbon against lower border of nasal alae. Bring a second strip into the nose and press downward.
- Continue this process, layering the gauze from inferior to superior until the naris is completely packed. Both ends of ribbon must protrude from the naris and should be secured with tape. If this does not stop the bleeding, consider bilateral nasal packing.
  - *Compressed sponge (Merocel):* Trim the sponge to fit snugly through the naris. Moisten the tip with surgical lubricant or topical antibiotic ointment. Firmly grasp the length of the sponge with bayonet forceps, spread the naris vertically with a nasal speculum and advance the sponge along the floor of the nasal cavity. Once wet with blood or a small amount of saline, the sponge expands to fill the nasal cavity and tamponade bleeding.

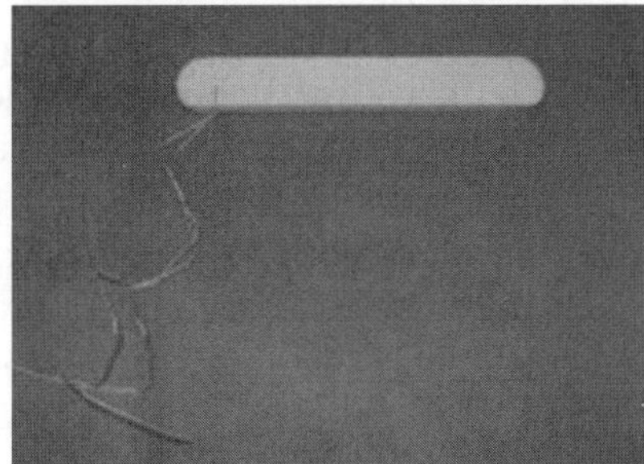

Fig. 7.28: Compressed sponge—Merocel

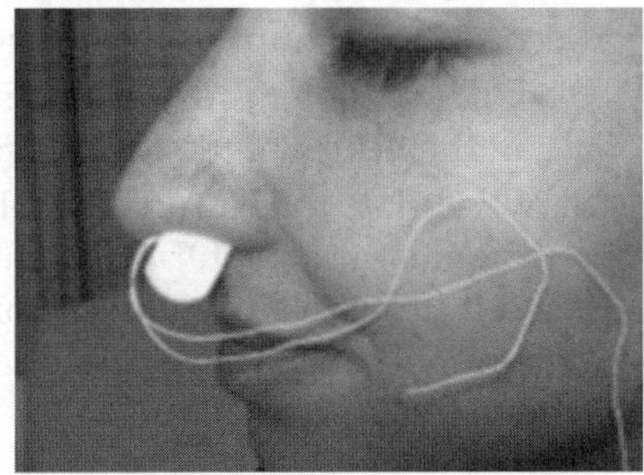

Fig. 7.29: Merocel placed in left nostril for anterior packing

- *Anterior epistaxis balloons (Rapid Rhino):* Anterior epistaxis balloons are available in different lengths. A carboxycellulose outer layer promotes platelet aggregation. The balloons are as efficacious as nasal tampons with superior ease and patient comfort on insertion and removal. To insert, soak the knit outer layer of the balloon with water, insert along the floor of the nasal cavity and inflate slowly with air until the bleeding stops.

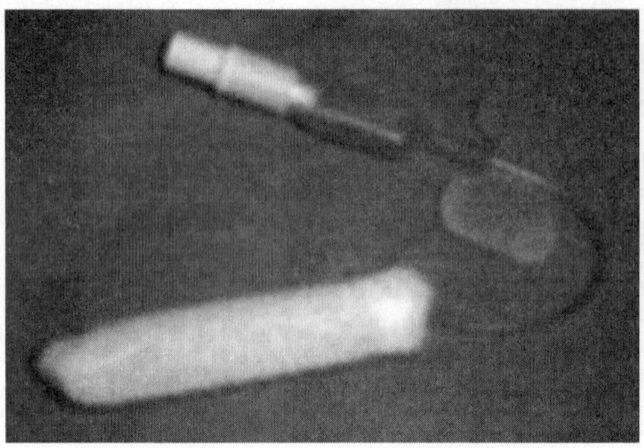

Fig. 7.30: Rapid Rhino—5.5 cm for anterior nasal packing

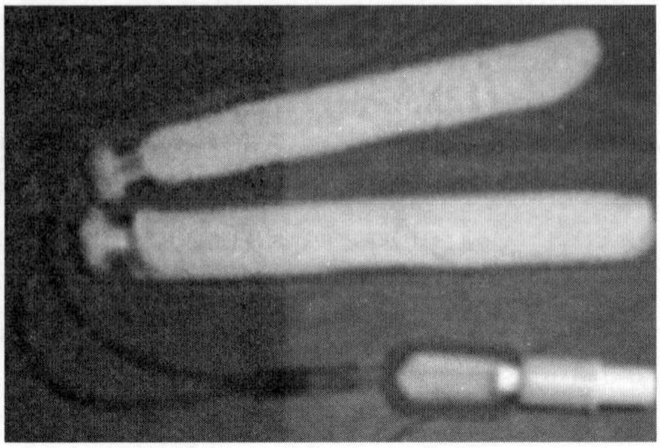

Fig. 7.31: Rapid Rhino bilateral—7.5 cm for anterior/posterior nasal packing

- Absorbable materials such as oxidized cellulose (Surgicel), gelatin foam (Gelfoam) and gelatin and thrombin combination (FloSeal) are suitable alternatives to nasal packing for anterior bleeds. They directly tamponade bleeding sites, increase clot formation and protect the nasal mucosa from desiccation or further trauma. They are easy to use, comfortable and conform to the irregularity of the nasal contours.
- *Posterior epistaxis balloons:* Posterior epistaxis balloons generally have separate anterior and posterior balloons.
  - After passing the posterior balloon through the naris and into the posterior nasal cavity, inflate it with 4–5 mL of sterile water and gently pull it forward to fit snugly in the posterior choana. After bleeding into the posterior pharynx has been controlled, fill the anterior balloon with sterile water until the bleeding completely stops.
  - Avoid overinflation because pressure necrosis or damage to the septum may result. Record the amount of fluid placed in each balloon.
  - If a Foley catheter is used, place a 12–16F catheter with a 30 mL balloon into the nose along the floor of the nasopharynx, until the tip is visible in the posterior pharynx.
  - Slowly inflate the balloon with 15 mL of sterile water, pull it anteriorly until it firmly sets against the posterior choanae and secure it in place with an umbilical clamp. Use a buttress clamp with cotton gauze to avoid pressure necrosis on the nasal alae or columella. Finally, an anterior nasal pack should be placed.

Medication

Child discharged from the hospital with anterior packing should receive follow-up care with an ENT specialist within 48–72 hour. Nasal packing prevents drainage of sinuses. Consider placing child on a broad-spectrum antibiotic to cover all likely pathogens in the context of the clinical setting. Oral analgesics should be prescribed to assure quality patient care.

Antibiotics

Consider giving child a penicillin or first-generation cephalosporin.

Amoxicillin (Biomox, Trimox)

Treats infections caused by susceptible organisms and used as prophylaxis in minor procedures.

Adult

250–500 mg PO q8h; not to exceed 3 g/d.

Pediatric

20–50 mg/kg/d PO q8h Reduces the efficacy of oral contraceptives. Documented hypersensitivity

Pregnancy

B-Fetal risk not confirmed in studies in humans but has been shown in some studies in animals.

Cephalexin (Keflex)

First-generation cephalosporin, which is primarily active against skin flora. Used for skin structure coverage and as prophylaxis in minor procedures.

Adult

250–1000 mg PO q6h; not to exceed 4 g/d.

Pediatric

25–50 mg/kg/d PO q6h; not to exceed 3 g/d. Coadministration with aminoglycosides increases nephrotoxic potential. Documented hypersensitivity.

Analgesics

Pain control is essential to quality patient care. It ensures patient comfort, promotes pulmonary toilet and enables physical therapy regimens. Most analgesics have sedating properties, which are beneficial for child who have painful skin lesions. Avoid NSAIDs and aspirin.

Complications

- Sinusitis
- Septal hematoma/perforation
- External nasal deformity
- Mucosal pressure necrosis
- Balloon migration
- Aspiration.

Prognosis

With proper treatment, prognosis is excellent.

Nursing Management

- Admit child with posterior packing. Elderly child may receive supplemental oxygen and be admitted to a monitored setting.
- Significant or uncontrolled bleeding from a posterior site may require operative management; this occurs in about 30% of cases. Interventional radiology embolization of involved arteries and surgical ligation of vessels are possible options in such instances.
- Child discharged with anterior packing should receive follow-up care with an ENT specialist within 48–72 hours. Nasal packing increases the risk of sinusitis or toxic shock syndrome.
- Child discharged with nasal packing should be prescribed a penicillin or first-generation cephalosporin. Oral analgesics should also be prescribed.
- Advise child to avoid aspirin, aspirin-containing products and NSAIDs.
- Child who take warfarin may generally continue their current regimen unchanged. Temporary discontinuation of warfarin or active reversal of coagulopathy is indicated only in cases of uncontrolled hemorrhage.
- Give child specific written follow-up instructions.

LOWER RESPIRATORY TRACT INFECTIONS

Introduction

The lower respiratory tract infection can also be applied to other types of infection including lung abscess, acute bronchitis and emphysema. Symptoms include shortness of breath, weakness, high fever, coughing and fatigue. Lower respiratory tract infections place a considerable strain on the health budget and are generally more serious than upper respiratory infections. Since 1993, there has been a slight reduction in the total number of deaths from lower respiratory tract infection. However in 2002, they were still the leading cause of deaths among all infectious diseases and they accounted for 3.9 million deaths worldwide and 6.9% of all deaths that year.

There are a number of acute and chronic infections that can affect the lower respiratory tract. The two most common infections are bronchitis and pneumonia. Influenza affects both the upper and lower respiratory tracts.

Antibiotics are often thought to be the first line treatment in lower respiratory tract infections; however, these are not indicated in viral infections. It is important to use appropriate antibiotic selection based on the infecting organism and to ensure this therapy changes with the evolving nature of these infections and the emerging resistance to conventional therapies. *H. influenzae* and *M. catarrhalis* are of increasing importance in both community acquired pneumonia (CAP) and acute exacerbation of chronic bronchitis (AECB) while the importance of *S. pneumonia* is declining. It has also become apparent the importance of atypical pathogens such as *C. pneumoniae, M. pneumoniae* and *L. pneumophila.*

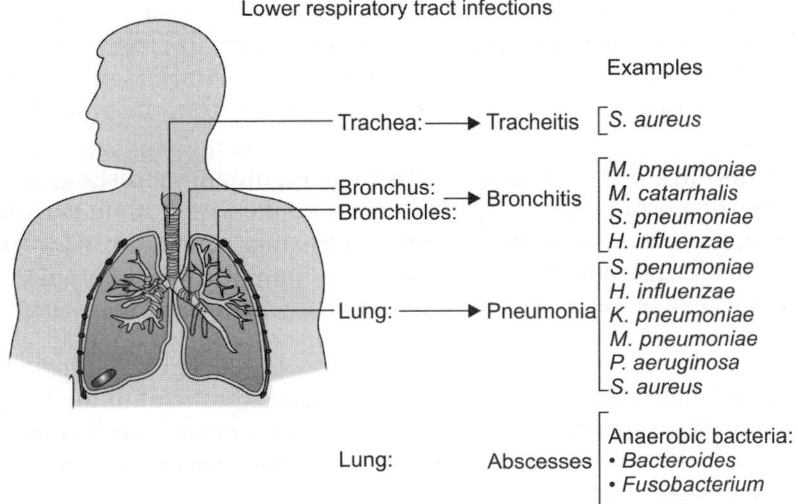

Fig. 7.32: Classification of lower respiratory tract infection

BRONCHITIS

Introduction

Bronchitis is a pulmonary disease caused by the onset of inflammation in the bronchial tubes, which are the air passages into the lungs. It causes a cough that often brings up mucus,

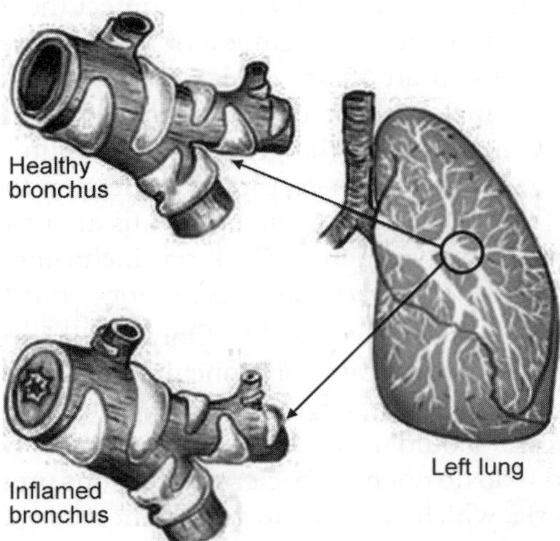

Fig. 7.33: Difference between normal and inflamed bronchus

as well as shortness of breath, wheezing and chest tightness. There are two main types of bronchitis: Acute and chronic.

Acute bronchitis is characterized by the development of a cough, with or without the production of sputum, mucus that is expectorated (coughed up) from the respiratory tract. Acute bronchitis often occurs during the course of an acute viral illness such as the common cold or influenza. Viruses cause about 90% of cases of acute bronchitis while bacteria account for less than 10%.

Chronic bronchitis, a type of chronic obstructive pulmonary disease, is characterized by the presence of a productive cough that lasts for 3 months or more per year for at least 2 years. Chronic bronchitis most often develops due to recurrent injury to the airways caused by inhaled irritants. Cigarette smoking is the most common cause, followed by air pollution and occupational exposure to irritants and cold air.

Definition

Bronchitis is an inflammation of the main air passages (bronchi) to the lungs. Coughing often brings up yellow or greenish mucus. There are two main types of bronchitis: acute and chronic. Acute bronchitis, often caused by the same viruses that cause colds, usually starts as a sore throat, runny nose or sinus infection.

Classification

- Acute bronchitis
- Chronic bronchitis

ACUTE BRONCHITIS

Introduction

Acute bronchitis is most often caused by viruses that infect the epithelium of the bronchi, resulting in inflammation and increased secretion of mucus. Cough, a common symptom of acute bronchitis, develops in an attempt to expel the excess mucus from the lungs. Other common symptoms include sore throat, runny nose, nasal congestion (coryza), low-grade fever, pleurisy, malaise and the production of sputum. Acute bronchitis often develops during the course of an upper respiratory infection (URI) such as the common cold or influenza. About 90% of cases of acute bronchitis are caused by viruses, including rhinoviruses, adenoviruses and influenza. Bacteria, including *Mycoplasma pneumoniae, Chlamydia pneumoniae* and *Bordetella pertussis*, account for about 10% of cases.

Most cases of acute bronchitis resolve quickly. Only about 5–10% of bronchitis cases are caused by a bacterial infection. Most cases of bronchitis are caused by a viral infection and are 'self-limited' and resolve themselves in a few weeks. As most cases of acute bronchitis are caused by viruses, antibiotics should not be used since they are only effective against bacteria. Using antibiotics in child who do not have bacterial infections promotes the development of antibiotic-resistant bacteria, which may lead to greater morbidity and mortality. Antibiotics should only be prescribed if microscopic examination of Gram stained sputum shows large numbers of bacteria present.

Definition

Acute bronchitis is an inflammation of the large bronchi (medium-sized airways) in the lungs that is usually caused by viruses or bacteria and may last several days or weeks.

Characteristic symptoms include cough, sputum (phlegm) production and shortness of breath and wheezing related to the obstruction of the inflamed airways. Diagnosis is by clinical examination and sometimes microbiological examination of the phlegm. Treatment for acute bronchitis is typically symptomatic. As viruses cause most cases of acute bronchitis, antibiotics should not be used unless microscopic examination of Gram stained sputum reveals large numbers of bacteria.

Cause

Acute bronchitis can be caused by contagious pathogens. In about half of instances of acute bronchitis a bacterial or viral pathogen is identified. Typical viruses include respiratory syncytial virus, rhinovirus, influenza and others.

- Damage caused by irritation of the airways leads to inflammation and leads to neutrophils infiltrating the lung tissue.
- Mucosal hypersecretion is promoted by a substance released by neutrophils.
- Further obstruction to the airways is caused by more goblet cells in the small airways. This is typical of chronic bronchitis.
- Although infection is not the reason or cause of chronic bronchitis it is seen to aid in sustaining the bronchitis.

Signs and Symptoms

Acute bronchitis, symptoms usually resolve within 7 to 10 days

- Fever and cough
- Shortness of breath (dyspnea)
- Wheezing
- 'Rattle' sensation in chest
- Tickle feeling in back of throat that leads to soreness
- Chest pain and tightness in the chest
- Poor sleep
- Chills (uncommon)
- Fatigue or malaise.

Diagnostic Evaluation

- A physical examination will often reveal decreased intensity of breath sounds, wheezing, rhonchi and prolonged expiration.
- Pulmonary function tests.
- A chest X-ray that reveals hyperinflation; collapse and consolidation of lung areas would support a diagnosis of pneumonia. Some conditions that predispose to bronchitis may be indicated by chest radiography.
- A sputum sample showing neutrophil granulocytes (inflammatory white blood cells) and culture showing that has pathogenic microorganisms such as streptococcus.
- A blood test would indicate inflammation (as indicated by a raised white blood cell count and elevated C-reactive protein).

- Arterial blood gas (ABG)
- Chest X-ray
- Pulse oximetry (oxygen saturation testing)
- Complete blood count (CBC)
- Chest CT scan.

Management

Treatment for acute bronchitis is primarily symptomatic. Non-steroidal anti-inflammatory drugs (NSAIDs) may be used to treat fever and sore throat. Decongestants can be useful in child with nasal congestion and expectorants may be used to loosen mucus and increase expulsion of sputum. Cough suppressants may be used if the cough interferes with sleep or is bothersome, although coughing may be useful in expelling sputum from the airways.

Antibiotics

Only about 5–10% of bronchitis cases are caused by a bacterial infection. Most cases of bronchitis are caused by a viral infection and are 'self-limited' and resolve themselves in a few weeks. Acute bronchitis should not be treated with antibiotics unless microscopic examination of the sputum reveals large numbers of bacteria. Treating non-bacterial illnesses with antibiotics leads to the promotion of antibiotic-resistant bacteria, which increase morbidity and mortality.

Antihistamines

Using over-the-counter antihistamines may be harmful in the self-treatment of bronchitis. An effect of antihistamines is to thicken mucus secretions. Expelling infected mucus via coughing can be beneficial in recovering from bronchitis. Expulsion of the mucus may be hindered if it is thickened. Antihistamines can help bacteria to persist and multiply in the lungs by increasing its residence time in a warm, moist environment of thickened mucus.

Using antihistamines along with an expectorant cough syrup may be doubly harmful encouraging the production of mucus and then thickening that which is produced. Using an expectorant cough syrup alone might be useful in flushing bacteria from the lungs. Using an antihistamine along with it works against the intention of using the expectorant.

Prognosis

Acute bronchitis usually lasts a few days or weeks. It may accompany or closely follow a cold or the flu, or may occur on its own. Bronchitis usually begins with a dry cough, including waking the sufferer at night. After a few days it progresses to a wetter or productive cough, which may be accompanied by fever, fatigue and headache. The fever, fatigue and malaise may last only a few days; but the wet cough may last up to several weeks.

Should the cough last longer than a month, some doctors may issue a referral to an otorhinolaryngologist (ear, nose and throat doctor) to see if a condition other than bronchitis is causing the irritation. It is possible that having irritated bronchial tubes for as long as a few months may inspire asthmatic conditions in some child. In addition, if one starts coughing mucus tinged with blood, one should see a doctor. In rare cases, doctors may conduct tests to see if the cause is a serious condition such as tuberculosis or lung cancer.

Preventive Measures

Smoking Cessation

Many physicians recommend that to help the bronchial tree heal faster and not make bronchitis worse, smokers should quit smoking completely to allow their lungs to recover from the layer of tar that builds up over time.

CHRONIC BRONCHITIS

Introduction

Chronic bronchitis, a type of chronic obstructive pulmonary disease, is defined by a productive cough that lasts for 3 months or more per year for at least 2 years. Other symptoms may include wheezing and shortness of breath, especially upon exertion. The cough is often worse soon after awakening and the sputum produced may have a yellow or green color and may be streaked with blood.

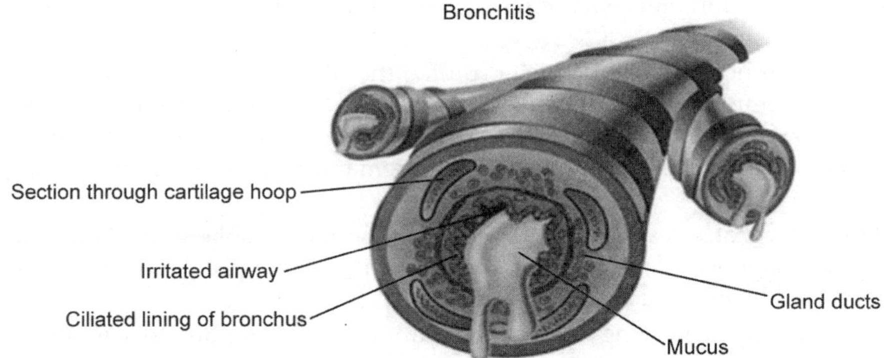

Fig. 7.34: Cross section view of chronic bronchitis

Definition

Chronic bronchitis is defined as a chronic inflammation of the bronchi (medium-size airways) in the lungs. It is generally considered one of the two forms of chronic obstructive pulmonary disease (COPD). It is defined clinically as a persistent cough that produces sputum (phlegm) and mucus, for at least three months in two consecutive years.

Causes

- Chronic bronchitis is caused by recurring injury or irritation to the respiratory epithelium of the bronchi, resulting in chronic inflammation, edema (swelling) and increased production of mucus by goblet cells. Airflow into and out of the lungs is partly blocked because of the swelling and extra mucus in the bronchi or due to reversible bronchospasm.
- Most cases of chronic bronchitis are caused by smoking cigarettes or other forms of tobacco.
- Chronic inhalation of irritating fumes or dust from occupational exposure or air pollution may also be causative.

- About 5% of the population has chronic bronchitis and it is two times more common in males than females.
- Tobacco smoking is the most common cause. Pneumoconiosis and long-term fume inhalation are other causes.

Signs and Symptoms

- Bronchitis may be indicated by an expectorating cough (also known as a productive cough, i.e. one that produces sputum).
- Shortness of breath (dyspnea) and wheezing.
- Occasionally chest pains, fever.
- Fatigue or malaise may also occur.
- Mucus is often green or yellowish green and also may be orange or pink, depending on the pathogen causing the inflammation.

Diagnostic Evaluation

- A physical examination will often reveal diminished breath sounds, wheezing and prolonged expiration.
- Pulmonary function tests, however, unlike the other common obstructive disorders, asthma and emphysema, bronchitis rarely causes a high residual volume. This is because the air flow obstruction found in bronchitis is due to increased resistance, which does not generally cause the airways to collapse prematurely and trap air in the lungs chronic bronchitis.
- A chest X-ray that reveals hyperinflation; collapse and consolidation of lung areas would support a diagnosis of pneumonia. Some conditions that predispose to bronchitis may be indicated by chest radiography.
- A sputum sample showing neutrophils granulocytes (inflammatory white blood cells) and culture showing that has pathogenic microorganisms such as streptococcus.
- A blood test would indicate inflammation (as indicated by a raised white blood cell count and elevated C-reactive protein).
- Neutrophils infiltrate the lung tissue, aided by damage to the airways caused by irritation.
- Damage caused by irritation of the airways leads to inflammation and leads to neutrophils being present.
- Mucosal hypersecretion is promoted by a substance released by neutrophils.

Management

Chronic bronchitis is treated symptomatically. Inflammation and edema of the respiratory epithelium may be reduced with inhaled corticosteroids. Wheezing and shortness of breath can be treated by reducing bronchospasm (reversible narrowing of smaller bronchi due to constriction of the smooth muscle) with bronchodilators such as inhaled β-Adrenergic agonists (e.g. albuterol) and inhaled Anticholinergic (e.g. pratropium bromide). Hypoxemia, too little oxygen in the blood, can be treated with supplemental oxygen. However, oxygen supplementation can result in decreased respiratory drive leading to increased blood levels of carbon dioxide and subsequent respiratory acidosis. The most effective method of preventing chronic bronchitis and other forms of COPD is to avoid smoking cigarettes and other forms of tobacco.

Antibiotics

Only about 5–10% of bronchitis cases are caused by a bacterial infection. Most cases of bronchitis are caused by a viral infection and are 'self-limited' and resolve themselves in a few weeks. For acute exacerbations of chronic bronchitis, if antibiotics are used, amoxicillin or doxycycline is recommended.

Bronchodilators

Ipratropium is an example of a bronchodilator that may be useful for people suffering from chronic obstructive pulmonary disease, such as chronic bronchitis.

Acute Exacerbations

Acute exacerbations of chronic bronchitis (AECB) are episodes of difficulty in breathing in a person with chronic bronchitis. During AECB, breathing becomes much more difficult because of further narrowing of the airways, in addition to increased secretion of mucus, which often is thicker than usual.

Treatment of AECB may include:

- Cough suppressants
- Inhaled bronchodilators
- Antibiotics are used if a bacterial infection is the suspected cause. However, antibiotics will not treat exacerbations caused by viruses.
- Corticosteroids
- Theophylline
- Oxygen therapy.

Protracted Bacterial Bronchitis

Protracted bacterial bronchitis is defined as a cough of more than 8 weeks, with a positive bronchoalveolar lavage (BAL), that resolves with antibiotics. It is usually caused by *streptococcus pneumoniae, haemophilus influenzae,* or *moraxella catarrhalis.*

Prevention

- Good handwashing is one of the best ways to avoid getting viruses and other respiratory infections.
- Since flu viruses have been shown to be a major cause of bronchitis, getting a flu shot may also help prevent acute bronchitis.
- Limit exposure to cold, damp environments.

Nursing Diagnosis and Intervention for Bronchitis

- Ineffective airway clearance
  - Related to: Increased production of secretions.
- Acute pain
  - Related to: The inflammation of the pleura.
- Impaired gas exchange
  - Related to: Airway obstruction by secretions, spasm of the bronchus.
- Ineffective breathing pattern
  - Related to: Bronchoconstriction, mucus.

- Imbalanced nutrition, less than body requirements
  - Related to: Dyspnea, anorexia, nausea, vomiting.
- Risk for infection
  - Related to: The settlement of secretions, chronic disease processes.
- Activity intolerance
  - Related to: Insufficiency of ventilation and oxygenation.
- Anxiety
  - Related to: Changes in health status.
- Knowledge deficit
  - Related to: The lack of information about the disease process and treatment at home.

Nursing Diagnosis Ineffective Airway Clearance Related

- Bronchoconstriction
- Increased mucus formation
- Ineffective cough
- Bronchopulmonary infection.

Goal: Achievement of client airway clearance

Nursing Interventions Ineffective Airway Clearance

- Give the patient 6 to 8 glasses of fluid/day unless there is a cor pulmonale.
- Teach and give encouragement for use of diaphragmatic breathing and coughing techniques.
- Assist in the provision of action nebulizer, metered dose inhalers.
- Perform postural drainage with percussion and vibration in the morning and evening according to the requirement.
- Instruct patient to avoid irritants such as cigarette smoke, aerosols, temperature extremes and smoke.
- Teach about the early signs of infection should be reported to your doctor immediately: Increased sputum, change in sputum color, viscosity of sputum, increased shortness of breath, chest tightness, fatigue.
- Give antibiotics as required.
- Give encouragement to child to immunize against influenzae and streptococcus pneumoniae.

Acute Pain Related to Inflammation and Tissue Damage

Goal: Improvement in comfort level

Intervention

- Carry out a number of actions that provide comfort (heat/cold; massage, position changes, break; foam mattresses, pillows buffer, splints; relaxation techniques, activity that distracts).
- Provide anti-inflammatory preparations, analgesics as recommended.
- Adjust treatment schedule to meet the needs of child to pain management.
- Encourage the patient to express his feelings about the nature of chronic pain and illness.

- Describe the pathophysiology of pain and helping child to realize that pain is often brought him to the method of unproven therapies.
- Assist in identifying a person's life that brings pain to the patient cases using unproven therapies.
- Perform an assessment of the subjective changes in pain.

Fatigue Related to an Increase in Disease Activity, Pain, Depression

Goal: Include action as part of the activities of daily living necessary for change.

Intervention

- Give an explanation of fatigue:
  - The relationship between disease activity and fatigue.
  - Explain the actions to provide comfort while executing.
  - Develop and maintain a sleep routine actions fatherly (warm water bath and relaxation techniques that facilitate sleep).
  - Explaining the importance of rest to reduce systemic stress, articular and emotional.
  - Explains how to use traditional techniques to save energy.
  - Identify the factors that lead to physical and emotional exhaustion.
- Facilitating the development schedule of the activity/rest right.
- Encourage child's adherence to treatment programs.
- Refer and thrust conditioning program.
- Encourage adequate nutrition including iron from food sources and supplements.

BRONCHIOLITIS

Definition

Bronchiolitis is inflammation of the bronchioles, the smallest air passages of the lungs. This inflammation is usually caused by viruses.

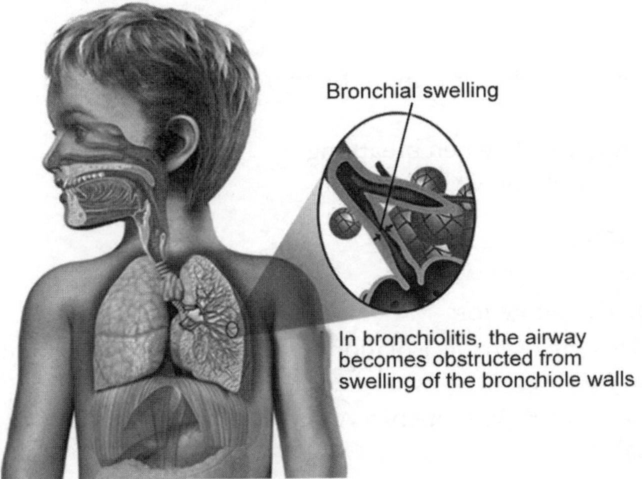

Fig. 7.35: Child with bronchiolitis

Causes

The American Academy of Pediatrics has published a clinical practice guideline for the Diagnosis and Management of Bronchiolitis, including a review of the evidence and recommendations.

- Bronchiolitis is usually caused by a viral infection, most commonly respiratory.
- Respiratory syncytial virus (RSV) infections are responsible for more than half of all cases of bronchiolitis.
- Other viruses associated with bronchiolitis include rhinovirus (the common cold virus), influenza (flu), human metapneumovirus, adenovirus, coronavirus and parainfluenza.
- Childcare attendance and exposure to cigarette smoke also can increase a child's risk for bronchiolitis.

Risk Factors

Environmental and social risk factors:

- Older siblings
- Nursery attendance
- Passive smoke, particularly maternal
- Overcrowding.

Signs and Symptoms

Bronchiolitis begins as a mild upper respiratory infection. Within 2 to 3 days, the child develops more breathing problems, including wheezing and a cough.

Symptoms Include

- Bluish skin due to lack of oxygen (cyanosis)—emergency treatment is needed
- Breathing difficulty including wheezing and shortness of breath
- Cough
- Fatigue
- Fever
- Muscles around the ribs sink in as the child tries to breathe in (called intercostal retractions)
- Infant's nostrils get wide when breathing
- Rapid breathing (tachypnea).

Diagnostic Evaluation

- Pulse oximetry.
- Nasopharyngeal aspirate for:
  - RSV rapid testing to enable isolation or cohort arrangements and to prevent further, unnecessary testing.
  - Viral cultures for RSV, influenza A and B, parainfluenza and adenovirus can also be undertaken.

Other investigations that are not recommended for typical acute bronchiolitis include:

- Electrolytes and renal function: Only perform if the child is dehydrated or on IV fluids.
- Blood and urine culture: Consider if pyrexia >38.5 °C or the child has a 'toxic' appearance.
- Arterial blood gases may be required in the severely ill child, especially in those who may need mechanical ventilation.

In a typical case, an infant under two years of age develops cough, wheeze and shortness of breath over one or two days. The diagnosis is made by clinical examination. Chest X-ray is sometimes useful to exclude pneumonia, but not indicated in routine cases.

Testing for specific viral cause (e.g. RSV by nasopharyngeal aspirate) can be done but has little effect on management. In a systematic review, RSV testing by direct immunofluorescence testing on nasopharyngeal aspirate had a sensitivity of 61% and specificity of 89%. Identification of RSV-positive child can be helpful for:

- Disease surveillance
- Grouping ('cohorting') child together in hospital wards as to prevent cross infection
- Predicting whether the disease course has peaked yet
- Reducing the need for other diagnostic procedures (by providing confidence that a cause has been identified).

Management

There is no effective specific treatment for bronchiolitis. Therapy is principally supportive.

Bronchodilators

Bronchodilator drugs such as salbutamol/albuterol or ipratropium are no longer recommended, but many clinicians offer a trial dose to see if there is any benefit (especially if there is a family history of asthma, since it can be difficult to clinically distinguish bronchiolitis from a viral-induced asthma).

Hypertonic Saline

There is some interest in the use of hypertonic saline in bronchiolitis. Initially recommended for use in cystic fibrosis child, it is speculated to increase hydration of secretions, thus facilitating their removal.

Complications

- Middle ear bacterial infection
- Development of asthma later (bronchial hyperactivity).

Preventive Measures

Vaccine

A vaccine is available for babies most at risk of developing severe and occasionally fatal, RSV infection. These will be very young infants born prematurely who have predisposing conditions such as chronic lung disease, congenital heart disease or children who are immunodeficient. It is usually given in secondary care.

Immunoprophylaxis

Recent years have seen the development of agents which provide passive immunity to RSV: RSV immunoglobulin (RSV-Ig) which has been superseded by palivizumab, a monoclonal antibody. It has been shown to reduce RSV-related hospitalization and intensive care admissions significantly. The Joint Committee on Vaccination and Immunization recommends that it should be used by those at high-risk of severe RSV disease:

- Children aged under 2 years with chronic lung disease, who have required at least 28 days of supplemental oxygen from birth or who are receiving home oxygen.
- Infants less than 6 months old with a left-to-right shunt, hemodynamically significant congenital heart disease or pulmonary hypertension.
- Children aged under 2 years with severe congenital immunodeficiency.

The first dose should be administered before the start of the RSV season.

Infection Control

Disease transmission should be limited by:

- Handwashing
- Use of gloves, aprons or gowns when in direct contact with the patient
- Isolation of infected child or nursing in cohorts, based on laboratory confirmation of RSV status.

Prognosis

- Most children with bronchiolitis make a full recovery.
- Mechanical ventilation is required for some child but one study found that the majority can be managed without.
- Most deaths occur in infants younger than 6 months or in those with underlying cardiac or pulmonary disease.
- The underlying mechanism by which RSV or other agents, such as rhinovirus, cause reactive airways disease is unknown.

PNEUMONIA

Introduction

The word pneumonia means 'infection of the lung.' While such infections were extremely dangerous in past generations, today most children can recover from them easily if they receive proper medical attention. Most cases of pneumonia follow a viral upper respiratory tract infection.

Pneumonia is a form of acute respiratory infection that affects the lungs. The lungs are made up of small sacs called alveoli, which fill with air when a healthy person breathes. When an individual has pneumonia, the alveoli are filled with pus and fluid, which makes breathing painful and limits oxygen intake.

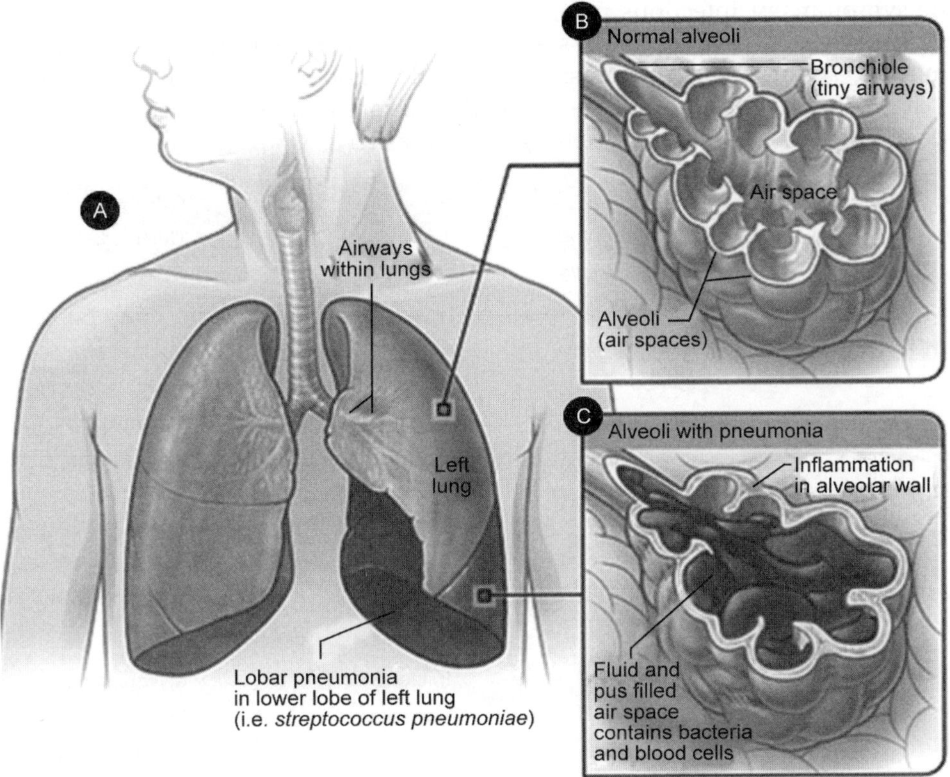

Fig. 7.36: Normal and pneumonia affected alveoli

Definition

Pneumonia is an inflammatory condition of the lung. It is often characterized as including inflammation of the parenchyma of the lung (alveoli) and abnormal alveolar filling with fluid (consolidation and exudation).

Causes

Pneumonia is caused by a number of infectious agents, including viruses, bacteria and fungi. The most common are:

- *Streptococcus pneumonia:* The most common cause of bacterial pneumonia in children.
- *Haemophilus influenzae type B (Hib):* The second most common cause of bacterial pneumonia.
- Respiratory syncytial virus is the most common viral cause of pneumonia.
- Infants are infected with HIV, Pneumocystis jiroveci is one of the commonest causes of pneumonia, responsible for at least one quarter of all pneumonia deaths in HIV-infected infants.

The symptoms of infectious pneumonia are caused by the invasion of the lungs by microorganisms and by the immune system's response to the infection. Although more than one hundred strains of microorganism can cause pneumonia, only a few are responsible for most cases. The most common causes of pneumonia are viruses and bacteria. Less common causes of infectious pneumonia are fungi and parasites.

Age	Bacteria	Viruses	Others
Neonate	*Group B streptococci*	CMV Herpes	Chlamydia
	E. coli, Klebsiella		
	Listera, MS aureus		
1–3 Months	*S. pneumoniae*	CMN, RSV	
	S. aureus	Influenza	
	S. influenzae	Parainfluenza	Chlamydia
4 months	*S. pneumoniae*	RSV	Mycoplasma
5 years	*S. aureus*	Adenovirus	
	H. influenzae	Influenza	
	Group A		
	Streptococcus		
	Klebsiella		
Over 5 years	*S. pneumoniae*	Influenza	Mycoplasma
	S. aureus	Varicella	Legionella spp
	H. influenzae		M. catarrhalis
	M. tuberculosis		

Mode of Transmission

Pneumonia can be spread in a number of ways. The viruses and bacteria that are commonly found in a child's nose or throat can infect the lungs if they are inhaled. They may also spread via air-borne droplets from a cough or sneeze. In addition, pneumonia may spread through blood, especially during and shortly after birth. More research needs to be done on the different pathogens causing pneumonia and the ways they are transmitted, as this is of critical importance for treatment and prevention.

Classification

Pneumonias can be classified in several ways. The primary system of classification is the combined clinical classification, which combines factors such as age, risk factors for certain microorganisms, the presence of underlying lung disease or systemic disease and whether the person has recently been hospitalized. Other classifications include according to the anatomic changes that found in the lungs during autopsies, based on the microbial cause and a radiological classification.

Types of Infectious Pneumonias

- Bacterial pneumonia
- Viral pneumonia

- Fungal pneumonia
- Parasitic pneumonia
- Atypical pneumonia
- Community-acquired pneumonia
- Healthcare-associated pneumonia
- Hospital-acquired pneumonia
- Ventilator-associated pneumonia
- Severe acute respiratory syndrome.

Pneumonias Caused by Infectious or Noninfectious Agents

- Aspiration pneumonia
- Lipid pneumonia
- Eosinophilic pneumonia
- Bronchiolitis obliterans organizing pneumonia.

Noninfectious Pneumonia

- Chemical pneumonia.

Community-acquired Pneumonia

Community-acquired pneumonia (CAP) is infectious pneumonia in a person who has not recently been hospitalized. CAP is the most common type of pneumonia. The most common causes of CAP vary depending on a person's age, but they include *Streptococcus pneumoniae*, viruses, the atypical bacteria and *Haemophilus influenzae*. Overall, *Streptococcus pneumoniae* is the most common cause of community-acquired pneumonia worldwide. Gram-negative bacteria cause CAP in certain at-risk populations. The term 'walking pneumonia' has been used to describe a type of community-acquired pneumonia of less severity (because the sufferer can continue to 'walk' rather than require hospitalization). Walking pneumonia is usually caused by the atypical bacterium, *Mycoplasma pneumoniae*.

Hospital-acquired Pneumonia

- Hospital-acquired pneumonia, also called nosocomial pneumonia, is pneumonia acquired during or after hospitalization for another illness or procedure with onset at least 72 hrs after admission. The causes, microbiology, treatment and prognosis are different from those of community-acquired pneumonia.
- Up to 5% of child admitted to a hospital for other causes subsequently develop pneumonia. Hospitalized child may have many risk factors for pneumonia, including mechanical ventilation, prolonged malnutrition, underlying heart and lung diseases, decreased amounts of stomach acid and immune disturbances. Additionally, the microorganisms a person is exposed to in a hospital are often different from those at home.
- Hospital-acquired microorganisms may include resistant bacteria such as Methicillin-resistant staphylococcus aureus (MRSA), Pseudomonas, Enterobacter and Serratia. Because individuals with hospital-acquired pneumonia usually have underlying illnesses and are exposed to more dangerous bacteria, it tends to be more deadly than

community-acquired pneumonia. Ventilator-associated pneumonia (VAP) is a subset of hospital-acquired pneumonia. VAP is pneumonia which occurs after at least 48 hours of intubation and mechanical ventilation.

Other types

- *Severe acute respiratory syndrome (SARS)*
  - SARS is a highly contagious and deadly type of pneumonia which first occurred in 2002 after initial outbreaks in China. SARS is caused by the SARS coronavirus, a previously unknown pathogen.
- *Bronchiolitis obliterans organizing pneumonia (BOOP)*
  - BOOP is caused by inflammation of the small airways of the lungs. It is also known as cryptogenic organizing pneumonitis (COP).
- *Eosinophilic pneumonia*
  - Eosinophilic pneumonia is invasion of the lung by eosinophils, a particular kind of white blood cell. Eosinophilic pneumonia often occurs in response to infection with a parasite or after exposure to certain types of environmental factors.
- *Chemical pneumonia*
  - Chemical pneumonia (usually called chemical pneumonitis) is caused by chemical toxicants such as pesticides, which may enter the body by inhalation or by skin contact. When the toxic substance is oil the pneumonia may be called lipoid pneumonia.
- *Aspiration pneumonia*
  - Aspiration pneumonia (or aspiration pneumonitis) is caused by aspirating foreign objects which are usually oral or gastric contents, either while eating, or after reflux or vomiting which results in bronchopneumonia. The resulting lung inflammation is not an infection but can contribute to one, since the material aspirated may contain anaerobic bacteria or other unusual causes of pneumonia. Aspiration is a leading cause of death among hospital and nursing home child, since they often cannot adequately protect their airways and may have otherwise impaired defenses.
- *Dust pneumonia*
  - Dust pneumonia describes disorders caused by excessive exposure to dust storms, particularly during the Dust Bowl in the United States. With dust pneumonia, dust settles all the way into the alveoli of the lungs, stopping the cilia from moving and preventing the lungs from ever clearing themselves.
- *Necrotizing pneumonia,* although overlapping with many other classifications, includes pneumonias that cause substantial necrosis of lung cells and sometimes even lung abscess. Implicated bacteria are extremely commonly anaerobic bacteria, with or without additional facultatively anaerobic ones like *Staphylococcus aureus, Klebsiella pneumoniae* and *streptococcus pyogenes*. Type 3 pneumococcus is uncommonly implicated.
- *Opportunistic pneumonia* includes those that frequently strike immunocompromised victims. Main pathogens are cytomegalovirus, *Pneumocystis jiroveci, Mycobacterium avium-intracellulare*, invasive aspergillosis, invasive *candidiasis*, as well as the 'usual bacteria' that strike immunocompetent people as well.

- *Double pneumonia* is a historical term for acute lung injury (ALI) or acute respiratory distress syndrome (ARDS). However, the term was and is used still, especially by lay people, to denote pneumonia affecting both lungs. Accordingly, the term 'double pneumonia' is more likely to be used to describe bilateral pneumonia than it is ALI or ARDS.

Signs and Symptoms

Mild Pneumonia in Children

Pneumonia that is caused by certain bacteria, including *Mycoplasma pneumoniae* and *Chlamydophila pneumoniae*, usually results in milder symptoms even in children. This type of pneumonia, known as atypical or walking pneumonia, it is more prevalent among school-age children. Children with walking pneumonia may not feel sick enough to stay home, but they could have the following symptoms:

- Dry cough
- Low-grade fever
- Headache
- Tiredness.

Moderate Pneumonia in Children

Viruses cause most cases of pneumonia in preschool children between four months and five years old. Affected children will usually have symptoms associated with other viruses, such as:

- Sore throat
- Cough
- Low-grade fever
- Nasal congestion
- Diarrhea
- Loss of appetite
- Lack of energy or tiredness.

Severe Pneumonia in Children

Bacterial pneumonia is more common among school-age children and teens. These types of pneumonia often develop more abruptly than a cold or virus and have more dramatic symptoms, such as:

- High fever
- Cough that produces yellowish or green mucus
- Sweating or chills
- Flushed skin
- A bluish tint to the lips or nail beds
- Wheezing
- Difficulty breathing.

Pneumonia in Newborns and Infants

Newborns and infants may not show typical signs of pneumonia infection. It may also be difficult to determine if toddlers have the illness because they may not be able to communicate how they feel as well as an older child can.

- Being limp or lethargic
- Crying more than usual
- Feeding poorly
- Being irritable or restless
- Vomiting.

Diagnostic Evaluation

- History collection.
- Physical examination, further investigations are needed to confirm the diagnosis. Information from a chest X-ray and blood tests are helpful and sputum cultures in some cases.
- *Chest X-ray*: Identifies structural distribution (e.g. lobar, bronchial); may also reveal multiple abscesses/infiltrates, empyema (staphylococcus); scattered or localized infiltration (bacterial); or diffuse/extensive nodular infiltrates (more often viral). In mycoplasmal pneumonia, chest X-ray may be clear.
- *Fiberoptic bronchoscopy*: May be both diagnostic (qualitative cultures) and therapeutic (re-expansion of lung segment).
- *ABGs/pulse oximetry*: Abnormalities may be present, depending on extent of lung involvement and underlying lung disease.
- *Gram stain/cultures*: Sputum collection; needle aspiration of empyema, pleural and transtracheal or transthoracic fluids; lung biopsies and blood cultures may be done to recover causative organism. More than one type of organism may be present; common bacteria include *Diplococcus pneumoniae, Staphylococcus aureus, a-hemolytic streptococcus, Haemophilus influenzae; cytomegalovirus (CMV).* Note: Sputum cultures may not identify all offending organisms. Blood cultures may show transient bacteremia.
- *CBC*: Leukocytosis usually present, although a low white blood cell (WBC) count may be present in viral infection, immunosuppressed conditions such as AIDS and overwhelming bacterial pneumonia. Erythrocyte sedimentation rate (ESR) is elevated.
- *Serologic studies,* e.g. viral or Legionella titers, cold agglutinins: Assist in differential diagnosis of specific organism.
- *Pulmonary function studies*: Volumes may be decreased (congestion and alveolar collapse); airway pressure may be increased and compliance decreased. Shunting is present (hypoxemia).
- *Electrolytes*: Sodium and chloride levels may be low.
- *Bilirubin*: May be increased.
- *Percutaneous aspiration/open biopsy of lung tissues*: May reveal typical intranuclear and cytoplasmic inclusions (CMV), characteristic giant cells (rubeola).

Management

Bacterial Pneumonia

- Antibiotics improve outcomes in those with bacterial pneumonia. Initially antibiotic choice depends on the characteristics of the person affected such as age, underlying health and location the infection was acquired.
- Where the 'atypical' forms of community-acquired pneumonia are becoming more common, macrolides (such as azithromycin) and doxycycline have displaced amoxicillin as first-line outpatient treatment for community-acquired pneumonia.
- The use of fluoroquinolones in uncomplicated cases is discouraged due to concerns of side effects and resistance. The duration of treatment has traditionally been seven to ten days, but there is increasing evidence that short courses (three to five days) are equivalent.
- Antibiotics recommended for hospital-acquired pneumonia include third and fourth-generation **cephalosporins, carbapenems, fluoroquinolones, aminoglycosides** and **vancomycin**. These antibiotics are often given intravenously and may be used in combination.

Viral Pneumonia

- No specific treatments exist for most types of viral pneumonia including SARS coronavirus, adenovirus, hantavirus and parainfluenza virus with the exception of influenza A and influenza B.
- Influenza A may be treated with rimantadine or amantadine while influenza A or B may be treated with oseltamivir or zanamivir.
- These are beneficial only if they are started within 48 hours of the onset of symptoms. Many strains of H5N1 influenza A, also known as avian influenza or 'bird flu,' have shown resistance to rimantadine and amantadine.

Aspiration Pneumonia

- There is no evidence to support the use of antibiotics in chemical pneumonitis without bacterial superinfection.
- If infection is present in aspiration pneumonia, the choice of antibiotic will depend on several factors, including the suspected causative organism and whether pneumonia was acquired in the community or developed in a hospital setting.
- Common options include clindamycin, a combination of a beta-lactam antibiotic and metronidazole, or an aminoglycoside.
- Corticosteroids are commonly used in aspiration pneumonia, but there is no evidence to support their use either.

Preventive Measures

There are several ways to prevent infectious pneumonia. Appropriately treating underlying illnesses (such as AIDS) can decrease a person's risk of pneumonia. Smoking cessation is important not only because it helps to limit lung damage, but also because cigarette smoke interferes with many of the body's natural defenses against pneumonia.

Research shows that there are several ways to prevent pneumonia in newborn infants. Testing pregnant women for Group B Streptococcus and Chlamydia trachomatis and then giving antibiotic treatment if needed, reduces pneumonia in infants. Suctioning the mouth and throat of infants with meconium-stained amniotic fluid decreases the rate of aspiration pneumonia.

Vaccination is important for preventing pneumonia in both children and adults. Vaccinations against *Haemophilus influenzae* and *Streptococcus pneumoniae* in the first year of life have greatly reduced the role these bacteria play in causing pneumonia in children. Vaccinating children against *Streptococcus pneumoniae* has also led to a decreased incidence of these infections in adults because many adults acquire infections from children. Hib vaccine is now widely used around the globe.

The childhood pneumococcal vaccine is still as of 2009 predominantly used in high-income countries, though this is changing. In 2009, Rwanda became the first low-income country to introduce pneumococcal conjugate vaccine into their national immunization program.

A vaccine against *Streptococcus pneumoniae* is also available for adults. In the US, it is currently recommended for all healthy individuals older than 65 and any adults with emphysema, congestive heart failure, diabetes mellitus, cirrhosis of the liver, alcoholism, cerebrospinal fluid leaks, or those who do not have a spleen. A repeat vaccination may also be required after five or ten years.

Influenza vaccines should be given yearly to the same individuals who receive vaccination against *Streptococcus pneumoniae*. In addition, health care workers, nursing home residents and pregnant women should receive the vaccine. When an influenza outbreak is occurring, medications such as amantadine, rimantadine, zanamivir and oseltamivir can help prevent influenza.

Nursing Management

Nursing Priorities

- Maintain/improve respiratory function.
- Prevent complications.
- Support recuperative process.
- Provide information about disease process, prognosis and treatment.

Nursing Diagnosis

- Ineffective airway clearance related to presence of secretions secondary to pneumonia.
- Ineffective breathing pattern related to presence of tracheobronchial secretions and nasal secretions.
- Impaired gas exchange related to alveolar capillary membrane changes secondary to inflammation.
- Risk for infection (spread) related to inadequate secondary defenses (decrease hemoglobin, hematocrit and immunosuppression).

Nursing Diagnosis

- Ineffective airway clearance.

Related to

- Tracheal bronchial inflammation, edema formation, increased sputum production
- Pleuritic pain
- Decreased energy, fatigue.

Desired Outcomes

- Identify/demonstrate behaviors to achieve airway clearance.
- Display patent airway with breath sounds clearing; absence of dyspnea, cyanosis.

Nursing interventions	Rationale
Assess the rate and depth of respirations and chest movement.	Tachypnea, shallow respirations and asymmetric chest movement are frequently present because of discomfort of moving chest wall and/or fluid in lung.
Auscultate lung fields, noting areas of decreased or absent airflow and adventitious breath sounds: Crackles, wheezes.	Decreased airflow occurs in areas with consolidated fluid. Bronchial breath sounds can also occur in these consolidated areas. Crackles, rhonchi and wheezes are heard on inspiration and/or expiration in response to fluid accumulation, thick secretions and airway spams and obstruction.
Elevate head of bed, change position frequently.	Doing so would lower the diaphragm and promote chest expansion, aeration of lung segments, mobilization and expectoration of secretions.
Teach and assist patient with proper deep-breathing exercises. Demonstrate proper splinting of chest and effective coughing while in upright position. Encourage him to do so often.	Deep breathing exercises facilitates maximum expansion of the lungs and smaller airways. Coughing is a reflex and a natural self-cleaning mechanism that assists the cilia to maintain patent airways. Splinting reduces chest discomfort and an upright position favors deeper and more forceful cough effort.
Suction as indicated: Frequent coughing, adventitious breath sounds, desaturation related to airway secretions.	Stimulates cough or mechanically clears airway in patient who is unable to do so because of ineffective cough or decreased level of consciousness.
Force fluids to at least 3000 mL/day (unless contraindicated, as in heart failure). Offer warm, rather than cold fluids.	Fluids, especially warm liquids, aid in mobilization and expectoration of secretions.
Assist and monitor effects of nebulizer treatment and other respiratory physiotherapy: Incentive spirometer, IPPB, percussion, postural drainage. Perform treatments between meals and limit fluids when appropriate.	Nebulizers and other respiratory therapy facilitate liquefaction and expectoration of secretions. Postural drainage may not be as effective in interstitial pneumonias or those causing alveolar exudate or destruction. Coordination of treatments and oral intake reduces likelihood of vomiting with coughing, expectorations.
Administer medications as indicated: Mucolytics, expectorants, bronchodilators, analgesics.	Aids in reduction of bronchospasm and mobilization of secretions. Analgesics are given to improve cough effort by reducing discomfort, but should be used cautiously because they can decrease cough effort and depress respirations.
Provide supplemental fluids: IV.	Room humidification has been found to provide minimal benefit and is thought to increase the risk of transmitting infection.
Monitor serial chest X-rays, ABGs, pulse oximetry readings.	Followers progress and effects of the disease process, therapeutic regimen and may facilitate necessary alterations in therapy.
Assist with bronchoscopy and/or thoracentesis, if indicated.	Occasionally needed to remove mucous plugs, drain purulent secretions, and/or prevent atelectasis.
Urge all bedridden and postoperative child to perform deep breathing and coughing exercises frequently.	To promote full aeration and drainage of secretions.

Impaired Gas Exchange

Related to

- Alveolar-capillary membrane changes (inflammatory effects)
- Altered oxygen-carrying capacity of blood/release at cellular level (fever, shifting oxyhemoglobin curve)
- Altered delivery of oxygen (hypoventilation).

Desired Outcomes

- Demonstrate improved ventilation and oxygenation of tissues by ABGs within patient's acceptable range and absence of symptoms of respiratory distress.
- Participate in actions to maximize oxygenation.

Nursing interventions	Rationale
Assess respiratory rate, depth and ease.	Manifestations of respiratory distress are dependent on/and indicative of the degree of lung involvement and underlying general health status.
Observe color of skin, mucous membranes and nailbeds, noting presence of peripheral cyanosis (nail beds) or central cyanosis (circumoral).	Cyanosis of nail beds may represent vasoconstriction or the body's response to fever/chills; however, cyanosis of earlobes, mucous membranes and skin around the mouth ('warm membranes') is indicative of systemic hypoxemia.
Assess mental status.	Restlessness, irritation, confusion and somnolence may reflect hypoxemia and decreased cerebral oxygenation.
Monitor heart rate and rhythm.	Tachycardia is usually present as a result of fever and/or dehydration but may represent a response to hypoxemia.
Monitor body temperature, as indicated. Assist with comfort measures to reduce fever and chills: Addition or removal of bedcovers, comfortable room temperature, tepid or cool water sponge bath.	High fever (common in bacterial pneumonia and influenza) greatly increases metabolic demands and oxygen consumption and alters cellular oxygenation.
Maintain bedrest. Encourage use of relaxation techniques and diversional activities.	Prevents over exhaustion and reduces oxygen demands to facilitate resolution of infection.
Elevate head and encourage frequent position changes, deep breathing and effective coughing.	These measures promote maximum chest expansion, mobilize secretions and improve ventilation.
Assess anxiety level and encourage verbalization of feelings and concerns.	Anxiety is a manifestation of psychological concerns and physiological responses to hypoxia. Providing reassurance and enhancing sense of security can reduce the psychological component, thereby decreasing oxygen demand and adverse physiological responses.
Observe for deterioration in condition, noting hypotension, copious amounts of bloody sputum, pallor, cyanosis, change in LOC, severe dyspnea and restlessness.	Shock and pulmonary edema are the most common causes of death in pneumonia and require immediate medical intervention.
Monitor ABGs, pulse oximetry.	Follows progress of disease process and facilitates alterations in pulmonary therapy.
Administer oxygen therapy by appropriate means: Nasal prongs, mask, Venturi mask.	The purpose of oxygen therapy is to maintain PaO_2 above 60 mm Hg. Oxygen is administered by the method that provides appropriate delivery within the patient's tolerance. Note: Child with underlying chronic lung diseases should be given oxygen cautiously.

CHILD WITH ASTHMA

Introduction

Asthma is a chronic condition in which the airways that carry air to the lungs are inflamed and narrowed. Inflamed airways are very sensitive and they tend to react to things in the environment called triggers, such as substances that are inhaled. When the airways react, they swell and narrow even more and also produce extra mucus, all of which make it harder for air to flow to the lungs. The muscles around the airways also tighten, which further restricts air flow.

Asthma can begin at any age (even in the very elderly), but most children have their first symptoms by age 5. Asthma is typically diagnosed with a medical exam and a test that measures the airflow in and out of the lungs. Children who are of preschool age or younger may not be able to complete the airflow test, which requires blowing very hard into a tube. And since infants and toddlers cannot describe how they feel, parents, other family members and caregivers need to be alert for symptom.

Definition

Asthma is a disorder caused by inflammation in the bronchi that lead to the lungs. This inflammation causes airways to tighten and narrow, which blocks air from flowing freely into the lungs, making it hard to breathe. Symptoms include wheezing, breathlessness, chest tightness, and cough, particularly at night or after exercise/activity.

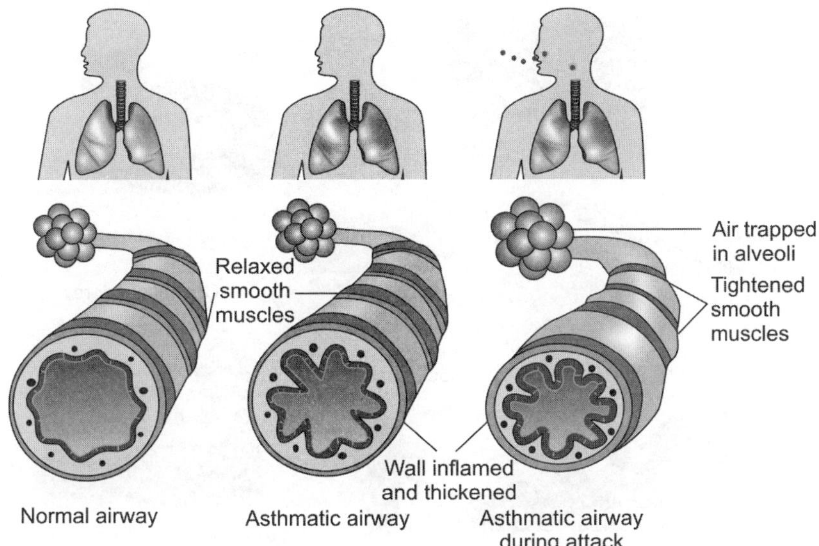

Fig. 7.37: Difference between normal and asthmatic bronchi

Classifications

Asthma is classified into four categories based on the symptom indicator of disease:

1. Mild intermittent asthma
2. Mild persistent asthma
3. Moderate persistent asthma
4. Severe persistent asthma

Table 7.5: Classification of asthma

	Symptoms		≤ 5 years of age	> 5 years of age	
	Daytime	**Nighttime**	**Exercise tolerance**	**PEF or FEV1**	**PEF variability**
Mild intermittent	≤ 2 per week	≤ 2 per month	Exercise tolerance	≥ 80%	< 20%
Mild persistent	> 2 per week but < 1 per day	> 2 per month	Exercise symptoms	≥ 80%	20–30%
Moderate persistent	Daily symptoms	> 1 per week	Frequent exercise symptoms	60–80%	> 30%
Severe persistent	Continual day symptoms	Frequent night symptoms	Exercise severely limited	≤ 60%	> 30%

Causes

Allergy influences both the persistence and severity of the disease. Genetic predisposition for the development of an IgE mediated response to common aeroallergens is the strongest predictor, 20–40% have no evidence of allergic disease.

Asthma triggers

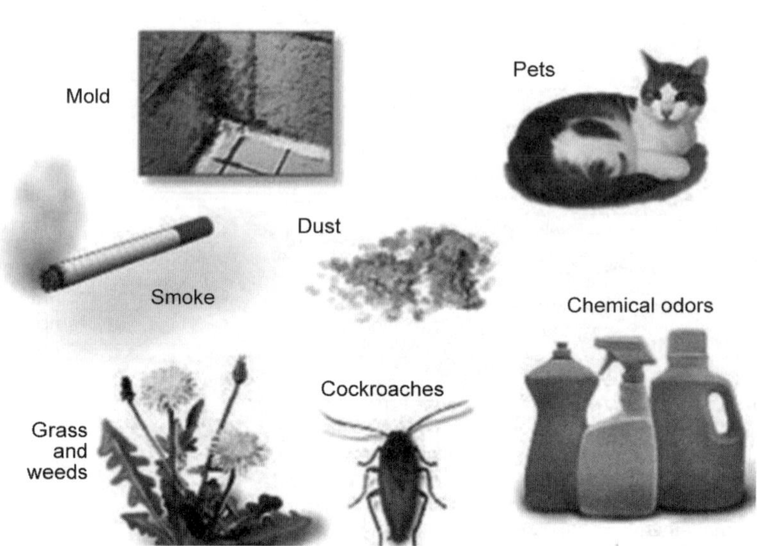

Trigger for Asthma

Allergens

- *Outdoor:* Trees, shrubs, weeds, grasses.
- *Indoor:* Dust or dust mites, mild, cockroach antigen
- *Irritant:* Tobacco, smoke, wood smoke, sprays
  - Exposure to occupational chemicals
  - Cold air

- Changes in weather or temperature
- *Environmental change:* Moving to new home, starting new school, etc.
- Cold and infections
- Animals
- *Medication:* Aspire, NSAIDs, antibiotic
- *Conditions:* Gastroesophageal reflux
- *Food allergies:* Suffix preservatives
- *Foods:* Nuts, milk/dairy products
- *Endocrine factors:* Menses, pregnancy, thyroid, disease.

Pathophysiology

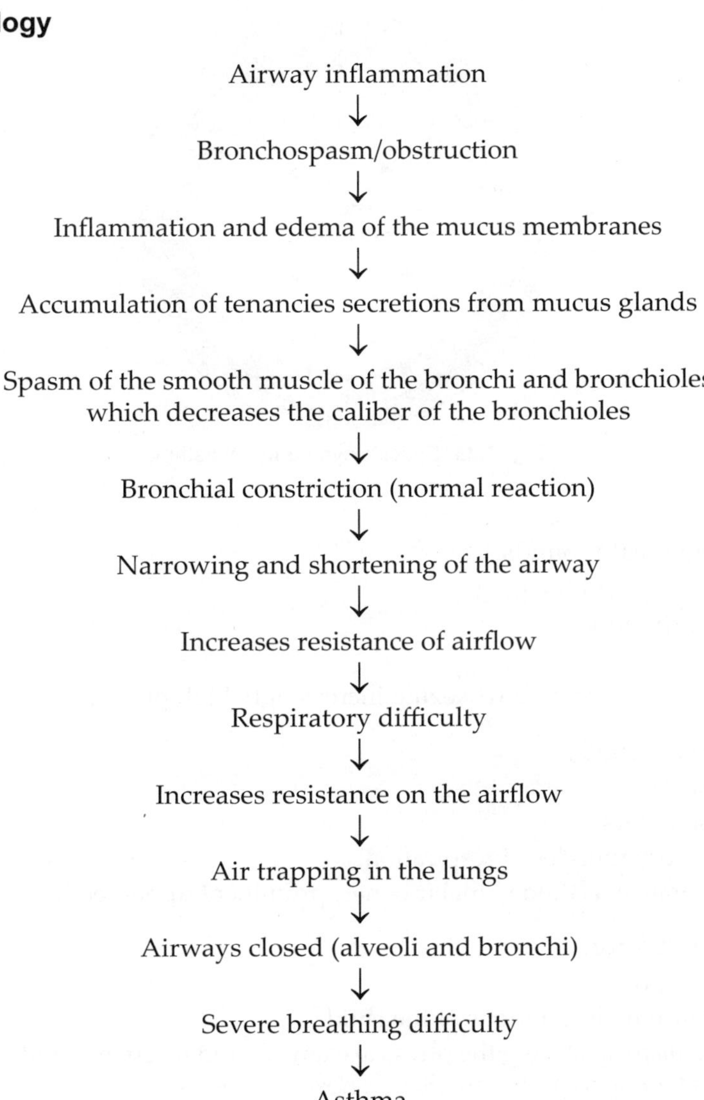

Signs and Symptoms

Cough

Hacking, paroxysmal, Irritative, Non predictor, Becomes rattling and productive of frothy, Cleat gelatinous sputum.

Respiratory Related Signs

Shortness of breath, prolonged expiratory phase, audible wheeze, malar flush and red ears, LPS deep, dark red color, may progress to cyanosis of nail beds or cyanosis. Restlessness sweating, older children-sit upright with shoulders in a hunched over position, hands on the bed or chair and arms braced. Speak with short, panting, broken phrases.

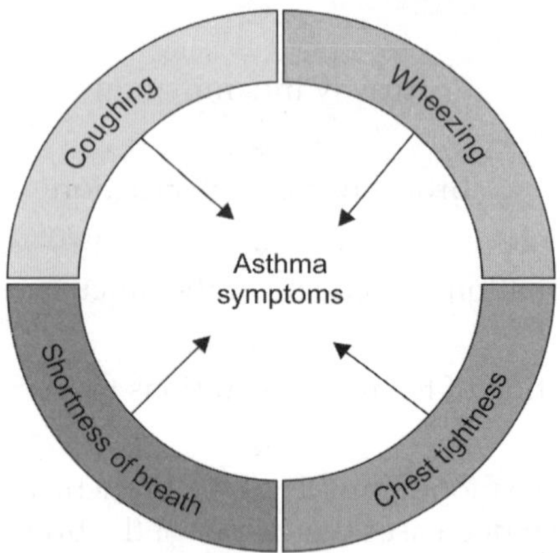

Fig. 7.38: Specific symptoms of asthma

Chest

- Coarse, loud breath sounds
- Wheezes throughout the lung
- Prolonged expiration
- Crackles
- Inspiratory and expiratory wheezing increasingly high pitched.

With Repeated Episodes

- Barrel chest
- Elevated shoulders
- Use of accessory muscles of respiration
- Facial appearance: Flattened malar bones, prominent upper teeth.

Diagnostic Evaluation

- History collection
- Specific clinical manifestations of the child
- *Physical examination:* During the physical exam should listen the child's heart and lungs sounds and look for signs of an allergic nose or eyes.

- Laboratory tests
- Radiographic examinations (X-ray and CT scan)
- Pulmonary function tests (PETs)
- Skin testing.

Management

The optimal treatment of asthma depends upon a number of factors, including the child's age, the severity and frequency of asthma attacks and the ability to properly use the prescribed medications. For the great majority of children, asthma treatment can control symptoms, allowing the child to participate fully in all activities, including sports.

Successful treatment of asthma involves three components:

- Controlling and avoiding asthma triggers
- Regularly monitoring asthma symptoms and lung function
- Understanding how and when to use medications to treat asthma.

Goal

Prevent disability, minimize physical and psychologic morbidity, assist in loving as normal and happy life as possible, facilitating the child's social adjustments.

Medication

There are three type of medication:

1. Long-term control medications reduce the inflammation in your airways that leads to symptoms.
2. Quick-relief inhalers (bronchodilators) quickly open swollen airways that are limiting breathing.
3. In some cases allergy medications are necessary.

Long-term Asthma Control Medications

These medications keep asthma under control on a day-to-day basis and make it less likely child have an asthma attack.

Types of long-term control medications include:

- *Inhaled corticosteroids:* These anti-inflammatory drugs include:
  - Fluticasone (Flonase, Flovent HFA)
  - Budesonide (Pulmicort Flexhaler, Rhinocort)
  - Flunisolide (Aerospan HFA)
  - Ciclesonide (Alvesco, Omnaris, Zetonna)
  - Beclomethasone (Qnasl, Qvar)
  - Mometasone (Asmanex) and fluticasone furoate (Arnuity Ellipta).
- *Leukotriene modifiers:* These oral medications include:
  - Montelukast (Singulair)
  - Zafirlukast (Accolate) and zileuton (Zyflo), this medicine relieve asthma symptoms up to 24 hours.

- *Long-acting beta agonists:* These inhaled medications, which include:
  - Salmeterol (Serevent)
  - Formoterol (Foradil, Perforomist), open the airways.
- *Combination inhalers:* These medications such as:
  - Fluticasone-salmeterol (Advair Diskus)
  - Budesonide-formoterol (Symbicort)
  - Formoterol-mometasone (Dulera) contains a long-acting beta agonist along with a corticosteroid.
- *Theophylline:* Theophylline (Theo–24, Elixophyllin, others) is a daily pill that helps keep the airways open (bronchodilator) by relaxing the muscles around the airways. It is not used as often now as in past years.

Quick-Relief (Rescue) Medications

These medications are used as needed for rapid, short-term symptom relief during an asthma attack or before exercise if your doctor recommends it.

Types of quick-relief medications include:

- *Short-acting beta agonists:* These inhaled, quick-relief bronchodilators act within minutes to rapidly ease symptoms during an asthma attack. They include albuterol (ProAir HFA, Ventolin HFA, others) and levalbuterol (Xopenex).

  Short-acting beta agonists can be taken using a portable, hand-held inhaler or a nebulizer, a machine that converts asthma medications to a fine mist—so that they can be inhaled through a face mask or a mouthpiece.

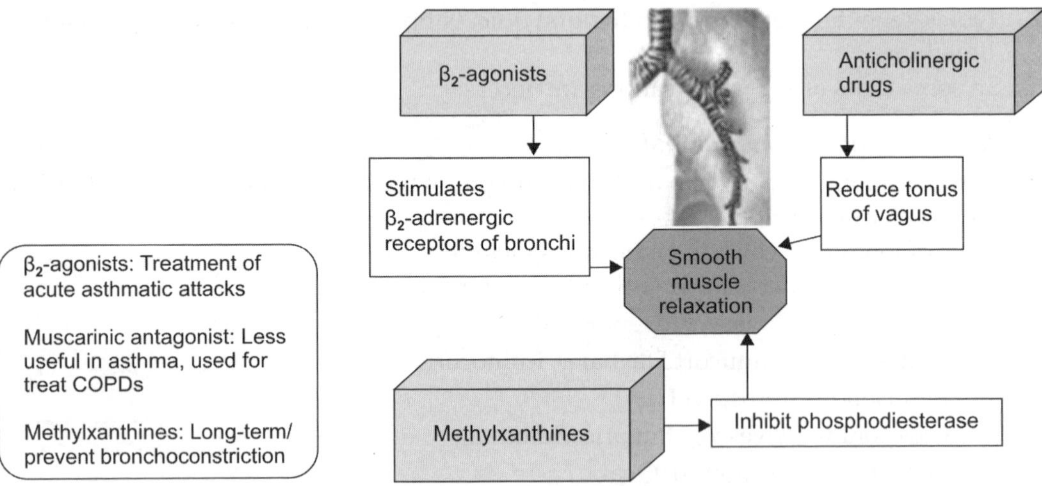

Fig. 7.39: Mode of action in bronchodilator

- *Ipratropium (Atrovent)*: Other bronchodilators, ipratropium acts quickly to immediately relax your airways, making it easier to breathe. Ipratropium is mostly used for emphysema and chronic bronchitis, but it is sometimes used to treat asthma attacks.
- *Oral and intravenous corticosteroids*: These medications which include prednisone and methylprednisolone relieve airway inflammation caused by severe asthma. They can

cause serious side effects when used long-term, so they are used only on a short-term basis to treat severe asthma symptoms.

- *Allergy medications* may help if your asthma is triggered or worsened by allergies. These include:
  - *Allergy shots (immunotherapy)*: Over time, allergy shots gradually reduce your immune system reaction to specific allergens. You generally receive shots once a week for a few months, then once a month for a period of three to five years.
  - *Omalizumab (Xolair)*: This medication, given as an injection every two to four weeks, is specifically for people who have allergies and severe asthma. It acts by altering the immune system.

Bronchial Thermoplasty

- This treatment which is not widely available is not right for everyone, it is used for severe asthma that does not improve with inhaled corticosteroids or other long-term asthma medications.
- Bronchial thermoplasty heats the insides of the airways in the lungs with an electrode, reducing the smooth muscle inside the airways. This limits the ability of the airways to tighten, making breathing easier and possibly reducing asthma attacks.

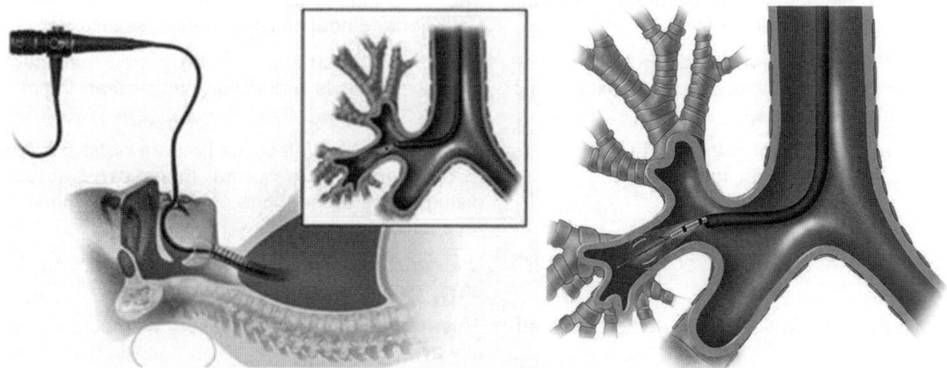

Fig. 7.40: Bronchial thermoplasty

Complications

- Status asthmaticus
- Severe respiratory failure
- Death.

Nursing Management

Nursing Priorities

- Maintain airway patency.
- Assist with measures to facilitate gas exchange.
- Enhance nutritional intake.
- Prevent complications and slow progression of condition.
- Provide information about disease process, prognosis and treatment regimen.

Nursing Diagnosis

- Ineffective airway clearance related to bronchoconstriction, increased mucus production and respiratory infection as evidenced by wheezing, dyspnea and cough.
- Ineffective breathing pattern related to presence of secretions as evidenced by productive cough and dyspnea.
- Impaired gas exchange related to ventilation perfusion imbalance as evidenced by dyspnea, tachypnea and tachycardia.
- Risk for activity intolerance related to decrease oxygenation.
- Fatigue related to physical exertion to maintain adequate ventilation as evidenced by use of accessory muscles to breathe.

Nursing Intervention

- Ineffective airway clearance related to bronchoconstriction, increased mucus production and respiratory infection as evidenced by wheezing, dyspnea and cough.

Nursing interventions	Rationale
• Keep the child adequately hydrated	Systemic hydration keeps secretion moist and easier to expectorate
• Teach and encourage the use of diaphragmatic breathing and coughing exercises.	These techniques help to improve ventilation and mobilize secretions without causing breathlessness and fatigue.
• Instruct parents to avoid bronchial irritants such as cigarette smoke, aerosols, extremes of temperature and fumes.	Bronchial irritants cause bronchoconstriction and increased mucus production, which then interfere with airway clearance.
• Teach early signs of infection that are to be reported to the clinician immediately.	Minor respiratory infections that are of no consequence to the person with normal lungs can produce fatal disturbances in the lungs of an asthmatic person. Early recognition is crucial.
• Assist and prepare child for postural drainage.	Uses gravity to help raise secretions so they can be more easily expectorated.
• Administer nebulization as per doctors ordered.	This ensures adequate delivery of medications to the airways.
• Administer medications as per doctors ordered.	Antibiotics may be prescribed to treat the infection.

- Ineffective breathing pattern related to presence of secretions as evidenced by productive cough and dyspnea.

Nursing interventions	Rationale
• Assess the child respiratory rate, depth and rhythm. Obtain pulse oximetry.	To obtain baseline data
• Monitor and record vital signs.	Increase in respiratory rate could mean worsening condition.
• Auscultate breath sounds and assess airway pattern	To check for the presence of adventitious breath sounds
• Elevate head of the bed and change position of the pattern every 2 hours.	To minimize difficulty in breathing.
• Encourage deep breathing and coughing exercises.	To maximize effort for expectoration.

Contd...

Contd...

Nursing interventions	Rationale
• Demonstrate diaphragmatic and pursed-lip breathing.	To decrease air trapping and for efficient breathing.
• Encourage increase in fluid intake	To prevent fatigue.
• Encourage opportunities for rest and limit physical activities.	To prevent situations that will aggravate the condition.
• Reinforce low salt, low fat diet as ordered.	To mobilize secretions.

- Impaired gas exchange related to ventilation perfusion imbalance as evidenced by dyspnea, tachypnea and tachycardia

Nursing interventions	Rationale
Assess vital signs, respiratory rate, depth and rhythm.	To obtain baseline data.
Vital signs monitor and record.	Serve to track important changes.
Auscultate breath sounds and assess airway pattern.	To check for the presence of adventitious breath sounds.
Elevate head of the bed and change position of the pattern every 2 hours.	To minimize difficulty in breathing and promote maximum lung expansion.
Encourage deep breathing and coughing exercises.	To maximize effort for expectoration.
Demonstrate diaphragmatic and pursed-lip breathing.	To decrease air trapping and for efficient breathing.
Encourage increase in fluid intake.	To prevent fatigue.
Encourage opportunities for rest and limit physical activities.	To prevent situations that will aggravate the condition.
Reinforce low salt, low fat diet as ordered.	To mobilize secretions.

- Risk for Activity Intolerance related to decrease oxygenation.

Nursing interventions	Rationale
Monitor vital sings of child.	For baseline data.
Assess motor function of asthmatic child.	To identify causative factors.
Note contributing factors to fatigue.	To identify precipitating factors.
Evaluate degree of deficit.	To identify severity.
Ascertain ability to stand and move about.	To identify necessity of assistive devices.
Assess emotional or psychological factors.	Stress and/or depression may increase the effects of illness.
Plan care with rest periods between activities.	To reduce fatigue.
Increase activity/exercise gradually such as assisting the child in doing PROM to active or full range of motions.	Minimizes muscle atrophy, promotes circulation, helps to prevent contractures.
Provide adequate rest periods.	To replenish energy.
Assist client in doing self-care needs.	To promote independence and increase activity tolerance.
Elevate arm and hand.	Promotes venous.
Place knees and hips in extended position.	Maintain the normal airflow.

STATUS ASTHMATICUS

Introduction

Status asthmaticus is an acute exacerbation of asthma that is unresponsive to treatment with bronchodilators. Status asthmaticus can vary from a mild to a severe form with bronchospasm, airway inflammation and mucus plugging that can cause difficulty breathing, carbon dioxide retention, hypoxemia and respiratory failure. Exposure to an allergen or trigger causes a characteristic form of airway inflammation in susceptible individuals, exemplified by mast cell degranulation, release of inflammatory mediators, infiltration by eosinophils and activated T-lymphocytes. Bronchospasm, mucus plugging and edema in the peripheral airways result in a no uniform pattern of airflow obstruction and increased airway resistance. With a decreased ability to expel air, hyperinflation results and eventually leads to severe ventilation/perfusion (V/Q) mismatch and increased dead space ventilation.

Definition

Status asthmaticus is defined as a significantly increasing the severe asthma that is not responsive to drugs that are usually effective like sympathomimitic drugs with or without theophylline.

Status asthmaticus is the condition of a child in progressive respiratory failure due to asthma, in whom conventional forms of therapy have failed.

Causes

- Atopy (hypersensitive reaction to allergens such as pollen and food)
- Viral infections are known to trigger
- Industrial and other air pollutants
- Whose mothers smoke, are more likely to develop asthma.
- Medications, such as beta-blockers, aspirin and nonsteroidal anti-inflammatory drugs (NSAIDs), are all known to trigger asthma in susceptible individuals.
- Gastroesophageal reflux disease (GERD).
- Other triggers include cold temperature and exercise.
- Aspiration syndromes, bronchiectasis, bronchiolitis, congenital lung malformations, cystic fibrosis, gastroesophageal reflux, heart failure, congestive, inhalation injury, pulmonary artery sling, respiratory syncytial virus infection, tracheomalacia, vascular ring, double aortic arch, foreign bodies in the esophagus and trachea.

Signs and Symptoms

Symptoms

- Dyspnea and cough
- Unable to speak properly
- Lack of proper sleep.

Diagnostic Evaluation

- History collection
- Physical examination.

Lab Studies

- Pulse oximetry, blood gas determination, serum electrolyte measurement, serum glucose, a complete blood count (CBC) and differential, blood theophylline, peak flow monitoring, chest radiography, indicated when only pneumonia, pneumothorax, pneumomediastinum or significant atelectasis is suspected.
- Pulmonary function testing is important; it should be performed in children who are old enough and who are capable of cooperating.
- Forced expiratory volume in 1 second (FEV1) is the most common test used to monitor degree of airway obstruction. In the acutely ill patient, peak flow monitoring is more commonly performed.
- On other pulmonary function tests (e.g. maximum expiratory flow rate, mid-maximum expiratory flow rate, forced vital capacity), findings may be diminished. Functional residual capacity and residual volume increase as a result of air trapping.

Therapy

Over reliance on aerosol, inhaler therapy, delayed use of systemic corticosteroids sedation, delayed admission to hospital or intensive care unit, scoring systems for assessment of severity of asthma.

Blood Investigation

Blood count and electrolyte estimation, cardiac monitoring is necessary because drugs like theophylline, adrenergic drugs and hypoxia may cause arrhythmias. Analysis of arterial blood gases for PaO_2, PCO_2 and pH is also indicated.

Evaluation of Asthma in Infants

- The clinical, roentgen graphic and blood gas findings of asthma are similar to bronchiolitis. Bronchiolitis is more common around 6 months of age particularly in winter season. Recurrences are rare. If the child respond to bronchodilators, it confirms the diagnosis of asthma.
- A child with recurrent attacks of coughing and wheezing associated with bacterial infections should be investigated for cystic fibrosis or immunological deficiently.
- Food allergy can also cause asthma
  - Skin test for IgE mediated sensitivity to food
  - Temporary elimination of suspected food particularly milk, wheat or egg can improve the condition
  - Challenge with implicated food after 3 weeks may be appropriate to confirm the diagnosis.
- Previous history of eczema can predispose to asthma
- Absolute eosinophils counts more than 400 cells/cu mm, especially more than 700 cells/cu mm and high IgE levels can predict continuous respiratory problems.
  - Mild eosinophilic–up to 1500
  - Moderate–1500 to 5000
  - Severe–More than 5000

Chest Radiography

- Homogenous opacity is present on the affected side with highest level in the axilla
- Intercostals spaces are widened
- Intercostals bulging may be present
- 1000 ml of fluid is required to shift the mediastinum to opposite side
  - *Mild effusion*: The fluid is present up to the 4th rib.
  - *Moderate effusion*: The fluid is present up to the 2nd rib.
  - *Massive effusion*: The fluid is present beyond the 2nd rib.

Diagnostic Thoracentesis is Necessary to Confirm the Diagnosis

Diagnostic aspiration of the fluid and its findings:

- The diagnosis of empyema is strongly supported by the presence of the following features:
  - Thick pus
  - Demonstration of bacteria
  - pH less than 7.3
  - Glucose concentration is less than 60 mg/dl
  - The protein concentration is more than 30 gm/dl
  - Culture of the fluid should be done
  - The cell count.

CT Scan

CT scan is very useful in identification and evaluation of the type of fluid. Empyema appears with a lent form shape at an obtuse angle with the chest wall separation of the two pleural layers, compression of the adjacent lung and uniform chest wall width with a sharp interface with the lung. Contrast enhancement may demonstrate thick and enhancing ring surrounding an empyema. Thick and enhancing empyema may be caused by *S. aureus* or other organisms.

Management

Therapeutic Procedures

Oxygen Therapy

It is indicated because patient is hypoxic in bronchial asthma. Patient is giver 2 to 3 liter/minutes in order to maintain O_2 level at 70–90 mm of Hg or O_2 saturation greater than 92%.

Fluid Therapy: Child is dehydrated due to

- Tachypnea
- Diuretic effect of theophylline
- Decreased intake
- Excessive working of respiratory muscles.

Bronchodilators

- *Epinephrine:* 0.01 ml/kg/dose to be given SC. If there is no response, it can be repeated after 20 minutes. And if there is no response with the second dose change of drug is necessary.

- *Terbutaline*: The better drug for parenteral use is terbutaline because it is a selective Beta-2 agonist with minimal cardiac stimulation and prolonged action. IV method can be used. Dose 10 μg/kg/min as a bolus does followed by 0.4 to 0.6 μg/kg/min as a continuous infusion, increasing it by 0.2 μg/kg/min to 3–6 μg/kg/min or 0.01 mg/kg/dose, maximum 0.3 mg to be given SC. If there is no response it can be repeated after 30 min.
- *Theophylline:* Intermittent therapy is preferable to continuous therapy. Dose of the intermittent therapy 45 mg/kg/dose to be given over 20 min IV 6th hourly. Continuous therapy: 5 mg/kg to be given as a bolus dose followed by 0.75 mg to 1.25 mg/kg/hour may be given.
- *Beta 2 agonists are best used as aerosols*. These can be used intermittently or continuously. The details of doses are given above.
- *Antimuscarinie*: Drugs like atropine sulfate can be used as inhalation. Dose: 0.05–0.1 mg/kg is safe, for adults and adolescents 0.02 mg/kg is more appropriate. If it is combined with beta agonists as nebulizers it is more effective rathan than using as a single drug. Ipratropium bromide can be used as nebulizer. It causes less side effects.

Dose

- 0.25 mg for children less than 6 years of age.
- 0.5 mg for children in between 7 and 12 years of age.
- *Corticosteroids*: Prednisolone is preferred to hydrocortisone because of the following:
  - *Advantages*: Less effect on mineral metabolism, lower cost and equally effective dose: 1–2 mg/kg/day to be given 6th hourly in divided doses.

Medication

The main stay of the treatment of empyema consists of

- Antimicrobial therapy
- Adequate drainage of infected material in the pleural space.

Antibiotic Therapy

Apropriate antibiotics to be used depending upon culture and sensitivity. Empirically antibiotics are used covering for both *S. aureus* and *S. pneumonia*. Beta lactamase resistant penicillin like oxacillin and an extended spectrum cephalosporin esuch as ceftriaxone are often used together as an initial therapy. Most antibiotics diffuse well into the pleural fluid. Duration on therapy for a period of 14 to 28 days course will be appropriate. Appropriate antibiotics depending on culture and sensitivity.

Infecting agent	Drugs	Dosage per kg
• Staphylococci	• Cloxacillin • Methicillin	100–200 mg in 3–6 divided doses 200–400 mg in 3–4 divided doses
• Haemophilus influenzae	• Cefotaxime • Ceftriaxone • Chloramphenicol	150–114 mg/kg in 3 divided doses 80–100 mg/kg in 1–2 divided doses 50–100 mg/kg in 4 divided doses
• Pneumococcus and streptococci	• Penicillin, G	1–4 lakhs/kg in 4 divided doses

Contd...

Contd...

Infecting agent	Drugs	Dosage per kg
• E. coli and Klebsiella	• Cefotaxime, dose mentioned above	
• Pseudomonas	• Ticarcillin • Ceftazidime • Tobramycin	

Closed tube drainage is indicated if the fluid is large in quantity or if the pleural space is having frank pus, after diagnostic thoracocentesis. Chest tubes should be positioned in a dependent part of the empyema and should be of sufficient diameter to prevent clogging. The tube should be connected to a underwater seal. Clinical and radiological improvement should be evident within 48 to 72 hours, if it is properly draining.

Nursing Management

- Admission to the pediatric intensive care unit (PICU).
- Oxygen can be provided via nasal cannula or facial masks.
- Beta agonist agents, including albuterol or salbutamol (Nebulizer: Dilute 0.5 mL [2.5 mg] of 0.5% inhalation solution in 1–2.5 mL of isotonic sodium chloride solution; administer 2.5–5 mg q4–6h diluted in 2–5 mL of sterile saline or water), terbutaline, isoproterenol and epinephrine are the mainstays of acute therapy of asthma. Many of these agents are administered by inhalation, although some may be administered intravenously.
- Corticosteroids are critical in the therapy of status asthmaticus and are used to decrease the intense airway inflammation in asthma.
- Among anticholinergic agents, atropine was used to treat asthma.
- Theophylline: Loading 20 mg/kg/dose, followed by 5 mg/kg/day.
- Ketamine is a pentachlorophenol (PCP) derivative shown to have bronchodilator effects because it directly relaxes smooth muscle and causes catecholamines to accumulate at the beta-receptors.
- Magnesium produces bronchodilator by competing with calcium at its binding sites.

Surgical Care: Thoracentesis or thoracostomy is indicated in pneumothorax.

- Antireflux and histamine 2 (H2)-receptor antagonist agents.
- Novel therapies to treat status asthmaticus.
- Helium/oxygen, a gas mixture with much lower density than oxygen/nitrogen mixtures, provides decreased airflow resistance.

Prognosis

Mortality and morbidity rates from empyema are high. Bad prognostic factors are:

- Inadequate antibiotic therapy
- Inadequate drainage
- Young age
- Severe infection.

Long-term sequelae are:
- Restrictive scar tissue or peel
- Decreased exercise tolerance
- Chest deformities
- Chronic restrictive pulmonary disease.

CYSTIC FIBROSIS

Introduction

Cystic fibrosis is one of the most common life-shortening; Cystic fibrosis (CF) is a genetic disorder that particularly affects the lungs and digestive system. Child who has it is more vulnerable to repeated lung infections.

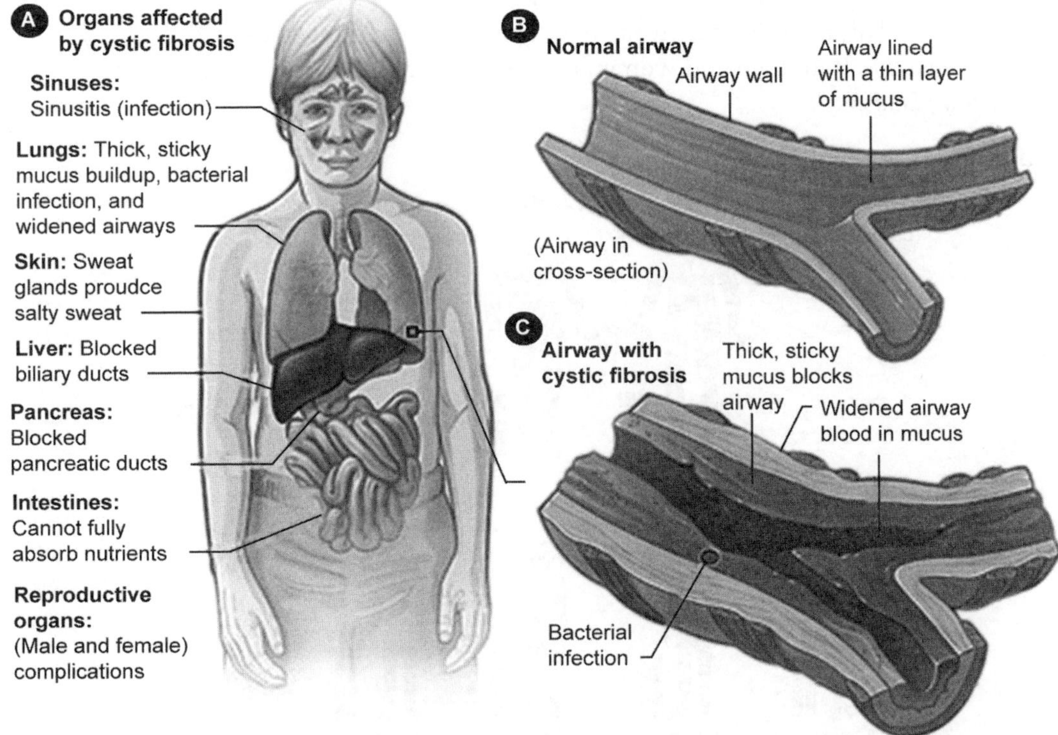

Fig. 7.41: Difference between healthy and cystic fibrosis trachea

CF is caused by a mutation in a gene called the cystic fibrosis transmembrane conductance regulator (CFTR). The product of this gene is a chloride ion channel important in creating sweat, digestive juices and mucus. Although most people without CF have two working copies (alleles) of the CFTR gene, only one is needed to prevent cystic fibrosis. CF develops when neither allele can produce a functional CFTR protein. Therefore, CF is considered an autosomal recessive disease.

Definition

Cystic fibrosis is defined as a hereditary disease affecting the exocrine (mucus) glands of the lungs, liver, pancreas and intestines, causing progressive disability due to multisystem failure.

Cystic fibrosis is a hereditary disease the symptoms of which usually appear shortly after birth. These symptoms include faulty digestion, breathing difficulties and respiratory infections due to mucus accumulation and excessive loss of salt in sweat. Cystic fibrosis (CF) affects mostly the lungs, pancreas, liver, intestines, sinuses and sex organs—*Encyclopedia*

Children with CF have an abnormality in the function of a cell protein called the CFTR. CFTR controls the flow of water and certain salts in and out of the body's cells. As the movement of salt and water in and out of cells is altered, mucus becomes thickened. The thickened mucus can affect many organs and body systems including:

- *Respiratory:* This includes sinuses and lungs.
- *Digestive*: This includes pancreas, liver, gallbladder and intestines.
- *Reproductive*: Both men and women may experience reproductive problems.
- *Sweat glands.*

Causes

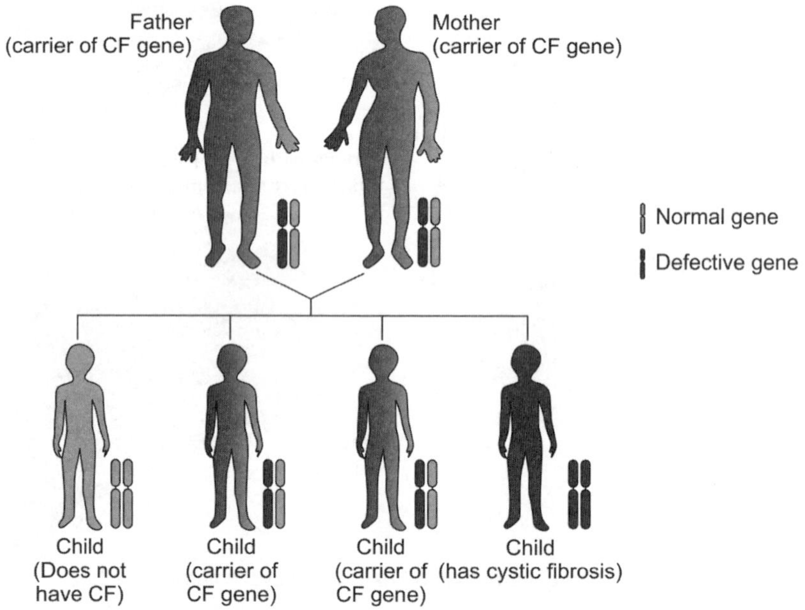

Fig. 7.42: Inheritance of cystic fibrosis (CF)

- In cystic fibrosis, a defect (mutation) in a gene changes a protein that regulates the movement of salt in and out of cells. The result is thick, sticky mucus in the respiratory, digestive and reproductive systems, as well as increased salt in sweat.
- Many different defects can occur in the gene. The type of gene mutation is associated with the severity of the condition.

- Children need to inherit one copy of the gene from each parent in order to have the disease. If children inherit only one copy, they will not develop cystic fibrosis, but will be carriers and possibly pass the gene to their own children.

Signs and Symptoms

Respiratory Signs and Symptoms

The thick and sticky mucus associated with cystic fibrosis clogs the tubes that carry air in and out of your lungs. This can cause:

- A persistent cough that produces thick (sputum) mucus
- Wheezing
- Breathlessness
- Exercise intolerance
- Repeated lung infections
- Inflamed nasal passages or a stuffy nose.

Digestive Signs and Symptoms

The thick mucus can also block tubes that carry digestive enzymes from your pancreas to your small intestine. Without these digestive enzymes, your intestines cannot fully absorb the nutrients in the food you eat. The result is often:

- Foul-smelling, greasy stools
- Poor weight gain and growth
- Intestinal blockage, particularly in newborns (meconium ileus)
- Severe constipation.

Pathophysiology

Cystic fibrosis occurs when there is a mutation in the CFTR gene. The protein created by this gene is anchored to the outer membrane of cells in the sweat glands, lungs, pancreas and other affected organs. The protein spans this membrane and acts as a channel connecting the inner part of the cell (cytoplasm) to the surrounding fluid.

In the airway this channel is primarily responsible for controlling the movement of chloride from inside to outside of the cell however in the sweat ducts it facilitates the movement of chloride from the sweat into the cytoplasm. When the CFTR protein does not work, chloride is trapped inside the cells in the airway and outside in the skin. Because chloride is negatively charged, positively charged ions also cannot cross into the cell because they are affected by the electrical attraction of the chloride ions. Sodium is the most common ion in the extracellular space and the combination of sodium and chloride creates the salt, which is lost in high amounts in the sweat of individuals with CF. This lost salt forms the basis for the sweat test.

How this malfunction of cells in cystic fibrosis causes the clinical manifestations of CF is not well understood. One theory suggests that the lack of chloride exodus through the CFTR protein leads to the accumulation of more viscous, nutrient-rich mucus in the lungs that allows bacteria to hide from the body's immune system. Another theory proposes that the CFTR protein failure leads to a paradoxical increase in sodium and chloride uptake, which, by leading to increased water reabsorption, creates dehydrated and thick mucus. Yet another theory focuses on abnormal chloride movement out of the cell, which also leads to dehydration of mucus, pancreatic secretions, biliary secretions, etc.

These theories all support the observation that the majority of the damage in CF is due to blockage of the narrow passages of affected organs with thickened secretions. These blockages lead to remodeling and infection in the lung, damage by accumulated digestive enzymes in the pancreas, blockage of the intestines by thick feces, etc.

Diagnostic Evaluation

Cystic fibrosis may be diagnosed by many different categories of testing including those such as:

- Newborn screening.
- *Sweat (chloride) test*: A test to measure the amount of chloride in the sweat. The test is done by placing a solution on the forearm (or the thigh, if the child is too small) and attaching electrodes. The skin is stimulated to sweat with a mild electric current, which does not cause pain or harm to your child. The sweat is collected onto a gauze pad and analyzed. Higher than normal amounts of chloride may suggest CF. The sweat test is not painful and usually causes only minor discomfort.
- *Genetic tests*: Blood or cells taken from a cheek scraping can be tested for mutations in the CFTR gene.

Diagnostic Procedures

- *Blood tests*: Blood tests, including pancreatic function tests, can look at infection and to see which organs may be affected.
- *Chest X-rays*: A diagnostic test that uses invisible electromagnetic energy beams to produce images of internal tissues, bones and organs onto film.
- *Pulmonary function tests*: Diagnostic tests that help to measure the lungs' ability to exchange oxygen and carbon dioxide appropriately. The tests are usually done with special machines that a child must breathe into.
- *Sputum cultures*: A diagnostic test done on the material that is coughed up from the lungs and into the mouth. A sputum culture is often done to find out if an infection is present.
- *Stool evaluations*: These are done to measure stool fat absorption.

Prenatal Diagnosis

Couples who are pregnant or who are planning a pregnancy can themselves be tested for CFTR gene mutations to determine the likelihood that their child will be born with cystic fibrosis. Testing is typically performed first on one or both parents and, if the risk of CF is found to be high, testing on the fetus can then be performed.

During pregnancy, testing can be performed on the placenta (chorionic villus sampling) or the fluid around the fetus (amniocentesis). However, chorionic villus sampling has a risk of fetal death of 1 in 100 and amniocentesis of 1 in 200, although a recent study has indicated this may actually be much lower, perhaps 1 in 1,600, so the benefits must be determined to outweigh these risks prior to going forward with testing. Alternatively, some couples choose to undergo third party reproduction with egg or sperm donors.

Management

Still now there is no treatment that can cure cystic fibrosis. However, many treatments exist for the symptoms and complications of this disease. The main goals of treatment for someone with cystic fibrosis are to prevent and treat infections, keep the airways and lungs as clear as possible and maintain adequate calories and nutrition.

The goals of treatment include:

- Preventing and controlling lung infections
- Loosening and removing mucus from the lungs
- Preventing and treating intestinal blockage
- Providing adequate nutrition.

Medications

- Antibiotics to treat and prevent lung infections
- Mucus-thinning drugs to help you cough up the mucus, which improves lung function
- Bronchodilators to help keep your airways open by relaxing the muscles around your bronchial tubes
- Oral pancreatic enzymes to help your digestive tract absorb nutrients.

Chest Physical Therapy

Loosening the thick mucus in the lungs makes it easier to cough up. Chest physical therapy helps loosen mucus. It is usually done from one to four times a day. A common technique is clapping with cupped hands on the front and back of the chest.

Pulmonary Rehabilitation

- Exercise training
- Nutritional counseling
- Breathing techniques
- Psychological counseling and group support.

Surgical and Other Procedures

- *Nasal polyp removal*: A surgery to remove nasal polyps that obstruct breathing.
- *Oxygen therapy*: The child blood-oxygen level declines, oxygen to prevent high blood pressure in the lungs (pulmonary hypertension).
- *Endoscopy and lavage*: Mucus may be suctioned from obstructed airways through an endoscope.
- *NG tube feeding*: Cystic fibrosis interferes with digestion; it cannot absorb nutrients from food very well. This tube may be threaded through your nose to your stomach or surgically implanted into the abdomen.
- *Bowel surgery*: A blockage develops in child bowel, you may need surgery to remove it. Intussusception, where a section of bowel has folded in on itself, also may require surgical repair.
- *Lung transplant*: If child have severe breathing problems, life-threatening lung complications or increasing resistance to antibiotics used to treat lung infections, lung transplantation may be an option. Because both lungs are affected by cystic fibrosis, both need to be replaced. CF does not recur in transplanted lung.

Complication

Respiratory System Complications

- *Damaged airways (bronchiectasis)*: Cystic fibrosis is one of the leading causes of bronchiectasis, a condition that damages the airways, making it harder to move air in and out of the lungs and clearing mucus from their airways (bronchial tubes).
- *Chronic infections*: Thick mucus in the lungs and sinuses provides an ideal breeding ground for bacteria and fungi. People with cystic fibrosis may have frequent bouts of bronchitis or pneumonia.
- *Growths in the nose (nasal polyps)*: Because the lining inside the nose is inflamed and swollen, it can develop soft, fleshy growths (polyps). Nasal polyps can obstruct your breathing during sleep.
- *Coughing up blood (hemoptysis)*: Over time, cystic fibrosis can cause thinning of the airway walls. As a result, teenagers and adults with cystic fibrosis may cough up blood.
- *Pneumothorax*: This condition, in which air collects in the space that separates the lungs from the chest wall, is also more common in older people with cystic fibrosis. Pneumothorax can cause chest pain and breathlessness.
- *Respiratory failure*: Over time, cystic fibrosis can damage lung tissue so badly that it no longer works. Lung function typically worsens gradually and it eventually can become life-threatening.

Digestive System Complications

- *Nutritional deficiencies*: Thick mucus can block the tubes that carry digestive enzymes from your pancreas to your intestines. Without these enzymes, your body cannot absorb protein, fats or fat-soluble vitamins.
- *Diabetes*: The pancreas produces insulin, which your body needs to use sugar. Cystic fibrosis increases the risk of diabetes. Nearly 20 percent of people with cystic fibrosis develop diabetes by age 30.
- *Blocked bile duct*: The tube that carries bile from your liver and gallbladder to your small intestine may become blocked and inflamed, leading to liver problems and sometimes gallstones.
- *Intestinal obstruction*: Intestinal obstruction can occur at any age. Children with cystic fibrosis are at higher risk of intussusception, a condition in which a section of the intestines folds in on itself like an accordion.
- *Distal intestinal obstruction syndrome (DIOS)*: DIOS is partial or complete obstruction where the small intestine meets the large intestine.

Reproductive System Complications

- Almost all men with cystic fibrosis are infertile because the tube that connects the testes and prostate gland (vas deferens) is either blocked with mucus or missing entirely.
- Certain fertility treatments and surgical procedures sometimes make it possible for men with cystic fibrosis to become fathers.
- Although women with cystic fibrosis may be less fertile than other women, it is possible for them to conceive and to have successful pregnancies. Still, pregnancy can worsen the signs and symptoms of cystic fibrosis.

Other Complications

- *Thinning of the bones (osteoporosis)*: Child with cystic fibrosis are at higher risk of developing a dangerous thinning of bones.
- *Electrolyte imbalances and dehydration*: Because child with cystic fibrosis have saltier sweat, the balance of minerals in their blood may be upset. Signs and symptoms include increased heart rate, fatigue, weakness and low blood pressure.

Nursing Management

- Give medications as ordered. Administer pancreatic enzymes with meals and snacks.
- Perform chest physiotherapy, including postural drainage and chest percussion several times a day as ordered.
- Administer oxygen therapy as ordered.
- Provide a well-balanced, high calorie, high protein diet for the patient.
- Make sure the patient receives plenty of fluids to prevent dehydration.
- Provide exercise and activity periods for the patient to promote health.
- Provide the young child with play periods and enlist the help of physical therapy department.
- Provide emotional support to the parents of children with cystic fibrosis.
- Be flexible with care and visiting hours during hospitalization to allow the child to continue school.
- Include the family in all phases of the child's care.

LUNG ABSCESS

Introduction

The lung abscesses are much less common in children than in adults, but can cause significant morbidity or mortality in children. Lung abscess is defined as necrosis of the pulmonary parenchyma caused by microbial infection. Similar with parapneumonic effusion or empyema, lung abscess is also a complication of complicated community acquired pneumonia (CAP).

The term 'necrotizing pneumonia' is used to distinguish pulmonary necrosis with multiple small abscesses from a larger cavitation, but they represent a same continuum. Pulmonary abscess can be classified as primary or secondary type. The primary lung abscess occurs in a previously healthy patient with no underlying medical disorders. The secondary lung abscess occurs in child with underlying or predisposing conditions that may be congenital (cystic fibrosis, immunodeficiency or structural abnormality as congenital cystic adenomatoid malformation (CCAM) and acquired (neuro-developmental abnormality and suppurative lung infection).

Definition

Lung abscess is defined as necrosis of the pulmonary tissue and formation of cavities containing necrotic debris or fluid caused by microbial infection. The formation of multiple small (< 2 cm) abscesses is occasionally referred to as necrotizing pneumonia or lung gangrene. Both lung abscess and necrotizing pneumonia are manifestations of a similar pathologic process.

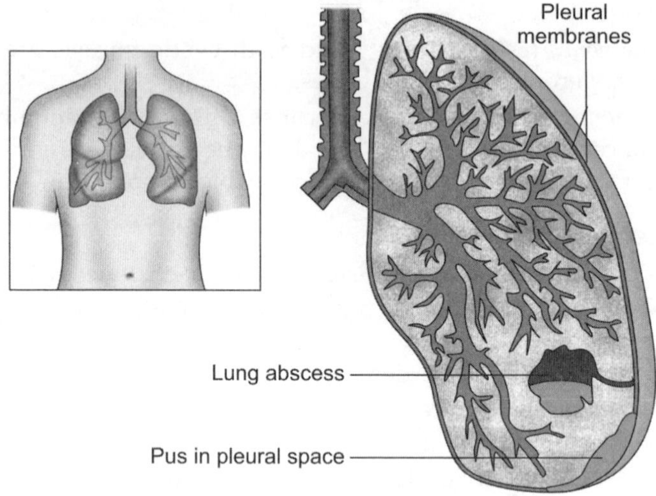

Fig. 7.43: Anatomical view of child with lung abscess

Types of Lung Abscess

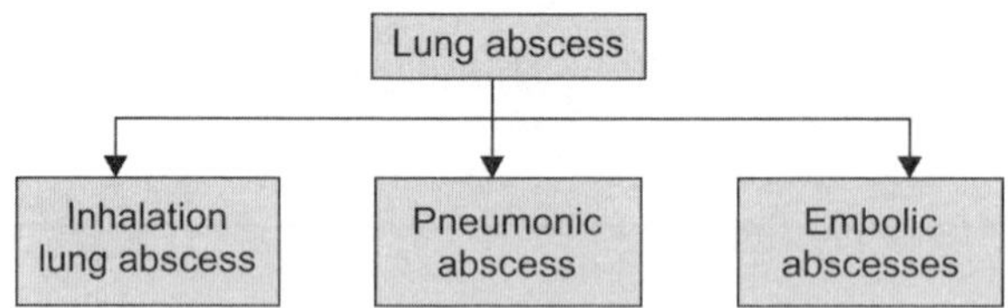

Fig. 7.44: Types of lung abscess

Causes

- *Streptococcus pneumonia* in primary lung abscess
- *Pseudomonas aeruginosa* was the most common pathogen in the secondary lung abscesses
- Chronic and persistent aspiration
- Seizure disorder
- Dental procedure and intubation.

Etiologies of pediatric lung abscess are complex:

- Both anaerobic and aerobic organisms can cause lung abscesses.
- Common isolated pathogens are listed *S. aureus* (especially CA-MRSA)
- *S. pyogenes, S. aureus* especially can progress to abscess.
- Aspiration of gastric content or bacterial of oropharynx is likely to cause lung abscess, especially the anaerobic bacteria.
- Abscesses in intubated child are usually due to nosocomial pathogens.
- Both bacterial and fungi can cause lung abscess in child with immunodeficiency.
- Mycoplasma pneumonia infection rarely cause lung abscess.

Signs and Symptoms

The most common symptoms of lung abscess in the pediatric population are cough, fever, tachypnea, chest pain, vomiting, sputum production and hemoptysis. Physical examinations may reveal tachypnea, a dull percussion note or reduced air entry in the lungs.

- High-grade fever, cough
- Chest pain
- Dyspnea
- Sputum production foul smell breaths and hemoptysis
- Blood stained purulent sputum
- Aspiration of foreign bodies
- Physical examination—dullness of percussion, decreased breath sounds.

Diagnostic Evaluation

- History collection
- Physical examination
- Blood investigations
- Increased neutrophils
- Chest radiograph
- CT scan—pulmonary masses
- Bronchoscopy—obstruction.

Management

Antibiotics Treatment

The lung abscesses in pediatric child can be effectively treated with antibiotics without surgical intervention, since most abscesses will be drained through the bronchial tree. The suggestions of empiric antibiotics are different as below:

Primary Lung Abscesses

- The antibiotics chosen for primary lung abscess should cover *Streptococcus pneumoniae, Staphylococcus aureus,* streptococcal species and Gram-negative bacilli of respiratory tract. 3rd cephalosporin plus clindamycin are the appropriate antibiotics regiment.
- Vancomycin can be substituted for clindamycin if patient is allergic to clindamycin or in those with clindamycin-resistant MRSA.

Secondary Lung Abscesses

The children who are predisposed to aspiration episode, the antibiotics should cover anaerobic pathogens.

- *Ampicillin-sulbactam or clindamycin:* Vancomycin can be substituted for clindamycin if patient is allergic to clindamycin or clindamycin-resistant MRSA.
- Piperacillin-tazobactam, ticarcillin-tazobactam or meropenem are appropriate for nosocomial aspiration episode. Vancomycin should be added if MRSA is the suspected pathogen.

- *Response to therapy:* The duration of antibiotics treatment is based on clinical response. Child with lung abscesses usually respond to antibiotics in 7–10 days.
- The recommended duration of antibiotics treatment varies from institution to institution. Some authors recommended that parental antibiotics may be given for 2–3 weeks followed by oral therapy for 4–8 weeks. However, it may be shortened to 4 weeks in presence of interventional radiology.

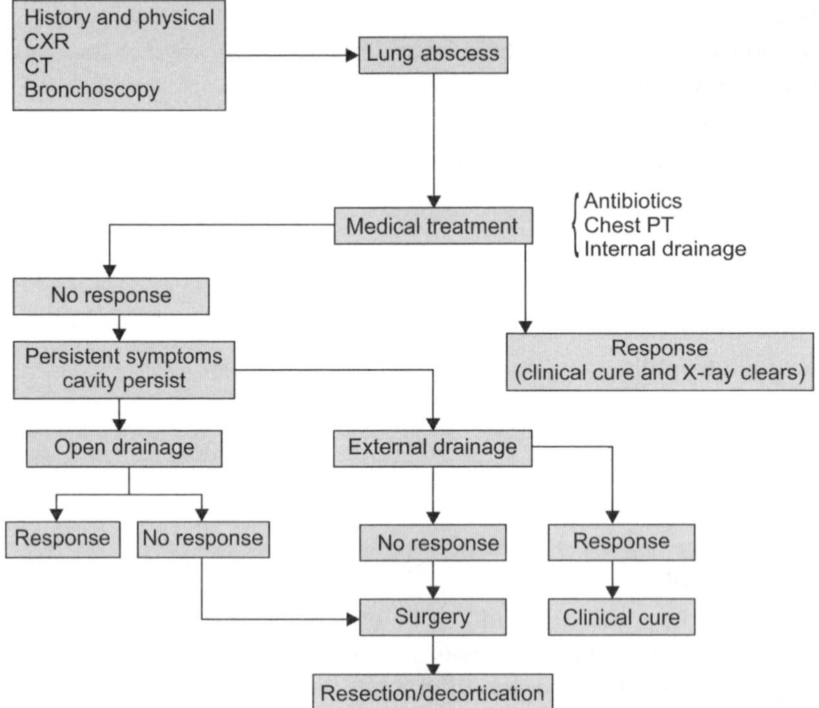

Fig. 7.45: Algorithm for lung abscess management

Surgical Intervention

Thoracoscopic surgery provides an alternative treatment option for pediatric lung abscesses and is reserved for child not responding to medical therapy and interventional radiology. Surgical intervention can provide a treatment option with favorable outcome for child who fail to response to medical therapy and drainage procedures. With advancement in radiology-guided techniques, intervention radiology has mostly replaced surgical intervention.

Usual indications of surgery include chronic abscess lasting longer than 3 months, persistent significant hemoptysis, bronchial stenosis, significant bronchiectasis and massive pulmonary necrosis. Surgical treatment is more necessary for immunocompromised child than for immunocompetent child. However, it may increase the risk of bronchoalveolar air leak.

The outcome of the thoracoscopic management is good, with few reported death and long-term complication. However, randomized control trials to compare outcome between radiological intervention and thoracoscopic management for pediatric lung abscess are needed.

Conclusion

Lung abscesses are uncommon in pediatrics. Medical treatment is still the mainstay for these child. With advancements in radiological intervention, early radiologic intervention can provide diagnostic and therapeutic benefit in some child. Surgery should be performed on those with poor response to medical treatment or radiologic intervention.

COMMON RESPIRATORY DISORDERS IN NEONATES, INFANTS AND YOUNG CHILDREN

Introduction

The symptoms and signs of respiratory distress vary and include nasal flaring; intercostal, subcostal and suprasternal retractions; weak breathing, irregular breathing, or a combination; tachypnea and apneic spells; cyanosis, pallor, mottling, delayed capillary refill, or a combination; and hypotension. In neonates, symptoms and signs may be apparent immediately on delivery or develop minutes or hours afterward.

Causes

Respiratory distress in neonates and infants has multiple causes (see Table 7.6: Respiratory disorders in neonates, infants and young children: causes of respiratory distress in neonates and infants).

Table 7.6: Causes of respiratory distress in neonates and infants

Category	Causes
Cardiac	**Right-to-left shunting with normal or increased pulmonary flow:** Transposition of the great vessels, total anomalous venous return, truncus arteriosus, hypoplastic left heart syndrome. **Right-to-left shunting with decreased pulmonary flow:** Pulmonary atresia, tetralogy of Fallot, critical pulmonic stenosis, tricuspid atresia, single ventricle with pulmonic stenosis, Ebstein's anomaly, persistent fetal circulation/persistent pulmonary hypertension.
Respiratory	**Upper tract:** Choanal atresia or stenosis, trachea-broncholaryngeal stenosis, compressive obstruction (e.g. vascular ring), tracheoesophageal anomalies (e.g. cleft, fistula). **Lower tract:** Respiratory distress syndrome, transient tachypnea of the newborn, meconium aspiration, pneumonia, sepsis, pneumothorax, congenital diaphragmatic hernia, pulmonary hypoplasia, cystic malformation of the lung, congenital deficiency of surfactant proteins B or C.
Neurologic	Intracranial hemorrhage or hypertension, over sedation (infant or maternal), diaphragmatic paralysis, neuromuscular disease, seizure disorder.
Hematologic	Methemoglobinemia, polycythemia, severe anemia.
Miscellaneous	Hypoglycemia, blood loss, metabolic disorders (e.g. acid-base disorders, hyperammonemia), hypovolemic shock.

Physiology

There are several significant differences in the physiology of the respiratory system in neonates and infants compared with that of older children and adults. These differences include:

- A more compliant collapsible chest wall
- More reliance on diaphragmatic excursions over intercostal muscles
- Collapsible extra thoracic airways.

Also, infants' smaller airway caliber gives increased airway resistance and absence of collateral ventilation increases tendency toward atelectasis. Yet, other principles of respiration are similar in adults and children.

Diagnostic Evaluation

History and Physical Examination

History in the neonate focuses on maternal and prenatal history, particularly gestational age, maternal infection or bleeding, meconium staining of amniotic fluid and oligohydramnios or polyhydramnios. Physical examination focuses on the heart and lungs. Chest wall asymmetry or sunken abdomen suggests diaphragmatic hernia. Asymmetric breath sounds suggest pneumothorax, pneumonia, or asthma. A displaced left apical impulse, heart murmur or both suggest a congenital heart defect. Assessment of BP and femoral pulses may identify circulatory collapse with or without congenital defects. Poor capillary refill reflects circulatory compromise.

In both neonates and infants, it is important to assess oxygenation and response to O_2 therapy by pulse oximetry or blood gases. Chest X-ray also is recommended.

APNEA OF PREMATURITY

Definition

Apnea of prematurity is defined as respiratory pauses > 20 sec or airflow interruption and respiratory pauses > 20 sec associated with bradycardia (< 80 beats/min), central cyanosis, or O_2 saturation < 85% in neonates born at < 37 week gestation and with no underlying disorders causing apnea.

Cause

Cause may be CNS immaturity (central) or airway obstruction. Diagnosis is by multichannel respiratory monitoring. Treatment is with respiratory stimulants for central apnea and head positioning for obstructive apnea. Prognosis is excellent; apnea resolves in most neonates by 37 week. About 25% of preterm infants have apnea of prematurity, which usually begins 2 to 3 days after birth and only rarely on the first day; apnea that develops > 14 days after birth in an otherwise healthy infant signifies a serious illness other than apnea of prematurity (e.g. sepsis). Risk increases with earlier gestational age.

Pathophysiology

Apnea of prematurity may be:

- Central apnea
- Obstructive apnea
- A mixed pattern (most common) apnea

Central apnea is caused by immaturity of medullary respiratory control centers; insufficient neural impulses from the respiratory centers in the medulla reach the respiratory muscles and the infant stops breathing. Hypoxemia and hypercarbia stimulate respiratory efforts.

Obstructive apnea is caused by obstructed airflow, neck flexion causing opposition of hypopharyngeal soft tissues, nasal occlusion, or reflex laryngospasm. Both types of apnea can cause hypoxemia, cyanosis and bradycardia if the apnea is prolonged. Among infants dying of SIDS, 18% have a history of prematurity, but apnea of prematurity does not seem to be a precursor to SIDS.

Diagnostic Evaluation

- Clinical evaluation
- Cardiorespiratory monitoring, physiologic parameter recordings
- Other causes (e.g. hypoglycemia, sepsis, intracranial hemorrhage, gastroesophageal reflux disease [GERD]) ruled out.

Although frequently attributable to immature respiratory control mechanisms, apnea of prematurity can be sign of major infectious, metabolic, thermoregulatory, respiratory, cardiac, GI and CNS dysfunction. Careful history, physical assessment and when necessary, testing should be done before accepting prematurity as cause of apnea.

Diagnosis of apnea usually is made by visual observation or by use of impedance-type cardiorespiratory monitors used continuously during assessment and ongoing care of preterm infants. Multichannel recordings of multiple physiologic parameters (e.g. chest wall movement, airflow, O_2 saturation, heart rate, brain electric activity) taken for up to 24 hours can be used as adjuncts for diagnosis and planning and monitoring treatment.

Management

- Stimulation
- Treatment of underlying disorder
- Respiratory stimulants (e.g. caffeine).

When apnea is noted, either by observation or monitor alarm, infants are stimulated, which may be all that is required; if breathing does not resume, bag-valve-mask or mouth-to-mouth-and-nose ventilation is provided. For infants at home, the physician is contacted if apnea occurs but ceases after stimulation; if intervention beyond stimulation is required, the infant should be rehospitalized and evaluated.

Frequent or severe episodes should be quickly and thoroughly evaluated and identifiable causes should be treated. If no infectious or other treatable underlying disorder is found, respiratory stimulants are indicated for treatment of frequent or severe episodes, characterized by hypoxemia, cyanosis, bradycardia, or a combination. Caffeine is the safest and most commonly used respiratory stimulant drug.

It can be given as caffeine base (loading dose 10 mg/kg followed by a maintenance dose of 2.5 mg/kg po q 24 h) or caffeine citrate, a caffeine salt that is 50% caffeine (loading dose 20 mg/kg followed by a maintenance dose of 5 to 10 mg/kg q 24 h). Caffeine is preferred because of ease of administration, less adverse effects, larger therapeutic window and less need to monitor drug levels.

Treatment continues until the infant is 34 to 35 week gestation and free from apnea requiring physical intervention for at least 5 to 7 days. Monitoring continues until the infant is free of apnea requiring intervention for 5 to 10 days.

The apnea continues despite respiratory stimulants, the infant may be given continuous positive airway pressure starting at 5 to 8 cm H_2O pressure. Intractable apneic spells require ventilator support. Discharge practices vary; some practitioners observe infants for 7 days after treatment has ended to ensure that apnea or bradycardia does not recur, whereas others discharge with caffeine if treatment seems effective.

Prevention

Hospitalized high-risk infants who have not had clinically significant cardiopulmonary events (e.g. apnea > 20 sec, apnea accompanied by central cyanosis, apnea associated with heart rate < 80 for > 5 sec) during continuous cardiorespiratory monitoring can be discharged home safely without a monitor. A home cardiorespiratory monitor may be prescribed to shorten the hospital stay for infants that are otherwise ready for discharge but are still having clinically significant cardiopulmonary events that reverse without intervention. Caffeine can be used as an adjunct to a home monitor to achieve this status. Parents should be taught how to properly use equipment, assess alarm situations, intervene (e.g. CPR) and keep a log of events. Round-the-clock telephone support and triage as well as outpatient follow-up regarding the decision to stop using the monitor should be provided. Monitors that store event information are preferred.

Infants should sleep on their back. The infant's head should be kept in the midline and the neck should be kept in the neutral position or slightly extended to prevent upper airway obstruction. All premature infants, especially those with apnea of prematurity, are at risk of apnea, bradycardia and O_2 desaturation while in a car seat and should undergo a car seat challenge test before discharge.

Prognosis

Most preterm infants stop having apneic spells by the time they reach about 37 week gestation. Apnea may continue for weeks in infants born at extremely early gestational ages (e.g. 23 to 27 week). Death is rare.

BACTERIAL TRACHEITIS (PSEUDOMEMBRANOUS CROUP)

Definition

Bacterial tracheitis is bacterial infection of the trachea. Bacterial tracheitis is uncommon and can affect children of any age. *Staphylococcus aureus* and group A β-hemolytic streptococci are involved most frequently. Onset is acute and is characterized by respiratory stridor, high fever and often copious purulent secretions. Rarely, bacterial tracheitis may develop as a complication of viral croup or endotracheal intubation. As in child with epiglottitis, the child may have marked toxicity and respiratory distress that may progress rapidly and may require intubation.

Diagnosis

Diagnosis is suspected clinically and can be confirmed by direct laryngoscopy, which reveals purulent secretions and inflammation in the subglottic area with a shaggy, purulent membrane or by lateral neck X-ray, which reveals subglottic narrowing that may be irregular as opposed to the symmetric tapering typical of croup.

Treatment

- Treatment in severe cases is the same as that of epiglottitis whenever possible, endotracheal intubation should be done in controlled circumstances by a person skilled in managing a pediatric airway.
- Initial antibiotics should cover *S. aureus* and streptococcal species; cefuroxime, some trade names Ceftin, Zinacef or an equivalent IV preparation may be appropriate, empirically unless methicillin-resistant staphylococcus is prevalent in the community, in which case vancomycin, some trade names Vancocin should be used.
- Therapy for critically ill children should be guided by a consultant knowledgeable in local susceptibility patterns. Once definitive microbial diagnosis is made, coverage is narrowed and continued for ≥ 10 days.

Complications

Complications include bronchopneumonia, sepsis and retropharyngeal cellulitis or abscess. Subglottic stenosis secondary to prolonged intubation is uncommon. Most children treated appropriately recover without sequelae.

BRONCHOPULMONARY DYSPLASIA (BPD)

Definition

BPD is chronic lung disease of the neonate that typically is caused by prolonged ventilation and is further defined by age of prematurity and extent of O_2 requirement. BPD is considered present when there is need for supplemental O_2 in premature infants who do not have other conditions requiring O_2 (e.g. pneumonia, congenital heart disease).

Causes

BPD has a multifactorial etiology. Significant risk factors include:

- Prolonged mechanical ventilation
- High concentrations of inspired O_2
- Infection
- Degree of prematurity.

Additional risk factors include:

- Pulmonary interstitial emphysema
- High peak inspiratory pressures
- Large end-tidal volumes
- Increased airway resistance
- Increased pulmonary artery pressures
- Male sex.

The lungs of premature infants are more vulnerable to the inflammatory changes that result from mechanical ventilation. The development of normal lung architecture is interrupted; fewer and larger alveoli develop and the interstitium is thickened.

Diagnosis

- National Institute of Child Health and Human Development (NICHD) criteria
- Characteristic X-ray findings.

BPD typically is suspected when a ventilated infant is unable to wean from O_2 therapy, mechanical ventilation or both. Infants typically develop worsening hypoxemia, hypercapnia and increasing O_2 requirements. Additionally, when an infant cannot be weaned within the expected time, possible underlying disorders, including patent ductus arteriosus and nursery-acquired pneumonia, should be sought.

Diagnosis the patient has to have required at least 28 days of > 21% O_2. Specific additional diagnostic criteria have been developed by the NICHD.

Chest X-ray initially shows diffuse haziness due to accumulation of exudative fluid; appearance then becomes multicystic or spongelike, with alternating areas of emphysema, pulmonary scarring and atelectasis. Alveolar epithelium may slough and macrophages, neutrophils and inflammatory mediators may be found in the tracheal aspirate.

Table 7.7: National Institute of Child Health and Human Development criteria for diagnosis of bronchopulmonary dysplasia (BPD)*

< 32 Wk Gestational Age†	≥ 32 Wk Gestational Age‡	Diagnosis
Breathing room air at 36 wk PMA or discharge, whichever comes first	Breathing room air by 56 days postnatal age or discharge, whichever comes first	Mild BPD
Need for < 30% O_2 at 36 wk PMA or discharge, whichever comes first	Need for < 30% O_2 at 56 days postnatal age or discharge, whichever comes first	Moderate BPD
Need for ≥ 30% O_2, positive pressure, or both at 35 wk PMA or discharge, whichever comes first	Need for ≥ 30% O_2, positive pressure, or both at 56 days postnatal age or discharge, whichever comes first	Severe BPD

*Note: These criteria are in addition to the baseline requirement of > 21% O_2 for at least 28 days.

†Assessed at 36 wk PMA.

‡Assessed at age 29 to 55 days.

PMA = Postmenstrual age.

Treatment

- Nutrition supplementation
- Fluid restriction
- Diuretics
- Inhaled bronchodilators
- O_2 supplementation as needed
- Respiratory syncytial virus (RSV) monoclonal antibody

Treatment is supportive and includes nutritional supplementation, fluid restriction, diuretics and perhaps inhaled bronchodilators. Respiratory infections must be diagnosed early and treated aggressively. Weaning from mechanical ventilation and supplemental O_2 should be accomplished as early as possible. Feedings should achieve an intake of 150 calories/kg/day; caloric requirements are increased because of the increased work of breathing and to aid lung healing and growth. Because pulmonary congestion and edema may develop, daily fluid intake is often restricted to about 120 to 140 mL/kg/day.

Diuretic therapy is sometimes used: Some trade names:

- Chlorothiazide
- Diuril
- Sodium diuril 10 to 20 mg/kg po bid plus spironolactone some trade names
- Aldactone 1 to 3 mg/kg once/day or split into twice-daily doses. Furosemide some trade names
- Lasix (1 to 2 mg/kg IV or IM or 1 to 4 mg/kg po q 12 to 24 h for neonates and q 8 h for older infants) may be used for short periods, but prolonged use causes hypercalciuria with resultant osteoporosis, fractures and renal calculi. If long-term diuretic use is required, chlorothiazide some trade names.

Weeks or months of additional ventilator support, supplemental O_2, or both may be required for advanced BPD. Ventilator pressures and fraction of inspired O_2 (FiO_2) should be reduced as rapidly as tolerated, but the infant should not be allowed to become hypoxemic. Arterial oxygenation should be continuously monitored with a pulse oximeter and maintained at ≥ 88% saturation. Respiratory acidosis may occur during ventilator weaning and treatment and is acceptable as long as the pH remains > 7.25 and the infant does not develop severe respiratory distress.

Prognosis

Prognosis varies with severity. Infants who still depend on mechanical ventilation at 36 wk gestation have a 20 to 30% mortality rate in infancy. Infants with BPD have a 3- to 4-fold increased rate of growth failure and neurodevelopmental problems. For several years, infants are at increased risk of lower respiratory tract infections (particularly viral pneumonia or bronchiolitis) and may quickly develop respiratory decompensation if pulmonary infection occurs. The threshold for hospitalization should be low if signs of a respiratory infection or respiratory distress develop.

CROUP (LARYNGOTRACHEOBRONCHITIS)

Definition

Croup is acute inflammation of the upper and lower respiratory tracts most commonly caused by parainfluenza virus type 1 infection. It is characterized by a barking cough and inspiratory stridor. Diagnosis is usually obvious clinically but can be made by anterioposterior neck X-ray. Treatment is antipyretics, hydration, nebulized racemic epinephrine and corticosteroids. Prognosis is excellent.

Incidence

Croup affects mainly children aged 6 months to 3 years.

Etiology

The parainfluenza viruses, especially type 1, are the major pathogens. Less common causes are respiratory syncytial virus (RSV) and influenza A and B viruses, followed by adenovirus, enterovirus, rhinovirus, measles virus and *Mycoplasma pneumoniae.* Croup caused by influenza may be particularly severe and may occur in a broader age range of children.

Seasonal outbreaks are common. Cases caused by parainfluenza viruses tend to occur in the fall; those caused by RSV and influenza viruses tend to occur in the winter and spring. Spread is usually through the air or by contact with infected secretions.

Pathophysiology

The infection causes inflammation of the larynx, trachea, bronchi, bronchioles and lung parenchyma. Obstruction caused by swelling and inflammatory exudates, develops and becomes pronounced in the subglottic region. Obstruction increases the work of breathing; rarely, tiring results in hypercapnia. Atelectasis may occur concurrently if the bronchioles become obstructed.

Signs and Symptoms

Croup is usually preceded by URI symptoms. A barking, often spasmodic, cough and hoarseness then occur, commonly at night; inspiratory stridor may be present as well. The child may awaken at night with respiratory distress, tachypnea and retractions. In severe cases, cyanosis with increasingly shallow respirations may develop as the child tires.

The obvious respiratory distress and harsh inspiratory stridor are the most dramatic physical findings. Auscultation reveals prolonged inspiration and stridor. Rales also may be present, indicating lower airway involvement. Breath sounds may be diminished with atelectasis. Fever is present in about half of children. The child's condition may seem to have improved in the morning but worsens again at night.

Recurrent episodes are often called spasmodic croup. Allergy or airway reactivity may play a role in spasmodic croup, but the clinical manifestations cannot be differentiated from those of viral croup. Also, spasmodic croup usually is initiated by a viral infection.

Diagnostic Evaluation

- Clinical presentation (e.g. barking cough, inspiratory stridor)
- Anterioposterior (AP) and lateral neck X-rays as needed.

Diagnosis is usually obvious by the barking nature of the cough. Similar inspiratory stridor can result from epiglottitis, bacterial tracheitis, foreign body, diphtheria and retropharyngeal abscess. Epiglottitis retropharyngeal abscess and bacterial tracheitis have a more rapid onset and cause a more toxic appearance, odynophagia and fewer upper respiratory tract symptoms. A foreign body may cause respiratory distress and a typical croupy cough, but fever and a preceding URI are absent. Diphtheria is excluded by a history of adequate immunization and is confirmed by identification of the organism in viral cultures of scrapings from typical grayish diphtheritic membrane.

If the diagnosis is unclear, child should have AP and lateral X-rays of the neck and chest; subepiglottic narrowing (steeple sign) seen on AP neck X-ray supports the diagnosis. Seriously ill child, in whom epiglottitis is a concern, should be examined in the operating room by appropriate specialists able to establish an airway. Child should have pulse oximetry and those with respiratory distress should have ABG measurement.

Treatment

- For out child, cool humidified air and possibly a single dose of oral corticosteroids
- For in child, humidified O_2, racemic epinephrine, some trade names

- Adrenalin
- Primatene mist and oral corticosteroids.

The illness usually lasts 3 to 4 days and resolves spontaneously. A mildly ill child may be cared for at home with hydration and antipyretics. Keeping the child comfortable is important, because fatigue and crying can aggravate the condition. Humidification devices (e.g. cold-steam vaporizers or humidifiers) may ameliorate upper airway drying and are frequently used at home by families but have not been shown to alter the course of the illness. The vast majority of children with croup recover completely.

Increasing or persistent respiratory distress, tachycardia, fatigue, cyanosis or hypoxemia, or dehydration indicates need for hospitalization. Pulse oximetry is helpful for assessing and monitoring severe cases. If O_2 saturation falls < 92%, humidified O_2 should be given and blood gases should be measured to assess CO_2 retention. A 30 to 40% inspired O_2 concentration is usually adequate. CO_2 retention ($PaCO_2$ > 45 mm Hg) generally indicates fatigue and the need for endotracheal intubation, as does inability to maintain oxygenation.

Nebulizer with Epinephrine

- Adrenalin
- Primatene mist 5 to 10 mg in 3 mL of saline q 2 h offers symptomatic improvement and relieves fatigue. However, the effects are transient; the course of the illness, the underlying viral infection and the PaO_2 are not altered by its use. Tachycardia and other adverse effects may occur.

High-dose Dexamethasone

- Decadron
- Dexasone
- Hexadrol (0.6 mg/kg IM or po once, maximum dose 10 mg) may benefit children early in the first 24 h of the disease. It can help prevent hospitalization or help the child who is hospitalized with moderate to severe croup. The viruses that most commonly cause croup do not usually predispose to secondary bacterial infection and antibiotics are rarely indicated.

MECONIUM ASPIRATION SYNDROME

Definition

Intrapartum meconium aspiration can cause inflammatory pneumonitis and mechanical bronchial obstruction, causing a syndrome of respiratory distress. Findings include tachypnea and rhonchi and cyanosis or desaturation. Diagnosis is suspected when there is respiratory distress after delivery through meconium-tinged amniotic fluid and is confirmed by chest X-ray. Treatment is vigorous suction immediately on delivery before neonates take their first breath, followed by respiratory support as needed. Prognosis depends on the underlying physiologic stressors.

Causes

Physiologic stress at the time of labor and delivery (e.g. due to hypoxia caused by umbilical cord compression or placental insufficiency or caused by infection) may cause the fetus to pass meconium into the amniotic fluid before delivery; meconium passage is noted in about 10 to 15% of births. During delivery, perhaps 5% of neonates with meconium passage aspirate the meconium, triggering lung injury and respiratory distress, termed meconium aspiration syndrome. Post-term infants delivered through reduced amniotic fluid volume are at risk of more severe disease because the less dilute meconium is more likely to cause airway obstruction.

Pathophysiology

The mechanisms by which aspiration induces the clinical syndrome probably include:

- Nonspecific cytokine release
- Airway obstruction
- Surfactant inactivation
- Chemical pneumonitis.

Underlying physiologic stressors also may contribute. If complete bronchial obstruction occurs, atelectasis results; partial blockage leads to air trapping on expiration, resulting in hyper expansion of the lungs and possibly pulmonary air leak with pneumomediastinum or pneumothorax. Persistent pulmonary hypertension can be associated with meconium aspiration as a comorbid condition or because of continuing hypoxia.

Neonates also may aspirate vernix caseosa, amniotic fluid, or blood of maternal or fetal origin during delivery and can develop respiratory distress and signs of aspiration pneumonia on chest X-ray. Treatment is supportive; if bacterial infection is suspected, cultures are taken and antibiotics are begun.

Signs and Symptoms

Signs include tachypnea, nasal flaring, retractions, cyanosis or desaturation, rales, rhonchi and greenish yellow staining of the umbilical cord, nail beds or skin. Meconium staining may be visible in the oropharynx and (on intubation) in the larynx and trachea. Neonates with air trapping may have a barrel-shaped chest and also symptoms and signs of pneumothorax, pulmonary interstitial emphysema and pneumomediastinum.

Diagnostic Evaluation

- Meconium passage
- Respiratory distress
- Characteristic X-ray findings.

Diagnosis is suspected when a neonate shows respiratory distress in the setting of meconium-tinged amniotic fluid and is confirmed by chest X-ray showing hyperinflation with variable areas of atelectasis and flattening of the diaphragm. Initial X-ray findings can be confused with the findings of transient tachypnea of the newborn. Fluid may be seen in the lung fissures or pleural spaces and air may be seen in the soft tissues or mediastinum. Because meconium may enhance bacterial growth and meconium aspiration syndrome is difficult to distinguish from bacterial pneumonia, cultures of blood and tracheal aspirate also should be taken.

Treatment

- Suctioning at birth before the first breath
- Endotracheal intubation as needed

- Mechanical ventilation as needed
- Supplemental O_2 as needed
- IV antibiotics.

Immediate treatment, indicated for all neonates delivered through meconium, is vigorous suctioning of the mouth and nasopharynx using a De Lee suction apparatus as soon as the head is delivered and before the neonate breathes and cries. If suction returns no meconium and the neonate appears vigorous, observation without further intervention is appropriate. If the neonate has labored or depressed respirations, poor muscle tone, or is bradycardia (< 100 beats/min), the trachea should be intubated with a 3.5- or 4.0-mm endotracheal tube.

A meconium aspirator connected to a suction apparatus is attached directly to the endotracheal tube, which then serves as the suction catheter. Suction is maintained while the endotracheal tube is removed. Reintubation and continuous positive airway pressure are indicated for continued respiratory distress, followed by mechanical ventilation and admission to the neonatal ICU as needed. Because positive pressure ventilation enhances risk of pulmonary air-leak syndrome, regular evaluation (including physical examination and chest X-ray) is important to detect these complications. These complications should be sought immediately in any intubated neonate whose BP, perfusion, or O_2 saturation suddenly worsens. Additional treatments may include surfactant for mechanically ventilated neonates with high O_2 requirements, which can decrease the need for extracorporeal membrane oxygenation and antibiotics (usually Ampicillin).

Prognosis

Prognosis is generally good, although it varies with the underlying physiologic stressors; overall mortality is slightly increased. Infants with meconium aspiration syndrome may be at greater risk of asthma in later life.

PERSISTENT PULMONARY HYPERTENSION OF THE NEWBORN

Definition

Persistent pulmonary hypertension of the newborn is the persistence of or reversion to pulmonary arteriolar constriction, causing a severe reduction in pulmonary blood flow and right-to-left shunting. Symptoms and signs include tachypnea, retractions and severe cyanosis or desaturation unresponsive to O_2.

Causes

The most common causes involve:

- *Perinatal asphyxia or hypoxia*: A history of meconium staining of amniotic fluid or meconium in the trachea is common. Hypoxia triggers reversion to or persistence of intense pulmonary arteriolar constriction, a normal state in the fetus.

Additional causes include:

- Premature ductus arteriosus or foramen ovale closure, which increases fetal pulmonary blood flow and may be triggered by maternal NSAID use
- Polycythemia, which obstructs blood flow

- Congenital diaphragmatic hernia, in which one lung is severely hypoplastic, forcing most of the pulmonary blood flow through the other lung
- Neonatal sepsis presumably because vasoconstrictive prostaglandins are produced by activation of the cyclo-oxygenase pathway by bacterial phospholipids.

Pathophysiology

Whatever the cause, elevated pressure in the pulmonary arteries causes abnormal smooth muscle development and hypertrophy in the walls of the small pulmonary arteries and arterioles and right-to-left shunting via the ductus arteriosus or a foramen ovale, resulting in intractable systemic hypoxemia. Both pulmonary and systemic resistances are high, which leads to an increased load on the heart. This load increase may result in right heart dilation, tricuspid insufficiency and right heart failure.

Signs and Symptoms

Symptoms and signs include tachypnea, retractions and severe cyanosis or desaturation unresponsive to supplemental O_2. In infants with a right-to-left shunt via a patent ductus arteriosus, oxygenation is higher in the right brachial artery than in the descending aorta; thus cyanosis may be differential (i.e. O_2 saturation in the lower extremities is 5% or lower than in the right upper extremity).

Diagnostic Evaluation

- Cyanosis unresponsive to O_2 therapy
- Echocardiogram
- X-ray to identify underlying disorders.

Diagnosis should be suspected in any near-term infant with arterial hypoxemia, cyanosis, or both, especially one with a suggestive history whose O_2 saturation does not improve with 100% O_2. Diagnosis is confirmed by echocardiogram, which can confirm the presence of elevated pressures in the pulmonary artery and simultaneously can exclude congenital heart disease. Lung fields on X-ray may be normal or may show changes due to the underlying disorder (e.g. meconium aspiration syndrome, neonatal pneumonia, congenital diaphragmatic hernia).

Treatment

- O_2 to dilate pulmonary vasculature and improve oxygenation
- Mechanical ventilation support
- Use of nitric oxide considered
- Extracorporeal membrane oxygenation as needed
- Circulatory support.

Treatment with O_2, which is a potent pulmonary vasodilator, is begun immediately to prevent disease progression. O_2 is delivered via bag and mask or mechanical ventilation; mechanical distention of alveoli aids vasodilation. FiO_2 should initially be 1 but can be titrated downward to maintain PaO_2 between 50 and 90 mm Hg to minimize lung injury.

Once PaO_2 is stabilized, weaning can be attempted by reducing FiO_2 in decrements of 2 to 3%, then reducing ventilator pressures; changes should be gradual, because a large drop in PaO_2 can cause recurrent pulmonary artery vasoconstriction. High-frequency oscillatory ventilation expands and ventilates the lungs while minimizing barotraumas and should be considered for infants with underlying lung disease in which atelectasis and ventilation/perfusion (V/Q) mismatch may exacerbate the hypoxemia of persistent pulmonary hypertension of the newborn.

Inhaled nitric oxide relaxes endothelial smooth muscle, dilating pulmonary arterioles, which increases pulmonary blood flow and rapidly improves oxygenation in as many as half of child. Initial dose is 20 ppm, titrated downward by effect. Extracorporeal membrane oxygenation may be used in newborns with severe hypoxic respiratory failure defined by an oxygenation index > 35 to 40 despite maximum respiratory support.

Normal fluid, electrolyte, glucose and Ca levels must be maintained. Infants should be kept in a neutral thermal environment and treated with antibiotics for possible sepsis until culture results are known. Inotropes and pressors may be required as part of circulatory support.

Prognosis

An oxygenation index (mean airway pressure [cm H_2O] × fraction of inspired O_2 [FiO_2] × 100/PaO_2) > 40 predicts mortality of > 50%. Overall mortality ranges from 10 to 80% and is directly related to the oxygenation index but also varies with underlying disorder. However, many survivors (perhaps 1/3) exhibit developmental delay, hearing deficits, functional disabilities, or a combination. This rate of disability may be no different from that of other infants with severe illness.

PULMONARY AIR-LEAK SYNDROMES

Definition

Pulmonary air-leak syndromes involve dissection of air out of the normal pulmonary airspaces. Air-leak syndromes include pulmonary interstitial emphysema, pneumomediastinum, pneumothorax, pneumopericardium, pneumoperitoneum and subcutaneous emphysema. Pneumothorax and pneumomediastinum occur in 1 to 2% of normal neonates, probably because large negative intrathoracic forces created when the neonate starts breathing occasionally disrupt alveolar epithelium, which allows air to move from the alveoli into extra-alveolar soft tissues or spaces.

Air leak is more common and severe among neonates with lung disease, who are at risk because of poor lung compliance and the need for high airway pressures (e.g. in respiratory distress) or because of air trapping (e.g. meconium aspiration syndrome), which leads to alveolar overdistention.

Diagnostic Evaluation

Many affected neonates are asymptomatic; diagnosis is suspected clinically or because of deterioration in O_2 status and is confirmed by X-ray. Treatment varies by type of air leak but in ventilated infants always involves lowering inspiratory pressures to lowest tolerated settings. High-frequency ventilators may be helpful but are of unproven benefit.

Classification

Pulmonary interstitial emphysema: Pulmonary interstitial emphysema is leakage of air from alveoli into the pulmonary interstitium, lymphatics, or subpleural space. It usually occurs in infants with poor lung compliance, such as those with respiratory distress syndrome who are being treated with mechanical ventilation, but it may occur spontaneously. One or both lungs may be involved and pathology may be focal or generalized within each lung. If dissection of air is widespread, respiratory status may acutely worsen because lung compliance suddenly is reduced.

Chest X-ray shows a variable number of cystic or linear lucencies in the lung fields. Some lucencies are elongated; others appear as enlarged subpleural cysts ranging from a few millimeters to several centimeters in diameter. Pulmonary interstitial emphysema may resolve dramatically over 1 or 2 days or persist on X-ray for weeks. Some infants with severe respiratory disease and pulmonary interstitial emphysema develop bronchopulmonary dysplasia and the cystic changes of long-standing pulmonary interstitial emphysema then merge into the X-ray picture of BPD.

Management

Treatment is mainly supportive. If one lung is significantly more involved than the other, the infant may be laid down on the side of the lung with the more severe pulmonary interstitial emphysema; this will help to compress the lung with pulmonary interstitial emphysema, thereby decreasing air leakage and perhaps improving ventilation of the normal (elevated) lung. If one lung is very severely affected and the other is mildly affected or uninvolved, differential bronchial intubation and ventilation of the less-involved lung also may be attempted; total atelectasis of the nonintubated lung soon results. Because only one lung is now being ventilated, ventilator settings and fraction of inspired O_2 may need to be altered. After 24 to 48 hours, the endotracheal tube is pulled back into the trachea, at which time the air leak may have stopped.

Pneumomediastinum

Pneumomediastinum is dissection of air into connective tissue of the mediastinum, the air may further dissect into the subcutaneous tissues of the neck and scalp. Pneumomediastinum usually causes no symptoms or signs, though subcutaneous air causes crepitus. Diagnosis is by X-ray; in an anteroposterior view, air may form a lucency around the heart, whereas on a lateral view, air lifts the lobes of the thymus away from the cardiac silhouette (spinnaker sail sign). No treatment is usually needed and the condition resolves spontaneously.

Pneumopericardium

Pneumopericardium is dissection of air into the pericardial sac. It affects mechanically ventilated infants almost exclusively. Most cases are asymptomatic, but if sufficient air accumulates, it can cause cardiac tamponade. Diagnosis is suspected if infants experience acute circulatory collapse and is confirmed by lucency around the heart on X-ray or by return of air on pericardiocentesis using angiocatheter and syringe. Treatment is pericardiocentesis followed by surgical insertion of a pericardial tube.

Pneumoperitoneum

Pneumoperitoneum is dissection of air into the peritoneum. It is generally not clinically significant but must be distinguished from pneumoperitoneum due to a ruptured abdominal viscus, which is a surgical emergency. Diagnosis is made by abdominal X-ray and physical examination. Clinical symptoms that include abdominal rigidity, absent bowel sounds and signs of sepsis suggest abdominal viscus injury.

Pneumothorax

Pneumothorax is dissection of air into the pleural space; sufficient accumulation of air causes tension pneumothorax. Although sometimes asymptomatic, pneumothorax typically causes worsening of tachypnea, grunting and cyanosis. Breath sounds decrease and the chest enlarges on the affected side. Tension pneumothorax causes cardiovascular collapse.

Diagnosis is suspected by deterioration of respiratory status, by transillumination of the chest with a fiberoptic probe, or both. Diagnosis is confirmed by chest X-ray or in the case of tension pneumothorax, return of air during thoracentesis.

Most small pneumothoraces resolve spontaneously, but larger and tension pneumothoraces require evacuation of the air in the pleural cavity. In tension pneumothorax, a scalp vein needle or an angiocatheter and syringe can be used to temporarily evacuate free air from the pleural space. Definitive treatment is insertion of an 8 or 10 French chest tube attached to continuous suction. Follow-up auscultation, transillumination and X-ray confirm that the tube is functioning properly.

RESPIRATORY DISTRESS SYNDROME (HYALINE MEMBRANE DISEASE)

Definition

Respiratory distress syndrome is caused by pulmonary surfactant deficiency in the lungs of neonates, most commonly in those born at < 37 week gestation. Risk increases with degree of prematurity. Symptoms and signs include grunting respirations, use of accessory muscles and nasal flaring appearing soon after birth. Diagnosis is clinical; prenatal risk can be assessed with tests of fetal lung maturity. Treatment is surfactant therapy and supportive care.

Causes

- Surfactant is not produced in adequate amounts until relatively late in gestation; thus, risk of respiratory distress syndrome (RDS) increases with greater prematurity. Other risk factors include multifetal pregnancies, maternal diabetes and being male and white.
- Risk decreases with fetal growth restriction, preeclampsia or eclampsia, maternal hypertension, prolonged rupture of membranes and maternal corticosteroid use.
- Rare cases are hereditary, caused by mutations in surfactant protein (SP-B and SP-C) and ATP-binding cassette transporter A3 (ABCA3) genes.

Pathophysiology

Pulmonary surfactant is a mixture of phospholipids and lipoproteins secreted by type II pneumocytes. It diminishes the surface tension of the water film that lines alveoli, thereby decreasing the tendency of alveoli to collapse and the work required to inflate them.

With surfactant deficiency, the lungs become diffusely atelectatic, triggering inflammation and pulmonary edema. Because blood passing through the atelectatic portions of lung is not oxygenated (forming a right-to-left intrapulmonary shunt), the infant becomes hypoxemic. Lung compliance is decreased, thereby increasing the work of breathing. In severe cases, the diaphragm, intercostal muscles fatigue, CO_2 retention and respiratory acidosis develop.

Signs and Symptoms

Signs and symptoms include rapid, labored and grunting respirations appearing immediately or within a few hours after delivery, with suprasternal and substernal retractions and flaring of the nasal alae. As atelectasis and respiratory failure progress, symptoms worsen, with cyanosis, lethargy, irregular breathing and apnea. Neonates weighing < 1000 g may have lungs so stiff that they are unable to initiate or sustain respirations in the delivery room. On examination, breath sounds are decreased. Peripheral pulses may be decreased with peripheral extremity edema and decreased urine output.

Diagnostic Evaluation

- Clinical presentation
- ABG (hypoxemia and hypercapnia)
- Chest X-ray
- Blood, CSF and tracheal aspirate cultures.

Diagnosis is by clinical presentation, including recognition of risk factors; ABGs showing hypoxemia and hypercapnia; and chest X-ray. Chest X-ray shows diffuse atelectasis classically described as having a ground-glass appearance with visible air bronchograms; appearance correlates loosely with clinical severity.

Treatment

- Surfactant
- Supplementary O_2 as needed
- Mechanical ventilation as needed.

Prognosis with treatment is excellent; mortality is < 10%. With adequate ventilatory support alone, surfactant production eventually begins and once production begins, RDS resolves within 4 or 5 days. However, in the meantime, severe hypoxemia can result in multiple organ failure and death.

Specific treatment is intratracheal surfactant therapy. This therapy requires endotracheal intubation, which also may be necessary to achieve adequate ventilation and oxygenation. Less premature infants (those > 1 kg) and those with lower O_2 requirements (fraction of inspired O_2 [FiO_2] < 40 to 50%) may respond well to supplemental O_2 alone or to treatment with nasal continuous positive airway pressure. A treatment strategy of early (within 20 to 30 min after birth) surfactant therapy is associated with significant decrease in duration of mechanical ventilation, lesser incidence of air leak syndromes and lower incidence of bronchopulmonary dysplasia.

Surfactant hastens recovery and decreases risk of pneumothorax, interstitial emphysema, intraventricular hemorrhage, bronchopulmonary dysplasia and neonatal mortality in the hospital and at 1 year. However, neonates who receive surfactant for established RDS have an increased risk of apnea of prematurity. Options for surfactant replacement include beractant.

Complications

Complications of RDS include intraventricular hemorrhage, periventricular white matter injury, tension pneumothorax, bronchopulmonary dysplasia, sepsis and neonatal death. Intracranial complications have been linked to hypoxemia, hypercarbia, hypotension, swings in arterial BP and low cerebral.

Prevention

When a fetus must be delivered between 24 week and 34 week, giving the mother 2 doses of betamethasone.

TRANSIENT TACHYPNEA OF THE NEWBORN (NEONATAL WET LUNG SYNDROME)

Introduction

Transient tachypnea of the newborn is respiratory distress caused by delayed resorption of fetal lung fluid. Transient tachypnea of the newborn affects premature infants, term infants delivered by cesarean section and infants born with respiratory depression, all of whom have delayed clearance of fetal lung fluid. For unknown reasons, maternal diabetes and asthma are also risk factors. The disorder can occur in preterm infants with respiratory distress syndrome and in term infants born through meconium-stained amniotic fluid.

Definition

Transient tachypnea of the newborn is suspected when the infant develops respiratory distress shortly after birth. Symptoms include tachypnea, intracostal and subcostal retractions, grunting, nasal flaring and possible cyanosis.

Diagnostic Evaluation

Pneumonia and sepsis may have similar manifestations, so chest X-ray, CBC and blood cultures usually are done. Chest X-ray shows hyperinflated lungs with streaky perihilar markings, giving the appearance of a shaggy heart border while the periphery of the lungs is clear. Fluid is often seen in the lung fissures.

Treatment

If initial findings are indeterminate or suggest infection, antibiotics (e.g. ampicillin, omnipen principen, gentamicin, garamycinare) given while awaiting culture results. Recovery usually occurs within 2 to 3 days. Treatment is supportive and involves giving O_2 by hood and monitoring ABGs or pulse oximetry. Rarely, extremely premature infants, those with neurologic depression at birth, or both require continuous positive airway pressure and occasionally even mechanical ventilation.

GASTROINTESTINAL (GI) SYSTEM

INTESTINAL (BOWEL) OBSTRUCTION

Definition

Bowel obstruction (or intestinal obstruction) is a mechanical or functional obstruction of the intestines, preventing the normal transit of the products of digestion. It can occur at any level distal to the duodenum of the small intestine and is a medical emergency. Although many cases are not treated surgically, it is a surgical problem.

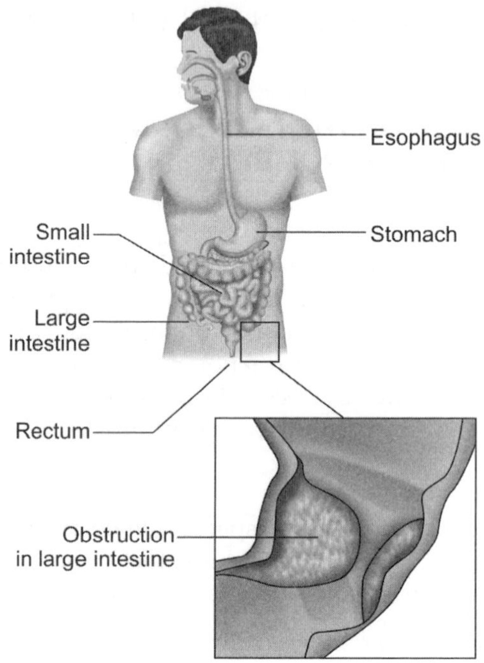

Fig. 7.46: Bowel obstruction

Bowel Obstruction in Children

Fetal and neonatal bowel obstructions are often caused by an intestinal atresia, where there is a narrowing or absence of a part of the intestine. These atresias are often discovered before birth via a sonogram and treated with using laparotomy after birth. If the area affected is small, then the surgeon may be able to remove the damaged portion and join the intestine back together. In instances where the narrowing is longer, or the area is damaged and cannot be used for a period of time, a temporary stoma may be placed.

Classification

- Small bowel obstruction
- Large bowel obstruction

Incidence

Malrotation of the bowel with midgut volvulus occurs at a rate of 1 case per 600 infants. Jejunoileal atresia and stenosis have a combined reported incidence of 1 case per 330–1500 live births. These conditions are common among child with maternal polyhydramnios; 38% have jejunal atresia and 15% have ileal atresia. Overall, the atresia is almost equally divided between the jejunum (51%) and ileum (49%). Jejunoileal atresia is twice as common as duodenal atresia and is more common than colonic atresia. Duodenal atresia and stenosis, collectively, are relatively rare causes of obstruction that occur at a rate of just 1 case per 10,000 live births. The incidence of alimentary tract duplications is 1 case per 4,500 populations.

Causes

Causes of small bowel obstruction include:

- Adhesions from previous abdominal surgery
- Hernias containing bowel
- Crohn's disease causing adhesions or inflammatory strictures
- Neoplasm's, benign or malignant
- Intussusception in children
- Volvulus
- Superior mesenteric artery syndrome, a compression of the duodenum by the superior mesenteric artery and the abdominal aorta
- Ischemic strictures
- Foreign bodies (e.g. gallstones in gallstone ileus, swallowed objects)
- Intestinal atresia
- Carcinoid rare, preferred location: Ileum.

Causes of large bowel obstruction include:

- Neoplasm
- Hernias
- Inflammatory bowel disease
- Colonic volvulus (sigmoid, cecal, transverse colon)
- Fecal impaction
- Colon atresia
- Benign strictures (diverticular disease)
- Endometriosis.

Causes of Acute Intestinal Obstructions

Intussusceptions

Intussusception is the most common cause of intestinal obstruction in infants and children aged 3 months to 6 years and is the second most common cause of acute abdomen in this age group.

It occurs when a proximal segment of the intestine (called intussusceptum) telescopes or invaginates into the lumen of another immediately adjacent distal segment (called intussuscipiens). The peak age of presentation is between 5 and 10 months. Intussusception is more common in males. Less than 1% of intussusceptions are found in neonates; however, cases have been reported in newborns and premature babies. Early diagnosis and prompt treatment prevent catastrophic complications.

In 95% of cases, the intussusception is in the ileocecal area. Ileoileal and colocolic intussusceptions are rare. Occasionally, an ileoileal intussusception of the terminal ileum may progress through the ileocecal valve, a condition known as ileoileocolic intussusception. Ileoileal intussusceptions are seen as a postoperative complication after extensive retroperitoneal dissections, as in surgery for neuroblastoma or Wilms tumors.

Incarcerated Hernias

Incarcerated hernias occur when the contents of a hernia sac cannot be reduced back into the abdominal cavity. Incarcerated hernias can be inguinal, femoral, or umbilical. Inguinal and femoral incarcerated hernias are most common in both sexes. The vast majority of inguinal hernias in children are indirect hernias.

Most direct hernias in the pediatric population occur following repair of an indirect hernia. Femoral hernias, which tend to incarcerate, are extremely rare in children and are the only hernias that occur in girls more often than boys. Incarceration represents the most common complication associated with inguinal hernias. In several large series, incarceration was reported in 6–18% of child. The incidence could be as high as 30% for infants younger than 2 months.

Umbilical hernias are very common in children, rarely incarcerate and often close spontaneously by age 5 years. Internal hernias are extremely rare and cause bowel obstruction in children. Hernias in the mesentery, mesocolon, mesosigmoid and Winslow foramen and defects in the falciform ligament have been described.

Malrotation of Bowel with Midgut Volvulus

Intestinal malrotation refers to errors of midgut rotation around the superior mesenteric artery axis and the subsequent fixation of the midgut in the peritoneal cavity. Nonrotation, incomplete rotation, reversed rotation and alterations of fixation including the internal hernias (mesocolic, paraduodenal) and the mobile cecum are among the many embryonic variants of the anomaly. Malrotation is always present in child with abdominal wall defects (gastroschisis, omphalocele) and child with congenital diaphragmatic hernia. It is often associated with other congenital and acquired lesions of the GI tract, such as Hirschsprung's disease, intussusception and atresia of the jejunum, duodenum and esophagus.

In children, the most common form of malrotation occurs when the process of rotation is incomplete and the ligament of treitz or the cecum is abnormally located or fixed. The mesenteric attachment of the midgut to the posterior abdominal wall is narrow and predisposes the midgut to twist around an axis formed by the superior mesenteric artery (midgut volvulus). Complete volvulus of the bowel for more than 1–2 hours can totally obstruct blood supply to the bowel, leading to complete necrosis of the involved segment.

Postoperative Adhesions

Adhesive small-bowel obstruction is an annoying surgical complication. Its incidence seems to be lower after laparoscopic procedures than after laparotomy. Postoperative adhesions are responsible for about 7% of the intestinal obstructions in infants and children. A single adhesion causes most obstructions, regardless of the nature of the previous illness or type of abdominal surgery. Onset of obstructive symptoms can range from 2 days to 10 years postsurgery, although most adhesions (> 50%) occur within the first 3–6 postoperative months and a few occur after 2 years.

Annular Pancreas

This rare condition involves a lesion that consists of a thin, flat ring of histologically normal pancreatic tissue that surrounds the descending duodenum in an anomalous position. Annular pancreas results from abnormal rotation of the ventral pancreatic bud and usually functions normally, barring development of pancreatitis or an obstruction of the duct of Wirsung. An annular pancreas can be asymptomatic or can cause external compression on the second portion of the duodenum, which creates a partial or complete obstruction. Annular pancreas is almost invariably associated with an intrinsic cause of duodenal obstruction (duodenal atresia).

Mesocolic Hernia

Mesocolic hernia is a malrotation abnormality. Nonfixed colonic and duodenal mesenteries lead to formation of potential hernia pouches, which transiently and recurrently entrap the bowel and cause partial obstructions. Their exact incidence is still unknown, but fortunately, they are rather rare. The internal hernias may be right-sided or left-sided and can sometimes incarcerate and strangulate. The mesocolic hernia is not a malrotation anomaly per se but occurs in the presence of a rotational anomaly. Mesocolic hernias can also occur as a consequence of retroperitoneal surgery in cases in which a mesenteric defect is not properly closed during the procedure.

Necrotizing Enterocolitis

Strictures from previous necrotizing enterocolitis (NEC) occur most often in premature infants. These strictures account for 15% of deaths in infants older than 1 week whose birth weights were less than 1500 g. In 11–36% of child, NEC can produce strictures that subsequently cause intestinal obstruction. Strictures usually occur within 1–6 months following an acute NEC episode. While the exact cause of NEC remains unknown, multiple factors probably lead to ischemic or hypoxemic insult of the intestinal mucosa, followed by bacterial invasion of the denuded mucosa with gram-negative septicemia and intestinal necrosis. The most common sites for these strictures are the terminal ileum and the colon.

Causes of Chronic Partial Intestinal Obstructions

Most chronic partial intestinal obstructions are due to anatomic abnormalities such as intestinal duplications, hernias and intestinal stenosis. Rarely, children may experience obstruction due to trichobezoar; this usually occurs in young females with trichotillomania (irresistible desire to pull out ones own hair) or trichophagia. When the trichobezoar has a long tail that extends beyond the stomach into the small intestine it is called Rapunzel syndrome.

Cecal Volvulus

Cecal volvulus is a rare disorder of nonfixation (i.e. a mobile cecum), rather than a complete malrotation. Cecal volvulus most commonly occurs as axial twisting of the cecum, ascending colon and terminal ileum. It has also been described in children who have undergone a malone antegrade continent enema (MACE) procedure, in which the cecal appendix is used as a tubular conduit between the abdominal wall and the cecum, creating a stoma through which the patient can get an antegrade enema to achieve 'social continence.'

Duplication Cysts

Duplications of the alimentary tract comprise a group of rare malformations that vary greatly in appearance, size, location and symptoms.

The three characteristics of alimentary tract duplications proposed by Ladd and Gross include:

1. Contiguity with and strong adherence to some part of the alimentary tract
2. A smooth muscle coat (usually in 2 layers)
3. A mucosal lining that consists of one or more types of cells normally observed in the alimentary tract.

Most duplication is truly enteric cysts; few of them actually represent attempts to double the alimentary tract. The intestinal epithelium may or may not correspond to the epithelium of the adjacent intestinal structure. Gastric mucosa is the most common ectopic tissue found. Intestinal obstruction, bleeding, infection and carcinomatous degeneration have been observed with these anomalies and early correct diagnosis is vital. Most symptoms are caused by the mass effect and the duplication causes either a partial or complete small-bowel obstruction.

Signs and Symptoms

Depending on the level of obstruction, bowel obstruction can present with:

- Abdominal pain and abdominal distension.
- Vomiting, fecal vomiting and constipation.
- Obstruction may be due to causes within the bowel lumen, within the wall of the bowel, or external to the bowel (such as compression, entrapment or volvulus).
- Bowel obstruction may be complicated by dehydration and electrolyte abnormalities due to vomiting; respiratory compromise from pressure on the diaphragm by a distended abdomen, or aspiration of vomitus; bowel ischemia or perforation from prolonged distension or pressure from a foreign body.
- In small bowel obstruction the pain tends to be colicky (cramping and intermittent) in nature, with spasms lasting a few minutes.
- The pain tends to be central and mid-abdominal. Vomiting occurs before constipation. In large bowel obstruction the pain is felt lower in the abdomen and the spasms last longer. Constipation occurs earlier and vomiting may be less prominent.
- Proximal obstruction of the large bowel may present as small bowel obstruction.

Diagnostic Evaluation

The main diagnostic tools are blood tests, X-rays of the abdomen, CT scanning and/or ultrasound. If a mass is identified, biopsy may determine the nature of the mass radiological signs of bowel obstruction include bowel distension and the presence of multiple (more than six) gas-fluid levels on supine and erect abdominal radiographs. Contrast enema or small bowel series or CT scan can be used to define the level of obstruction, whether the obstruction is partial or complete and to help define the cause of the obstruction.

Management

Some causes of bowel obstruction may resolve spontaneously; many require operative treatment. In adults, frequently the surgical intervention and the treatment of the causative lesion are required. In malignant large bowel obstruction, endoscopically placed self-expanding metal stents may be used to temporarily relieve the obstruction as a bridge to surgery, or as palliation.

SMALL BOWEL OBSTRUCTION (SBO)

Introduction

In the small bowel obstructions it is often said that 'ever let the sun rise or set on small-bowel obstruction' because they are sometimes fatal if treatment is delayed. This traditional surgical canon is no longer followed, largely because of improvements in radiologic imaging of small bowel obstruction, which allow confident distinction between simple obstructions, that can be treated conservatively and obstructions associated with surgical emergencies (volvulus, closed-loop obstructions, ischemic bowel, incarcerated hernias, etc.). A small flexible tube may be inserted from the nose into the stomach to help decompress the dilated bowel. This tube is uncomfortable but does relieve the abdominal cramps, distension and vomiting. Intravenous therapy is utilized and the urine output is monitored with a catheter in the bladder.

Definition

An obstruction can occur when there is no open passageway for food or digested food waste to move through the bowel, or intestine. It can occur anywhere in the small or large intestine and there can be a partial or complete blockage.

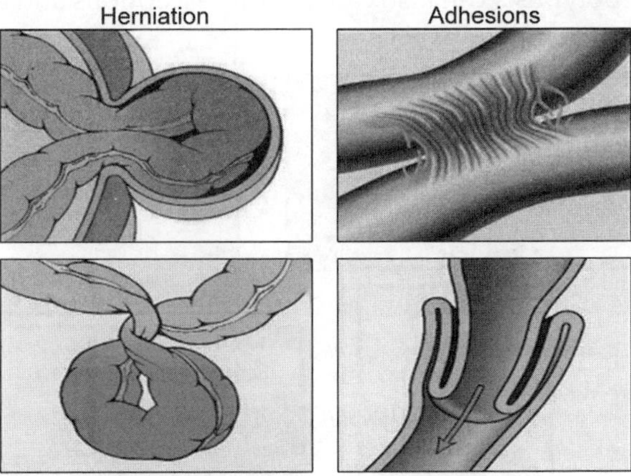

Fig. 7.47: Small bowel obstructions

Classification

Many different pathologic processes can cause small-bowel obstructions. These processes can be divided into acute intestinal obstructions and chronic partial intestinal obstructions. These conditions can be further subdivided into those that present in the immediate postnatal period and those occur later in childhood.

- Acute intestinal obstructions
- Chronic partial intestinal obstructions.

Etiology (Causes)

Small bowel obstruction caused by Crohn's disease, peritoneal carcinomatosis, sclerosing peritonitis, radiation enteritis and postpartum bowel obstruction are typically treated conservatively, i.e. without surgery. Conversely, a small bowel obstruction in a 'virgin abdomen' (an abdomen that has not seen an operation) is almost never treated conservatively.

Types of Small Bowel Obstructions

Intussusception

- Although the cause of intussusception is unknown in 90–95% of children, a viral etiology is suspected because of its seasonal predisposition for spring and autumn, as well as higher incidence of adenoid hypertrophy in children who suffered intussusceptions.
- Gastroenteritis, rotavirus infection or allergic stimuli is believed to cause intestinal lymphoid tissue to swell and become a lead point to pull the mass into adjacent proximal intestine. In child younger than 1 month and older than 3 years, pathologic lesions serve as the lead points that produce the condition.
- Intussusception is a well-described complication of child with Meckel diverticulum, Waugh syndrome, cocaine abuse, laxative use and even antibiotic use, presumably due to motility derangements caused by some of these agents.
- In Henoch-Schönlein purpura, mucosal hematomas are thought to act as lead points.
- Peutz-Jeghers syndrome is a rare cause of intussusception in older children; in this condition, hamartomatous polyps act as the lead point. Similarly, familial polyposis coli and juvenile polyposis can also cause intussusceptions and a vermiform appendix may occasionally cause the disease.

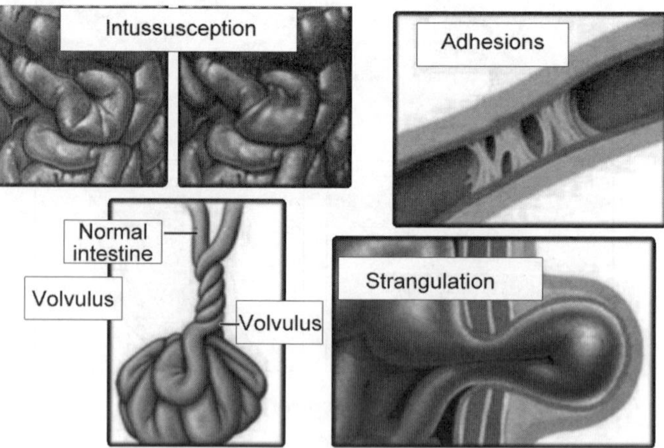

Fig. 7.48: Types of small bowel obstructions

- Familial cases of intussusception have been described.
- Suspect intestinal lymphomas in all children older than 6 years with intussusception.
- As mentioned above, extensive retroperitoneal dissections are known to predispose children to postoperative intussusceptions, probably because of intestinal dysmotility in these child.
- Blunt abdominal trauma has also been known to cause intussusception.

Incarcerated Hernia

- During the third month of gestation, the abdominal peritoneum protrudes at the internal inguinal ring and extends to the scrotum to form a diverticulum known as the processus vaginalis. In females, this diverticulum is called the canal of Nuck and extends through the internal inguinal ring to the labia majora.
- At birth, the processus vaginalis is open and in communication with the peritoneal cavity in about 80% of babies. Closure takes place progressively during the first 2 years of life, with an estimated 20–30% incidence of patency at age 2 years and then little further decline. This patent processus vaginalis becomes a hernia only when it contains abdominal viscera.
- Incarcerated or nonreducible hernias may contain small bowel, cecal appendix (Amyand hernia), omentum or rarely, Meckel diverticulum (Littre hernia). In girls, the ovary, fallopian tube or both is usually incarcerated. When a part of the bladder wall or the colonic wall is contained in the hernia sac, it is called a sliding hernia.
- Umbilical hernias are the result of an incompletely closed umbilical ring. Most spontaneously resolve by age 2 years (80%).

Malrotation of the Bowel with Midgut Volvulus

The primitive gut, which forms during the fourth week of embryonal life, is divided into the foregut, midgut and hindgut. The largest of these, the midgut, is the only portion that undergoes rotation by herniating extraembryonically into the umbilical cord and rotating 270° in a counterclockwise direction around the superior mesenteric artery on its journey back to the abdominal cavity by 11 weeks' gestation. This produces the normal C-shaped configuration of the duodenum and results in the cecum coming to rest in the right lower quadrant of the abdomen.

For unknown reasons, midgut rotation can arrest at any point, most commonly rotating 180° and leaving the cecocolic loop in the right upper quadrant. Dense peritoneal bands (i.e. Ladd bands) cross from the malpositioned right colon across the duodenum to the right lateral abdominal wall. This configuration leaves a narrow mesenteric root and creates a predisposition to clockwise torsion of the midgut, while the Ladd bands themselves can obstruct the duodenum.

The extent of atresia and the appearance of the atretic intestinal segment vary according to the timing and degree of the disruption of the mesenteric blood supply. Small-bowel atresia variably reduces the size of the colon. The volume of intestinal secretions and amniotic fluid that passes through the colon in fetal life determines its size in the newborn. Atresia blocks this fluid flow through the colon, thus limiting colon growth; however, passage of meconium does not rule out intestinal atresia because the vascular insult that leads to the atresia may occur after the recanalization phase of the intestinal development.

Postoperative Adhesive Small-bowel Obstruction

- *Duplication cysts*: The embryogenesis of rectal duplications has been attributed to the pinching off of diverticula that are present in the 8-week-old to 9-week-old embryo. The reported association of spinal abnormalities makes the split notochord mechanism another probable origin of rectal duplications.
- *Annular pancreas*: Annular pancreas occurs when the ventral pancreatic bud fails to rotate behind the duodenum, leaving pancreatic tissue fully encircling the second portion of the duodenum. This results in a nondistensible ring of pancreatic parenchyma and a functional stenosis.
- *Necrotizing enterocolitis*: The primary infectious process likely results in enteroinvasion, release of inflammatory mediators, toxin production, ileus, gas production, bowel distension, increased intraluminal pressure and vascular compromise, which causes loss of mucosal integrity and bacterial translocation, which results in a systemic inflammatory response.
  - Mesocolic hernia
  - Cecal volvulus
  - Meconium disease
  - Myocardial infarction (MI) is caused by intestinal and pancreatic dysfunction, which results from the autosomal recessive disease cystic fibrosis (CF). MI is the result of the accumulation of sticky and inspissated intraluminal meconium.
  - Meconium plug syndrome or meconium obstruction does not appear to be associated with CF or Hirschsprung disease in extremely low birth weight infants.

Duodenal Atresia and Stenosis

Duodenal atresia and stenosis are believed to be caused by failure of recanalization or vacuolization of the duodenum after the embryologic cord stage, when the lumen is completely obliterated. The three basic morphologic features of duodenal atresias are as follows:

- Type I atresias are characterized by luminal webs or membranes.
- Type II is characterized by a complete atresia connected by a fibrous cord.
- Type III is characterized by complete atresia with a mesenteric gap between the affected intestinal segments.

Signs and Symptoms

Small-bowel obstructions in pediatric child are uncommon but should be suspected in any child with persistent vomiting, distention and abdominal pain, because delayed diagnosis and treatment can lead to devastating consequences. Infants and young children with intestinal obstruction present with pain, irritability, vomiting and abdominal distension. Small-bowel obstructions progress to decreased or no bowel movements. Undiagnosed or improperly managed obstructions can progress to vascular compromise, which causes bowel ischemia, necrosis, perforation, sepsis and death.

Abdominal Pain

- Pain is common. Caregivers may describe an infant or small child with abdominal pain as irritable or inconsolable.

- Pain from a small-bowel obstruction is usually colicky. It is described as cramplike and episodic, persisting a few minutes at a time.
- A child with obstructive pain may be unable to remain immobile on the examining table.
- Constant pain occurs later in the disease course, when strangulation, perforation, or both have occurred.

Nausea and Vomiting

- Vomiting is a classic symptom of mechanical obstruction.
- Emesis caused by a proximal obstruction is usually of gastric content, or bilious if the obstruction is distal to the ampulla of Vater; in distal ileal obstructions, vomit is feculent.
  - *Anorexia*: Anorexia is an early and frequent sign.
  - *Diarrhea*: Diarrhea may occur early in the course of the obstruction.
  - *Obstipation*: This is a late sign of complete obstruction.
  - *Fever*: Fever can occur late in the disease process and is associated with bowel strangulation and necrosis.

Clinical Assessment

Obtain as much history as possible from the child. Younger children for example, are likely to recall recent events, whereas adults remember more remote events. Physicians should seek an accurate chronology of the disorder. Asking when the child was last completely healthy may provide a more accurate assessment of the child's pathophysiology.

Bilious vomiting in the neonate should be considered secondary to a mechanical obstruction until proven otherwise and every newborn with this symptom warrants an emergent surgical evaluation.

Diagnostic Evaluation

Laboratory Investigation

The following laboratory tests may be useful in child with small-bowel obstruction:

- Serum electrolyte level
  - BUN level
  - Creatinine level
  - Glucose level
  - CBC count
  - Urinalysis
  - ABG level
  - Stool for occult blood.

Routine laboratory studies usually do not help establish a diagnosis of malrotation with midgut volvulus, although leukocytosis with a left shift may develop late in the disease process. Potassium is an intracellular ion; thus, child with incarcerated hernias or other conditions that lead to ischemic bowel may present with hyperkalemia.

Imaging Studies

Plain abdominal radiography should be the initial radiologic study in suspected cases of small-bowel obstruction.

- Obtain flat decubitus and upright radiographs of the abdomen.
- Study radiographs for signs of dilated small-bowel loops and air-fluid levels produced by the layering of air and intestinal content.
- Absent colonic or rectal gas also indicates a complete bowel obstruction.
- The pattern of bowel gas on plain radiography can help differentiate between proximal and distal bowel obstructions. Drawing an imaginary line from the right upper quadrant to the left lower one is helpful in establishing the level of the obstruction. The jejunum corresponds to the left upper three fifths of the small bowel, whereas the right lower two fifths of it represent the ileum.
- When intestinal perforation is suspected and the child cannot be placed in an upright position, a left lateral decubitus film with horizontal beam is helpful in diagnosing free intraperitoneal air because it facilitates identification of free air around the hepatic density.
- Contrast studies such as upper GI series and contrast enemas can help determine obstruction location. Contrast studies also reveal whether the obstruction is intrinsic or extrinsic to the bowel. Remember to always use hydrosoluble contrast to avoid severe barium peritonitis in child with a perforation.
- Abdominal CT scanning should not be obtained when the diagnosis is evident on radiography because this would only delay treatment and subject the child to unnecessary radiation. CT scanning helps identify causes of chronic partial obstructions, as well as abscesses, tumors and other causes of acute abdominal pain.
- Ultrasonographic examinations reveal many intestinal abnormalities, including tumors, mesenteric cysts and intussusceptions.

Management

Medical Management

General Principles in Small-bowel Obstruction Treatment

Stabilize the patient and monitor ABCs. Replace fluids with diligent intravenous resuscitation, using isotonic sodium chloride solution or lactated Ringer solution. Early bowel decompression with an nasogastric (NG) tube decreases the chance of bowel necrosis and perforation. Administer broad-spectrum antibiotics when necrosis or perforation is suspected.

Intussusception

Stabilize the patient's ABCs and replace large fluid losses. Administer nothing by mouth (NPO) to the child and place an NG tube to decompress the obstruction from above. The use of antibiotics is appropriate for management of bacterial translocation. Barium, water, or air enema reduction is appropriate after surgical consultation if symptom duration is less than 24 hours and if the patient has no signs of peritonitis.

Enemas successfully reduce 80–95% of all intussusceptions, with better success rates in short-duration intussusceptions. Children whose symptoms persist longer than 24 hours, or have signs of peritonitis, should not be considered candidates for enema reduction. Stabilize these children and immediately transport them to the operating room because untreated intussusception is almost always fatal. The recurrence rate is higher after radiographic than after surgical reduction. Surgery is also indicated for child whose intussusception cannot be reduced after 2 enema attempts.

Adhesive Small-bowel Obstruction

Only about 6–7% of children with adhesive small-bowel obstruction require immediate laparotomy. Approximately one half of these child respond to medical treatment, which includes NPO, intravenous fluids, NG decompression and antibiotics. Children younger than 1 year tend to respond poorly to conservative management. No single agent or treatment has proven effective in preventing adhesion formation after a laparotomy.

The use of water-soluble contrast via NG tube may decrease the need for surgery in some child. Water-soluble contrast media (Gastrografin) cause redistribution of intravascular and extracellular fluid into the intestinal lumen because of their hyperosmolarity. As a result, these media decrease intestinal wall edema and act as a direct stimulant to intestinal peristalsis

Incarcerated Hernia

Stabilize the patient's ABCs and focus on replacing the large fluid losses. Nonoperative reduction of a nonstrangulated hernia is possible in approximately 95–98% of cases. Facilitate the reduction by sedating the patient and placing the patient in a mild Trendelenburg position. Gentle traction on the hernia and the contents of the sac usually suffices to reduce the volume and rapidly retract the contents of the sac into the abdominal cavity. The only contraindication to nonoperative reduction is a long-standing incarceration with evidence of peritoneal irritation. Antibiotic therapy is usually unwarranted, but critically ill infants with perforation and peritonitis require coverage for aerobic gram-negative organisms and anaerobic infections.

Necrotizing Enterocolitis (NEC)

NEC management involves cessation of enteral feeds, gastric decompression on low continuous suction with a sump-type tube, fluid management to correct hypovolemia, parenteral nutrition with a centrally located intravenous catheter once fluid resuscitation is complete and antibiotic therapy. Direct antimicrobial therapy is aimed at enteric bacteria (e.g. *Escherichia coli, Klebsiella species, Enterococcus species, anaerobic colonic flora,* [*Clostridia* species]). Serial abdominal examinations are preferably performed by the same examiner. Obtain radiographs of the abdomen, including cross-table lateral films, every 6–8 hours for the first 48 hours. Obtain blood, urine, sputum and CSF cultures, if indicated.

Meconium Disease

Treatment of MI requires evacuating the meconium. Nonsurgical methods relieve the obstructions of more than 50% of child. The therapy of choice for uncomplicated MI is nonoperative hyperosmolar enema (Gastrografin or Omnipaque), with enterotomy and irrigation reserved for enema failures. Dilute Gastrografin with N-acetylcysteine may also be administered using an NG tube from above to help loosen the meconium. Distal intestinal obstruction syndrome may be treated in the same way. Complicated cases (meconium peritonitis, meconium pseudocyst, perforation, intestinal atresia) require exploration and bowel resection with primary anastomosis or stoma creation. Meconium plug syndrome is usually relieved with rectal stimulation (suppositories, washouts, or contrast enemas).

Medication

Bowel obstructions often require surgical interventions, but start antibiotic administration in the emergency department (ED) first. Antibiotic coverage must include gram-negative aerobic and gram-negative anaerobic organisms.

Surgical Management

Intussusception: Intussusception can be reduced by radiographic means in 80–95% of child. Surgical reduction is indicated when symptoms have been present for more than 24 hours, in the presence of shock that cannot be corrected, when a lead point has been identified, when necrosis or perforation are present, or if the intussusception is irreducible by radiographic means.

Incarcerated hernia: After reducing the hernia, elective repair is possible 24–48 hours after the edema subsides. For child whose hernias cannot be reduced and for child with strangulation, immediate surgery is mandatory to prevent the incarceration from progressing to perforation and frank peritonitis.

Malrotation of the Bowel with Midgut Volvulus

Preserving intestinal viability requires rapid diagnosis and surgery for malrotation with midgut volvulus. Initiate NG suction and intravenous hydration when entertaining the possibility of midgut volvulus. If abdominal plain radiographic findings confirm the diagnosis, defer contrast studies and take the child directly to the operating room.

A Ladd procedure is the preferred treatment. It includes evisceration and inspection of the mesenteric root, derotation of the volvulus (which has always been reported to occur in a clockwise direction), lysis of Ladd bands with kocherization of the duodenum along the right abdominal gutter, opening of the visceral peritoneum that covers the mesentery and replacing the small bowel into the right side of the abdomen and the large bowel into the left side (in a position of nonrotation). It also includes an appendectomy (usually an inversion appendectomy) because the cecum and appendix are located in an unusual place. The procedure can also be laparoscopically performed.

Any frankly necrotic bowel should be resected and end-to-end anastomosis performed unless the peritoneal cavity is grossly contaminated or the condition of the patient does not allow it; in such cases, stomas should be created.

Postoperative adhesive small-bowel obstruction: A possible diagnosis of adhesive small-bowel obstruction requires prompt surgical consultation because delay can lead to intestinal necrosis. Child usually present with a single-point obstruction. Adhesiolysis is the treatment of choice. This can be achieved laparoscopically or with laparotomy. Some child requires bowel resection because of perforation or necrosis.

Duplication Cysts

The treatment for duplications is surgical excision, even in an asymptomatic patient who is incidentally diagnosed. The prevalence of gastric mucosa suggests that the duplications should not be left indefinitely. The procedure may depend on the location of the cyst. In esophageal duplications, the cyst is excised and a mucosectomy is performed if the muscular layer shared with the esophagus is left behind. The entire muscular wall can be excised with the cyst, taking care not to penetrate the esophageal mucosa.

Duplications of the small intestine usually require resection and anastomosis. In rectal duplications, only the mucosal lining usually needs to be excised because the duplication and normal rectum share the muscularis layer. If malignant degeneration is suspected, total excision including the normal rectum may be necessary. Infected duplications may require initial drainage, followed by a staged resection. Laparoscopically assisted resection of ileocecal duplications is safe and effective.

Annular pancreas: Surgical management is similar to that of duodenal atresia. Diamond-shaped duodenoduodenostomy is the preferred approach (Kimura procedure).

Necrotizing enterocolitis: Indications for surgery include pneumoperitoneum, fixed dilated bowel loop, abdominal wall discoloration, or children whose conditions deteriorate or show no improvement with conservative therapy. Portal venous air suggests extensive intestinal necrosis but does not indicate that celiotomy is necessary.

Mesocolic hernia: Surgically reduce the hernia and repair the potential hernia pouch, either electively (for reducible hernias) or emergently (for incarcerated hernias.) Cecal volvulus: Surgical reduction of the cecal volvulus and pexy to the lateral peritoneal wall is usually required, in addition to fluid resuscitation, bowel decompression and ABC monitoring.

Jejunoileal Atresia and Stenosis

Surgical resection of the atretic segment is followed by end-to-end anastomosis. The proximal dilated bowel may need to be tapered to fit the smaller distal intestine. Care should be taken to preserve as much intestinal length as possible in order to prevent short bowel syndrome, mainly in child with multiple atresias. These have classically been repaired through transverse supraumbilical incision, although single jejunoileal atresias have been successfully approached through a smaller periumbilical incision (as the one described for hypertrophic pyloric stenosis).

Meconium ileus: Surgical management by either primary resection and anastomosis or an ileostomy is sometimes required. Duodenal atresia and stenosis: The usual treatment for duodenal atresia is a linear or diamond-shaped duodenoduodenostomy (Kimura procedure). Duodenojejunostomy is another option. A duodenal web is much rarer and can be treated with duodenotomy and excision of the web, with or without duodenoplasty.

Nursing Management

- Child with partial small-bowel obstructions can be nonoperatively treated with adequate fluid resuscitation and nasoenteric suctioning.
- Child who do not respond to nonoperative treatment within 12–24 hours require surgical treatment.
- After nonoperative hernia reduction, elective repair may be accomplished 24–48 hours after the edema subsides.
- Admit any child with an intussusception that is successfully reduced with a barium enema for observation because this condition has a high reoccurrence rate, especially in the first 24 hours.

- Close follow-up observation is mandatory for child whose partial small-bowel obstructions are nonoperatively treated and who are stable for discharge.
- Instruct parents that they must take their child immediately to an ED if the child's symptoms (e.g. vomiting, pain) recur.

Complications

- Bowel necrosis
- Bowel perforation
- Sepsis
- Shock
- Abscess
- Short bowel syndrome with malabsorption and malnutrition
- Death
- Testicular infarction and atrophy, lesion to the testicular vessels or vas deferens, hernia recurrence (complications of incarcerated hernias).

Prognosis

The prognosis of small-bowel obstruction depends on the location and source of obstruction and on the extent of bowel necrosis. With early diagnosis and treatment, the prognosis is good; however, mortality rates may reach 65% if more than 75% of the small bowel is necrotic at the time of laparotomy.

HIRSCHSPRUNG'S DISEASE (HD)

Introduction

Hirschsprung's (HIRSH-sproongz) disease is a condition that affects the large intestine (colon) and causes problems with passing stool. Hirschsprung's disease is present when a

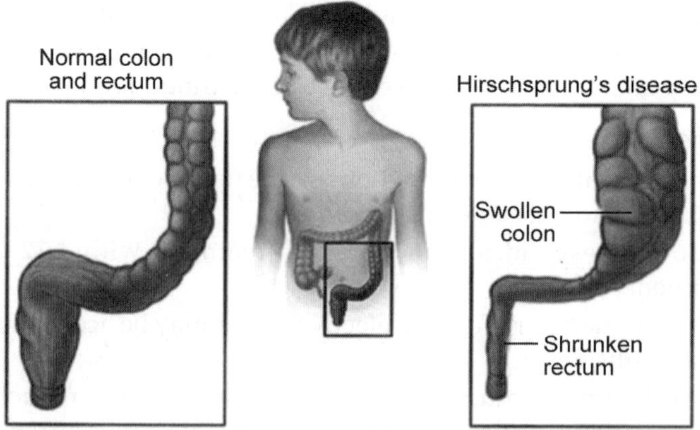

Fig. 7.49: Difference between normal and Hirschsprung's diseases

baby is born (congenital) and results from missing nerve cells in the muscles of part or the baby's entire colon.

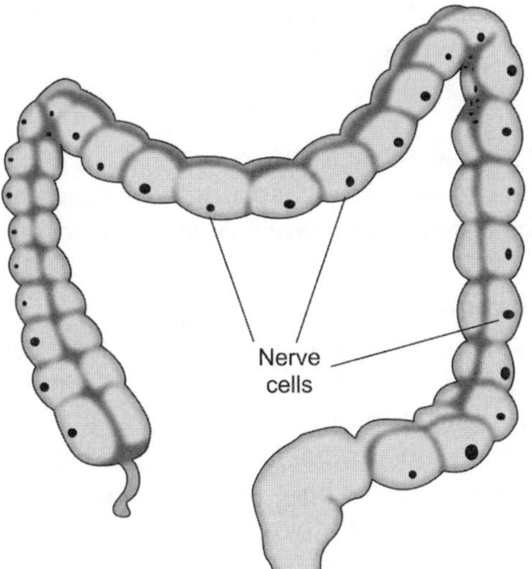

Fig. 7.50: Healthy large intestine: Nerve cells are found throughout the intestine

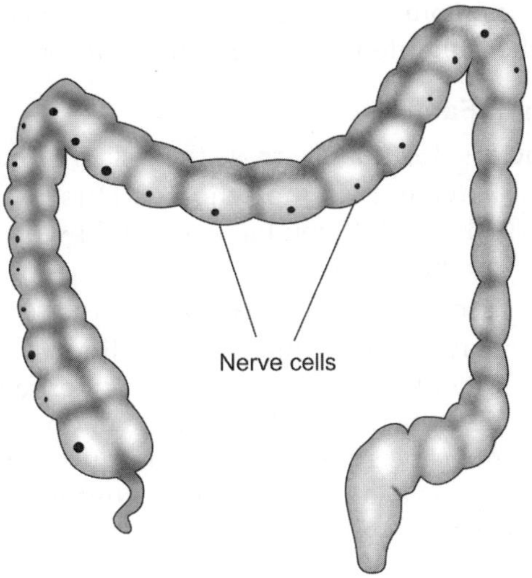

Fig. 7.51: HD large intestine: Nerve cells are missing from the last part of the intestine

Definition

Hirschsprung's disease is a developmental disorder of the enteric nervous system and is characterized by an absence of ganglion cells in the distal colon resulting in a functional obstruction. The large intestine is also sometimes called the colon. The word bowel can refer to the large and small intestines. HD usually occurs in children. It causes constipation, which means that bowel movements are difficult. Some children with HD cannot have bowel movements at all. The stool creates.

Children with Hirschsprung's disease are missing the nerve cells (ganglion cells) within the wall of their colon or rectum. These cells are responsible for the normal wave-like motion of the bowel (peristalsis). When they are missing the stool stops and an obstruction occurs. The length of affected bowel varies. The most common transition point is in the upper rectum or the sigmoid colon.

Hirschsprung's disease is a congenital disease. That means a person is born with it. The disease may also be hereditary, which means a parent can pass it to a child.

Cause

It is not clear what causes Hirschsprung's disease. It sometimes occurs in families and may in some cases be associated with a genetic mutation.

Constipation

- Normally, muscles in the intestine push stool to the anus, where stool leaves the body.
- Special nerve cells in the intestine, called ganglion cells make the muscles push.
- A person with HD does not have these nerve cells in the last part of the large intestine.

Hereditary

Hirschsprung's disease causes about 25% of all newborn intestinal blockages. It occurs five times more often in males than in females. Hirschsprung's disease is sometimes linked to other inherited or congenital conditions, such as Down syndrome.

Risk Factors

Factors that may increase the risk of Hirschsprung's disease include:

- Having a sibling who has Hirschsprung's disease. Hirschsprung's disease can be inherited. If you have one child who has the condition, future biological children also might be at risk.
- Being male, Hirschsprung's disease is more common in males.
- Having other inherited conditions. Hirschsprung's disease is associated with certain inherited conditions, such as inherited heart problems and Down syndrome. It may also be associated with multiple endocrine neoplasias, type IIB—a syndrome that causes noncancerous tumors in the mucous membranes and adrenal glands (located above the kidneys) and cancer of the thyroid gland (located at the base of the neck). Roughly a third of children who have Hirschsprung's disease have other abnormalities.

Pathophysiology

Congenital aganglionosis of the distal bowel defines Hirschsprung disease. Aganglionosis begins with the anus, which is always involved and continues proximally for a variable distance. Both the myenteric (Auerbach) plexus and the submucosal (Meissner) plexus are absent, resulting in reduced bowel peristalsis and function. The precise mechanism underlying the development of Hirschsprung disease is unknown.

Enteric ganglion cells are derived from the neural crest. During normal development, neuroblasts will be found in the small intestine by the 7th week of gestation and will reach the colon by the 12th week of gestation. One possible etiology for Hirschsprung's disease is a defect in the migration of these neuroblasts down their path to the distal intestine. Alternatively, normal migration may occur with a failure of neuroblasts to survive, proliferate, or differentiate in the distal aganglionic segment. Abnormal distribution in affected intestine of components required for neuronal growth and development, such as fibronectin, laminin, neural cell adhesion molecule (NCAM) and neurotrophic factors may be responsible for this theory.

Additionally, the observation that the smooth muscle cells of aganglionic colon are electrically inactive when undergoing electrophysiologic studies also points to a myogenic component in the development of Hirschsprung's disease. Finally, abnormalities in the interstitial cells of Cajal, pacemaker cells connecting enteric nerves and intestinal smooth muscle have also been postulated as an important contributing factor.

Signs and Symptoms

Symptoms of HD usually show up in very young children. But sometimes they do not appear until the person is a teenager or an adult. The symptoms are a little different for different ages.

In infants, the primary symptom is not passing meconium, an infant's first bowel movement, within the first 24 to 48 hours of life. Other symptoms include:

- Vomiting and abdominal distention as a newborn
- Chronic constipation
- More rarely diarrhea, fever and distention (symptoms associated with enterocolitis–inflammation of the small intestine and colon).

Symptoms in Newborns

Newborns with HD do not have their first bowel movement when they should. These babies may also throw up green liquid called bile after eating and their abdomens may swell. Discomfort from gas or constipation might make them fussy. Sometimes, babies with HD develop infections in their intestines.

- Difficulty with bowel movements
- Failure to pass meconium shortly after birth
- Failure to pass a first stool within 24–48 hours after birth
- Infrequent but explosive stools
- Jaundice
- Poor feeding
- Poor weight gain
- Vomiting
- Watery diarrhea (in the newborn).

Symptoms in Older Children

Most children with HD have always had severe problems with constipation. Some also have more diarrhea than usual. Children with HD might also have anemia, a shortage of red blood cells, because blood is lost in the stool. Also, many babies with HD grow and develop more slowly than they should.

- Constipation that gradually gets worse
- Fecal impaction
- Malnutrition
- Slow growth
- Swollen belly.

Symptoms in Teenagers and Adults

Like younger children, teenagers and adults with HD usually have had severe constipation all their lives. They might also have anemia. Those with anemia look pale and tire easily.

Diagnostic Evaluation

Physical Examination

Neonatal Period

- They may have abdominal distention (which is tympanic on percussion) and symptoms of intestinal obstruction.
- They may present with acute enterocolitis in this age group and (rarely) with neonatal meconium plug syndrome or appendicitis.

Older Infants and Children

- They have chronic constipation.
- There may be marked abdominal distention with palpable dilated loops of colon.
- Rectal examination often reveals an empty rectum and may result in the forceful expulsion of fecal material as examination is completed.
- More rarely, older children can present with malnourishment and possibly enterocolitis.

Other Test

- Barium enema (BAR-ee-um EN-uh-muh) X-ray
- Manometry (ma-NOM-eh-tree)
- Biopsy (BY-op-see)

Barium Enema X-ray

An X-ray is a black-and-white picture of the inside of the body. The picture is taken with a special machine that uses a small amount of radiation. For a barium enema X-ray, the doctor puts barium through the anus into the intestine before taking the picture. Barium is a liquid that makes the intestine show up better on the X-ray.

In some cases, instead of barium another liquid, called Gastrografin, may be used. Gastrografin is also sometimes used in newborns to help remove a hard first stool. Gastrografin causes water to be pulled into the intestine and the extra water softens the stool.

In places where the nerve cells are missing, the intestine looks too narrow. If a narrow large intestine shows on the X-ray, the doctor knows HD might be the problem. More tests will help the doctor know for sure.

Manometry and Biopsy

Manometry: The doctor inflates a small balloon inside the rectum. Normally, the anal muscle will relax. If it does not, HD may be the problem. This test is most often done in older children and adults.

Biopsy: This is the most accurate test for HD. The doctor removes and looks at a tiny piece of the intestine under a microscope. If the nerve cells are missing, HD is the problem.

Rectal biopsy: The definitive diagnosis rests on histology of a rectal biopsy. Tissue is obtained either by suction anal biopsy or by transanal wedge resection. Suction biopsy is best performed 2–2.5 cm above the dentate line, on the posterior wall to reduce the risk of perforation. The specimen is examined for the presence or absence of ganglion cells in the myenteric plexus. This may be difficult in short segments or with skip lesions and acetylcholine staining may be helpful.

Management

Medical Management

The general goals of medical care are 3-fold:

1. To treat the complications of unrecognized or untreated Hirschsprung's disease
2. To institute temporary measures until definitive reconstructive surgery can take place
3. To manage bowel function after reconstructive surgery.

Management of complications of recognized aganglionosis is directed toward reestablishing normal fluid and electrolyte balance, preventing bowel overdistension (with possible perforation) and managing complications, such as sepsis. Thus, intravenous hydration, nasogastric decompression and as indicated, administration of intravenous antibiotics remain the cornerstones of initial medical management.

- Colonic lavage, consisting of mechanical irrigation with a large-bore rectal tube and large volumes of irrigant, may be required.
- Balanced salt solutions may help prevent electrolyte imbalances.
- Nasogastric decompression, intravenous fluids, antibiotics and colonic lavage may also need to be used in postoperative child who develop enterocolitis as a complication. Sodium cromoglycate, a mast cell stabilizer, has been reported to be of benefit in these child as well.
- Routine colonic irrigation and prophylactic antibiotic therapy have been proposed as a means of decreasing the risk of enterocolitis.
- Injecting the nonrelaxing internal sphincter mechanism with botulinum toxin has been shown to induce more normal patterns of bowel movements in postoperative child with enterocolitis.

Medication

The goals of pharmacotherapy are to eradicate infection, to reduce morbidity and to prevent complications.

Antibiotics

Empiric antimicrobial therapy must be comprehensive and cover all likely pathogens in the context of this clinical setting. Antibiotic selection should be guided by blood culture sensitivity whenever feasible.

Ampicillin (Marcillin, Omnipen, Principen)

Bactericidal activity against susceptible organisms. Alternative to amoxicillin when unable to take medication orally.

- Adult Dose = 1–2 g IV q6h
- Pediatric Dose = 25 mg/kg IV q6h.

Gentamicin (Garamycin, Jenamicin)

Aminoglycoside antibiotic for gram-negative coverage. Used in combination with both an agent against gram-positive organisms and one that covers anaerobes. Not the DOC. Consider if penicillins or other less-toxic drugs are contraindicated, when clinically indicated and in mixed infections caused by susceptible staphylococci and gram-negative organisms. Dosing regimens are numerous; adjust dose based on CrCl and changes in volume of distribution. May be administered IV/IM.

- Adult Dose = 5–7 mg/kg/d IV
- Pediatric Dose = 2.5 mg/kg IV q8h.

Metronidazole (Flagyl)

Imidazole ring-based antibiotic active against various anaerobic bacteria and protozoa. Used in combination with other antimicrobial agents (except for Clostridium difficile enterocolitis).

- Adult Dose = 500 mg PO/IV q6–8h
- Pediatric Dose = 7.5 mg/kg IV q6h.

May increase toxicity of anticoagulants, lithium and phenytoin; cimetidine may increase toxicity; disulfiramlike.

Botulinum Toxin Type A (BOTOX®)

Binds to receptor sites on motor nerve terminals and inhibits release of acetylcholine, which in turn inhibits transmission of impulses in neuromuscular tissue.

- Adult Dose = 1.25–2.5 U IM; may repeat q3–4 months
- Pediatric Dose = > 12 years: Administer as in adults
- < 12 years: 0.25–1 U IM; may repeat q3–4 months

Surgical Management

Surgical management of Hirschsprung's disease begins with the initial diagnosis, which often requires a full-thickness rectal biopsy. Traditionally, treatment also includes creating a diverting colostomy at the time of diagnosis and once the child grows and weighs more than 10 kg, the definitive repair is performed.

This standard of treatment was developed in the 1950s after reports of relatively high leak and stricture rates with the single stage procedure were initially described by Swenson. However, with the advent of safer anesthesia and more advanced hemodynamic monitoring, a primary pull-through procedure without a diverting colostomy is increasingly being performed. Contraindications to a one-stage procedure include massively dilated proximal bowel, severe enterocolitis, perforation, malnutrition and inability to accurately determine the transition zone by frozen section.

For neonates who are first treated with a diverting colostomy, the transition zone is identified and the colostomy is placed proximal to this area. The presence of ganglion cells at the colostomy site must be unequivocally confirmed by a frozen-section biopsy. Either a loop or end stoma is appropriate, usually based on the surgeon's preference.

A number of definitive procedures have been used, all of which have demonstrated excellent results in experienced hands. The three most commonly performed repairs are the Swenson, Duhamel and Soave procedures. Regardless of the pull-through procedure chosen, cleaning the colon before definitive repair is necessary.

Swenson Procedure

- The Swenson procedure was the original pull-through procedure used to treat Hirschsprung's disease.
- The aganglionic segment is resected down to the sigmoid colon and the remaining rectum and an oblique anastomosis is performed between the normal colon and the low rectum.

Duhamel Procedure

- The Duhamel procedure was first described in 1956 as a modification to the Swenson procedure.
- Key points are that a retrorectal approach is used and a significant portion of aganglionic rectum is retained.

- The aganglionic bowel is resected down to the rectum and the rectum is oversewn. The proximal bowel is then brought through the retrorectal space (between the rectum and sacrum) and an end-to-side anastomosis is performed on the remaining rectum.

Soave (Anorectal) Procedure

- The Soave procedure was introduced in the 1960s and consists of removing the mucosa and submucosa of the rectum and pulling the ganglionic bowel through the aganglionic muscular cuff of the rectum.
- The original operation did not include a formal anastomosis, relying on scar tissue formation between the pull-through segment and the surrounding aganglionic bowel. The procedure has since been modified by Boley to include a primary anastomosis at the anus.

Anorectal Myomectomy

- For children (and occasionally adults) with ultrashort-segment Hirschsprung's disease, removing a strip of posterior midline rectal wall is an alternative surgical option.
- The procedure removes a 1 cm wide strip of extramucosal rectal wall beginning immediately proximal to the dentate line and extending to the normal ganglionic rectum proximally.
- The mucosa and submucosa are preserved and closed.

Procedures for Long-segment Hirschsprung's Disease

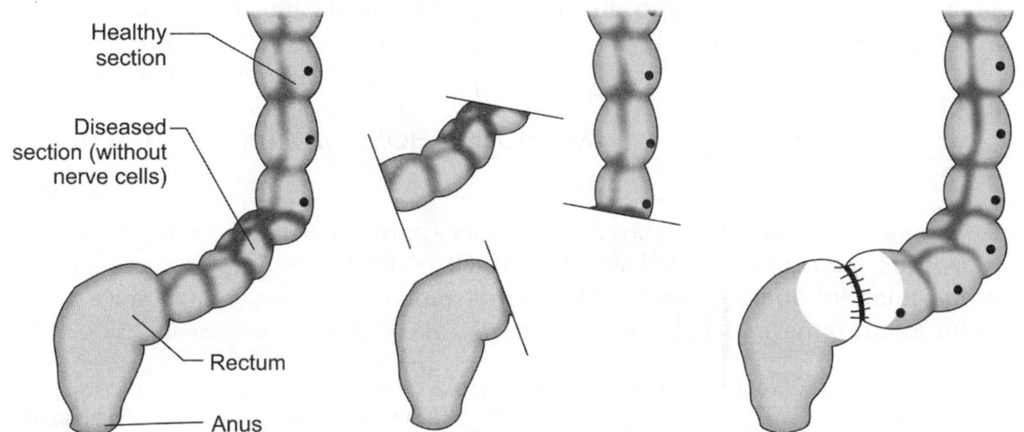

Before surgery: The diseased section is the part of the intestine that does not work.

Step 1: The surge removes the diseased section.

Step 2: The healthy section is attached to the rectum or anus.

- Child with total colonic involvement require modified procedures to bypass the aganglionic colon yet preserve the absorptive surface area and allow for proper growth and nutritional support.

- Most procedures include a side-to-side anastomosis of the ganglionic/propulsive small bowel to a short segment of the aganglionic/absorptive colon.
- Whether a short right colonic patch or a small bowel-to-rectal wall, Duhamel anastomosis is created, it is perhaps less important than maintaining a short patch length (< 10 cm).
- Long-segment anastomoses, such as the Martin procedure, are no longer advocated.
  - A laparoscopic approach to the surgical treatment of Hirschsprung's disease was first described in 1999 by Georgeson. The transition zone is first identified laparoscopically, followed by mobilization of the rectum below the peritoneal reflection. A transanal mucosal dissection is performed, followed by prolapsing of the rectum through the anus and anastomosis. Functional outcomes appear to be equivalent to open techniques based on short-term results.
  - The possibility of stem cell transplantation into the aganglionic gut and the reactivation of dormant stem cells in the gut to regenerate the enteric nervous system are being actively investigated. Experiments have demonstrated that neural crest stem cells (NCSC) are present, even in the adult gut and are capable of proliferation and differentiation. In addition, researchers have been able to inject neural crest stem cells and later identify them in the native rectum. Whether or not injected stem cells or reactivated native progenitor cells will have the capability to recreate a functional enteric nervous system remains to be elucidated.

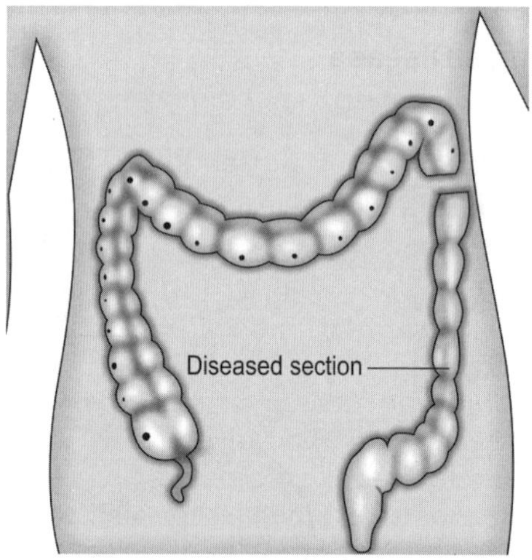

Step 1: The surgeon takes out most of the diseased part of the intestine.

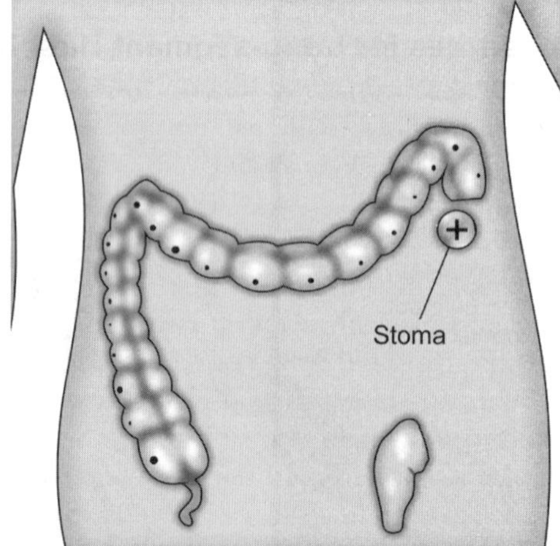

Step 2: The surgeon attaches the healthy part of the intestine to the stoma (a hole in the abdomen).

Pull-through Surgery

HD is treated with surgery. The surgery is called a pull-through operation. There are three common ways to do a pull-through and they are called the Swenson, the Soave and the Duhamel procedures. Each is done a little differently, but all involve taking out the part of the intestine that does not work and connecting the healthy part that is left to the anus. After pull-through surgery, the child has a working intestine.

Colostomy and Ileostomy

The pull-through can be done right after the diagnosis. However, children who have been very sick may first need surgery called an ostomy. This surgery helps the child get healthy before having the pull-through. Some doctors do an ostomy in every child before doing the pull-through.

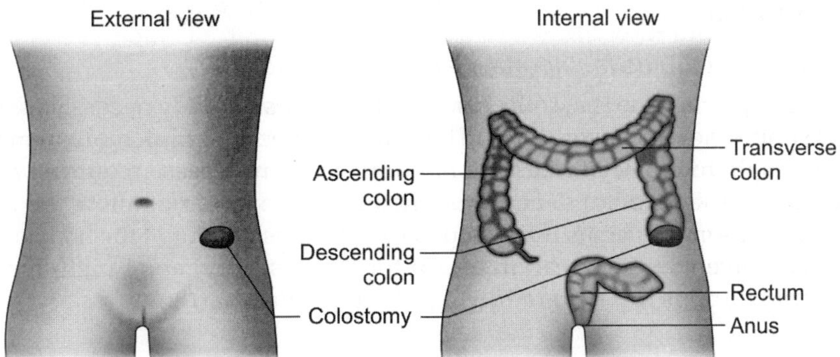

Fig. 7.52: Bowel resection and colostomy

In an ostomy, the doctor takes out the diseased part of the intestine. Then he cuts a small hole in the baby's abdomen. The hole is called a stoma. He connects the top part of the intestine to the stoma. Stool leaves the body through the stoma while the bottom part of the intestine heals. Stool goes into a bag attached to the skin around the stoma. She should need to empty this bag several times a day.

If the doctor removes the entire large intestine and connects the small intestine to the stoma, the surgery is called an ileostomy. If the doctor leaves part of the large intestine and connects that to the stoma, the surgery is called a colostomy.

Later, the doctor will do the pull-through surgery. In that disconnects the intestine from the stoma and attaches it just above the anus. The stoma is not needed any more, so the doctor either sews it up during surgery or waits about 6 weeks to make sure that the pull-through worked.

Nursing Management

Postoperative Care

Ostomy Care

Most babies are more comfortable after having an ostomy because they can pass gas more easily and are not constipated anymore. Older children will be more comfortable too, but they may have some trouble getting used to an ostomy. They will need to learn how to take care of the stoma and how to change the bag that collects stool. They may be worried about being different from their friends. Most children can lead a normal life after surgery.

Adjusting after Pull-through

After a pull-through, 9 out of 10 children pass stool normally. Some children may have diarrhea for a while and babies may develop a nasty diaper rash. Eventually the stool will become more solid and the child will need to go to the bathroom less often. Toilet training may be delayed, as the child learns how to use the bottom muscles only after pull-through surgery. Older children might stain their underwear for a while after the surgery. It is not their fault. They cannot control this problem, but it improves with time. Some children become constipated because 1 in 10 children with HD has difficulty moving stool through the part of the colon without nerve cells. A mild laxative may also be helpful.

Diet and Nutrition

Drinking Plenty of Liquids is Important after Surgery for HD

One job of the large intestine is to collect the water and salts the body needs. Since your child's intestine is shorter now, it absorbs less. The child will need to drink more to make sure his body gets enough fluids. An infant who has long-segment disease requiring an ileostomy may need special tube feedings. The shortened intestine does not allow the bloodstream enough time to absorb nutrients from food before it is pushed out of the body as stool. Tube feedings that deliver nutrients can make up for what is lost. Eating high-fiber foods like cereal and bran muffins can help reduce constipation and diarrhea.

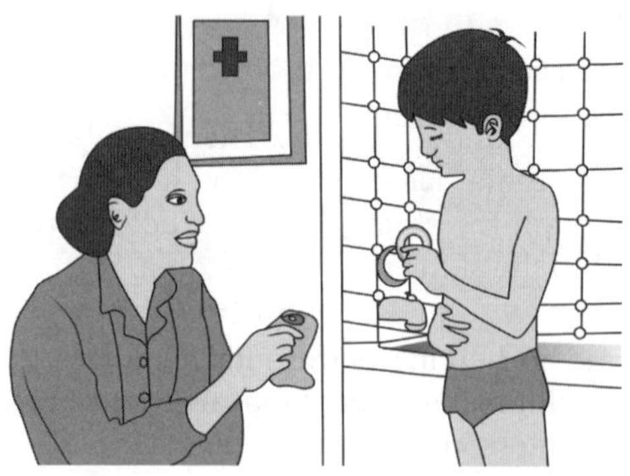

Fig. 7.53: Maintain the personal hygiene

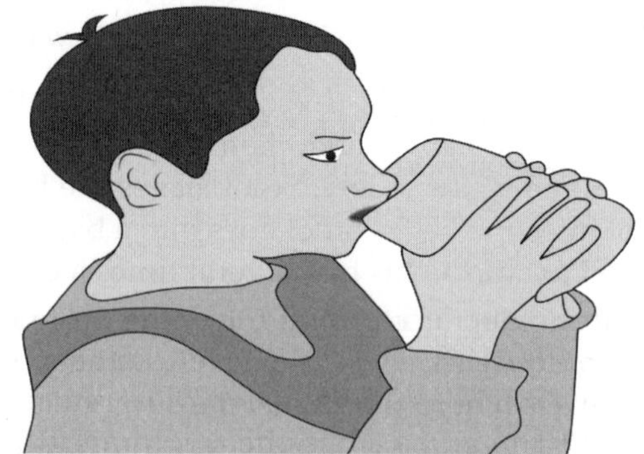

Fig. 7.54: Allow the child to drink the plenty of water

Diet Management

- The patient should have nothing by mouth before the operation.
- Institute tube feeding or formula/breast milk once bowel function resumes.
- High-fiber diets and diets containing fresh fruits and vegetables may optimize postoperative bowel function in certain child.

Daily Activity

Limit physical activity for about 6 weeks to allow the wound to heal properly (applies more to older children).

Complication

Infection

Infections can be very dangerous for a child with Hirschsprung's disease. Infection of the large and small intestines is called enterocolitis. It can happen before or after surgery to treat Hirschsprung's disease. Here are some of the signs to look for:

- Fever
- Swollen abdomen
- Vomiting
- Diarrhea
- Bleeding from the rectum
- Sluggishness.

Long-segment HD

Sometimes HD affects most or all of the large intestine, plus some of the small intestine. Children with long-segment HD can be treated with pull-through surgery, but there is a risk of complications such as infection, diarrhea and diaper rash afterward. Parents need to pay close attention to their child's health. Also, since some, most, or the entire intestine is removed, drinking a lot of fluid is important.

Conclusion

- HD is a disease of the large intestine.
- HD develops in children before they are born. It is not caused by anything the mother did while pregnant.
- Symptoms of HD include:
  - Delayed first bowel movement in newborns
  - Swollen abdomen and vomiting
  - Constipation since birth
  - Slow growth and development
  - Anemia
- Children with HD may get an infection, called enterocolitis, which can cause fever and diarrhea.
- HD is a serious disease that needs to be treated right away. HD is treated with pull-through surgery or sometimes, ostomy.
- After treatment, most children with HD lead normal lives.

MALABSORPTION SYNDROMES

Introduction

Malabsorption syndromes encompass numerous clinical entities that result in chronic diarrhea, abdominal distention and failure to thrive. Clinical malabsorption can be broken down into several distinct conditions, both congenital and acquired, that affect one or more of the different steps in the intestinal hydrolysis and subsequent transport of nutrients.

Incidence

Genetically Determined Syndromes

The prevalence of celiac disease in the United States is around 1% of the general population and has increased over time. Celiac disease in its entirety (i.e. including the forms without overt malabsorption) is by far the most common inherited malabsorption syndrome. Cystic fibrosis is the second most common malabsorption syndrome. Other congenital disorders are rare, with the exception of adult-type hypolactasia, which has a prevalence that varies greatly among different ethnic groups.

Acquired Syndromes

- The Cow's milk and soy milk protein allergies are common, especially in infants and young children. The prevalence of milk protein allergy, of which enteropathy is one of the presenting clinical symptoms, is estimated to be around 3%.
- A transient and common form of malabsorption in infants results from acute-onset enteritis (mostly viral, specifically rotavirus), which causes transient lactose intolerance.
- Although toddler's (or unspecific) diarrhea accounts for approximately 7.5% of referrals to pediatric gastroenterologists, it should not be considered a malabsorption syndrome because, by definition, no digestive or absorptive processes are impaired.
- Secondary malabsorption syndromes that result from liver, pancreas and intestinal diseases are uncommon. The manifestations vary according to the severity of each disease and the extent of intestinal mucosal injury.
- Neonates and young infants with malabsorption syndromes are at particularly high risk for chronic diarrhea and malnutrition.
- Symptoms of a congenital disease are usually apparent shortly after birth (the exception being adult-onset lactase deficiency, which appears only after age 6–8 years) or after a short hiatus once a particular substance is ingested in substantial amounts. Protein sensitivity syndromes to milk or soy protein usually present in infants younger than 3 months, but solid food protein sensitivity syndromes are also known to occur in older child.

Causes

See the table: 7.8.

Types

- Selective Malabsorption, (as seen in lactose malabsorption)
- Partial Malabsorption, (as observed in A-beta-lipoproteinemia)
- Total Malabsorption (as in celiac disease)

Table 7.8: Causes of malabsorption syndrome

Due to infective agents	Due to structural defects
• Whipple's disease	• Blind loops
• Intestinal tuberculosis	• Inflammatory bowel diseases commonly in Crohn's disease
• HIV related malabsorption	• Intestinal hurry from postgastrectomy; postvagotomy, gastrojejunostomy
• Tropical sprue	• Fistulae, diverticulae and strictures
• Traveller's diarrhea	• Infiltrative conditions such as amyloidosis, lymphoma, Eosinophilic gastroenteropathy

Contd...

Contd...

Due to infective agents	Due to structural defects
• Parasites e.g. Giardia lamblia, fish tape worm (B_{12} malabsorption); roundworm, hookworm (Ancylostoma duodenale and Necator americanus)	• Radiation enteritis
	• Systemic sclerosis and collagen vascular diseases
	• Short gut syndrome
Due to mucosal abnormality	**Due to enzyme deficiencies**
• Celiac/Celiac disease	• Lactase deficiency inducing lactose intolerance (constitutional, secondary or rarely congenital)
• Cows' milk intolerance	• Sucrose intolerance
• Soya milk intolerance	• Intestinal disaccharidase deficiency
• Fructose malabsorption	• Intestinal enteropeptidase deficiency
Due to digestive failure	**Due to other systemic diseases affecting GI tract**
• Pancreatic insufficiencies:	• Hypothyroidism and hyperthyroidism
– Cystic fibrosis	• addison's disease
– Chronic pancreatitis	• diabetes mellitus
– Carcinoma of pancreas	• hyperparathyroidism and Hypoparathyroidism
– Zollinger-Ellison syndrome	• Carcinoid syndrome
• Bile salt malabsorption	• Malnutrition
– Terminal ileal disease	• abeta-lipoproteinemia
– Obstructive jaundice	
– Bacterial overgrowth	

Other Types

Carbohydrate Malabsorption

Starch molecules are primarily digested by salivary and pancreatic amylase, but glucoamylase in the intestinal brush boarder also assists in digestion. Pancreatic insufficiency impedes the digestion of large starch molecules. Absence or reduction of the brush border disaccharidases causes selective carbohydrate malabsorption.

Transient reduction of these enzymes is common after an infection in the intestine, particularly a viral infection, because intestinal villi and microvilli may be damaged. Glucoamylase and maltase are most resistant to the depleting effects of mucosal injury that result from infection, whereas lactase is the most sensitive because of its predominant distribution near the tips of the villi. Lack of sucrose and isomaltase is, by far, the most frequent congenital enzyme deficiency. This enzyme deficiency is inherited in an autosomal recessive manner. Congenital lactase deficiency is exceedingly rare, but adult-type lactase deficiency (also called adult-type hypolactasia) is very common in some ethnic groups. A congenital deficiency in the glucose galactose transporter (SGLT–1) is inherited in an autosomal recessive manner.

Take care when diagnosing lactose or complex carbohydrate intolerance because many complex carbohydrates are broken down into glucose. Small bowel bacterial overgrowth of normal flora alters the intraluminal metabolism of carbohydrates and results in their malabsorption. This entity should also be suspected in children with diarrhea-predominant irritable bowel syndrome. Bacteria ferment carbohydrates into smaller osmotically active molecules and organic acids. Increased osmolarity causes fluid from systemic circulation to enter the intestinal lumen, resulting in diarrhea. Organic acids stimulate motility and may directly injure the intestinal mucosa. Fermentation eliminates the reducing substances and lowers the pH of the stool.

The production of lactate and short-chain fatty acids in the human colon can result in systemic acidosis. In particular, a syndrome of D-lactic acidosis may develop when specific bacteria that are capable of producing this uncommon and poorly cleared D-isomer of lactate exist in the intestinal flora.

Protein Malabsorption

- Protein malabsorption is a fairly common result of exocrine pancreatic enzyme deficiency, as occurs in child with cystic fibrosis.
- Protein malabsorption that results from congenital enterokinase deficiency is well described but rare. Loss of protein in the stool (i.e. protein-losing enteropathy), is often caused by the leakage of protein from the serum due to inflammation of the mucosa, as in Crohn's disease, celiac disease and protein sensitivity syndromes.
- Congenital lymphangiectasia, a developmental disorder in which dilation and dysfunction of intestinal lymphatics occurs, often in association with limb edema (Milroy disease), may present with severe protein-losing enteropathy without mucosal injury.

Vitamin Malabsorption

- Malabsorption of vitamin B_{12} and folate is associated with tropical spruce, a disorder that is acquired after travel to tropical areas.
- Vitamin B_{12} is absorbed in the ileum and absorption requires an intrinsic factor made in the gastric parietal cell.
- Intrinsic factor deficiency that results from atrophic gastritis or absence (from resection) or disease of the terminal ileum (the predominant site of active B_{12}) results in vitamin B_{12} malabsorption.

Signs and Symptoms

The following are important to assess in child with possible malabsorption syndromes:

GI Tract Symptoms

- GI tract symptoms are common in child with malabsorption syndromes and symptoms range from mild abdominal gaseous distention to severe abdominal pain and vomiting.
- Chronic or recurrent diarrhea is by far the most common symptom. Abdominal distention and watery diarrhea, with or without mild abdominal pain, associated with skin irritation in the perianal area due to acidic stools are characteristic of carbohydrate malabsorption syndromes.

- Periodic nausea, abdominal distention and pain
- Diarrhea is common in child with chronic Giardia infections.
- Vomiting, with moderate-to-severe abdominal pain and bloody stools, is characteristic of protein sensitivity syndromes or other causes of intestinal injury (e.g. inflammatory bowel disease).
- Recurrent abdominal pain has been implicated as a symptom of dietary disorders, although psychological variables that relate to an elevated anxiety level have clouded the certainty of this relationship.
- Malabsorption syndromes can definitely cause abdominal pain or irritability (particularly seen in celiac disease).
- Failure to identify the cause of malabsorption can result in the misdiagnosis of a physiologic syndrome as a behavioral disorder. Some dietary items may cause symptoms only when they are taken alone or with other specific dietary items.
  - Poor appetite is common in food sensitivity syndromes.
  - The child becomes conditioned to refuse foods that cause inflammatory reactions of the intestine.
  - Malabsorption syndromes not associated with inflammatory reactions typically cause an increase in appetite (e.g. cystic fibrosis), unless the associated abdominal gaseous distention hampers intake and induces early satiety.

Stool Characteristics

The toddler's diarrhea often has loose stools with undigested food particles. This should not be taken to imply the presence of true malabsorption.

- Frequent loose watery stools may indicate carbohydrate intolerance.
- Pasty or loose foul-smelling stools indicate fat malabsorption, also termed Steatorrhea.
- This symptom is commonly seen in Giardia infections, enterokinase deficiency, hepatic and pancreatic dysfunction and protein sensitivity syndromes.
- Bloody stools are seen in child with protein sensitivity syndromes and not in disaccharidase and pancreatic enzyme deficiencies or in child with giardiasis.

Other Symptoms

- Systemic symptoms, including weakness.
- Fatigue and failure to thrive, are systemic consequences of chronically poor nutrient absorption.
- Malabsorption of carbohydrates, fats, or proteins can cause failure to thrive, whereas folate and B_{12} malabsorption result in macrocytic anemia.
- Child with abeta-lipoproteinemia develop retinitis pigmentosa.
- Ataxia because of chronic fat-soluble vitamin malabsorption and deficiency (vitamins A and E).

Diagnostic Evaluation

There is no specific test for malabsorption. As for most medical conditions, investigation is guided by symptoms and signs. Moreover, tests for pancreatic function are complex and vary widely between centers.

History Collection

Diet history: Obtain a complete history of the patient's diet, including the amount and type of fluids, solid foods and formula ingested. Caregivers should keep a detailed journal of the patient's diet and symptoms for a minimum of 1 week. The proper amount of fluid for most young children is around 100 mL/kg/d. Fluid intake that exceeds this amount may result in looser stools, which causes a referral for a suspected but nonexistent malabsorption.

Fat is important for slowing the movement of food through the intestine via hormonal mechanisms. Fat intake of less than 3 g/kg/d may contribute to toddler's diarrhea, especially in the setting of excessive free fluid and carbohydrate intake (e.g. as occurs with large amounts of fruit juice intake). Thus, history is important in differentiating the common toddler's diarrhea from the rarer malabsorption syndromes.

Physical Assessment

In the absence of GI tract symptoms, malabsorption syndromes should be considered during the workup for failure to thrive, malnutrition, poor weight gain, or delayed puberty. Signs of malnutrition discovered during physical examination, such as reduced muscle and fat mass, atrophic tongue changes, or enlarged liver or spleen, have been reported in children with chronic malabsorption. Malabsorption syndromes should be suspected in infants with weight loss or little weight gain since birth and in infants with low weight and weight-for-height percentiles. By definition, toddler's diarrhea does not cause failure to thrive, unless anxious parents intervene by imposing unnecessary dietary restrictions that result in lower caloric intake.

Dehydration caused by a diarrhea that is induced by a malabsorption syndrome is not common, but, when it occurs, dehydration can cause serious morbidity and mortality. Assess each patient for signs, symptoms and severity of dehydration. Lethargy, depressed consciousness, sunken anterior fontanel, dry mucous membranes, sunken eyes, poor skin turgor and delayed capillary refill are all signs of dehydration. Borborygmi, a significant increase in peristaltic activity, can be detected audibly and with tactile palpation. This is associated with decreased intestinal transient time. Large numbers of stools result in a constant wet diaper in young children. Failure to properly dry the buttocks and perianal area results in erythema, skin irritation and skin breakdown, with evidence of bleeding seen in the diaper or in stool. Protein sensitivity may be associated with an eczematous rash.

Blood Tests

- Routine blood tests may reveal anemia, high ESR or low albumin; which has high sensitivity for presence of organic disease. In this setting, microcytic anemia usually implies iron deficiency and macrocytosis can be from impaired folic acid or B_{12} absorption or both. Low cholesterol or triglyceride may give clue toward fat malabsorption as low calcium and phosphate toward osteomalacia from low vitamin D.
- Specific vitamins like vitamin D or micronutrient like zinc levels can be checked. Fat soluble vitamins (A, D, E and K) are affected in fat malabsorption. Prolonged prothrombin time can be from vitamin K deficiency.
- Serological studies specific tests are carried out to determine underlying cause. IgA tissue transglutamate or IgA antiendomysium assay for gluten sensitive enteropathy.

Laboratory Studies

Stool Analysis

The presence of reducing substances indicates that carbohydrates have not been properly absorbed. One common mistake, especially with the use of superabsorbent diapers, is to test the solid portion of the stool instead of the liquid portion. Furthermore, in stools that are not fresh, bacterial hydrolysis, removal of the reducing substances and artifactual reduction of pH occur. Acidic stool has a pH level of less than 5.5. This indicates carbohydrate malabsorption, even in the absence of reducing substances.

Normally, stool bile acids should not be detected. If bile acid malabsorption is suspected, quantitative conjugated and unconjugated bile acids may be measured in stool, although this test is not routinely available and is not used in routine clinical practice.

Microscopy is particularly useful in diarrhea, may show protozoa like giardia, ova, cyst and other infective agents.

- Fecal fat study to diagnose steatorrhoea is less frequently performed nowadays.
- Low elastase is indicative of pancreatic insufficiency. Chymotrypsin and pancreolauryl can be assessed as well.

Urinalysis

Urine examination may reveal an unusually high concentration of the malabsorbed substance because, in many cases, the kidney and the gut use the same transporter. In glucose-galactose malabsorption, the urinary glucose level is typically elevated when the serum glucose level is within reference range because of congenital malfunction of SGLT–1. Levels of urinary 4-hydroxyphenylacetic acid have been demonstrated to be elevated in the urine of children with bacterial overgrowth syndrome.

Radiological Studies

- Barium follow through is useful in delineating small intestinal anatomy.
- Barium enema may be undertaken to see colonic or ileal lesions.
- CT abdomen is useful in ruling out structural abnormality, done in pancreatic protocol when visualising pancreas.
- Magnetic resonance cholangiopancreatography (MRCP) to complement or as an alternative to ERCP.

Diagnostic Procedures

Substance Tolerance Test

Attempt to isolate the substance that is causing the malabsorption. Resolution of diarrhea after the suspected substance is removed from the diet and resumption of the diarrhea when the substance is reintroduced are specific signs that the particular substance is not adequately absorbed. If diarrhea does not resolve when the particular substance is removed from the diet, this does not necessarily indicate intolerance to the substance.

Malabsorption of certain nutrients can result in secondary intestinal damage and secondary malabsorption, which may no longer be related to the malabsorbed substance. Thus, this technique has low sensitivity until mucosal injury has had a chance to heal. Challenging the patient with the suspected malabsorbed substance once the diarrhea has resolved, provides a more sensitive test.

Carbohydrate Malabsorption Tolerance Test

Carbohydrate malabsorption results in bacterial fermentation. This biochemical process releases hydrogen gas that is absorbed into the blood and excreted by the lungs. Under normal conditions, fermenting bacteria reside in the large intestine. When the bacteria in the large intestine ferment the carbohydrate load, an increase in the level of exhaled hydrogen is detected. The amount of carbohydrate administered is typically 2 g/kg, with a maximum dose of 50 g. When testing for lactose tolerance, using a more physiologic amount (e.g. 12.5–25 g) may be preferable.

An increase in the exhaled hydrogen concentration following ingestion of an oral carbohydrate load (> 20 ppm) indicates carbohydrate malabsorption. Bacterial overgrowth in the small intestine results in an additional early rise in the exhaled hydrogen concentration. Antibiotic administration within the 2 weeks prior to the test may cause false-negative results in this test.

D-xylose Absorption Test

Another time-honored test for carbohydrate malabsorption is the D-xylose absorption test. Xylose is a pentose that is passively absorbed by the jejunal mucosa. A standard dose of 5 g or, alternatively, 14.5 g/m^2 (maximum dose of 25 g) of D-xylose is orally administered as a 10% solution in water. The test result is positive in the following instances:

- *Children who weigh less than 30 kg:* Serum level at 1 hour after ingestion is less than 25 mg/dL
- *Children who weigh more than 30 kg:* The 5-hour urinary excretion is less than 15%.

A positive test result suggests malabsorption due to proximal small bowel mucosal lesion (enteropathy). Beware of false-positive results (e.g. from delayed gastric emptying, small bowel bacterial overgrowth and accelerated transit time).

Mucosal Biopsy

This test is fundamental in obtaining a definitive diagnosis in many circumstances, such as common celiac disease. Almost all pediatric gastroenterology centers obtain biopsies of the duodenal mucosa during an upper endoscopy. Moderate villous atrophy may be seen in protein-sensitive enteropathies, giardia infection or bile acid malabsorption. Histologic examination of the biopsy tissue may reveal the mucosal inclusions seen in abetalipoproteinemia, eosinophilic gastroenteritis, Wolman disease or congenital microvillous atrophy, for which electron microscopy is needed. Functional assays of the biopsy tissue assess carbohydrate disaccharidase enzymes.

Histologic Findings

Biopsy of the small intestine remains the criterion standard for the diagnosis of celiac disease. The classic features include villous atrophy, infiltration of the epithelium by cytotoxic intraepithelial T lymphocytes and crypt hyperplasia. However, the spectrum can range from a simple intraepithelial lymphocytosis without villous blunting or crypt hyperplasia to total villous atrophy with severe crypt hyperplasia.

Management

- The treatment of malabsorption syndromes depends on the specific entity being considered and thus widely varies. Although several new possibilities of gluten predigestion and detoxification and ways of increasing intestinal barrier tightness to gluten penetration are currently under active investigation and offer promising results, the only current therapeutic option for celiac disease remains the gluten-free diet, which is a diet completely devoid of wheat, barley and rye.

- Chronic diarrhea due to proximal small bowel bacterial overgrowth is treated with oral broad-spectrum antibiotics, particularly those with anaerobic coverage (e.g. metronidazole). More recently, rifaximin has also been found to be very effective in adults. Because this entity often occurs in individuals who have an anatomic or functional predisposition (e.g. short gut, motility disorders), repeated courses are typically needed.
- In children with chronic diarrhea secondary to bile acid malabsorption, the use of cholestyramine (Questran) to bind bile acids may help to reduce the duration and severity of the diarrhea. Any loss of pancreatic enzymes can be replaced with oral supplements.
- Immunosuppressive medications can be used to control autoimmune enteropathy and should be prescribed only by a specialist. Children with malabsorption secondary to food allergic enteropathy need to be on an elimination diet, avoiding offending food antigens. Their identification is often the result of empiric trials because food allergic enteropathies cannot be diagnosed by immunoglobulin E (IgE) measurement, either by radioallergosorbent assay test (RAST) or skin prick tests.

Medication

Digestive Enzymes

Pancreatic enzyme deficiency may occur because of steatorrhea, secondary to malabsorption. Pancrelipase (ultrase, pancreas, creon) assists in digestion of protein, starch and fat. It contains lipase, protease and amylase.

Pediatric dose: Adjust dose according to severity of pancreatic enzyme deficiency and fat content of stools 500–1500 U/kg (based on lipase content) enteric-coated tab per meal; not to exceed 2500 IU/kg/dose, because colitis with strictures (fibrosing colonopathy) may occur at higher doses. Drugs that increase gastric pH (e.g. H_2 antagonists) may increase effects of pancreatic enzymes by inhibiting destruction of ingested pancreatic enzymes.

Bile Acid–binding Agents

These agents are used in combination with antibiotics for bile acid malabsorption syndromes. Bacteria overgrowth may cause diarrhea by deconjugation and dehydroxylation of bile acids. Primary bile acid malabsorption may also occur.

Cholestyramine (Questran)

Binds bile acids, thus reducing damage to the intestinal mucosa. Also reduces induction of colonic fluid secretion. Forms a nonabsorbable complex with bile acids in the intestine, which in turn inhibits enterohepatic reuptake of intestinal bile salts.

Pediatric Dose: 2–4 g/d PO divided bid/qid for 8–10 d inhibits absorption of numerous drugs including warfarin, thyroid hormone, amiodarone, NSAIDs, methotrexate, digitalis glycosides, glipizide, phenytoin, phenobarbital, imipramine, niacin, methyldopa, tetracyclines, clofibrate, hydrocortisone, penicillin G and fat-soluble vitamins.

Antibiotics: Metronidazole may be considered and provides anaerobic coverage. Although the use of rifaximin in children for the indication of small intestinal bacterial overgrowth is not US Food and Drug Administration (FDA) approved, this antibiotic is virtually nonabsorbed (< 0.4%) and has been proven useful in the treatment of small intestinal bacterial overgrowth in adults.

- *Metronidazole (Flagyl)*: DOC for documented small bowel bacterial overgrowth. Provides good anaerobic coverage.
- *Adult Dose*: 500 mg PO bid/tid
- *Pediatric Dose*: 10–20 mg/kg/d PO divided bid/tid.

Nursing Management

Diet Management

Carbohydrate intolerance initiate treatment in child with severe acquired carbohydrate intolerance by eliminating all dietary carbohydrates until the diarrhea is resolved. Then, slowly reintroduce carbohydrates. In infants, use a glucose polymer (polycose)-based formula (e.g. pregestimil). Once the diarrhea has resolved, slowly reintroduce fructose into the diet as the only enteral carbohydrate source.

Begin with 14 g fructose/L formula and gradually advance in 14 g increments to a maximum of 56 g fructose/L formula. Once this goal is reached, slowly replace fructose with polycose until 56 g polycose/L formula is tolerated. Once 56 g polycose/L formula is tolerated, begin introducing pregestimil, a lactose-free formula. For older children, eliminate simple carbohydrates and lactose from the diet until the diarrhea is resolved. Simple sugars, including fruit juices, should be avoided for several weeks. If after several weeks of a relatively carbohydrate-free diet symptoms return when carbohydrates are reintroduced, the child most likely has a congenital defect in carbohydrate transport or digestion.

Fat Intolerance

MCT oil is used to treat child with poor weight gain that results from fat malabsorption. MCT oil does not require traditional fat metabolism and, thus, is more easily absorbed directly into the enterocyte and is transported through the portal vein to the liver. Fat-soluble vitamin supplements are required for child with fat malabsorption or short gut syndrome. Supplements in child with fat malabsorption should also include linoleic and linolenic fatty acids. Child with short gut syndrome may not be able to effectively absorb formula until mucosal hyperplasia has increased the mucosal absorption area. During this period of adaptation, appropriate parenteral nutrition may be needed to maintain optimal nutritional status.

- Child with a malabsorption syndrome shows any symptoms of dehydration or malnutrition admit the patient to a medical care facility and immediately initiate treatment with parenteral fluid and nutrition supplements.
- Treatment for severe acquired carbohydrate malabsorption requires admission to a medical care facility for enteral nutrition with a low-carbohydrate formula and administration of parenteral dextrose.
- Strict follow-up monitoring with the primary care pediatrician is necessary to reevaluate diet therapy efficacy and compliance.

- The availability of sensitive and specific serological testing for celiac disease, namely the antitissue transglutaminase and the newer antideamidated gliadin peptides antibodies, allows the screening of first-degree relatives of child, in whom the prevalence of celiac disease is higher.
- Asymptomatic subjects with positive results and celiac disease that is eventually confirmed by biopsy findings can then initiate a gluten-free diet, thus preventing all malabsorptive symptoms.

Prognosis

The malabsorption syndromes are transient, whereas others simply require a change in diet. Most disorders that cause secondary malabsorption are progressive and, because of systemic complications, result in a limited lifespan in child. For example, child with abetalipoproteinemia can die in early adulthood because of cardiac abnormalities, whereas child with severe autoimmune enteropathies or microvillus inclusion disease have a very poor prognosis without intestinal transplantation.

Outcome in child with short gut syndrome varies. The long-term prognosis depends primarily on the amount of time, parenteral nutrition is required. The complications of parenteral nutrition and the lack of trophic stimulation of intestinal mucosal growth impede recovery. Delayed intestinal autonomy depends on the characteristics of the residual intestine length, presence of the ileocecal valve and colon and motor function. Bacterial overgrowth compromises intestinal adaptation and increases the risk of liver disorders.

INFLAMMATORY CONDITIONS: ULCERATIVE COLITIS/ INFLAMMATORY BOWEL DISEASE

Definition

Ulcerative colitis (UC) is an inflammatory bowel disease (IBD) that occurs in the colon. It is characterized by the inflammation and ulceration of the innermost lining of the colon and

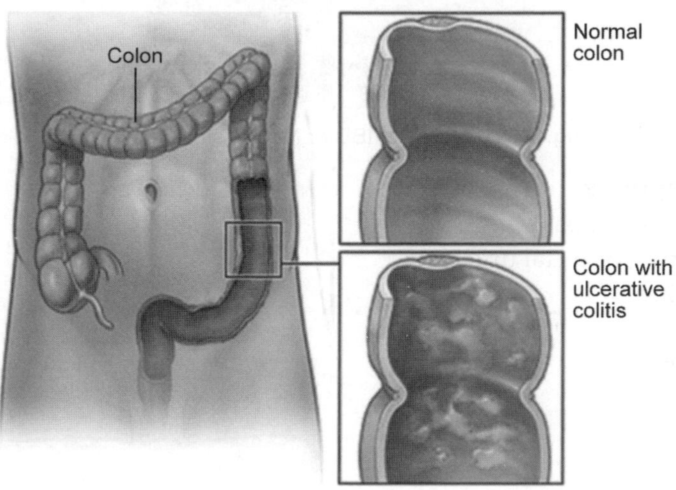

most commonly affects the left side of the colon and the rectum. UC is usually found in people ages 15 to 40 years; however, younger children sometimes develop UC.

Incidence

Early studies tended to show a higher prevalence of UC in white Americans than in black Americans. Over time, this trend seems to be decreasing, with recent incidence rates nearly the same. Asian Americans appear to have low incidences. Several studies have shown that the incidence of IBD in white Americans is up to 4 times higher in Jewish people than in other racial or ethnic groups. No sex predilection for UC is reported.

- In most studies, incidence of UC peaks between adolescence and early adulthood (i.e. in people aged 15–30 years).
- A smaller peak occurs in child aged 60–80 years.
- UC occurs less frequently in children younger than 5 years than in others.

Causes

The specific cause of ulcerative colitis is unknown, it has been suggested that the following factors may increase the risk of developing ulcerative colitis:

- *Heredity:* Having an immediate family member (such as a parent or sibling) with ulcerative colitis increases the risk.
- *Immune system:* A child's immune system may overreact to normal intestinal bacteria causing the inflammation.
- Disease causing bacteria and viruses.

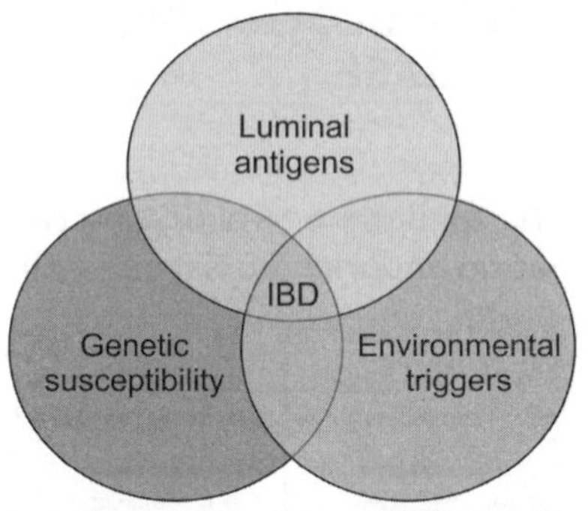

Fig. 7.55: Causes of IBD or Meckel's diverticulum

Signs and Symptoms

- Cramps/abdominal pain
- Bloody diarrhea or rectal urgency
- Rectal bleeding
- High fever
- Loss of appetite
- Weight loss
- Anemia
- Constipation
- Poor growth.

Pathophysiology

UC is characterized by accumulations of polymorphonuclear neutrophils in the crypts of the colon (crypt abscesses) with epithelial ulceration, edema and hemorrhage. These changes may represent the final common pathway of a heterogeneous group of diseases relating to genetic and environmental factors.

The mucosal immune system of the large intestine is continuously exposed to a wide array of antigens from ingested food products and from the billions of bacteria that live there. When activated, the cells of the mucosal immune system release cytokines that recruit inflammatory cells to the tissue and perpetuate the inflammatory response. In child with IBD, the inflammatory response to luminal antigens may be exaggerated over that in healthy individuals or they may not respond normally to down-regulation. The patient's genetic background likely determines when and how the inflammatory cells of the mucosal immune system react to the environment.

Diagnostic Evaluation

Blood Test

- CBC commonly reveals a mild anemia, which can be due to chronic blood loss (i.e. microcytic, hypochromic) or may represent chronic disease (i.e. normocytic). In cases of fulminant colitis, severe anemia may be present.
- Erythrocyte sedimentation rate (ESR) and C-reactive protein (CRP) level are frequently elevated during active disease.
- Result for antineutrophil cytoplasmic antibody with a perinuclear staining pattern (p-ANCA) are positive in up to 80% of child with UC and in up to 20% of child with Crohn' disease (CD).
- Serum albumin levels may be low in fulminant colitis.

Stool Test

- Obtain stool cultures to rule out infectious colitis. Obtain an assay for *E. coli* H7:0157 if the patient's symptoms are consistent with hemolytic uremic syndrome.
- Obtain a stool assay for *C. difficile* toxins A and B because *C. difficile* colitis can mimic UC or it may be responsible for a flare. Evaluation for toxin A or toxin B alone is inadequate for an accurate diagnosis of *C. difficile* infection.

Other Test

- Liver dysfunction may indicate sclerosing cholangitis or autoimmune hepatitis.
- An abdominal obstruction series (i.e. supine and upright abdominal radiography) is useful to evaluate for air-fluid levels, dilated loops of bowel, evidence of obstruction, or possible toxic megacolon. No pathognomonic findings for UC on this type of study are reported.
- Barium enema study is useful to evaluate the colon for stricture and for mucosal abnormalities, especially when colonoscopy cannot be performed. Barium enema studies may also demonstrate source of bleeding other than UC, such as a polyp.
- An upper GI series with small-bowel follow-through is used to evaluate for small-bowel inflammation that would support a diagnosis of CD rather than UC.

- CT scanning of the abdomen is useful to evaluate for bowel-wall thickening and obstruction. If present, abscesses and fistulae imply a diagnosis of CD rather than UC.
- Radionuclide-tagged WBC scanning can be used to demonstrate small-bowel inflammation that differentiates CD from UC.
- MRI of the abdomen is increasingly used to evaluate the large and small bowel for inflammatory changes and to look for transmural versus mucosal inflammation.

Complications

- Toxic megacolon is the most serious acute complication of UC and is reported to occur in up to 5% of child, but it is rare in young child.
- Colonic malignancy is a clinically significant complication in child with UC.
- Extraintestinal manifestations are common in UC.
- Approximately 25–35% of child with IBD have at least 1 extraintestinal manifestation.

Management

The goals of therapy such as:

- Control the inflammatory process to reduce or eliminate the symptoms
- Obtain long-term remission
- Promote normal growth and development
- Allow as normal life style as possible.

Medical Management

The general goals for managing IBD in children are to achieve the best possible clinical and laboratory control of the disease with the least adverse effects while permitting the patient to function as normally as possible.

Hospitalization is necessary when maximal outpatient therapy is unsuccessful or when child develop severe disease:

- *5-Aminosalicylate (5-ASA)*: The mainstay of outpatient management is anti-inflammatory therapy with 5-ASA preparations.
- Sulfasalazine (azulfidine) was the first 5-ASA preparation available for the treatment of UC.
- Asacol tablets must be swallowed whole, which limits its use in young children.
- *Corticosteroids*: Corticosteroids (e.g. prednisone) are effective in controlling acute flares of disease but less effective at maintaining long-term remission and a number of adverse effects make their long-term use undesirable.
- *Immunomodulatory agents*: Immunomodulatory agents are purine analogs that inhibit purine ribonucleotide synthesis and cell proliferation. Immunosuppressive agents also inhibit the immune response of natural killer cells and cytotoxic T-cells.
- *Intravenous corticosteroids*: Intravenous corticosteroids (e.g. methylprednisolone) may be effective in inducing remission when oral steroids are ineffective.
- *Cyclosporine*: Cyclosporine (cyclosporin A) is a potent inhibitor of the inflammatory cascade that primarily acts by inhibiting interleukin (IL)-2 productions, though it also decreases the recruitment of cytotoxic T-cells and blocks other inflammatory cytokines.

- *Infliximab*: Infliximab is a monoclonal antibody against tumor necrosis factor (TNF)-alpha, a proinflammatory cytokine that occurs early in the inflammatory cascade.

Nutritional Management

- Child with fulminant disease, possible obstruction, or possible toxic megacolon should ingest nothing by mouth (NPO) until their condition is stable.
- Child should avoid poorly digested foods, such as uncooked vegetables, seeds, nuts and high roughage, especially child with stricture or narrowing.

Surgical Management

Surgery is indicated for UC when medical and nutritional therapies fail to prevent complication. Surgical option includes a Subtotal Colostomy and Ileostomy that leaves a rectal stump as a blind pouch.

In case of children, segmental intestinal resection are preformed for small bowel obstruction, stricture or fistulas. Partial colonic resection is not curative and the disease often recurs.

Nursing Management

- Continued guidance of families in terms of dietary management
- Coping with factors that increase stress and emotional liability
- Adjusting to a disease of remission and exacerbations
- When indicated, preparing the child and parents for the possibility of diversionary bowel surgery
- Encourage child to take small, frequent meals or snacks rather then three large meals a day
- Provide high protein, high caloric food such as eggnog, milkshakes, cream soups, pudding, custards
- Provide mouth care before going to meals that relieve the discomfort of mouth care
- Provide psychological support to the parents
- Provide medication in time.

CHILD WITH APPENDICITIS

Introduction

Appendicitis, the most common pediatric surgical emergency, is caused by inflammation of the vermiform appendix. Four of 1,000 children younger than age 14 years will be diagnosed with appendicitis. The diagnosis of appendicitis can be difficult in children because the classic symptoms are often not present. A delay in the diagnosis of appendicitis is associated with rupture and associated complications, especially in young children. Improvements in rupture rates have been made with advanced radiologic imaging. Appendicitis is a clinical diagnosis with imaging used to confirm equivocal cases.

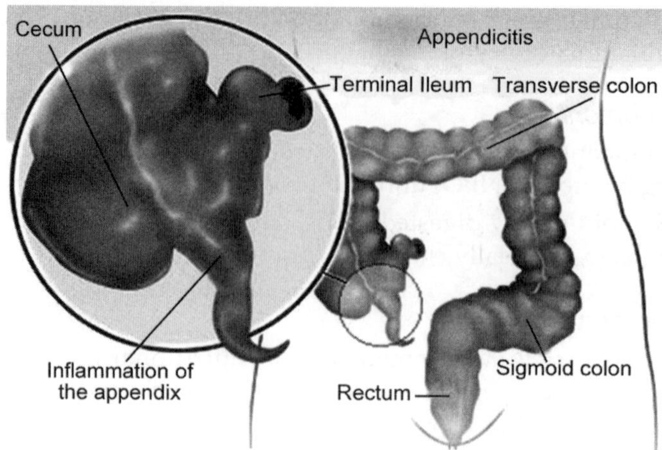

Fig. 7.56: Anatomical view of appendicitis

Definition

Appendicitis is defined as an inflammation of the vermiform appendix. Common symptoms of appendicitis include abdominal pain, fever and vomiting.

Incidence

Appendicitis has an incidence of 70,000 pediatric cases per year in the United States. Appendicitis has an incidence of 1–2 cases per 10,000 children per year between birth and age 4 years. The incidence increases to 25 cases per 10,000 children per year between age 10 and 17 years.

The rate of appendiceal perforation is 80–100% for children younger than 3 years compared to less than 10–20% of children aged 10–17 years. The mortality rate for children with appendicitis ranges from 0.1–1%. Delay in diagnosis increases perforation rate.

The male-to-female ratio of appendicitis is approximately 1.4:1. Appendicitis occurs in all age groups. The diagnosis of appendicitis in a younger child is more difficult and often the condition is more advanced.

Causes

Appendicitis results from a luminal obstruction. This obstruction can be caused by fecaliths, lymphoid hyperplasia, foreign bodies, or parasites. Children and adults have also developed appendicitis following severe blunt abdominal trauma.

Signs and Symptoms

These often include:

- Loss of appetite
- Nausea
- Vomiting
- Low-grade fever
- Inability to pass gas
- Abdominal swelling
- Constipation or diarrhea.

Understanding the typical clinical manifestations of appendicitis is essential in order to make an early and accurate diagnosis prior to perforation.

The classic history of anorexia and periumbilical pain, followed by right lower quadrant (RLQ) pain, fever and vomiting, is observed in fewer than 60% of child. The clinician is more likely to make the diagnosis by maintaining a high-degree of suspicion and a broad differential diagnosis and looking for the atypical case rather than the classic appendicitis. Vomiting, RLQ pain, focal tenderness and guarding are significantly associated with appendicitis.

- At McBurney's point, local tenderness with pressure and some rigidity of the lower portion of the right rectus muscle. McBurney's point is located halfway between the umbilicus and the anterior spine of the ilium
- Rebound tenderness may be present; location of appendix dictates amount of tenderness, muscle spasm and occurrence of constipation or diarrhea.
- Rovsing's sign (elicited by palpating left lower quadrant, which paradoxically causes pain in right lower quadrant).

Diagnostic Evaluation

Physical Assessment

- Children vary in their ability to cooperate with the physical examination. It is important to tailor the physical examination with respect to the child's age and developmental stage. It is also important to exclude extra-abdominal causes of abdominal pain, such as urinary tract infection (UTI) or pneumonia.

Note the following assessment:

- In early appendicitis, children may have focal tenderness in the RLQ without significant guarding or peritoneal signs.
- Observation of the child's interaction and gait prior to the examination can be extremely helpful. If able to stand, asking a child to hop is helpful in assessing for peritoneal irritation. If the child is unwilling to stand, shaking the bed or pelvis can also evaluate for peritoneal signs.
- A child with advanced appendicitis typically prefers to lie still due to peritoneal irritation.
- The child may have localized guarding or rebound tenderness.
- Typically, maximal tenderness can be found at McBurney's point, which is halfway between the umbilicus and the anterior superior iliac spine in the RLQ.
- On examination, bowel sounds may be decreased.
- Roving sign is pain in the RLQ in response to palpation of the left lower quadrant (LLQ), suggestive of peritoneal irritation.
- The psoas sign is elicited by placing the child on the left side and hyperextending the right hip.
- The obturator sign is determined by internal rotation of the flexed right thigh. Pain on movement may be caused by an inflammatory mass overlying the psoas muscle.
- A mass may be palpable in the RLQ if the appendix is perforated.
- An external genitourinary (GU) examination is helpful to rule out testicular or scrotal tenderness in males and hematocolpos in pubertal females.

- A rectal examination should be performed last and may reveal impacted stool, right-sided tenderness, or a mass. Be sure to perform a rectal examination (inspection, palpation and digital examination) in children who have any abdominal tenderness, a history of constipation, a history of rectal bleeding, trauma, or suspected physical abuse. A retrocecal appendix may cause exquisite tenderness on rectal examination.
- A pelvic examination should be considered in sexually active females to evaluate for tenderness (adnexal and/or cervical motion tenderness), masses, bleeding, or discharge.

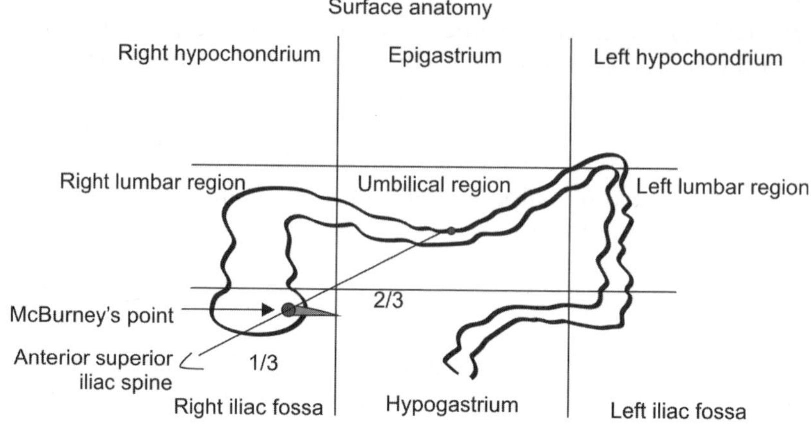

Fig. 7.57: Anatomical view of McBurney's points to assess the appendicitis

Laboratory Studies

- CBC with differential and urinalysis. Electrolytes may be useful if concern of dehydration or diabetic ketoacidosis.
- Liver function tests and amylase and lipase levels may additionally be helpful if other diagnoses are considered.
- The WBC count is neither sensitive nor specific for appendicitis. The WBC count is elevated in approximately 70–90% of child with acute appendicitis, but it also is elevated in many other abdominal conditions.

Urinalysis

- It is useful for detecting urinary tract disease, such as infection or renal stones.
- Pyuria can be present in children with appendicitis.
- Irritation of the bladder or ureter by an inflamed appendix may result in a few WBCs in the urine, but the presence of more than 20 WBCs/hpf suggests a urinary tract infection or vaginitis.
- Possible causes of hematuria include renal stones; urinary tract infection.
- Henoch-Schönlein purpura (HSP); or hemolytic uremic syndrome (HUS), in this case related to hemolysis and not red blood cells by microscopy.
- Grossly abnormal urinalysis findings may suggest another cause of abdominal pain.
- C-reactive protein (CRP) is a nonspecific inflammatory marker.
- A normal CRP does not exclude appendicitis, especially early in the illness.

Liver Function Tests

- Serum amylase level and serum lipase level may be helpful when the etiology of the abdominal pain is unclear.
- Electrolytes and renal function tests are more helpful in the management than in the diagnosis of appendicitis.
- Indications for assessing electrolytes include a significant history of vomiting or clinical suspicion of dehydration.

Imaging Studies

Plain radiographs rarely add to the diagnosis because they are typically normal in appendicitis. Abdominal radiographs should be obtained in any patient with an examination concerning for intestinal obstruction or with peritoneal signs. The presence of a calcified appendiceal fecalith occurs in fewer than 10% of cases. Note the image.

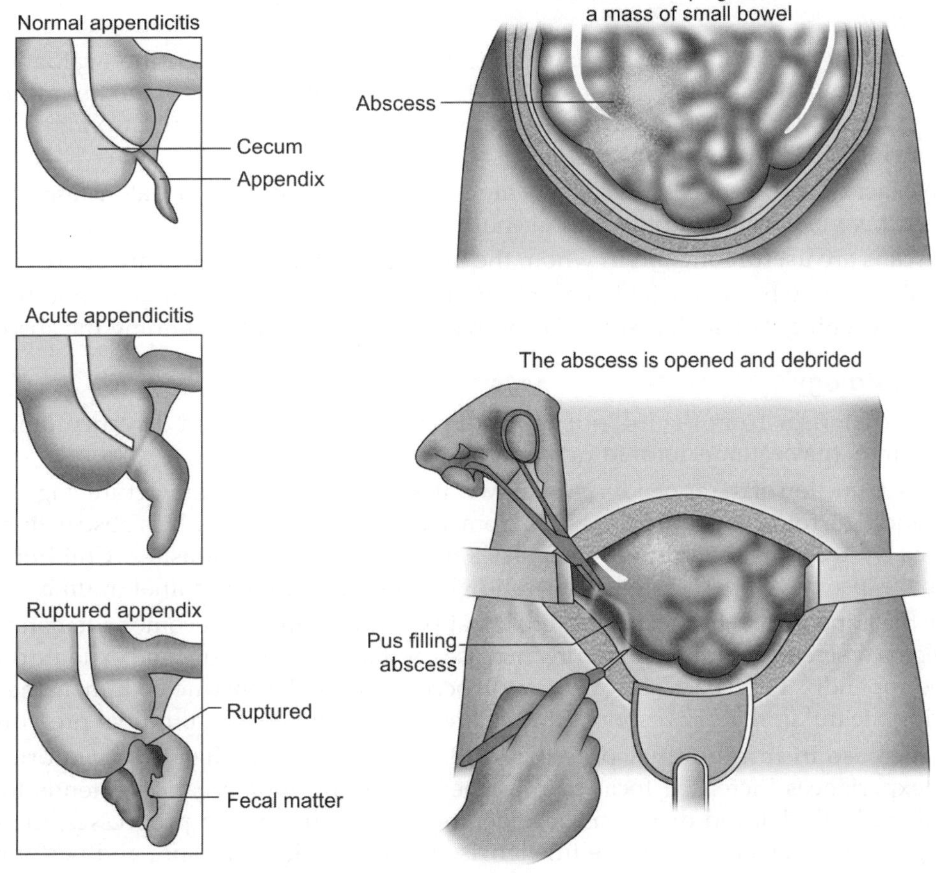

Fig. 7.58: Perforated appendicitis

Ultrasonography

- Ultrasonography is the preferred imaging modality in the evaluation of acute appendicitis in pediatrics when available.

- Ultrasonography advantages include noninvasiveness, no contrast or radiation exposure and minimal pain. One disadvantage is that the examination is operator-dependent and children with larger body mass indexes (BMIs) are difficult to examine.
- Specific findings can support the diagnosis. The finding of a noncompressible dilated appendix is a strong indicator of nonperforated appendicitis. After perforation, ultrasonography can identify a periappendiceal phlegmon or abscess formation. Additional findings that can support the diagnosis of appendicitis include the presence of appendicoliths, fluid in the appendiceal lumen, focal tenderness over the inflamed appendix and a transverse diameter of 6 mm or more.
- Ultrasonography is especially helpful in adolescent females, as it is useful in diagnosing alternate pathology, such as a tubo-ovarian abscess, ovarian torsion and ovarian cyst.
- An ultrasonographic image that does not identify the appendix should not be interpreted as normal, but it should prompt further investigation if clinical suspicion remains.

CT Scanning

- In children, numerous studies have investigated the use of CT in the evaluation of pediatric appendicitis. CT scanning appears to have its greatest value among child with large BMIs for which ultrasonography is difficult or when ultrasonography is inconclusive.
- No exact CT protocol is best; some centers use intravenous contrast alone and others use intravenous contrast plus enteral contrast.
- CT scans are useful for child in whom the ultrasonographic findings are equivocal.
- A CT scan may be beneficial in complicated cases with abscess formation and bowel-wall thickening. For such cases, oral contrast is most helpful for defining the abscess.

Pathophysiology

The appendix arises from the inferior tip of the cecum as a long, thin diverticulum. For most children, the cecum is located in the right lower quadrant.

The exact function of the appendix is unknown. It is a highly lymphatic structure, suggesting an immunologic role. Appendicitis results from a luminal obstruction. This obstruction can be caused by fecaliths, lymphoid hyperplasia, foreign bodies or parasites. Children and adults have also developed appendicitis following severe blunt abdominal trauma.

Once the appendiceal lumen is blocked, the appendiceal mucosa becomes edematous. A cycle begins where intraluminal pressure increases, inflammation ensues and exudate drains from the appendix. Fecal bacterial overgrowth occurs within the obstructed lumen, thereby enhancing the inflammatory response and further increasing the intraluminal pressure.

The increase in intraluminal pressure leads to a dull generalized discomfort. The patient experiences increased focal pain as the transmural inflammation extends to the peritoneum. With delayed diagnosis of appendicitis, the obstruction progresses, the wall of the appendix stretches due to the further rise in intraluminal pressure and perforation occurs.

When the inflammatory fluid and bacterial contents are released into the abdominal cavity, peritonitis develops. Concomitantly, the patient complains of more intense and generalized abdominal pain.

In the younger child, the omentum is less well developed and less likely to wall off a perforation, at last making:

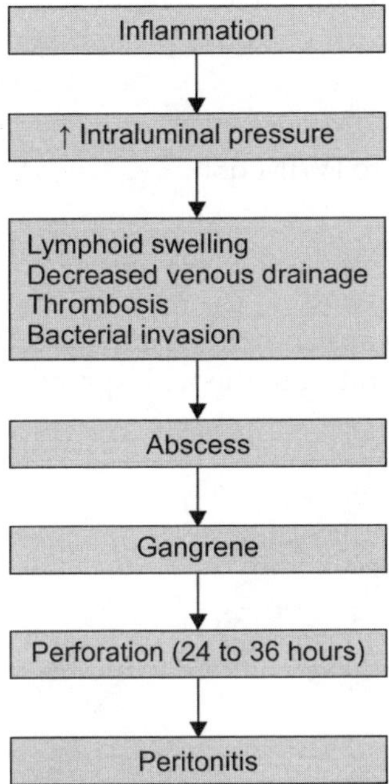

Fig. 7.59: Pathophysiology of appendicitis

Management

Medication

Preoperative antibiotics are given to children with suspected appendicitis and stopped after surgery if no perforation exists. Child presenting with perforated appendicitis may be volume depleted and require aggressive fluid resuscitation.

The combination of ampicillin, clindamycin and gentamicin is administered to treat infection from aerobic and anaerobic organisms. Alternative regimens include ampicillin and sulbactam, cefoxitin, cefotetan, piperacillin and tazobactam, ticarcillin and clavulanate and imipenem and cilastatin.

Antibiotics

Regimens should cover the most commonly encountered organisms, such as *E. coli, Bacteroides, Klebsiella, Enterococci* and *Pseudomonas* species.

Ampicillin (Omnipen, Principen)

Bactericidal activity against susceptible organisms. Alternative to amoxicillin when unable to take medication orally.

Adult dose: 1–2 g IV/IM q4–8h.

Pediatric dose: 100–200 mg/kg/d IV/IM divided q4–6h.

Gentamicin (Garamycin)

Aminoglycoside with activity against gram-negative bacteria including *pseudomonas* species. Also produces a synergistic effect when used in conjunction with a beta-lactam against *Enterococci*. Interferes with bacterial protein synthesis by binding to the 30S and 50S ribosomal subunits.

Adult dose: 1–1.5 mg/kg/dose IV/IM q8–24h.

Pediatric dose: 1.5–2.5 mg/kg/dose IV/IM q8h.

Surgical Management

Appendectomy

- The definitive treatment for appendicitis is appendectomy. Historically, appendectomy had a 10–20% false-positive rate, but the widespread use of imaging studies has reduced this rate.

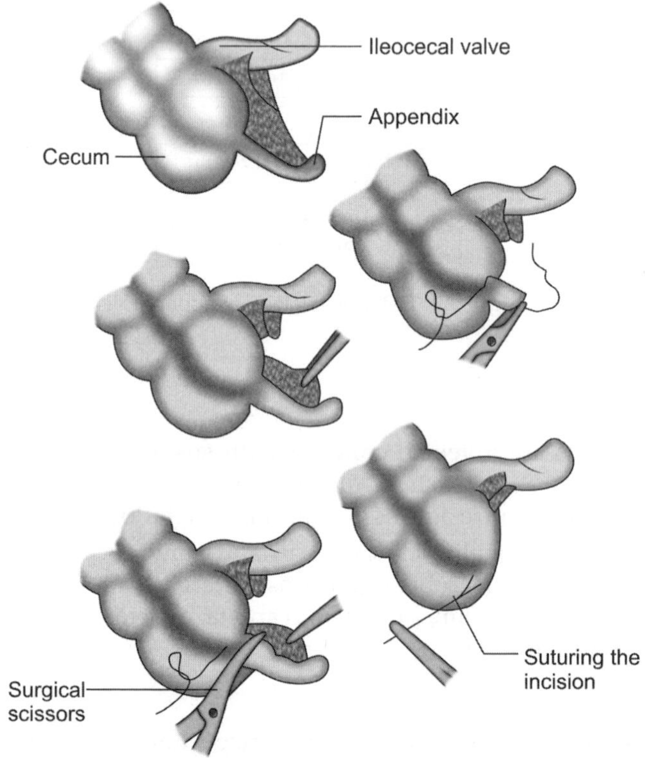

Fig. 7.60: Appendectomy

- Child with perforated appendicitis can be divided into 2 cohorts; those whose perforation is discovered in the operating room during appendectomy and those with preoperative evidence of perforation, most commonly seen on CT scans or ultrasounds. Increasingly, the approach in the latter group is conservative (nonoperative) management, with percutaneous drainage if possible and surgery after 8–12 weeks (i.e. interval appendectomy).

- Child discovered to have perforated appendicitis during appendectomy should be treated in the same fashion as those with nonperforated appendicitis. The surgeon should complete the appendectomy in a normal fashion.

The Laparoscopic Appendectomy

The laparoscopic appendectomy is being performed, perforation alone is not a reason for conversion to open appendectomy. However, if an abscess is encountered and drained, placement of a drain in the abscess cavity should be considered. In addition, when an open appendectomy is being performed on a patient with a perforated appendix, the high incidence of wound infection should be considered in terms of skin closure.

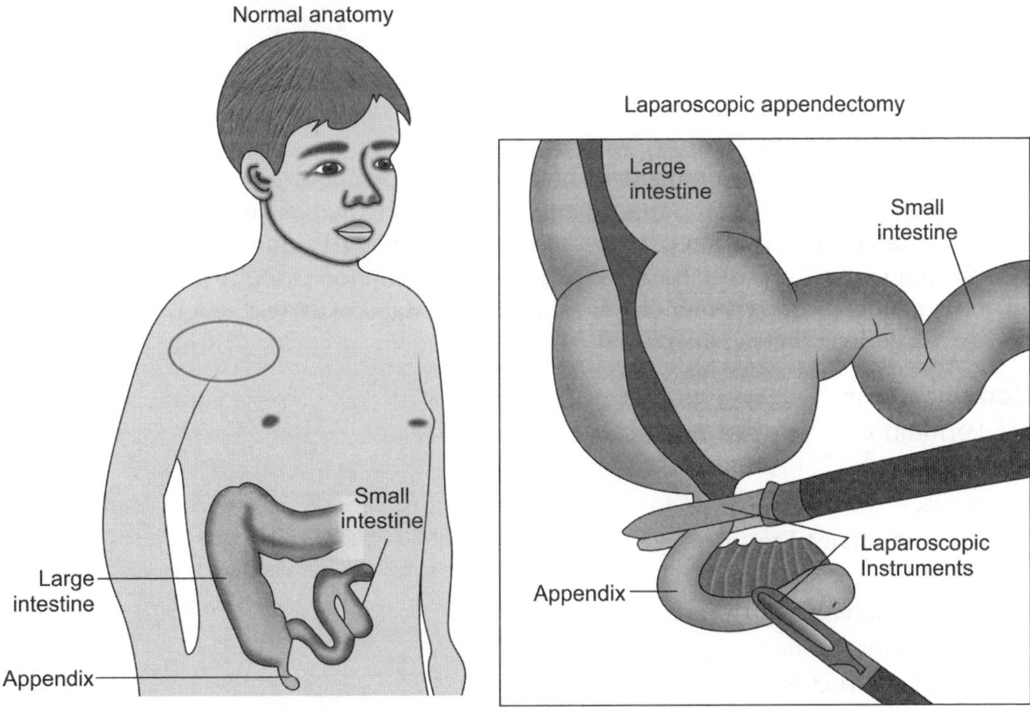

Fig. 7.61: The laparoscopic appendectomy

In rare instances, the inflammation can be so severe that the appendix cannot be safely identified and removed. To avoid unnecessary morbidity, drainage procedures with subsequent interval appendectomy.

Nursing Management

Nursing Priorities

- Prevent complications
- Promote comfort
- Provide information about the upcoming surgical procedure, prognosis, treatment needs and potential complications.

Nursing Diagnoses

- Acute pain
- (Risk for) Deficient fluid volume—preoperative vomiting, postoperative restrictions (NPO after surgery), hypermetabolic state, fever, healing process.
- Risk for infection—risk factors may include: Inadequate primary defenses, ruptured or perforated appendix, peritonitis, abscess formation and surgical incision.
- Deficient knowledge.

Nursing Intervention

- Nursing goals include relieving pain, preventing fluid volume deficit, reducing anxiety, eliminating infection due to the potential or actual disruption of the GI tract, maintaining skin integrity and attaining optimal nutrition.
- Preoperatively, prepare patient for surgery, start IV line, administer antibiotic and insert nasogastric tube (if evidence of paralytic ileus). Do not administer an enema or laxative (could cause perforation).
- Postoperatively, place patient in high Fowler's position, give narcotic analgesic as ordered, administer oral fluids when tolerated, give food as desired on day of surgery (if tolerated). If dehydrated before surgery, administer IV fluids.
- If a drain is left in place at the area of the incision, monitor carefully for signs of intestinal obstruction, secondary hemorrhage, or secondary abscesses (e.g. fever, tachycardia, and increased leukocyte count).

Complications

- Perforation
- Sepsis
- Shock
- Postoperative adhesions
- Infertility
- Wound dehiscence
- Wound infection
- Bowel obstruction.

MECKEL'S DIVERTICULUM (ULCERATIVE COLITIS)

Introduction

Meckel's diverticulum is an outpouching or bulge in the lower part of the small intestine. The bulge is congenital (present at birth) and is a leftover of the umbilical cord. Meckel's diverticulum is the most common congenital defect of the gastrointestinal tract. It occurs in about 2–3 percent of the general population.

Meckel's diverticulum is a true intestinal diverticulum that results from the failure of the vitelline duct to obliterate during the fifth week of fetal development. The embryologic origin and usual location of Meckel's diverticulum are explained by the development of the midgut. During the first few weeks of fetal life, the primitive yolk sac divides into two portions, the larger forming primitive gut while the smaller continuing as a yolk sac near the placenta. The two portions remain connected by a tube contained within the umbilical cord and this tube is called as omphalomesenteric or vitelline duct. Ordinarily, it becomes obliterated by the seventh week.

Definition

Meckel's diverticulum is defined as a pouch of extra tissue in the wall of the small intestine. It is the most common birth defect of the gastrointestinal tract.

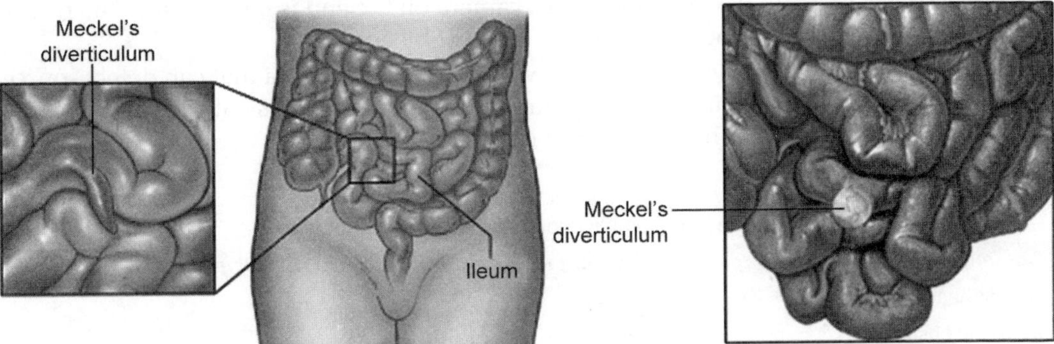

Fig. 7.62: Anatomical view of child with Meckel's diverticulum

Causes

- Genetic and environmental factors.
- Meckel's diverticulum occurs more often in males than females.
- Complications are also more likely to develop in male children under 2 years old.

Signs and Symptoms

Meckel's diverticulum that is infected or inflammation can cause:

- Blood in the stool
- Cramping abdominal pain
- Vomiting
- Fever
- Constipation.

Meckel's diverticulitis can cause sudden and severe symptoms that mimic appendicitis such as:

- Pain in lower abdomen that worsens with sneezing
- Coughing and deep breathing
- Loss of appetite
- Mild fever.

Diagnostic Evaluation

- History collection
- Physical examination
- Ultrasonography could demonstrate omphaloenteric duct remnants or cysts

- Blood test
  - Hematocrit
  - Hemoglobin
- Stool smear for invisible blood (stool occult blood test)
- CT scan
- *Technetium scan*: Radioactive technetium is injected into the body. This substance is absorbed by stomach cells in the diverticulum and can be detected by a special camera.
- *Colonoscopy*: A small, flexible tube with a camera on the end is inserted into the rectum and colon to look for blockages and the cause of bleeding.
- *Wireless capsule endoscopy*: The patient swallows a small camera that can detect sources of bleeding in the small intestine. If your child is too young to swallow a pill, it can be placed in the stomach while your child is asleep.

Complication

Table 7.9: Complications of Meckel's diverticulum

Complications	Percentage of symptomatic Meckel's diverticulum (%)
Hemorrhage	20–30
Intestinal obstruction	20–25
Diverticulitis	10–20
Umbilical anomalies	≤10
Neoplasm	0.5–2

Management

Meckel's Diverticulectomy

A Meckel's diverticulectomy is a surgical procedure done to remove a small pouch from the lining of the small intestine. This pouch is a birth defect called the Meckel's diverticulum. Surgery to remove the diverticulum should be recommended, if bleeding develops at the time of procedure, the Meckel's diverticulum and surrounding small intestine are removed and the ends of the remaining intestines are sewn together.

This can be done either through open abdominal surgery or laparoscopically (a narrow tube with a camera is inserted through a small incision and the Meckel's diverticulum is repaired through another small incision).

Indication for Surgery

- Symptomatic Meckel's diverticulum
- Hemorrhage
- Intestinal obstruction
- Diverticulitis
- Umbilicoileal fistulas
- Diverticula longer than 2 cm
- Diverticula with narrow necks
- Diverticula with fibrous bands

- Suspected ectopic gastric tissue
- Inflamed, thickened diverticulum.

WORM INFESTATION

Introduction

Worm infestation constitutes an important limitation on growth and development of children. In children with borderline nutritional status, worms can precipitate nutritional failure. Knowing size, shape of worms, larvae and eggs was important when treatment for each worm was different. With availability of broad spectrum antihelminthic drugs, it is not necessary that one should know morphology in details. Instead we should concentrate on the clinical pattern and drug details. Knowledge of breaking the life cycle is important from prevention point of view.

Causes of Worm Infection in Children

A few common causes of worm infection include:

- *Coming in contact with infected surface*: The worms and their eggs are capable of surviving up to two weeks without feeding. Some of the most common places where child may contract worm infestation are:
  - Soil containing worms or eggs—in playground or outdoor play
  - Touching pets or their excrement infected with worms
- *Inadequate handwashing*: It is difficult to keep child away from putting things in their mouth. If child is suffering from worms, there will be itching around anus, particularly in case of pin worms. During scratching, the eggs of the worms come in contact with the skin on hand, which wherever touched tends to spread. The worse scenario is when child put that hand back in the mouth, such as for thumb sucking or pleasure. Read more about children.
- *Poor hygiene*: Unwashed bedding, undergarments, filth in the room, all present breeding room for worms and their eggs. Someone who has not washed hands properly can also pose a risk for others as worm eggs can stay on fingernails which can be passed to child through touching.
- *Consuming infected food or water*: It is very important to wash vegetables and fruits before consumption as worm eggs can be on them. Raw or under-cooked food also carries a risk of worm infestation. Contaminated water is again a very common source of worm infestation.

Types of Worm Infections

Most common types of worm infections that trouble children:

- *Tapeworms*: These are flat, ribbon-like worms that can grow up to 15–30 ft and thrive in the intestine.
- *Roundworms*: They resemble earthworms and can grow up to the size of 30–35 cm.
- *Pinworms or thread-worms*: As the name suggests, thread-worms appear to be fine white cottony threads and live in intestine and around anus of the individual.
- *Hookworms*: These are commonly contracted through coming in touch with the contaminated soil and later enter intestine.

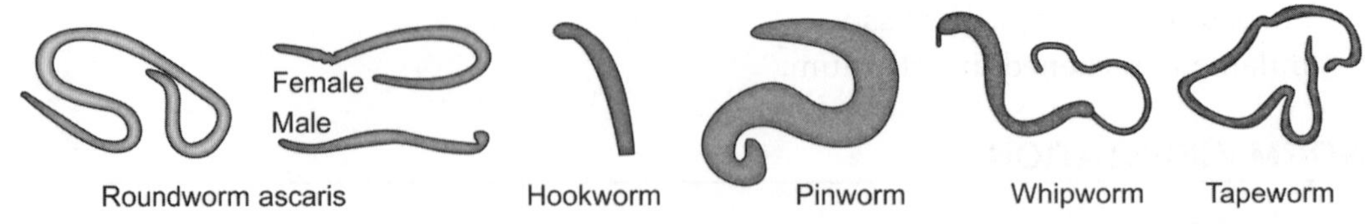

Fig. 7.63: Types of worms

Signs and Symptoms

Tapeworm Infection

- Nausea and vomiting.
- *Loss of appetite, sometimes eating too frequently and weight loss*: These usually appear in case of infection by tapeworms. Malnutrition may also be seen.
- *Jaundice*: This is more common in tapeworm infections.

Threadworm Infection

- Itching around anus is a common complaint in children who have thread-worm infection. Thread-worms creep out during night and lay eggs near anus which can trigger itching.
- Trouble sleeping (due to itching).
- *Painful urination*: This is typical in thread-worm infestation.

Roundworm Infection

- *Diarrhea, passing worms with stools*: If roundworm infection persists, then mature worms may be passed out from stools.
- *Fever and dry cough*: These are spotted within 4–16 days after coming in contact with the roundworm eggs.

Hookworm Infection

- *Coughing, wheezing*: Such respiratory troubles may crop up when the hookworm larvae attack lungs.
- *Anemia, fatigue*: These symptoms can be seen in case of severe hookworm infection.

Diagnostic Evaluation

- A microscope is used to find ova or larvae in the stools.
- To measure a child's worm load, count all the ova in a fecal smear. Less than 20 ova in a standard fecal smear is a light worm load. Between 20 to 40 ova is a moderate load. More than 40 ova is a heavy load. Threadworms are diagnosed by perianal smear by scotch tape collected in the early morning.

Management

The treatment of worm infection is quite simple and often required a course of anti-parasitic medicine to be followed. Antiworm medications or deworming treatments are easily available as over-the-counter medications, but exercise caution when administering medicines to your child. Since worm infections can hinder growth and development of your kid, it is best to obtain professional advice from the physician.

Table 7.10: Anti-worm medications or deworming treatments

Sr. No.	Worms	Mebendazole	Pyrantel	Piperazine
1	Ascaris (Roundworms)	4+ 3 days	4+ Single dose	2+ 2 days
2	Enterobius (Threadworms)	4+ Single dose	4+ Single dose	3+ 7 days
3	Ancylostoma (Hookworms)	4+ 3 days	4+ 3 days	-- --
4	Trichuris (Whipworms)	4+ 3 days	3+ --	2+ --

(4 + = 90–100%, 3 + = 80–89%, 2 + = 70–79%, 1 + = 70%)

Preventive Measures of Worm Infection in Children

Hygiene here is crucial. Teach children basic hygiene habits and educate them about worms entering their body and making them sick.

- Inculcate the habit of frequently and thoroughly washing the hands with a good antibacterial soap
- It is a good idea to introduce hand sanitizer to the apple of your eyes
- Teach your kid to drink clean, filtered or boiled water. Practice the same at home
- Make sure your kids change their undergarments daily
- Wash their bedding, pillow covers, blanket, etc. regularly
- Sterilize your toddler's toys
- Encourage your kid to play in dry areas and not splash in muddy puddles as these horde millions of germs
- Make sure that your veggies and meat are thoroughly cooked before you serve them to your kid
- Keep your kid's nails well-trimmed. Show them how dirt collects under long fingernails and must be kept clean
- Washing hands thoroughly before eating anything should be the rule
- Teach potty hygiene
- Do not share towels and undergarments
- Teach your kid to shower regularly. Practice thorough cleaning of private parts
- Clean your house thoroughly and with proper disinfectants
- Allow plenty of sunshine in your kid's room. Some worms are sensitive to light and nothing better than letting the sun do this job.

CARDIOVASCULAR SYSTEM (CVS)

RHEUMATIC FEVER

Introduction

Rheumatic fever causes chronic progressive damage to the heart and its valves. Until 1960, it was a leading cause of death in children and a common cause of structural heart disease.

The disease has been known for many centuries. Baillou (1538–1616) first distinguished acute arthritis from gout. Sydenham (1624–1668) described chorea but did not associate it with acute rheumatic fever (ARF). In 1812, Charles Wells associated rheumatism with carditis and provided the first description of the subcutaneous nodules. In 1836, Jean-Baptiste Bouillaud and in 1889, Walter Cheadle published classic works on the subject.

The association between sore throat and rheumatic fever was not made until 1880. The connection with scarlet fever was made in the early 1900s. In 1944, the Jones criteria were formulated to assist disease identification. These criteria, with some modification, remain in use today. The most recent advance is the recognition that there is genetic predisposition to development of acute rheumatic fever, though the exact reason is still a matter of research.

Definition

Rheumatic fever is a sequela of a previous group A streptococcal infection, usually of the upper respiratory tract. This is an autoimmune response secondary to molecular mimicry following group A streptococcal pharyngitis.

The disease involves the heart, joints, central nervous system (CNS), skin and subcutaneous tissues. It is characterized by an exudative and proliferative inflammatory lesion of the connective tissue, especially that of the heart, joints, blood vessels and subcutaneous tissue.

Incidence

The incidence is low in most parts of the country but is variable. In a study published in 2006, Martin and Barbadora showed that the disease remains a problem in western Pennsylvania with 121 new cases from 1994–2003. Consistent with earlier reports, most Child were children and most had carditis. Curiously, most studies report that rheumatic fever is very unusual if not rare in developed countries, but remains a major problem in developing nations. Acute rheumatic fever is common among American Samoans in Hawaii.

Incidence of streptococcal infection virulence of the bacterial strain and M protein subtypes determine the incidence of rheumatic fever in the population. As a sequela of beta-streptococcal exposure, acute rheumatic fever occurs during the school-aged years when streptococcal pharyngitis is most prevalent. Similarly, prevalence is higher in the colder months of the year when streptococcal pharyngitis is most likely to occur.

Causes

Rheumatic fever can occur after an infection of the throat with a bacterium called *Streptococcus pyogenes*, or group A streptococcus. Group A streptococcus infections of the throat cause strep throat or, less commonly, scarlet fever. Group A streptococcus infections of the skin or other parts of the body rarely trigger rheumatic fever.

Signs and Symptoms

Common Symptoms

Arthritis

Pain and swelling of the joints (arthritis) is the most common symptom of rheumatic fever, affecting three out of four people. The larger joints, such as the knees, ankles, elbows and

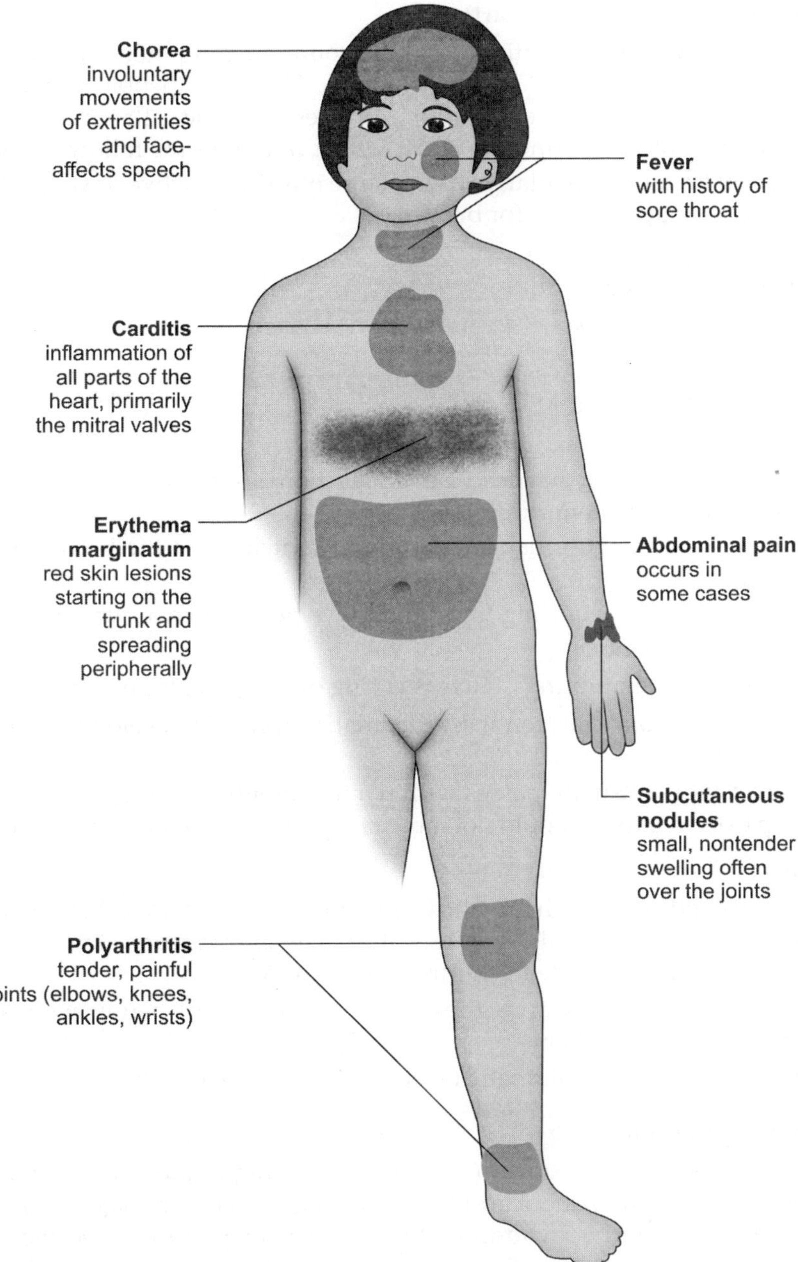

Fig. 7.64: Specific signs and symptoms of rheumatic fever

wrists are usually affected, typically on both sides of the body. Several joints are usually affected at the same time. The symptoms of arthritis should pass within four to six weeks as the inflammation settles, without causing any permanent damage.

Carditis (Inflammation of the Heart)

Inflammation of the heart (carditis) is another common and potentially serious symptom of rheumatic fever. Carditis occurs in an estimated 30–60% of people with rheumatic fever and is more common in younger children. As a result of the inflammation, the heart has difficulty pumping blood around the body, which can cause the following symptoms:

- Shortness of breath, particularly when you're physically active or when sleeping (it can often wake you up, gasping for breath)
- Persistent cough
- Rapid heartbeat (tachycardia)
- Feeling tired all the time
- Chest pain

Carditis can persist for several months, but it should improve over time.

Sydenham's Chorea

Sydenham's chorea is a term that describes a collection of symptoms related to inflammation of the nerves. These symptoms are:

- Involuntary and uncontrollable jerking and twitching of the body—most often, the hands and feet
- Difficulty with tasks requiring fine hand movements, such as writing
- Problems with balance
- Unusual emotional outbursts, such as crying or laughing for no apparent reason.

Around in one in four children with rheumatic fever will develop Sydenham's chorea, but it is rare in adults.

Sydenham's chorea usually passes within a few months, although in some cases it can persist for up to two years. It should not cause any permanent damage to the nervous system.

Skin Rash

Around 1 in 10 children with rheumatic fever will develop a skin rash, known as erythema marginatum. The rash is usually painless, non-itchy and spreads slowly over the child's body. It may only be noticeable in children with fair skin.

The rash usually comes and goes over the course of a few weeks or months, before disappearing altogether.

It is rare for adults with rheumatic fever to develop a skin rash.

Physical Assessment

Diagnosis of acute rheumatic fever (ARF) requires a high index of suspicion. Guidelines of diagnosis used by the American Heart Association include major and minor criteria (i.e. modified Jones criteria). In addition to evidence of a previous streptococcal infection, the diagnosis requires two major Jones criteria or one major plus two minor Jones criteria.

Major Criteria

- *Carditis*: This occurs in as many as 40% of child and may include cardiomegaly new murmur, congestive heart failure and pericarditis with or without a rub and valvular disease.

- *Migratory polyarthritis*: This condition occurs in 75% of child and is polyarticular, fleeting and involves the large joints. Note that one group of authors has suggested that atypical cases may only involve small joints.
- *Subcutaneous nodules (i.e. Aschoff bodies)*: These nodules occur in 10% of child and are edematous, fragmented collagen fibers. They are firm, painless nodules on the extensor surfaces of the wrists, elbows and knees.
- *Erythema marginatum*: This condition occurs in about 5% of child. The rash is serpiginous and long lasting.
- *Chorea (also known as Sydenham chorea and 'St Vitus dance')*: This characteristic movement disorder occurs in 5–10% of cases. Sydenham chorea consists of rapid, purposeless movements of the face and upper extremities. Onset may be delayed for several months and may cease when the patient is asleep. Note that a murmur in a patient with Sydenham's predicts carditis with a high degree of probability.

Minor Criteria

- Clinical findings include arthralgia, fever and previous history of ARF.
- Laboratory findings include elevated acute-phase reactants (e.g. erythrocyte sedimentation rate, C-reactive protein), a prolonged PR interval and supporting evidence of antecedent group A streptococcal infections (i.e. positive throat culture or rapid streptococcal screen and an elevated or rising streptococcal antibody titer).

Table 7.11: Modified Jones criteria for assessment of rheumatic fever

Major criteria	Minor criteria
Pancarditis (pericarditis, endocarditis, myocarditis)	Fever
Polyarthritis	Arthralgia
Sydenham chorea	Prolonged PR interval
Subcutaneous nodules	Increased ESR or CRP*
Erythema marginatum	Leukocytosis

*Erythrocyte sedimentation rate or C-reactive protein

Two major or 1 major and 2 minor must be present to diagnose rheumatic fever

Diagnostic Evaluation

Laboratory Studies

- No specific confirmatory laboratory tests exist for acute rheumatic fever. However, several laboratory findings indicate continuing rheumatic inflammation. Some are part of the Jones minor criteria.
- Streptococcal antibody tests disclose preceding streptococcal infection.
- The CDC has stated that a rapid antigen test in the appropriate clinical setting is sufficient to make the diagnosis of active GABHS infection and begin treatment.
- Isolate group A streptococci via throat culture. A significant percentage will result in a culture positive for group A beta-hemolytic streptococcus (GABHS). However, a culture positive for GABHS does not definitively prove active infection. Some children are carriers.

- Acute-phase reactants (e.g. erythrocyte sedimentation rate [ESR], C-reactive protein [CRP] in serum and leukocytosis) may show an increase in serum complement, mucoproteins, alpha–2 and gamma globulins. Anemia is usually caused by suppression of erythropoiesis.
- PR-interval prolongation is present in approximately 25% of all cases and is neither specific for nor diagnostic of acute rheumatic fever.
- Although there are a few small studies that show the contrary, troponins have not been shown to be helpful in making the diagnosis because ischemia and necrosis are not the major cardiac problems.
- Synovial fluid analysis may demonstrate an elevated white blood cell count with no crystals or organisms.

Imaging Studies

- Echocardiography may be helpful in establishing carditis. Some suggest it may be performed in all suspected cases.
- Chest radiography should be performed to determine presence of cardiomegaly and congestive heart failure.

Management

Medication

Medical therapy for acute rheumatic fever involves the following areas:

- Treat group A streptococcal infection regardless of organism detection.
- Steroids and salicylates are useful in the control of pain and inflammation.
- Heart failure may require digitalis, fluid and sodium restriction, diuretics and oxygen.
- Administer prophylaxis against GABHS infections to child who has developed ARF. Most authorities suggest that prophylaxis be given for 5 years. For those who have rheumatic carditis, some authorities suggest lifelong prophylaxis.
- Phenobarbital and haloperidol may be helpful in controlling chorea.
- Note that clinical trials for a 6-valent and a 26-valent vaccine are likely to take place in the near future. Phase I trials have been very promising.

Antimicrobials

Because of the direct link between ARF and group A beta-streptococcal infection, the first step in treatment is the eradication of the organism. Antibiotic regimens used for prevention of recurrence are mentioned briefly under further outpatient care.

Penicillin G Benzathine

Interferes with synthesis of cell wall mucopeptide during active multiplication, resulting in bactericidal activity against susceptible bacteria. Because of its prolonged blood level, several authors believe this to be the DOC. Others prefer daily injections.

Adult Dose: 2.4 million U IM once.

Pediatric Dose: Infants and children <60 lb (27 kg): 600,000 U IM once. Children > 60 lb (27 kg): 1.2 million U IM once Combination of 900,000 U benzathine penicillin and 300,000 U procaine penicillin (Bicillin C-R) may be used in smaller children.

Penicillin G Procaine (Crysticillin, Wycillin)

Long-acting parenteral penicillin (IM only) indicated in the treatment of moderately severe infections caused by penicillin G-sensitive microorganisms. Some prefer 10-d therapy. Administer by deep IM injection only into the upper outer quadrant of the buttock. In infants and small children, the midlateral aspect of the thigh may be the best site for administration.

Adult Dose: 2.4 million U IM once.

Pediatric Dose: Infants and children < 30 lb: 600,000 U IM.
Children 30–60 lb: 900,000 to 1.2 million U IM.

Amoxicillin

Inhibits the biosynthesis of the cell-wall mucopeptide and is effective during the stage of active multiplication. Inadequate concentrations may produce only bacteriostatic effects. Penicillin VK is the oral alternative for the treatment of rheumatic fever. Some authors suggest that once-daily amoxicillin is as effective and can be recommended as an alternative because compliance is likely to be better.

Adult Dose: 500 mg PO q6h for 10 days.

Pediatric Dose: < 12 years: 25–50 mg/kg/d PO divided tid/qid; not to exceed 3 g/days
> 12 years: Administer as in adults.

Erythromycin

DOC for child allergic to penicillin; inhibits RNA-dependent protein synthesis, possibly by stimulating the dissociation of peptidyl tRNA from ribosomes, which inhibits bacterial growth. In children, age, weight and severity of infection determine the proper dosage. When bid dosing is desired, one-half the daily dose may be administered q12h. For more severe infections, the dose may be doubled.

Adult Dose: 1 g/d PO divided bid for 10 d

Pediatric Dose: 30–50 mg/kg/d PO divided bid

Nursing Management

Most child with acute rheumatic fever (ARF) will be managed as in child by a multidisciplinary team of pediatrics, internal medicine, cardiology, infectious disease and rheumatology specialists.

Several regimens exist to prevent recurrences 'secondary prevention.' Duration of prophylaxis is determined by the number of previous attacks, time since last attack, the risk of exposure to streptococcal infections, patient age and very importantly presence or absence of cardiac involvement. Although the emergency medicine physician is not likely to be the prescriber of such a regimen, it is worth knowing what our colleagues may prescribe.

- Penicillin is still the drug of choice and may be given daily by mouth or monthly by intramuscular injection. Macrolides are acceptable in penicillin-allergic child.
- Those who have had carditis should be treated well into adulthood and may require lifelong prophylaxis.
- Those without carditis may be treated until they reach their 20s and after at least 5 years have elapsed since the past episode. Duration may increase if child in this group is at risk for exposure to streptococcal infection.

Complications

- Carditis
- Mitral stenosis
- Mitral regurgitation
- Aortic stenosis
- Congestive heart failure (CHF).

Prognosis

- Sequelae are limited to the heart and are dependent upon the severity of the carditis during the acute attack.

CONGESTIVE HEART FAILURE (CHF)

Definition

Congestive heart failure (CHF) is defined as heart fail to pump enough blood out to rest of the body to meet the body's demand for energy. This can be due to either a heart that pumps well but is very insufficient (due to a structural problem), or it can be a result of a weak heart muscle that does not pump a normal amount of blood to the body.

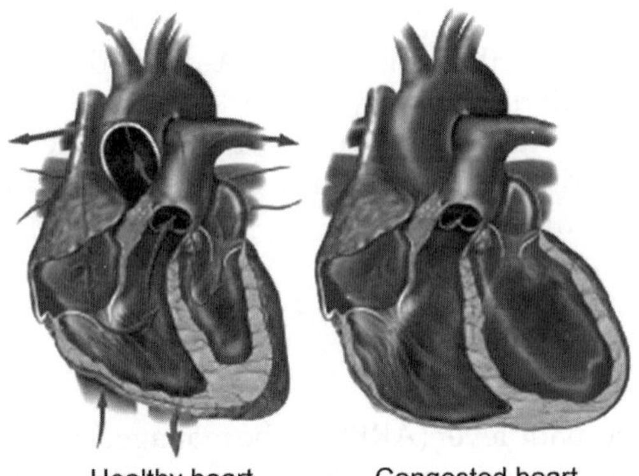

Fig. 7.65: Anatomical difference between normal and congested heart

Types

- Right side congestive cardiac failure
- Left side congestive cardiac failure.

Causes

Common problems caused by CHF include:

- The right side of the heart receives blood from the body's veins. If this side is not pumping as well as it should, blood returning to the heart backs up in the veins. When this happens, fluid collects in the body tissues. In babies and children, you may see this fluid as swelling (edema) or puffiness around your child's eyes, hands, feet and belly.

- The left side of the heart receives blood from the lungs. When the left side is not pumping well, fluid backs up into the lungs. If this happens, you may notice that your child's breathing becomes noisy, difficult and faster.
- Both sides of the heart can be connected with a hole that allows blood to pass through in an abnormal way. Like problems with the left side of the heart, this can lead to extra fluid in the lungs. This may cause breathing problems. It may also make it harder for your child to feed and gain weight.

Other Causes

- Various forms of congenital heart disease such as ventricular septal defect (VSD), patent ductus arteriosus (PDA) or common atrioventricular (AV) canal
- Heart valve disease caused by past rheumatic fever or other infections
- Infections of the heart valves and/or heart muscle (endocarditis)
- Cardiac arrhythmias (irregular heartbeats)
- Cardiomyopathy or another primary disease of the heart muscle
- Coronary artery disease
- Kawasaki's disease
- Inflammation of heart muscle (myocarditis).

Signs and Symptoms

- Failure to gain weight in infancy. Some babies will have normal length, but low weight for age
- Shortness of breath or labored breathing
- Fatigue
- Needing to take frequent rest breaks while playing with friends
- Falling asleep when feeding or becoming too tired to eat during infancy
- Cough and congestion in the lungs
- Sweating.

Pathophysiology

Congestive heart failure can affect the right side, left side or both sides of the heart.

The right side of the heart begins to function less efficiently, it is unable to pump much blood into the vessels of the lungs. Because of the congestion in the right side of the heart, blood flow begins to back up into the veins. Eventually, swelling may be noticed in the feet, ankles, eyelids and abdomen due to fluid retention. These symptoms are much more common in adults with CHF than in children. In children, congestion in the liver often is a better measure of right-sided failure than visible signs of swelling.

When the left side of the heart fails, it is unable to pump blood to the body efficiently. Blood begins to back up into the vessels in the lungs and the lungs become stressed. Breathing becomes faster and more difficult. Also, the body does not receive enough blood to meet its needs, resulting in fatigue and poor growth. In babies, most symptoms may occur with feeding or crying when the infant may have labored breathing and sweating.

Diagnostic Evaluation

- History collection and physical examination
- Blood tests
- *Chest X-ray*: A chest X-ray can be very useful to determine if the heart is enlarged and if there is extra blood flow or fluid in the lungs. This can be very important in determining the progression of congestive heart failure.
- *Electrocardiogram (ECG or EKG)*: A test that records the electrical activity of the heart, shows abnormal rhythms (arrhythmias or dysrhythmias) and detects problems with the heart muscle.
- *Echocardiogram (echo)*: A noninvasive test that uses sound waves to produce a study of the motion of the heart's chambers and valves. The echo sound waves create an image on the monitor as an ultrasound transducer is passed over the heart. This can very effectively show both the structure and function of the heart.
- Cardiac catheterization.
- Cardiac MRI provides a useful means to evaluate heart function.

Management

Medical Management

- Angiotensin-converting enzyme (ACE) inhibitors, which lower blood pressure
- Beta-blockers, which lower blood pressure and heart rate
- Digoxin, which makes the heart beat slower and with more force.

There are several types of medications used to treat congestive heart failure.

- A diuretic like furosemide (Lasix), which helps the kidneys to eliminate extra fluid in the lungs, is often the first medicine given both in babies and older children.
- Lower the blood pressure like an ACE inhibitor (Captopril), or more recently, beta blockers (Propranolol) are used. Theoretically, lowering the blood pressure will decrease the workload of the heart by decreasing the amount of pressure against which it has to pump.
- Digoxin is used to help make the heart squeeze better and help pump blood more efficiently. Since weight gain is a major challenge for infants with congestive heart failure, giving babies high calorie formula or fortified breast milk can help give the extra nutrition they require.
- Babies will need to have extra nutrition given to them via a tube that goes directly from the nose to the stomach, a nasogastric feeding tube. This is good for babies who work hard or get very tired from feeding in order to prevent them from using up all the extra calories needed for growth.
- Older children with significant heart failure can also benefit from nasogastric feeding to give them more calories and energy to do their usual activities.
- Oxygen can worsen blood flow to the lungs in babies with large ventricular septal defects but may be helpful as a buffer to children with weak hearts.

Nursing Management

Nursing assessment of the child's condition:

- Observe and record information relevant to the child's growth and development
- Observe and record child's level of exercise tolerance
- Observe child's skin and mucous membranes for color and temperature changes
- Observe for clubbing of the fingers, especially the thumb nails, with thickening and shininess of the terminal phalanges-may occur in cyanotic children by 2–3 months of age.
- Observe for chest deformities
- Observe for respiratory pattern
- Palpate the child's pulses in all extremities
- Auscultate the child's heart
- Record vital signs.

Nursing Diagnosis

- Impaired gas exchange related to altered pulmonary blood flow or oxygen deprivation
- Altered cardiac output related to specific anatomic defect
- Activity intolerance related to decreased oxygenation in blood and tissues
- *Altered nutrition:* Less than body requirements related to the excessive energy demands required by increased cardiac workload
- Increased potential for infection related to poor nutritional status
- Anxiety related to diagnostic procedures and hospitalization
- Developmental delay related to decreased energy, inadequate nutrition, physical limitations and social isolation
- Alteration in parenting related to parental perception of the child as vulnerable.

Nursing Interventions

Provide adequate nutritional and fluid intake to maintain the growth and developmental needs of the child

- Feed in semi-erect position
- Provide small frequent feedings
- Provide foods with high nutritional value
- Determine child's likes and dislikes
- Strict input and output
- Daily weight

Prevent infection

- Prevent exposure to communicable diseases
- Immunizations should be up-to-date
- Handwashing should be observed
- Be certain that the child receives prophylactic medication for infective endocarditis.

Reduce the workload of the heart since decreased activity and expenditure of energy will decrease oxygen requirements

- Uninterrupted rest
- Avoid unnecessary activities
- Prevent excessive crying
- Provide diversional activities
- Prevent constipation
- Relieve the respiratory distress associated with increased pulmonary blood flow or oxygen deprivation
  - Determine degree of respiratory distress
  - Include specific information in nursing record
  - Position child at 45 degree angle to decrease pressure of the viscera on the diaphragm and increase lung volume
  - Pin diapers loosely and provide loose-fitting pajamas for older children
  - Feed slowly
  - Tilt infant's head slightly
  - Suction the nose and throat if unable to cough out secretions
  - Provide oxygen therapy as needed
  - Improve oxygenation so that the body functions may be maintained
  - Provide effective oxygen environment
  - Observe response to oxygen therapy
  - Observe response to oxygen weaning therapy
    - Relieve hypoxic spells associated with cyanotic types of congenital heart disease
    - Observe for 'tet' spells
    - Encourage fluid intake
    - Obtain vital signs.

INFECTIVE ENDOCARDITIS

Introduction

An infective endocarditis (IE) otherwise called bacterial endocarditis (BE) is an infection caused by bacteria that enter the bloodstream and settle in the heart lining, a heart valve or a blood vessel.

Endocarditis is an infection of the inner lining of your heart (endocardium). It is generally occurs when bacteria or other germs from another part of your body, such as your mouth, spread through your bloodstream and attach to damaged areas in your heart. Left untreated, endocarditis can damage or destroy your heart valves and can lead to life-threatening complications.

Definition

Infective endocarditis is defined as an inflammation of the inner tissues (endocardium—such as its valves) of the heart. It is caused by infectious agents or pathogens.

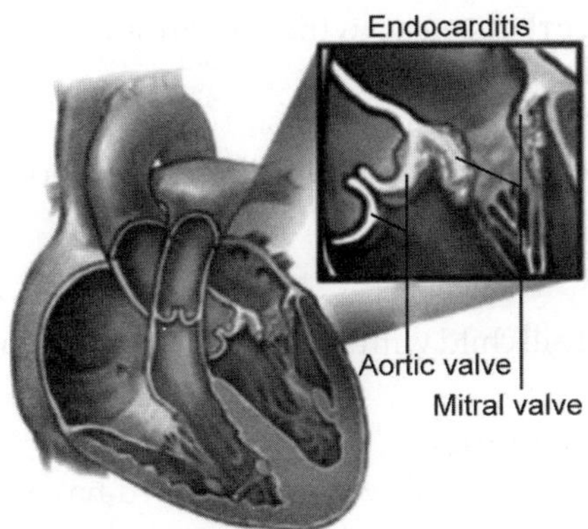

Fig. 7.66: Anatomical view of infective endocarditis

Types

- Subacute bacterial endocarditis (SBE) is often due to streptococci of low virulence (mainly viridans streptococci) and mild to moderate illness which progresses slowly over weeks and months and has low propensity to hematogenously seed extracardiac sites.
- Acute bacterial endocarditis (ABE) is a fulminant illness over days to weeks and is more likely due to *Staphylococcus aureus* which has much greater virulence, or disease-producing capacity and frequently causes metastatic infection.

Causes

Staphylococcus Aureus

The most common cause of IE overall (acute and subacute); most common with prosthetic valves, acute IE and IE related to intravenous drug abuse.

Coagulase-negative *S. aureus* causes subacute disease similar to *Streptococcus viridans*. Accounts for 30% of IE associated with prosthetic valves.

Streptococci

- *S. viridans*: 50–60% of subacute IE cases.
- *Group D streptococci*: Usually subacute and the third most common cause of IE.
- *Streptococcus intermedius*: Acute and subacute infection. Causes 15% of all cases of IE.
- *Group A, C and G streptococci*: Acute IE is similar to that with *S. aureus*. High mortality (up to 70%).
- *Group B streptococci*: Acute disease, high mortality often requiring valve replacement. Occurs in pregnancy and the elderly particularly.

Risk Factors

- Artificial heart valves
- Intracardiac devices, such as implantable cardioverter-defibrillators
- Unrepaired cyanotic congenital heart defects
- History of infective endocarditis

- Chronic rheumatic heart disease, which is an autoimmune response to repeated *Streptococcus pyogenes* infection
- Age-related degenerative valvular lesions
- Hemodialysis, a medical procedure that filters the blood of individuals with kidney failure.

Signs and Symptoms

- *Fever*: Elderly, chronically ill child with subacute IE may not have fever but the majorities do.
- *Heart murmurs*:
  - Most patients have a murmur.
  - The exception is right-sided IE where one third have murmurs.
  - Only 15% have the classic 'changing murmur'.
  - The most common murmur is aortic regurgitation.
- *Petechiae*:
  - Conjunctivae.
  - Hands and feet (dorsum).
  - Chest and abdominal wall.
  - Oral mucosae and soft palate.
- *Splinter or subungual hemorrhages*: Linear and red.
- *Osler's nodes*: Small tender red-to-purple nodules on the pulp of the terminal phalanges of the fingers and toes.
- *Clubbing*: Only 10% of cases and usually in long-standing subacute IE.
- *Roth's spots*: Retinal hemorrhages with pale centres.
- *Janeway's lesions*: Irregular painless erythematous macules on the thenar and hypothenar eminence (usually with acute IE and *S. aureus*).
- *Arthritis*:
  - With subacute IE, usually asymmetric and up to three joints affected (fluid sterile).
  - Acute IE can give acute septic monoarticular arthritis.

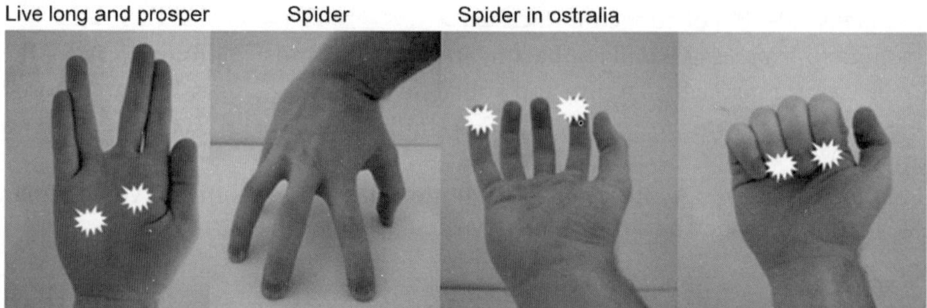

- *Splenomegaly*: Most often observed in long-standing subacute disease and often persists after treatment.

The Valves Most Commonly Affected by IE

- Mitral valve
- Aortic valve

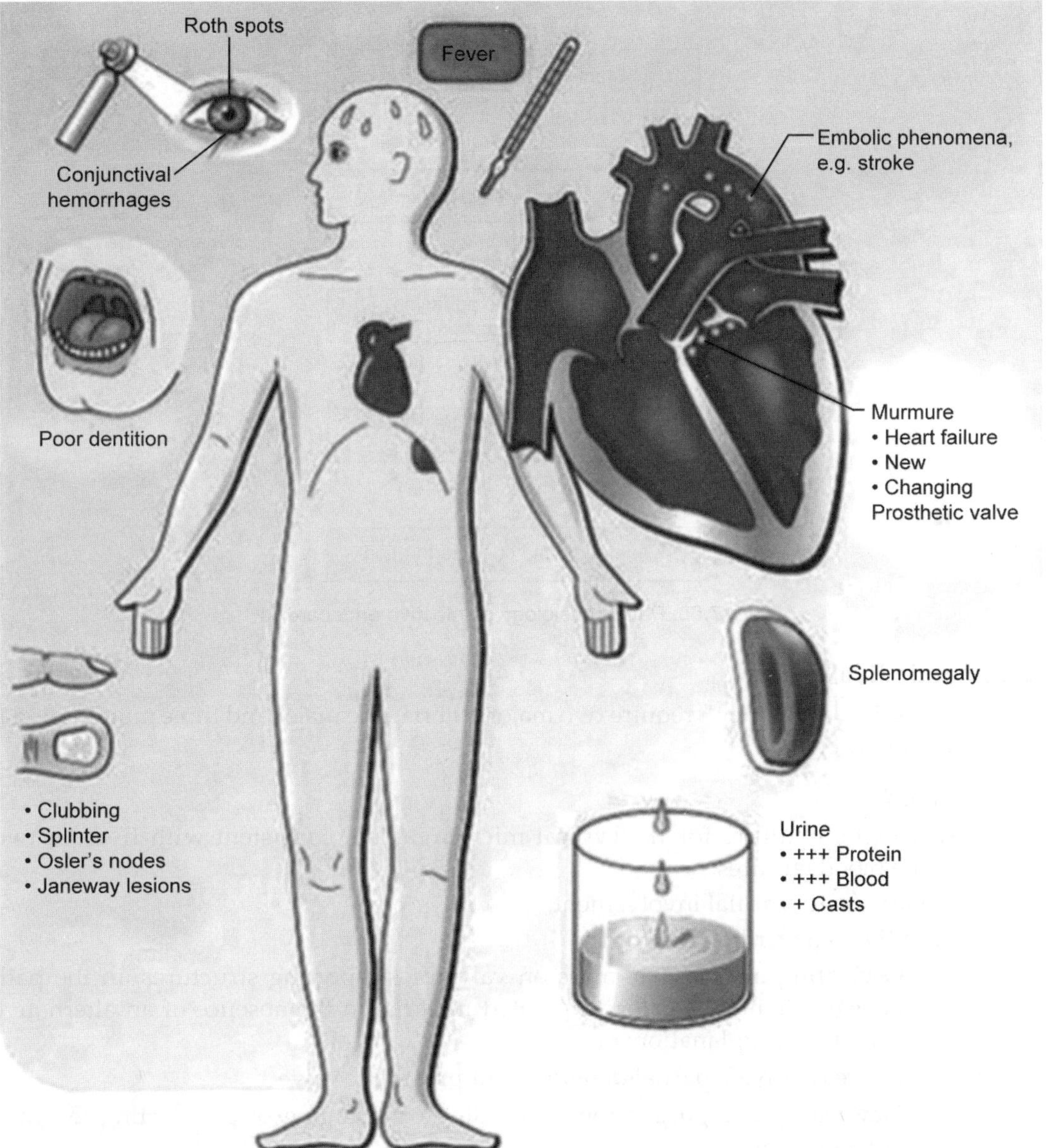

Fig. 7.67: Signs and symptoms of IE

- Combined mitral and aortic valve
- Tricuspid valve
- Pulmonary valve—rare.

Pathophysiology

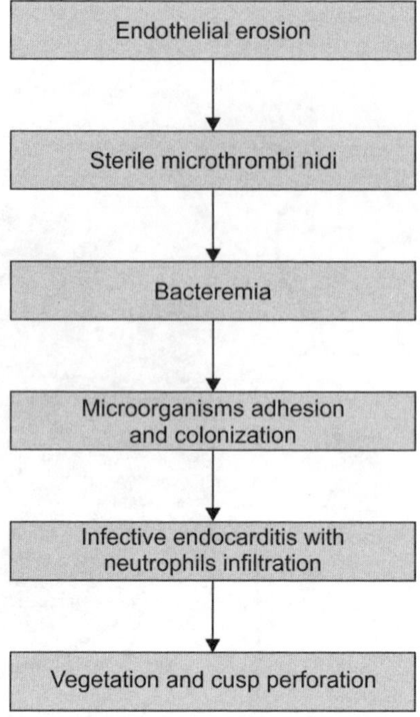

Fig. 7.68: Pathophysiology of infective endocarditis

Diagnostic Evaluation

Clinical criteria for definite IE require two major criteria, one major and three minor criteria, or five minor criteria.

Major Criteria

- Positive blood culture for IE: Typical microorganism consistent with IE from two separate blood cultures.
- Evidence of endocardial involvement:
  - Positive echocardiogram for IE:
    - Oscillating intracardiac mass on valve or supporting structures, in the path of regurgitant jets, or on implanted material in the absence of an alternative anatomical explanation; or
    - Abscess or New partial dehiscence of prosthetic valve
    - New valvular regurgitation (worsening or changing of pre-existing murmur not sufficient).

Minor Criteria

- *Predisposition:* Predisposing heart condition or intravenous drug use.
- *Fever:* Temperature > 38 °C.

- *Vascular phenomena:* Major arterial emboli, septic pulmonary infarcts, mycotic aneurysm, intracranial hemorrhage, conjunctival hemorrhages and Janeway's lesions.
- *Immunological phenomena:* Glomerulonephritis, Osler's nodes, Roth's spots and rheumatoid factor.
- *Microbiological phenomena:* Positive blood culture but does not meet a major criterion as noted above or serological evidence of active infection with organism consistent with IE.
- *Polymerase chain reaction (PCR):* Broad-range PCR of 16S (polymerase chain reaction using broad-range primers targeting the bacterial DNA that codes for the 16S ribosomal subunit).
- Echocardiographic findings consistent with IE but do not meet a major criterion as noted above.
- *Chest X-ray:* As part of the initial assessment.

Blood Test

Blood culture-negative IE (BCNIE) refers to IE in which no causative microorganism can be grown using the usual blood culture methods.

Echocardiography

- Echocardiography must be performed as soon as possible (ideally within 24 hours) in all patients with suspected IE.

Serological Examination

- In patients with blood culture-negative IE, serological testing for Coxiella and Bartonella species should be performed.
- Consider brucellosis in patients with negative blood cultures and a risk of exposure (dietary, occupational or travel).
- Candida antibody and antigen tests should not be used to diagnose candidal IE because there is currently no evidence to support their use and therefore relying on these tests may lead to inappropriate treatment.

Investigation of Excised Heart Valves

- Samples of valve or other infected tissue removed at the time of surgery should be sent for microbiological and histopathological investigation.
- Samples of excised heart valve (or tissue from embolectomy) from cases of culture-negative IE should be referred for broad-range bacterial PCR and sequencing.

Management

The following principles of management of infective endocarditis:

- Selection of the antibiotic agents is based on the sensitivity of the offending organism to antibiotics
- Bactericidal rather than bacteriostatic antibiotics are preferable
- Intermittent intravenous antibiotic administration to achieve high concentration of the antibiotic is recommended; a bactericidal level of 1:8 or greater should be achieved

- Prolonged (4–8 weeks) treatment to ensure eradication of the organism is generally required
- Documentation of cessation of bacteremia prior to discontinuation of antibiotics is suggested
- Surgery may be necessary in some cases as detailed below.

Staphylococcal Endocarditis

Intravenous therapy for four weeks is recommended for staphylococcal NVE, which should be extended to at least six weeks in patients with intracardiac prostheses, secondary lung abscesses and osteomyelitis. Routine switch to oral antimicrobials is not recommended.

- Meticillin-susceptible staphylococci: Flucloxacillin.
- Meticillin-resistant: Vancomycin and rifampicin.
- Meticillin-resistant, vancomycin-resistant: Daptomycin and rifampicin or gentamicin.

Streptococcal Endocarditis

- Benzylpenicillin monotherapy; ceftriaxone monotherapy; benzylpenicillin and gentamicin; ceftriaxone and gentamicin.
- Treatment of streptococci in patients with significant penicillin allergy: vancomycin and gentamicin; teicoplanin and gentamicin.

Enterococcal Endocarditis

- Amoxicillin or penicillin and gentamicin; vancomycin and gentamicin; teicoplanin and gentamicin; amoxicillin (for amoxicillin-susceptible and high-level gentamicin resistant isolates).

HACEK Endocarditis

- Treatment should be with a B-lactamase-stable cephalosporin or amoxicillin if the isolate is susceptible.
- Gentamicin should only be added for the first two weeks of therapy.
- Ciprofloxacin can be considered as an alternative agent.
- NVE should receive four weeks and PVE six weeks of treatment.

Bartonella

- Amoxicillin and gentamicin (if penicillin-allergic then use tetracycline).
- Doxycycline and gentamicin.

Fungal Endocarditis

Antifungal agents used include fluconazole, voriconazole, amphotericin, micafungin, caspofungin, anidulafungin, posaconazole and flucytosine. Itraconazole should not be used.

Candidal Endocarditis

Initial treatment should be with an echinocandin or amphotericin. Surgical valve replacement is recommended.

Aspergillus Endocarditis

Initial treatment should be with voriconazole. Surgical valve replacement is mandatory for survival.

Surgical Management

A surgical opinion should be sought at the earliest opportunity for every patient with endocarditis affecting intracardiac prosthetic material. Antibiotics are the standard treatment for native valve IE, with surgery primarily reserved for patients with heart failure or inadequate response to antibiotic treatment.

The timing and indications for surgical intervention to prevent systemic embolism in IE remain controversial. A trial to compare clinical outcomes of early surgery and conventional treatment in patients with left-sided IE, severe valve disease and large vegetations found that early surgery in patients with IE and large vegetations significantly reduced mortality from embolic events by effectively decreasing the risk of systemic embolism.

Complications

These are an inherent part of the progression of the disease. Potential complications of IE include:

- Myocardial infarction, pericarditis, cardiac arrhythmias.
- Heart valve insufficiency.
- Congestive heart failure.
- Sinus of Valsalva aneurysm.
- Aortic root or myocardial abscesses.
- Arterial emboli, infarctions, mycotic aneurysms.
- Arthritis, myelitis.
- Glomerulonephritis, acute kidney injury.
- Stroke syndromes.
- Mesenteric or splenic abscess or infarction.

Prognosis

Although novel diagnostic and therapeutic strategies have emerged, the overall one-year mortality has not improved and remains at 30%. However, the prognosis varies markedly according to a variety of factors.

MYOCARDITIS

Introduction

Myocarditis is an inflammatory disorder of the myocardium with necrosis of the myocytes and associated inflammatory infiltrate. It is usually caused by a viral infection, particularly adenovirus and enterovirus infections (e.g. coxsackievirus), although many infectious organisms commonly seen in infants and children have been implicated. Occasionally, myocarditis may be a manifestation of drug hypersensitivity (as depicted in the histologic image below) or toxicity.

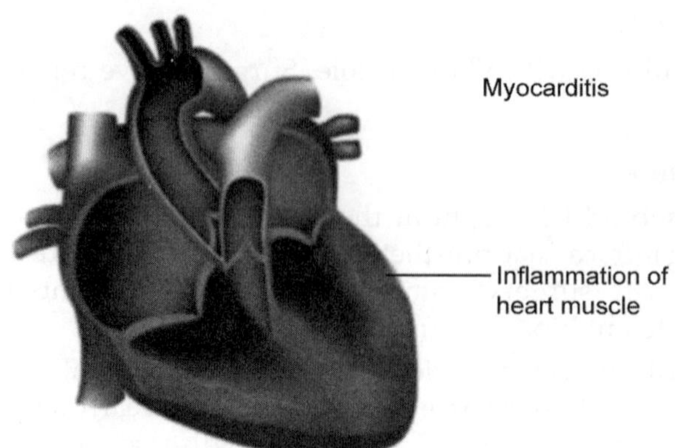

- *Active myocarditis:* Characterized by abundant inflammatory cells and myocardial necrosis.
- *Borderline myocarditis:* Characterized by an inflammatory response that is too sparse for this type to be labeled as active myocarditis; degeneration of myocytes not demonstrated with light microscopy.
- Nonmyocarditis.

Definition

Myocarditis is an inflammatory lesion of the cardiac muscle. Myocarditis can occur when any infectious disease, but currently myocarditis is most often seen in viral infections. To non-communicable factors that cause myocarditis are some medicines (antibiotics, sulfonamides, hydrochlorothiazide methyldopa and others), serum and vaccines. Myocarditis occurs in systemic diseases of connective tissue, for example, in systemic lupus erythematosus and other systemic vasculitis.

Incidence

Myocarditis is a rare disease. The World Health Organization (WHO) reports that incidence of cardiovascular involvement after enteroviral infection is 1–4%, depending on the causative organism. Incidence widely varies among countries and is related to hygiene and socioeconomic conditions. Availability of medical services and immunizations also affect incidence. Occasional epidemics of viral infections have been reported with an associated higher incidence of myocarditis. Enteroviruses (e.g. coxsackievirus, echovirus) and adenoviruses, particularly types 2 and 5, are the most commonly involved organisms.

Causes

Myocarditis is uncommon and can be caused by a viral infection or a self-directed immune response (this is when the person's own immune system attacks the body, such as in autoimmune diseases like rheumatoid arthritis or lupus). Some autoimmune diseases can affect the heart and cause myocarditis. Rare cases have also been associated with a variety of infections, toxic injuries, adverse drug reactions and even cancer.

Infecting Organisms

Adenovirus and Epstein-Barr virus have been considered the most common viruses that cause myocarditis. However, studies have found that, using polymerase chain reaction

(PCR) for the diagnosis, parvovirus B19 and human herpesvirus-6 are the most frequent pathogens in child with acute myocarditis.

Infecting organisms include the following:

- Coxsackievirus types A and B (especially type B)
- Adenovirus (most commonly types 2 and 5)
- Cytomegalovirus
- Echovirus
- Epstein-Barr virus
- Hepatitis C virus
- Herpes virus
- Human immunodeficiency virus
- Influenza and parainfluenza
- Measles
- Mumps, associated with endocardial fibroelastosis (EFE)
- Parvovirus B19
- Poliomyelitis virus
- Rubella
- Varicella.

Signs and Symptoms

Heart failure: This is the most common presenting picture in all ages. The condition of child who presents with heart failure may rapidly deteriorate even with supportive care. Neonates and young children have higher mortality rates than older child. Rapid supportive care with blood pressure support, afterload reduction and control of arrhythmia may prevent early death.

Chest pain: Although rare in young children, this may be the initial presentation for older children, adolescents and adults. Chest pain may be due to myocardial ischemia or concurrent pericarditis.

Arrhythmia: Child can present with any type of dysrhythmia, including atrioventricular conduction disturbances. Sinus tachycardia is typical and the rate is faster than expected for the degree of fever present, which is typically low-grade. Junctional tachycardia is also seen and can be difficult to control medically.

Dilated cardiomyopathy: The debate continues over whether myocarditis progresses to dilated cardiomyopathy. Many investigators believe that dilated cardiomyopathy is a direct result of a previously burned-out myocarditis episode.

Acute symptoms in infants include the following:

- Irritability
- Lethargy
- Periodic episodes of pallor
- Fever
- Hypothermia
- Tachypnea
- Anorexia
- Failure to thrive.

Older children present with similar symptoms and may experience lack of energy and general malaise. Parents may refer to a recent, nonspecific, flulike illness, GI symptoms, poor feeding or rapid breathing.

Pathophysiology

Myocarditis generally results in a decrease in myocardial function, with concomitant enlargement of the heart and an increase in the end-diastolic volume caused by increased preload. Normally, the heart compensates for dilation with an increase in contractility (Starling law), but because of inflammation and muscle damage, a heart affected with myocarditis is unable to respond to the increase in volume.

In addition, inflammatory mediators, such as cytokines and adhesion molecules, as well as apoptotic mechanisms are activated. The progressive increase in left ventricular end-diastolic volume increases left atrial, pulmonary venous and arterial pressures, resulting in increasing hydrostatic forces. These increased forces lead to both pulmonary edema and congestive heart failure. Without treatment, this process may progress to end-stage cardiac failure and death.

Diagnostic Evaluation

Physical Examination

Signs of diminished cardiac output, such as tachycardia, weak pulse, cool extremities, decreased capillary refill and pale or mottled skin may be present. Heart sounds may be muffled, especially in the presence of pericarditis. An S_3 may be present and a heart murmur caused by atrioventricular valve regurgitation may be heard. Hepatomegaly may be present in younger children. Rales may be heard in older children. Jugular venous distention and edema of the lower extremities may be present.

Neonates

- Neonates may seem irritable, be in respiratory distress and exhibit signs of sepsis.
- Somnolence, hypotonia and seizures can be associated if the CNS is involved.
- Hypothermia or hyperthermia, oliguria, elevated liver enzymes and elevated BUN and creatinine levels caused by direct viral damage, low cardiac output, or both may be present.

Infants

- Signs include failure to thrive, anorexia, tachypnea, tachycardia, wheezing and diaphoresis with feeding.
- In severe cases, low cardiac output may progress to acidosis and death.
- End-organ damage may develop because of direct viral infestation or because of low cardiac output.
- CNS involvement may also develop.

Adolescents

- Presentation may be similar to that of younger children but with a more prominent decrease in exercise tolerance, lack of energy, malaise, chest pain, low-grade fever, arrhythmia and cough.
- End-organ damage and low cardiac output may be present.

The following studies are indicated for viral myocarditis:

CBC count with differential

- Acute anemia of any origin may cause heart failure and chronic anemia exacerbates heart failure; both respond to blood transfusion.
- The presence of lymphocytosis or neutropenia supports diagnosis of a viral infection.
  - *Blood cultures:* Ruling out any bacterial infection is important.
  - *Sedimentation rate and C-reactive protein:* These nonspecific markers of inflammation are usually elevated. However, a normal value does not rule out myocarditis, particularly in the presence of congestive heart failure, which may lower the sedimentation rate.
  - *Viral cultures:* Nasopharyngeal and rectal swabs may help identify etiology.
  - *Viral titers:* A 4-fold increase in a specific titer from the acute to convalescent phase is strong evidence of infection.

Imaging Studies

Echocardiography

- This is the most cost-effective test used for evaluation of myocardial function.
- It is sensitive but not specific.

Findings include the following:

- Global hypokinesis (the most common finding)
- Increased left ventricular end diastolic and systolic dimensions
- Left ventricular dysfunction, primarily systolic with decreased ejection fraction and shortening fraction
- Segmental wall motion abnormalities
- Pericardial effusion.

Chest radiography

- Cardiomegaly and pulmonary edema may be depicted.
- Incidentally noted cardiomegaly on chest radiography may be the initial presentation.

MRI Scan

MRI with gadolinium is a newer technology to evaluate the cardiac muscle inflammation via a special protocol for myopericarditis.

Other Investigation

Electrocardiography (ECG)

- In some child with mild cardiac involvement, ECG changes may be the only abnormal findings suggestive of myocarditis.
- Low-voltage QRS (< 5 mm throughout the limb leads) is the classic pattern. Pseudoinfarction patterns with pathologic Q waves and poor progression of R waves in the precordial leads may also be present.

Diagnostic Procedures

- Biopsy is the criterion standard for the diagnosis of myocarditis. Myocardial biopsy findings establish diagnosis and classify disease stage.
- Biopsy is a relatively safe and effective way to sample heart muscle in older children; however, a risk of perforation in sick or younger infants is observed.
- The use of endomyocardial biopsy is controversial because of the possibility of a high false-negative result rate and because no proven therapy is available, even when a positive biopsy finding is obtained.
- Some advocate using radionuclide imaging techniques as screening tools before considering endomyocardial biopsy.
- Biopsy specimens may be useful for PCR diagnosis of viral etiology.

Management

Medical Management

In the acute phase of viral myocarditis, the patient should be admitted to the hospital, even if only mild signs of respiratory distress or congestive heart failure are present. Rapid progression to overt heart failure, hemodynamic collapse, or both may occur. Medical care is aimed at minimizing hemodynamic demands of the body. No specific proven therapy is available to prevent the myocardial damage, but maintenance of tissue perfusion is the goal to avoid further complications. Normal arterial blood oxygen levels should be maintained with supplemental oxygen as needed.

Surgical Management

Extracorporeal membrane oxygenation (ECMO) has been used as an interim treatment to provide rest to the heart and as a bridge for transplant in selected child with good results.

Medication

Inotropic agents are used when cardiac output cannot be maintained by less invasive measures. Dopamine, dobutamine, inamrinone (formerly amrinone) and milrinone are the most commonly used vasopressors. Afterload reduction is most important in treating acute myocarditis and is used when hypotension is not present.

This decreases the workload for the compromised myocardium and can allow child to recover from the acute phase of illness. Agents that reduce afterload improve cardiac output by decreasing systemic arterial resistance. Intravenous medications such as nitroprusside, inamrinone and milrinone can be replaced with oral ACE inhibitors when the patient stabilizes.

The use of immunosuppressive agents for the treatment of viral myocarditis is still controversial. Some animal studies revealed an exacerbation of viral cytotoxicity when treated with immunosuppressive agents. Other small series in humans have shown that the conditions of child improve when the child is treated with these agents. The Multicenter Myocarditis Treatment Trial aimed to establish differences in outcome among three treatment modalities. A total of 111 children were randomized into one of the three following groups:

- Prednisone/azathioprine
- Prednisone/cyclosporine
- Conventional therapy without immunosuppression.

Cardiac Glycosides

These agents may improve left ventricular function by increasing myocardial contraction by inhibiting the sodium/potassium adenosine triphosphatase (ATPase) pump. This leads to sodium accumulation within the myocyte, which stimulates the sodium-calcium exchange. The increased intracellular calcium increases the force of contraction.

Digoxin (Lanoxin)

Cardiac glycoside with direct inotropic effects in addition to indirect effects on the cardiovascular system. Acts directly on cardiac muscle, increasing myocardial systolic contractions. Its indirect actions result in increased carotid sinus nerve activity and enhanced sympathetic withdrawal for any given increase in mean arterial pressure.

Furosemide (Lasix)

This loop diuretic is the diuretic of choice in pediatric child. Increases excretion of water by interfering with chloride-binding cotransport system, which, in turn, inhibits sodium and chloride reabsorption in ascending loop of Henle and distal renal tubule.

Adult Dose: 20–80 mg/d PO/IV/IM divided q6–12h.

Pediatric Dose: 0.5–2 mg/kg/dose PO/IV/IM up to tid.

Nursing Management

- Discharge child with viral myocarditis when stable on oral medications.
- Monitor medication doses and adverse effects.
- Serial echocardiography is useful in monitoring ventricular function.
- Medications include the following, when indicated:
  - Digitalis
  - Afterload reduction agents
  - Diuretics
  - Antiarrhythmics
  - Anticoagulants.

Preventive Measures

- Limit patient activity until recovered.
- Avoid negative inotropes.
- Be aware of the possibility of further decrease in ventricular function.

Complications

- Arrhythmia
- Congestive heart failure
- Thromboembolism
- Further decrease in ventricular function
- Dilated cardiomyopathy.

Prognosis

The studies give a wide spectrum of mortality and morbidity statistics. With suspected coxsackievirus B, mortality rate is higher in newborns (75%) than in older infants and children (10–25%). Complete recovery of ventricular function has been reported in as many as 50% of children. Some children develop chronic myocarditis (ongoing or resolving), dilated cardiomyopathy, or both. Those who develop dilated cardiomyopathy may require a heart transplant.

PERICARDITIS

Definition

Pericarditis is the both viral and bacterial infections may involve the pericardium (pericarditis), although viral pericarditis is more common than bacterial pericarditis in both children and adults. Awareness of this disease has increased because of the introduction of noninvasive diagnostic techniques, such as echocardiography and CT scanning. Although it is usually benign, the disease can be severe and even lethal, especially in children with immunosuppression. The infection may also involve the myocardium (myopericarditis).

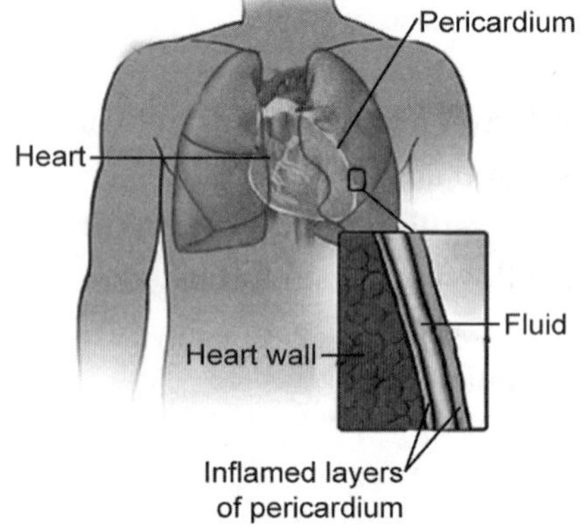

Child with Pericarditis heart

Causes

A specific etiologic agent is not identified. These cases are often considered viral in origin. Common viral causes include the following:

- Coxsackievirus B (most common cause)
- Echovirus
- Adenovirus
- Influenza virus
- Mumps virus
- Varicella virus
- Epstein-Barr virus
- Cytomegalovirus

- Viral hepatitis B
- Human immunodeficiency virus (HIV)
- Human herpesvirus 6
- Parvovirus B19
- Postimmunization (vaccinia)
- Hepatitis C virus.

Signs and Symptoms

Fever and chest pain are usual presenting symptoms.

- Low-to-moderate fever usually occurs but may be absent at the time of presentation.
- Pain in the chest or left shoulder is often present and is aggravated or relieved by changes in physical position. Child usually feel better in a sitting position.
- The pain is usually substernal and accompanied by a sensation of chest constriction.
- Any movement of the chest, including respiratory motion, increases the pain.
- Sitting up and leaning forward may reduce the pain. Therefore, a child may refuse to lie down for examination.
- Palm pressure applied to the sternum markedly increases the pain.

A hacking cough is occasionally a presenting symptom.

- The cough varies with position.
- Sitting up and leaning forward improves the cough.

Preceding symptoms of viral illness are present in 40–75% of children and include the following:

- Fever
- Runny nose
- Cough
- Diarrhea
- Rash.

Pathophysiology

The pericardium consists of two layers: The visceral pericardium (epicardium) and the parietal pericardium. These layers enclose the pericardial cavity (a potential space) between them. A small volume of serous fluid (< 30 mL in adults) lubricates this cavity. Inflammation of the pericardium secondary to a viral infection increases the volume of serous fluid (pericardial effusion). Studies show that persistent pericarditis triggers an autoimmune reaction to the myopericardial cells.

Diagnostic Evaluation

Laboratory Studies

- The CBC count is usually within the reference range but may show relative lymphocytosis.
- Obtain a blood culture to help exclude bacterial infection.
- Obtain nasopharyngeal aspirate and stool samples for viral isolation and obtain blood samples for acute and convalescent viral titers.

- Other blood tests (e.g. blood gas analysis and electrolyte, BUN and glucose tests) may be required for acute-stage management.
- Recently, elevated troponin I levels have been reported in young adults with pericarditis, especially with effusion. This may indicate the coexistence of varying degrees of underlying myocarditis.

Imaging Studies

Chest Radiography

- Radiography demonstrates cardiomegaly, depending on the amount of fluid and presence of underlying myocarditis.
- A typical saclike appearance of the cardiac silhouette is characteristic of large effusions.
- Chamber enlargement is not observed.
- Pulmonary venous congestion is not a feature of pericarditis, although coexistent myocarditis and heart failure may cause such congestion.
- Chest radiograph of a boy with viral pericarditis is seen below.

Other Investigation

Electrocardiography

Generalized elevation of the ST segment in leads with an upright T-wave is the typical pattern of pericarditis, although this finding may not be apparent. Low-voltage QRS complexes may occur in the presence of a large effusion. However, an adult study showed greater frequency of low P-wave and T-wave voltages than low QRS voltages.

Diagnostic Procedures

Pericardiocentesis

This procedure is required for all children who have clinical evidence of cardiac tamponade or suspected bacterial pericarditis and for some children with immunocompromise. Pericardiocentesis is also used as a diagnostic test in child with a pericardial effusion of unknown cause. The volume of fluid present should be sufficient to allow for the removal of a reasonable portion for diagnostic purposes. Place the child in a half-sitting position (roughly 45°), with sedation or anesthesia as needed. If anesthesia is used, avoid agents that precipitously decrease systemic pressure because circulatory collapse can ensue.

Pericardioscopy and Epicardial Biopsy

This new diagnostic procedure seldom applies to an episode of viral pericarditis. Instead, it is used to macroscopically visualize alterations of both the epicardium and the pericardium. The macropathology of the epicarditis and pericarditis can be observed in vivo. The prerequisite is documentation of a large pericardial effusion (> 150 mL by the cubic model) with an echocardiographically documented effusion of type C.

This procedure requires a separation of at least 5 mm between the epicardial and pericardial layers in diastole at the anterior side of the heart when echocardiographic imaging is performed from the subxiphoidal or third intercostal space. After the pericardial effusion is punctured, introduce a 9 ft sheath using a guidewire under echocardiographic or fluoroscopic control.

- Aspirate the fluid and infuse 100–150 mL of saline warmed to body temperature into the pericardial sac.
- Use a flexible 8-ft fiberglass instrument (e.g. Vantec, Baxter, Storz) and a rigid 110°, 8 ft endoscope (Storz) to visualize the pericardium and epicardium and to document the findings on videotape.
- The macropathology is endoscopically inspected. Fibrinous strands or increased vascular injection can be observed in viral, autoimmune, or idiopathic pericarditis or in idiopathic perimyocarditis. In the last 3 forms of pericardial effusion, only inflammatory cells are observed when the pericardial fluid is analyzed.

Management

Medical Management

Management is conservative (expectant) and symptom specific.

- Bed rest and the use of anti-inflammatory agents are mainstays of initial therapy.
- Aggressive pain control may be necessary in some child, although most cases respond to salicylates or nonsteroidal anti-inflammatory drugs (NSAIDs).
- Corticosteroid therapy is rarely indicated. Consider this option only when NSAIDs are unsuccessful and a bacterial etiology has clearly been excluded. Although corticosteroid therapy might dramatically reduce symptoms, no convincing evidence of any long-term benefits has been reported. Moreover, corticosteroid therapy may increase the risk of recurrence.
- A prospective randomized trial reported a significant reduction in the rate of recurrence with colchicine therapy in child with a first episode of acute pericarditis. However, this study involved mainly adult child with a wide spectrum of etiologies and diarrhea necessitated discontinuation of colchicine in numerous children.
- Resolution of effusion may occur within several days to weeks after initiating anti-inflammatory drugs; However, child should be closely observed for the development of pericardial tamponade as a part of their initial care.
- Pericardiocentesis is indicated when the etiology is in doubt and is essential in suspected tamponade.
- Occasionally, intravenous immunoglobulin has been used to treat child who develops chronic pericarditis with satisfactory results.

Medication

The bed rest and use of anti-inflammatory agents are the mainstays of initial therapy. Aggressive pain control may be necessary in some children; however, most cases respond to salicylates or NSAIDs. Although corticosteroid therapy is rarely indicated, consider this course when NSAIDs are unsuccessful and when a bacterial etiology is clearly excluded.

Corticosteroids may dramatically reduce symptoms, but no convincing evidence suggests any long-term benefit. Anti-inflammatory therapy (e.g. with aspirin, indomethacin) may continue for several months. After therapy is discontinued, 15–30% of children may have a relapse.

The optimal method for prevention is not fully established, but accepted modalities include NSAIDs, corticosteroids, immunosuppressive agents and pericardiectomy. Colchicine has also been used in some children with a good response.

Surgical Management

- Place a pericardial drainage catheter.
- Pericardiectomy, the surgical creation of a pericardial window needed in refractory cases to facilitate open drainage, is rarely required to manage chronic recurrent cases. Recently, video-assisted thoracoscopic window has been used in adult child for diagnosis and management of pericardial effusions.

Nursing Management

- Provide comfort, rest and sleep
- Monitor the vital of the child
- Maintain the intake and output chart
- Reevaluate recurrent cases
- Continue anti-inflammatory therapy, such as aspirin or indomethacin, for at least several months to monitor the patient's progress.
- Do not confuse tamponade with CHF. Medications used to treat heart failure (e.g. digoxin) may slow the heart rate. Because tachycardia represents the only effective compensatory mechanism available to the patient for maintaining cardiac output, slowing the rate may cause acute cardiovascular collapse.
- Administration of diuretics or afterload-reducing agents can also lead to cardiovascular collapse. Administration of diuretics, certain anesthetic agents that relax the peripheral vascular bed or afterload-reducing agents can also lead to cardiovascular collapse.

  After therapy is discontinued, 15–30% of children have a relapse.
  - The optimal method for prevention is not fully established.
  - Accepted modalities include NSAIDs, corticosteroids, immunosuppressive agents and pericardiectomy.
  - Colchicine has also been tried in some children, with a good response.

Prognosis

- Almost all children recover completely if no serious acute complication occurs.
- Constrictive pericarditis rarely occurs after viral pericarditis.

HEMATOLOGICAL SYSTEM: CHILD WITH BLOOD DISORDERS

CHILD WITH ANEMIA

Introduction

Anemia is one of the more common blood disorders, occurs when the level of healthy red blood cells (RBCs) in the body becomes too low. This can lead to health problems because RBCs contain hemoglobin, which carries oxygen to the body's tissues. Anemia can cause a variety of complications, including fatigue and stress on bodily organs.

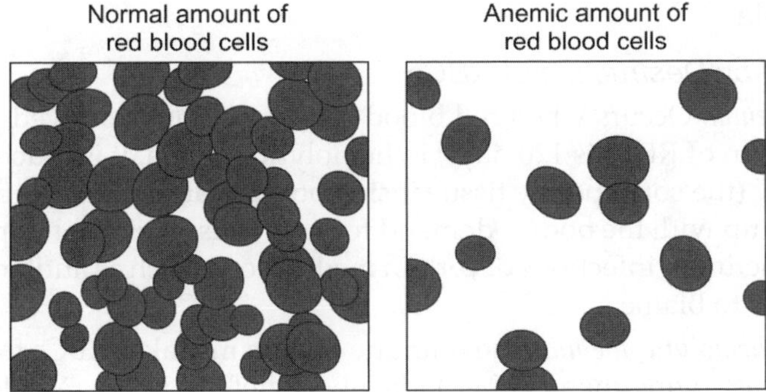

Fig. 7.69: Anatomical difference between normal and anemic RBC cells

Causes

Anemia can be caused by many things, but the three main bodily mechanisms that produce it are:

- Excessive destruction of RBCs
- Blood loss
- Inadequate production of RBCs.

Among many other causes, anemia can result from inherited disorders, nutritional problems (such as an iron or vitamin deficiency), infections, some kinds of cancer, or exposure to a drug or toxin.

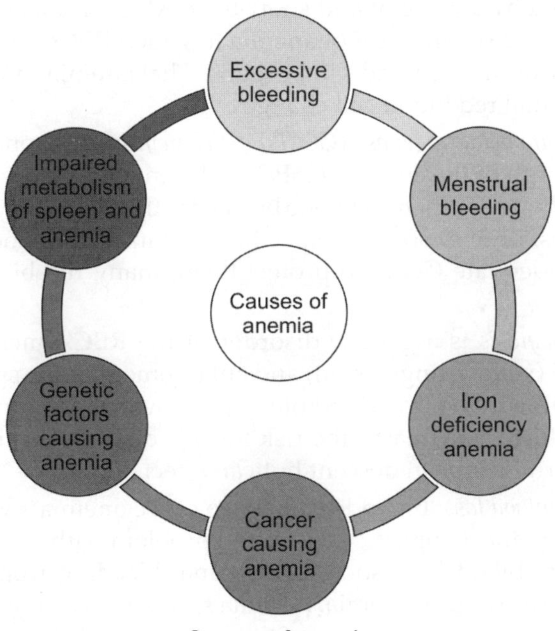

Causes of anemia

Types of Anemia

Anemia Caused by Destruction of RBCs

- *Hemolytic anemia*: Occurs when red blood cells are being destroyed prematurely. (The normal lifespan of RBCs is 120 days; in hemolytic anemia, it is much shorter.) And the bone marrow (the soft, spongy tissue inside bones that makes new blood cells) simply can not keep up with the body's demand for new cells. This can happen for a variety of reasons. Sometimes, infections or certain medications, such as antibiotics or antiseizure medicines are to blame.
- *Autoimmune hemolytic anemia*: The immune system mistakes RBCs for foreign invaders and begins destroying them. Other kids inherit defects in the red blood cells that lead to anemia; common forms of inherited hemolytic anemia include sickle cell anemia, thalassemia, glucose-6-phosphate dehydrogenase (G6PD) deficiency and hereditary spherocytosis.
- *Sickle cell anemia* is a severe form of anemia found most commonly in people of African heritage, although it can affect those of Caucasian, Saudi Arabian, Indian and Mediterranean descent. In this condition, the hemoglobin forms long rods when it gives up its oxygen, stretching red blood cells into abnormal sickle shapes. This leads to premature destruction of RBCs, chronically low levels of hemoglobin and recurring episodes of pain, as well as problems that can affect virtually every other organ system in the body. About 1 out of every 625 African-American children is born with this form of anemia.
- *Thalassemia*, which usually affects people of Mediterranean, African and Southeast Asian descent, is marked by abnormal and short-lived RBCs. Thalassemia major, also called Cooley's anemia, is a severe form of anemia in which RBCs are rapidly destroyed and iron is deposited in the skin and vital organs. Thalassemia minor involves only mild anemia and minimal red blood cell changes.
- *Glucose–6-phosphate dehydrogenase (G6PD) deficiency*: In this condition, the RBCs either do not make enough of the enzyme G6PD or the enzyme that is produced is abnormal and does not work well. When someone born with this deficiency has an infection, takes certain medicines, or is exposed to specific substances, the body's RBCs suffer extra stress. Without adequate G6PD to protect them, many red blood cells are destroyed prematurely.
- *Hereditary spherocytosis* is a genetic disorder of the RBC's membrane that can cause anemia, jaundice (yellow-tinged skin) and enlargement of the spleen. The RBCs have a smaller surface area than normal red blood cells, which can cause them to break open easily. A family history increases the risk for this disorder, which is most common in people of northern European descent but can affect all races.
- *Anemia caused by blood loss*: Blood loss can also cause anemia—whether it is because of excessive bleeding due to injury, surgery, or a problem with the blood's clotting ability. Slower, long-term blood loss, such as intestinal bleeding from inflammatory bowel disease (IBD), can also cause anemia. Anemia sometimes results from heavy menstrual periods in teen girls and women. Any of these factors will also increase the body's need for iron because iron is needed to make new RBCs.

Anemia Caused by Inadequate Production of RBCs

Aplastic anemia occurs when the bone marrow can not make enough RBCs. This can be due to a viral infection, or exposure to certain toxic chemicals, radiation, or medications (such as antibiotics, antiseizure drugs, or cancer treatments). Some childhood cancers can also cause aplastic anemia, as can certain chronic diseases that affect the ability of the bone marrow to make blood cells.

High-levels of hemoglobin and RBCs help fetal blood carry enough oxygen to developing babies in the relatively oxygen-poor environment in utero. After the child is born, more oxygen is available and the baby's hemoglobin level normally drops to a low point at about 2 months of age, a condition known as **physiologic anemia** of infancy. This temporary and expected drop in the blood count is considered normal and no treatment is required because the infant's body soon starts making RBCs on its own.

Anemia also occurs when the body is not able to produce enough healthy RBCs because of an iron deficiency. Iron is essential to hemoglobin production. Poor dietary iron intake (or excessive loss of iron from the body) can lead to **iron deficiency anemia,** the most common cause of anemia in kids. Iron deficiency anemia can affect kids at any age, but is most common in those younger than 2 years old. Young children who drink excessive amounts of milk are at increased risk for iron deficiency. Girls going through puberty also have a particularly high risk for iron deficiency anemia because of the onset of menstruation; the monthly blood loss increases the amount of iron they need to consume in their diets.

Signs and Symptoms

Symptoms common to many types of anemia include the following:

- Easy fatigue and loss of energy
- Unusually rapid heartbeat, particularly with exercise
- Shortness of breath and headache, particularly with exercise
- Difficulty concentrating
- Dizziness
- Pale skin
- Leg cramps
- Insomnia.

If the anemia is caused by excessive destruction of RBCs, symptoms also may include jaundice, a yellowing of the whites of the eyes, an enlarged spleen and dark tea-colored urine. In infants and preschoolers, iron deficiency anemia can result in developmental delays and behavioral disturbances, such as decreased motor activity and problems with social interaction and attention to tasks. Research indicates that developmental problems may last into and beyond school age if the iron deficiency is not properly treated.

Diagnostic Evaluation

In many cases, doctors do not diagnose anemia until they run blood tests as part of a routine physical examination. A complete blood count (CBC) may indicate that there are fewer RBCs than normal. Other diagnostic tests may include:

- *Blood smear examination*: Blood is smeared on a glass slide for microscopic examination of RBCs, which can sometimes indicate the cause of the anemia.

- *Iron tests*: These include total serum iron and ferritin tests, which can help to determine whether anemia is due to iron deficiency.
- *Hemoglobin electrophoresis*: Used to identify various abnormal hemoglobins in the blood and to diagnose sickle cell anemia, the thalassemias and other inherited forms of anemia.
- *Bone marrow aspiration and biopsy*: This test can help determine whether cell production is happening normally in the bone marrow. It is the only way to diagnose aplastic anemia definitively and is also used if a disease affecting the bone marrow (such as leukemia) could be causing of the anemia.
- *Reticulocyte count*: A measure of young RBCs, this helps to determine if RBC production is at normal levels.

In addition to running these tests, your doctor may ask about a family history of anemia and your child's symptoms and medications. This may lead the doctor to perform other tests to look for specific diseases that might be causing the anemia.

Management

Treatment for anemia depends on its cause. It is important not to assume that any symptoms your child may be having are due to iron deficiency. Be sure to have your child checked by a doctor. If your child has iron deficiency anemia, the doctor may prescribe medication as drops (for infants) or as a liquid or tablet (for older kids), which usually must be taken for as long as 3 months to rebuild the body's store of iron. The doctor also may recommend adding certain iron-rich foods to your child's diet or reducing milk intake.

Teenage girls are anemic and have heavy or irregular menstrual periods; her doctor may prescribe hormonal treatment to help regulate the bleeding. Folic acid and vitamin B_{12} supplements may be prescribed if the anemia is traced to a deficiency of these nutrients, although this is rare in children.

- Transfusions of normal red blood cells taken from a donor
- Removal of the spleen or treatment with medications to prevent blood cells from being removed from circulation or destroyed too rapidly
- Medications to fight infection or stimulate the bone marrow to make more blood cells.

In some cases of sickle cell anemia, thalassemia and aplastic anemia, bone marrow transplantation may be used. In this procedure, bone marrow cells taken from a donor are injected into the child's vein; they then travel through the bloodstream to the bone marrow and begin producing new blood cells.

Nursing Management

- The type, cause and severity of your child's anemia will determine what kind of care is needed. Rest assured, though, that kids often tolerate anemia much better than adults.
- In general, a child with significant anemia may tire more easily than other kids and therefore need to limit activity levels. Make sure that your child's teachers and other caregivers are aware of the condition.
- If iron deficiency is the cause, follow the doctor's directions about dietary changes and taking any iron supplements.
- If the spleen is enlarged, your child may be prohibited from playing contact sports because of the risk that the spleen could rupture or hemorrhage if your child is hurt.

Certain forms of anemia, such as sickle cell anemia, require other more specific kinds of care and treatment.

Preventive Measures

Currently, there is no way to prevent anemia due to genetic defects affecting the production of RBCs or hemoglobin. However, you can help prevent iron deficiency, the most common form of anemia. Before following any of these suggestions, be sure to talk them over with your doctor.

Cow's Milk Consumption

- During the first 6 months of life, babies are usually protected against developing iron deficiency by the stores of iron built up in their bodies before birth. But after month 6, they often do not get enough iron through breast milk alone or regular cow's milk (which contains less iron than fortified infant formula).
- Regular cow's milk can cause some infants to lose iron from their intestines and drinking lots of it can make a baby less interested in eating other foods that are better sources of iron. For these reasons, regular cow's milk is not recommended for children until they reach 1 year of age and are eating an iron-rich diet.
- In addition, they should not drink more than 24–32 ounces (709–946 ml) of milk each day. If you cannot get your child to eat more iron-rich foods, speak with your doctor about giving your child an iron supplement.

Iron-fortified Cereal and Formula

- These products can help ensure that your baby is getting enough iron, especially during the transition from breast milk or formula to solid foods.

Well-balanced Diet

- Make sure that child regularly eat foods that contain iron.
- Good choices include iron-fortified grains and cereals, red meat, egg yolks, leafy green vegetables, yellow vegetables and fruits, potato skins, tomatoes, molasses and raisins.
- If child is a vegetarian, you will need to make an extra effort to ensure sufficient iron sources because iron found in meat, poultry and fish is more easily absorbed than iron found in plant-based and iron-fortified foods.
- Be aware of certain food combinations can inhibit or promote absorption of iron. For example, drinking coffee or tea (including iced tea) with a meal can significantly lower the amount of iron absorbed. On the other hand, vitamin C helps the body absorb iron.

IRON DEFICIENCY ANEMIA

Introduction

Iron deficiency (ID) and iron-deficiency anemia (IDA) continue to be of worldwide concern. Among children in the developing world, iron is the most common single-nutrient deficiency. In industrialized nations, despite a demonstrable decline in prevalence, IDA remains a common cause of anemia in young children. However, even more important than anemia itself is the indication that the more common ID without anemia may also adversely affect long-term neurodevelopment and behavior and that some of these effects may be irreversible.

Definition

Anemia is a condition in which the body does not have enough healthy red blood cells. Red blood cells bring oxygen to body tissues. There are many types of anemia. Iron deficiency anemia is a decrease in the number of red blood cells in the blood due to a lack of iron.

Causes

Iron deficiency anemia is the most common form of anemia. You get iron through certain foods and your body also reuses iron from old red blood cells.

Iron deficiency (too little iron) may be caused by:

- An iron-poor diet (this is the most common cause)
- Body not being able to absorb iron very well, even though you are eating enough iron
- Long-term, slow blood loss—usually through menstrual periods or bleeding in the digestive tract
- Rapid growth (in the first year of life and in adolescence), when more iron is needed.

The risk of developing iron deficiency anemia is increased in:

- Infants younger than 12 months who drink cow's milk rather than breast milk or iron-fortified formula
- Young children who drink a lot of cow's milk rather than eating foods that supply the body with more iron.

Iron deficiency anemia most commonly affects babies 9–24 months old. All babies should have a screening test for iron deficiency at this age. Babies born prematurely may need to be tested earlier.

Iron deficiency in children also can be related to lead poisoning.

Signs and Symptoms

- Blue-tinged or very pale whites of eyes
- Blood in the stools
- Brittle nails
- Decreased appetite (especially in children)
- Fatigue
- Headache
- Irritability
- Pale skin color (pallor)
- Shortness of breath
- Sore tongue
- Unusual food cravings (called pica)
- Weakness.

Note: There may be no symptoms if anemia is mild.

Diagnostic Evaluation

The health care provider will perform a physical exam. A blood sample is taken and sent to a laboratory for examination. Iron-deficient red blood cells appear small and pale when looked at under a microscope.

Specific tests that may be done include:

- Hematocrit
- Serum ferritin reveals the amount of iron stored in your body
- Serum iron shows how much iron is in your blood
- Total iron binding capacity (TIBC) to measure the ability of a protein called transferrin to carry iron in the blood.

A measurement called iron saturation often can give a good assessment of whether you have enough iron in your body.

Management

- Treatment involves iron supplements (ferrous sulfate), which are taken by mouth.
- The iron is best absorbed on an empty stomach, but many people need to take the supplements with food to avoid stomach upset.
- If you cannot tolerate iron supplements by mouth, iron may be given by injection into a muscle or through a vein (IV). Milk and antacids can interfere with iron absorption and should not be taken at the same time as iron supplements.
- Iron-rich foods include raisins, meats (especially liver), fish, poultry, egg yolks, legumes (peas and beans) and whole-grain bread.

Prognosis

With treatment, the outcome is likely to be good. In most cases, the blood counts will return to normal in 2 months. It is essential to determine the cause of the iron deficiency. If it is being caused by blood loss other than monthly menstruation, further investigation will be needed.

He should continue taking iron supplements for another 6 to 12 months after blood counts return to normal, or as your health care provider recommends. This will help the body rebuild its iron storage.

Iron supplementation improves learning, memory and cognitive test performance in adolescents who have low levels of iron. Iron supplementation also improves the performance of athletes with anemia and iron deficiency.

Complications

- Iron deficiency anemia can affect school performance.
- Low iron levels are an important cause of decreased attention span, reduced alertness and learning difficulties, both in young children and adolescents.
- Excess amounts of lead may be absorbed by people with iron deficiency.

Prevention

The American Academy of Pediatrics (AAP) recommends that all infants should be fed breastmilk or iron-fortified formula for at least 12 months. The AAP does not recommend giving cow's milk to children under 1 year old. Diet is the most important way to prevent and treat iron deficiency.

Good sources of iron include:

Sources of Iron	
• Apricots	• Fish
• Kale and other greens	• Molasses
• Oatmeal	• Peanut butter
• Prunes	• Soybeans
• Raisins	• Turkey
• Spinach	• Baby formula with iron
• Tuna	• Breast milk (the iron is very easily used by the child)
• Chicken and other meats	• Infant cereals and other iron-fortified cereals
• Dried beans and lentils	• Liver
• Eggs	• Prune juice

MEGALOBLASTIC ANEMIA

Introduction

Megaloblastic anemia is an uncommon problem in childhood that is most frequently associated with vitamin deficiency or gastrointestinal disease. The megaloblastic effect is characterized by a regenerative macrocytic anemia with nuclear dysmaturity, where the nucleus appears immature relative to the cytoplasm because of impaired DNA synthesis.

DNA synthesis is impaired because of inadequate amounts of metabolically active folate derivatives necessary for DNA base synthesis. Megaloblastic changes affect all 3 hematopoietic cell lines. Thrombocytopenia, leukopenia and anemia are all observed to varying extents.

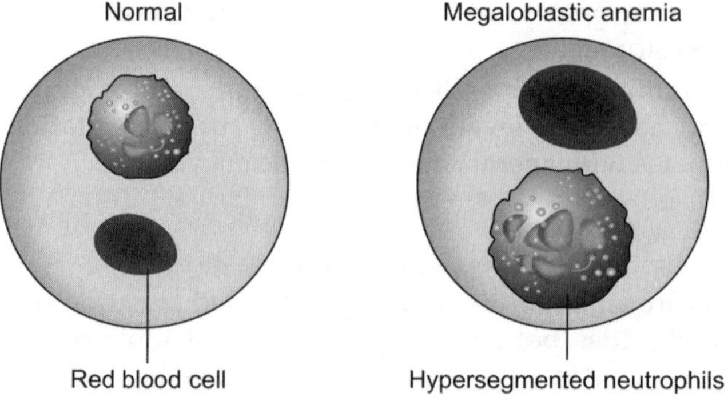

Fig. 7.70: Anatomical difference between normal cell and megaloblastic anemia

The two most common causes of megaloblastic anemia are vitamin B_{12} deficiency (cobalamin) and folinic acid deficiency. Although their clinical settings differ considerably, no hematologic finding can distinguish between the two conditions. Other less common causes include the use of metabolic inhibitors such as methotrexate and 6-mercaptopurine and certain rare inborn errors, such as thiamine-responsive megaloblastic anemia, Lesch-Nyhan syndrome and hereditary orotic aciduria.

Definition

Megaloblastic anemia is a type of anemia characterized by very large red blood cells. In addition to the cells being large, the inner contents of each cell are not completely developed. This malformation causes the bone marrow to produce fewer cells and sometimes the cells die earlier than the 120-day life expectancy. Instead of being round or disk-shaped, the red blood cells can be oval.

Incidence

The prevalence of megaloblastic anemia in childhood has not been established, vitamin B_{12} deficiency is a worldwide problem, particularly in the newborn period due to the combined effects of poor maternal diet and congenital deficiencies of transcobalamin. Pernicious anemia is a common cause of megaloblastic anemia especially in persons of European or African descent. Dietary vitamin B_{12} deficiency is a serious problem in India, Mexico, Central America, South America and some areas of Africa. The increase in vegetarianism is related to an increase in vitamin B_{12} deficiency, especially concerning in breastfed infants of vitamin B_{12}–deficient mothers.

Causes

Megaloblastic anemia is caused by lack of vitamin B_{12} or lack of folic acid.

- Acquired causes of insufficient B_{12} include the following:
  - Inadequate intake in diet
  - Inadequate absorption
    - Deficient intrinsic factor (IF)
    - Deficient absorption from ileum
  - Impaired transport from the intestine
- Acquired causes of insufficient folate include the following:
  - Inadequate dietary intake
  - Inadequate absorption from the proximal small intestine
  - Medications associated with folate deficiency include the following:
    - Sulfonamide antibiotics may interfere with folate metabolism, particularly when they are used on a long-term basis.
    - Other antifolate antimetabolite drugs may also cause megaloblastic changes.
    - Megaloblastic changes are observed with some frequency with antineoplastic agents, such as methotrexate. Imuran may also cause megaloblastic changes.
  - Increased metabolic demand (e.g. chronic hemolysis such as sickle cell disease)
- Imerslund-Grasbeck syndrome of proteinuria and excretion of cobalamin and IF is a rare disorder but is an important cause of B_{12} deficiency that arises in early childhood.

Signs and Symptoms

The following are the most common symptoms of megaloblastic anemia. However, each child may experience symptoms differently. Symptoms may include:

- Abnormal paleness or lack of color of the skin
- Decreased appetite
- Irritability
- Lack of energy or tiring easily (fatigue)
- Diarrhea
- Difficulty walking
- Numbness or tingling in hands and feet
- Smooth and tender tongue
- Weak muscles.

The symptoms of megaloblastic anemia may resemble other blood conditions or medical problems.

Pathophysiology

Megaloblastic anemia is caused by various DNA synthesis defects. In folate deficiency, purine biosynthesis is affected because folic acid is essential in this process. Folic acid is essential for purine biosynthesis. Folic acid absorbed from the diet must be activated to produce active tetrahydrofolic acid (THF). THF is necessary for single carbon transfers in the synthesis of pyrimidine nucleotides. Without adequate levels of biologically active THF, the ability to repair and replicate DNA is decreased. Vitamin B_{12} is a cofactor for the activation of folic acid in a step that also converts homocysteine to methionine. In the case of inadequate folic acid intake, THF production is depleted and DNA synthesis is slowed. The effect on hematopoiesis is to reduce the rate of cell production, resulting in pancytopenia. In the cells that are produced, the effect created is an arrest of nuclear maturation. In other words, the cells that are produced have immature nuclei compared to the degree of maturation of the cytoplasm.

Diagnostic Evaluation

Family History Collection

- Congenital absence or deficiency of carrier proteins is a common cause of vitamin B_{12} deficiency. These deficiencies occur in families. Obtaining an extended family history is usually necessary to detect other affected family members. These conditions often manifest during infancy and early childhood and are rare but important causes of megaloblastic anemia because myelopathy and developmental delays occur without treatment.
- Evaluate for Imerslund-Grasbeck syndrome of proteinuria and excretion of cobalamin and intrinsic factor (IF).

Physical Examination

- The physical examination is largely directed by the findings of the history. Common findings include glossitis, stomatitis, hyperpigmentation and weight loss.
- Look for physical evidence of anemia, thrombocytopenia and neutropenia. Pancytopenia can be observed in megaloblastic anemia, but it should raise the suspicion of a possible malignancy.

- Evaluate for lymphadenopathy, hepatosplenomegaly and abdominal or retroperitoneal masses as evidence of a malignancy.
- Carefully document the neurologic status of a child with megaloblastic anemia. Document altered mental or neurologic status. Vibratory sensation in the extremities is frequently affected in B_{12} deficiency. These changes may reflect neurotoxicity from deficient B_{12} levels. Once documented, these symptoms can be monitored to determine the degree of resolution once the child is B_{12} replete.

Laboratory Studies

The following studies are indicated in megaloblastic anemia:

- CBC count with a manual differential:
  - CBC count reveals macrocytic red cell indices and evaluates for other cytopenias.
  - The manual differential is essential to rule out the possibility of circulating blast cells, which may be present in a patient with leukemia who presents with pancytopenia.
- Reticulocyte count: The reticulocyte count is important in the assessment of red cell production.
- Serum and RBC folate levels:
  - RBC folate level is the best measure of metabolically active folate and includes 5 methyl tetrahydrofolate (THF) in the assay.
  - Serum folate measures the circulating pool of folate but does not accurately reflect the amount of THF present in the tissues.
- Bone marrow evaluation: Consider bone marrow evaluation for any child with more than one abnormal cell line on the CBC. It can help to rule out other disorders such as leukemia, myelodysplasia and aplastic anemia.
- Additional laboratory studies: A platelet count may be indicated.

Procedures

- When B_{12} deficiency is suspected, a Shilling test may be performed to determine whether congenital absence of a binding protein is present. However, the classical nuclear medicine Shilling test is not commonly available due to the unavailability of the radiolabeled B_{12}.
- The Shilling test may be modified to avoid radiolabeled B_{12} by measuring B_{12} levels before and after a known B_{12} dose, followed by a similar test using B_{12} with accompanying IF. A comparison of B_{12} levels allows detection of a deficiency of either IF or IF-binding protein.
- Shilling test findings that reveal elevation of the B_{12} level with oral B_{12} indicates dietary insufficiency.
- Shilling test findings that reveal improved B_{12} levels with oral B_{12} and IF indicates the absence of IF, which is pernicious anemia.
- Shilling test findings that reveal no improvement with IF indicates either no absorption in the ileum or transport carrier protein deficiency.

Management

Treatment of megaloblastic anemia depends on the underlying cause.

Folate Deficiency

- Folate deficiency due to dietary deficiency or increased demands is best treated with folate supplements.
- Folate deficiency caused by the use of sulfa drugs or other antifolate medications may be addressed by folate supplementation or by reducing or eliminating the drug.
- Folate deficiency due to celiac sprue requires treatment of the underlying disorder and folate supplements.

B_{12} Deficiency

- B_{12} deficiency is often more complex because of the nature of B_{12} deficiency in childhood.
- B_{12} supplements can be administered orally, even for intrinsic factor (IF) deficiency, using higher doses.
- Often, B_{12} deficiency must be treated with parenteral supplements if high-dose oral B_{12} supplements are unsuccessful.
- For those children with congenital disorders that lead to B_{12} deficiency, supplementation is a lifelong necessity; therefore, concern regarding a regimen that is tolerable over time is essential to maintaining compliance.
- Recent data, albeit from small trials, suggests that oral B_{12} supplementation is as effective as parenteral supplementation in patients with nutritional deficiency. Patients with IF deficiency or who have undergone intestinal surgery should be considered for parenteral therapy because of impaired secretion or absorption of IF.

Surgical Management

A carefully monitor for the onset of megaloblastic anemia due to impaired absorption of B_{12} or folic acid following surgical illnesses that involve the stomach, jejunum, or ileum.

Medication

Vitamins

Vitamins are organic substances required by the body in small amounts for various metabolic processes. Vitamins may be synthesized in small or insufficient amounts in the body or not synthesized at all, thus requiring supplementation. Use folic acid and vitamin B_{12} supplements as indicated.

Folic Acid

It is a member of the vitamin B group. Folic acid is reduced in the body to THF, which is a coenzyme for various metabolic processes including purine and pyrimidine nucleotides synthesis essential for DNA. Important cofactor for enzymes used in production of red blood cells.

Adult: One mg PO/IM/SC qd initially until symptoms resolve, then 0.4 mg/d PO.

Pediatric

- *Infants*: 15 mcg/kg/d PO/IM/SC; alternatively, 50 mcg/d
- *7–13 years*: 1 mg/d PO/IM/SC initially, then 0.1–0.15 mg/d
- *> 13 years*: Administer as in adults.

Cyanocobalamin (Crystamine, Crysti 1000, Cyomin, Nascobal)

Deoxyadenosylcobalamin and hydroxocobalamin are active forms of vitamin B_{12} in humans. Vitamin B_{12} is synthesized by microbes but not humans or plants. Vitamin B_{12} deficiency may result from IF deficiency (pernicious anemia), partial or total gastrectomy, or diseases of the distal ileum.

Adult

100–1000 mcg IM qd for 1–2 wk, followed by 100–1000 mcg IM once every mo for life. Alternatively, 500 mcg (i.e. 1 spray) intranasally in 1 nostril qwk.

Pediatric

10–50 mcg/d IM for 5–10 d, followed by 100–250 mcg/dose q2–4 wk.

Diet Management

- A diet rich in green, leafy vegetables is essential for normal intake of folic acid.
- Because vitamin B_{12} is contained exclusively in animal products (meat), vitamin supplementation is the only means of appropriate vitamin B_{12} intake in humans choosing vegetarian diets.

Foods that are naturally rich in folate include the following:

- Orange juice
- Oranges
- Romaine lettuce
- Spinach
- Liver
- Rice
- Barley
- Sprouts
- Wheat germ
- Soy beans
- Green, leafy vegetables
- Beans
- Peanuts
- Broccoli
- Asparagus
- Peas
- Lentils
- Chick peas (garbanzo beans)

Foods that are fortified with folic acid include the following:

- Breakfast cereals
- Breads
- Enriched pasta
- Enriched rice

Foods that are rich in vitamin B_{12} include the following:

- Meat
- Poultry
- Milk
- Shellfish and some fish
- Eggs
- Cheese.

Complications

Neurologic complications are frequent problems in patients with megaloblastic anemia due to B_{12} deficiency. These may be observed in any age group and may be at least partially reversible with repletion of the B_{12} deficit.

Prognosis

- Prognosis depends on the underlying cause of the megaloblastic anemia and the degree of compliance with therapy.
- Folic acid deficiency is relatively easy to treat; patients usually respond to added folate in their diet.
- Vitamin B_{12} deficiency may be a more significant concern because some patients may need to use parenteral vitamin B_{12} injections, with which they may not readily comply.
- Vitamin B_{12} deficiency may be associated with severe abnormalities of neural function that may be long lasting and persist even with appropriate vitamin B_{12} therapy.

SICKLE CELL ANEMIA

Definition

Sickle cell disease is an inherited blood disorder characterized by defective hemoglobin (a protein in red blood cells that carries oxygen to the tissues of the body). The resulting abnormal hemoglobin causes a normocytic, hemolytic anemia with multiple diversely shaped RBCs that are susceptible to morphologically changing into a sickle shape.

These sickled cells produce obstruction in small vessels, leading to ischemia and necrosis of distal tissue. Pain as a consequence of musculoskeletal ischemia is the most common reason

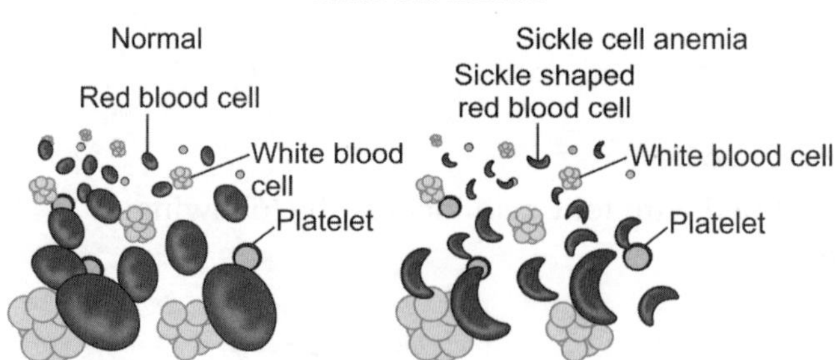

Fig. 7.71: Anatomical difference between normal RBC and sickle shape RBC

for affected patients to visit the ED. Serious complications from visceral ischemia and impaired immunity are also common. There are a number of types of hemoglobinopathies, which can cause sickling of red cells. This article focuses on homozygous hemoglobin SS disease.

Incidence

The clinical course of sickle cell disease is one of chronic illness precipitated by multiple acute exacerbations that can become life threatening at any time. Approximately 50% of patients survive beyond the fifth decade. Deaths during an acute crisis may occur in patients who are clinically free of organ failure. Infection is the leading cause of death in children. Strokes and trauma are the leading causes of death in patients aged 10–20 years. Children in this age range also die from acute chest syndrome, splenic sequestration crisis and aplastic crisis. Older patients most often die of acute chest crisis.

Types

- *Sickle cell trait*: The child is carrying a single defective gene. Some of their hemoglobin is the destructive HbS, but they also have some normal hemoglobin, HbA. This is referred to as HbAS. Children with sickle cell trait are usually without symptoms of the disease. Mild anemia may occur and red cells tend to be small. Under intense stressful conditions, exhaustion, hypoxia (low oxygen), and/or severe infection, the sickling of the defective hemoglobin may occur and result in some complications associated with the sickle cell disease. Most children with the sickle cell trait lead normal lives.
- *Sickle cell anemia*: The child has most or all of the normal hemoglobin (HbA) replaced with the sickle hemoglobin (HbS). This is referred to as HbSS. It is the most common and most severe form of the sickle cell variations. These children suffer from a variety of complications due to the shape and thickness of the sickled cells. Severe and chronic anemia is also a common characteristic for children with HbSS.
- *Sickle cell-hemoglobin SC disease*: The child has one copy of both HbS and HbC. This is often referred to as HbSC. Hemoglobin C causes red blood cells, called target cells, to develop. Having just some hemoglobin C and normal hemoglobin, a person will not have any symptoms of anemia, but can develop it and eye and hip complications later in life. However, if the sickle hemoglobin S is combined with the target cell, some mild to moderate anemia occurs. These children often suffer some of the complications associated with HbSS, sickle cell disease, but to a milder degree. Vaso-occlusive crises (the flow of blood is blocked because the sickled cells have become stuck in the blood vessels), organ damage from repeated sickling and anemia and high-risk for infection are all similar traits for HbSS and HbSC.
- *Sickle cell-hemoglobin E disease*: This variation is similar to sickle cell-C disease except that an element has been replaced in the hemoglobin molecule. This variation is most often also seen in Southeast Asia populations. Some children with hemoglobin E disease are without symptoms. However, under certain conditions, such as exhaustion, hypoxia, severe infection, and/or iron deficiency, some mild to moderate anemia may occur.
- *Hemoglobin S-beta-thalassemia*: This involves an inheritance of both the thalassemia and sickle cell genes. The disorder produces symptoms of moderate anemia and many of the same conditions associated with sickle cell disease. While this disorder more often has milder symptoms than sickle cell disease, it may also produce exacerbations as severe as those of sickle cell disease.

Causes

A specific cause is often not identified. Sickle cell is an inherited disease caused by a genetic defect. If a child inherits one gene from the mother and one from the father, he or she will be born with sickle cell disease. A person who has only one gene is healthy and said to be a 'carrier' of the disease. They may also be described as having 'sickle cell trait.' A carrier has an increased chance of having a child with sickle cell disease.

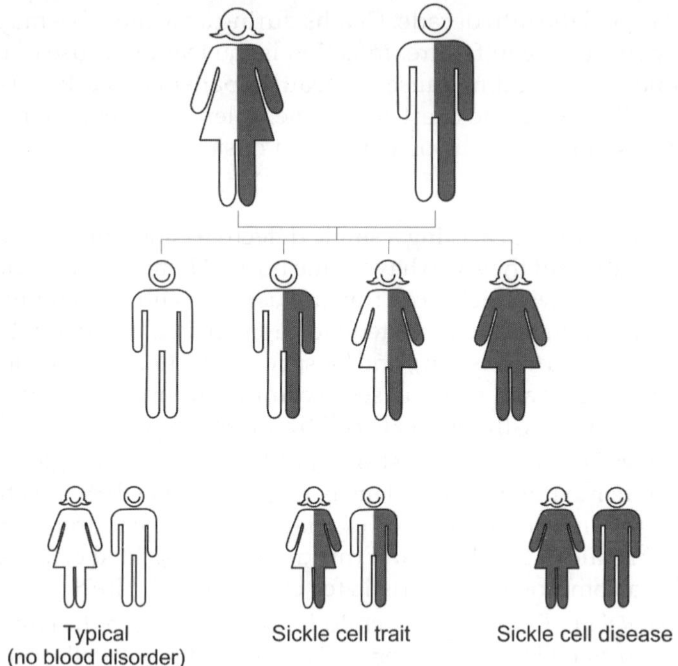

Fig. 7.72: Sickle cell trait

Signs and Symptoms

Sickle cell disease (SCD) usually manifests early in childhood. Complaints may include the following:

- Acute and chronic pain in any body part
- vaso-occlusive crisis
- Bone pain
- Anemia: Universally present, chronic and hemolytic in nature
- Aplastic crisis
- Splenic sequestration
- Infection: Organisms that pose the greatest danger include encapsulated respiratory bacteria, particularly *Streptococcus pneumonia*; adult infections are predominately with gram-negative organisms, especially *Salmonella*
- Growth retardation, delayed sexual maturation, being underweight
- *Hand-foot syndrome*: This is a dactylitis presenting as bilateral painful and swollen hands and/or feet in children

- *Acute chest syndrome:* Young children present with chest pain, fever, cough, tachypnea, leukocytosis and pulmonary infiltrates in the upper lobes; adults are usually afebrile, dyspneic with severe chest pain, with multilobar/lower lobe disease
- *Pulmonary hypertension:* Increasingly recognized as a serious complication of SCD
- *Avascular necrosis of the femoral or humeral head:* This is due to vascular occlusion
- *CNS involvement:* Most severe manifestation is stroke
- *Ophthalmologic involvement:* Ptosis, retinal vascular changes, proliferative retinitis
- *Cardiac involvement:* Dilation of both ventricles and the left atrium
- *GI involvement:* Cholelithiasis is common in children; liver may become involved
- *GU involvement:* Kidneys lose concentrating capacity; priapism is a well-recognized complication of SCD
- *Dermatologic involvement:* Leg ulcers are a chronic painful problem.

Triggers of vaso-occlusive crisis include the following:

- *Hypoxemia:* May be due to acute chest syndrome or respiratory complications
- *Dehydration:* Acidosis results in a shift of the oxygen dissociation curve
- Changes in body temperature (e.g. an increase due to fever or a decrease due to environmental temperature change).

Pathophysiology

Sickle cell disease results from a single amino acid substitution (valine for glutamate) in position 6 of the beta-globin chain of hemoglobin. In homozygotes, this genetic alteration

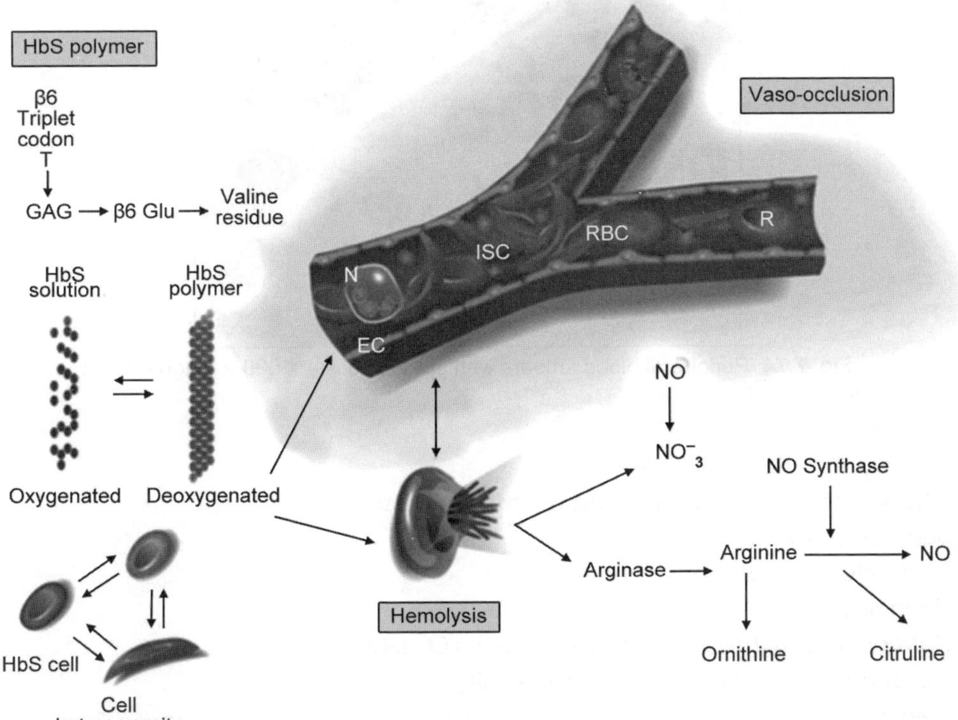

Fig. 7.73: Pathophysiology of sickle cell anemia

yields an unstable RBC with a shortened survival. Hypoxia or hemoconcentration causes the cells to become sickle shaped. The abnormal morphology and other cellular characteristics lead to sludging and thrombosis in small vessels with consequent tissue ischemia. These processes are shown in the image.

Diagnostic Evaluation

Laboratory Studies

Newborn screening for sickle hemoglobinopathies is mandated in 50 states. Therefore, most patients presenting to the ED have a known diagnosis. Specific diagnosis is confirmed with hemoglobin electrophoresis performed in specialized reference laboratories.

Baseline Abnormalities

The patient with homozygous sickle cell disease typically has a hemoglobin level of 5–9 g/dL, with a hematocrit level decreased to 17–29%. The total leukocyte count is elevated to 12,000–20,000 cells/mm^3 (12–20 × 109/L), with a predominance of neutrophils. The platelet count is increased and the sedimentation rate is low. The reticulocyte count is usually elevated, but it may vary depending on the extent of baseline hemolysis. Peripheral blood smears demonstrate target cells, elongated cells and characteristic sickle erythrocytes. These findings are shown in the images.

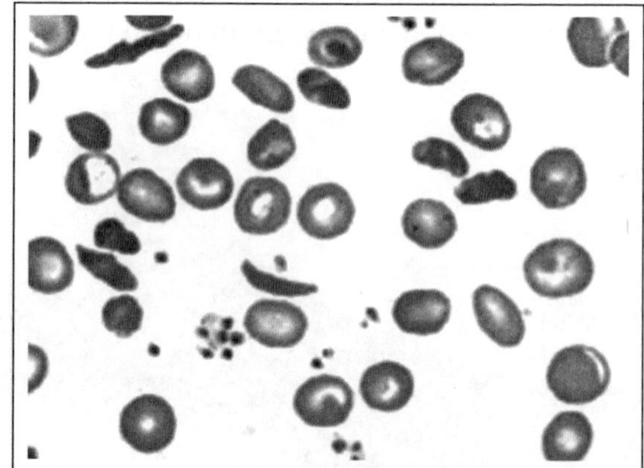

Fig. 7.74: Peripheral blood smears with sickled cells at 1000 × magnification

Laboratory Studies

- Hemoglobin electrophoresis
- CBC count with differential and reticulocyte count
- Serum electrolytes
- Hemoglobin solubility testing
- Peripheral blood smear
- Pulmonary function tests (transcutaneous O_2 saturation)
- Renal function (creatine, BUN, urinalysis)
- Hepatobiliary function tests, (ALT, fractionated bilirubin)

- *CSF examination:* Consider lumber puncture (LP) in febrile children who appear toxic and in those with neurologic findings (e.g. neck stiffness, + Brudzinski/Kernig signs, focal deficits); consider CT scanning before performing LP
- Blood cultures
- ABGs
- Secretory phospholipase A2 (sPLA2).

Imaging Studies

- *Radiography:* Chest X-rays should be performed in patients with respiratory symptoms
- *MRI:* Useful for early detection of bone marrow changes due to acute and chronic bone marrow infarction, marrow hyperplasia, osteomyelitis and osteonecrosis
- *CT scanning:* May demonstrate subtle regions of osteonecrosis not apparent on plain radiographs in patients who are unable to have an MRI and to exclude renal medullary carcinoma in patients presenting with hematuria
- *Nuclear medicine scanning:* Bone scanning detects early stages of osteonecrosis. In WBC, scanning is used for diagnosing osteomyelitis
- *Transcranial Doppler ultrasonography:* Can identify children with SCD at high-risk for stroke
- *Abdominal ultrasonography:* Can be used to rule out cholecystitis, cholelithiasis, or an ectopic pregnancy and to measure spleen and liver size
- *Echocardiography:* Identifies patients with pulmonary hypertension
- *Transcranial near-infrared spectroscopy or cerebral oximetry:* Can be used as a screening tool for low cerebral venous oxygen saturation in children with SCD.

Management

Treatment strategies include the following seven goals:

1. Management of vaso-occlusive crisis
2. Management of chronic pain syndromes
3. Management of chronic hemolytic anemia
4. Prevention and treatment of infections
5. Management of the complications and the various organ damage syndromes associated with the disease
6. Prevention of stroke
7. Detection and treatment of pulmonary hypertension.

Medication

Pharmacotherapy

- *Antimetabolites:* Hydroxyurea
- Opioid analgesics (e.g. oxycodone/ASA, methadone, morphine sulfate, oxycodone/APAP, fentanyl, nalbuphine, codeine, APAP/codeine)
- Nonsteroidal analgesics (e.g. ketorolac, ASA, APAP, ibuprofen)
- Antibiotics (e.g. cefuroxime, amoxicillin/clavulanate, penicillin VK, ceftriaxone, azithromycin, cefaclor)

- Vaccines (e.g. PCV7, PPV23, meningococcal, influenza, recommended scheduled childhood/adult vaccinations)
- Vitamins (e.g. folic acid).

Nonpharmacologic Therapy

- *Stem cell transplantation:* Can be curative
- *Transfusions:* For sudden, severe anemia due to acute splenic sequestration, parvovirus B19 infection, or hyperhemolytic crises
- Physical therapy
- Heat and cold application
- Acupuncture and acupressure
- Toxic epidermal necrolysis syndrome (TENS).

Combination of Pharmacotherapy and Nonpharmacotherapy

- *Vigorous hydration (plus analgesics):* For vaso-occlusive crisis
- *Oxygen, antibiotics, analgesics, incentive spirometry, simple transfusion and bronchodilators:* For treatment of acute chest syndrome.

Preventive Measures

Genetic testing can identify parents at risk for having a child with sickle cell disease. If both parents have the sickle cell trait, the chance that a child will have sickle cell disease is 25%. If one parent is carrying the trait and the other actually has disease, the odds increase to 50% that their child will inherit the disease. Screening and genetic counseling theoretically have the potential to drastically reduce the prevalence of SS disease. This promise has not been realized. Some authors have recommended ED screening or referral for patients unaware of their status as a possible heterozygote.

Complications

Complications of sickle cell anemia include:

- Long-term anemia may lead to delayed healing and delayed growth and development
- Pain crisis, or sickle crisis
- *Acute chest syndrome*: Multiple episodes of acute chest syndrome can cause permanent lung damage
- *Splenic sequestration (pooling):* The spleen can become damaged and scarred after repeated episodes of splenic sequestration. Most children, by age 8, either have had their spleen removed or have permanent damage from repeated splenic sequestration. The risk of infection is a major concern for children without a working spleen. Infection is the major cause of death in children younger than age 5.
- *Stroke:* If there is a blockage of the blood vessels to the brain, a stroke may occur. Serious long-term problems may result. A child who has had a stroke is more likely to have another one.
- Priapism that is not promptly treated, can result in impotence or the inability to have an erection.

- Any major organ may be affected by sickle cell disease. The following may result:
  - Frequent infections
  - Leg ulcers or serious sores
  - Bone damage
  - Gallstones
  - Kidney damage
  - Eye damage.

Prognosis

The child with sickle cell disease can be faced with a myriad of potentially life-threatening and unpredictable complications. Most patients and families with a good understanding of the disease process have good outcomes due to compliance with medication regimens and an overall healthy attitude that promotes well-being.

APLASTIC ANEMIA

Introduction

Mr Paul Ehrlich introduced the concept of aplastic anemia in 1888 when he studied the case of a pregnant woman who died of bone marrow failure. However, it was not until 1904 that Anatole Chauffard named this disorder aplastic anemia. Aplastic anemia is a condition in which the bone marrow does not make enough blood cells. Bone marrow is the soft, tissue in the center of bones that is responsible for producing blood cells and platelets.

Three Basic Types of Blood Cells

- *Red blood cells (RBCs)* are also called erythrocytes. They make up almost half of blood. Red blood cells are filled with the protein hemoglobin that picks up oxygen in the lungs and brings it to cells all around the body.
- *White blood cells (WBCs)* are also called leukocytes. They fight disease and infection by attacking and killing germs that get into the body. There are several kinds of white blood cells, each of which fights a different kind of germ.
- *Platelets* are also called thrombocytes. They are small pieces of cells that help blood clot and stop bleeding.

Definition

Aplastic anemia is a syndrome of bone marrow failure characterized by peripheral pancytopenia and marrow hypoplasia and mild macrocytosis is observed in association with stress erythropoiesis and an elevated fetal hemoglobin levels.

Causes

Congenital or Inherited Causes of Aplastic Anemia (20%)

- Patients usually have dysmorphic features or physical stigmata. On occasion, marrow failure may be the initial presenting feature.
- Fanconi anemia
- Dyskeratosis congenital
- Cartilage-hair hypoplasia

- Pearson syndrome
- Amegakaryocytic thrombocytopenia (thrombocytopenia-absent radius [TAR] syndrome)
- Shwachman-Diamond syndrome
- Dubowitz syndrome
- Diamond-Blackfan syndrome
- Familial aplastic anemia.

Acquired Causes of Aplastic Anemia (80%)

- Idiopathic factors
- Infectious causes, such as hepatitis viruses, Epstein-Barr virus (EBV), human immunodeficiency virus (HIV), parvovirus and mycobacteria.

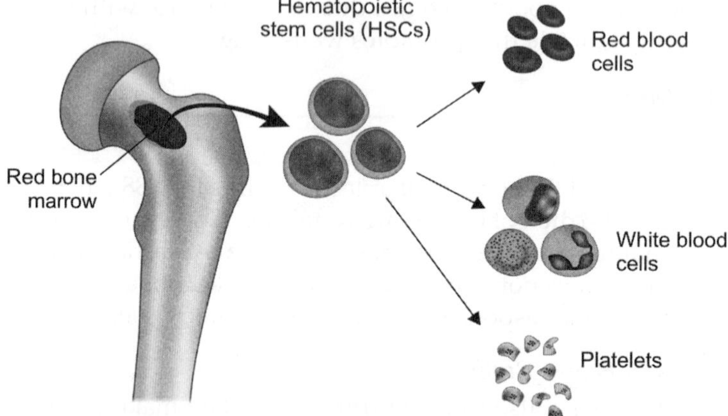

Fig. 7.75: Normal anatomy of blood cells formation

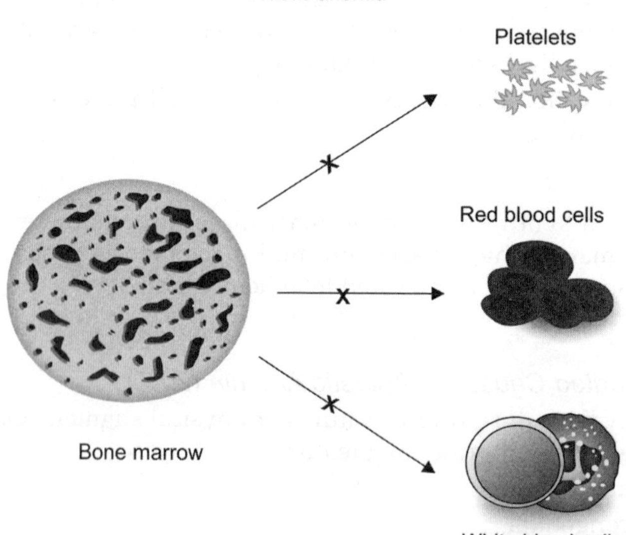

Fig. 7.76: Anatomical view of aplastic anemia

- Toxic exposure to radiation and chemicals, such as benzene
- Drugs and elements, such as chloramphenicol, phenylbutazone and gold may cause aplasia of the marrow. The immune mechanism does not account for the marrow failure in idiosyncratic drug reactions. In such cases, direct toxicity may occur, perhaps due to genetically determined differences in metabolic detoxification pathways. For example, the null phenotype of certain glutathione transferases is overrepresented among patients with aplastic anemia.

Signs and Symptoms

The clinical presentation of patients with aplastic anemia includes symptoms related to the decrease in bone-marrow production of hematopoietic cells. The onset is insidious and the initial symptom is related to anemia or bleeding, although fever or infections are also often noted at presentation.

Low Red Blood Cell Count (Anemia)

- Fatigue
- Pallor (paleness)
- Rapid heart rate
- Shortness of breath with exercise
- Weakness
- Lightheadedness upon standing.

Low White Blood Cell Count (Leukopenia)

- Increased risk of infection.

Low Platelet Count (Thrombocytopenia) can Result in Bleeding

- Bleeding gums
- Easy bruising
- Frequent or severe infections
- Nose bleeds
- Rash, small pinpoint red marks on the skin (petechiae).

Diagnostic Evaluation

Laboratory Studies

- Blood tests
  - Low red cell count (anemia)
  - Low white blood cell count (leukopenia)
  - Low reticulocyte count (reticulocytes are immature red blood cell)
  - Low platelet count (thrombocytopenia).
- *Bone marrow aspirate and biopsy*: To rule out other causes of pancytopenia (i.e. neoplastic infiltration or significant myelofibrosis).
- *History of iatrogenic exposure to cytotoxic chemotherapy*: Can cause transient bone marrow suppression
- X-rays, computed tomography (CT) scans

- *Ultrasound imaging tests*: Enlarged lymph nodes (sign of lymphoma), kidneys and bones in arms and hands (abnormal in Fanconi anemia)
- *Chest X-ray*: Infections
- *Liver tests*: Liver diseases
- *Viral studies*: Viral infections.

Medication

Treatments for aplastic anemia may include observation for mild cases, blood transfusions and medications for more-serious cases and in severe cases, bone marrow transplantation. The goals of pharmacotherapy in cases of aplastic anemia are to reduce morbidity, prevent complications and eradicate malignancy.

Blood Transfusions

- Child with aplastic anemia require transfusion support until the diagnosis is established and until specific therapy can be instituted.

Stem Cell Transplant

A stem cell transplant to rebuild the bone marrow with stem cells from a donor may offer the only successful treatment option for people with severe aplastic anemia. A stem cell transplant, which is also called a bone marrow transplant, is generally the treatment of choice for people who are younger and have a matching donor most often a sibling.

Treatment of Infections

Infections are a major cause of mortality.

- Risk factors include prolonged neutropenia and the indwelling catheters used for specific therapy. Fungal infections, especially those due to *Aspergillus* species pose a major risk.
- Empirical antibiotic therapy should be broad based, with gram-negative and staphylococcal coverage based on local microbial sensitivities. Especially consider including anti-pseudomonal coverage at the start of treatment for patients with febrile neutropenia and consider early introduction of antifungal agents for those with persistent fever.
- Cytokine support with granulocyte colony-stimulating factor (G-CSF) and granulocyte-macrophage colony-stimulating factor (GM-CSF) may be considered in refractory infections, although this therapy should be weighed against cost and efficacy.

Diet Management

The diet for the patient with aplastic anemia who has neutropenia or who is receiving immunosuppressive therapy should be tailored carefully to exclude raw meats, dairy products, or fruits and vegetables that are likely to be colonized with bacteria, fungus, or molds. Furthermore, a salt-limited diet is recommended during therapy with steroids.

Daily Activity of Child

- The patient should avoid any activity that increases the risk of trauma during periods of thrombocytopenia.
- The risk of community-acquired infections increases during periods of neutropenia.

Complications

- Complications of aplastic anemia
  - Infections
  - Bleeding
- Complications of BMT
  - Graft-versus-host disease (GVHD) is a complication that can occur after a stem cell or bone marrow transplant.
  - Graft failure

Prognosis

The outcome of patients with aplastic anemia has substantially improved because of improved supportive care. The natural history of aplastic anemia suggests that as many as one fifth of patients may spontaneously recover with supportive care; however, observational and/or supportive care therapy alone is rarely indicated. The estimated 5-year survival rate for the typical patient receiving immunosuppression is 75%. The rate for those receiving a BMT from a matched sibling donor is greater than 90%. However, in case of immunosuppression, relapse and late clonal disease are risks.

THALASSEMIA

Introduction

Thalassemia intermedia is a term used to define a group of patients with β thalassemia in whom the clinical severity of the disease is somewhere between the mild symptoms of the β thalassemia trait and the severe manifestations of β thalassemia major. The diagnosis is a clinical one that is based on the patient maintaining a satisfactory hemoglobin (Hb) level of at least 6–7 g/dL at the time of diagnosis without the need for regular blood transfusions.

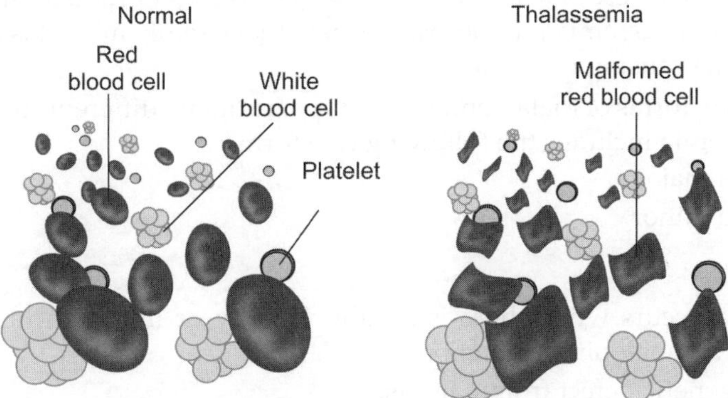

Fig. 7.77: Anatomical difference between normal and thalassemia blood cells

Definition

Thalassemia is an inherited blood disorder in which the body makes an abnormal form of hemoglobin. Hemoglobin is the protein molecule in red blood cells that carries oxygen. The disorder results in excessive destruction of red blood cells, which leads to anemia.

Types

The two main forms of thalassemia are alpha-thalassemia and beta-thalassemia. In alpha-thalassemia, at least one of the alpha globin genes has a mutation or abnormality. In beta-thalassemia, the beta globin genes are affected.

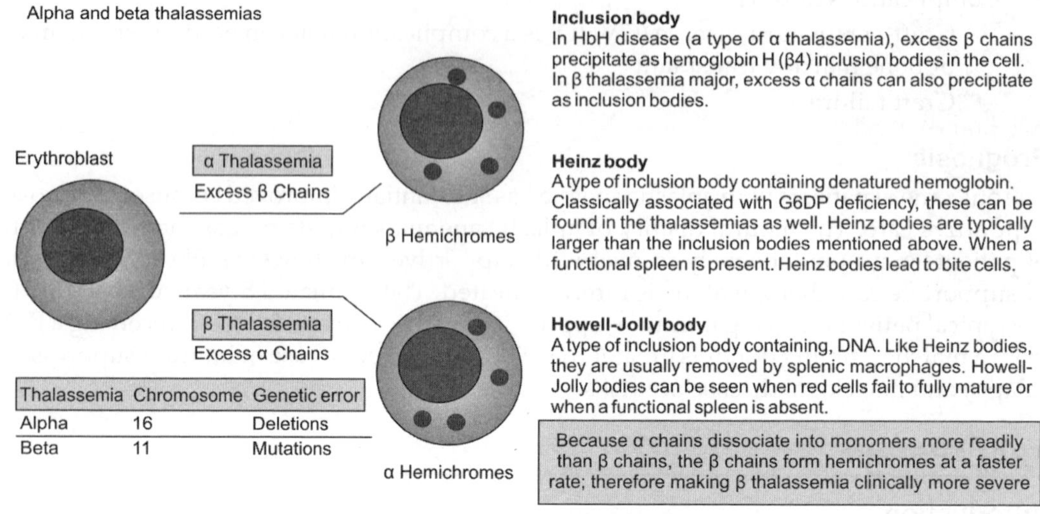

Fig. 7.78: Types of thalassemia

- *Alpha thalassemia:* The alpha thalassemias are caused by deletions or changes in one or more of the alpha globin genes. The alpha globin protein is produced by four genes instead of the usual two. Deletions may be on the same chromosome or there may one deletion on each chromosome.
- *Beta thalassemia:* It occurs when similar gene defects affect production of the beta globin protein. Beta thalassemia (also known as beta thalassemia minor) is an inherited form of thalassemia causing mild anemia.

There are many forms of thalassemia. Each type has many different subtypes. Both alpha and beta thalassemia includes the following two forms:

1. Thalassemia major
2. Thalassemia minor

Causes

- Thalassemia occurs when there is an abnormality or mutation in one of the genes involved in hemoglobin production.
- Inherit the genetic defect from parents.

Signs and Symptoms

Symptoms will depend on the type of thalassemia:

- *Thalassemia minor:* Thalassemia minor usually does not cause any symptoms. If it does, it causes minor anemia.
- *Betathalassemia:* Betathalassemia comes in two serious types, which are thalassemia major, or Cooley's anemia and thalassemia intermedia.

The symptoms of thalassemia major generally appear before a child's second birthday. The severe anemia related to this condition can be life-threatening.

Other signs and symptoms include:

- Fussiness
- Paleness
- Frequent infections
- A poor appetite
- Failure to thrive
- Jaundice, which is a yellowing of the skin or the whites of the eyes
- Enlarged organs.

Diagnostic Evaluation

- A severe form of thalassemia intermedia must be differentiated from β thalassemia major; this is mainly a clinical differentiation based on close monitoring to determine whether the patient's Hb level can be maintained at 6–7 g/dL without blood transfusions.
- CBC count and differential reveal anemia with marked hypochromasia and microcytosis. An Hb level below 7–8 g/dL indicates a severe case; whether the thalassemia is major or intermedia can be determined only after adequate monitoring.
- Hb electrophoresis shows an abnormal pattern.
- Iron studies should be performed, either as baseline in anticipation of iron overload in the future or for diagnosis and management of this condition when suspected.
- Serum transferrin saturation may provide some information about the patient's iron status however, it lacks sensitivity.
- Liver function tests are needed at diagnosis and during follow-up, especially in patients who are receiving blood transfusions.

Management

Medical management

The treatment of most cases of thalassemia intermedia involves close monitoring and observation. Patients with satisfactory hemoglobin (Hb), levels are frequently monitored. These patients usually require blood transfusions only on certain occasions, such as the presence of intercurrent infections, hypersplenism, or other illnesses.

Medication

There is no specific medications are available for the treatment of thalassemia intermedia. Most patients with severe disease are prone to developing megaloblastic anemia due to folate deficiency for several reasons, including poor absorption, low dietary intake, and, most importantly, the extreme demand of the very active bone marrow for folic acid. For this reason, most patients benefit from a low dose of folate.

Child with iron overload should be treated with chelation therapy (orally or parenterally). The drugs of choice at the present time are the oral agent deferasirox and deferoxamine administered subcutaneously by infusion pump 5 times per week. It can be administered while the patient sleeps. Low-dose vitamin C with each infusion of deferoxamine is beneficial in enhancing iron chelation. Combination therapy with more than one agent has proved to be effective in certain situations.

Surgical Management

Splenectomy is frequently recommended for patients who are no longer able to maintain an adequate Hb level. It is usually performed to restore the Hb steady state in patients who are not receiving blood transfusions and frequently succeeds in averting the need for regular transfusions.

Diet Management

A well-balanced diet with adequate folic acid supply is a necessity. Foods with high iron content should be avoided, particularly meat because heme iron is especially well-absorbed. Vitamin C assists absorption of dietary iron; patients should avoid coingesting vitamin C and iron-rich foods. Alternatively, drinking tea with iron-rich foods helps chelate some of the iron before it is absorbed in the bowels.

Daily Activity

Child with thalassemia intermedia should be able to tolerate most daily activities. However, once the anemia worsens, exercise intolerance develops and may represent a warning sign indicating the need for initiation of blood transfusions. Massive splenomegaly has been observed in severe cases and is a cause for limiting the patient's activity for fear of injury to the abdomen causing rupture of the spleen. Regular transfusions decrease the size of the spleen in most instances, allowing splenectomy to be avoided whenever possible.

Nursing Management

- Most medical care in thalassemia intermedia is provided in an outpatient setting.
- Inpatient care is reserved for surgical procedures such as splenectomy or resection of large extramedullary hematopoietic tumorlike masses compressing vital organs, infectious complications, or in rare severe cases that are treated by a bone marrow transplant.
- Frequent outpatient visits are needed in the early stages to monitor hematologic parameters, activity, exercise tolerance, growth and development of bone changes.
- Once the patient requires regular transfusions, monthly outpatient visits for blood transfusions and laboratory work for monitoring iron load status are usually required.
- Guidelines for transfusion in neonates and older children have been established.
- While receiving chelation therapy, patients should have eye examinations and hearing tests as part of monitoring for the complications of therapy.

Prognosis

Child with milder cases have good prognosis; however, after several years of stable disease, many patients develop the severe form and become transfusion dependent. Patients with the severe forms have the same prognosis as those with thalassemia major.

HEMOPHILIA IN CHILDREN

Introduction

Hemophilia is an inherited bleeding disorder in which the blood does not clot normally due to a lack of clotting protein. People with hemophilia bleed for a longer time than others after an injury.

The most common type of hemophilia, caused by a lack of clotting factor VIII, is called Hemophilia A or classic hemophilia. The second most common type is caused by a lack of clotting factor IX and is called Hemophilia B or Christmas disease, named for Stephen Christmas, the first person diagnosed with the factor IX deficiency. Hemophilia A and B almost always occur in boys. A third, very rare type of hemophilia, called Hemophilia C, is caused by a lack of clotting factor XI and can occur in both girls and boys.

Children with hemophilia may qualify for coverage of medical expenses through California Children's Services and the Genetically Handicapped Persons' Program and if severely disabled, for financial support from the Social Security Administration. A social worker at the Hemophilia Treatment Center can refer you to the appropriate resources.

Definition

Hemophilia is a coagulation disorder arising from a genetic defect of the X chromosome, the defect can either be inherited or result from spontaneous gene mutation. In each type of hemophilia (hemophilias A, B and C), a critical coagulation protein is missing, causing individuals to bleed for long periods of time before clotting occurs. Depending on the degree of the disorder in the affected individual, uncontrolled bleeding may occur spontaneously with initiating event, or occur after specific events such as surgery, dental procedures, immunizations, or injury.

Types

There are two types of inherited hemophilia, type A and type B. Hemophilia A is much more common than hemophilia B. With hemophilia A, clotting factor VIII (eight) is lower than normal. With hemophilia B, clotting factor IX (nine) is lower than normal.

- *Hemophilia A:* Caused by a missing or reduced amount of the blood clotting protein Factor VIII.
- *Hemophilia B:* Caused by a missing or reduced amount of the blood clotting protein Factor IX.

Hemophilia

Hemophilia may occur in mild, moderate and severe forms, based on both the child's symptoms and the level or amount of clotting factor in the blood.

- *Mild Hemophilia:* A child with mild hemophilia has 6 percent to 49 percent factor level and usually has problems with bleeding only after serious injury, trauma or surgery. In many cases, mild hemophilia is not discovered until a major injury, surgery or tooth extraction results in unusual bleeding. The first episode may not occur until adulthood.
- *Moderate Hemophilia:* A child with moderate hemophilia has 1 percent to 5 percent factor level and has bleeding episodes after injuries, major trauma or surgery. He also may experience occasional bleeding without obvious cause. These are called spontaneous bleeding episodes.
- Severe Hemophilia: A child with severe hemophilia has less than 1 percent factor level and has bleeding following an injury or surgery and may have frequent spontaneous bleeding episodes into the joints and muscles.

Levels

There are three levels of hemophilia. These are based on the amount of clotting factor or the kind of bleeding episodes your child has. A bleeding episode is bleeding that is prolonged, usually lasting more than several minutes. Bleeding episodes can occur with or without injury. A bleeding episode that happens without an injury is called a spontaneous bleeding episode.

- *Mild:* A child has some clotting factor activity in his blood. He may have severe (very bad) bleeding only after a major surgery or serious injury. Your child's hemophilia may not be discovered until he has a tooth pulled, or has surgery or a bad injury.
- *Moderate:* A child has little clotting factor activity in his blood. He likely will have severe bleeding when he has an injury or surgery. He may also have episodes of spontaneous bleeding that occur suddenly.
- *Severe:* A child has very little clotting factor activity in his blood. He will have bleeding following an injury. He may also have frequent spontaneous bleeding, usually into his joints and muscles.

Causes

Hemophilia types A and B are inherited bleeding diseases passed on to children from defective genes located on the X chromosome. Females have two X chromosomes (XX), while males have one X and one Y chromosome (XY). Males (XY) have hemophilia when the gene for clotting factor VIII (Hemophilia A) or clotting factor IX (Hemophilia B) on the single X chromosome is affected.

A female carrier of hemophilia has the hemophilia gene on one of her X chromosomes and the normal gene on her other X chromosome. When a woman who is a carrier of the hemophilia gene becomes pregnant, there is a 50% chance that the child will get the X chromosome with the hemophilia gene. If the gene is passed onto the daughter, she will be a carrier.

If the father has hemophilia and the mother does not carry the hemophilia gene, then none of her sons will have hemophilia disease (because the mother has donated a normal X chromosome and the father has donated a normal Y chromosome). However in this scenario, all of the daughters will be carriers because the mom donates her normal X chromosome and the father has donated his abnormal X chromosome with the abnormal gene present.

Signs and Symptoms

The most common symptom of hemophilia is bleeding, especially into the joints and muscles. When a child with hemophilia is injured, he does not bleed faster than a child without hemophilia. He bleeds longer. He may also start bleeding again several days after an injury or surgery. Small cuts or surface bruises usually are not a problem, but deeper injuries may result in bleeding episodes that can cause serious problems and lead to permanent disability unless treated promptly.

The most common symptom of hemophilia is excessive, uncontrollable bleeding. Patients with hemophilia do not bleed faster than normal children; they bleed for a longer time. The severity of symptoms in children with hemophilia depends on the severity of the disease.

Severe Hemophilia

Severe hemophilia is when factor VIII or factor IX clotting factor activity is less than 1%.

- Spontaneous bleeding can occur unrelated to injury and is most dangerous when it occurs in the head
- Joint bleeding is common.

Moderate Hemophilia

Moderate hemophilia is when factor VIII or IX clotting factor activity is 1–5%.

- Bleeding episodes are usually related to injury
- Joint bleeding can occur.

Mild Hemophilia

Mild hemophilia is when factor VIII or IX clotting factor activity is 6–40%.

- Episodes of bleeding are usually related to surgery or dental extractions
- Joint bleeding is uncommon.

Other symptoms of hemophilia include:

- Bruising
- Soft tissue bleeding
- Bleeding from the nose, gums or mouth
- Pain, swelling and limited mobility in the joints and muscles
- Blood found in the urine or stool, or vomiting blood
- Excessive bleeding following circumcision.

Pathophysiology

Hemophilia in Children (Factor VIII Deficiency)

Hemophilia is a common bleeding disorder in children (it is the most common hereditary coagulation disorder). Hemostasis is the process of stopping bleeding and this process needs three main elements: Contraction of vascular wall, platelets and *clotting factors (coagulation factors)* which are 13 in number. Absence or deficiency of one of these clotting factors will lead to failure to stop the bleeding. Hemophilia A (the commonest type) is the deficiency of factor 8 (VIII) which is known as the anti-hemophilic globulin.

Diagnostic Evaluation

Hemophilia is an inherited genetic condition, meaning it is passed down through families. It is caused by a defect in the gene that determines how the body makes factors VIII, IX, or XI. These genes are located on the X chromosome, making hemophilia an X-linked recessive disease.

- Various diagnostic tests are available to measure, under carefully controlled conditions, the length of time it takes to produce certain components of the final fibrin clot. The activated partial thromboplastin time (APTT) is performed and will typically be prolonged while a prothrombin time (PT) will likely be normal. Factor assays, measurement methods performed by the clinical laboratory, can determine the

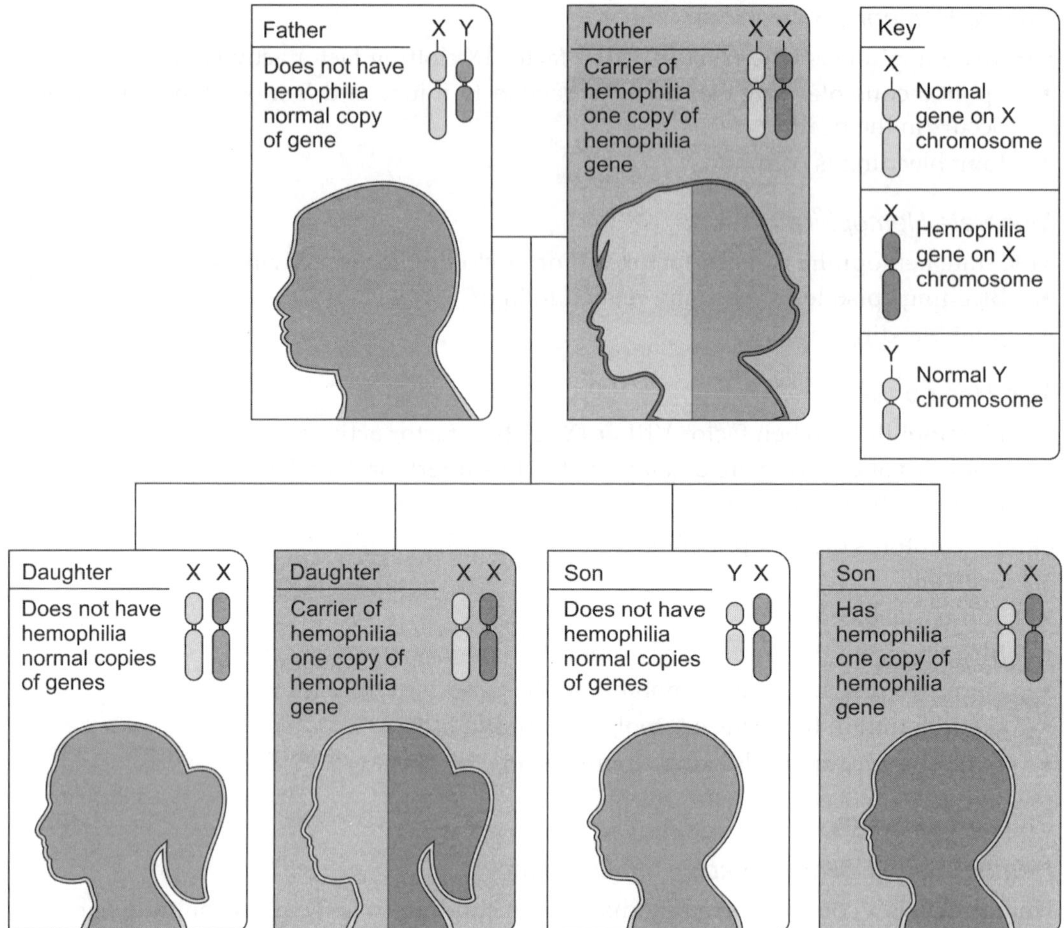

Fig. 7.79: Inheritance of hemophilia

percentage of factors VIII and IX present compared to normal percentages. This information helps to confirm a diagnosis of hemophilia and identifies the type and severity of hemophilia present.

- Families with a history of hemophilia can also have tests done during a pregnancy to determine whether the fetus will have hemophilia. Chorionic villous sampling is a test that examines proteins for deficiencies or defects that are characteristic of hemophilia. The test can be performed at 10 to 14 weeks; test performance is associated with a 1 percent risk of miscarriage.
- **Amniocentesis** is a method of withdrawing amniotic fluid from the placenta to allow examination of fetal cell DNA shed into the amniotic fluid, helping to identify genetic mutations. Amniocentesis can be performed at 15 to 18 weeks gestation and is associated with a one in 200 risk of miscarriage.

Inheritance

The type of inheritance of hemophilia is called X-linked recessive. This causes the disease to be more common in boys who inerit it from their mothers. The mother acts as a carrier (she has one abnormal gene and another normal one).

Management

- *First aid*: The first treatment for any bleeding episode is called **RICE**. You and anyone else who cares for your child must know how to do all of these if your child starts bleeding. If these measures do not stop the bleeding, other treatments will be needed. Prompt use of RICE may reduce the amount of bleeding and decrease the pain that goes with it
  - **R = Rest:** Have your child sit or lie quietly until the bleeding episode ends.
  - **I = Ice:** Apply an icepack to the bleeding area. Do not apply ice directly to the skin. A package of frozen peas or other small vegetables in a thin towel can be used instead of an ice pack.
  - **C = Compression:** Apply pressure to the bleeding site. A bleeding joint can be wrapped with an elastic compression bandage such as an ace bandage. Ask your caregiver for more information about elastic bandages.
  - **E = Elevate:** Position your child so the bleeding area of his body is raised. Raise the area above the level of his heart if possible.
- *IV access*: Your child may need a central venous line (CVL) device. This is needed if an intravenous (IV) catheter (plastic tube) or needle cannot be easily placed in a vein in his hand, arm, or foot. This may also be done if he needs frequent IV infusions of blood products such as clotting factor. These IV access devices are surgically placed into a large vein, usually in the upper chest. Your child may have a CVL, also called a broviac line that is partially under his skin. He may have an implanted port, which is completely under his skin. Ask your caregiver for more information about these CVL devices.

Medication

- *Antifibrinolytic proteins*: These are also known as local blood clotting agents. They help protect clots and hold them in place. They may be used to stop bleeding in the mouth, nose, or abdomen.
- *Desmopressin*: This medicine may be used to treat hemophilia A. It works by increasing the amount of clotting factor VIII in your child's blood.
- *Rehabilitation*: Physical activities and sports will help build strong muscles to protect your child's joints. Ask your child's caregiver which exercises and sports your child can do safely.
- *Replacement therapy*: Certain blood products, called factor concentrates, may be given to your child. They replace the missing clotting factor in your child's blood. Replacement clotting factor is given so that your child's blood will be able to clot and to stop any bleeding. Clotting factor can come from human blood or be man-made. You may be taught how to give clotting factor to your child at home.
- *Demand therapy*: This is when your child receives clotting factor to stop a bleeding episode.

- *Preventive therapy*: Preventive or prophylaxis (PRO-fi-lak-sis) therapy is treatment given to prevent future bleeding episodes. This therapy is often used for the goal of preventing injury to your child's joints. Your child may be started on prophylaxis therapy as early as 1 to 2 years of age, or after one or more joint bleeds.
- *Surgery*: Surgery may be done to repair any damage caused by bleeding into joints. Ask your caregiver about what kind of surgery your child may need.

Prognosis

The type and severity of hemophilia makes it difficult to generalize a prognosis, however, for individuals with mild hemophilia, the prognosis is quite good. Those with more severe hemophilia can also live relatively normal lives with careful management and avoidance of injury. Many individuals achieve normal life expectancy. Without treatment of bleeding episodes, severe muscle and joint pain and eventually permanent damage can occur. Much depends upon the physical activity level of the individual and the possibility of accidental injuries or surgeries required for other conditions, which cannot be predicted.

POLYCYTHEMIA

Introduction

Polycythemia is characterized by an increase in the red blood cell (RBC) compartment in the peripheral blood and is measured by an increase in the RBC count, the hemoglobin content and the hematocrit level above reference ranges adjusted for age, sex, race and altitude. Polycythemia is categorized as primary or secondary due to intrinsic or extrinsic changes, respectively, to erythroid progenitors and RBCs. Both primary and secondary polycythemia can be congenital or acquired in origin.

Definition

Polycythemia is characterized by an increase in absolute quantity of red cells or total RBC volume. In contrast, relative polycythemia (pseudoerythrocytosis) is secondary to fluid loss or decreased fluid intake resulting in hemoconcentration.

Polycythemia is a rare blood disorder that occurs when there are too many red blood cells circulating in the bloodstream. Red blood cells carry oxygen from the lungs to all parts of the body. Polycythemia causes the blood to thicken, making it more difficult for the blood to flow through the body to the organs.

Types

Two basic categories of polycythemia are recognized:

1. *Primary polycythemias* due to factors intrinsic to red cell precursors, including primary familial and congenital polycythemia (PFCP), idiopathic erythrocytosis and polycythemia vera (PV).
2. *Secondary polycythemias* are caused by factors extrinsic to red cell precursors and include a *physiologic-approproriate erythropoietin (EPO)* production in response to tissue hypoxia and physiologic-inappropriate erythropoietin production not in response to tissue hypoxia.

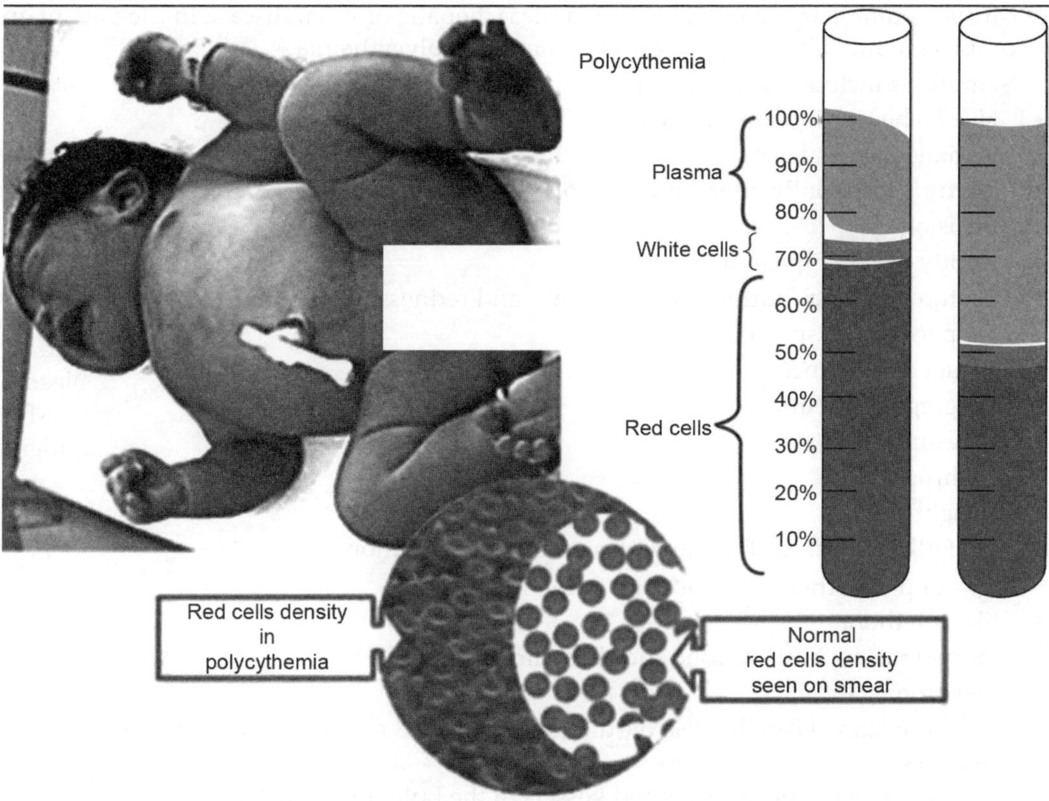

Fig. 7.80: Anatomical view of difference between normal RBC and polycythemia RBC

Causes

- High-altitude erythrocytosis
- *Pulmonary disease:* Chronic obstructive pulmonary disease, diffuse pulmonary infiltrates, kyphoscoliosis, chronic cor pulmonale
- Cyanotic heart disease
- *Hypoventilation syndromes:* Obstructive sleep apnea
- *Epo-secreting tumors:* Renal cell carcinoma, hepatocellular carcinoma
- *Polycythemia of the newborn:* Usually results from a poor intrauterine environment or hypoxic insult during labor or delivery
- *Congenital causes:* High-affinity hemoglobin and 2,3-Bisphosphoglycerate (2,3-BPG) deficiency.

Signs and Symptoms

The clinical features associated with polycythemia are a direct result of the increase in red cell mass, which causes an expansion of blood volume. Signs of hyperviscosity and increased metabolism accompany polycythemia. A thorough history must be obtained for a history of cardiac, pulmonary (including sleep apnea), hepatic or renal disease in the patient and a complete family history for evidence of familial polycythemia.

Symptoms include the following:
- Headache, vertigo, insomnia
- Weakness or malaise
- Pruritus (especially after exposure to warm water)
- Bruising
- Ruddy or red appearance
- Erythromelalgia (burning pain, warmth and redness of extremities)
- Diaphoresis/dyspnea
- Visual disturbance
- Ringing in the ears
- Paresthesias
- Arthropathies
- Weight loss
- GI: Fullness, thirst, abdominal discomfort, constipation.

Signs of polycythemia include the following:
- Skin plethora
- Hypertension, both systolic and diastolic
- Hepatomegaly
- Splenomegaly: Usually feels hard and smooth and occurs in more than two thirds of patients
- Conjunctival plethora (engorged vessels in the bulbar conjunctiva)
- Ecchymosis
- Cardiac hypertrophy (rarely observed).

Pathophysiology

Primary polycythemia is due to factors intrinsic to red cell precursors caused by acquired and inherited mutations. It includes the diagnoses of primary familial and congenital polycythemia, idiopathic erythrocytosis and polycythemia vera. Polycythemia vera, also known as polycythemia rubra vera, is a chronic clonal myleoproliferative disorder characterized by clonal proliferation of myeloid cells. Currently, the diagnosis of polycythemia vera is based on the 2008 World Health Organization (WHO) criteria, which has integrated molecular diagnostics into the evaluation and screening for polycythemia vera. A diagnosis of polycythemia vera is made when both major and one minor criterion are present or when the first major criterion is present with any two minor criteria. The current criteria include the following.

Diagnostic Evaluation

Major Criteria

Hemoglobin level of more than 18.5 g/dL in men (>16.5 g/dL in women) or other evidence of increased red cell volume or hemoglobin or hematocrit level higher than 99th percentile of method-specific reference range for age, sex, altitude, of residence or hemoglobin level of more than 17 g/dL in men (> 15 g/dL in women) if associated with a documented and sustained increase of at least 2 g/dL from an individual's baseline value that cannot be attributed to correction of iron deficiency or elevated red cell mass greater than 25% above mean normal predicted value.

Minor Criteria

- Bone marrow trilineage myeloproliferation
- Subnormal serum EPO levels
- Endogenous erythroid colony growth
- Earlier diagnostic criteria for polycythemia vera included the following (based on the Polycythemia Vera Study Group Diagnostic Criteria):
  - Red cell mass greater than 36 mL/kg for men and greater than 32 mL/kg for women
  - Arterial oxygen saturation greater than 92%
  - Splenomegaly or 2 of the following:
    - Thrombocytosis greater than 400 × 109/L
    - Leukocytosis greater than 12 × 109/L
    - Leukocyte alkaline phosphatase activity greater than 100 U/L in adults (reference range, 30–120 U/L) without fever or infection
    - Serum vitamin B_{12} greater than 900 pg/mL (reference range, 130–785 pg/mL)
    - Unsaturated vitamin B_{12} binding capacity greater than 2200 pg/mL.

Laboratory Studies

- *CBC count:* Leukocytosis and thrombocytosis are commonly observed but not universal in patients with polycythemia. Leukocytes are greater than 12 × 109/L; platelets are greater than 400 × 109/L. Large platelets are often observed. Platelets can be morphologically and qualitatively abnormal. Red cell mass is greater than 36 mL/kg in men and greater than 32 mL/kg in women. RBCs often have anisocytosis, basophilic stippling and polychromatophilia.
- *Serum erythropoietin (Epo):* Elevated serum Epo levels can be used to distinguish polycythemia vera (PV) from secondary polycythemia. Elevated Epo levels are observed in secondary polycythemia. Low Epo levels suggest primary familial and congenital polycythemia (PFCP) or polycythemia vera, but Epo levels may be normal.
- *Hemoglobin:* Hemoglobin analysis is indicated in patients with inadequately high serum Epo levels. Oxygen dissociation curves and hemoglobin electrophoresis can be used to assess for high oxygen affinity mutants and 2,3-Bisphosphoglycerate deficiency (2, 3-BPG) deficiency.
  - *Serum B_{12}:* Serum B_{12} levels are greater than 900 pg/mL (reference range, 130–785 pg/mL), resulting from transcobalamin release from an increased granulocytic mass.
  - *Leukocyte alkaline phosphatase:* Activity is greater than 100 U/L (reference range adult levels, 30–120 U/L) because levels vary for age; check pediatric age-specific controls.

- *Uric acid:* Uric acid levels are increased (reference range adult levels, 2–8 mg/dL). Because levels vary for age, check pediatric age-specific controls. The uric acid level can be within the reference range.
  - Elevated sedimentation rate
  - Spurious hyperkalemia
  - Increased blood viscosity
  - Artifactual prolongation of coagulation studies
  - Endogenous erythroid colony formation: In vitro, this is characteristic for polycythemia vera; however, its specificity and sensitivity limits its use for diagnosis.

Other Tests

The need for bone marrow biopsy is still controversial. Biopsy is not a part of the diagnostic criteria. It may be helpful when trying to differentiate polycythemia vera from other myeloproliferative disorders and to assess the degree of fibrosis. Cytogenetics are not routinely performed but should be used if the diagnosis is questionable and if the differential includes malignancy, myelodysplastic syndrome, or other myeloproliferative disorders.

Histologic Findings

If a bone marrow biopsy is performed, the marrow in polycythemia vera is typically hypercellular, including all marrow elements and displaced marrow fat. The number of megakaryocytes is usually increased with wide variation in size. Stainable iron is decreased or absent, and, later in the disease course, fibrosis and marrow reticulin fibers are increased.

Management

Medical Management

Treatment of secondary polycythemia depends on its cause. Supplemental oxygen can be provided for individuals with chronic hypoxia. Other therapies can be directed toward treating the cause of polycythemia (for example, appropriate treatment of heart failure or chronic lung disease).

Primary Polycythemia

The goals of therapy are to maximize survival while minimizing the complications of therapy as well as of the disease itself. Phlebotomy and myelosuppressive chemotherapy are the cornerstones of therapy and have produced a median survival time of 9–14 years after the beginning of treatment.

Secondary Polycythemia

Phlebotomy is used for symptomatic hyperviscosity. The goal is to treat the underlying cause of polycythemia.

Surgical Management

Surgery is not typically indicated. Occasionally, splenectomy is performed late in the course of the disease if massive splenomegaly causes adverse effects, such as early satiety, anemia, or thrombocytopenia from sequestration. Please note that these patients have a high-risk of complications during surgical procedures.

Complications

- *Vascular occlusive events*: Splenic infarcts, thrombosis (cerebral, portal vein, pulmonary embolus)
- Hemorrhage
- Marrow fibrosis resulting in pancytopenia
- *Malignancy*: Acute myelogenous leukemia (AML), chronic lymphocytic leukemia (CLL), chronic myelogenous leukemia (CML), lymphoma
- *Hyperuricemia*: Renal stones, nephropathy, gout
- Budd-Chiari syndrome.

Prognosis

The median survival time for patients with polycythemia vera (PV) is 18 months for untreated patients and 9–14 years for treated patients.

THROMBOCYTOPENIA OR IDIOPATHIC THROMBOCYTOPENIA PURPURA (ITP)

Introduction

Thrombocytopenia is a condition in which there are a few platelets, the blood cells that prevent bleeding. Many things can cause thrombocytopenia in children, most commonly infections (especially viral infections) and destruction of platelets by the immune system (called immune thrombocytopenia or ITP).

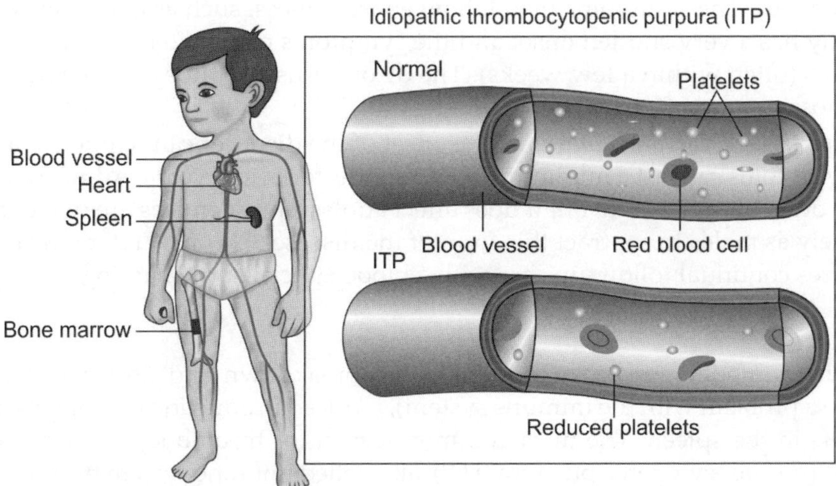

Fig. 7.81: Anatomical view of difference between normal and ITP cells

Idiopathic thrombocytopenic purpura is a blood disorder characterized by an abnormal decrease in the number of platelets in the blood. Platelets are cells in the blood that help stop bleeding. A decrease in platelets can result in easy bruising, bleeding gums and internal bleeding.

- 'Idiopathic' means the cause is unknown.
- 'Thrombocytopenia' means a decreased number of platelets in the blood.
- 'Purpura' refers to the purple discoloring of the skin, as with a bruise.

Definition

Idiopathic thrombocytopenic purpura (ITP), also known as primary immune thrombocytopenic purpura and autoimmune thrombocytopenic purpura, is defined as isolated thrombocytopenia with normal bone marrow and the absence of other causes of thrombocytopenia. The two distinct clinical syndromes manifest as an acute condition in children and a chronic condition in adults. ITP is a decrease in the number of circulating platelets in the absence of toxic exposure or a disease associated with a low platelet count.

Incidence

Hemorrhage represents the most serious complication; intracranial hemorrhage is the most significant. The mortality rate from hemorrhage is approximately 1% in children and 5% in adults. In patients with severe thrombocytopenia, predicted 5-year mortality rates from bleeding are significantly raised in patients older than 60 years versus patients younger than 40 years, 47.8% versus 2.2%, respectively. Older age and previous history of hemorrhage increase the risk of severe bleeding in adult ITP. Spontaneous remission occurs in more than 80% of cases in children but is uncommon in adults.

Types

- *Acute thrombocytopenic purpura:* This is most commonly seen in young children (2 to 6 years old). The symptoms may follow a viral illness, such as chickenpox. Acute ITP usually has a very sudden onset and the symptoms usually disappear in less than six months (often within a few weeks). The disorder usually does not recur. Acute ITP is the most common form of the disorder.
- *Chronic thrombocytopenic purpura*: The onset of the disorder can happen at any age and the symptoms can last a minimum of six months to several years. Adults have this form more often than children, but it does affect adolescents. Females are two to three times as likely as males to contract this form of the disease. Chronic ITP can recur often and requires continual follow-up care with a blood specialist (hematologist).

Causes

Causes of thrombocytopenia include increased breakdown and destruction of platelets (related to a problem with the immune system), reduced production of platelets or trapping of platelets in the spleen. The most common reason for thrombocytopenia in children is idiopathic thrombocytopenic purpura (ITP), also called immune system thrombocytopenia. Idiopathic means unknown cause.

Signs and Symptoms

- The symptoms of bleeding (e.g. type, severity, duration) and on symptoms that may exclude other causes of thrombocytopenia.
- Elicit risk factors for HIV and systemic symptoms linked to other illnesses or to medications (e.g. heparin, alcohol, quinidine/quinine, sulfonamides) that may cause thrombocytopenia.
- Address risk factors for increased bleeding, such as GI disease, CNS disease, urologic disease, or active lifestyle, as these may determine the aggressiveness of management.

Common signs, symptoms and precipitating factors include the following:

- Abrupt onset (childhood ITP)
- Gradual onset (adult ITP)
- Purpura
- Menorrhagia
- Epistaxis
- Gingival bleeding
- Recent live virus immunization (childhood ITP)
- Recent viral illness (childhood ITP)
- Bruising tendency.

Pathophysiology

Platelets, or thrombocytes, are blood cells produced in the bone marrow. Platelets circulate in the blood for approximately 8 to 10 days. At any given time, about two-thirds of all platelets are present in the blood stream while one-third remains in the spleen. New platelets are always being made in the bone marrow.

The main function of platelets is to prevent bleeding. A normal platelet count ranges from 150,000 to 400,000 per microliter of blood. A microliter is a unit of volume equal to one-millionth of a liter.

If child has a low platelet count, he may bruise easily and bleed from superficial surfaces. For example, he may get nosebleeds.

- Child's platelet count is less than 50,000 per microliter, he will bruise more easily than normal.
- Child's platelet count is less than 20,000 per microliter, he may develop spontaneous bleeding.

Diagnostic Evaluation

Physical Examination

Evaluate the type and the severity of bleeding and try to exclude other causes of bleeding. Seek evidence of liver disease, thrombosis, autoimmune diseases (e.g. nephritis, cutaneous vasculitis, arthritis) and infection, particularly HIV.

Common physical findings include the following:

- Nonpalpable petechiae, which mostly occur in dependent regions
- Hemorrhagic bullae on mucous membranes

- Purpura
- Gingival bleeding
- Signs of GI bleeding
- Menometrorrhagia, menorrhagia
- Retinal hemorrhages
- Evidence of intracranial hemorrhage with possible neurologic symptoms
- *Nonpalpable spleen:* The prevalence of palpable spleen in patients with ITP is approximately the same as that in the non-ITP population (i.e. 3% in adults, 12% in children).
- Spontaneous bleeding when platelet count is less than 20,000/mm^3.

CBC (complete blood count)

- Isolated thrombocytopenia is the key finding regarding laboratory evaluation.
- Truly giant platelets on peripheral smear suggest congenital thrombocytopenia.
- The WBC count and hemoglobin typically are normal, unless severe hemorrhage has occurred.

Coagulation studies are normal and a bleeding time is not useful.

Imaging Studies

A CT scan of the head is warranted if concern exists regarding intracranial hemorrhage.

Management

Prehospital Care

- Prehospital care focuses on the ABCs, which include providing oxygen, controlling severe hemorrhage and initiating intravenous (IV) fluids to maintain hemodynamic stability.
- Prehospital airway control may be necessary for a large intracranial hemorrhage.
- EMS providers should be aware of the potential for serious bleeding complications in patients with idiopathic thrombocytopenic purpura (ITP).

The two most common forms of treatment are:

- *Steroids,* which help prevent bleeding by decreasing the rate of platelet destruction. Steroids will give effective result in an increase in platelet counts seen within 2 to 3 weeks. Side effects may include irritability, stomach irritation, weight gain, hypertension and acne.
- *Intravenous gamma globulin (IVGG),* a protein that contains many antibodies and also slows the destruction of platelets. IVGG works more quickly than steroids (within 24 to 48 hours).

Other treatments for ITP may include:

- *Rh immune globulin:* This medication temporarily stops the spleen from destroying platelets. The child must be Rh positive and have a spleen for this medication to be effective.
- *Medication changes:* If medication is the suspected cause of child's ITP, discontinuation or changing the medication may be necessary.

- *Infection treatment:* If infection is the cause for ITP, then treatment of the infection may result in higher platelet counts.
- *Splenectomy:* In some cases of child's spleen need to be removed since this is the site of platelet destruction. This is considered more often in older children with chronic ITP to decrease the rate of platelet destruction.
- *Hormone therapy:* Teenage girls may need to take hormones to stop their menstrual cycle when their platelets are low if excessive bleeding occurs.

The following is a short list of medicines that should not be given to your child with ITP:

- Aspirin and all compounds that contain it. These include: Ecotrin, Midol and 'blue' Alka-Seltzer
- Antihistamines
- Non-steroidal anti-inflammatory drugs (NSAIDs), such as Motrin, Nuprin, Advil and Indocin
- Vitamin E
- Cod liver oil.

Nursing Management

- Rule out other potential causes of thrombocytopenia.
- Emergency splenectomy may be necessary if severe bleeding complications due to thrombocytopenia do not respond to medical therapy.
- Observe for life-threatening bleeding.
- Consult with a hematologist, as further treatments (e.g. steroids, IVIg, platelet transfusion) may be indicated.
- Close follow-up care with a hematologist is required.
- Elective splenectomy may be necessary if medical therapy fails.
- Instruct patients to return for follow-up in order to assess for a potentially reduced platelet count.
- Emphasize close outpatient follow-up care.
- Because of the increased risk of bleeding, instruct patients to avoid aspirin products.

Complications

Complications of idiopathic thrombocytopenic purpura may include the following:

- Intracranial or other major hemorrhage
- Severe blood loss
- Adverse effects of corticosteroids
- Pneumococcal infections if the patient must have a splenectomy.

Prognosis

- Children
  - Approximately 83% of children have a spontaneous remission and 89% of children eventually recover.
  - More than 50% of patients recover within 4–8 weeks.
  - Approximately 2% of patients die.

DISSEMINATED INTRAVASCULAR COAGULATION (DIC)

Introduction

Disseminated intravascular coagulation (DIC) otherwise called as disseminated intravascular coagulopathy or consumptive coagulopathy, in this pathological process characterized by the widespread activation of the clotting cascade that results in the formation of blood clots in the small blood vessels throughout the body.

This is life-threatening condition that prevents blood from clotting normally. The blood clots reduce blood flow and can block blood from reaching bodily organs. This increased clotting can use up the blood's platelets and clotting factors. Fewer platelets and clotting factors available result in excessive bleeding.

Definition

Disseminated intravascular coagulation is a condition in which small blood clots develop throughout the bloodstream, blocking small blood vessels. The increased clotting depletes the platelets and clotting factors needed to control bleeding, causing excessive bleeding.

Disseminated intravascular coagulation (DIC) is characterized by systemic activation of blood coagulation, which results in generation and deposition of fibrin, leading to microvascular thrombi in various organs and contributing to multiple organ dysfunction syndrome. Consumption and subsequent exhaustion of coagulation proteins and platelets (from ongoing activation of coagulation) may induce severe bleeding, though micro clot formation may occur in the absence of severe clotting factor depletion and bleeding.

Causes

DIC can occur in the following conditions:

- Solid tumors and blood cancers (especially acute promyelocytic leukemia)

Obstetric Complications

- Abruptio placenta
- Pre-eclampsia or eclampsia
- Amniotic fluid embolism
- Retained intrauterine fetal demise
- Septic abortion.

Massive Tissue Injury

- Severe trauma
- Burns
- Hyperthermia
- Rhabdomyolysis
- Extensive surgery.

Sepsis or Severe Infection

- Bacterial (Gram-negative and Gram-positive sepsis)
- Viral, fungal, or protozoan infections

- Transfusion reactions (i.e. ABO incompatibility hemolytic reactions)
- Severe allergic or toxic reactions (i.e. snake or viper venom)
- Giant hemangiomas (Kasabach-Merritt syndrome)
- Large aortic aneurysms.

Risk Factors for DIC

- Blood transfusion reaction
- Cancer, especially certain types of leukemia
- Inflammation of the pancreas (pancreatitis)
- Infection in the blood, especially by bacteria or fungus
- Liver disease
- Pregnancy complications (such as placenta that is left behind after delivery)
- Recent surgery or anesthesia
- Severe tissue injury (as in burns and head injury)
- Large hemangioma (a blood vessel that is not formed properly).

Signs and Symptoms

- Bleeding, possibly from many sites in the body
- Blood clots
- Bruising
- Drop in blood pressure
- Rectal or vaginal bleeding
- Red dots on the surface of the skin.

Pathophysiology

Based on causes, the activation of the coagulation cascade yields thrombin that converts fibrinogen to fibrin; the stable fibrin clot being the final product of hemostasis. The fibrinolytic system then functions to break down fibrinogen and fibrin.

Activation of the fibrinolytic system generates plasmin (in the presence of thrombin), which is responsible for the lysis of fibrin clots. The breakdown of fibrinogen and fibrin results in polypeptides called fibrin or fibrin split products (FSPs). In a state of homeostasis, the presence of plasmin is critical, as it is the central proteolytic enzyme of coagulation and is also necessary for the breakdown of clots, or fibrinolysis.

In DIC, the processes of coagulation and fibrinolysis are dysregulated and the result is widespread clotting with resultant bleeding.

Regardless of the triggering event of DIC, once initiated, the pathophysiology of DIC is similar in all conditions. One critical mediator of DIC is the release of a transmembrane glycoprotein called tissue factor (TF).

TF is present on the surface of many cell types (including endothelial cells, macrophages and monocytes) and is not normally in contact with the general circulation, but is exposed to the circulation after vascular damage. For example, TF is released in response to exposure to cytokines (particularly interleukin), tumor necrosis factor, and endotoxin.

This plays a major role in the development of DIC in septic conditions. TF is also abundant in tissues of the lungs, brain and placenta. This helps to explain why DIC readily develops in patients with extensive trauma. Upon exposure to blood and platelets, TF binds with activated factor VIIa (normally present in trace amounts in the blood), forming the extrinsic tenase complex. This complex further activates factor IX and X to IXa and Xa, respectively, leading to the common coagulation pathway and the subsequent formation of thrombin and fibrin.

The release of endotoxin is the mechanism by which Gram-negative sepsis provokes DIC. In acute promyelocytic leukemia, treatment causes the destruction of leukemic granulocyte precursors, resulting in the release of large amounts of proteolytic enzymes from their storage granules, causing microvascular damage. Other malignancies may enhance the expression of various oncogenes that result in the release of TF and plasminogen activator inhibitor–1 (PAI–1), which prevents fibrinolysis.

Excess circulating thrombin results from the excess activation of the coagulation cascade. The excess thrombin cleaves fibrinogen, which ultimately leaves behind multiple fibrin clots in the circulation. These excess clots trap platelets to become larger clots, which leads to microvascular and macrovascular thrombosis. This lodging of clots in the microcirculation, in the large vessels and in the organs is what leads to the ischemia, impaired organ perfusion and end-organ damage that occurs with DIC.

Diagnostic Evaluation

- Complete blood count (CBC) with blood smear exam
- Fibrin degradation products
- Partial thromboplastin time (PTT)
- Prothrombin time (PT)
- Serum fibrinogen.

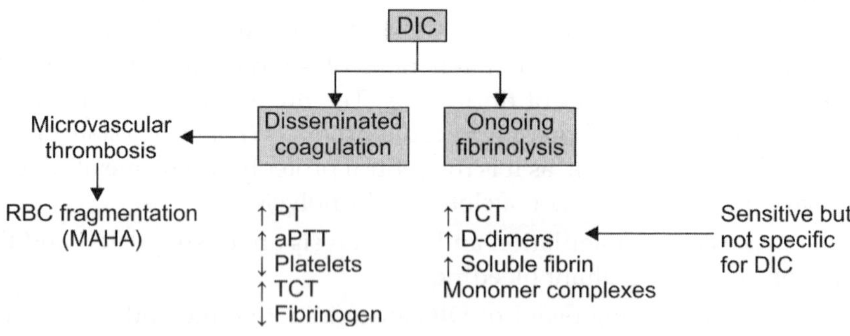

Fig. 7.82: Laboratory test value

Management

DIC that develops suddenly is life threatening and is treated as an emergency. Platelets and clotting factors are transfused to replace those depleted and to stop bleeding. Heparin may be used to slow the clotting in people who have more chronic, milder DIC in which clotting is more of a problem than bleeding.

Supportive treatments may include:

- Plasma transfusions to replace blood clotting factors if a large amount of bleeding is occurring
- Blood thinner medicine (heparin) to prevent blood clotting if a large amount of clotting is occurring.

Complications

- Bleeding
- Lack of blood flow to the arms, legs, or vital organs
- Stroke.

CHILD WITH PURPURA

Introduction

Bleeding under the skin or into mucosal membranes is called purpura and may be an innocent finding related to mild childhood trauma or may be the presenting sign of a life threatening disease. Purpura can be subdivided based on size into petechiae and ecchymosis. Pinpoint areas (less than 2 mm) of hemorrhage, which are reddish-purple lesions are called petechiae, while larger confluent lesions are referred to as ecchymosis. Ecchymosis are commonly called bruises. In some cases, ecchymosis may be tender or raised. In contrast to other erythematous or vascular skin lesions, purpuric lesions do not blanch when pressure is applied to the skin.

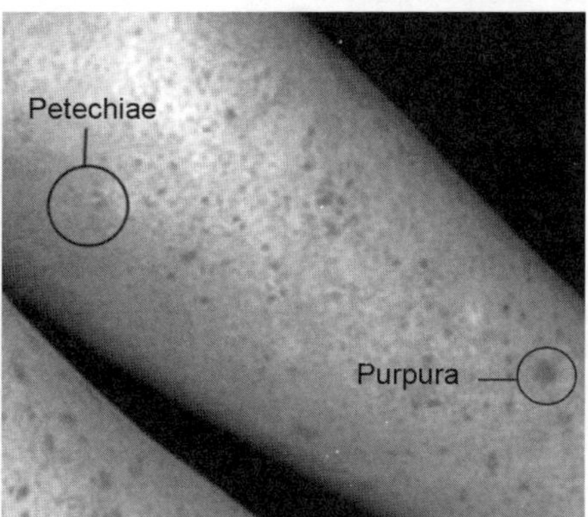

Fig. 7.83: Structural difference between petechiae and purpura

Definition

The term 'purpura' describes a purplish discoloration of the skin produced by small bleeding vessels near the surface. Purpura may also occur in the mucous membranes, especially of the mouth and in the internal organs. When purpura spots are very small (< 1 cm in diameter), they are called petechiae or petechial hemorrhages. Larger, deeper purpura are referred to as ecchymosis or bruising.

Henoch-Schonlein purpura (HSP) is a disease involving inflammation of small blood vessels. It most commonly occurs in children. The inflammation causes blood vessels in the skin, intestines, kidneys and joints to start leaking. The main symptom is a rash with numerous small bruises, which have a raised appearance, over the legs or buttocks.

Types

Purpura may occur with either normal platelet counts (non-thrombocytopenic purpuras) or decreased platelet counts (thrombocytopenic purpuras). Platelets help maintain the integrity of the capillary lining as well as being important in the clotting process. As a general rule, purpura indicates a problem of the platelet system whilst a deficiency of clotting factors will cause hematomas or haemarthrosis as in hemophilia. Nevertheless, clotting factor deficiency must be considered.

- Purpura may occur with normal platelet counts (non-thrombocytopenic purpuras)
- Decreased platelet counts (thrombocytopenic purpuras).

Causes

Non-thrombocytopenic Purpura

Congenital causes, such as:

- Hereditary haemorrhagic telangiectasia (Osler-Weber-Rendu syndrome).
- Connective tissue diseases, such as Ehlers-Danlos syndrome and pseudoxanthoma elasticum.
- Congenital cytomegalovirus (CMV) and congenital rubella.

Acquired causes, such as severe infections:

- Septicemia, meningococcal infections, measles.
- Allergic causes, such as Henoch-Schönlein purpura, connective tissue disorders (e.g. systemic lupus erythematosus (SLE), rheumatoid arthritis).
- Drug-induced causes, such as steroids and sulfonamides.
- Other causes, such as senile purpura, trauma, scurvy, dependent purpura with venous hypertension and factitial purpura.

Thrombocytopenic Purpura

Causes include:

- Impaired platelet production, such as:
  - Generalized bone marrow failure (e.g. leukemia, aplastic anemia, myeloma, marrow infiltration by solid tumors).
  - Selective reduction in megakaryocytic (e.g. drugs such as cotrimoxazole, chemicals, viral infections).
- Excessive platelet destruction, such as:
  - Immune problems (e.g. immune thrombocytopenia, secondary immune thrombocytopenia-SLE, viral infections, drugs-post-transfusion purpura).

  - Coagulation problems (e.g. disseminated intravascular coagulation (DIC), immune thrombocytopenia, hemolytic uremic syndrome).
- Sequestration of the platelets as occurs in splenomegaly.
- Dilutional loss as might be seen following massive transfusion of stored blood.

Signs and Symptoms

The classic symptoms of HSP are rash, joint pain and swelling, abdominal pain, and/or related kidney disease, including blood in urine. Before these symptoms begin, patients may have 2 to 3 weeks of fever, headache and muscular aches and pains. Rarely, other organs, such as the brain, heart, or lungs, may be affected.

- *Skin rash:* The rash looks like small bruises or small reddish-purple spots. It is usually seen on the buttocks, on the legs and around the elbows.
- *Swelling:* Many children with HSP also have swelling over the backs of the feet and hands and the scrotum in boys.
- *Pain in the joints:* Such as the knees and ankles.
- Stomach pain.
- Blood in the stool (poo) or urine

Diagnostic Evaluation

- CBC, ESR, platelets. The platelet count is fundamental. Leukemia or related diseases may produce anemia and leukocytopenia. ESR may indicate an inflammatory process. It is very nonspecific.
- LFTs to check for liver disease.
- A coagulation screen will screen for clotting factor deficiencies.
- If the patient is on warfarin, check INR.
- Plasma electrophoresis may show hypergammaglobulinemia, paraproteinemia and cryoglobulinemia.
- Autoantibody screen for connective tissue disorders.

Management

Administer the Acetaminophen or nonsteroidal anti-inflammatory drugs (NSAIDs), such as ibuprofen and naproxen for joint pain. In some cases, corticosteroid medication may be used. The rash and joint pain will usually go away after four to six weeks without causing any permanent damage. Bouts of the rash may recur in approximately one-third of cases, but they are usually milder, do not involve joint and abdominal symptoms and they clear up on their own.

CHILDHOOD LEUKEMIA

Introduction

Leukemia is the most common cancer in children and teens, accounting for almost 1 out of 3 cancers. Most childhood leukemia is acute lymphocytic leukemia (ALL). Most of the remaining cases are acute myeloid leukemia (AML). Chronic leukemia are rare in children.

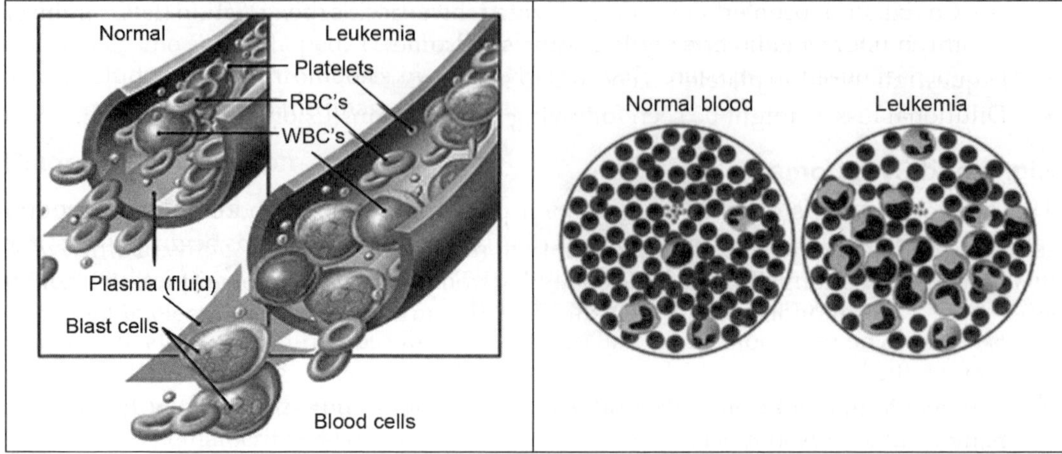

Fig. 7.84: Anatomical difference between normal and leukemia cell

Definition

Leukemia is cancer of the blood cells. Blood cells and platelets are produced in the bone marrow. In leukemia, white bloods cells fail to mature properly. These immature cells continue to reproduce at a rapid rate, crowding out healthy cells and producing a host of symptoms.

Acute leukemia is defined as a malignant clonal proliferation of lymphoid or myeloid precursor cells, of unknown etiology, leading to replacement of normal hematopoiesis by blasts comprising 25 percent or more of bone marrow cells and infiltration of lymph nodes, spleen, liver or other organs. For therapeutic purposes, the acute leukemia is broadly classified as either lymphoid (ALL) or myeloid (AML).

Incidence

The incidence in the West varies from 3.5 to 13 per 100,000 per year. Roughly 75 percent of cases occur in adults. The male to female ratio is 1.3:1. Their ratio in children and adults is 4:1 for ALL and 1:6 for AML.

Types of Childhood Leukemia

- Acute lymphoblastic leukemia (ALL), also called acute lymphocytic leukemia. ALL accounts for three out of every four cases of childhood leukemia.
- Acute myelogenous leukemia (AML). AML is the next most common type of childhood leukemia.
- Hybrid or mixed lineage leukemia. This is a rare leukemia with features of both ALL and AML.
- Chronic myelogenous leukemia (CML). CML is rare in children.
- Chronic lymphocytic leukemia (CLL). CLL is very rare in children.
- Juvenile myelomonocytic leukemia (JMML). This is a rare type that is neither chronic nor acute and occurs most often in children under age of 4 years.

Signs and Symptoms

Table 7.12: Signs and symptoms of leukemia

Signs	Symptoms
• Pallor due to anemia	• General malaise, fatigue and lethargy
• Signs of bleeding tendency such as petechiae, purpura, bruising, etc.	• Prolonged or recurrent episodes of fever
• Signs related to severe infection	• Irritability and/or protracted crying
• Lymphadenopathy	• Growth restriction and/or failure to thrive
• Hepatosplenomegaly	• Shortness of breath and/or reduced exercise tolerance
• Expiratory wheeze (due to mediastinal mass)	• Dizziness and palpitations
• Cranial nerve lesions or other focal CNS pathology	• Bleeding diathesis, particularly causing epistaxis, bleeding gums and/or easy bruising
• Testicular enlargement	• Muscular or bony pain, particularly in the legs
	• Troublesome constipation
	• Prolonged cough
	• Headache
	• Nausea and vomiting, particularly if central nervous system (CNS) infiltration is present
	• Repeated or severe common childhood infections

The risk for childhood leukemia increases if your child has:

- An inherited disorder such as Li-Fraumeni syndrome, Down syndrome, or Klinefelter syndrome
- An inherited immune system problem such as ataxia telangiectasia
- A brother or sister with leukemia, especially an identical twin
- A history of being exposed to high levels of radiation, chemotherapy, or chemicals such as benzene (a solvent)
- A history of immune system suppression, such as for an organ transplant.

Diagnostic Evaluation

Blood Test

Total white blood count (WBC) is often as 100,000/cm. However, it is normal or low in nearly one-half of the cases. Hemoglobin level and platelet count are usually decreased at presentation, marrow examination is essential for the diagnosis of acute leukemias and also to confirm complete remission and relapse.

In addition to morphological evaluation, the cells are also subjected to cytochemistry, electron microscopy, immunophenotyping, cytogenetics and molecular studies. Rapid turnover of cells causes elevated serum Lactate dehydrogenase (S-LDH) uric acid and alkaline phosphatase. Coagulation tests may show evidence of DIC, especially in AML-M3.

Cerebrospinal Fluid (CSF) Examination

Cerebrospinal fluid (CSF) examination is mandatory in all patients of ALL to evaluate CNS involvement at presentation and follow-up. To diagnose childhood leukemia, the doctor will take a thorough medical history and perform a physical exam. Tests are used to diagnose childhood leukemia as well as classify its type.

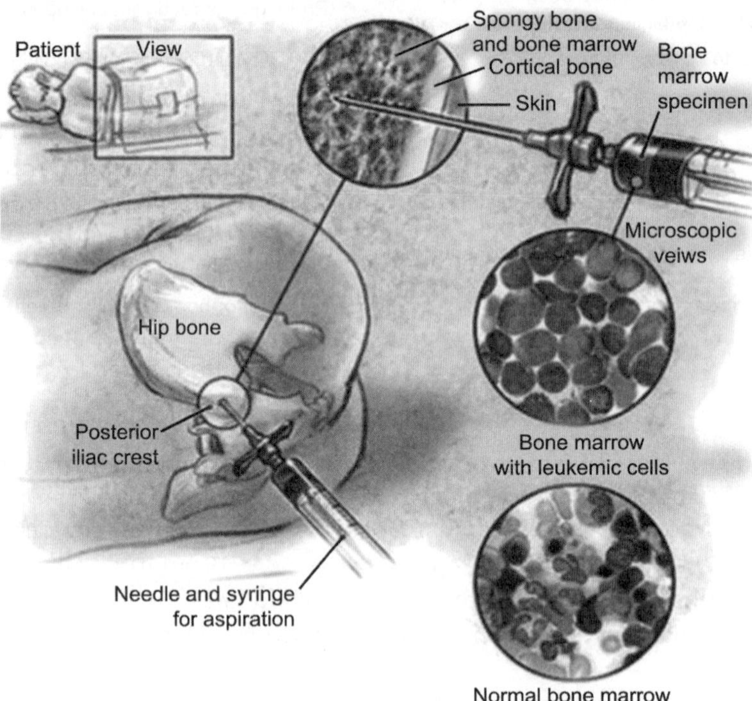

Fig. 7.85: Bone marrow aspiration and biopsy

Initial Tests

- Blood tests to measure the number of blood cells and see how they appear.
- Bone marrow aspiration and biopsy

  It is usually taken from the pelvic bone, to confirm a diagnosis of leukemia.
- Lumbar puncture, or spinal tap, to check for spread of leukemia cells in the fluid that bathes the brain and spinal cord.

A pathologist examines cells from the blood tests under a microscope. This specialist also checks bone marrow samples for the number of blood-forming cells and fat cells. Other tests may be done to help determine which type of leukemia your child may have. These tests also help the doctors know how likely the leukemia is to respond to treatment.

Management

Chemotherapy can reduce it by 3 to 5 logs. Hence, the patient still has 10 leukemic cells when the marrow examination shows complete remission. To achieve long-term cure, the patient therefore needs further treatment. The initial high dose chemotherapy given to reduce the leukemic cells below the level of morphological detection is called induction. This is followed by another course of chemotherapy meant to further attenuate the leukemic burden-consolidation or early intensification. Low dose oral therapy given for eighteen months to 2 years is called maintenance therapy. High dose therapy given more than six months after induction is termed as late intensification.

Chemotherapy

Acute Lymphoblastic Leukemia (ALL)

Combination chemotherapy remains the primary therapeutic modality with evolving indications for limited radiation therapy. Current treatment for ALL is divided into four phases:

- *Remission induction* although prednisolone and vincristine are capable of producing remission in approximately 80 percent patients, it is now clear that it is inadequate. The addition of a third agent, either Lasparaginase or daunorubicin, raises the induction rate to 90 percent and significantly prolongs remission. The addition of a fourth induction agent usually the anthracycline, improves remission duration even in patients with poor risk features.
- *Central nervous system prophylaxis* the concept of CNS prevention therapy is based on the assumption that undetectable CNS leukemia is present at the time of diagnosis. In high-risk patients cranial irradiation and intrathecal methotrexate prevent CNS relapse. However, long-term ALL survivors have adverse effects of CNS irradiation on neurological and intellectual functions. The combination of intrathecal and moderate dose of intravenous methotrexate, maintenance triple intrathecal therapy (methotrexate, cytarabine and hydrocortisone) and high-dose methotrexate alone appear to provide equivalent protection to that offered by cranial irradiation,
- *Consolidation* the cranial prophylaxis is followed by another dose of chemotherapy meant to decrease the leukemic burden to the minimum. The drugs used for consolidation are a combination of drugs used for induction and maintenance therapy.
- *Maintenance* methotrexate and 6-mercaptopurine are the two drugs most frequently administered. This therapy is continued for 2 years in order to eradicate the dormant leukemic cells. The dosage of these drugs should be adjusted to maintain the total leukocyte count between 1000–3000/cmm.

Acute Myeloid Leukemia (AML)

Induction therapy is the mainstay of the treatment. It consists of a combination of cytarabine (100 to 200 mg/m^2/day for 7 days) and an anthracycline (dauno-mycin 30 mg/m^2/day for three days). The addition of a third agent (thioguanine or epipodophyllotoxin) may add to the result. The overall complete remission rate is 85 percent after a single course of therapy. About 5 percent are currently refractory to therapy and 5 percent succumb to infection and hemorrhage during remission induction.

- Intensive treatment with high-dose cytarabine containing combinations
- Myeloablative therapy followed by allogenic or autologous BMT. Allogenic BMT offers the best antileukemic activity thus far. The application of modern immunotherapy in

the course of treatment may be beneficial in the near future. The five year survival with chemotherapy alone is 15 to 20 percent.

Chemotherapy alone is able to prolong survival without achieving cure in a majority of the patients with AML. Allogenic BMT provides cure for up to 50 percent for AML patients treated with this modality.

Prognosis

Survival in ALL has improved from 1 percent in 1965 to 50 percent in mid 70's and up to 70 percent in mid 80's. A variety of prognostic factors have been identified in acute leukemia. Total WBC count at presentation and age are the most important ones. Patients with high WBC count (> 20,000) and age (< 3 or > 10 years) do poorly.

Complications

Early Complication

These may cause a life-threatening leukemia:

- Neutropenia-overwhelming sepsis (usually Gram-negative) +/- disseminated intravascular coagulation
- Thrombocytopenia—bleeding, pulmonary or gastrointestinal (GI) hemorrhage, stroke
- Electrolyte imbalance—hyperkalemia and hyperphosphatemia (due to blast cell lysis)
- Acute kidney injury (secondary to hyperuricemia)
- Acute airway obstruction (secondary to mediastinal thymic mass)
- Leukostasis—stroke, acute pulmonary edema, heart failure
- CNS involvement—stroke, seizures.

During Treatment (Complication)

- Tumor-lysis syndrome
- Renal or hepatic impairment
- Profound immunosuppression leading to sepsis (febrile Neutropenia)
- Thromboembolism
- Alopecia
- Mucositis causing severe mouth pain
- Hyperemesis
- GI erosion/bleeding.

Late Complication

- Growth hormone deficiency and short stature (where cranial irradiation has been applied)
- Neurological problems including headache, motor, coordination and cognitive impairment, seizures (again following cranial irradiation)
- Peripheral neuropathy (due to vincristine)
- Obesity
- Congestive cardiac failure (due to toxicity of some chemotherapeutic agents, e.g. doxorubicin)

- Cognitive impairment
- Infertility
- Psychosocial impairment
- Second malignancy.

Nursing Management

Nurses will care for child during treatment:

- Check child to make sure he is comfortable
- Using the soft bendable tube in child's chest, called the central line, to give medicines or to withdraw blood
- Giving chemotherapy medicines to treat child's cancer
- Giving any other care child may need while he is being treated
- Health Teaching will helping child and family
- Talking with child's health care team.

NEUROLOGICAL SYSTEM

MENINGITIS

Introduction

Meningitis is an inflammation of the meninges, the membranes that cover the brain and spinal cord. Most cases are caused by bacteria or viruses, but some can be due to certain medications or illnesses.

Definition

Meningitis is an inflammation of the lining around the brain and spinal cord caused by bacteria or viruses. Meningitis is classified as septic or aseptic. The aseptic form may be viral or secondary to lymphoma, leukemia, or human immunodeficiency virus (HIV). The septic form is caused by bacteria, such as *Streptococcus pneumoniae* and *Neisseria meningitidis*.

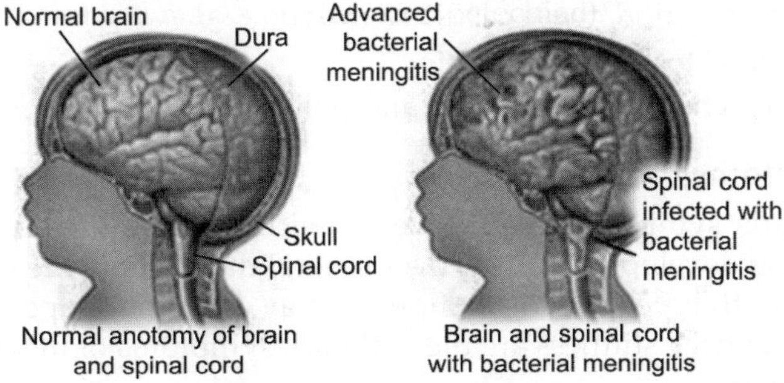

Fig. 7.86: Anatomical difference between normal and meningitis brain

Meningitis is inflammation of the protective membranes covering the brain and spinal cord, known collectively as the meninges. The inflammation may be caused by infection with viruses, bacteria, or other microorganisms and less commonly by certain drugs. Meningitis can be life-threatening because of the inflammation's proximity to the brain and spinal cord; therefore the condition is classified as a medical emergency.

Incidence

In a recent survey by the Hib and Pneumococcal Working Group, the incidence of meningitis in 2000 varied from regions across the world. The overall incidence of pneumococcal meningitis was 17 cases per 100,000, with the highest incidence in Africa at 38 cases per 100,000 and the lowest incidence in Europe at 6 cases per 100,000. The overall death rate was 10 cases per 100,000.

Types

- Bacterial meningitis
- Tuberculosis meningitis
- Aseptic meningitis
- Viral meningitis
- Parasitic meningitis
- Non-infectious meningitis.

Causes

Bacterial and Viral

The types of bacteria can cause bacterial meningitis.

In newborns the most common causes are:

- Group B streptococcus
- Escherichia coli
- Listeria monocytogenes.

In older kids

- Streptococcus pneumoniae (Pneumococcus)
- Neisseria meningitidis (meningococcus) are more often the causes.
- Haemophilus influenza type b (Hib), also can cause the illness but because of widespread childhood immunization, these cases are rarer.

The viruses can lead to viral meningitis

- Enteroviruses (such as coxsackievirus and poliovirus) and the herpesvirus.

Signs and Symptoms

Bacterial meningitis symptoms may develop within hours or days. Viral meningitis symptoms may also develop quickly or over several days. There are more common signs and symptoms of both types. Not all symptoms may appear or appear in the same order. Fever, headache and neck stiffness are the hallmark symptoms of meningitis.

- High-grade fever
- Severe and persistent headache
- Neck stiffness and pain that makes it difficult to touch your chin to your chest
- Nausea and vomiting
- Confusion and disorientation (acting 'goofy')

- Drowsiness or sluggishness
- photophobia (eye sensitivity to light)
- Poor appetite
- More severe symptoms include seizure and coma.

The warning sign	
Early symptoms Develop within 8 hours of infection	(See the rash test, right)
• Cold hands/feet	• Sensitivity to light
• Leg pain	• Severe headache
• Unusually pale or mottled skin	• Fever
Classic signs Take 13–22 hours to develop	• Stiff neck and joints
• Purple rash	• Drowsiness or coma

Other Potential Signs and Symptoms of Meningococcal Disease

These are additional signs and symptoms of meningococcal infection that has entered the bloodstream:

- Abnormal skin color
- Stomach cramps
- Ice-cold hands and feet
- Skin rash
- Muscle ache or joint pain
- Rapid breathing
- Chills.

Pathophysiology

Brain surrounded by pus (the yellow-greyish coat around the brain, under the dura lifted by the forceps), the result of bacterial meningitis. A brain autopsy demonstrating signs of meningitis. The forceps (center) are retracting the dura mater (white). Underneath the dura mater are the leptomeninges, which appear to be edematous and have multiple small hemorrhagic foci (red).

The causative organism enters the bloodstream, crosses the blood–brain barrier and triggers an inflammatory reaction in the meninges. Independent of the causative agent, inflammation of the subarachnoid and pia mater occurs. Increased intracranial pressure (ICP) results.

Meningeal infections generally originate in one of two ways: Either through the bloodstream from other infections (cellulitis) or by direct extension (after a traumatic injury to the facial bones).

Bacterial or meningococcal meningitis also occurs as an opportunistic infection in patients with acquired immunodeficiency syndrome (AIDS) and as a complication of Lyme disease. Bacterial meningitis is the most significant form. The common bacterial pathogens are

N. meningitidis (meningococcal meningitis) and *S. pneumoniae*, accounting for 80% of cases of meningitis in adults. *Haemophilus influenzae* was once a common cause of meningitis in children, but, because of vaccination, infection with this organism is now rare in developed countries.

Diagnostic Evaluation

- Physical examination to look for symptoms of meningitis
- A blood test to check for bacteria or viruses
- A lumbar puncture where a sample of fluid is taken from the spine and checked for bacteria or viruses
- A computerized tomography (CT) scan to check for any problems with the brain, such as swelling
- CSF Analysis.

Table 7.13: CSF findings in different forms of meningitis

Type of meningitis	Glucose	Protein	Cells
Acute bacterial	Low	High	PMNs, often > 300/mm^3
Acute viral	Normal	Normal or high	Mononuclear, < 300/mm^3
Tuberculosis	Low	High	Mononuclear and PMNs, < 300/mm^3
Fungal	Low	High	< 300/mm^3
Malignant	Low	High	Usually mononuclear

Lumbar Puncture

A lumbar puncture is done by positioning the patient, usually lying on the side, applying local anesthetic and inserting a needle into the dural sac (a sac around the spinal cord) to collect cerebrospinal fluid (CSF). When this has been achieved, the 'opening pressure' of the CSF is measured using a manometer. The pressure is normally between 6 and 18 cm water (H_2O) in bacterial meningitis the pressure is typically elevated. The initial appearance

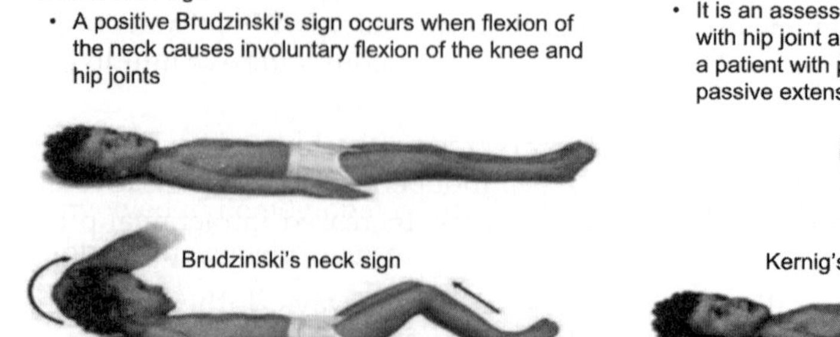

Fig. 7.87: Physical assessment of Brudzinski's signs and Kernig's signs

of the fluid may prove an indication of the nature of the infection: Cloudy CSF indicates higher levels of protein, white and red blood cells and bacteria and therefore may suggest bacterial meningitis.

A Blood Culture

A sample of blood is cultured in the laboratory to determine if there are bacteria present (normally, no bacteria should be present in the blood). The results of the blood culture can also help determine which antibiotic is best. The results of a blood culture are generally not available for 48 to 72 hours.

Management

The treatment for meningitis depends upon whether the meningitis is caused by a virus or a bacterium. However, this distinction may not be clear until the culture results are available (usually 48 to 72 hours after they are obtained). In many cases, children are treated as if they have bacterial meningitis until bacterial meningitis is definitively excluded. The reason for this is that there is a significant risk of serious illness or even death if the child has bacterial meningitis and treatment is delayed for a prolonged period of time.

Bacterial Meningitis

Bacterial meningitis is a life-threatening illness that requires hospitalization and treatment with intravenous antibiotics. The child will be monitored closely for signs of complications. Depending upon the severity of the illness, the child may also need supportive treatments to aid breathing, maintain blood pressure, prevent excessive bleeding and keep the child hydrated.

Antibiotics Therapy

Treatment with antibiotics is usually started immediately after the blood tests and lumbar puncture are performed. Treatment is administered intravenously. Oral antibiotics are not recommended. The concentration of antibiotics necessary to treat bacterial meningitis cannot be achieved with oral administration. Bacterial meningitis and septicemia are treated with antibiotics intravenously (through a vein in the arm).

Length of Treatment

The length of antibiotic treatment depends upon the results of the bacterial cultures.

- If the cultures are negative and the child has improved, antibiotics may be discontinued after 48 to 72 hours.
- If the cultures are positive, the length of treatment depends upon the bacteria that is identified and whether there are complications. The treatment course may range from several days to several weeks.

Corticosteroid Drugs: Such as dexamethasone, may also be used to reduce inflammation in the brain.

Viral Meningitis

In most cases, there is no medication that can eliminate the virus causing viral meningitis. Instead, treatment is supportive, meaning that it is given to support the child while he or she recovers. This generally includes rest, encouraging the child to drink an adequate amount of fluid (when alert enough to do so), providing intravenous fluids (if unable to drink enough fluid) and medications to treat fever and/or headache (e.g. acetaminophen or ibuprofen).

Nursing Management

Nursing Diagnosis

The following are possible nursing diagnosis for patients with bacterial meningitis:

- Risk for infection transmission related to contagious nature of organism
- Acute pain related to headache, fever, neck pain secondary to meningeal irritaiton
- Acute pain related to nuchal rigidity, muscle aches, immobility and increased sensitivity to external stimuli secondary to infectious process
- Impaired physical mobility related to intravenous infusion, nuchal rigidity and restraining devices
- Activity intolerance related to fatigue and malaise secondary to infection
- Risk for impaired skin integrity related to immobility, dehydration and diaphoresis
- Risk for injury related to restlessness and disorientation secondary to meningeal irritation
- Interrupted family process related to critical nature of situation and uncertain prognosis
- Anxiety related to treatment and risk of death
- Risk for ineffective therapeutic regimen management.

Nursing Intervention

Related nursing interventions include the following:

- Assess neurologic status and vital signs constantly. Determine oxygenation from arterial blood gas values and pulse oximetry.
- Insert cuffed endotracheal tube (or tracheostomy) and POSI-position patient on mechanical ventilation as prescribed.
- Assess blood pressure (usually monitored using an arterial line) for incipient shock, which precedes cardiac or respiratory failure.
- Rapid IV fluid replacement may be prescribed, but take care not to overhydrate patient because of risk of cerebral edema.
- Reduce high fever to decrease load on heart and brain from oxygen demands.
- Protect the patient from injury secondary to seizure activity or altered level of consciousness (LOC).
- Monitor daily body weight; serum electrolytes; and urine volume, specific gravity and osmolality, especially if syndrome of inappropriate antidiuretic hormone (SIADH) is suspected.
- Prevent complications associated with immobility, such as pressure ulcers and pneumonia.
- Institute infection control precautions until 24 hours after initiation of antibiotic therapy (oral and nasal discharge is considered infectious).
- Inform family about patient's condition and permit family to see patient at appropriate intervals.

Prevention

Several measures can help to reduce the risk of developing bacterial and viral meningitis.

Vaccines

Several routine childhood vaccines reduce the risk of developing bacterial meningitis, including the pneumococcal, meningococcal and Haemophilus influenzae type b (Hib) vaccines. These are discussed in detail separately. Vaccines are also available to prevent certain types of viral infections that may cause meningitis or other central nervous system infections, including polio, influenza, varicella, measles and mumps.

Preventive Antibiotics

Preventive antibiotics are recommended for close contacts of anyone infected with meningococcal infection, even if the contact was previously vaccinated. Close contact is defined as a person who lives with the child or who spent ≥4 hours with the child for at least five of the seven days before the child developed symptoms.

Preventive antibiotics may also be necessary for close contacts of anyone infected with Hib bacterial infection. However, this only applies for those households in which there is a person with invasive Hib disease and at least one household member who is a child younger than 48 months of age and did not receive all of the vaccinations against Hib or an individual who has a weakened immune system (even if that person was vaccinated against Hib).

Infection Control

Families of children with meningitis should take care to avoid becoming infected. This includes washing hands after touching the child or changing diapers and before eating or preparing food. Utensils and cups should not be shared, the child's mouth should be covered during a cough and the child should not be kissed on the mouth. These measures should be continued until the child no longer has symptoms (e.g. fever, diarrhea, rash).

Prognosis

A child's prognosis after an episode of meningitis depends upon the cause (type of bacterium or virus), the severity of the illness and the age of the child.

Bacterial Meningitis

A majority of children with bacterial meningitis recover completely with no long-term complications. The child should begin to improve within 24 to 36 hours after starting antibiotics. However, fever may persist for four to six days or longer.

- Meningitis can damage the brain and cause long-term complications, including deafness, developmental delay or learning disabilities, spastic or paralyzed muscles and seizures.
- To determine if a child's hearing was affected by the illness, hearing testing is usually performed around the time of discharge from the hospital. Young children should also be monitored closely for signs of developmental delay (e.g. not walking, talking, etc. at expected time).
- Bacterial meningitis is fatal in a small number of cases; between 2001 and 2006, approximately 4 percent of children in the United States with bacterial meningitis died.

Viral Meningitis

Most children with viral meningitis recover with no long-term complications. Symptoms usually begin to improve within one week, although some children will have fatigue, irritability, decreased concentration, muscle weakness and spasm and difficulty with coordination for several weeks or more. Death is uncommon in children with viral meningitis.

ENCEPHALITIS

Introduction

Encephalitis is an uncommon but potentially devastating neurological syndrome with different etiologies including direct central nervous system infection with different agents (most commonly viral) and those mediated by the immune system. Whilst there have been several recent publications and guidelines on the management of bacterial central nervous system infections in adults and children, viral infections have been relatively neglected whereas acute encephalitis is most commonly a viral infection with parenchymal damage varying from mild to profound.

Definition

Encephalitis, an inflammation of the brain parenchyma, presents as diffuse and/or focal neuropsychological dysfunction. From an epidemiologic and pathophysiologic perspective, encephalitis is distinct from meningitis, though on clinical evaluation with signs and symptoms of meningeal inflammation, such as photophobia, headache, or a stiff neck.

Encephalitis is a term used to describe inflammation of the brain. The inflammation causes the brain to swell, which leads to changes in the child's neurological condition, including mental confusion, changes in mental status (sometimes even coma) and seizures.

Incidences

Encephalitis literally means an inflammation of the brain, but it usually refers to brain inflammation caused by a virus. It is a rare disease that occurs in approximately 0.5 per 100,000 individuals most commonly in children, the elderly and people with weakened immune systems (e.g. those with HIV/AIDS or cancer).

Although several thousand cases of encephalitis (also called acute viral encephalitis or aseptic encephalitis) are reported to the Centers for Disease Control and Prevention (CDC) every year, experts suspect that many more may go unreported because the symptoms are so mild.

Causes

- The etiology of encephalitis is usually infectious, but may be noninfectious, such as the demyelinating process in acute disseminated encephalitis.
- *Infectious etiologies:* Viral agents, such as HSV type 1 and 2 (almost exclusively in neonates), measles virus, mumps and rubella are spread through person-to-person contact. Human herpesvirus 6 may also be a causative agent.
  - Important animal vectors include mosquitoes, ticks (arbovirus) and warm-blooded mammals (rabies, lymphocytic choriomeningitis).

- Bacterial pathogens, such as *Mycoplasma* species and those causing rickettsial or catscratch disease, are rare and invariably involve inflammation of the meninges out of proportion to their encephalitic components.
- Encephalitis due to parasites and fungi other than *Toxoplasma gondii* is beyond the scope of this article.

- The CDC confirmed that West Nile virus can be transmitted by means of an organ transplant and via blood transfusions.

Signs and Symptoms

Symptoms in milder cases of encephalitis usually include:

- Hyperthermia
- Headache
- Poor appetite
- Loss of energy
- A general sick feeling
- Fatigue or weakness.

Symptoms that relate to the central nervous system including:

- Severe headache
- Nausea and vomiting
- Stiff neck
- Confusion
- Disorientation
- Personality changes
- Convulsions (seizures)
- Problems with speech or hearing
- Hallucinations
- Memory loss
- Drowsiness
- Coma.

Signs and symptoms in infants and young children may also include:

- Bulging in the soft spots (fontanels) of the skull in infants
- Nausea and vomiting
- Body stiffness
- Inconsolable crying
- Poor feeding or not waking for a feeding
- Irritability.

Pathophysiology

Portals of entry are virus specific. Many viruses are transmitted by humans, although most cases of HSE are thought to be reactivation of the herpes simplex virus (HSV) lying dormant in the trigeminal ganglia. Mosquitoes or ticks inoculate arbovirus and rabies virus is transferred via animal bite. With some viruses, such as varicella-zoster virus (VZV) and cytomegalovirus (CMV), an immunocompromised host is a key risk factor.

In general, the virus replicates outside the CNS and gains entry either by hematogenous spread or by traveling along neural (rabies, HSV, VZV) and olfactory (HSV) pathways. The etiology of slow virus infections, such as those implicated in the measles-related subacute sclerosing panencephalitis (SSPE) and progressive multifocal leukoencephalopathy (PML), is poorly understood.

Once across the blood-brain barrier, the virus enters neural cells, with resultant disruption in cell functioning, perivascular congestion, hemorrhage and inflammatory response diffusely affecting gray matter disproportionately to white matter. Focal pathology is the result of neuron cell membrane receptors found only in specific portions of the brain and accounts for regional tropism found with some viruses. For example, HSV has a predilection for the inferior and medial temporal lobes.

Although most histologic features are nonspecific, brain biopsies are the diagnostic criterion standard for rabies. Presence of Negri bodies in the hippocampus and cerebellum are pathognomonic of rabies, as are HSV Cowdry type A inclusions with hemorrhagic necrosis in the temporal and orbitofrontal lobes.

In contrast to viruses that invade gray matter directly, acute disseminated encephalitis and postinfectious encephalomyelitis (PIE), secondary to measles (most common), Epstein-Barr virus (EBV) and CMV, are immune-mediated processes, which result in multifocal demyelination of perivenous white matter.

Diagnostic Evaluation

Physical Examination

- The signs of encephalitis may be diffuse or focal (80% of patients with HSE present with focal findings) as follows:
  - Altered mental status and/or personality changes (most common)
  - Focal findings, such as hemiparesis, focal seizures and autonomic dysfunction
  - Movement disorders (St Louis encephalitis)
  - Ataxia
  - Cranial nerve defects
  - Dysphagia (Rabies may account for foaming at the mouth and hydrophobia.)
  - Meningismus (less common and less pronounced than in meningitis)
  - Unilateral sensorimotor dysfunction (PIE)
- HSV infection in the neonate (aged 1–45 days)
  - Herpetic skin lesions over the presenting surface from birth or with breaks in the skin, such as those resulting from fetal scalp monitors
  - Keratoconjunctivitis
  - Oropharyngeal involvement, particularly buccal mucosa and tongue
  - Encephalitis symptoms, such as seizures, irritability, change in level of attentiveness, bulging fontanels
  - Additional signs of disseminated HSV, such as shock, jaundice and hepatomegaly
- Toxoplasma encephalopathy: In immunosuppressed patients, 75% present with a focal neuropathology, about one half with encephalopathic changes.

Laboratory Studies

- *Complete blood count (CBC) with differential:* Findings are usually within the reference range.
- *Serum electrolytes:* These are usually within the reference range. Syndrome of inappropriate secretion of antidiuretic hormone (SIADH) occurs in 25% of patients with St Louis encephalitis.)
- *Serum glucose level:* Use this level as a baseline for determining normal CSF glucose values. The result may be low if glycogen stores are depleted or high in infected patients with diabetes mellitus.
- *BUN/creatinine and liver function tests (LFTs):* Assess organ function and the need to adjust the antibiotic dose.
- *Platelet test and a coagulation profile:* These are indicated in patients with chronic alcohol use, liver disease, or if disseminated intravascular coagulation (DIC) is suspected. The patient may require platelets or fresh-frozen plasma (FFP) before lumbar puncture (LP).
- *Urinary electrolyte test:* Perform this assessment if SIADH is suspected.
- *Urine and/or serum toxicology screening:* Perform 1 or both of these tests, if indicated.

Imaging Studies

- Perform head CT, with and without contrast agent, in virtually all patients with encephalitis before LP to search for evidence of elevated intracerebral pressure (ICP), obstructive hydrocephalus, or mass effect. It is helpful also in differential diagnosis. MRI is more likely to show abnormalities earlier in disease course than head CT.
- In HSE, an MRI may show several foci of increased T2 signal intensity in medial temporal lobes and inferior frontal gray matter. Head CT may show petechial hemorrhage in the same areas.
- EEE and tick-borne encephalitis may show similar increased signal intensity in the basal ganglia and thalami.
- In toxoplasmosis, contrast-enhanced head CT typically reveals several nodular or ring-enhancing lesions. Because lesions may be missed without contrast, MRI should be performed in patients for whom use of contrast material is contraindicated.

Management

Prehospital Care

Evaluate and treat for shock or hypotension. Administer a crystalloid infusion until the patient is euvolemic. Consider airway protection in patients with an altered mental status. Consider seizure precautions. Treat seizures according to usual protocol (i.e. lorazepam 0.1 mg/kg given intravenously [IV]). Stabilize alert patients with normal vital signs by administering oxygen, securing IV access and providing rapid transport to the hospital.

Emergency Department Care

The important exceptions of HSE and varicella-zoster encephalitis, the viral encephalitides are not treatable beyond supportive care. Treatments for *T. gondii* and CMV encephalitis are available but generally not initiated in the ED.

- The goal of treatment for acutely ill patients is administration of the first dose or doses acyclovir with or without antibiotics or steroids as quickly as possible.
  - The standard for acute bacterial meningitis is the initiation of treatment within 30 minutes of arrival.
  - Consider instituting an emergency triage protocol to identify patients at risk for HSE.
- Collect laboratory samples and blood cultures before the start of IV therapy. Even in uncomplicated cases of encephalitis, most authorities recommend a neuroimaging study (e.g. MRI or, if not available, a contrast-enhanced head CT scan) before LP.
- Signs of hydrocephalus and increased ICP
  - General measures: Manage fever and pain, control straining and coughing and avoid seizures and systemic hypotension.
  - In otherwise stable patients, elevating the head and monitoring neurologic status usually are sufficient.
  - When more aggressive maneuvers are indicated, some authorities favor the early use of diuresis (e.g. furosemide 20 mg IV, mannitol 1 g/kg IV) provided circulatory volume is protected. Dexamethasone 10 mg IV q6h helps in managing edema surrounding space-occupying lesions. Hyperventilation ($PaCO_2$ 30 mm Hg) may cause a disproportional decrease in cerebral blood flow (CBF), but it is used to control increasing ICP on an emergency basis.
  - Intraventricular ICP monitoring is controversial because some authorities believe dangerous focal edema with a pressure gradient between the temporal lobe and the subtentorial space usually is not detected by the monitor, leading to a false sense of security. In fact, monitor placement may potentially aggravate a pressure gradient.
- Look for and treat systemic complications, particularly in HSE and JE, such as hypotension or shock, hypoxemia, hyponatremia (SIADH) and exacerbation of chronic diseases.
- Empiric adult emergency treatment for HSV meningoencephalitis and VZV encephalitis is acyclovir 10 mg/kg (infuse over 1 h) q8h for 14–21 days. Give acyclovir 10–15 mg/kg IV q8h for neonatal HSV; for HSV encephalitis in the pediatric population, give acyclovir 10 mg/kg IV q8h.
- In HIV-positive patients, consider foscarnet, given increased incidence of acyclovir-resistant HSV and HZV.

Follow-up Therapy

This therapy may include:

- *Physical therapy* to improve strength, flexibility, balance, motor coordination and mobility
- *Occupational therapy* to develop everyday skills and to use adaptive products that help with everyday activities
- *Speech therapy* to relearn muscle control and coordination to produce speech
- *Psychotherapy* to learn coping strategies and new behavioral skills to improve mood disorders or address personality changes with medication management if necessary.

Preventive Measures

Encephalitis can not be prevented, but you can try to avoid the illnesses that may lead to it. Many common childhood illnesses are largely preventable through immunization, so follow the immunization schedule recommended by your child's doctor. Kids should also avoid contact with anyone who already has encephalitis.

In areas where encephalitis can be transmitted by insect bites, especially mosquitoes, child should:

- Avoid being outside at dawn and dusk (when mosquitoes are most active).
- Wear protective clothing like long sleeves and long pants.
- Use insect repellent.
- Waste and stagnated water around your home should be drained, including buckets, birdbaths, flowerpots and tire swings because these are breeding grounds for mosquitoes.

To Avoid Tick Bites

- Limit the children to contact with soil, leaves and vegetation.
- Shoul offer the long-sleeved, light-colored shirts and long pants when outdoors.
- Check your kids and your pets frequently for ticks.

Prognosis

The prognosis depends the virulence of the virus and on variables associated with the patient's health status, such as extremes of age, immune status and preexisting neurologic conditions.

- Rabies, EEE, JE and untreated HSE have high rates of mortality and severe morbidity, including mental retardation, hemiplegia and seizures.
- Increased mortality and morbidity rates are found in patients who are older than 60 years and have St Louis encephalitis or West Nile encephalitis (WNE). Long-term sequelae with St Louis encephalitis include behavioral disorders, memory loss and seizures.
- WEE is associated with relatively low mortality and morbidity rates, although developmental delay, seizure disorder and paralysis occur in children and postencephalitic parkinsonism occurs in adults.
- CE usually is a milder disease, with most patients making a full recovery, though 25% of those with severe disease continue to have focal neurologic dysfunction.

The mortality rate in treated HSE averages 20% and is correlated with mental status changes at time of first dose of acyclovir. Approximately 40% of survivors have minor-to-major learning disabilities, memory impairment, neuropsychiatric abnormalities, epilepsy, fine-motor-control deficits and dysarthria.

CONVULSIVE DISORDERS

Convulsion/Seizures

Introduction

A *convulsion* is a medical condition where body muscles contract and relax rapidly and repeatedly, resulting in an uncontrolled shaking of the body. Because a convulsion is often a symptom of an epileptical seizure, the term convulsion is sometimes used as a synonym for seizure. However, not all epileptic seizures lead to convulsions and not all convulsions are caused by epileptic seizures. Convulsions are also consistent with an electric shock. For non-epileptic convulsions, see non-epileptic seizures.

Convulsions may also be referred to as 'fits' in some instances.

Definition of Convulsions

Convulsions are when a person's body shakes rapidly and uncontrollably. During convulsions, the person's muscles contract and relax repeatedly. The term 'convulsion' is often used interchangeably with 'seizure,' although there are many types of seizures, some of which have subtle or mild symptoms instead of convulsions. Seizures of all types are caused by disorganized and sudden electrical activity in the brain.

Types

- Epilepsy
- Fever (febrile) convulsions in children

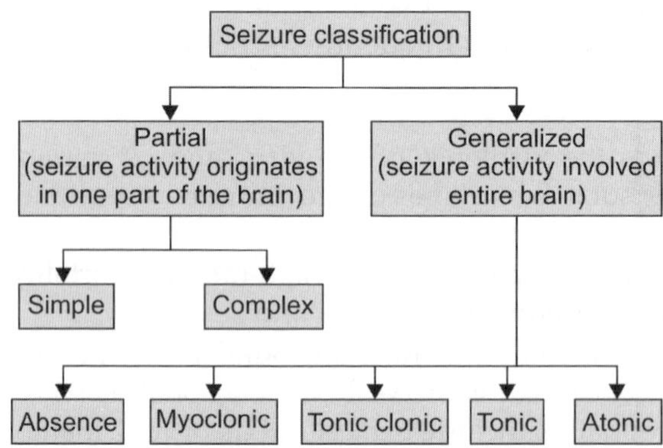

Fig. 7.88: Types of seizures

- Generalized tonic clonic seizure
- Partial (focal) seizure
- Petit mal (absence) seizure
- Seizure.

Generalized Tonic Clonic Seizure

Definition of Generalized Tonic Clonic Seizure

A generalized tonic clonic seizure is a seizure involving the entire body. It is also called a grand mal seizure. Such seizures usually involve muscle rigidity, violent muscle contractions and loss of consciousness. Generalized tonic clonic seizures are the type of seizure that most people associate with the term 'seizure,' convulsion, or epilepsy. They may occur in people of any age, as a single episode, or as part of a repeated, chronic condition (epilepsy).

Definition of Partial (Focal) Seizure

All seizures are caused by abnormal electrical disturbances in the brain. Partial (focal) seizures occur when this electrical activity remains in a limited area of the brain. The seizures may sometimes turn into generalized seizures, which affect the whole brain. This is called secondary generalization.

Partial seizures can be further characterized as:

- Simple—not affecting awareness or memory
- Complex—affecting awareness or memory of events before, during and immediately after the seizure and affecting behavior.

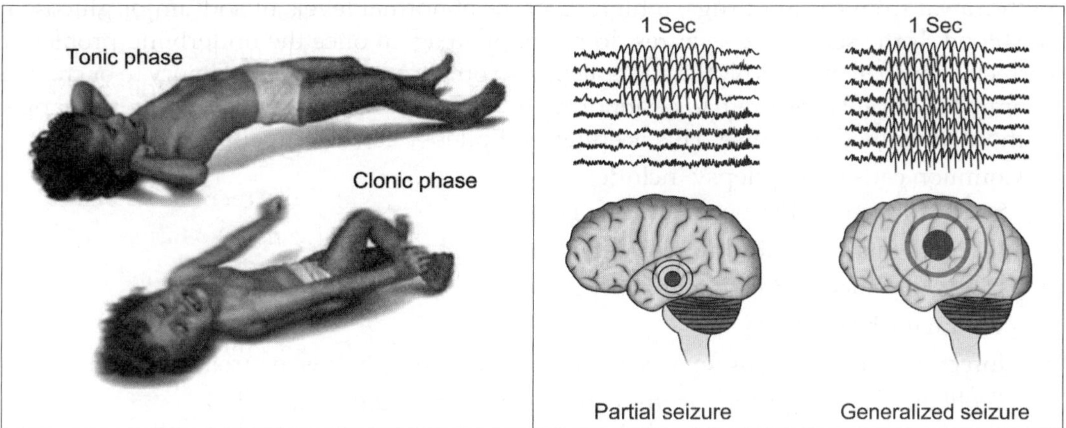

Fig. 7.89: Tonic, clonic seizure and partial, generalized seizure

Grand Mal Seizure

A febrile seizure is a generalized tonic clonic (grand mal) seizure that occurs in some children as a response to a fever. Febrile seizures are usually associated with rapidly rising fevers and usually occur early in the fever rather than later.

EPILEPSY

Introduction

The vagus nerves branch of the brain on either side of the head and travel down the neck, along the esophagus to the intestinal tract. They are the longest nerves in the body and affect swallowing and speech. The vagus nerves also connect to parts of the brain involved in seizures. In many seizure disorders, electrical stimulation of the vagus nerves may afford relief of symptoms.

Definition of Epilepsy

Epilepsy is a brain disorder involving repeated, spontaneous seizures of any type. Seizures ('fits,' convulsions) are episodes of disturbed brain function that cause changes in attention or behavior. They are caused by abnormally excited electrical signals in the brain.

Incidence

Epilepsy may be idiopathic, which means the cause cannot be identified. These seizures usually begin between ages 5 and 20, but they can happen at any age. People with this condition have no other neurological problems, but sometimes have a family history of seizures or epilepsy.

Causes and Risk Factors

Seizures ('fits,' convulsions) are episodes of disturbed brain function that cause changes in attention or behavior. They are caused by abnormally excited electrical signals in the brain.

Sometimes a seizure is related to a temporary condition, such as exposure to drugs, withdrawal from certain drugs, a high fever, or abnormal levels of sodium or glucose in the blood. If the seizure or seizures do not happen again once the underlying problem is corrected, the person does NOT have epilepsy. In other cases, permanent injury to or changes in brain tissue cause the brain to be abnormally excitable. In these cases, the seizures happen without an immediate cause. This is epilepsy. Epilepsy can affect people of any age.

Common causes of epilepsy include:

- Stroke or transient ischemic attack (TIA)
- Illnesses that cause the brain to deteriorate
- Dementia, such as Alzheimer's disease
- Traumatic brain injury
- Infections (including brain abscess, meningitis, encephalitis, neurosyphilis and AIDS)
- Problems that are present from before birth (congenital brain defects)
- Injuries near the time of birth (in this case, seizures usually begin in infancy or early childhood)
- Kidney failure or liver failure
- Metabolic diseases that children may be born with (such as phenylketonuria)
- Tumors or other structural brain lesions (such as hematomas or abnormal blood vessels).

Signs and Symptoms

The severity of symptoms can vary greatly, from simple staring spells to loss of consciousness and violent convulsions. For most people with epilepsy, each seizure is similar to previous ones. The type of seizure a person has depends on a variety of things, such as the part of the brain affected and the underlying cause of the seizure.

An aura consisting of a strange sensation (such as tingling, smelling an odor that is not actually there, or emotional changes) occurs in some people prior to each seizure.

A detailed description of the symptoms associated with a specific type of seizure:

- Absence (petit mal) seizure
- Generalized tonic clonic (grand mal) seizure
- Partial (focal) seizure.

Diagnostic Evaluation

A physical examination (including a detailed neurologic examination) may be normal, or it may show abnormal brain function related to specific areas of the brain. Persons with epilepsy will often have abnormal electrical activity seen on an electroencephalograph (EEG). An EEG is a reading of the electrical activity in the brain. In some cases, the test may show where in the brain the seizures start. EEGs can often be normal in between seizures, so it may be necessary to perform a longer test.

Various blood tests and other tests to rule out temporary and reversible causes of seizures, may include:

- Blood chemistry
- Blood sugar
- CBC (complete blood count)
- CSF (cerebrospinal fluid) analysis
- Kidney function tests
- Liver function tests
- Tests for infectious diseases.

Tests for the cause and location of the problem may include:

- EEG
- Head CT or MRI scan
- Lumbar puncture (spinal tap).

Management

Treatment of seizures, an underlying cause for recurrent seizures (such as infection) has been identified and treated, seizures may stop. Treatment may include surgery to remove a tumor, an abnormal or bleeding blood vessel, or other brain problems.

Medication to prevent seizures, called anticonvulsants, may reduce the number of future seizures. These drugs are taken by mouth.

- The type of medicine you take depends on what type of seizures you are having. The dosage may need to be adjusted from time to time.
- Some seizure types respond well to one medication and may respond poorly (or even be made worse) by others. Some medications need to be monitored for side effects and blood levels.
- It is very important that you take your medication on time and at the correct dose. Most people taking these drugs need regular checkups and regular blood tests to make sure they are receiving the correct dosage.
- You should not stop taking or change medications without talking to your doctor first.

The factors increase the risk for a seizure in a person with epilepsy.

- Certain prescribed medications
- Emotional stress
- Illness, especially infection
- Lack of sleep
- Pregnancy
- Skipping doses of epilepsy medications
- Use of alcohol or other recreational drugs.

Epilepsy that does not get better after two or three seizure drugs have been tried is called 'medically refractory epilepsy.'

- Some patients with this type of epilepsy may benefit from brain surgery to remove the abnormal brain cells that are causing the seizures.
- Others may be helped by a vagal nerve stimulator. This is a device that is implanted in the chest (similar to a heart pacemaker). This stimulator can help reduce the number of seizures, but rarely stops the seizures completely.

The children are placed on a special diet to help prevent seizures. The most popular one is the ketogenic diet. A diet low in carbohydrates, such as the Atkins diet, may also be helpful in some adults. Persons with epilepsy should wear medical alert jewelry so that prompt medical treatment can be obtained if a seizure occurs.

Complications

- Difficulty learning
- Inhaling fluid into the lungs, which can cause aspiration pneumonia
- Injury from falls, bumps, or self-inflicted bites during a seizure
- Injury from having a seizure while driving or operating machinery
- Many epilepsy medications cause birth defects—women wishing to become pregnant should alert their doctor in advance in order to adjust medications
- Permanent brain damage (stroke or other damage)
- Prolonged seizures or numerous seizures without complete recovery between them (status epilepticus)
- Side effects of medications.

Prevention

There is no known way to prevent epilepsy. However, proper diet and sleep and staying away from illegal drugs and alcohol, may decrease the likelihood of triggering seizures in people with epilepsy.

Reduce the risk of head injury by wearing helmets during risky activities; this can help lessen the chance of developing epilepsy. Persons with uncontrolled seizures should not drive. Each state has a different law that determines which people with a history of seizures are allowed to drive. If you have uncontrolled seizures, you should also avoid activities where loss of awareness would cause great danger, such as climbing to high places, biking and swimming alone.

Nursing Management

Nursing Priorities

- Prevent or control seizure activity.
- Protect patient from injury.
- Maintain airway or respiratory function.
- Promote positive self-esteem.
- Provide information about disease process, prognosis and treatment needs.

Goals

- Seizures activity controlled.
- Complications or injury prevented.

- Capable or competent self-image displayed.
- Disease process or prognosis, therapeutic regimen and limitations understood.
- Plan in place to meet needs after discharge.

Nursing Diagnosis

- Risk for Trauma
- Risk for Suffocation
- Risk for Ineffective Airway Clearance
- Risk for Ineffective Breathing Pattern
- Low Self-Esteem
- Knowledge deficit.

Nursing Intervention

Nursing Management of Child with Partial Seizures

In this condition some of the symptoms can be very frightening, the nurse should stay with the patient and offer reassurance that the seizure will pass. Because the simple partial seizure is a warning of a stronger seizure, the nurse should assess the immediate environment to ensure that, should the patient fall, any potential hazards are removed that could cause injury.

Nursing Management of Complex Partial Seizures

Complex partial seizures can be difficult to manage. If the seizure starts as only a warning, nursing management should be the same as for simple partial seizures. However, should the patient fall to the floor management should be as follows:

- Assess the patient for any signs of injury. Check also for limb displacement, as this may indicate the patient has a fracture
- Patients' behavior may change if they think they are being restrained. Therefore, nurses must consider their own personal safety
- Talk in a calm, reassuring voice
- If the patient gets up from the floor and starts to walk off before the automatisms start, be prepared to go along as well. If it is known that the patient is likely to remove his or her personal clothing, grab a blanket or towel to minimize any embarrassment to the patient on recovery.

Nursing Management of Generalized Seizures

Tonic clonic seizures are severe and can be frightening to an onlooker, but nurses should bear in mind how frightening they must also be to the patient. The following procedures should be taken when managing such patients:

- Communicate with the patient throughout the seizure
- Continually give reassurance that the seizure will stop and that the patient will not be left alone
- Protect the patient's head from banging on the floor while the convulsive movements are occurring and loosen any tight clothing
- Try to turn the patient into the recovery position
- Do not force anything into the patient's mouth as this could damage teeth and gums.

If, initially, it is not possible to turn the patient into the recovery position, it is crucial that this is done as soon as the limbs relax and that the airway is checked before the stertorous breathing phase begins. Doing so will allow any excess saliva to drain freely. Do not restrain patients who are moving about; simply continue observation.

Conclusion

Epilepsy is a very complex condition, affecting large numbers of the population. Nurses must be familiar with the different types of seizure and know how to manage them to ensure patients are given appropriate care and medication. Around 70 percent will be free of seizures if they have the correct diagnosis and treatment.

FEBRILE SEIZURES

Definition

A febrile seizure is a convulsion in a child triggered by a fever. These convulsions occur without any brain or spinal cord infection or other nervous system (neurologic) cause.

Incidence

About 3–5% of otherwise healthy children between ages 9 months and 5 years will have a seizure caused by a fever. Toddlers are most commonly affected. Febrile seizures often run in families. Most febrile seizures occur in the first 24 hours of an illness and not necessarily when the fever is highest. The seizure is often the first sign of a fever.

Causes and Risk Factors

Febrile seizures are usually triggered by fevers from:

- Ear infections
- Roseola
- Upper respiratory infections caused by a virus.

Meningitis causes less than 0.1% of febrile seizures but should always be considered, especially in children less than 1 year old, or those who still look ill when the fever comes down.

A child is likely to have more than one febrile seizure if:

- There is a family history of febrile seizures
- The first seizure happened before age 12 months
- The seizure occurred with a fever below 102 °F.

Signs and Symptoms

A febrile seizure may be as mild as the child's eyes rolling or limbs stiffening. Often a fever triggers a full-blown convulsion that involves the whole body. Febrile seizures may begin with the sudden contraction of muscles on both sides of a child's body—usually the muscles of the face, trunk, arms and legs. The child may cry or moan from the force of the muscle contraction. The contraction continues for several seconds, or tens of seconds. The child will fall, if standing and may pass urine. The child may vomit or bite the tongue. Sometimes children do not breathe and may begin to turn blue. Finally, the contraction is broken by brief moments of relaxation. The child's body begins to jerk rhythmically. The child does not respond to the parent's voice.

A simple febrile seizure stops by itself within a few seconds to 10 minutes. It is usually followed by a brief period of drowsiness or confusion. A complex febrile seizure lasts longer than 15 minutes, is in just one part of the body, or occurs again during the same illness. Febrile seizures are different than tremors or disorientation that can also occur with fevers. The movements are the same as in a grand mal seizure.

Signs and Tests

The health care provider may diagnose febrile seizure if the child has a grand mal seizure but does not have a history of seizure disorders (epilepsy). In infants and young children, it is important to rule out other causes of a first-time seizure, especially meningitis.

In a typical febrile seizure, the examination usually shows no abnormalities other than the illness causing the fever. Typically, the child will not need a full seizure workup (which includes an EEG, head CT and lumbar puncture (spinal tap).

To avoid having to undergo a seizure workup:

- The child must be developmentally normal.
- The child must have had a generalized seizure, meaning that the seizure was in more than one part of the child's body and not confined to one part of the body.
- The seizure must not have lasted longer than 15 minutes.
- The child must not have had more than one febrile seizure in 24 hours.
- The child must have a normal neurologic exam performed by a health care provider.

Management

During the seizure, leave your child on the floor.

- Need to slide a blanket under the child if the floor is hard.
- Move him only if he is in a dangerous location.
- Remove objects that may injure him.
- Loosen any tight clothing, especially around the neck. If possible, open or remove clothes from the waist up.
- If child vomits, or if saliva and mucus build up in the mouth, turn him on his side or stomach. This is also important if it looks like the tongue is getting in the way of breathing.

Do not try to force anything into his mouth to prevent him from biting the tongue, as this increases the risk of injury. Do not try to restrain your child or try to stop the seizure movements.

Focus your attention on bringing the fever down:

- Insert an acetaminophen suppository (if you have some) into the child's rectum.
- Do not try to give anything by mouth.
- Apply cool washcloths to the forehead and neck. Sponge the rest of the body with lukewarm (not cold) water. Cold water or alcohol may make the fever worse.
- After the seizure is over and your child is awake, give the normal dose of ibuprofen or acetaminophen.

After the seizure, the most important step is to identify the cause of the fever.

Prognosis

The first febrile seizure is a frightening moment for parents. Most parents are afraid that their child will die or have brain damage. However, simple febrile seizures are harmless.

There is no evidence that they cause death, brain damage, epilepsy, mental retardation, a decrease in IQ, or learning difficulties.

A small number of children who have had a febrile seizure do go on to develop epilepsy, but not because of the febrile seizures. Children who would develop epilepsy anyway will sometimes have their first seizures during fevers. These are usually prolonged, complex seizures. Nervous system (neurologic) problems and a family history of epilepsy make it more likely that the child will develop epilepsy. The number of febrile seizures is not related to future epilepsy.

About a third of children who have had a febrile seizure will have another one with a fever. Of those who do have a second seizure, about half will have a third seizure. Few children have more than three febrile seizures in their lifetime. Most children outgrow febrile seizures by age 5.

Complications

- Pneumonia
- Complications if a serious infection, such as meningitis
- Injury from falling down or bumping into objects
- Injury from long or complicated seizures
- Seizures not caused by fever
- Side effects of medications used to treat and prevent seizures (if prescribed).

Prevention

The febrile seizures can be the first sign of illness, it is often not possible to prevent them. A febrile seizure does not mean that your child is not getting the proper care. Occasionally, a health care provider will prescribe diazepam to prevent or treat febrile seizures that occur more than once. However, no medication is completely effective in preventing febrile seizures.

CRANIOCEREBRAL TRAUMA

Brain Injury

Introduction

Traumatic brain injury (TBI) is one of the leading causes of acquired disability and death in infants and children. Falls and motor vehicle collisions are common unintentional causes, whereas child abuse in infants and young children and assaults in adolescents are unfortunate inflicted causes of traumatic brain injury. Management focuses on limiting progression of the 'primary' brain injury and minimizing 'secondary' brain injury (discussed below). Research has revealed important age-dependent responses following pediatric traumatic brain injury.

Definition

Traumatic brain injury (TBI), otherwise known as intracranial injury, occurs when an external force traumatically injures the brain. it can be classified based on severity, mechanism (closed or penetrating head injury), or other features (e.g. occurring in a specific location or over a widespread area). Head injury usually refers to TBI, but is a broader category because it can involve damage to structures other than the brain, such as the scalp and skull.

Causes of Brain Injury

- Repetitive injury is a major cause of morbidity and mortality in infants and young children.
- Unintentional injuries in this age group occur as a result of falls and motor vehicle collisions.
- Falls become the predominant mechanism of injury by the toddler age.
- Among motor vehicle related injuries in this age group, motor-pedestrian injuries are more common than motor vehicle occupant injuries.
- School-aged children exhibit a rise in bicycle-related injuries whereas adolescents experience a rise in motor vehicle injuries, sports-related repetitive injuries and assaults.
- Children appear to experience age-dependent pathology following pediatric traumatic brain injury. Subdural hematomas and diffuse injury, such as diffuse cerebral swelling, are more common than focal injuries, such as contusions, in infants and young children.
- Hypoxic-ischemic injuries appear to be less common in unintentional traumatic brain injuries.

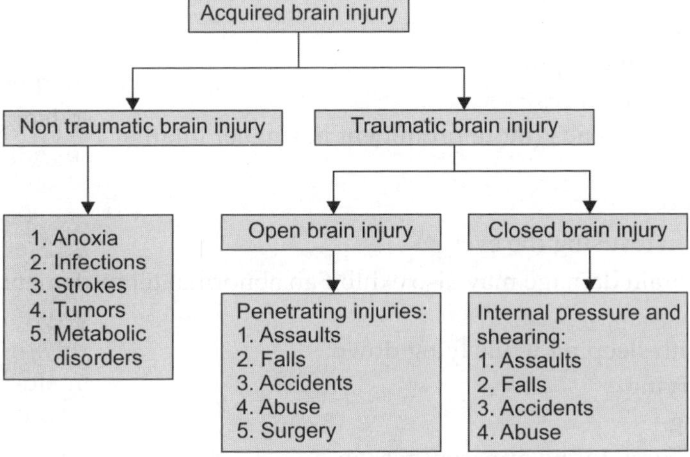

Fig. 7.90: Causes of brain injury

Types of Injuries

- Scalp injury
- Skull fracture (e.g. basilar skull fracture)
- Concussion
- Contusion
- Intracranial and/or subarachnoid hemorrhage
- Epidural and/or subdural hematoma
- Intraventricular hemorrhage.

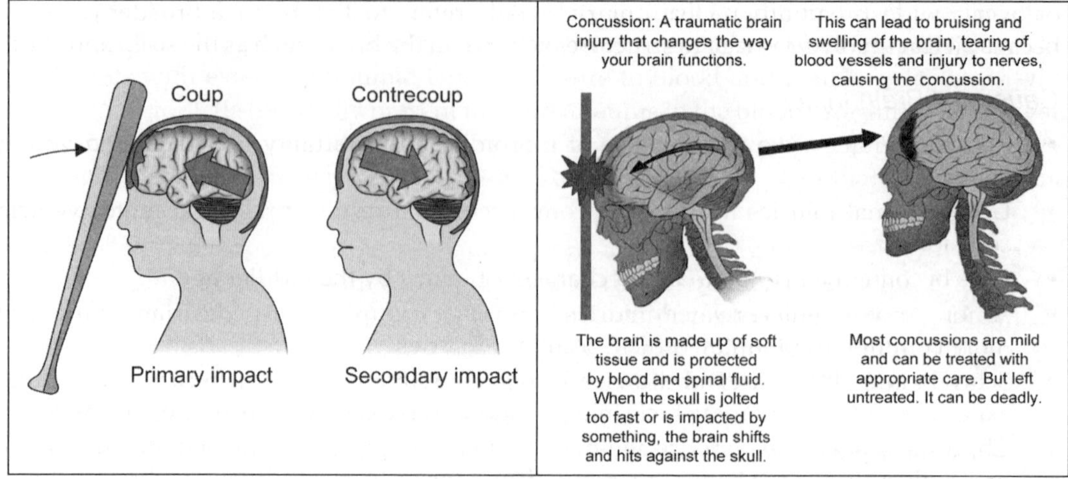

Fig. 7.91: Types of brain injury

Signs and Symptoms

Common symptoms and signs shortly after birth include:

- Elargeded forehead
- Abnormally-shaped spine
- Distorted facial features
- Unusually small heads (more prominent in smaller infants)
- Seizures
- Neck stiffness
- Difficulties in focusing the eyes.

Infants with brain damage may also exhibit an abnormal temperament, with symptoms including:

- Troubles with sleeping while lying down
- Excessive crying
- Poor feeding
- Excessively fussy for no apparent reason.

Cognitive Symptoms

Cognitive symptoms are usually identified as the child grows older and possibly misses normal developmental steps. The most common symptoms include difficulties with:

- Attention and concentration
- Memory and processing information
- Processing language
- Controlling impulses
- Communication.

Physical Symptoms

As the infant grows older, additional physical symptoms may manifest. Some physical symptoms may be difficult to diagnose (such as headaches). Some of the more obvious symptoms include:

- Extreme fatigue
- Sleeping disorders
- Light sensitivity
- Paralysis
- Tremors.

Other physical symptoms include missing developmental milestones, such as:

- Crawling
- Pulling themselves up without assistance
- Walking
- Running
- Hopping or skipping
- Walking up and down stairs without assistance
- Feeding themselves without assistance
- Tying shoes, drawing and coloring without assistance
- Sitting up alone without assistance
- Getting dressed without assistance
- Holding things without dropping them and with a firm grasp.

Pathophysiology

Primary Brain Injury

Primary injury to the brain occurs as an immediate consequence of the force of the trauma. Contact, linear forces as a result of direct blows to the head generate focal injuries, such as intracranial hemorrhages and contusions. Intracranial hemorrhage resulting from trauma typically occurs in four locations: Epidural, subdural, subarachnoid and intraparenchymal.

Features of Intracranial Hemorrhage

Contusions are bruises of the brain parenchyma as a result of blunt head injury that causes the brain surface to impact the bony ridges of the skull. Injury patterns include acceleration-deceleration injuries where the brain strikes the skull in a 'coup-contracoup' fashion, with the 'coup' contusion occurring at the site of impact and the 'contracoup' contusion located directly opposite the site of impact. Clinical symptoms relate to the severity and location of injury. Contusions may lead to local edema and ischemia with resultant neurologic deterioration, increased intracranial pressure (ICP) and intracranial hypertension and brain herniation.

Acceleration-deceleration injuries can also generate inertial, angular forces resulting in physical shearing or tearing of axons termed 'primary' axotomy. Rotational forces on the brain during acceleration-deceleration injuries cause widespread damage to axons in the white matter of the brain and should be suspected in a child when the degree of neurologic deterioration is associated with a relatively unremarkable CT scan.

Secondary Brain Injury

Secondary brain injury develops in the initial minutes to weeks following primary brain injury and occurs in two forms. The first form of secondary brain injury is potentiated by a myriad of physiologic and metabolic alterations including hypoxemia, hypotension, elevated intracranial pressure (ICP) and intracranial hypertension, hypercarbia or hypocarbia, hyperglycemia or hypoglycemia, electrolyte abnormalities, enlarging hematomas, coagulopathy, seizures and hyperthermia. This form of secondary brain injury is potentially avoidable and is amenable to treatment. Currently, the primary focus in the acute management of traumatic brain injury is to prevent and ameliorate these events that promote secondary brain injury.

Diagnostic Evaluation

Glasgow Coma Scale

Intracranial injuries resulting in increased ICP and intracranial hypertension may initially present with headache and vomiting but may rapidly progress to altered mental status and obtundation. The Glasgow Coma Scale (GCS) is classically used to evaluate injury severity with a score of 8 or less suggestive of severe brain injury.

Table 7.14: Glasgow coma scale

Behavior	Response	Score
Eye opening response	Spontaneously	4
	To speech	3
	To pain	2
	No response	1
Best verbal response	Oriented to time, place and person	5
	Confused	4
	Inappropriate words	3
	Incomprehensible sounds	2
	No response	1
Best motor response	Obeys commands	6
	Moves to localized pain	5
	Flexion withdrawal from pain	4
	Abnormal flexion (decorticate)	3
	Abnormal extension (decerebrate)	2
	No response	1
Total score	Best response	15
	Comatose client	8 or less
	Totally unresponsive	3

As the ICP continues to rise with subsequent intracranial hypertension, herniation syndromes may develop with classical clinical findings of the Cushing triad: Irregular respirations, bradycardia and hypertension. Neurogenic posturing and seizures may also occur in addition to changes in cranial nerve exam due to brainstem compression. Signs of occult traumatic brain injury with no history of trauma include the presence of retinal hemorrhages on ophthalmalogic examination that herald findings concerning for intentional trauma, commonly associated with subdural hematomas in 'shaken baby' or 'shaken-impact' syndrome. Additionally, findings of papilledema following unintentional or intentional trauma signify intracranial hypertension, necessitating emergent further evaluation.

CT Scan

Various modalities including CT scanning and MRI are used to diagnose traumatic brain injury. CT scanning provides rapid images of the skull and brain and is the first imaging modality used to diagnose skull fractures and intracranial pathology such as an epidural hematoma with mass effect. Evidence of elevated ICP may include midline shift due to mass effect and the loss of ventricular space, which are some of the features that herald impending herniation.

MRI Scan

MRI provides more detailed imaging and is used to confirm the diagnosis of traumatic brain injury and better visualizes posterior fossa lesions. However, MRI is typically not obtained during the initial period due to its lengthy imaging requirements. For those with severe brain injury or GCS of 8 or less and suspected intracranial hypertension, either an intraparenchymal or intraventricular ICP monitor is placed, with the latter being advantageous for draining CSF in the case of intracranial hypertension.

Management

Initial intervention for patients with traumatic brain injury focuses on detection of primary injury and prevention or treatment of secondary brain injury. Secondary brain injury exacerbated by hypoxemia, hypotension, elevated ICP leading to intracranial hypertension, hypercarbia or hypocarbia, hyperglycemia or hypoglycemia, electrolyte abnormalities, enlarging hematomas, coagulopathy, seizures and hyperthermia is treatable.

The primary goal in the acute management of the pediatric patient with severe traumatic brain injury is to prevent or ameliorate factors that promote secondary brain injury. In 2003, the Society of Critical Care Medicine published guidelines for the acute management of severe traumatic brain injury for the pediatric population based on a review of the pediatric traumatic brain injury literature and previously established adult guidelines. A brief synopsis of the guidelines is shown below, but the reader is urged to read the actual guidelines for complete details. At all times during the treatment of intracranial hypertension, repeating CT scanning may be warranted if the patient is not improving.

CSF Drainage

Ventricular drains have long been used for the drainage of CSF in patients with hydrocephalus. With the advent of ventricular ICP monitoring, ventricular drainage for patients with intracranial hypertension has also been commonly used. With removal of CSF, total intracranial volume is reduced, which may lead to decreased ICP and improvement of CPP.

Neuromuscular Blockade

If initial maneuvers are unsuccessful in controlling intracranial hypertension, neuromuscular blockade should be considered. Benefits of neuromuscular blockade include the prevention of shivering, which decreases metabolic demand and oxygen consumption; improved cerebral venous drainage through decreased intrathoracic pressure; and ease of ventilation and oxygenation by elimination of ventilator-patient asynchrony. Concerns regarding neuromuscular blockade include, but are not limited to, masking of seizure activity, nosocomial pneumonia due to ineffective pulmonary drainage, increased stress and ICP related to inadequate sedation and analgesia and the inability to perform a clinical neurologic examination to monitor the patient's course.

Hyperosmolar Therapy

Mannitol has long been successfully used to treat intracranial hypertension, especially following traumatic brain injury in adults. Mannitol is an osmolar agent with rapid onset of action via two distinct mechanisms. Initial effects of mannitol result from reduction of blood viscosity and a reflex decrease in vessel diameter to maintain cerebral blood flow through autoregulation. This decrease in vessel diameter contributes to decreasing total cerebral blood volume and ICP.

Because mannitol is a potent diuretic, hypovolemia can also occur leading to hypotension and a decrease in CPP. More recently, hypertonic saline has been shown to be an effective therapy for intracranial hypertension following pediatric traumatic brain injury. Hypertonic saline, typically 3% saline, has an osmolar mechanism of action similar to that of mannitol, without the diuretic effects. Added theoretical benefits of hypertonic saline include improved vasoregulation, cardiac output, immune modulation and plasma volume expansion. Pediatric patients with severe traumatic brain injury appear to tolerate a higher osmolar load with the use of hypertonic saline rather than mannitol. Patients using hypertonic saline have tolerated serum osmolalities as much as 360 mOsm/L, although some of the patients developed reversible renal insufficiency. However, reversible renal insufficiency has been noted with the use of hypertonic saline when serum osmolality approached 320 mOsm/L; thus, caution should be used.

Risks of hypertonic saline administration include, but are not limited to, rebound intracranial hypertension after withdrawal of therapy, central pontine myelinolysis with rapidly increasing serum sodium levels, subarachnoid hemorrhage due to rapid shrinkage of the brain and tearing of bridging vessels and renal failure.

Hyperventilation

Hyperventilation has the potential to reduce intracranial hypertension via reflex vasoconstriction in the presence of hypocapnia. The vasoconstriction leads to decreased cerebral blood flow, decreased cerebral blood volume and a subsequent decrease in ICP. Hyperventilation is one of the fastest methods to lower ICP in a child with impending herniation. In cases of refractory intracranial hypertension despite all of the above treatments (sedation, analgesia, head elevation, CSF drainage, neuromuscular blockade and hyperosmolar therapy), mild hyperventilation ($PaCO_2$ of 30–35 mm Hg) may be beneficial in decreasing ICP.

Barbiturates

The administration of high-dose barbiturate therapy, such as pentobarbital, is used for refractory intracranial hypertension. This class of medications suppresses the cerebral metabolic rate. With continuous electroencephalographic monitoring, barbiturate infusions may be titrated to achieve burst suppression. The minimum dose required to control refractory intracranial hypertension is recommended, as barbiturates may cause myocardial depression, decreased systemic vascular resistance and hypotension. Furthermore, the ability to perform neurological examination is lost when barbiturates are used to control ICP. Prolonged barbiturate therapy may result in immune suppression leading to sepsis and ileus with subsequent feeding intolerance.

Decompressive Craniectomy

When refractory intracranial hypertension persists despite medical therapy, decompressive craniectomy is a surgical option for refractory cerebral swelling. Decompressive craniectomy typically involves either unilateral frontal-temporal-parietal or bilateral frontal craniectomy. Patients typically undergo this procedure within the first 48 hours of initial injury. Potential complications from decompressive craniectomy include, but are not limited to, hemorrhage and exacerbation of cerebral edema.

Seizure

Seizures should be aggressively treated because they can potentially cause hyperthermia, intracranial hypertension and brain damage. Although prophylactic anticonvulsants may be a treatment option to prevent early post-traumatic seizures (occurring within 1 week following injury) in infants and young children, prophylactic anticonvulsants are not recommended for preventing late post-traumatic seizures (> 1 week) because this has not been associated with improved outcome.

Conclusion

Although various interventions are used to maintain adequate CPP and treat intracranial hypertension in children with severe traumatic brain injury, the hallmark of a successful therapy is improved long-term outcome. Because traumatic brain injury remains a significant burden in the pediatric population, intense investigation is of paramount importance to discover therapies that ultimately will reduce morbidity and mortality and improve long-term outcomes.

HEAD TRAUMA (INJURY)

Introduction

Trauma is a leading cause of death in children older than 1 year in the United States, with head trauma representing 80% or more of the injuries. In approximately 5% of head trauma cases, patients die at the site of the accident. Head trauma has a high emotional, psychosocial and economic impact because these patients often have comparatively long hospital stays and 5–10% require discharge to a long-term care facility.

The anatomical differences of the child's brain render it more susceptible than the adult brain to certain types of injuries following head trauma. The head is larger in proportion to the body surface area and stability is dependent on the ligamentous rather than bony structure. The pediatric brain has a higher water content, 88% versus 77% in adult, which makes the brain softer and more prone to acceleration-deceleration injury. The water content is inversely related to the myelinization process. The unmyelinated brain is more susceptible to shear injuries. Infants and young children tolerate intracranial pressure (ICP) increases better because of open sutures.

Types of Injury

Scalp Injury

Often observed with traumatic brain injuries, scalp injury can overlie other intracranial pathology; therefore, it requires careful exploration for foreign bodies or underlying skull fractures. Bleeding associated with scalp lacerations could be significant enough to cause hypotension and shock in a small infant. Caput succedaneum and cephalohematoma are observed with birth-related head trauma. Caput succedaneum involves molding of the neonatal head and crosses the suture lines, whereas cephalohematoma involves subperiosteal bleeding and is limited by the suture lines.

Skull Fracture

Skull fractures are linear, comminuted, depressed and diastatic. In children, 90% of the fractures are linear and tend to be more diastatic; thus, the radiographic appearance is more impressive. An open fracture is a fracture overlaid by a laceration. The presence of cerebrospinal fluid (CSF) in the wound indicates a violation of the dura and warrants further exploration. Location of the fracture is important because it may cross the path of a major vessel and be associated with an intracranial bleed. Depressed skull fracture is defined as displacement of the inner table of the skull by more than one thickness of the bone. One third of depressed fractures are simple, one third are associated with dural laceration and one fourth have cortical lacerations.

Basilar Skull Fracture

This is present in 6–14% of pediatric patients with head trauma and is suggested by a history of a blow to the back of the head. Loss of consciousness, seizures and neurologic deficits may or may not be present. Children with basilar skull fracture usually have prolonged nausea, vomiting and general malaise, most likely because of the vicinity of the fracture to the emesis and vestibular brainstem centers. Physical findings, such as battle sign, raccoon eyes and CSF otorrhea and rhinorrhea are pathognomonic; ocular nerve entrapment may occur in 1–10% of patients.

Concussion

A transient loss of consciousness, concussion occurs as the result of head trauma. Patients often have normal findings on neurologic examination; the diagnosis is usually a retrospective one. Infants and young children have a higher incidence of post-traumatic seizures and most often increased delayed somnolence and vomiting; older children have a history of post-traumatic amnesia. Waxing and waning of mental status in the absence of any morphologic changes is also characteristic of concussion and is more often observed in older children.

Contusion

Caused by a direct injury to the head, a contusion is an area of bruising or tearing of the brain tissue. The temporal and frontal lobes are the most vulnerable areas because of their anatomical relationship with the bony protuberances of calvaria. The typical presentation is of progressive neurologic deterioration secondary to local cerebral edema, infarcts, and/or late-developing hematomas.

Epidural Hematoma with Acute Neurologic Deterioration

Developing between the skull and the dura and secondary to the laceration of an artery or vein, epidural hematomas of arterial origin peak in size 6–8 hours after the injury. Epidural hematomas of venous origin may grow over 24 or more hours. Common locations are the temporal, frontal and occipital lobes. An overlying skull fracture may be present. Patients may present with the classic lucid interval between the initial loss of consciousness and subsequent neurologic deterioration, but this is less frequent in the pediatric population. When neurologic deterioration with hemiparesis, unconsciousness, posturing and pupillary changes develops, it is due to the expansion of hematoma and exhaustion of compensatory mechanisms, with subsequent compression of the temporal lobe and/or brain stem.

Subdural Hematoma

- Located between the dura and the cortex, subdural hematoma results from tearing of the bridging veins across the dura or laceration of the cortical arteries during acceleration-deceleration forces; it is usually associated with severe parenchymal injury and the presentation is that of profound and progressive neurologic deterioration.
- Subdural hematoma may develop secondary to birth trauma, in which case the presentation is within 12 hours of life and includes seizures, full fontanel, anisocoria and respiratory distress.
- Subdural hematoma is also a feature of shaken baby syndrome; the usual presentation is of new-onset seizures, increased head circumference, poorly thriving infant and tense fontanel. Focal neurologic deficits are usually absent.

Penetrating Injuries

Resulting from various sources, penetrating injuries should be considered neurosurgical emergencies because rapid deterioration and fatal hemorrhages may ensue.

Intraventricular Hemorrhage

This type of hemorrhage is usually the result of minor trauma and resolves spontaneously. Large hemorrhages could lead to obstructive hydrocephalus, especially when they are located at the level of the foramen of Monroe and the aqueduct of Sylvius, in which case surgical intervention is required.

Subarachnoid Hemorrhage

The most common form of hemorrhage associated with head trauma, subarachnoid hemorrhage, results from disruption of the small vessels on the cerebral cortex. The usual location is along the falx cerebri or tentorium and the outer cortical surface. Common symptoms include nausea, vomiting, headache, restlessness, fever and nuchal rigidity caused by blood in the subarachnoid space.

Diffuse Axonal Injury

A result of rapid acceleration-deceleration forces, this type of injury causes disruption of the small axonal pathways. The most commonly affected areas are the basal ganglia, thalamus, deep hemispheric nuclei and corpus callosum. Their increased vulnerability to shear injuries is attributed to a different momentum of these structures from the rest of the brain at the time of the injury. Patients usually present with various states of altered mentation and often remain in a vegetative state for long periods. A marked discrepancy between the highly abnormal neurologic examination findings and the lack of findings on CT scanning is observed. Occasionally, small petechial hemorrhages may be present. Prognosis for full recovery is often poor.

Physical

Head trauma patients often have multiple organ injuries. Assessment of patients with severe head injuries involves a primary and a secondary survey. The primary survey is a focused physical examination directed at identifying and treating life-threatening conditions present in a trauma patient and by this, preventing secondary brain injury. The secondary survey of patients with head trauma is a detailed examination and assessment of the system with the goal of identifying all traumatic injuries and directing further treatment.

Causes

The most head injuries occur secondary to motor vehicle accidents, falls, assaults, recreational activities and child abuse. The percentage of each contributing factor differs between studies and the distribution varies according to age, group and sex. A few factors such as seizure disorder, attention deficit disorder and alcohol and drug use enhance the vulnerability of the child or adolescent to this type of trauma. Infants and young children are more vulnerable to abuse because of their dependency on adults.

Diagnostic Evaluation

Laboratory Studies

The following laboratory studies may be indicated in patients with head trauma:

- A CBC count, including platelets, provides a baseline hematocrit and should be monitored serially, especially when bleeding is suspected in patients with head trauma.
- Blood chemistry, including an amylase and lipase, provides information regarding other organ injury.
- Coagulation profile, prothrombin time (PT)/activated partial thromboplastin time (aPTT) and fibrinogen should be obtained in patients with head trauma because they may have an underlying or trauma-triggered coagulopathy.
- Type and cross is useful in anticipation of need for transfusion, especially in patients with multiple traumas.
- ABG provides information regarding oxygenation and ventilation and results direct further treatment.
- A blood or urine toxicology screen should be obtained in addition to the routine panel, especially in patients who have altered mental status, seizures and an unclear history.
- Wound cultures from lacerations or open skull fractures should be taken; findings might help guide further therapy when infection is suspected.

Management

Medical Management

The goal of medical care of patients with head trauma is to recognize and treat life-threatening conditions and to eliminate or minimize the role of secondary injury. Guidelines for the treatment of patients with head trauma have been established. Patients with severe head trauma are at increased risk of developing cerebral edema, respiratory failure and herniation secondary to the increased intracranial pressure (ICP); therefore, frequent serial assessments of the neurologic status must be performed. The Brain Trauma Foundation has developed guidelines regarding the medical management of patients with severe head injury. These guidelines suggest that cardiopulmonary resuscitation should be the foundation upon which treatment of intracranial hypertension must be based. They also state that, in the absence of any obvious signs of increased ICP, no prophylactic treatment should be initiated because this may directly interfere with the optimal resuscitation process.

Medication

Medical therapy is directed at controlling the intracranial pressure (ICP) with sedatives and neuromuscular blockers, diuretics, lidocaine and anticonvulsants.

Nondepolarizing Neuromuscular Blockers

These are used in combination with a sedative as part of the rapid sequence intubation process or to achieve control of the ICP.

Airway Management

A stable airway should be obtained to provide adequate oxygenation and ventilation. If endotracheal intubation is required, adequate sedation and paralysis must be assured to avoid further increase in ICP. Rapid sequence induction and endotracheal intubation are generally recommended. Stabilization of the cervical spine should be achieved in every patient with severe head trauma. Nasal intubation or nasogastric tube placement should be avoided, especially for patients in whom basilar skull fracture is suspected. Breathing may be impaired because of neurological or thoracic injuries. Patients with significant head injury and altered mentation should be supplemented with 100% oxygen and should be supported with positive pressure ventilation. Endotracheal intubation should be performed in cases in which the patient has difficulty maintaining the airway because of large secretions, poor gag reflex, coma, or the need prolonged ventilatory support.

Cardiovascular Management

Achieving normotension and euvolemia is the goal in cardiovascular management. Cerebral perfusion pressure (CPP), defined as the mean arterial blood pressure (MAP) minus the ICP (CPP = MAP-ICP), is the physiologic variable that defines the pressure gradient driving the cerebral blood flow (CBF) and metabolite delivery; it is therefore closely related to ischemia. Several clinical studies suggest that maintaining CPP at 70–80 mm Hg may be the critical threshold. Adequate volume resuscitation with isotonic solutions should be conducted to maintain adequate filling pressures, normal cardiac output and ultimately normotension (MAP > 90 mm Hg). More recent adult and pediatric studies have shown that the use of hypertonic solution in the resuscitation process is superior to that of lactated Ringer solution or isotonic sodium chloride solution. Patients who have received hypertonic sodium chloride solution have improved blood pressure response, overall decreased fluid requirement, fewer interventions in controlling the ICP, fewer complications and improved survival.

Increased ICP and Cerebral Perfusion Management

Medical management of increased ICP includes elevating the head end of the bed to 30° and maintaining head and neck in midline position. Sedation and paralysis are used to prevent agitation and increased muscular activity that may increase the ICP. If neuromuscular blockers are used, monitoring the ICP and having an electroencephalogram in place is necessary. The use of loop or osmotic diuretics (e.g. furosemide, mannitol) is directed mostly at decreasing CSF production and improving cerebral compliance and CBF by decreasing the cerebral blood volume

Bleeding Management

A disseminated intravascular coagulopathy is present in one third of head trauma patients and requires aggressive management and correction with replacement factors in order to decrease the risk of further intracranial bleeding and allow surgical intervention when necessary.

Seizure Management

Post-traumatic seizures present in 10% of pediatric patients with head trauma may affect the outcome adversely by increasing the ICP, increasing the metabolic demands of the brain and causing hypoxia and/or hypoventilation in a spontaneously breathing patient. Short-acting benzodiazepines (e.g. lorazepam, diazepam) may be used to control the seizure and phenytoin or phenobarbital should be used for maintenance anticonvulsant.

Surgical Management

Surgical treatment in patients with head trauma includes the following:

- Surgical decompression is required in the presence of a rapidly expanding epidural or subdural hematoma that causes an increase in ICP and focal compression.
- The craniotomy and surgical drainage of an epidural hematoma and repair of vessels should be done immediately if signs of increased ICP, altered mentation, focal neurologic signs, pupillary changes, or a midline shift are present.
- Conservative management with close monitoring in a pediatric ICU (PICU) is acceptable if no focal neurologic signs, altered mentation, or pressure effects with midline shift are present and the hematoma is less than 2 cm.
- Patients with subdural hematoma with midline shift or altered mental status should have the hematoma emergently drained.
- Patients with small subdural hematoma with no midline shift or pressure effects should be managed conservatively with close monitoring.
- Surgical drainage of subdural hematoma is not required in most cases.

Complications

Complications in head trauma may include the following:

- Seizures are more commonly observed with contusions (subdural hematoma more so than epidural hematoma), depressed skull fracture and severe head injury.

- Leptomeningeal cyst or growing fracture represents extrusion of leptomeninges and brain tissue through a dural defect.
- Meningitis could develop secondary to basilar skull fracture.
- Cranial nerve injury may develop secondary to basilar skull fracture. Oculomotor palsy is due to injury of cranial nerves VI, III, or IV. Trauma to nerve VII leads to facial nerve palsy. Hearing loss may occur because of injury of cranial nerve VIII.
- Post-traumatic syndrome may develop following mild-to-moderate head trauma and consists of irritability, inability to concentrate, nervousness and occasionally behavioral or cognitive impairment.
- Cortical blindness, described as an acute loss of vision following head trauma, usually resolves spontaneously within 24 hours. Several mechanisms have been implicated, including acute cerebral edema and transient vasospasm. Cortical blindness is now considered to result from minor transient alterations in the brain function triggered by the traumatic event.
- Trauma-induced migraine may begin from minutes to hours following the injury and may last from hours to days. Beta-blockers are the drugs of choice for this complication.
- Hydrocephalus results from either an obstruction caused by an intraventricular hemorrhage or decreased reabsorption of cerebrospinal fluid (CSF) due to proteinaceous obstruction of the arachnoid villi.
- Neurogenic pulmonary edema is thought to be due to medullary ischemia that leads to increased sympathetic tone with subsequent increase in pulmonary vascular pressure and a shift in blood distribution from the systemic to pulmonary bed.
- Pulmonary infections are often present in patients with head trauma because of either an initial aspiration process or prolonged mechanical ventilation.

ENDOCRINE SYSTEM

ENDOCRINE DISORDERS

Introduction

The endocrine system is a complex collection of hormone-producing glands that control basic body functions such as metabolism, growth and sexual development. Many of the hormones produced by the endocrine glands interact with each other to maintain balance.

The amount of hormones produced by each gland is carefully balanced. Too much or too little of a certain hormone can have effects throughout the body and cause various endocrine disorders. Although many endocrine disorders that affect adults can affect children, the disorders may produce different symptoms in children.

Endocrinology is the study of hormones. Hormones travel in the blood and control many important body functions by delivering signals between the cells. Insulin, for example, is a hormone that moves food energy from the blood into muscle, fat and liver cells. If your child's body does not make enough insulin or becomes resistant to its effects, your child may develop diabetes. Diabetes is a lifelong condition in which the body does not properly control the amount of sugar in the blood.

Metabolism is the chemical activity that occurs in cells, releasing energy from nutrients or using energy to create other substances, such as proteins. The basal metabolic rate (BMR) is a measurement of energy required to keep the body functioning at rest. Measured in calories, metabolic rates increase with exertion, stress, fear and illness.

Major glands in the endocrine system are:

- Hypothalamus
- Pituitary
- Thyroid
- Parathyroids
- Adrenals
- Pineal body
- Reproductive glands.

Which include the ovaries and testes, the pancreas is also part of this hormone-secreting system, even though it is also associated with the digestive system because it also produces and secretes digestive enzymes.

The endocrine system is a network of glands that produce and release hormones that help control many important body functions, especially the body's ability to change calories into energy that powers cells and organs. The endocrine system influences how your heart beats, how your bones and tissues grow, even your ability to make a baby. It plays a vital role in whether or not you develop diabetes, thyroid disease, growth disorders, sexual dysfunction and a host of other hormone-related disorders.

Glands of the Endocrine System

Each gland of the endocrine system releases specific hormones into your bloodstream. These hormones travel through your blood to other cells and help control or coordinate many body processes.

Endocrine Glands Include

- *Adrenal glands:* Two glands that sit on top of the kidneys that release the hormone cortisol.
- *Hypothalamus:* A part of the lower middle brain that tells the pituitary gland when to release hormones.
- *Ovaries:* The female reproductive organs that release eggs and produce sex hormones.
- *Islet cells in the pancreas:* Cells in the pancreas control the release of the hormones insulin and glucagon.
- *Parathyroid:* Four tiny glands in the neck that play a role in bone development.
- *Pineal gland:* A gland found near the center of the brain that may be linked to sleep patterns.
- *Pituitary gland:* A gland found at the base of brain behind the sinuses. It is often called the 'master gland' because it influences many other glands, especially the thyroid. Problems with the pituitary gland can affect bone growth, a woman's menstrual cycles and the release of breast milk.
- *Testes:* The male reproductive glands that produce sperm and sex hormones.
- *Thymus:* A gland in the upper chest that helps develops the body's immune system early in life.
- *Thyroid:* A butterfly-shaped gland in the front of the neck that controls metabolism.

Even the slightest hiccup with the function of one or more of these glands can throw off the delicate balance of hormones in your body and lead to an endocrine disorder, or endocrine disease.

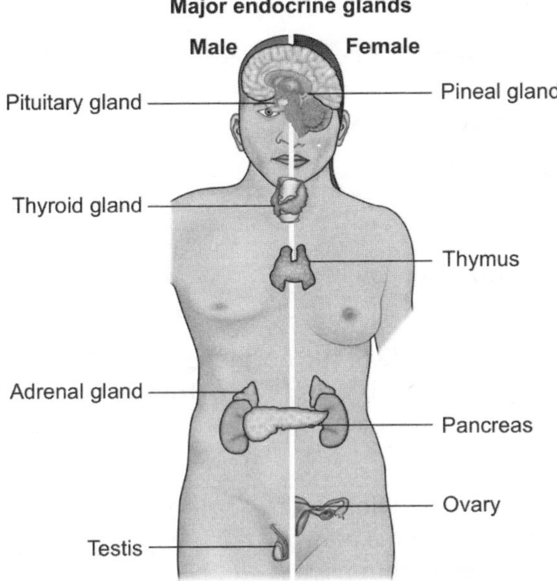

Fig. 7.92: Anatomy of endocrine system

Causes of Endocrine Disorder

- A problem with the endocrine feedback system
- Disease
- Failure of a gland to stimulate another gland to release hormones
- A genetic disorder, such as multiple endocrine neoplasia (MEN) or congenital hypothyroidism
- Infection
- Injury to an endocrine gland
- Tumor of an endocrine gland.

Hormones

The word hormone is derived from the Greek 'hormao' meaning 'I excite or arouse'. Hormones communicate this effect by their unique chemical structures recognized by specific receptors on their target cells, by their patterns of secretion and their concentrations in the general or localized circulation.

Functions of Hormones

- Reproduction and sexual differentiation
- Development and growth
- Maintenance of the internal environment
- Regulation of metabolism and nutrient supply

- The endocrine system keeps our bodies in balance, maintaining homeostasis and guiding proper growth and development
- A single hormone may affect more than one of these functions and each function may be controlled by several hormones.

Types of Endocrine Disorders
- Diabetes insipidus
- Diabetes mellitus—IDDM, NIDDM
- Hyper and hypo thyroidism
- Phenylketonuria
- Galactosemia.

Other types of endocrine disorders include:

Adrenal Insufficiency

The adrenal gland releases too little of the hormone cortisol and sometimes, aldosterone. Symptoms include fatigue, stomach upset, dehydration, and skin changes. Addison's disease is a type of adrenal insufficiency.

Cushing's Disease

Overproduction of a pituitary gland hormone leads to an overactive adrenal gland. A similar condition called Cushing's syndrome may occur in people, particularly children, who take high-doses of corticosteroid medications.

Gigantism (Acromegaly)

If the pituitary gland produces too much growth hormone, a child's bones and body parts may grow abnormally fast. If growth hormone levels are too low, a child can stop growing in height.

Hyperthyroidism

The thyroid gland produces too much thyroid hormone, leading to weight loss, fast heart rate, sweating and nervousness. The most common cause for an overactive thyroid is an autoimmune called Grave's disease.

PITUITARY DISORDERS

Introduction

The pituitary gland is a tiny organ, the size of a pea, found at the base of the brain. As the 'master gland' of the body, it produces many hormones that travel throughout the body, directing certain processes or stimulating (causing) other glands to produce other hormones. The pituitary gland makes or stores many different hormones.

The following hormones are made in the anterior (front part) of the pituitary gland:

- *Prolactin:* Prolactin stimulates breast milk production after childbirth. It also affects sex hormone levels from ovaries in women and from testes (testicles) in men, as well as fertility.
- *Growth hormone (GH):* GH stimulates growth in childhood and is important for maintaining a healthy body composition and well-being in adults. In adults, GH is

important for maintaining muscle mass and bone mass. It also affects fat distribution in the body.

- *Adrenocorticotropin (ACTH):* ACTH stimulates the production of cortisol by the adrenal glands—small glands that sit on top of the kidneys. Cortisol, a 'stress hormone,' is vital to our survival. It helps maintain blood pressure and blood glucose (sugar) levels and is produced in larger amounts when we are under stress especially after illness or injury. Read about having too much ACTH.

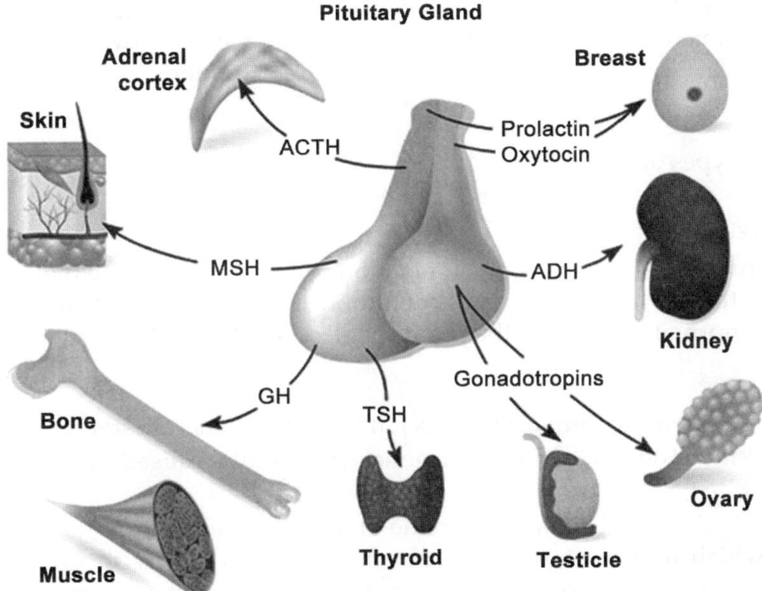

Fig. 7.93: Anatomical view of pituitary gland

- *Thyroid-stimulating hormone (TSH):* TSH stimulates the thyroid gland to produce thyroid hormones, which regulate the body's metabolism, energy balance, growth and nervous system activity. Read about TSH-secreting tumors.
- *Luteinizing hormone (LH):* LH stimulates testosterone production in men and egg release (ovulation) in women.
- *Follicle-stimulating hormone (FSH):* FSH promotes sperm production in men and stimulates the ovaries to produce estrogen and develop eggs in women. LH and FSH work together to enable normal function of the ovaries and testes.

The following hormones are stored in the posterior (back part) of the pituitary gland:

- *Antidiuretic hormone (ADH):* ADH, also called vasopressin, regulates water balance in the body. It conserves body water by reducing the amount of water lost in urine.
- *Oxytocin:* Oxytocin causes milk to flow from the breasts in breastfeeding women and may also help labor to progress.

Types of Disorders

- Pituitary tumors in children
- Growth hormone deficiency in children
  - Hypopituitarism
  - Hyperpituitarism

PITUITARY TUMORS

Introduction

The most frequent type of pituitary disorder is a pituitary gland tumor. These tumors are fairly common in adults. They are not brain tumors and are almost always benign (that is, not cancer). In fact, cancerous tumors of this sort are extremely rare.

Types

There are two types of tumors:

1. Secretory
2. Non-secretory

Secretory tumors produce too much of a hormone normally made by the pituitary and non-secretory tumors do not. Both types of tumors can cause problems if they are large and interfere with normal function of the pituitary gland and/or nearby structures in the brain.

Causes

The problems caused by pituitary tumors fall into three general categories:

1. *Hypersecretion:* Too much of any hormone in the body is caused by a secretory pituitary tumor.
2. *Hyposecretion:* Too little of any hormone in the body can be caused by a large pituitary tumor, which interferes with the pituitary gland's ability to produce hormones. Hyposecretion can also result from surgery or radiation of a tumor.
3. *Tumor mass effects:* As a pituitary tumor grows and presses against the pituitary gland or other areas in the brain, it may cause headaches, vision problems, or other health effects.

Injuries, certain medications, bleeding inside or close to the pituitary and other conditions can also affect the pituitary gland. Loss of normal pituitary function also can occur after major head trauma.

Signs and Symptoms

In general, the symptoms seen with pituitary tumors are related to a disturbance in production of a specific hormone or group of hormones and relate to the role the hormones play in maintaining health and development. The symptoms of pituitary tumors vary depending on the size and location of the tumor and whether the tumor presses on other organs or affects the secretion of hormones. For instance, pituitary tumors may press on the optic nerve, causing problems with vision.

- Headaches
- Vision problems
- Changes in menstrual cycles in women

- Impotence, which is the inability to achieve or maintain an erection in men and is caused by hormone changes
- Infertility, meaning the inability to have children
- Inappropriate production of breast milk
- Cushing's syndrome, a combination of weight gain, high blood pressure, diabetes and easy bruising that is caused by overproduction of ACTH
- Acromegaly, the enlargement of the extremities or limbs and thickening of the skull and jaw caused by too much growth hormone
- Unexplained tiredness
- Mood changes
- Irritability.

Diagnostic Evaluation

Blood and urine tests can be used to determine hormone levels. MRI or CT scans can detect tumors in the pituitary gland.

- *Blood and urine tests:* These can determine whether child have an overproduction or deficiency of hormones.
- *Brain imaging:* A CT scan or MRI scan of child brain can help the doctors to judge the location and size of a pituitary tumor.
- *Vision testing:* This can determine if a pituitary tumor has impaired child sight or peripheral vision.

Pituitary cancer is most likely to spread to the:

- Brain
- Spinal cord
- Meninges (brain and spinal cord covering)
- Nearby bone.

It is very rare for pituitary cancer to spread to the lungs, heart, or liver.

Management

Medical Management

A pituitary tumor is overproducing a hormone, there are medications that can help. The drugs bromocriptine (Parlodel) and cabergoline (Dostinex) are used to treat tumors that secrete prolactin. Octreotide (Sandostatin) or pegvisomant (Somavert) can be used to treat tumors that make growth hormone. Octreotide can also be used to treat pituitary tumors that secrete thyroid-stimulating hormone.

The medications used to treat pituitary tumors are continually being evaluated. Talking with your doctor is often the best way to learn about the medications you have been prescribed, their purpose and their potential side effects or interactions with other medications.

Hormone Therapy for Hyposecretion

Sometimes tumors cause a lack of a hormone. Other times, the lack of a hormone is caused by the treatment you have for pituitary tumors. Surgery or radiation therapy, for example, can lead to permanent loss of hormone secretion. In these cases, hormone replacement therapy is an important part of treatment.

Some types of hormones are necessary for survival. These hormones must be replaced immediately.

- *TSH, or thyroid stimulating hormone:* Regulates thyroid hormone production, which, in turn, regulates metabolism. If a problem with TSH secretion is causing low thyroid hormone levels, you may also need to start thyroid hormone replacement.
- *Antidiruetic hormone (ADH), or vasopressin:* Controls the body's water balance.

Hormone Replacement Therapy (HRT)

HRT is often necessary for patients with a pituitary tumor when the gland is not making enough of a hormone due to the disease. This may include replacement of:

- Thyroid hormones
- Adrenal hormones
- Growth hormone
- Testosterone in men
- Estrogen in women

Surgical Management

The most common form of surgery to remove pituitary tumors is trans-sphenoidal microsurgery. A neurosurgeon approaches the pituitary gland tumor through the nose, in the sphenoid sinus cavity. Using this natural pathway, the surgeon does not need to operate on your skull. With a surgical microscope and special instruments, the surgical goal is to safely remove the tumor without damaging the surrounding pituitary gland.

Radiation Therapy

Radiation therapy uses high-energy X-rays to destroy tumors. It can be used after surgery or alone if surgery is not an option. Radiation therapy can be beneficial if a tumor persists or returns after surgery and causes signs and symptoms that medications do not relieve. Methods of radiation therapy include:

- *Gamma Knife stereotactic radiosurgery:* Often delivered as a single high-dose, this focuses radiation beams on the tumor without an incision. It delivers radiation beams the size and shape of the tumor into the tumor with the aid of special brain-imaging techniques. Minimal radiation comes in contact with healthy tissue surrounding the tumor, decreasing the risk of damage to normal tissue.
- *External beam radiation:* This delivers radiation in small increments over time. A series of treatments, usually five times a week over a four- to six-week period, is performed on an outpatient basis. While this therapy is often effective, it may take years to fully control the tumor growth and hormone production. Radiation therapy may also damage remaining normal pituitary cells and normal brain tissue, particularly near the pituitary gland.
- *Proton beam therapy:* Another radiation option, this type uses positively charged ions (protons) rather than X-rays. Unlike X-rays, proton beams stop after releasing their energy within their target. The beams can be finely controlled and can be used on tumors with less risk to healthy tissues. This type of therapy requires special equipment and is not widely available.

GROWTH HORMONE DEFICIENCY IN CHILDREN

HYPOPITUITARISM

Definition

Hypopituitarism (an underactive pituitary gland) is rare in children. When a child has hypopituitarism, the pituitary gland has lost its ability to make one, some or all pituitary hormones. The condition is often permanent, but very treatable.

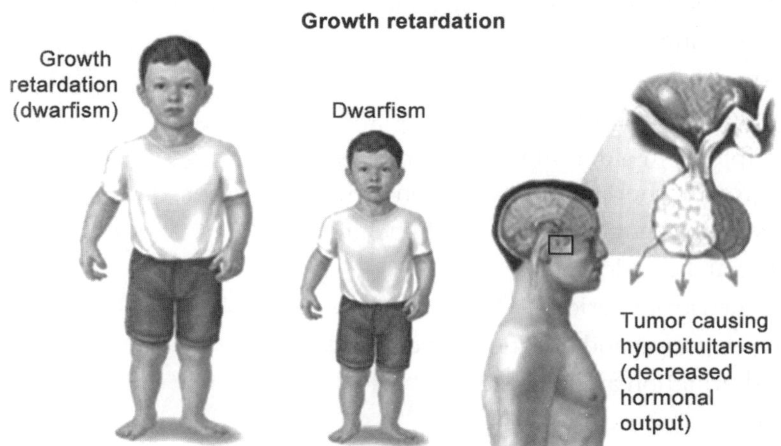

Fig. 7.94: Hypopituitarism child

Causes

Hypopituitarism may be congenital (a condition present at birth) and caused by:

- Birth trauma (injury)
- Genetic (inherited) disorders
- Central nervous system (CNS) defects
- Defective, underdeveloped, or absent pituitary gland.

Hypopituitarism can also be acquired (a condition that develops later in life) and may be caused by:

- Radiation to the head
- Tumors in the brain
- Other disorders, such as tuberculosis or sarcoidosis, which infiltrate the gland, can result in a reduction in function.

Tumor

A tumor can cause hypopituitarism. The tumor may grow in the pituitary gland or outside the gland, compressing the normal tissue. Parents worry that the tumor may be cancer, but that is unlikely.

Rare Causes

- An infection in the brain
- A traumatic brain injury
- Radiation to the brain
- Bleeding into the pituitary gland.

Signs and Symptoms

Common symptoms in newborns:

- Symptoms of low blood sugar, sluggishness, jitteriness, seizures
- Frequent urination
- Penis is small
- Skin is yellow (jaundice).

Common symptoms in older infants and children:

- Stunted growth, short stature (based on growth curve chart)
- Weight gain does not match growth in height
- Delayed sexual development
- Irregular menstrual periods
- Tooth development and eruption are delayed
- Thirst and urination are increased
- Fatigue, low tolerance for stress.

Diagnostic Evaluation

- *History and physical examination:* A head-to-toe physical exam. This includes the genitalia/private areas to determine if puberty is happening. If we need a blood test, you may be asked to return for a morning blood draw.
- *Morning blood test:* Measure hormone levels in the blood sample. The morning is the best time for this because hormone levels go up and down throughout the day. This blood test may be all that is needed.
- *Imaging study:* MRI scan to see inside the head, if needed. The scan can show us a tumor or other developmental abnormality in the pituitary gland—without exposing the child to radiation. Medicine lets the child sleep comfortably while we get the pictures.
- *Ophthalmology referral/eye exam:* The child's vision or about septo-optic dysplasia.
- *Bone study:* X-ray (of the hand and wrist) in diagnosis and as we manage the condition. The images tell us about the skeleton's development.

Management

Hormone Replacement

Hormone replacement therapy mimics the body's natural production. The medicines can be continued as long as needed, during childhood and adulthood. These medications are tolerated very well when the right amounts of hormones are replaced.

The following are examples of hormone replacement therapy:

- *Levothyroxine for hypothyroidism:* The child takes a tablet of levothyroxine each day.
- *Synthetic growth hormone for growth deficiency:* The child needs an injection of synthetic growth hormone every day. The needle is very small.
- *Hydrocortisone for adrenal insufficiency:* The child takes a tablet two to three times a day. To deal with illness, surgery or dehydration, the child needs a 'stress dose' (determined by the doctor) plus the regular daily medicine. The child should wear a medical alert bracelet or necklace. Sometimes prednisone or dexamethasone can be used instead of hydrocortisone.
- *Replacements for sex hormones:* Boys take testosterone. Girls take estrogen. Testosterone can be injections 1–2 times monthly or topical daily. Estrogen can be oral daily or a topical patch changed a few times each week. When puberty development is nearly complete, girls may use an estrogen/progesterone combination.
- *Replacements for antidiuretic hormone:* Nasal spray or tablets of desmopressin/DDAVP that melt in the mouth or can be swallowed work for children. (Some are used once a day, some more often; everyone is different). Infants with diabetes insipidus can receive chlorothiazide; this oral drug helps lower the infant's large urine output.

HYPERPITUITARISM

Introduction

The pituitary gland is a tiny pea-sized endocrine gland located in a bony cavity in the base of the brain. It plays a major role in regulating a wide range of biological functions.

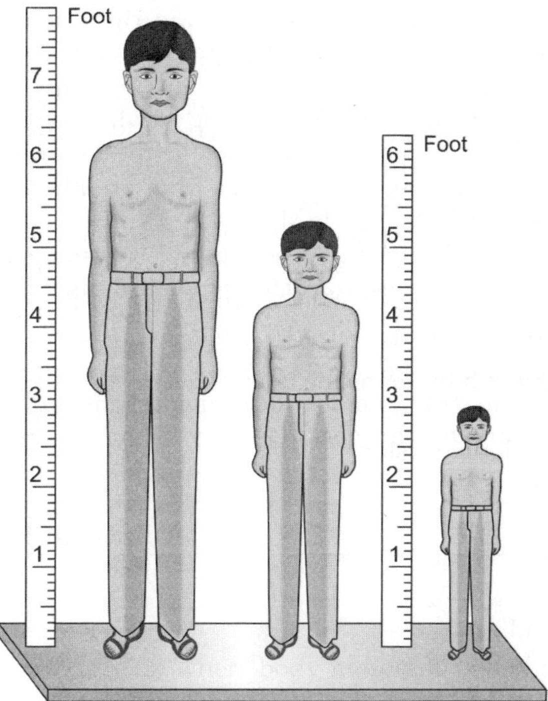

Fig. 7.95: Child with hyperpituitarism (acromegaly and gigantism)

It secretes a number of hormones involved in metabolism, growth, blood pressure and sexual maturation and function. Blood vessels connect the pituitary gland to a part of the brain known as the hypothalamus. The brain tells the pituitary to increase or decrease the secretion of certain hormones.

When the pituitary gland is overactive, it secretes excessive amounts of some hormones, usually due to the presence of a benign (noncancerous) tumor. Overactivity of the pituitary gland is called hyperpituitarism.

Definition

Hyperpituitarism also called acromegaly and gigantism. Hypersecretion of pituitary hormones secondary to macroadenomas can interfere with other pituitary hormone functions, resulting in target organ hormone deficiencies. Acromegaly occurs after epiphyseal closure, causing bone thickening and transverse growth and visceromegaly.

Hyperpituitarism can cause:

- Excessive hair growth in women
- Large hands, feet, forehead and face
- Skin discoloration
- Tongue problems.

Causes

- A pituitary tumor that is benign (adenoma) is most commonly the cause of overproduction of HGH.
- In rare cases, a tumor in the area of the brain right behind the pituitary gland (hypothalamus) might over stimulate HGH production.
- Benign tumors are the most frequent cause of an overactive pituitary. Generally it is not known why these tumors occur. Depending on which types of cells are affected, the pituitary gland will start to secrete excessive amounts of one or two hormones.
- In some cases, pituitary tumors may result from an inherited condition known as multiple endocrine neoplasia type 1 (MEN1).
- This disorder also causes benign tumors of the pancreas and parathyroid glands. In rare cases, a cancerous tumor or a disorder of the hypothalamus may be the underlying cause.

Signs and Symptoms

Symptoms of excess growth hormone include:

- Headache
- Visual field loss or double vision
- Excessive sweating
- Hoarseness
- Milk secretion from breast
- Sleep Apnea
- Carpal Tunnel Syndrome
- Joint pain and limitation of motion
- Muscle weakness
- Numbness or tingling of skin.

Diagnostic Evaluation

- Physical examination (to include visual-field exams) and child history. (large, 'doughy' hands; large feet; large face; enlarged jaw; tongue problems; big forehead; darkened skin in armpits; widely spaced teeth; oily, tough skin; skin pigmentation changes—darker or lighter; excessive hair growth in females; high blood pressure; goiter (enlarged thyroid); kyphosis or loss of disc spaces of the spine; osteoporosis; osteoarthritis).
- Blood tests will reveal elevated quantities of HGH which are not completely decreased by glucose administration.
- In the blood, elevated amounts of somatomedin-C (IGF–1) are measured.
- Computed tomography scans and MRI or magnetic resonance imaging, can identify a pituitary tumor.
- Increased bone mass detection using X-rays.

Management

Medical Management

Drugs may be used to shrink large tumors before surgery or in cases where surgery is not an option. Medication to reduce prolactin levels is usually the preferred treatment for patients with a prolactinoma. Dopamine inhibits prolactin secretion. Bromocriptine and cabergoline are dopamine agonists (drugs that behave like dopamine) and can shrink prolactinomas and return secretions of prolactin to normal levels.

Child with acromegaly may be treated with somatostatin analogs to lower growth hormone levels and shrink tumors. Dopamine agonists may also be used alone or in combination with somatostatin analogs.

Surgical Management

A procedure called a trans sphenoidal adenomectomy is usually recommended for patients with acromegaly or Cushing's disease. The surgeon makes a small incision through the nose or upper lip to reach the pituitary and remove the tumor. Although this procedure is very delicate, it has a success rate higher than 80% when performed by experienced surgeons. Trans sphenoidal surgery is most effective for small tumors (under 10 mm in diameter). Potential drawbacks include long-term dependence on pituitary hormone replacement therapy and cerebrospinal fluid leakage.

Radiation Therapy

Radiation may be used to treat patients who cannot undergo surgery or who have some residual tumor tissue after surgery and do not respond to medication.

There are two approaches to radiation: Conventional and stereotactic therapies.

1. Conventional radiation therapy is administered in small doses over a period of 4 to 6 weeks. One drawback is that radiation treatments can damage normal tissue surrounding the tumor.
2. Stereotactic therapy provides a high-dose beam of radiation targeted at the tumor. It may be completed in one session, resulting in less damage to surrounding tissue. Most patients that undergo radiation treatment require hormone replacement therapy due to a gradual decline in the secretion of other pituitary hormones.

Nursing management of pituitary disorders:

- Monitor vital signs blood pressure, heart rate and rhythm every 2 hours.
- Assess lung and heart sounds 4 hourly.
- Watch for chest pain or dyspnea because hypothyroidism can develop chronic arteriosclerosis.
- Monitor weight daily because ADH from pituitary gland regulates fluid retention and excretion in the body.
- Administer human growth hormone as prescribed.
- Somatropin should be injected subcutaneously on a daily basis, preferably in the evening.
- Teach patients that thyroid replacement therapy must be taken for lifetime and administered in the morning on an empty stomach because thyroid medications can cause insomnia if taken at night.
- Teaching patient to never miss any dose of medication without consulting with physician.
- Provide high protein, low calorie fiber food.
- Provide iodine rich diet, which is easily accomplished with iodized salt.
- Instruct patient to avoid constipation and provide stool softeners.
- Monitor laboratory test for hormonal deficiencies until the patient completes hormone replacement therapy.
- Administer replacement fluids, electrolytes and glucose as prescribed by physician to maintain normal serum levels.
- Monitor intake and output to ensure the balance is equal due to hormone regulation.
- Monitor physical and mental status and encourage patient to express their feelings.
- Instruct the patient when sleeping with head elevation position to reduce trauma to the eye.
- Teach the parents to change child positions slowly and to notify health care provider immediately if they develop an increased or irregular pulse, palpitations, nervousness, heat intolerance, diarrhea, sweating or irritability.

DIABETES INSIPIDUS

Introduction

Diabetes insipidus is a rare disorder of vasopressin (also called the antidiuretic hormone or ADH), a hormone that helps the kidneys regulate the amount of water in the body. Normally, the pituitary gland releases vasopressin to decrease the amount of urine the kidneys send to the bladder, thus keeping you from getting dehydrated.

Diabetes insipidus is a rare condition where the body cannot retain enough water. It occurs in approximately one in 25,000 people and can affect anyone of any age. It is more common in adults. Diabetes insipidus is very different from diabetes mellitus, which is often just referred to as diabetes. Diabetes mellitus is far more common and occurs when there is too much glucose (sugar) in the blood. It is possible for someone with diabetes mellitus to also develop diabetes insipidus although this is extremely rare.

Definition

Diabetes insipidus is a condition that results from insufficient production of the antidiuretic hormone (ADH), or vasopressin. ADH helps the kidneys and body conserve the correct amount of water. For this reason, it is also called 'water diabetes.'

Normally, ADH controls the kidneys' concentration of urine. It is secreted by the hypothalamus (a small gland located at the base of the brain), stored in the pituitary gland and then released into the bloodstream. ADH is secreted to concentrate the urine and decrease the amount of urine output, which helps prevent dehydration. Diabetes insipidus typically increases thirst and causes excessive production of dilute urine.

Diabetes insipidus (DI) is a condition characterized by excessive thirst and excretion of large amounts of severely diluted urine, with reduction of fluid intake having no effect on the latter. There are several different types of DI, each with a different cause.

Incidence

Diabetes insipidus is uncommon, with a prevalence of 1 case per 25,000 people.

- Mortality is rare in adults as long as water is available.
- Severe dehydration, hypernatremia, fever, cardiovascular collapse and death can ensue in children, elderly people, or in those with complicating illnesses.
- No significant sex differences in central or nephrogenic diabetes insipidus exist.
- Male and female prevalence are equal.

Etiology

- ADH fails to properly regulate your body's levels of water
- A tumor (cancerous or non-cancerous) in or around your hypothalamus, or pituitary gland
- A head injury
- An infection or illness affecting the brain, such as meningitis (infection of the meninges, the membranes in your brain)
- Surgery to the pituitary gland
- An inherited kidney problem
- Kidney conditions, such as Pyelonephritis (infection of your kidneys caused by bacteria).

Certain Medications such as

- Lithium and tetracycline, which can reduce the sensitivity of the nephrons. Lithium is sometimes prescribed to treat bipolar disorder (mood disorder with extreme mood swings)
- Tetracycline is an antibiotic that is sometimes used to treat common skin conditions, such as acne.

Types

- Neurogenic diabetes insipidus (or) central diabetes insipidus
- Nephrogenic diabetes insipidus
- Gestational diabetes insipidus
- Primary polydipsia.

Neurogenic Diabetes Insipidus (DI)

Insufficient production or secretion of ADH, resulting from damage to the hypothalamus or pituitary gland. Typical causes include injuries to the brain and rare genetic disorders. The most common type is Neurogenic DI, caused by a deficiency of arginine vasopressin (AVP), also known as antidiuretic hormone (ADH).

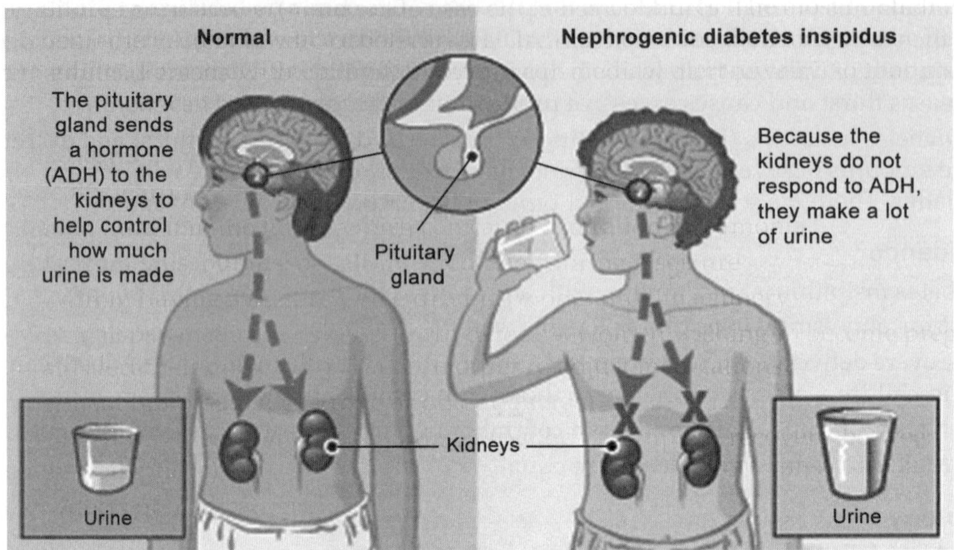

Fig. 7.96: Nephrogenic diabetes insipidus

Nephrogenic Diabetes Insipidus (DI)

The second common type of DI is nephrogenic diabetes insipidus, which is caused by an insensitivity of the kidneys to ADH. It can also be an iatrogenic artifact of drug use and nephrogenic diabetes insipidus occurs when there is enough ADH in the body, but the kidneys fail to respond to it. It can run in families or it can be caused by kidney damage. Diabetes insipidus can be treated by correcting the amount of urine that is produced by the body although the condition usually requires life-long treatment.

Gestational Diabetes Insipidus

Gestational diabetes insipidus occurs only during pregnancy and when an enzyme made by the placenta the system of blood vessels and other tissue that allows the exchange of nutrients and waste products between a mother and her baby destroys ADH in the mother.

Primary Polydipsia

This condition also known as dipsogenic diabetes insipidus or psychogenic polydipsia can cause excretion of large volumes of dilute urine. Rather than a problem with ADH production or damage, the underlying cause is intake of excessive fluids. Prolonged excessive water intake by itself can damage the kidneys and suppress ADH, making your body unable to concentrate urine. Primary polydipsia can be the result of abnormal thirst caused by damage to the thirst-regulating mechanism, situated in the hypothalamus. Primary polydipsia can also be caused by mental illness.

Signs and Symptoms

Each child may experience symptoms differently. Common symptoms may include:

- Excessive thirst
- Excessive urine production
- Dehydration.

Infants with diabetes insipidus may also exhibit the following symptoms:

- Irritability
- Poor feeding
- Failure to grow
- High fevers.

Pathophysiology

The amount of water in the body is regulated by a hormone which is known as antidiuretic hormone (ADH), or vasopressin. ADH is made by a part of the brain called the hypothalamus and is stored just below the brain, in the pituitary gland, until it is needed.

Based on etiological factors

↓

When the amount of water in the body becomes too low

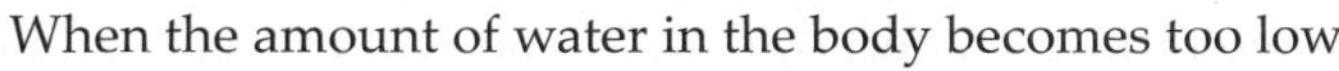

↓

Normally ADH is released from the pituitary gland. This helps to retain water in the body by stopping the kidneys from producing urine.

↓

Deficiencies of ADH, does not stop the kidneys from producing urine and allows too much water to be passed from the body.

↓

This results in symptoms such as needing to pass large quantities of urine often and feeling extremely thirsty all the time.

↓

Diabetes insipidus

Diagnostic Evaluation

- Urinalysis:
  - Dilute urine with a low specific gravity. Urine osmolarity and electrolyte levels are typically low.
- Blood Test: Level of ADH in blood
- Magnetic Resonance Imaging (MRI)
- Water deprivation test

- A water deprivation test, child will not be allowed to drink any liquid for several hours, to see whether or not you still continue to produce excess urine. If child have diabetes insipidus, you will continue to pass large amounts of dilute urine, compared with most people who would pass only a small amount of concentrated urine.

- Antidiuretic hormone (ADH) test
  - The endocrinologist will give the child a small-dose of ADH, usually as an injection. This will show how your body reacts to the hormone and can help to identify which type of diabetes insipidus you have. If the dose of ADH causes you to stop producing urine, it is likely that your condition is due to a shortage of ADH. If this is the case, child may be diagnosed with cranial diabetes insipidus.

Management (Gestational DI)

- Desmopressin
- Carbamazepine
- *Anti-convulsive medication:* It has also had some success in this type of DI. Also gestational DI tends to abate on its own 4 to 6 weeks following labor, though some women may develop it again in subsequent pregnancies. In dipsogenic DI, desmopressin is not usually an option.
- *Nephrogenic DI:* Desmopressin will be ineffective in nephrogenic DI. Instead, the diuretic hydrochlorothiazide (HCT or HCTZ) or indomethacin can improve nephrogenic diabetes insipidus.
  - *Prevent dehydration:* As long as you take your medication and have access to water when the medication's effects wear off, you will prevent serious problems. Plan ahead by carrying water with you wherever you go and keep a supply of medication in your travel bag, at work or at school.
  - *Wear a medical alert bracelet or carry a medical alert card in your wallet.* If you have a medical emergency, a health care professional will recognize immediately your need for special treatment.

Nursing Management

- Obtain history of onset of signs and symptoms of clinical manifestations
- Assess the level of weight loss
- Height and weight measurements
- Blood pressure measurements
- Thyroid examination
- Examination of hands, fingers, feet and toes for circulatory abnormalities
- Blood tests for ADH
- Family history of diabetes, cardiovascular disease and stroke
- Prior infections and medical conditions
- A list of current medications, including:
  - Prescription medications
  - Over-the-counter medications
  - Vitamin, mineral or herbal supplements.
- Smoking history, including encouragement to stop smoking (if applicable).

DIABETES MELLITUS (IDDM AND NIDDM)

Introduction

Diabetes mellitus is a metabolic disorder where in human body does not produce or properly uses insulin, a hormone that is required to convert sugar, starches and other food into energy. Diabetes mellitus is characterized by constant high levels of blood glucose (sugar). Human body has to maintain the blood glucose level at a very narrow range, which is done with insulin and glucagon. The function of glucagon is causing the liver to release glucose from its cells into the blood, for the production of energy.

Definition

Diabetes mellitus is a group of metabolic diseases characterized by high blood sugar (glucose) levels, which result from defects in insulin secretion, or action, or both. In patients with diabetes, the absence or insufficient production of insulin causes hyperglycemia.

—*Wongs*

Diabetes mellitus is a group of metabolic diseases characterized by high blood sugar (glucose) levels that result from defects in insulin secretion, or action, or both. Diabetes mellitus, commonly referred to as diabetes (as it will be in this article) was first identified as a disease associated with 'sweet urine'.

—*Wikipedia*

Incidence

The American Diabetes Association reported in 2009 that there are 23.6 million children and adults in the United States—7.8% of the population, who have diabetes. While an estimated 17.9 million in the US alone have been diagnosed with diabetes, nearly one in four (5.7 million) diabetics are unaware that they have the disease.

Etiology

Genetic and acquired, include autoimmune reactions. Autoimmune destruction the islets of Langerhans in the pancreas (which secrete insulin) results.

Classification

Four types of diabetes are recognized:

1. Type 1 diabetes mellitus or insulin-dependent (IDDM) or juvenile diabetes
2. Type 2 diabetes mellitus or non-insulin-dependent (NIDDM)
3. *Gestational diabetes:* Pregnant women who have never had diabetes before but who have high blood sugar (glucose) levels during pregnancy are said to have gestational diabetes. Gestational diabetes affects about 4% of all pregnant women and is usually of type 2.
4. *Pre-diabetes:* Termed 'America's largest health care epidemic,' pre-diabetes is a condition that occurs when a person's blood glucose levels are higher than normal but not high enough for a diagnosis of type 2 diabetes. As of 2009 there are 57 million Americans who have pre-diabetes.

Type 1 Diabetes Mellitus (Juvenile Diabetes)

Type 1 diabetes mellitus is characterized by loss of the insulin-producing beta cells of the islets of Langerhans in the pancreas, leading to a deficiency of insulin. There is no known preventative measure that can be taken against type 1 diabetes, which comprises up to 10% of diabetes mellitus cases. Type 1 diabetes can affect children or adults but was traditionally termed 'juvenile diabetes' because it represents a majority of cases of diabetes affecting children.

Type 1 diabetes in children is a condition in which your child's pancreas no longer produces the insulin your child needs to survive and you will need to replace the missing insulin. Type 1 diabetes in children used to be known as juvenile diabetes or insulin-dependent diabetes.

Type 2 Diabetes Mellitus

Type 2 diabetes mellitus is due to insulin resistance or reduced insulin sensitivity, combined with reduced insulin secretion. The defective responsiveness of body tissues to insulin almost certainly involves the insulin receptor in cell membranes. Type 2 diabetes is the most common type.

Type 2 diabetes may go unnoticed for years because visible symptoms are typically mild, non-existent or sporadic and usually there are no ketoacidotic episodes. However, severe long-term complications can result from unnoticed type 2 diabetes, including renal failure due to diabetic nephropathy, vascular disease (including coronary artery disease), vision damage due to diabetic retinopathy, loss of sensation or pain due to diabetic neuropathy, liver damage from non-alcoholic steatohepatitis and heart failure from diabetic cardiomyopathy.

Causes

There is no way to prevent the type 1 diabetes. Although there is a genetic predisposition to develop this disease, only about 30 percent of children with type 1 diabetes (previously known as insulin-dependent diabetes) have any close relatives with the disease.

The destruction of the cells that make insulin results from a process in which the body's immune system views these cells as foreign invaders and mounts an immune response against them. This autoimmune process starts years before the first symptoms of diabetes show up. The trigger for this process may be viruses or other agents in the environment.

Genetic Issues

Clear evidence suggests a genetic component in type 1 diabetes mellitus. Monozygotic twins have a 60% lifetime concordance for developing type 1 diabetes mellitus, although only 30% do so within 10 years after the first twin is diagnosed. In contrast, dizygotic twins have only an 8% risk of concordance, which is similar to the risk among other siblings.

The frequency of diabetes development in children with a mother who has diabetes is 2–3%; this figure increases to 5–6% for children with a father who has type 1 diabetes mellitus. The risk to children rises to almost 30% if both parents are diabetic.

Environmental Factors

Environmental factors are important, because even identical twins have only a 30–60% concordance for type 1 diabetes mellitus and because incidence rates vary in genetically similar populations under different living conditions. No single factor has been identified, but infections and diet are considered the 2 most likely environmental candidates.

Viral infections may be the most important environmental factor in the development of type 1 diabetes mellitus, probably by initiating or modifying an autoimmune process. Instances have been reported of a direct toxic effect of infection in congenital rubella. One survey suggests enteroviral infection during pregnancy carries an increased risk of type 1 diabetes mellitus in the offspring. Paradoxically, type 1 diabetes mellitus incidence is higher in areas where the overall burden of infectious disease is lower.

- Dietary factors are also relevant. Breastfed infants have a lower risk for type 1 diabetes and a direct relationship is observed between per capita cow's milk consumption and the incidence of diabetes. Some cow's milk proteins (e.g. bovine serum albumin) have antigenic similarities to an islet cell antigen.
- Nitrosamines, chemicals found in smoked foods and some water supplies, are known to cause type 1 diabetes mellitus in animal models; however, no definite link has been made with humans.
- The known association of increasing incidence of type 1 diabetes mellitus with distance from the equator may now have an explanation. Reduced exposure to ultraviolet (UV) light and lower vitamin D levels, both of which are more likely found in the higher latitudes, are associated with an increased risk of type 1 diabetes mellitus.

Other Causes

Additional factors in the development of type 1 diabetes mellitus include the following:

- Congenital absence of the pancreas or islet cells
- Pancreatectomy
- Pancreatic damage (i.e. cystic fibrosis, chronic pancreatitis, thalassemia major, hemochromatosis, hemolytic-uremic syndrome)
- Wolfram syndrome (diabetes insipidus, diabetes mellitus, optic atrophy, deafness)
- Chromosomal disorders such as Down syndrome, Klinefelter, or Prader-Willi syndrome (the risk is said to be around 1% in Down and Turner syndromes).

Pathophysiology

Based on etiological factors

↓

Insufficient insulin secretion

↓

Cells respond poorly to the effects of insulin (insulin insensitivity or resistance), or insulin itself defective

↓

Glucose will not be absorbed properly by those body cells that require it or it will be stored appropriately in the liver and muscles

↓

Increased blood glucose level, poor protein synthesis and other metabolic derangements, such as acidosis

↓

Hyperglycemia

Signs and Symptoms

Symptoms may develop quite rapidly (weeks or months) in type 1 diabetes, particularly in children. However, in type 2 diabetes the symptoms develop much more slowly polyuria, polydipsia and polyphagia, weight loss (despite normal or increased eating) and irreducible fatigue glycosuria, blurred vision-prolonged high blood glucose causes glucose absorption, which leads to changes in the shape of the lenses of the eyes, resulting in vision changes, nausea; vomiting.

Diagnostic Evaluation

- Family history of diabetes
- Presence of symptoms
- Glycosuria on routine examination
- Ketonuria
- Fasting plasma glucose level at or above 126 mg/dL (7.0 mmol/L).
- Plasma glucose at or above 200 mg/dL (11.1 mmol/L) two hours after a 75 g oral glucose load as in a glucose tolerance test.
- Random plasma glucose at or above 200 mg/dL (11.1 mmol/L).

Management

- *Fluid therapy in DKA:* Treat dehydration, increase peripheral perfusion and replace sodium and potassium loss due to osmotic diuresis.
- *Insulin therapy:* To reduce hyperglycemia.
- Subcutaneous insulin may be given twice a day.
- Dosage needs are based on the childs size, diet and level of activity. Dose are adjusted through daily monitoring of blood glucose level.
- Insulin pump therapy can be given in some cases. Balanced diet with controlled carbohydrates and adequate protein and fat to meet energy and growth requirements.

Dietary Management

Since children with diabetes have the same nutritional needs for growth and development as other children, they do not need to be on a special diet. Child's meal plan is one of the most important parts of managing diabetes. It can also be one of the most challenging for children and their families. Dietitians who are diabetes educators work with children and their families to assist in making meal planning healthful and to accommodate the child's and family's individual food preferences and meal schedule.

A good diet for children with diabetes at all ages is the same as that recommended for everyone.

Nursing Management

- Obtain history of onset of signs and symptoms of clinical manifestations
- Assess the level of weight loss
- Check for sores that are slow to heal
- Identity any fruit smell to breath acetone breath due to ketosis
- Height and weight measurements

- Blood pressure measurements
- Thyroid examination
- Examination of hands, fingers, feet and toes for circulatory abnormalities
- Blood tests for fasting blood sugar, A1c and cholesterol
- Family history of diabetes, cardiovascular disease and stroke
- Prior infections and medical conditions
- A list of current medications, including:
  - Prescription medications
  - Over-the-counter medications
  - Vitamin, mineral or herbal supplements
- Smoking history, including encouragement to stop smoking (if applicable)
- Signs of complications with pregnancy or trying to get pregnant for women patients
- Eating and exercise habits
- Vision abnormalities, to check for eye health issues
- Urination abnormalities, which can indicate kidney disease.

Nursing Intervention

- Fluid volume deficit related to osmotic diuresis and vomiting
- Altered nutrition: Less than body requirements due to metabolism catabolism due to lack of insulin
- Knowledge deficit related to insulin management
- Knowledge deficit related to blood glucose monitoring
- Risk for injury related to hypoglycemia
- Fear and anxiety of child and family related to diagnosis, treatment and management procedures.

Complication

- Hyperglycemia
- Hypoglycemia
- Diabetic Ketoacidosis (DKA)
- Skeletal and joint abnormalities
- Growth failure
- Retinopathy
- Neuropathy
- Nephropathy
- Cardiopathy.

HYPERTHYROIDISM (GRAVES' DISEASE)

Introduction

The thyroid gland is one of the seven major glands that make up the endocrine system. Endocrine glands produce hormones that are transported by the blood system to all parts of the body. These hormones regulate many of the bodies processes, such as reproduction, growth rate, metabolism, etc. The thyroid gland consists of two lobes and is situated in the neck on either side of the windpipe.

It is responsible for the production of the thyroid hormones, thyroxin (known as T_4) and triiodothyronine (T_3). Thyroid hormones regulate the body's metabolic rate and as this involves the digestive, circulatory and nervous systems, it becomes obvious that a disorder of the thyroid gland can produce many different clinical signs. These include fast heart beat and symptoms of palpitations, nervous system tremor and anxiety symptoms, digestive system hypermotility (diarrhea) and weight loss.

Definition

Hyperthyroidism is the term for overactive tissue within the thyroid gland, resulting in overproduction and thus an excess of circulating free thyroid hormones thyroxine (T_4), triiodothyronine (T_3), or both. Thyroid hormone is important at a cellular level, affecting nearly every type of tissue in the body.

Causes

Functional thyroid tissue producing an excess of thyroid hormone occurs in a number of clinical conditions.

The major causes:

- Graves' disease (the most common etiology with 70–80%)
- Toxic thyroid adenoma
- Toxic multinodular goiter
- *Thyroiditis:* There are a number of different kinds of thyroiditis including Hashimoto's (immune mediated) and subacute (DeQuervain's). These may be initially aassociated with secretion of excess thyroid hormone, but usually progress to gland dysfunction and thus, to hormone deficiency and hypothyroidism.
- Oral consumption of excess thyroid hormone tablets (termed 'Hamburger hyperthyroidism').
- Amiodarone, an anti-arrhythmic drug is structurally similar to thyroxin and may cause both under- or over activity of the thyroid.
- Postpartum thyroiditis (PPT) occurs in about 7% of women during the year after they give birth. PPT typically has several phases, the first of which is hyperthyroidism.

Pathophysiology

Based on etiological factors

↓

Hypothalamus produces thyrotropin-releasing hormone (TRH)

↓

Stimulates the anterior pituitary gland to secrete thyroid-stimulating hormone (TSH)

↓

Thyroid gland to release thyroid hormone

↓

Thyroid hormone concentration is regulated by negative feedback by circulating free hormone. The secretion of TRH is also partially regulated by higher cortical centers.

↓

The thyroid gland produces the parathormone thyroxin (T_4), kidneys to its active form, triiodothyronine (T_3). The thyroid gland also produces a small amount of T_3 directly.

↓

Unbound T_4 and T_3 levels best correlate with the patient's clinical status.

↓

Hyperthyroidism

Signs and Symptoms

Major clinical signs include:

- Weight loss (often accompanied by an increased appetite)
- Anxiety
- Intolerance to heat, fatigue
- Hair loss, weakness
- Hyperactivity, irritability
- Apathy, depression
- Polyuria, polydipsia
- Delirium, tremor
- Pre-orbital myxedema and sweating.

Additional symptoms such as:

- Palpitations and arrhythmias (notably atrial fibrillation)
- Shortness of breath (dyspnea)
- Loss of libido, nausea, vomiting and diarrhea.
- Long-term untreated hyperthyroidism can lead to osteoporosis
- In the elderly, these classical symptoms may not be present.

Neurological manifestations can include:

- Tremors, chorea, myopathy
- Periodic paralysis
- Myasthenia gravis
- Thyrotoxicosis are pseudotumor cerebral, amyotrophic lateral sclerosis
- Guillain-Barré-like syndrome.

Thyrotoxic Crisis

Thyrotoxic crisis (or thyroid storm) is a rare but severe complication of hyperthyroidism, which may occur when a thyrotoxic patient becomes very sick or physically stressed. Its symptoms can include: An increase in body temperature to over 40 degrees celsius (104 degrees Fahrenheit), tachycardia, arrhythmia, vomiting, diarrhea, dehydration, coma and death.

Diagnostic Evaluation

History Collection

- Weight loss
- Patients typically report an average loss of approximately 15% of their prior weight.

- Basal metabolic rate is increased with a stimulation of lipolysis and lipogenesis.
- Palpitations

Physical Examination

- Fever
- Tachycardia (often out of proportion to the fever)
- Diaphoresis (often profuse)
- Dehydration secondary to GI losses and diaphoresis
- Warm, moist skin
- Widened pulse pressure
- Congestive heart failure (may be a high output failure)
- Thyromegaly
  - Nontender, diffuse enlargement in Graves disease
  - Tender, diffusely enlarged gland in thyroiditis
  - Thyroid nodules, either single or multinodular goiter.
- Exophthalmos
- Shock
- Atrial fibrillation
  - Typically in elderly patients
  - May be refractory to attempted rate control with digitalis
  - Converts after antithyroid therapy in 20–50% of patients.
- Myopathy
- *Thyroid bruit:* Relatively specific for thyrotoxicosis
- Fine, resting tremor.

Blood Tests

Measuring the level of thyroid-stimulating hormone (TSH) in the blood is usually all that is required. A low TSH indicates that the pituitary gland is being inhibited by increased levels of T_4 and/or T_3 in the blood and is therefore a reliable marker of hyperthyroidism.

Measuring Specific Antibodies

Anti-TSH-receptor antibodies in Graves' disease, or anti-thyroid-peroxidase in Hashimoto's thyroiditism common cause of hypothyroidism—may also contribute to the diagnosis.

- Thyroid scintigraphy is a useful test to distinguish between causes of hyperthyroidism and this entity from thyroiditis.
- FNA Biopsy (Fine Needle Aspiration).
- Ultrasound testing and other radioactive scans can be done to determine whether these nodules are cancerous or not.

Management

Medical Management

Thyrostatics medication (Temporary medical therapy): Thyrostatics are believed to work by inhibiting the iodination of thyroglobulin by thyroperoxidase and thus, the formation of tetra-iodothyronine (T_4). Propylthiouracil also works outside the thyroid gland, preventing conversion of (mostly inactive) T_4 to the active form T_3.

- Carbimazole
- Methimazole
- Propylthiouracil
- Levothyroxine supplementation.

Beta-blockers

Beta blockers are a class of drug which offset this effect, reducing rapid pulse associated with the sensation of palpitations and decreasing tremor and anxiety. This does not help the underlying problem of excess thyroid hormone.

- Propranolol
- Metoprolol

Surgical Management

Surgical or Radioisotope Therapy

Graves' disease patients who cannot tolerate medicines for one reason or another, patients who are allergic to iodine, or patients who refuse radioiodine option for surgical intervention.

- Partial thyroidectomies
- Radioisotope therapy.

HYPOTHYROIDISM

Introduction

This arises when too little thyroid hormone is produced and circulated in the blood stream. This is caused by inflammation of the gland, autoimmune thyroiditis (which is probably an inherited condition), or the wasting away of the gland itself for reasons at present unknown. In the past it was thought that thyroid problems could be due to an iodine deficient diet (iodine is an essential component of the thyroid hormones).

Definition

Hypothyroidism is the disease state in humans and in animals caused by insufficient production of thyroid hormone by the thyroid gland. Cretinism is a form of hypothyroidism found in infants.

Causes

The most common cause of hypothyroidism is:

- Inflammation of the thyroid gland, which damages the gland's cells.
- Autoimmune or Hashimoto's thyroiditis, in which the immune system attacks the thyroid gland, is the most common example of this. Some women develop hypothyroidism after pregnancy (often referred to as 'postpartum thyroiditis').

Other common causes of hypothyroidism include:

- Congenital (birth) defects
- Radiation treatments to the neck to treat different cancers, which may also damage the thyroid gland

- Radioactive iodine used to treat an overactive thyroid (hyperthyroidism)
- Surgical removal of part or all of the thyroid gland, done to treat other thyroid problems
- Viral thyroiditis, which may case hyperthyroidism and is often followed by temporary or permanent hypothyroidism.

Types

Type	Origin	Description
Primary	Thyroid gland	The most common forms include Hashimoto's thyroiditis (an autoimmune disease) and radioiodine therapy for hyperthyroidism
Secondary	Pituitary gland	Occurs if the pituitary gland does not create enough thyroid stimulating hormones (TSH) to induce the thyroid gland to produce enough thyroxine and triiodothyronine. Although not every case of secondary hypothyroidism has a clear-cut cause, it is usually caused by damage to the pituitary gland, as by a tumor, radiation, or surgery
Tertiary	Hypothalamus	Results when the hypothalamus fails to produce sufficient thyrotropin-releasing hormone (TRH). TRH prompts the pituitary gland to produce thyrotropin

Signs and Symptoms

Early Symptoms

- Being more sensitive to cold
- Constipation
- Depression
- Fatigue or feeling slowed down
- Heavier menstrual periods
- Joint or muscle pain
- Paleness or dry skin
- Thin, brittle hair or fingernails
- Weakness
- Weight gain (unintentional).

Late Symptoms, If Left Untreated

- Decreased taste and smell
- Hoarseness
- Puffy face, hands and feet
- Slow speech
- Thickening of the skin
- Thinning of eyebrows.

Diagnostic Evaluation

A physical examination may reveal a smaller-than-normal thyroid gland, although sometimes the gland is normal size or even enlarged (goiter). The examination may also reveal:

- Brittle nails
- Coarse facial features

- Pale or dry skin, which may be cool to the touch
- Swelling of the arms and legs
- Thin and brittle hair.

A chest X-ray may show an enlarged heart.

Laboratory tests to determine thyroid function include:

- Serum TSH
- T_4 test

Lab tests may also reveal:

- Anemia on a complete blood count (CBC)
- Increased cholesterol levels
- Increased liver enzymes
- Increased prolactin
- Low sodium.

Management

Hypothyroidism is treated with the levorotatory forms of thyroxine (L-T_4) and triiodothyronine (L-T_3). Both synthetic and animal-derived thyroid tablets are available and can be prescribed for patients in need of additional thyroid hormone. Thyroid hormone is taken daily and doctors can monitor blood levels to help assure proper dosing. There are several different treatment protocols in thyroid replacement therapy:

T_4 Only

This treatment involves supplementation of levothyroxine alone, in a synthetic form. It is currently the standard treatment in mainstream medicine.

T_4 and T_3 in Combination

This treatment protocol involves administering both synthetic L-T_4 and L-T_3 simultaneously in combination.

Desiccated Thyroid Extract

Desiccated thyroid extract is an animal-based thyroid extract, most commonly from a porcine source. It is also a combination therapy, containing natural forms of L-T_4 and L-T_3.

Nursing Management

- Advice the parents Do Not stop taking the medication when you feel better. Continue taking the medication exactly as directed by your doctor.
- Advice the parents if you change brands of thyroid medicine, let your doctor know. Your levels may need to be checked.
- Advice the parents about dietary changes can change the way your body absorbs the thyroid medicine.
- Thyroid medicine works best on an empty stomach and when taken 1 hour before any other medications.
- Advice the parents Do Not take thyroid hormone with calcium, iron, multivitamins, alumin hydroxide antacids, colestipol, or other medicines that bind bile acids, or fiber supplements.

Complication

Myxedema coma, the most severe form of hypothyroidism, is rare. It may be caused by an infection, illness, exposure to cold, or certain medications in people with untreated hypothyroidism.

Symptoms and signs of myxedema coma include:

- Below normal temperature
- Decreased breathing
- Low blood pressure
- Low blood sugar
- Unresponsiveness

Other complications are:

- Heart disease
- Increased risk of infection
- Infertility
- Miscarriage

People with untreated hypothyroidism are at increased risk for:

- Giving birth to a baby with birth defects
- Heart disease because of higher levels of LDL ('bad') cholesterol
- Heart failure.

PHENYLKETONURIA (PKU)

Introduction

Phenylketonuria (PKU) is an autosomal recessive genetic disorder characterized by a deficiency in the enzyme hepatic phenylalanine hydroxylase. This enzyme is necessary to metabolize the amino acid phenylalanine to the amino acid tyrosine.

PAH is deficient, phenylalanine accumulates and is converted into phenylpyruvate (also known as phenylketone), which is detected in the urine. Untreated condition can cause problems with brain development, leading to progressive mental retardation, brain damage and seizures. However, PKU is one of the few genetic diseases that can be controlled by diet. A diet low in phenylalanine and high in tyrosine can be a very effective treatment. There is no cure.

Definition

Phenylketonuria (PKU) is a genetic disorder that is characterized by an inability of the body to utilize the essential amino acid, phenylalanine. Amino acids are the building blocks for body proteins. 'Essential' amino acids can only be obtained from the food we eat as our body does not normally produce them.

Incidence

- PKU and the other causes of hyperphenylalaninemia affect about one of every 10,000 to 20,000 Caucasian or Oriental births. The incidence in African Americans is far less. These disorders are equally frequent in males and females.

- PKU is about 1 in 15,000 births, but the incidence varies widely in different human populations from 1 in 4,500 births.

Causes

- PKU and the other causes of hyperphenylalaninemia are inherited in a recessive fashion. This means an affected person inherited two traits for the disorder (e.g. one from each parent).
- Phenylketonuria is caused by autosomal recessive inheritance due to mutations in the enzyme phenylalanine hydroxylase.
- The enzyme locus is on chromosome arm 12q. More than 100 mutations are known and mutation frequency varies among ethnic groups.
- Genotype and phenotype are broadly related (i.e. reproducible mild vs severe mutations), but unrelated individuals with identical mutations have some degree of variability in phenylalanine tolerance.

Pathophysiology

Based on etiological factors (Hyperphenylalaninemia)

↓

Deficiency of the enzyme

↓

Phenylalanine hydroxylase

↓

Deficiency is inherited in an autosomal recessive manner

↓

Elevated phenylalanine levels

↓

Cause mental retardation is not known, phenylketonuria

Signs and Symptoms

Infants with PKU appear normal at birth:

- Blue eyes
- Fairer hair and skin than other family members
- Vomiting
- Irritability
- An eczema-like rash
- A mousy odor to the urine.

Signs of Nervous System Function Problems

- Increased muscle tone
- More active muscle tendon reflexes
- Severe brain problems occur
- Mental retardation and seizures.

Untreated Children Include

- Microcephaly (small head)
- Prominent cheek and upper jaw bones with widely spaced teeth
- Poor development of tooth enamel
- Decreased body growth.

Diagnostic Evaluation

Screening for Phenylketonuria (PKU) includes the following:

- Follow-up with abnormal newborn screening results in accordance with local regulations.
- Low-grade elevations of phenylalanine may require repeat screening.
- More significant elevations may require definitive testing and/or referral to a metabolic treatment facility experienced with phenylketonuria.
- Late diagnoses are usually made during amino acid analysis of individuals who are developmentally abnormal.

A qualified laboratory should measure plasma phenylalanine and tyrosine.

A qualified laboratory should perform urine analysis of biopterin and neoptrins in order to rule out defects of biopterin synthesis or recycling.

Imaging Studies

MRI Scan

- Cranial MRI studies may be indicated in older individuals who have abandoned the diet and are experiencing deficits in motor or cognitive function.
- Areas of demyelination are common. These areas appear to be related to both higher phenylalanine levels in the blood and brain and to poorer cognitive outcome.

Magnetic resonance spectroscopy (MRS): Preliminary indications suggest that brain phenylalanine levels can be measured by MRS and that these levels may be more predictive of outcome than blood phenylalanine levels. However, this work is done in only a few centers and some controversy surrounds whether state-of-the-art technology makes it a useful clinical tool.

Management

Medical Management

Most patients with phenylketonuria (PKU) are treated in a specialty metabolic clinic, usually under the auspices of a genetics or pediatric endocrinology clinic. Treatment consists of dietary restriction of phenylalanine with tyrosine supplementation. The extent of phenylalanine restriction necessary for normal outcome remains controversial.

- Phenylalanine levels are followed at regular intervals, from 1–2 times weekly in neonates to once per month in older children and adults. Most US facilities recommend that phenylalanine levels be maintained from 2–6 mg/dL (120–360 mmol/L).
- 10 mg/kg PO qd initially; dosage ranges from 5–20 mg/kg/d; dissolve tab in 4–8 oz of water or apple juice and drink contents within 15 min of dissolving (tab may not dissolve completely, but swallowing small pieces floating on top of water or juice is normal and safe); administer with food to increase absorption.

Nursing Management

- The mainstay of the diet consists of phenylalanine restriction and supplementation of other essential amino acids, vitamins, minerals and energy intake, using medical foods and low-protein foods.
- Aspartame must also be eliminated. Phenylalanine is one of the primary components of aspartame. It is found in many artificially sweetened foods and soft drinks, as well as some vitamins and medicines. A 12-oz can of aspartame-sweetened diet drink contains approximately 105 mg of phenylalanine (i.e. 25–50% of the usual daily intake).
- The age at which the diet may be discontinued is somewhat controversial. Most US facilities no longer recommend discontinuation of the diet at any age.
- Most newborns with phenylketonuria require 40–60 mg/kg/d of dietary phenylalanine to maintain normal growth. Breastfeeding is usually possible and should not be stopped unless instructed to do so by a local health official or treatment facility. As growth slows, the phenylalanine requirement falls and older children and adults tolerate 200–400 mg/d.
- Providing some natural phenylalanine is essential in order to prevent deficiency of this essential amino acid. The diet requires elimination of all high-protein foods, such as meat, dairy, nuts and legumes. Starches, including bread, potatoes, corn and beans also must be restricted (a slice of bread or small order of fries contains approximately 120–150 mg phenylalanine).
- Essential amino acids, vitamins and minerals must be supplemented using medical foods. Currently, most are consumed as a powder dissolved in liquid (i.e. formula). Newer supplements, including capsules, amino acid bars and amino acids cooked into foods, are becoming available.
- Because most patients prefer a standard American diet, most teens and older children (in our clinic) cheat by failing to limit quantities of high-protein, non-meat foods, such as potatoes (e.g. fries, chips, mashed potatoes), pasta, bread and pizza crust (minus the cheese); however, few teens who were well managed as children cheat by consuming meat.

GALACTOSEMIA

Introduction

Galactosemia was first 'discovered' in 1908. Von Ruess, in a 1908 publication entitled, 'Sugar Excretion in Infancy,' reported on a breast-fed infant with failure to thrive, enlargement of the liver and spleen and 'galactosuria'. This infant ceased to excrete galactose through the urine when milk products were removed from the diet.

Galactosemia is a genetic disorder that is characterized by the patient's inability to metabolize sugar (galactose) into glucose. Glucose is readily usable by the body but galactose needs an enzyme called GALT to turn it into a sugar that the body can use. In nearly all people with this condition the body lacks the enzyme that is used in this process. When it is not broken down, the galactose remains in the body and the levels build up. Higher levels of galactose can act as a poison and have serious consequences for the health of the patient. Poor mental and physical growth and serious liver and kidney problems are just a few of the possible effects of this disorder.

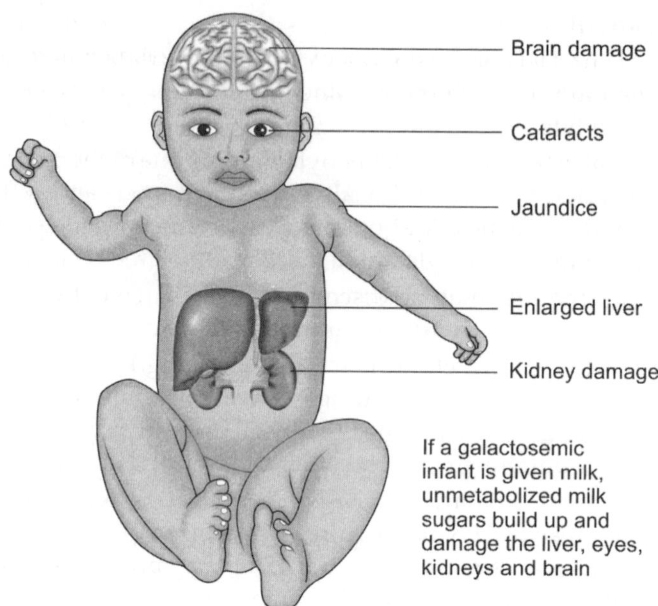

Galactosemia is a fairly rare disease that can affect about one in every eighty thousand or so babies although some figure put this much higher. The statistics do tend to vary depending on the source but this will give you a rough idea. Galactosemia is an inherited disease that is passed on by both parents being carriers.

Definition

Galactosemia is a genetic disorder that is characterized by the patient's inability to metabolize sugar (galactose) into glucose. Glucose is readily usable by the body but galactose needs an enzyme called GALT to turn it into a sugar that the body can use. In nearly all people with this condition the body lacks the enzyme that is used in this process. When it is not broken down, the galactose remains in the body and the levels build up.

Incidence

It is about 1 per 60,000 births (classic type). It is much rarer in Japan and much more common in Italy, specifically the traveler region. Galactosemia is also very common within the Irish Traveller population.

Causes

- Hereditary
- Lactose in food (broken down by the enzyme lactase into glucose and galactose.) with galactosemia
- Toxic levels of galactose in the blood, resulting in hepatomegaly (an enlarged liver), cirrhosis, renal failure, cataracts, brain damage
- Ovarian failure
- Without treatment, mortality in infants with galactosemia is about 75%.

There are three forms of the disease:

1. Galactose–1 phosphate uridyl transferase deficiency (classic galactosemia, the most common and most severe form)
2. Deficiency of galactose kinase
3. Deficiency of galactose–6-phosphate epimerase

People with galactosemia are unable to fully break down the simple sugar galactose. Galactose makes up half of lactose, the sugar found in milk. The other sugar is glucose.

If an infant with galactosemia is given milk, substances made from galactose build up in the infant's system. These substances damage the liver, brain, kidneys and eyes.

Persons with galactosemia cannot tolerate any form of milk (human or animal). They must be careful about eating other foods containing galactose.

Signs and Symptoms

Signs include:

- Amino acids in the urine and/or blood plasma (aminoaciduria)
- Enlarged liver (hepatomegaly)
- Fluid in the abdomen (ascites)
- Low blood sugar (hypoglycemia).

Newborn screening in many states will test for this condition.

Infants with galactosemia can develop symptoms in the first few days of life if they eat formula or breast milk that contains lactose. The symptoms may be due to a serious blood infection with the bacteria *E. coli*.

- Convulsions
- Irritability
- Lethargy
- Poor feeding (baby refuses to eat formula containing milk)
- Poor weight gain
- Yellow skin and whites of the eyes (jaundice)
- Vomiting

Pathophysiology

Based on etiological factors (hereditary)

↓

Lack of a liver enzyme (GALT)

↓

Galactose cannot be broken down into glucose and it remain in the body as galactose (toxic form)

↓

The cells and becomes toxic

↓

The body then produces abnormal chemicals

↓

Which causes the symptoms seen in infants with untreated galactosemia

Diagnostic Evaluation

Newborn Screening

Symptoms of lethargy, vomiting, diarrhea, failure to thrive and jaundice. None of these symptoms are specific to galactosemia, often leading to diagnostic delays. Luckily, most infants are diagnosed on newborn screening.

Blood Test

Tests include:

- Blood culture for bacteria infection (*E. coli* sepsis)
- Enzyme activity in the red blood cells
- Ketones in the urine
- Prenatal diagnosis by directly measuring the enzyme galactose–1-phosphate uridyl transferase
- 'Reducing substances' in the infant's urine and normal or low blood sugar while the infant is being fed breast milk or a formula containing lactose
- Prenatal diagnosis is also feasible by direct measurement of the enzyme.

Urine Test

- A person with galactosemia does not have one of these enzymes. This causes high levels of galactose in the blood or urine.

Management

Child with this condition must avoid all milk, milk-containing products (including dry milk) and other foods that contain galactose for life. It is essential to read product labels and be an informed consumer.

Infants can be fed with:

- Soya formula
- Meat-based formula or Nutramigen (a protein hydrolysate formula)
- Another lactose-free formula

Calcium supplements are recommended.

- Treatment for galactosemia is the elimination of galactose and lactose from the diet throughout life. A person with galactosemia will never be able to properly digest foods containing galactose.
- There is no chemical or drug substitute for the missing enzyme at this time. An infant diagnosed with galactosemia will simply be changed to a soy-based formula that does not contain galactose.
- Galactosemia is often confused with lactose intolerance, but please keep in mind that galactosemia is a disease. A person with galactosemia will not 'grow out of' it.

Prevention

It is helpful to know your family history. If you have a family history of galactosemia and want to have children, genetic counseling will help you make decisions about pregnancy and prenatal testing. Once the diagnosis of galactosemia is made, genetic counseling is recommended for other members of the family. Many states screen all newborns for galactosemia. If parents learn that the test indicates possible galactosemia, they should promptly stop giving their infant milk products and ask their health care provider about having a blood test done for galactosemia.

ADRENAL DISORDERS

Introduction

Adrenal glands otherwise called suprarenal glands or triangular glands located on top of both kidneys. An adrenal gland is made of two parts: the outer region, called the adrenal cortex and the inner region, called the adrenal medulla. The adrenal glands work interactively with the hypothalamus and pituitary gland, as well as secrete hormones that affect metabolism, blood chemicals and certain body characteristics. Adrenal glands also secrete hormones that help a person cope with both physical and emotional stress.

Hormones secreted by the adrenal glands include the following:

Adrenal Cortex

- Corticosteroid hormones (hydrocortisone or cortisol) help control the body's use of fats, proteins and carbohydrates, suppress inflammatory reactions in the body and affect the immune system function.
- Aldosterone inhibits the level of sodium excreted into the urine and maintains blood volume and blood pressure.
- Androgenic steroids (androgen hormones) have an effect on the development of male characteristics.

Adrenal Medulla

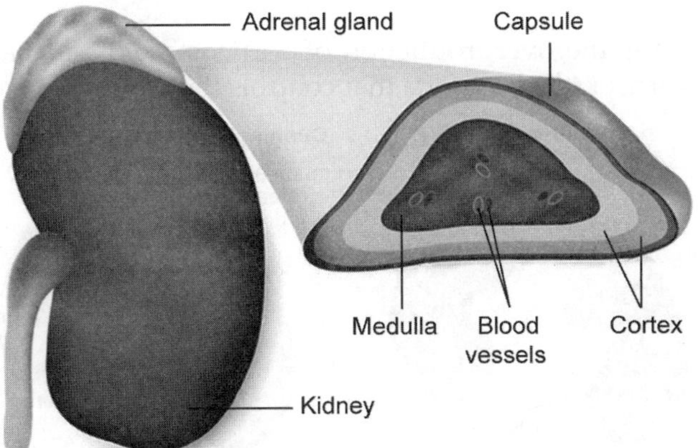

Fig. 7.97: Anatomy of adrenal gland

- Epinephrine (adrenaline) increases the heart rate and force of heart contractions, facilitates blood flow to the muscles and brain, causes relaxation of smooth muscles, helps with conversion of glycogen to glucose in the liver and other activities.

- Norepinephrine (nor-adrenaline) has little effect on smooth muscle, metabolic processes and cardiac output, but has strong vasoconstrictive effects (narrowing of the blood vessels), thus, increasing blood pressure.

Types of Disorders and Its Symptoms

- Adrenal carcinomas
- Cushing's syndrome
- Hyperaldosteronism
- Congenital adrenal hyperplasia (CAH)
- Pheochromocytoma
- Addison's disease

Adrenal Carcinomas

A cancer of the adrenal gland is rare in children, especially after the age of 5 years. The symptoms your child has may change depending on exactly what is happening. Generally there will be a lump, pain or a feeling of fullness in the abdomen. Child may also complain about pain in his back.

Symptoms often seen with increased cortisol or other hormone production include:

- A fatty hump on the back just below the neck, also called a 'buffalo hump'
- A flushed, round face and big cheeks
- Obesity
- Short stature and stunted growth
- The appearance of male characteristics in girls, such as increased body hair, pubic hair, acne, a deep voice and an enlarged clitoris.
- Increased production of the steroid hormone aldosterone, child will often see symptoms of low potassium in the blood, such as muscle cramps and weakness.

Cushing's Syndrome

Cushing's syndrome is the overproduction of corticosteroids; it may be caused by an overproduction of cortisol (the hormone that controls the adrenal gland) by the pituitary

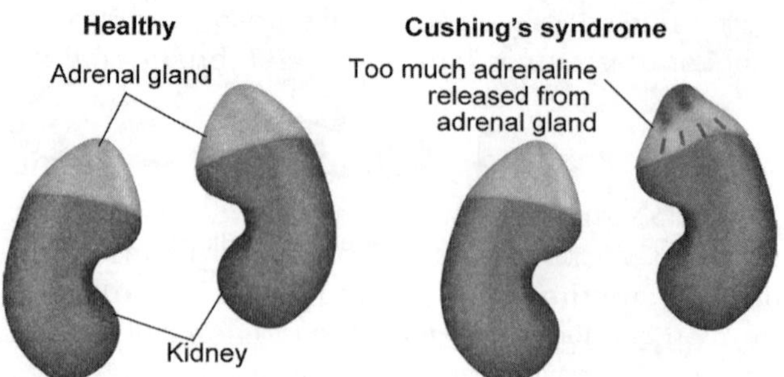

Fig. 7.98: Difference between normal and Cushing's syndrome kidney

gland. Occurs when the adrenal glands produce too much cortisol, which is the hormone that is connected to stress. It can be caused by taking certain medications. Less common causes include tumors that may either be cancerous or benign.

Signs and Symptoms

- Obesity in the upper body along with a round face and neck, yet thin arms and legs
- Skin problems including acne or reddish-blue streaks on the abdomen or in the area under their arms
- High blood pressure
- Weakness in the muscles and bones
- Moodiness or depression
- Increased blood sugar levels
- Slowing growth rates.

Diagnostic Evaluation

- *X-ray:* A diagnostic test which uses invisible electromagnetic energy beams to produce images of internal tissues, bones and organs onto film.
- 24-hour urinary test (urine is collected over a 24-hour period to measure corticosteroid hormones).
- *Computerized tomography scan (also called a CT or CAT scan):* A diagnostic imaging procedure that uses a combination of X-rays and computer technology to produce cross-sectional images (often called slices), both horizontally and vertically, of the body
- *Magnetic resonance imaging (MRI):* A diagnostic procedure that uses a combination of large magnets, radiofrequencies and a computer to produce detailed images of organs and structures within the body.
- Dexamethasone suppression test (to differentiate whether the excess production of corticotropins originates from the pituitary gland or tumors elsewhere).
- Corticotropin-releasing hormone (CRH) stimulation test (to differentiate whether the cause is a pituitary tumor or an adrenal tumor).

Hyperaldosteronism

Hyperaldosteronism is when the body makes too much aldosterone. Aldosterone is important in keeping sodium and potassium levels in balance, which controls blood pressure and fluids in the blood. The main symptom will be high blood pressure. Others include muscle cramping and frequent urination, especially during the night, as well as headaches and generalized weakness.

Congenital Adrenal Hyperplasia (CAH)

Congenital adrenal hyperplasia (CAH) is a common genetic disorder that is usually seen at birth. It prevents the body from making enough cortisol. Those with CAH may have other hormone imbalances. CAH has a wide variety of responses. For many, the disease may never be diagnosed because it does not cause notable symptoms. Milder forms may be diagnosed in either children or adults. The more severe forms usually are found during childhood.

Symptoms of the milder form include shorter than average height, early puberty, acne, irregular menstrual periods after puberty and extra facial hair in women. The more severe form has symptoms that include dehydration, low blood pressure and blood sugars, shorter than average height, early signs of puberty, irregular periods after puberty and excess facial hair in women.

In girls, there may be differences in external genitals. This is usually seen at birth and may need to be corrected through surgery.

Pheochromocytoma

Pheochromocytoma is a rare tumor of adrenal gland tissue that causes too much adrenaline to be excreted. Most of the time these tumors are not cancerous. The most common symptom is high blood pressure.

Others include:

- Increased heart rate
- Headaches
- Sweating
- Anxiety and/or panic attacks
- Shaking hands
- Pale skin
- Blurry vision
- Unplanned or unexplained weight loss
- Constipation
- Pain in the abdomen
- High blood sugar.

Addison's Disease

Addison's disease is a relatively rare disorder that happens when the adrenal glands do not make cortisol. A lack of aldosterone is also often evident. This is an autoimmune disease in which the immune system mistakenly sees the adrenal glands as an invader and attacks them. This results in damage to the glands and too little cortisol.

There can be some variation in the symptoms depending on the exact cause of the disease.

- These can include weight loss, weakness, fatigue, nausea and vomiting.
- Other possible symptoms are a decrease in blood pressure, patches of darkened skin, a craving for salt, dizziness when the child stands up and depression.
- Although not directly a disorder of the adrenal glands, some medications can stop (or suppress) their function.
- This is seen when children are taking steroid medications such as prednisone, hydrocortisone or dexamethasone for asthma or other health problems.

Usually the dose of steroids is tapered off slowly over several weeks and then stopped. If the dosing stops suddenly, the adrenal glands may not be able to get back to full hormone production for several weeks or even months.

Diagnostic Evaluation

- The child medical history
- Complete physical examination and laboratory tests.
- One or more of a group of three screening tests. One looks for cortisol levels in saliva, while another measures the level of cortisol found in urine over a 24-hour period.

- The third one uses a synthetic steroid known as dexamethasone to see if it stops or lessens cortisol production in the body.
- X-rays of glands may be used to find or rule out tumors.

Management

The primary treatment for **adrenocortical carcinoma** is surgery to remove the tumor. Depending on the results, chemotherapy often follows.

- Cushing's syndrome treatment will vary based on the cause. If a prescribed medication is creating the release of extra cortisol, doctor may change either the dosage of the current medication or try a different medicine. If it is caused by the body making too much of the hormone, then oral medication, surgery or radiation may be used.
- Congenital adrenal hyperplasia (CAH) is a disease that cannot be cured, but can be controlled. Usually this requires taking medication to replace the hormones the body is not making. Doctor will decide if medicine needs to be taken routinely or only when symptoms occur.
- Pheochromocytomas are usually treated by surgically removing the tumor. Most of the time, this improves blood pressure levels.
- Replacement of cortisol and/or aldosterone is the preferred treatment for Addison's disease. Child may also need to add salt to her diet.
- Medications that block the effect of aldosterone are the main treatment for Hyperaldosteronism. If there is a noncancerous tumor on only one adrenal gland, surgery to remove that tumor is often effective.
- Children's Medical Center uses a multidisciplinary approach to caring for child. This allows us to offer our patients care from multiple specialists and experts, in a single appointment, at one location. If child has symptoms of an adrenal disorder, contact us. We provide the comprehensive and individualized care necessary to put child back on the path to a healthy life.

DEVELOPMENTAL PROBLEM

CHILD WITH DISABILITIES (OR) HANDICAPPED CHILDREN

Introduction

Children who are mentally retarded, hard of hearing, deaf, speech impaired, visually handicapped, seriously emotionally disturbed, orthopedically impaired, other health impaired, deaf-blind, multi-handicapped, or as having specific learning disabilities, who because of those impairments need special education and related services.

Definition

A disability otherwise called as a 'handicap' because of environmental or attitudinal barriers that limit the opportunity for a person to participate fully. Negative attitudes or inaccessible entrances to building are examples of handicaps.

The term is used to refer to individual functioning, including physical impairment, sensory impairment, cognitive impairment, intellectual impairment, mental illness and various types of chronic disease.

Types

- Temporary total disability
- Temporary partial disability
- Permanent disability
  - Extrinsic handicap, e.g. Amputation (accident)
  - Internship handicap, e.g. Congenital handicap.

Types of Physical Disabilities

- Paraplegia
- Quadriplegia
- Multiple sclerosis (MS)
- Hemiplegia
- Cerebral palsy
- Absent limb/reduced limb function
- Dystrophy
- Polio.

Types of Other Disabilities

Intellectual or Learning Disabilities

Child with an intellectual, learning, or cognitive disability have a reduced capacity to learn tasks or process information. A learning disability may make it difficult for a person to take in information and communicate what they know. Learning difficulties can cause difficulties in reading, writing, or mathematics. Learning disabilities and Attention Deficit Disorder together affect between 3% and 10% of the population.

Psychiatric Disabilities

A psychiatric disability (or mental illness) can develop at any age and is often not apparent to other people. Psychiatric disabilities are often the most misunderstood disabilities in the community and peoples' attitudes may be based on prejudice and myth (e.g. schizophrenics are potentially violent).

Mental illnesses can include stress-related conditions, major depression, bipolar disorder (formally called manic-depressive illness), anxiety and schizophrenia. Depression is the most common non-psychotic mental illness (psychosis being a disorder which features the loss of contact with reality).

Visual Impairments

Visual impairments can be caused by a multitude of factors, including disease, accidents and congenital illnesses. There is a difference between the needs of visually impaired individuals and blind people.

Hearing Impairments

Deafness and hearing loss can be caused by a wide range of factors, including physical damage, disease during pregnancy, or exposure to very loud noises. There is a distinction between people who are deaf and those who have a hearing impairment. Those hearing up to three years of age (when language begins to develop) often have comparatively good speech and lip-reading ability.

Neurological Disabilities

A neurological disability is associated with damage to the nervous system that results in the loss of some physical or mental functions. A neurological disability may affect a person's capacity to move or manipulate things or the way they act or express their feelings. The way they think and process information may also be significantly influenced. The brain and the spine are the areas of the body most closely associated with neurology. Heart attacks, serious infections and lack of oxygen to the brain may also result in a neurological disability.
According to the Persons with Disabilities (PWD) Act, 1995, 'disability' includes:

- Blindness, low vision
- Leprosy
- Hearing impairment
- Locomotor disability
- Mental retardation and mental illness.

Major categories of the WHO 1980 disability classification

- Behavior disabilities
- Communication disabilities
- Personal care disabilities
- Locomotor disabilities
- Body disposition disabilities
- Dexterity disabilities
- Situational disabilities
- Particular skill disabilities
- Other activity restriction

Causes

The main causes of disability in children are:

- Muscular skeletal trauma
- Post traumatic
- Head injury, birth injury
- Communicable disease
- Infection in early childhood
- Early motherhood
- Nutritional deficiencies
- Insufficient or inaccessible health care services
- Inadequate sanitation
- Inter-family marriages

Management of Handicapped Children

Management of handicapped children requires multidisciplinary approach. Early diagnosis and treatment. The aim of management is to safeguard against or halt the progression of the disease process from impairment to disability and handicap.

The Approaches Should Include

The approaches should include careful history, thorough physical examination and necessary investigations for early detection of handicapped conditions are improvement. Regular medical supervision and developmental assessment help to identify the abnormal condition early in initial stage by MCH or school health services. Treatment of particular handicapped condition by medical or surgical management. E.g. cataract, otitismedia, leprosy, accidental injury, rickets, congenital anomalies.

Correction of Deformity

Visual or hearing problems could be corrected by spectacles or hearing aids. Physiotherapy and exercise to improve physical conditions. Occupational therapy according to the child's ability and that should be provided. Speech therapy to improve communication ability. Prosthetics, e.g. provision of artificial limb in a child with amputated leg.

Special Care

The Special care for mentally handicapped children with love, warmth, patience, tolerance, discipline and avoidance of criticism. Counseling and guidance to the parents and family members for continuation of care of the children with emotional, educational and social support. Referal for services (Govt, NGOs) for assistance of aids and appliances, for special training and education, rehabilitation and support services like pension, scholarship, special allowances.

Rehabilitation of Handicapped Children

Process of rehabilitation should involve the following aspects: Medical rehabilitation includes restoration of functions by prosthesis, artificial limbs, etc. Social rehabilitation includes restoration of family and social relationship by replacement in the family.

Educational and rehabilitation includes specialized training and educational facilities, e.g. Braille for blind, sign language for deaf and dumb. Psychological rehabilitation includes restoration of personal dignity and confidence during the period of growth and development and in adult life. Vocational rehabilitation includes restoration of the capacity to earn a livelihood. The handicapped child needs to be trained for an independent living with special training and education. These include day care centers, special school, (for blind, deaf and dumb) vocational training centers, special hospitals for crippled children.

These available welfare services of Govt. of India provide support services to the handicapped individuals. Non-govt. organization are also working along with Govt. Institutions for training, vocational guidance, counseling, manpower development, research, assistance for supply of aids and appliances to the handicapped and dissemination of informations. The Ministry of Welfare, Govt. of India has introduced a comprehensive Bill in the parliament known as 'Persons with disabilities' (equal opportunities, protection of right and full participation) Bill, 1995. It deals with preventive and promotional aspects of rehabilitation.

National Institute for Orthopedically Handicapped, Kolkota National Institute for Mentally Handicapped, Secunderabad National Institute for Visually Handicapped, New Delhi and Dehradun. Ali Yavar Jung National Institute for the Hearing Handicapped, Mumbai National Institute for Rehabilitation, Training and Research.

Social Work Intervention

Historically, the service delivery for the disabled was concentrated in the voluntary sector. Social welfare services in the field of medicine and rehabilitation were undertaken as missionary activities and as a part of their generally programs of social and economic development. As a result, a large number of societies in the non-governmental sectors were established, depending mainly on public support and donations, which would look after sick and infirm, the destitute and disabled.

There are more than 1000 voluntary organizations in India working in the field of welfare of the handicapped out of which about 350 receive grants from the government of India. The state governments have their own schemes of financial assistance to NGOs.

National Institutes for Disabled

- There are four national Institutes in each major area of disabilities under the ministry of welfare. They are:
  - The National Institute for the Orthopedically Handicapped, Kolkata (1978), The National Institute for the Visually Handicapped, Dehradun.
  - The National Institute for the Mentally Handicapped, Secunderabad (1984)
  - The Ali Yavar Jung National Institute for the Hearing Handicapped, Mumbai (1983)
  - Disabilities: How social workers help.
- Social workers and other professionals also help the people with disabilities and their families in a variety of settings such as:
  - Hospitals and long-term care facilities, schools, child welfare agencies and mental health centers.
  - Rehabilitation
- Rehabilitative services are often provided by specialized institutions. There are many social work professionals involved in rehabilitation of disabilities which include:
  - Early detection, diagnosis and intervention
  - Medical care and treatment
  - Social psychological and other types of counseling and assistance
  - Training in self-care activities, including mobility, communication and daily living skill, with special provisions as needed, e.g. for the hearing impaired, the visually impaired and the mentally retarded
  - Provision of technical and mobility aids and other devices
  - Specialized educational services
  - Community care
  - Vocational rehabilitation services (including vocational guidance, vocational training, placement in open or sheltered employment
  - Community-based rehabilitation
- Many persons with disabilities are either denied employment or given only menial and measly remunerated jobs. In times of unemployment and economic distress, disabled persons are usually the first to be fired and the last to be hired. This is true even though it can be demonstrated that with proper assessment, training and placement, the great majority of disabled persons can perform a large range of tasks in accordance with the

prevailing work norms. And this makes them not disabled but differently-abled. This is what is meant by disabilities and social work concern.

Nursing Management of Handicapped Children

Nursing assessment: Complete assessment include detailed history, thorough physical and neurological examination, special investigations, review of developmental screening, assessment of parent and child interaction and family coping, socioeconomic status, available support facilities, etc.

Nursing Diagnosis

- Ineffective family coping related to handicapped condition.
- Anxiety of the parents and family members
- Imbalanced nutritional status less than body requirements.
- Potential for infection, self-care deficit, bathing, feeding, dressing, toileting, hygienic care.
- Physical mobility impaired
- Activity intolerance
- Disturbed sleep pattern
- Sensory distribution, visual/auditory
- Knowledge deficit related to continued care of handicapped children.

Nursing Interventions

Nursing interventions: Handicapped children can be cared in the general hospitals, special health care setting and community health care centers in primary level and at home. Day care centers, special school, (for blind, deaf and dumb) vocational training centers, occupational therapy also can provide various services to these children. The goal is to bring close to normality as possible, physically, mentally and socially.

Nurses are key person for home-based or hospital-based care to guide and assist the parents and family members to promote optimum health of the handicapped children. Assist family to strengthen effective relationship and bondage to prevent children from becoming socially handicapped. Create awareness in the society about the prevention of handicaps, the abilities of the handicapped child and the potentialities present in him.

LEARNING DISABILITY

Introduction

A growing concern for parents lack of awareness about 'learning disability' or dyslexia is one of the reasons for our inability to identify great talents and potential in children. It is generally reported that fifteen per cent of the world's children have learning difficulties. Either the parents are no aware of it, or they do not know who to approach for help. Or, they shy away from help because of the stigma attached to their children, if they have to be sent to special schools. Even though children are the victims of this problem, burden is on those who are caring for them, especially parents. So parents should become aware of this emerging concern and help their children through early identification and management.

Definition of Learning Disability

The term 'Learning Disability' refers to a broad range of disorders that impair an individual's academic and functional abilities. These abilities are generally those of speaking, listening, reading, writing, spelling, reason and the ability to organize information. These children find difficulty in managing academic work. They may also be slow learners. They would score poor marks.

Learning disability (LD) affects the brain's ability to receive, process, analyze, or store information making it difficult for a student to learn as quickly as a normal boy or girl. These children are not intellectually weak. They posses different skills like music, sports, art, acting, innovating, drawing, craft and driving. Many eminent people like Winston Churchill, Einstein, Isaac Newton, Thomas Alva Edison and popular hollywood actors like Tom Cruise were dyslexic during their childhood. If these children are not identified and remedied, we will be guilty of losing eminent people. Many times, because of the punishment given by teachers and parents, such children use their skills in a negative way becoming criminals and antisocial elements.

Signs that Appear in Preschool

- Delay in understanding or using spoken language
- Difficulty in understanding simple instructions
- Lengthy pause before naming objects and colors
- Limited awareness or interest in books
- Difficulty in coloring or drawing
- Problems with motor coordination
- Short attention span (would not sit through one storybook).

Symptoms in School-age Children

- Difficulty in understanding and following instructions
- Trouble in remembering what someone tell them
- Failing to master reading, spelling, writing, and/or math skills and therefore fails to do schoolwork.
- Difficulty in telling the difference between 'right' and 'left', problems identifying words or a tendency to reverse letters, numbers or words (e.g. confusing 'b' with 'd', 18 with 81, or 'on' with 'no'.)
- Lacking motor coordination when walking, playing sports, holding a pencil or trying to tie a shoelace.
- Frequently loses or misplaces homework, schoolbooks or other items
- Unable to understand the concept of time, confused by the difference between 'yesterday,' 'today' and 'tomorrow'.

Specific Learning Disabilities

Reading disability (ICD-10 and DSM-IV codes: F81.0/315.00): Of all students with specific learning disabilities, 70–80% have deficits in reading.

The term 'dyslexia' is often used as a synonym for reading disability. A reading disability can affect any part of the reading process, including difficulty with accurate and/or fluent word recognition, work decoding, reading rate, prosody (oral reading with expression) and reading comprehension.

Disorders of Speaking and Listening

Difficulties that often co-occur with learning disabilities include difficulty with memory, social skills and executive functions such as organizational skills and time management). Auditory processing disorder: Difficulties in processing auditory information include difficulty comprehending more than one task at a time and a relatively stronger ability to learn visually.

Diagnostic Evaluation

Diagnosis Learning Disabilities

Learning disabilities are often detected in the first years of school, as a child learns to talk, read and write. Teachers are often the first to notice a problem. But a real diagnosis requires a formal evaluation by a specialist, preferable a pediatric psychologist or psychiatrist with expertize in the field. These evaluations usually are not made until a child is 5 to 7 years old and are repeated as the child gets older. Schools or doctors usually refer children for a diagnosis. Even if you notice a problem sooner, specialists generally agree that it is impossible to draw firm conclusions from preschoolers, because learning styles and speeds are so varied in the early years.

Management

Ten tips for parents to manage the situation:

1. Learn as much as you can about child's particular type of learning disability.
2. Talk to your child's teachers and principal about what resources they may have for accommodating your child's specific learning needs.
3. Raising a child with a learning problem is stressful. It can take a toll on parents and other siblings, who may be jealous of the extra attention the child receives. Many families find help through support groups or counseling. Numerous organizations offer a range of assistance for dealing with learning disabilities, from educational information to online chat rooms to referrals for counseling.
4. If there is a local support group for helping parents who have learning disability children, join it and attend meeting. You can share research, practical advice, your experiences and moral support. Plus, your child might make friends with some of the other children who are going through some of the same experiences.
5. If you do not have a local support group, look online for newsgroups and mailing lists to join.
6. Help your child with his/her homework every night. This has three benefits: you will be able to observe how your child learns best, your child will learn the material better as you help him/her to focus and his/her self-esteem will be booster.
7. Some types of LD result in a child losing his/her capacity to understand humor or sarcasm. In that case, speak plainly with him/her and always explain any jokes that he/she does not in order to reduce frustration at not being in on the jokes that he/she does not 'get' in order to reduce frustration at not being in on the joke.
8. Outside of learning, find what child is especially good at and nurture that talent, whether it is in the area of sports, art, dancing, or computer work. This will help raise self-esteem

and may also elevate child in the eyes of his/her peers – which also plays an important part in a child's self-worth.

9. Enlist child's help in doing chores around the house and be sure to break larger tasks into smaller steps.
10. Consider counseling if child seems overly sad, frustrated or angry and is having difficulty dealing with those feelings on his/her own. The counselor may also teach your child some social skills to help him/her make and keep friends.

Organization

- Teach child how to make 'to do' lists and prioritize their homework.
- Set aside a regular time each week for organizing workspace, belongings, schoolwork and activities, make a game of it or provide a reward.
- Give child a task that requires organization: grocery-shopping required for a recipe, planning a birthday party on a budget, using a map to figure out the route from one place to another, etc.

Critical Thinking

- Play games of strategy
- Talk about current events and ideas with multiple points of view
- Encourage all sorts of age—appropriate reading and writing.

Emotional Support

- Praise the child for the positive qualities he/she exhibits during the whole process of doing homework.
- Engage the child in social problem-solving: How to resolve conflicts with friends, teachers and kids who may be bothering them at school?
- Encourage activities that your child enjoys and excels in.
- Keep open lines of communication so that your child feels comfortable discussing feelings learn to regulate theirs.
- Let your children know that you enjoy their company by planning and talking with them. It is important not to ignore other children in the family.
- Research has shown that a set of personal characteristics, attitudes and behaviors can help persons with learning disabilities to achieve successful life-outcomes. Unfortunately, we often concentrate our efforts primarily on academic/educational areas, paying little attention to the development of this personal attitude. It is essential to direct greater efforts toward fostering the development of these success attributes, at least to the same degree that we strive to improve academic skills. Fostering the success attributes is one of the ways that parents can help their children with learning disabilities grow up to more successful in their lives.

MENTAL RETARDATION

Introduction

Mental retardation (MR) is a generalized disorder, characterized by significantly impaired cognitive functioning and deficits in two or more adaptive behaviors with onset before the age of 18. It has historically been defined as an Intelligence Quotient score under 70. Once focused almost entirely on cognition, the definition now includes both a component relating to mental functioning and one relating to individuals' functional skills in their environment.

Intellectual disability (ID) otherwise called mental retardation, is characterized by below-average intelligence or mental ability and a lack of skills necessary for day-to-day living. People with intellectual disabilities can and do learn new skills, but they learn them more slowly. There are varying degrees of intellectual disability, from mild to profound.

The term 'mental retardation' is a diagnostic term denoting the group of disconnected categories of mental functioning such as 'idiot', 'imbecile' and 'moron' derived from early IQ tests, which acquired pejorative connotations in popular discourse. The term 'mental retardation' acquired pejorative and shameful connotations over the last few decades due to the use of 'retarded' as an insult.

This may have contributed to its replacement with euphemisms such as 'mentally challenged' or 'intellectual disability'. While 'developmental disability' may be considered to subsume other disorders (see below), 'developmental disability' and 'developmental delay' (for people under the age of 18), are generally considered more acceptable terms than 'mental retardation'.

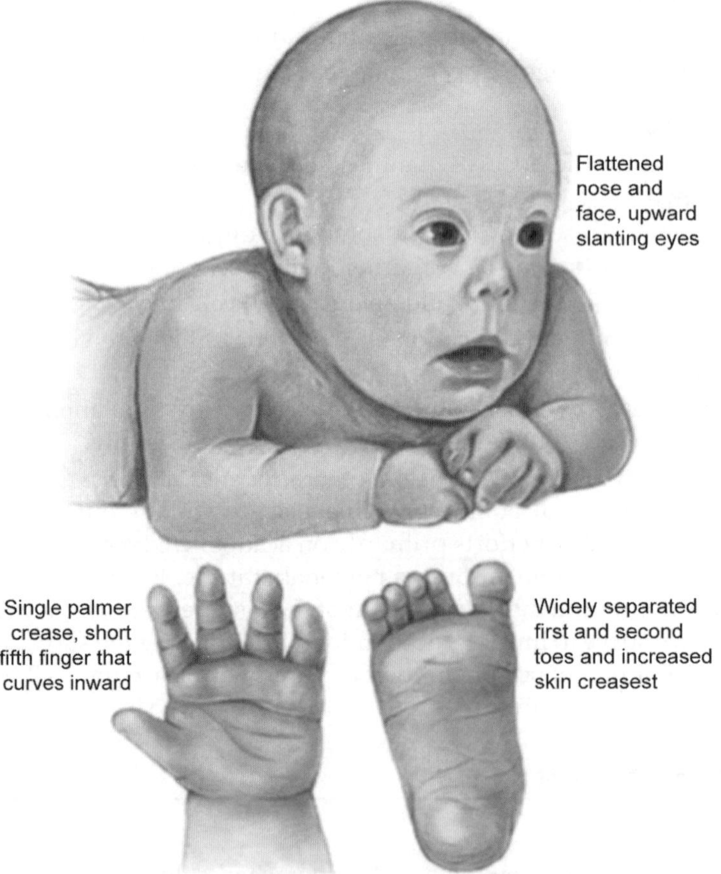

Fig. 7.99: Anatomical changes in mentally retarded (MR) child

Definition

The most commonly used definition of mental retardation is a 'significant sub average general intellectual functioning existing concurrently with deficits in adaptive behavior and manifested during the developmental period,' as stated by the American Association on Mental Deficiency. This can be translated as having an IQ below average (< 70), causing problems communicating with others and learning the skills necessary for daily living and work and it is apparent before the age of 18 years.

Incidence

Mental retardation (MR) is a common finding, affecting about 3% of the population.

Classification

Mental Retardation is Usually Classified by the Child's IQ (DSM-IV-TR)

- *Mild:* IQ of 55–69. About 85% of children with mental retardation are in this range and are further classified as being educable. These children may be able to learn to read and write at the 4th or 5th grade level, live relatively independently and work with special training.
- *Moderate:* IQ of 40–54. Also described as being trainable. 10% of children with mental retardation are in this group. These children may have academic potential at the kindergarten or 1st grade level and may have limited ability to read and will usually need some support and supervision in daily living activities (like with a supportive family or supervised group home) and work (with special training).
- *Severe:* IQ of 25–39. Five percent of children with mental retardation are in this group. Children with this level of mental retardation are unlikely to be able to learn to read or write, but may be able to be toilet trained and learn to dress with assistance. They usually require total supervision and support for daily living activities.
- *Profound:* IQ of < 24. Less then one percent of children with mental retardation are in this group.

A newer classification system was developed in 1992 that is based not on IQ scores, but rather on the amount of support and supervision that the individual needs: intermittent, limited, extensive and pervasive.

Table 7.15: Types of MR according to DSM-IV-TR and American Association on Mental Retardation (AAMR)

DSM–IV–TR		AAMR	
Mild	55 to 69	Mild	51 to 75
Moderate	40 to 54	Severe	< 50
Severe	25 to 39	These levels are based on more natural criteria, i.e.	
Profound	< 24	the increased likelihood of:	
The vast majority of children have MR in the mild range		• An identifiable cause	
Actual number score vary +/–5 points		• Comorbid health, behavior and psychiatric disorders	
		• The inability to benefit from formal academic training	
		• Parental burn-out	
		• A need for guardianship as an adult in persons with severe MR	

Signs and Symptoms

Children with mental retardation may learn to sit up, to crawl, or to walk later than other children, or they may learn to talk later. Both adults and children with mental retardation may also exhibit the following characteristics:

- Delays in language development
- Deficits in memory skills
- Difficulty learning social rules
- Difficulty with problem-solving skills
- Delays in the development of adaptive behaviors such as self-help or self-care skills
- Lack of social inhibitors.

The limitations of cognitive functioning will cause a child with mental retardation to learn and develop more slowly than a typical child. Children may take longer to learn language, develop social skills and take care of their personal needs such as dressing or eating. Learning will take them longer, require more repetition and skills may need to be adapted to their learning level. Nevertheless, virtually every child is able to learn, develop and become participating members of the community.

In early childhood mild mental retardation (IQ 50–69) may not be obvious and may not be identified until children begin school. Even when poor academic performance is recognized, it may take expert assessment to distinguish mild mental retardation from learning disability or emotional/behavioral disorders. As individuals with mild mental retardation reach adulthood, many learn to live independently and maintain gainful employment. Moderate mental retardation (IQ 35–49) is nearly always apparent within the first years of life. Children with moderate mental retardation will require considerable supports in school, at home and in the community in order to participate fully. As adults they may live with their parents, in a supportive group home, or even semi-independently with significant supportive services to help them, for example, manage their finances.

Causes

There are many different causes of why a child has mental retardation and they are usually grouped into prenatal, perinatal (around the time of birth) and postnatal causes. These include, but are not limited to:

Prenatal Causes

- Chromosomal disorders, including Fragile X Syndrome
- Gene defects
- Exposure to toxins or infections during pregnancy.

Perinatal Causes

- Prematurity complications
- Infection

Postnatal Causes

- Infections
- Lead poisoning or other toxins

- Metabolic disorders
- Head trauma

Testing to identify a cause for a child's mental retardation depends on which conditions are suspected and will vary greatly from child to child. Testing may be limited to chromosomal analysis for Down syndrome or Fragile X Syndrome, or more extensive testing may be done, including an MRI of the brain and metabolic screens for others. Testing will also include psychological tests to evaluate their IQ and level of functioning.

Some common causes include:

- Down syndrome, the most common cause of moderate to severe mental retardation.
- Fragile X syndrome, the most common inherited cause of mental retardation.
- Rett's syndrome, a progressive disorder that affects only females.

The symptoms of a child with mental retardation can vary greatly, depending on the cause and its severity. In general, most children without physical clues (such as infants with Down syndrome) are suspected of having mental retardation when they fail to meet age appropriate developmental milestones. Some children with mild mental retardation are not identified until they begin school.

Diagnostic Evaluation

According to the latest edition of the Diagnostic and Statistical Manual of Mental Disorders (DSM-IV), three criteria must be met for a diagnosis of mental retardation: an IQ below 70, significant limitations in two or more areas of adaptive behavior (as measured by an adaptive behavior rating scale, i.e. communication, self-help skills, interpersonal skills and more) and evidence that the limitations became apparent before the age of 18.

IQ Below 70

The following ranges, based on Standard Scores of intelligence tests, reflect the categories of the American Association of Mental Retardation, the Diagnostic and Statistical Manual of Mental Disorders-IV-TR and the International Classification of Diseases–10: Since the diagnosis is not based only on IQ scores, but must also take into consideration a person's adaptive functioning, the diagnosis is not made rigidly. It encompasses intellectual scores, adaptive functioning scores from an adaptive behavior rating scale based on descriptions of known abilities provided by someone familiar with the person and also the observations of the assessment examiner who is able to find out directly from the person what he or she can understand, communicate and the like.

Class	IQ
Profound mental retardation	Below 20
Severe mental retardation	20–34
Moderate mental retardation	35–49
Mild mental retardation	50–69
Borderline intellectual functioning	70–84

Management

Currently there is no 'cure' for an established disability, though with appropriate support and teaching, most individuals can learn to do many things. These 'goals' may take a much longer amount of time for them to accomplish, but the ultimate goal is independence. This may be anything from independence in tooth brushing to an independent residence. People with developmental disabilities learn throughout their lives and can obtain many new skills even late in life with the help of their families, caregivers, clinicians and the people who coordinate the efforts of all of these people.

There is no specific medication for mental retardation, many people with developmental disabilities have further medical complications and may take several medications. For example autistic children with developmental delay may utilize anti-psychotics or mood stabilizers to help with behavior.

Use of psychotropic medications such as benzodiazepines in people with mental retardation requires monitoring and vigilance as side effects occur commonly and are often misdiagnosed as behavioral and psychiatric problems.

Treatments depend on the underlying cause, but in general, there is not a cure for mental retardation. Treatments are aimed at teaching skills necessary to maximize how independent they can be.

Children with mental retardation can have other conditions too, including autism, ADHD, anxiety disorders, depression, obsessive compulsive disorder, cerebral palsy, epilepsy, hydrocephalus and spina bifida and they may have behavioral problems. If present, these comorbid conditions should be treated too.

Preventive Measures

There is no certain way to prevent mental retardation. Improved health care, prenatal testing and public health education are making it possible to avoid some cases of mental retardation. People who want to become parents can get genetic counseling to determine the likelihood of mental retardation from an inherited disorder. Medical tests such as amniocentesis, chorionic villus sampling and ultrasonography can help detect inherited metabolic and chromosomal disorders linked to mental retardation. Vaccinations can prevent pregnant women from getting infections such as German measles that can harm developing fetuses.

Immunization against diseases such as measles and HIV prevents many of the illnesses that can cause mental retardation. In addition, all children should undergo routine developmental screening as part of their pediatric care. Screening is particularly critical for those children who may be neglected or undernourished or may live in disease-producing conditions.

Newborn screening and immediate treatment for PKU and hyperthyroidism can usually catch these disorders early enough to prevent retardation.

Preventing toxoplasmosis and avoiding drugs and alcohol during pregnancy also help prevent mental retardation. Screening blood tests for newborns can detect some disorders at birth, allowing for earlier treatment. It is also important to protect babies from lead poisoning and head injuries.

- Amniocentesis is a test in which a long, thin needle is inserted in the mother's uterus to obtain a sample of the amniotic fluid from the sac that surrounds the fetus. The fetal cells in the fluid are then examined for genetic defects.

- Chorionic villus sampling is a test in which a small tube is inserted through the cervix and a small piece of the placenta supporting the fetus is removed for genetic testing.
- Ultrasonography is a painless test that uses high-frequency sound waves to record and show the shape of the fetus in the mother's uterus.

Prognosis

The child with mild to moderate mental retardation is frequently able to achieve some self-sufficiency and to lead happy and fulfilling lives. To reach these goals, they need appropriate and consistent educational, community, social, family and vocational supports. The outlook is less promising for those with severe to profound retardation. Studies have shown that these persons have a shortened life expectancy. The diseases that are usually associated with severe retardation may cause the shorter life span. People with Down syndrome will develop the brain changes that characterize Alzheimer's disease in later life and may develop the clinical symptoms of this disease as well.

DYSLEXIA

Introduction

'Dyslexia is a specific learning disability that is neurobiological in origin. It is characterized by difficulties with accurate and/or fluent word recognition and by poor spelling and decoding abilities. These difficulties typically result from a deficit in the phonological component of language that is often unexpected in relation to other cognitive abilities and the provision of effective classroom instruction. Secondary consequences may include problems in reading comprehension and reduced reading experience that can impede growth of vocabulary and background knowledge.'

A common assumption about dyslexia is that letters or words appear reversed, i.e. 'was' appears like 'saw.' This type of problem can be a part of dyslexia, but reversals are very common among kids up until first or second grade, not just kids with dyslexia. The major problem for kids with dyslexia is in phonemic awareness, phonics and rapid word recognition.

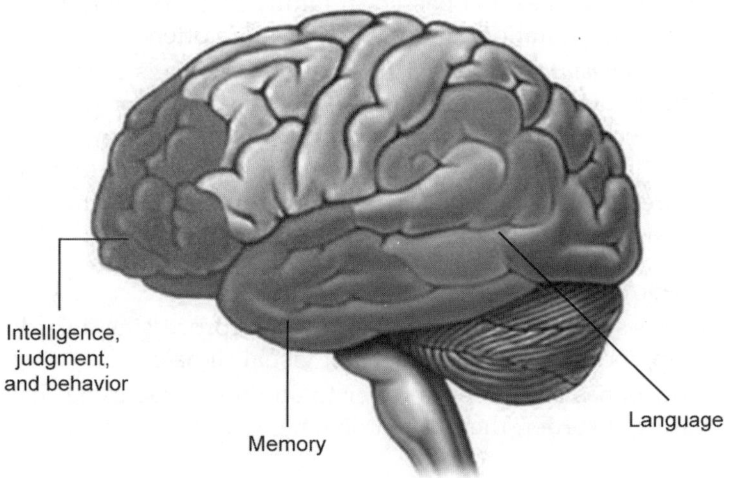

Fig. 7.100: Anatomical view of brain

Definition

Dyslexia is a disability that can hinder a person's ability to read, write and spell. It is a common learning disability in children and lasts throughout life. The severity of dyslexia can vary from mild to severe.

A dyslexic child will have trouble connecting the sound made by a specific letter or deciphering the sounds of all the letters together that form a word. Given these challenges, children with dyslexia often also have trouble with basic skills like writing, spelling, speaking and math.

Causes

Children with dyslexia have difficulty in learning to read despite traditional instruction, at least average intelligence and adequate motivation and opportunity to learn. It is thought to be caused by impairment in the brain's ability to process phonemes (the smallest units of speech that make words different from each other). It does not result from vision or hearing problems. It is not due to mental retardation, brain damage, or a lack of intelligence.

The causes of dyslexia vary with the type. In primary dyslexia, much research focuses on the hereditary factors. Researchers have recently identified specific genes identified as possibly contributing to the signs and symptoms of dyslexia. This research is very important because this may permit the identification of those children at risk for developing dyslexia and allow for earlier educational interventions and better outcomes.

Types

- *Primary dyslexia:* This is the most common type of dyslexia and is a dysfunction of, rather than damage to, the left side of the brain (cerebral cortex) and does not change with age. There is variability in the severity of the disability for individuals with this type of dyslexia and most who receive an appropriate educational intervention will be academically successful throughout their lives. Unfortunately there are others who continue to struggle significantly with reading, writing and spelling throughout their adult lives. Primary dyslexia is passed in family lines through genes (hereditary) or through new genetic mutations and it is found more often in boys than in girls.
- *Secondary or developmental dyslexia:* This type of dyslexia is caused by problems with brain development during the early stages of fetal development. Developmental dyslexia diminishes as the child matures. It is also more common in boys.
- *Trauma dyslexia:* This type of dyslexia usually occurs after some form of brain trauma or injury to the area of the brain that controls reading and writing. It is rarely seen in today's school-age population.

Other Types of Learning Disability Include

- Visual dyslexia is sometimes used to refer to visual processing disorder, a condition in which the brain does not properly interpret visual signals.
- Auditory dyslexia has been used to refer to auditory processing disorder. Similar to visual processing disorder, there are problems with the brain's processing of sounds and speech.
- Dysgraphia refers to the child's difficulty holding and controlling a pencil so that the correct markings can be made on the paper.

Signs and Symptoms of Dyslexia

- Delayed early language development
- Problems recognizing the differences between similar sounds or segmenting words
- Slow learning of new vocabulary words
- Difficulty copying from the board or a book
- Children may become withdrawn and appear to be depressed
- They may begin to act out, drawing attention away from their learning difficulty
- Problems with self-esteem can arise and peer and sibling interactions can become strained
- These children may lose their interest in school-related activities and appear to be unmotivated or lazy
- The emotional symptoms and signs are just as important as the academic and require equal attention.

Table 7.16: Signs and symptoms of dyslexia

Dyslexia symptoms by age		
Under 5	**5 to 13**	**13 and up**
Trouble recognizing the alphabet or alphabet sounds	Struggling with math word problems	Trouble with time management
Mixing up letters when pronouncing word, i.e. saying biving board instead of diving board	Problems recalling simple facts and numbers	Trouble understanding phrases, jokes or idioms
Problem with learning new vocabulary words	Trouble with using writing tools, i.e. pens	Problems reading aloud
Trouble learning familiar word sequences, i.e. the name of the months in a year or the days of the week	Trouble with understanding spelling rules, i.e. 'I' before 'E' except after 'C'	Reading below grade level, even with average intelligence
	Trouble following directions in order	Trouble learning a different language
	Trouble with understanding new knowledge	Problems with retelling the main points of a story

Diagnostic Evaluation

Dyslexia is a difficult to diagnose. There are many factors the psychologist or other health professional reviews to diagnose the disability. The testing determines the child's functional reading level and compares it to reading potential, which is evaluated by an intelligence test. All aspects of the reading process are examined to pinpoint where the breakdown is occurring. The testing further assesses how a child takes in and processes information and what the child does with the information. The tests determine whether a child learns better by

- Hearing information (auditory)
- Looking at information (visual)
- Doing something (kinesthetic).

They also assess whether a child performs better when allowed to give information (output), by saying something (oral), or by doing something with their hands (tactile-kinesthetic). The tests also evaluate how all of these sensory systems (modalities) work in conjunction with each other.

The tests administered are standardized and are considered highly reliable.

- The child should not feel as if there is something wrong because testing is occurring.
- Many of the tests use a game-type or puzzle format which can help make the child feel more comfortable.
- Children should get a good night's sleep prior to the testing and have a good breakfast.
- If the testing is done in a school setting, the teacher can prepare the child by talking about the person who will come and do special work with the child.
- With young children, the psychologist may visit the child's classroom before the testing so that the child is familiar with him.
- Whether or not the testing is done at school, the parent may want to talk to their child about a new person coming to work with them. However, parents should not try to coach the child concerning the testing. It is recommended that parents not be present during the testing.

A standard battery of tests can include the following:

- Wechsler Intelligence Scale for Children—Third Edition (WISC-III)
- Kaufman Assessment Battery for Children (KABC)
- Stanford-Binet Intelligence Scale
- Woodcock-Johnson Psycho-Educational Battery
- Peabody Individual Achievement Tests—Revised (PIAT)
- Wechsler Individual Achievement Tests (WIAT)
- Kaufman Tests of Educational Achievement (KTEA)
- Bender Gestalt Test of Visual Motor Perception
- Beery Developmental Test of Visual—Motor Integration
- Motor-Free Visual Perception Test
- Visual Aural Digit Span Test (VADS)
- Test of Auditory Perception (TAPS)
- Test of Visual Perception (TVPS)
- Peabody Picture Vocabulary Test—Revised
- Expressive One-Word Picture Vocabulary Test.

Management

An appropriate treatment plan will focus on strengthening the child's weaknesses while utilizing the strengths. A direct approach may include a systematic study of phonics. Techniques designed to help all the senses work together efficiently can also be used. Computers are powerful tools for these children and should be utilized as much as possible. The child should be taught compensation and coping skills. Attention should be given to optimum learning conditions and alternative avenues for student performance.

Perhaps the most important aspect of any treatment plan is attitude. Children will be influenced by the attitudes of the adults around them. Dyslexia should not become an excuse for a child to avoid written work. Because the academic demands on a child with dyslexia may be great and the child may tire easily, work increments should be broken down into appropriate chunks. Frequent breaks should be built into class and homework time. Reinforcement should be given for efforts as well as achievements.

Alternatives to traditional written assignments should be explored and utilized. Teachers are learning to deliver information to students in a variety of ways that are not only more interesting but helpful to students who may learn best by different techniques. Interactive technology is providing interesting ways for students to get feedback on what they have learned, in contrast to traditional paper-pencil tasks.

Prognosis

The prognosis for children with dyslexia is variable and dependent on the cause. In the case of primary dyslexia, the earlier the diagnosis is made and intervention started, the better the outcome. It is also important to focus on the child's self-esteem, since dealing with dyslexia can be extremely frustrating.

HEARING AND VISION IMPAIRMENT

Hearing Impairment

Introduction

Hearing impairment can affect a child's ability to develop communication, language and social skills. The earlier children with hearing loss start getting services, the more likely they are to reach their full potential.

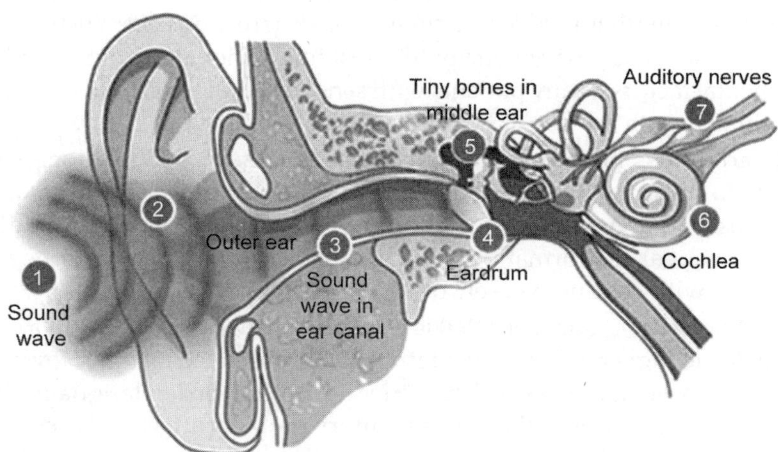

Fig. 7.101: Anatomy and physiology of ear

Definition

Children learn to communicate by imitating the sounds they hear. If they have a hearing loss that is undetected and untreated, they can miss much of the speech and language around them. This results in delayed speech/language development, social problems and academic difficulties.

Types

A hearing loss can be classified as a conductive, sensory, neural, or mixed hearing loss, based on the anatomic location of the problem (site of lesion, i.e. middle or inner ear). A hearing loss may also be labeled as unilateral or bilateral, depending on whether the loss is in one (unilateral) or both (bilateral) ears. The degree of loss might be the same in both ears (symmetrical hearing loss) or it could be different for each ear (asymmetrical hearing loss).

- Conductive hearing loss is characterized by an obstruction to air conduction that prevents the proper transmission of sound waves through the external auditory canal and/or the middle ear. It is marked by an almost equal loss of all frequencies. The auricle (pinna), external acoustic canal, tympanic membrane, or bones of the middle ear may be dysfunctional. Conductive hearing loss may be congenital or caused by trauma, severe otitis media, otosclerosis, neoplasms, or atresia of the ear canal. Some conductive hearing loss can be treated surgically with tympanoplasty or stapedectomy and the use of hearing aids and assistive listening devices may also be beneficial.
- Sensorineural hearing loss occurs when the sensory receptors of the inner ear are dysfunctional. Sensorineural deafness is a lack of sound perception caused by a defect in the cochlea and/or the auditory division of the vestibulocochlear nerve. This type of hearing loss is more common than conductive hearing loss and is typically irreversible. It tends to be unevenly distributed, with greater loss at higher frequencies. Sensorineural hearing loss may result from congenital malformation of the inner ear, intense noise, trauma, viral infections, ototoxic drugs (e.g. cisplatin, salicylates, loop diuretics), fractures of the temporal bone, meningitis, Ménière's disease, cochlear otosclerosis, aging (i.e. presbycusis), or genetic predisposition, either alone or in combination with environmental factors. Many patients with sensorineural hearing loss can be habilitated or rehabilitated with the use of hearing aids.
- Mixed hearing loss have both conductive and sensory dysfunction. Mixed hearing loss is due to disorders that can affect the middle and inner ear simultaneously, such as otosclerosis involving the ossicles and the cochlea, head trauma, middle ear tumors and some inner ear malformations. Trauma resulting in temporal bone fractures may be associated with conductive, sensorineural and mixed hearing loss.
- Auditory Processing Disorder (APD) is a deficit in neural processing of auditory stimuli that is not due to higher order language, cognitive, or related factors. However, APD may lead to or be associated with difficulties in higher order language, learning and communication functions. This type of auditory problem affects more complex auditory processes, such as understanding speech when there is background noise. The results of hearing sensitivity and physiological tests, such as otoacoustic emissions (OAE) and auditory brainstem response (ABR) are normal in children with a central auditory disorder.

Causes

- Congenital (present at birth) hearing loss
- Acquired (occurring after birth). These hearing losses may be sensorineural, conductive or mixed.

Congenital Causes

The term congenital hearing loss implies that the hearing loss is present at birth. It can include hereditary hearing loss or hearing loss due to other factors present either in utero (prenatal) or at the time of birth.

- Genetic factors are thought to cause more than 50% of all incidents of congenital hearing loss in children. Genetic hearing loss may be autosomal dominant, autosomal recessive, or X-linked (related to the sex chromosome).
- In autosomal dominant hearing loss, one parent who carries the dominant gene for hearing loss and typically has a hearing loss passes it on to the child. In this case there is at least a 50% probability that the child will also have a hearing loss. The probability is higher if both parents have the dominant gene (and typically both have a hearing loss) or if both grandparents on one side of the family have hearing loss due to genetic causes. Because at least one parent usually has a hearing loss, there is prior expectation that the child may have a hearing loss.
- In autosomal recessive hearing loss, both parents who typically have normal hearing, carry a recessive gene. In this case the probability of the child having a hearing loss is 25%. Because both parents usually have normal hearing and because no other family members have hearing loss, there is no prior expectation that the child may have a hearing loss.
- In X-linked hearing loss, the mother carries the recessive trait for hearing loss on the sex chromosome and passes it on to males, but not to females.
- There are some genetic syndromes, in which, hearing loss is one of the known characteristics. Some examples are Down syndrome (abnormality on a gene), Usher syndrome (autosomal recessive), Treacher Collins syndrome (autosomal dominant), Crouzon syndrome (autosomal dominant) and Alport syndrome (X-linked).

Acquired Causes

Acquired hearing loss is a hearing loss which appears after birth, at any time in one's life, perhaps as a result of a disease, a condition, or an injury. The following are examples of conditions that can cause acquired hearing loss in children are:

- Ear infections (otitis media) (link to specific section above)
- Ototoxic (damaging to the auditory system) drugs
- Meningitis
- Measles
- Encephalitis
- Chicken pox
- Influenza
- Mumps

- Head injury
- Noise exposure

Other Causes of Congenital Hearing Loss

Other causes of hearing loss that are not hereditary in nature include prenatal infections, illnesses, toxins consumed by the mother during pregnancy or other conditions occurring at the time of birth or shortly thereafter. These conditions typically cause sensorineural hearing loss ranging from mild to profound in degree. Examples include:

- Intrauterine infections including rubella (German measles), cytomegalovirus and herpes simplex virus
- Complications associated with the Rh factor in the blood
- Prematurity
- Maternal diabetes
- Toxemia during pregnancy
- Lack of oxygen (anoxia)

Signs and Symptoms

Indications that newborn and infant baby can hear include:

- *Newborn to eight weeks of age:* Startles or widens their eyes at sudden noises nearby and is woken or stirred from sleep by noise
- *Eight weeks to four months:* Looks towards direction of sound and may quieted while listening
- *Six to 12 months:* Turns head towards known voices or sounds, starts to babble
- *12 to 18 months:* Knows the names of favourite toys, begins to imitate simple words and sounds
- *18 to 24 months:* It has a small vocabulary of single words and can understand simple directions such as 'Give mummy the ball'
- *Two-and-a-half to three-and-a-half years:* It has clear speech with a good vocabulary.

Newborn and Infants

- Does not startle at loud noises.
- Does not turn to the source of a sound after 6 months of age.
- Does not say single words, such as 'dada' or 'mama' by 1 year of age.
- Turns head when he or she sees you but not if you only call out his or her name. This sometimes is mistaken for not paying attention or just ignoring, but could be the result of a partial or complete hearing loss.
- Seems to hear some sounds but not others.

Older Children

- Speech is delayed
- Speech is not clear
- Does not follow directions. This sometimes is mistaken for not paying attention or just ignoring, but could be the result of a partial or complete hearing loss.
- Turns the TV volume up too high.

Pathophysiology

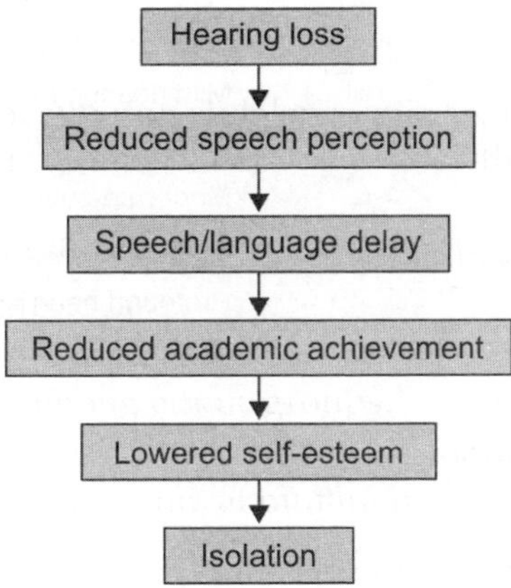

Fig. 7.102: Pathophysiology of hearing loss

Diagnostic Evaluation

A child with undetected hearing loss may not be able to develop normal speech and language or acquire the cognitive abilities (knowing, thinking and judging) needed for learning. Children whose hearing loss is not identified until, for example, 2 or 3 years of age may suffer from permanent impairment of speech, language and learning.

The type of tests used to diagnose hearing loss depends on the age of the child, but can include:

- *Objective tests,* such as auditory brainstem response testing, which measure the electrical activity in the brain in response to a sound
- *Simple tests* such as shaking a rattle nearby and observing the child's response (behavioural observation audiometry)
- *Tests with an audiometer*: A machine that produces sounds such as beeps and whistles. Whether or not the child can hear certain sounds helps to pinpoint their degree of hearing loss.

Degree of Hearing Loss

- **Deaf/Deafness** refers to a person who has a profound hearing loss and uses sign language.
- **Hard of hearing** refers to a person with a hearing loss who relies on residual hearing to communicate through speaking and lip-reading.
- **Hearing impaired** is a general term used to describe any deviation from normal hearing, whether permanent or fluctuating and ranging from mild hearing loss to profound deafness.
- **Residual hearing** refers to the hearing that remains after a person has experienced a hearing loss. It is suggested that greater the hearing loss, the lesser the residual hearing.

The level of severity of hearing loss, as used in this guideline, is defined as follows:

Table 7.17: The level of severity of hearing loss by Clark, 1981

–10 to 15 dB HL	Normal hearing
16–25 dB HL	Slight hearing loss
26–40 dB HL	Mild hearing loss
41–55 dB HL	Moderate hearing loss
56–70 dB HL	Moderate-severe hearing loss
71–90 dB HL	Severe hearing loss
> 90 dB HL	Profound hearing loss

Management

Interventions for most infants and young children with hearing loss are primarily focused on the following goals:

- Preventing or reducing the communication problems that typically accompany early hearing loss.
- Improving the child's ability to hear.
- Facilitating family support and confidence in parenting a child with a hearing loss.

Interventions focused on developing a child's communication skills and abilities differ according to the type of communication approach that will be used by the child and family. Communication approach options for young children with hearing loss range from sign language alone to auditory/verbal (spoken language) or various combination approaches. Often parents must make an initial decision about a communication approach soon after their child has been diagnosed with a hearing loss.

Treatment depends on the cause and severity of hearing loss, but can include:

- Antibiotics for otitis media
- Removal of the foreign object or wax plug
- Hearing aids to amplify sounds
- A cochlear implant may be considered in the case of severe or profound hearing loss
- Vibrotactile aids, which translate sound into vibrations felt through the skin
- Speech therapy
- Assistance from a specialist teacher of the deaf to help the child make the most of their residual hearing.

Aural rehabilitation following cochlear device and auditory brainstem implantation:

- Aural rehabilitation following implantation of cochlear and auditory brainstem devices is considered an integral part of the overall management of implant patients.
- Although programs vary widely, both with regard to treating disciplines and to the duration and scope of treatment, the general consensus is that some type of post-implantation aural therapy maximizes the benefit of the device.
- Sound recognition and speech intelligibility are evaluated prior to and just after implantation. Hearing capabilities are assessed by an audiologist, both with and without the assistance of a hearing aid.

- A speech-language pathologist evaluates and categorizes the patient's pre-implantation speech and language skills.

Post-cochlear implantation rehabilitation programs generally include the following components:

- Sound awareness (e.g. recognition of novel auditory signals)
- Visual/auditory processing, including speech-reading training (e.g. lip-reading, facial expression, gestures and body language)
- Speech recognition
- Mechanical training (e.g. use of the device and telephone)
- Voice, speech production and language therapy.

Nursing Management

Nursing Intervention for Auditory (hearing) Loss

- Keep background noise to a minimum. Turn off television and radio when communicating with client. Background noise significantly interferes with hearing in the hearing-impaired client.
- Stand or sit directly in front of client when communicating. Make sure adequate light is on nurse's face, avoid chewing gum or covering mouth or face with hands while speaking, establish eye contact and use nonverbal gestures. These measures make it easier to read lips and see nonverbal communication, which is a large component of all communication.
- Speak distinctly in lower voice tones if possible. Do not over-enunciate or shout at client. In many kinds of hearing loss, clients lose the ability to hear higher-pitched tones but can still hear lower-pitched tones. Over-enunciating makes it difficult to read lips. Shouting makes the words less clear and may be painful.
- If necessary, provide a communication board or personnel who knows the sign language. Alternative forms of communication help decrease social isolation.
- Try inserting the ear pieces of the stethoscope into the client's ears and talking into diaphragm. Stethoscopes magnify sound and can help some clients hear better.
- Refer to appropriate resources such as a speech and hearing clinic; audiologist; or ear, nose and throat physician. Refer children early for help. Hearing loss can be treated with medical or surgical interventions or use of a hearing aid. Research demonstrates the positive effects of early diagnosis and intervention on the social and cognitive development of hearing impaired children.
- Encourage client to wear hearing aid, but understand if he or she chooses to leave hearing aid out. Hearing aids amplify all noise and loud noises in the environment can be amplified to an unbearable volume.
- Observe emotional needs and encourage expression of feelings. Hearing impairments may cause frustration, anger, fear and self-imposed isolation.

VISION IMPAIRMENT

Introduction

Vision impairment means lots of different things. It can range from no vision (blindness) or very low vision to not being able to see particular colors. Vision impairment can happen at any age. Most vision conditions in children will stay the same through their life. Some conditions might result in vision problems for only a short time, but others might get worse over time, resulting in much poorer vision or blindness as the child gets older.

Definition

Vision impairment is a condition that prevents normal vision in one or both eyes. There are many problems with vision such as being near or short sighted (myopic), long sighted (hypermetropic), having normal vision in one eye only (monocular) or a turned eye (strabismus). Sometimes strabismus will be called a squint.

Blindness

A child has no vision in one or both eyes. This may be due to damage to the eye, nerves or brain, or because the child does not have an eye.

Types

- Near-sightedness (myopic)
- Long-sighted (hypermetropic)

Less familiar visual impairments include:

- **Strabismus,** where the eyes look in different directions and do not focus simultaneously on a single point
- **Congenital cataracts,** where the lens of the eye is cloudy
- **Retinopathy of prematurity,** which may occur in premature babies when the light-sensitive retina has not developed sufficiently before birth
- **Retinitis pigmentosa,** a rare inherited disease that slowly destroys the retina
- **Coloboma,** where a portion of the structure of the eye is missing
- **Optic nerve hypoplasia,** which is caused by underdeveloped fibers in the optic nerve and which affects depth perception, sensitivity to light and acuity of vision
- **Cortical visual impairment (CVI),** which is caused by damage to the part of the brain related to vision, not to the eyes themselves.

Causes

The most common causes of vision impairment are:

- Neurological conditions that affect the parts of the brain that control sight (cortical vision impairment)
- Genetic conditions like albinism and retinitis pigmentosa
- Illnesses that happen to some very premature babies or babies that have particular problems during their birth
- Conditions like pediatric glaucoma, cataracts and cancer for example, retinoblastoma
- Infections by particular viruses during pregnancy for example, rubella, cytomegalovirus, sexually transmitted infection, toxoplasmosis and so on.

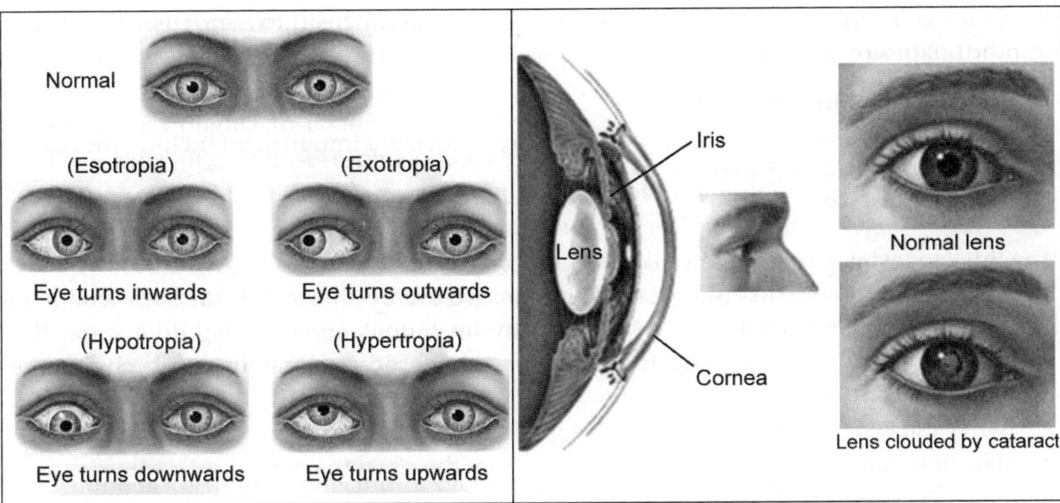

Fig. 7.103: Child with strabismus

Fig. 7.104: Child with congenital cataract

Signs and Symptoms

Other signs that a baby might have a problem with his vision are if his:

- Eyes move quickly from side to side (nystagmus), jerk or wander randomly
- Eyes do not follow your face or an object, or he does not seem to make eye contact with family and friends
- Eyes do not react to bright light being turned on in the room
- Pupils seem white or cloudy rather than black
- Eyes do not line up but look towards his nose or turn outwards.

An older child might:

- Hold things up close to her face
- Rub her eyes a lot
- Turn or tilt her head or cover one eye when looking at things up close
- Get tired after looking at things up close—for example, reading, drawing or playing handheld games
- Seem to see better during the day than at night
- Say she has tired eyes
- Seem to have misaligned eyes or a squint
- Seem clumsy–for example, she might knock things over or trip often.

Diagnostic Evaluation

An ophthalmologist, optometrist, pediatrician or other specialist may examine a child between birth and 3 months, between 6 months to 1 year, around 3 years or 5 years of age.

Types of Diagnosis

- Diagnosis begins with complete history and family history of visual impairment in the patient.

- External examination of the eye including lids, conjunctiva, cornea, iris, lens, etc. are the next step.

Tests for Visual Impairment

The tests that are used to diagnose visual acuity and visual impairment include the Snellen test, visual field test and so forth.

Snellen Test

The Snellen test is also known as the visual acuity test.

- The Snellen's chart is used. It contains progressively shortening random letters and numbers and is placed 6 meters away from the patient.
- The patient is asked to read the letters with each eye separately and both together. Ability to read the letters at each size determines the visual acuity.
- After the test a score is obtained. It is made up of two numbers.
- The first number represent how far away from the chart the patient was when he or she was able to successfully read the letters on the chart.
- The second number represents how far away a person with healthy vision should be able to read the chart.
- Healthy vision scores 6/6. If the score is 6/60, it means that the patient can only read something 6 meters away what a person with healthy eyesight can read 60 meters away.
- Being partially sighted, or sight impaired means if level of sight loss is moderate and blindness, or severe sight impairment means when level of vision loss is so severe that a person is unable to complete any activities that require eyesight.

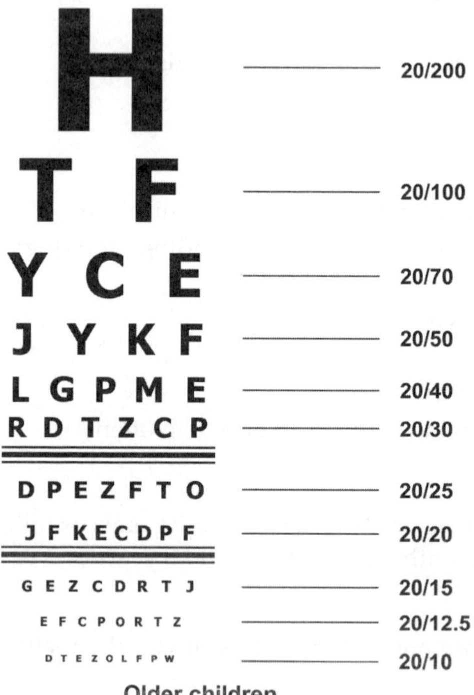

Older children

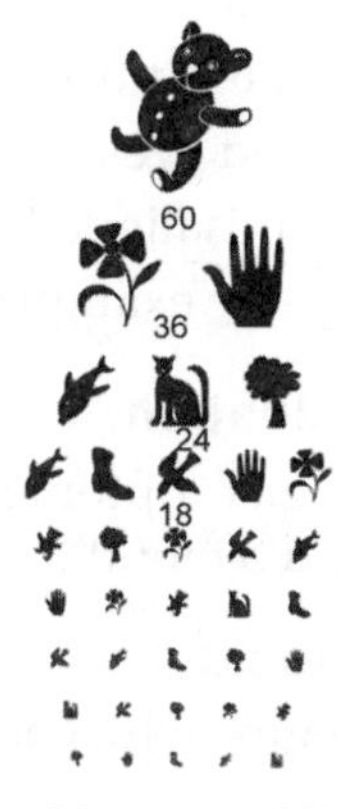

Younger child

- Partial sight or sight impairment is defined as 3/60 to 6/60 visions or having a combination of moderate visual acuity (up to 6/24) and a reduced field of vision.
- Blindness is defined as having poor visual acuity (less than 3/60) but having a full field of vision or having poor visual acuity (between 3/60 and 6/60) and a severe reduction in the vision field or having average visual acuity (6/60 or above) and an severely reduced field of vision.

Visual Field Test

- Visual field is the range of vision that a person can see without tilting or turning one's head. This measures the peripheral vision of the eyes.
- The test uses a device strapped over the patient's eyes. Lights are flashed on and off in the patient's peripheral vision.
- He or she is then asked to press a button every time they see a light. Any gap of field of vision is detected.

Tonometry Test

This test uses specialized instruments to determine fluid pressure inside the eye to evaluate for glaucoma.

Ocular Motility Assessment

This tests if there is squint of other problems in the movement of the eyeballs.

Other Tests

- Other tests like visually evoked potential (VEP)
- Electroretinogram (ERG)
- Electro-oculogram (EOG) are sometimes prescribed to test if the signals from the eye are travelling adequately to the brain.

Management

- **Antibiotics or antiviral drugs to help treat eye infections**
- **Corrective lenses (glasses or contact lenses):** These are used to treat refractive errors—such as nearsightedness (myopia), farsightedness (hyperopia) and astigmatism.
- *Patch therapy and other interventions for amblyopia:* Amblyopia can be caused by misalignment of the eyes, farsightedness or astigmatism or cataracts. The earlier the treatment is started, the faster the recovery. If amblyopia is not treated before the age of eight, vision loss may be less responsive to treatment. Amblyopia is a reduction in vision that happens when the brain disregards the image received from an eye. That means treating amblyopia calls for retraining the brain as well as the eye by forcing the brain to process visual images from the problem eye. Sometimes this can be accomplished just with corrective lenses (eyeglasses). Usually, though, doctors 'disable' the healthy, stronger eye by putting a patch over it or using eye drops to blur vision. This method forces the 'lazy' eye to work, thus strengthening its vision. It also makes the brain form new connections with that eye rather than the one that it had been relying on. If a cataract

is present, it may require surgery. If strabismus is the cause, it should be corrected after the vision has been equalized between the eyes.

- *Corrective lenses for strabismus:* Strabismus is a misalignment of one eye so that its line of vision is not directed at the same point as the other eye. It is caused by an imbalance in the muscles that control the eye's position or sometimes by near sighted vision. If left untreated, strabismus can lead to amblyopia and possibly permanent vision loss. Strabismus is treated by correcting of any refractive error with glasses, an eye patch to equalize vision, and, in some cases, surgery to alter the way the muscles pull the eye. The surgery may have to be repeated several times. Another option is injected medication to weaken an overactive eye muscle. If nonsurgical approaches do not work, then surgery may be performed on eye muscles to straighten the eyes. A set of eye exercises may be advised to correct faulty visual habits.

Surgical Management

Surgery to Remove Cataracts

Cataracts are one of the most curable causes of vision loss in early childhood and should be treated as promptly as possible in order to prevent blindness. A cataract not only blurs the image that the eye takes in, but it also interrupts the development of the visual pathways in the brain. A critical period of visual development takes place between birth and three to four months of age. If the brain does not receive clear visual messages from both eyes because of a cataract, then blindness may occur. The preferred method of treatment of cataracts in infants is to remove them surgically. After the surgery, the child must wear contact lenses or glasses to replace the eye's natural lens, or receive a lens implant. If the child is dependable about wearing lenses or glasses, then vision progresses normally. But that may be difficult with younger children, who may not like wearing contact lenses all the time.

Laser Surgery or Cryotherapy (Freezing) for Retinopathy

A major risk factor for developing retinopathy of prematurity (ROP) is birth weight of 2.75 pounds or less, generally born before 31 weeks of pregnancy. The smaller the baby, the higher the likelihood that the infant will have ROP, which usually affects both eyes. Each year approximately 15,000 premature, low-birth-weight infants in the US develop ROP.

Rehabilitation

- Vision aids
- Occupational therapy to help with learning activities of daily living, fine motor skills and age appropriate play.
- Orientation and mobility training (O and M) which helps your child learn such things as:
  - *Sensory awareness*: Gaining information about the world through hearing, smell and touch
  - *Spatial concepts:* Realizing that objects exist even if not heard or felt and understanding the relationships which exist between objects in the environment
  - *Searching skills:* Locating items or places efficiently
  - *Independent movement:* This includes crawling, rolling and walking.

OTHER CONDITION

FLUID AND ELECTROLYTE IMBALANCE

Introduction

Fluid and electrolyte therapy is an essential component of the care of hospitalized children and a thorough understanding of the changing requirements of growing children is fundamental in appreciating the many important pharmacokinetic changes that occur from birth to adulthood. While there are many factors that contribute to the fluid and electrolyte needs of children, approaching this therapy in a systematic, organized fashion can help pharmacists meet ongoing as well as changing needs of the patient. Organizing fluid therapy into maintenance, deficit and replacement requirements and then monitoring the patient for response to therapy makes fluid therapy manageable.

Definition

An electrolyte imbalance is defined as a deficiency or an overabundance of minerals in the body. For example, hyperkalemia and hypercalcemia are indicative of excess amounts of potassium and calcium, respectively, which can disrupt the overall balance and functioning of the nerves, cardiovascular system and muscles.

Types

Potassium

Potassium is the major positive ion (cation) found inside of cells. The chemical notation for potassium is K^+. The proper level of potassium is essential for normal cell function. Among the many functions of potassium in the body are regulation of the heartbeat and the function of the muscles. A seriously abnormal increase in potassium (hyperkalemia) or decrease in potassium (hypokalemia) can profoundly affect the nervous system and increases the chance of irregular heartbeats (arrhythmias), which, when extreme, can be fatal.

- *Hyperkalemia:* Increased potassium is known as hyperkalemia. Potassium is normally excreted by the kidneys, so disorders that decrease the function of the kidneys can result in hyperkalemia. Certain medications may also predispose an individual to hyperkalemia.
- *Hypokalemia:* Decreased potassium, can arise due to kidney diseases; excessive losses due to heavy sweating, vomiting, diarrhea, eating disorders, certain medications, or other causes.

Sodium

Sodium is the major positive ion (cation) in fluid outside of cells. The chemical notation for sodium is Na^+. When combined with chloride, the resulting substance is table salt. Excess sodium (such as that obtained from dietary sources) is excreted in the urine. Sodium regulates the total amount of water in the body and the transmission of sodium into and out of individual cells also plays a role in critical body functions. Many processes in the body, especially in the brain, nervous system and muscles, require electrical signals for communication. The movement of sodium is critical in the generation of these electrical signals. Therefore, too much or too little sodium can cause cells to malfunction and extremes in the blood sodium levels (too much or too little) can be fatal.

- *Hypernatremia:* Increased sodium in the blood occurs whenever there is excess sodium in relation to water. There are numerous causes of hypernatremia; these may include kidney disease, too little water intake, and loss of water due to diarrhea and/or vomiting.
- *Hyponatremia:* A decreased concentration of sodium occurs whenever there is a relative increase in the amount of body water relative to sodium. This happens with some diseases of the liver and kidney, in patients with congestive heart failure, in burn victims and in numerous other conditions.

A normal blood sodium level is 135–145 milliEquivalents/Liter (mEq/L), or in international units, 135–145 millimoles/Liter (mmol/L).

Chloride

Chloride is the major anion (negatively charged ion) found in the fluid outside of cells and in the blood. An anion is the negatively charged part of certain substances such as table salt (sodium chloride or NaCl) when dissolved in liquid. Chloride plays a role in helping the body maintain a normal balance of fluids.

The balance of chloride ion (Cl^-) is closely regulated by the body. Significant increases or decreases in chloride can have deleterious or even fatal consequences:

- *Hyperchloremia:* Increased chloride Elevations in chloride may be seen in diarrhea, certain kidney diseases and sometimes in overactivity of the parathyroid glands.
- *Hypochloremia:* Decreased chloride is normally lost in the urine, sweat and stomach secretions. Excessive loss can occur from heavy sweating, vomiting and adrenal gland and kidney disease.

Bicarbonate

The bicarbonate ion acts as a buffer to maintain the normal levels of acidity (pH) in blood and other fluids in the body. Bicarbonate levels are measured to monitor the acidity of the blood and body fluids. The acidity is affected by foods or medications that we ingest and the function of the kidneys and lungs. The chemical notation for bicarbonate on most lab reports is HCO_3^- or represented as the concentration of carbon dioxide (CO_2). The normal serum range for bicarbonate is 22–30 mmol/L.

The bicarbonate test is usually performed along with tests for other blood electrolytes. Disruptions in the normal bicarbonate level may be due to diseases that interfere with respiratory function, kidney diseases, metabolic conditions.

Causes

Electrolyte imbalance in children can be caused by vomiting, diarrhea, sweating, certain medications or kidney problems. Any illness or medical concern that results in the body losing more fluids than it is taking in can result in an electrolyte imbalance. Dehydration in children can be common due to illness or as a reaction to food. Children can also sweat excessively during a fever or activity, which means water, is quickly evaporating from the body.

Electrolyte imbalances can be caused by medical conditions including:

- Addison's disease (deceased production of hormones by the adrenal glands)
- Alcoholism, which causes the breakdown of muscle fibers, resulting in potassium being released into the bloodstream

- Diabetes
- Diarrhea
- Heat exhaustion
- Kidney disease
- Vomiting

Electrolyte imbalances may be caused by medications including:

- Angiotensin-converting enzyme (ACE) inhibitors
- Calcium supplements
- Certain hormones that are potassium-sparing (lead to the retention of potassium by the kidneys)
- Diuretics, which promote fluid excretion by the kidneys
- Potassium supplements.

Serious or Life-threatening Causes of Electrolyte Imbalances

In some cases, electrolyte imbalances may be a symptom of a serious or life-threatening condition that should be immediately evaluated in an emergency setting. These include:

- Dehydration
- Shock.

Signs and Symptoms

General Symptoms

- Dizziness
- Fatigue
- Nausea with or without vomiting
- Trembling.

Electrolyte imbalance symptoms related to other body systems including:

- Constipation
- Dark urine
- Decreased urine output
- Dry mouth and foul breath
- Dry skin
- Lack of perspiration
- Muscle weakness
- Stiff or aching joints.

Life-threatening symptoms including:

- Change in mental status or sudden behavior change such as confusion, delirium, lethargy, hallucinations or delusions
- Poor skin elasticity
- Rapid heart rate (tachycardia)
- Sunken eyes.

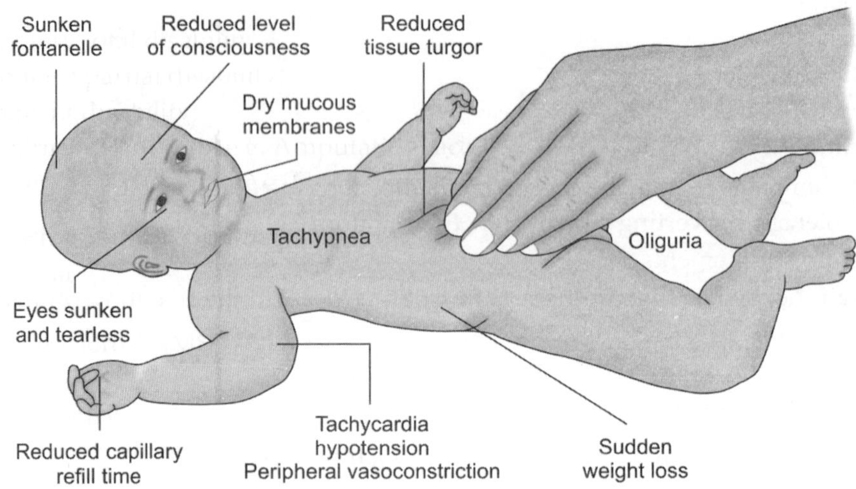

Fig. 7.105: Signs and symptoms of imbalance fluid and electrolyte child

Diagnostic Evaluation

- History collection
- Physical examination.

Complications

An electrolyte imbalance can be due to serious diseases, failure to seek treatment can result in serious complications and permanent damage. Once the underlying cause is diagnosed, it is important for you to follow the treatment plan that you and your health care professional design specifically for you to reduce the risk of potential complications including:

- Cerebral edema (swelling of the brain)
- Overheating
- Seizures or convulsions
- Shock
- Unconsciousness and coma.

Management

Fluid Therapy

Physiologic differences also play a role in fluid therapy. The changes that take place as a child grows have a great effect on fluid requirements, making special attention to fluid therapy essential in pediatric pharmacotherapy. *There are three classifications of fluid therapy:*

1. Maintenance fluid therapy
2. Deficit fluid therapy
3. Replacement fluid therapy

When choosing the type of fluid and volume to be administered, nurse carefully should consider the each component of fluid therapy.

Maintenance Fluids

Maintenance fluids are given to compensate for ongoing losses and are required for all patients. Maintenance fluids are frequently given through an intravenous line, but can also be given orally if the patient is able to tolerate oral therapy. Sensible losses, which include urine output and fecal water, make up the majority of ongoing losses, with additional contributions from insensible losses such as respiration and perspiration.

Deficit Fluids

Fluids lost prior to medical care are termed 'deficit fluids.' Examples of clinical situations where a patient would present with a deficit fluid include gastrointestinal illness with vomiting and diarrhea, traumatic injuries with significant blood loss and inadequate intake of fluids over a period of time.

Deficit fluids, like maintenance fluids, are most easily handled by approaching the needs of the patient in a systematic manner. Clinical signs of dehydration should be taken into consideration first, as they can provide useful insight into the fluid needs of the patient. One clinical sign of dehydration which can be of use is weight loss. Most young children visit their pediatricians frequently and a relatively recent pre-illness weight will be on record. Other clinical signs include increased thirst, dry mucous membranes and decreased urine output.

Table 7.18: Degree of dehydration

	Mild dehydration	Moderate dehydration	Severe dehydration
Older child	3% (30 mL/kg)	6% (60 mL/kg)	9% (90 mL/kg)
Infant	5% (50 mL/kg)	10% (100 mL/kg)	15% (150 mL/kg)

Table 7.19: Clinical signs of dehydration

Clinical sign	Mild dehydration	Moderate dehydration	Severe dehydration
Weight loss (%)	3–5	6–9	≥ 10
Behavior	Normal	Normal to listless	Normal to lethargic or comatose
Thirst	Slight	Moderate	Intense
Mucous membranes	May be normal	Dry	Dry
Anterior fontanelle	Flat	Sunken	Sunken
Eyes	Normal	Sunken	Deeply sunken
Skin turgor	Normal	Decreased	Decreased
Blood pressure	Normal	Normal	Normal to decreased
Heart rate	Normal rate	Increased	Increased
Urine output	Decreased	Markedly decreased	Anuria
Data from provisional committee on quality improvement, subcommittee on acute gastroenteritis.			

Child with hypotonic or isotonic dehydration are given fluids using the same technique to calculate fluid amount and rate rehydration is divided into three phases. In phase I, a bolus of fluid is given in order to restore blood volume to ensure adequate perfusion of critical organs, such as the brain. Bolus fluids should be isotonic; either normal saline or lactated ringers solution is used at a volume of 20 mL per kg, given over 60 minutes. Repeat boluses are given if necessary to maintain adequate perfusion. Isotonic fluids are used because they provide rapid volume expansion in the plasma and extracellular fluid.

Table 7.20: Method for calculating rehydration fluid in isotonic or hypotonic dehydration

Dehydration phase	Fluid volume	Example 10 kg child with 1 kg weight loss (deficit = 1000 mL)
Phase I Emergency phase	20 mL/kg May repeat if necessary	200 mL (remaining deficit = 800 mL)
Phase II First 8 hours	1/2 remaining deficit + 1/3 daily maintenance	400 mL + 333 mL = 733 mL = 92 mL/hr
Phase III Next 16 hours	1/2 remaining deficit + 2/3 daily maintenance	400 mL + 666 mL = 1066 mL = 67 mL/hr

Replacement Fluids

Replacement fluids are defined as those given to meet ongoing losses due to medical treatment. Examples of clinical situations where replacement fluids are needed include patients with chest tubes in place, uncontrolled vomiting, continuing diarrhea, or externalized cerebrospinal fluid shunts. Each of these examples demonstrates a situation where there is an ongoing loss which would not be met by administering only maintenance fluids. Replacement fluids differ from deficit fluids in that they are ongoing, as opposed to a loss of fluid that occurred prior to receiving medical treatment.

Nursing Management

- Fluid volume deficit related to restricted oral fluid intake before, during and after surgery; blood loss; and loss of fluid associated with vomiting, nasogastric tube drainage, and/or profuse wound drainage
- Hypokalemia, hypochloremia and metabolic alkalosis related to loss of electrolytes and hydrochloric acid associated with vomiting and nasogastric tube drainage
- Fluid volume excess or water intoxication related to vigorous fluid therapy during and immediately following surgery and an increased secretion of antidiuretic hormone (output of ADH is stimulated by trauma, pain and anesthetic agents).

Nursing Intervention

Goal: Fluid and electrolyte deficits resolved

Outcomes

- There are no signs of dehydration
- Mucosa of the mouth and lips moist
- Fluid balance.

Intervention

- Observation of vital signs
- Observation for signs of dehydration
- Measure the input and output of fluid (fluid balance)
- Provide and encourage the family to drink a lot more than 2000–2500 cc per day
- Collaboration with physicians in fluid therapy, electrolyte laboratory examination
- Collaboration with a team of nutrition in low-sodium fluids.

CHILD WITH BURNS

Introduction

Burns are one of the most common household injuries, especially among children. The term 'burn' means more than the burning sensation associated with this injury. Burns are characterized by severe skin damage that causes the affected skin cells to die.

Definition

A burn is tissue damage caused by heat, chemicals, electricity, sunlight or nuclear radiation. The most common burns are those caused by scalds, building fires and flammable liquids and gases.

- First-degree burns affect only the outer layer (the epidermis) of the skin.
- Second-degree burns damage the epidermis and the layer beneath it (the dermis).
- Third-degree burns involve damage or complete destruction of the skin to its full depth and damage to underlying tissues.

Types of Burns

- **First-degree burns**, such as sunburns are minor and heal quickly. First-degree burns result in reddened skin.
- **Second-degree burns** are serious injuries that require medical attention. Symptoms of second-degree burns include blistered, peeling skin.
- **Third-degree burns** are severe and require immediate, professional medical attention. You will likely notice dry/charred, white, yellow or bright red tissue. Although the severely burned area may not be blistered, it often is surrounded by blistered areas.

Causes

- Thermal burns caused by flames, heat contact and scalding
- Electrical burns
- Chemical injuries
- Freezing injuries
- Traumatic wounds
- Purpura fulmanins (hemorrhagic skin condition)
- Pyoderma gangrenous (ulcerating skin condition)

- Intravenous infiltration
- Exfoliative dermatosis, including erythema multiform, Stevens-Johnson Syndrome, toxic epidermal necrolysis syndrome (TENS), phemphigus and scaled skin syndrome.

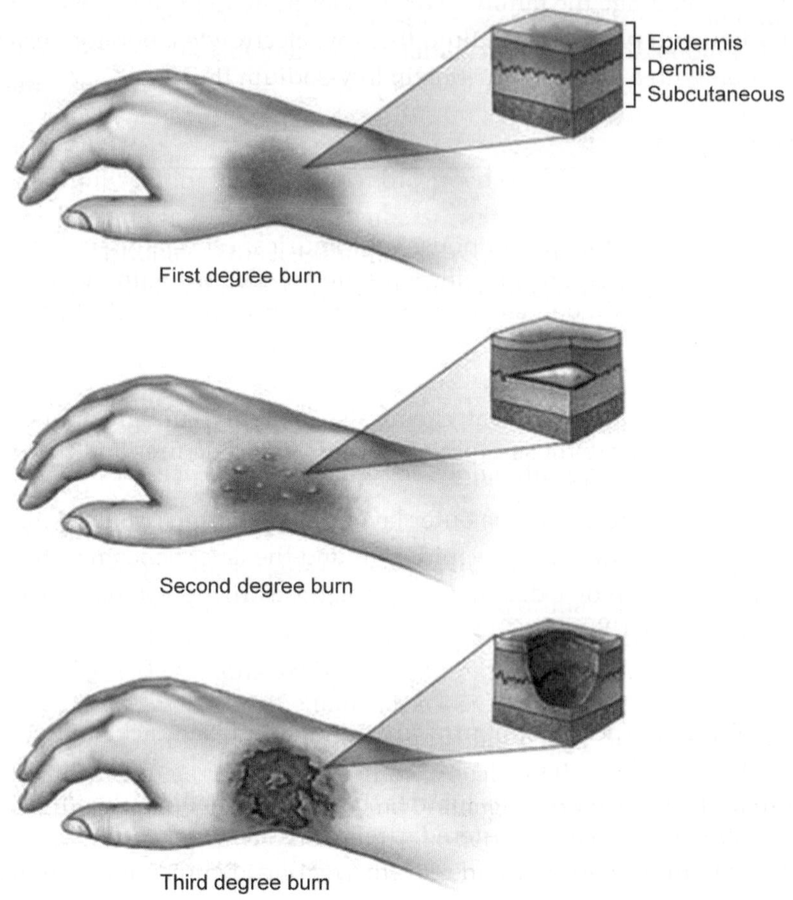

Fig. 7.106:Types of burns in children

Diagnostic Evaluation

- History collection
- Physical examination
  - Burns depth assessment may be difficult, the table below aids accurate estimation of burn depth.
  - Suspicion of deep partial thickness or full thickness burns warrants referral.

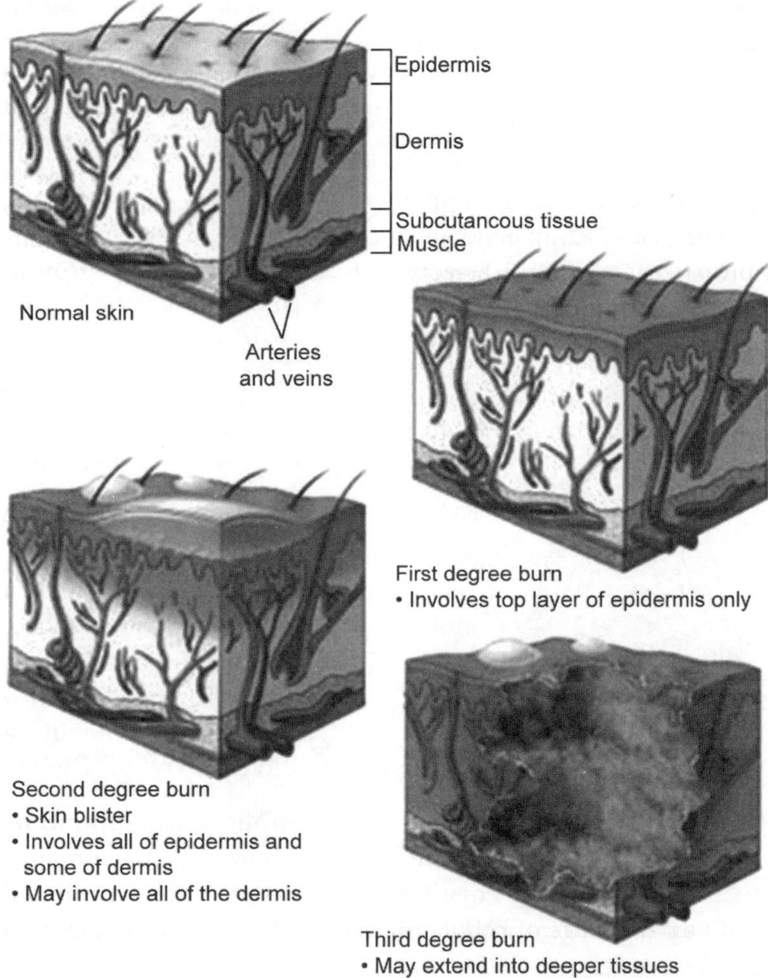

Fig. 7.107: Anatomical view of degree of burns

Depth of burns	Cause	Surface/color	Pain sensation
Superficial	Sun, flash, minor scald	Dry, minor blisters, erythema, brisk capillary return	Painful
Superficial partial thickness (superficial dermal)	Scald	Moist, reddened with broken blisters, brisk capillary return	Painful
Deep partial thickness (deep dermal)	Scald, minor flame contact	Moist white slough, red mottled, sluggish capillary return	Painless
Full thickness	Flame, severe scald or flame contact	Dry, charred whitish. Absent capillary return	Painless

Management

Burn First Aid

- Stop the burning process.
- Run cool water over the burn.
- Do not use ice directly on the burn wound.
- Do not apply home remedies/ointments.
- Cover the burn with a clean bandage or cloth.
- Take Ibuprofen or Acetaminophen for pain.
- Seek medical attention if needed.

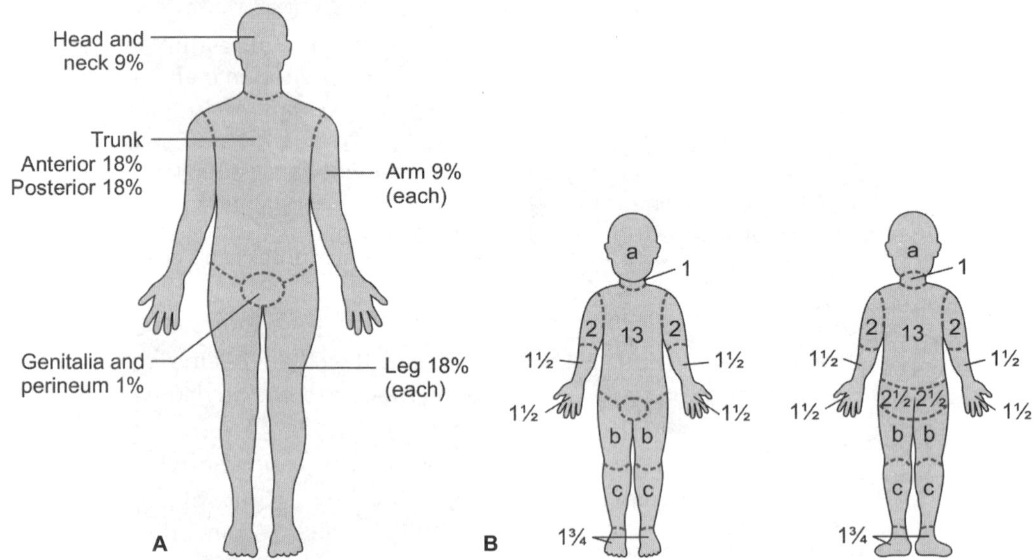

Relative percentage of body surface area (% BSA) affected by growth

(A) Rule of nines (for adult) and (B) Lund Browder chart (for children) for estimating extent of burns

	Age				
Body part	**0 year**	**1 year**	**5 year**	**10 year**	**15 year**
a = 1/2 of heasd	9½	8½	6½	5½	4½
b = 1/2 of 1 thigh	2¾	3¼	4	4¼	4½
c = 1/2 of 1 lower leg	2½	2½	2¾	3	3¼

Fig. 7.108: (A) Rule of nines for adult (B) Lund and Browder chart for children

Management of Minor Burns

- Clean burns with soap and water, or a dilute water-based disinfectant to remove loose skin.
- Blisters smaller than 1 cm in diameter (or smaller than the patients little finger nail) should be left intact to minimize the risk of infection.

- Larger blisters or those in an awkward position (in danger of bursting) should be aspirated under aseptic technique.
- Non-adhesive dressing with gauze padding is usually effective; however, biological dressings are better, especially for children.
- Dressings should be examined at 48 hours to reassess the burn, including depth.
- Dressings on superficial partial-thickness burns can be changed after 3–5 days in the absence of infection.
- If infection occurs, daily wound inspection and dressing change is required. The patient should be prescribed seven days of flucloxacillin first-line or erythromycin. Clarithromycin should be used if the patient is intolerant of erythromycin.
- Ensure adequate analgesia and assess the need for tetanus prophylaxis.

Management of Major Burns

The initial treatment of burns needs to include the following possible injuries:
- Direct thermal injury producing upper airway edema and obstruction.
- Inhalation of products of combustion (carbon particles) and toxic fumes, leading to chemical tracheobronchitis, edema and pneumonia.
- Carbon monoxide (CO) poisoning.

Immediate Management

Airway

The airway above the glottis is very susceptible to obstruction because of exposure to heat. The clinical presentation of inhalation injury may be subtle and often does not appear in the first 24 hours.

Clinical indications of inhalation injury include
- Face and/or neck burns
- Singeing of the eyebrows and around the nose
- Carbon deposits and acute inflammatory changes in the oropharynx
- Carbon particles seen in sputum
- Hoarseness
- History of impaired awareness, e.g. alcohol or head injury, and/or confinement in a burning environment
- Explosion, with burns to head and torso
- Carboxyhemoglobin level greater than 10% if the patient is involved in a fire.

Management of acute inhalation injury:
- Early management may require endotracheal intubation and mechanical ventilation
- Transfer to a burn center
- Stridor is an indication for immediate endotracheal intubation
- Circumferential burns of the neck may lead to swelling of the tissues around the airway and so require early intubation.

Intravenous access and fluid replacement

- Large-caliber intravenous lines must be established immediately in a peripheral vein.
- Any adult with burns affecting more than 15% of the total body surface area burned (where superficial burns are disregarded) or a child with more than 10% of the total body surface area burned requires fluid replacement.
- Replacement fluids required in the first 24 hours from the time of injury aim to maintain a good urine output—0.5–1 mL/kg in adults, 1–2 mL/kg in children:
- *Adults:*
  - For partial-thickness and full-thickness burns, or those with associated inhalation injury, use 4 mL of Hartmann's solution/kg body weight/% total body surface area (superficial burns are discounted here).
  - Half of this calculated volume is given in the first eight hours and the other half is given over the following 16 hours.
- *Children:*
  - Replacement fluid as above plus maintenance (0.45% saline with 5% dextrose) which should be titrated against nasogastric feeds or oral intake.
  - 100 mL/kg for first 10 kg body weight plus 50 mL/kg for the next 10 kg body weight plus 20 mL/kg for each extra kg.
- *Ensure adequate analgesia:* Strong opiates should be used.
- Prevent hypothermia.

Medical Management

- *Antibiotics:* Should be reserved for the treatment of infection.
- *Tetanus:* Determination of immunization status is very important.
- *Full-thickness burns:* Require excision and grafting unless they are less than 1 cm in diameter. Grafting is required within three weeks in order to minimize scarring. Therefore, early referral is essential.

Skin Grafting

There are two types of skin grafts. An autologous skin graft transfers skin from one part of the body to another while an allograft transfers skin from another person, sometimes even a cadaver. Scientists typically take cells from the epidermal layer of skin and then grow them into large sheets of cells in the laboratory. They do not yet know how to grow the lower, dermal layer of skin in the lab. For this reason, surgeons, after removing burned skin, first cover the area with an artificial material and then add the cell sheets on top. This procedure helps encourage the growth of new skin.

Complications

- Respiratory distress from smoke inhalation or a severe chest burn
- Fluid loss, hypovolemia and shock
- Infection
- Increased metabolic rate leading to acute weight loss

- Increased plasma viscosity and thrombosis
- Vascular insufficiency and distal ischemia from a circumferential burn of limb or digit
- Muscle damage from an electrical burn may be severe even with minimal skin injury; rhabdomyolysis may cause acute kidney failure
- Poisoning from inhalation of noxious gases released by burning (e.g. cyanide poisoning due to smouldering plastics)
- Hemoglobinuria and renal damage
- Scarring and possible psychological consequences. Hypertrophic scarring is more common following deeper burns treated by surgery and skin grafting than with superficial burns.

Preventive Measures

Infants and young children are the most vulnerable to burns. Preventive measures parents can take at home include:
- Keep children out of the kitchen while cooking.
- Turn pot handles toward the back of the stove.
- Place a fire extinguisher in or near the kitchen.
- Test smoke detectors once a month.
- Replace smoke detectors every 10 years.
- Keep water heater temperature under 120 degrees Fahrenheit.
- Measure bath water temperature before use.
- Lock up matches and lighters.
- Install electrical outlet covers.
- Check and discard electrical cords with exposed wires.
- Keep chemicals out of reach and wear gloves during chemical use.
- Wear sunscreen every day and avoid peak sunlight.
- Ensure all smoking products are stubbed out completely.
- Clean out dryer lint traps regularly.

PROBLEMS WITH LOCOMOTION

POLIOMYELITIS

Introduction

Poliomyelitis (polio) is a highly infectious viral disease, which mainly affects young children. The virus is transmitted by person-to-person spread mainly through the fecal-oral route or, less frequently, by a common vehicle (e.g. contaminated water or food) and multiplies in the intestine, from where it can invade the nervous system and can cause paralysis.

Initial symptoms of polio include fever, fatigue, headache, vomiting, stiffness in the neck and pain in the limbs. In a small proportion of cases, the disease causes paralysis, which is often permanent. There is no cure for polio, it can only be prevented by immunization.

—*WHO*

Definition

Poliomyelitis is an acute infection caused by a poliovirus (an enterovirus). Manifestations include a nonspecific minor illness (abortive poliomyelitis), sometimes aseptic meningitis without paralysis (no paralytic poliomyelitis), and, less often, flaccid weakness of various muscle groups (paralytic poliomyelitis). Diagnosis is clinical, although laboratory diagnosis is possible. Treatment is supportive.

Types of Polio

There are three types of polio infections:

1. *Subclinical:* Approximately 95 percent of polio cases are subclinical and patients may not experience any symptoms. This form of polio does not affect the central nervous system (the brain and spinal cord).
2. *Non-paralytic:* This form, which does affect the central nervous system, produces only mild symptoms and does not result in paralysis.
3. *Paralytic:* This is the rarest and most serious form of polio, which produces full or partial paralysis in the patient. There are three types of paralytic polio: spinal polio (affects the spine), bulbar polio (affects the brainstem) and bulbospinal polio (affects the spine and brainstem).

Post-polio syndrome is a complication that can occur after a person has caught and recovered from poliovirus. Symptoms of the syndrome can appear up to 35 years after the polio infection.

Causes of Polio

Poliovirus is often transmitted from person-to-person through fecal matter. People living in areas with limited access to running water or flush toilets often get the virus from drinking water contaminated by human waste that contains the virus.

The virus spreads by:

- Direct person-to-person contact
- Contact with infected mucus or phlegm from the nose or mouth
- Contact with infected feces.

Signs and Symptoms

Subclinical Polio

If child do have symptoms, they usually last for 72 hours or less and may include:

- Headache
- Sore, red throat
- Slight fever
- Vomiting
- General discomfort.

Non-Paralytic Polio

The symptoms of nonparalytic polio may last for a couple of days to a week or two and includes:

- Fever
- Sore throat in the absence of upper respiratory infection

- Headache
- Vomiting
- Fatigue
- Abnormal reflexes
- Problems swallowing and/or breathing
- Back and neck pain and stiffness, particularly neck stiffness with forward flexion of the neck
- Arm and leg pain or stiffness
- Muscle tenderness and spasms.

Paralytic Polio

- Loss of reflexes
- Severe spasms and muscle pain
- Loose and floppy limbs, sometimes on just one side of the body, this is due to the weakness which results from the involvement of the spine
- Sudden paralysis (temporary or permanent)
- Deformed limbs (especially the hips, ankles and feet due to prolonged weakenss and the lack of appropriate orthopedic bracing.

Post-Polio Syndrome

The symptoms of post-polio syndrome are:

- Continuing muscle and joint weakness
- Muscle pain that gets worse
- Becoming easily exhausted or fatigued
- Muscle wasting, also called muscle atrophy
- Trouble in breathing and/or swallowing
- Sleep-related breathing problems (sleep apnea)
- Becoming easily cold or
- New onset of weakness in previously uninvolved muscles.

Diagnostic Evaluation

- Lumbar puncture
- Viral culture (stool, throat and CSF)
- Reverse transcriptase–PCR of blood or CSF
- Serologic testing for poliovirus serotypes, enteroviruses and West Nile virus.

Management

Treatment may include:

- Antibiotics for urinary tract infections
- Moist heat (heating pads, warm towels) to reduce muscle pain and spasms
- Painkillers to reduce headache, muscle pain and spasms (narcotics are not usually given because they increase the risk of breathing trouble)
- Physical therapy, braces or corrective shoes, or orthopedic surgery to help recover muscle strength and function.

Preventive Measures

All infants and children should be immunized with poliomyelitis vaccine. The American Academy of Pediatrics recommends vaccination at ages 2 months, 4 months and 6 to 18 months and a booster dose at age 4 to 6 years. Childhood vaccination produces immunity in > 95% of recipients.

Salk inactivated poliovirus vaccine (IPV) is preferred to Sabin live-attenuated oral polio vaccine (OPV), which causes paralytic poliomyelitis in about 1 case per 2,400,000 doses and is thus no longer available in the US. Serious adverse effects have not been associated with IPV. As part of the Global Polio Eradication Initiative, all countries are to implement routine IPV vaccination programs by the end of 2016.

Adults are not routinely vaccinated. Nonimmunized adults traveling to endemic or epidemic areas should receive primary vaccination with IPV, including 2 doses given 4 to 8 weeks apart and a 3rd dose given 6 to 12 months later. At least 1 dose is given before travel. Immunized adults traveling to endemic or epidemic areas should be given 1 dose of IPV. Immuno compromised patients and their household contacts should not be given OPV.

Nursing Management

Nursing Diagnosis for Poliomyelitis

- *Imbalanced Nutrition:* Less than body requirements related to anorexia, nausea and vomiting
- Ineffective thermoregulation related to the infection process
- Ineffective airway clearance related to muscle paralysis
- Ineffective breathing pattern related to muscle paralysis
- Acute pain related to the infection that attacks the nerve
- Impaired physical mobility related to paralysis
- *Anxiety:* In children and families related to disease conditions.

Nursing Intervention

- Provide complete bed rest.
- Physiotherapy may be necessary.
- Place the child on firm mattress with support for feet, change position frequently.
- Moist heat application to decrease muscular pain.
- Encourage oral intake of food and fluid.
- Catheterization of distended bladder may be necessary.
- Antibacterial prophylaxis may be ordered.
- Good disposal of stool because it is infectious.
- In bulbar polio therapy is directed at suctioning of pharynx, postural drainage, IV fluid.
- Tracheostomy
- Oxygen therapy
- Prolong rehabilitation may be necessary including braces, splint or surgery.

(For more details see the topic in Unit 5 Communicable Diseases)

OSTEOMYELITIS

Introduction

Osteomyelitis can be described as the inflammation of bone and bone marrow and it usually indicates the presence of an infection. Although the term of osteomyelitis among children usually expresses acute hematogenous osteomyelitis, it may occur as sub-acute and rarely as chronic. Although bacteria are the main cause for it, fungi, parasites and other microorganisms can also be responsible.

Definition

Osteomyelitis is defined as an infection in the bone. Infection is more common in the long bones of the body, but it can affect any bone in the body. Osteomyelitis can occur in children of any age, but is more common in premature infants.

Types and Stages of Bone Infection

Acute osteomyelitis is usually in children. Acute osteomyelitis occur in sudden onset and it is easier to treat and overall turns out better than chronic osteomyelitis. In children, osteomyelitis usually shows up in arm or leg bones.

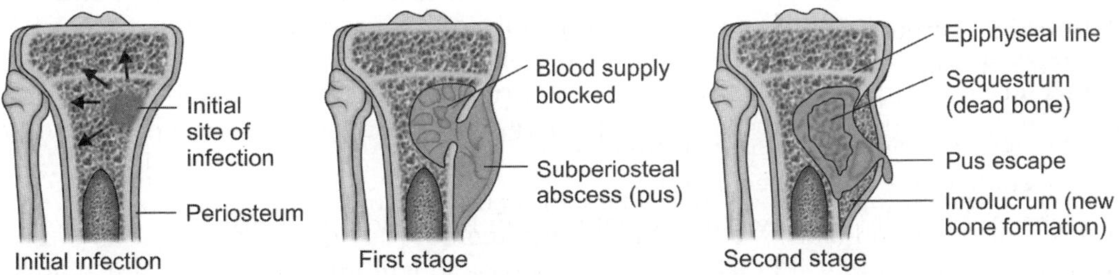

Fig. 7.109: Stages of bone infection

Acute or chronic osteomyelitis can be occur in adults people with diabetes, HIV, or peripheral vascular disease are more prone to chronic osteomyelitis, which persists or recurs, despite treatment. Whether chronic or acute, osteomyelitis often affects an adult's pelvis or vertebrae of the spine. It can also occur in the feet, especially in a person with diabetes.

Causes

The most common type of bacteria is called *staphylococcus aureus*. Fungi can also cause osteomyelitis. The bacteria and fungi can enter the body in a variety of ways including, but not limited to the following:

- Infected wounds
- Open fractures in which broken bones penetrate through the skin
- Foreign object penetrating the skin
- Infected joints
- Infection that spreads from another source inside the body, such as ear infections
- Trauma.

Risk Factors for Osteomyelitis

- Diabetes (most cases of osteomyelitis stem from diabetes)
- Sickle cell disease
- HIV or AIDS
- Rheumatoid arthritis
- Intravenous drug use
- Alcoholism
- Long-term use of steroids
- Hemodialysis
- Poor blood supply
- Recent injury.

Signs and Symptoms

- Tenderness or pain in the infected area
- The child may have limited use or may not use the infected extremity at all
- The child typically will guard or protect this area from being touched or seen
- Swelling and Redness in the infected area
- Warmth around the infected area and fever.

Additional symptoms that may be associated with this disease include:

- Excessive sweating
- Chills
- Lower back pain (if the spine is involved)
- Swelling of the ankles, feet and legs
- Changes in gait (walking pattern that is a painful, yielding a limp).

Pathophysiology

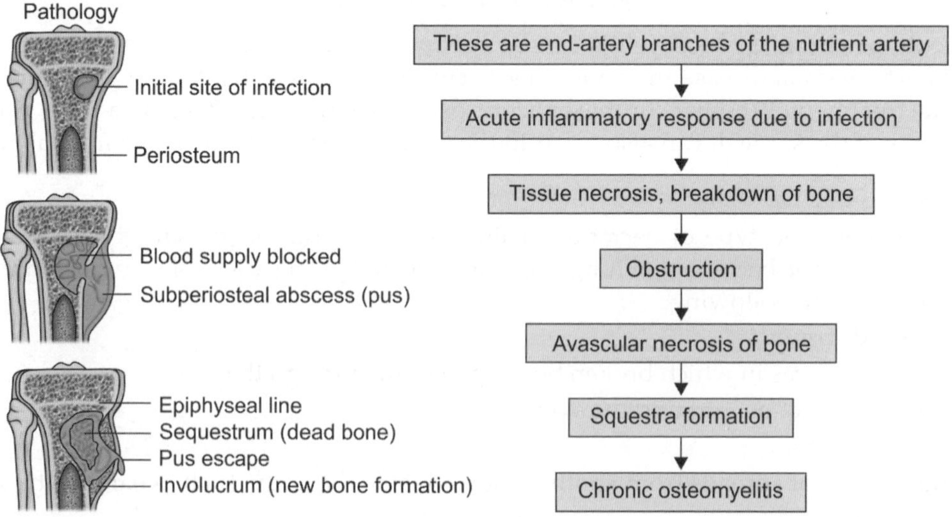

Fig. 7.110: Pathophysiology of osteomyelitis

Diagnostic Evaluation

- A complete medical history of the child
- Physical examination
- Diagnostic tests
- A complete prenatal and birth history of the child.

Diagnostic Procedures may Include

- *X-rays:* A diagnostic test that uses invisible electromagnetic energy beams to produce images of internal tissues, bones and organs onto film.
- *Bone scans:* A nuclear imaging method to evaluate any degenerative and/or arthritic changes in the joints; to detect bone diseases and tumors; to determine the cause of bone pain or inflammation.
- Magnetic resonance imaging (MRIs).
- *Blood tests:* These include a complete blood count (CBC), the erythrocyte sedimentation rate (ESR), C-reactive protein (CRP) and blood cultures.
- A bone biopsy is necessary to confirm a diagnosis of osteomyelitis.

Management

The goal of treatment is to relieve the pain and completely treat the infection. Treatment may include one, or a combination, of the following:

- Antibiotics to fight the infection
- Pain medications
- Surgery to clean out the infected area in and around the bone.

In most cases, the infection is cured with antibiotic medication. In severe cases of osteomyelitis, the infection can be very destructive to the bone, surrounding muscles, tendons and blood vessels, resulting in long-term or chronic infection. Amputation of the infected limb is rare.

Surgical Management

The most common treatments for osteomyelitis are surgery to remove portions of bone that are infected or dead followed by antibiotics. Hospitalization is usually necessary.

Depending on the severity of the infection, osteomyelitis surgery may include one or more of the following procedures:

- *Drain the infected area:* Opening up the area around child infected bone and surgeon will drain any pus or fluid that has accumulated in response to the infection.
- *Remove diseased bone and tissue:* In a procedure called debridement, the surgeon removes as much of the diseased bone as possible and takes a small margin of healthy bone to ensure that all the infected areas have been removed. Surrounding tissue that shows signs of infection also may be removed.
- *Amputate the limb:* As a last resort, surgeons may amputate the affected limb to stop the infection from spreading further.

Table 7.21: Treatment approach in acute osteomyelitis

Patient characteristics	Possible pathogen	Antibiotics selection
Empirical treatment	*Staphylococcus aureus* *Haemophilus influenzae* type b	Nafcillin/clindamycin/vancomycin (MRSA*) cefuroxime/cefotaxime/ceftriaxone/ chloramphenicol
Newborn	*S. aureus* Group B *streptococcus* Gram negative enteric bacteria	Nafcillin* cefotaxime/gentamicin
< 5 years	*S. aureus* *Streptococci* *H. influenzae* type	Nafcillin+, cefotaxime/ceftriaxone OR cefuroxime OR ampicillin-sulbactam
> 5 years	Gram positive cocci	Nafcillin OR Clindamycin OR Cefazolin
Sickle cell anemia	*S. aureus* Coliform bacteria	Nafcillin/clindamycin + cefotaxime/ceftriaxone
Puncture injuries Partially broken	*S. aureus* Anaerobe bacteria	Clindamycin
Immunosuppressed patients	MRSA *Pseudomonas aeruginasa*	Vancomycin + ceftazidime ticarcillin-clavulanate
Puncture foot injury	*P. aeruginasa*	Ceftazidime/mezlosilin + aminoglycosides and surgical debridement
Remained in the hospital for a long time preterm	MRSA, resistant gram negative bacteria, antifungal agents.	Vancomycin, carbapenems, Fungus

*MRSA methicillin-resistant *staphylococcus aureus*

Table 7.22: Antibiotics doses in acute osteomyelitis

Medicine	Dose (mg/kg/day)	Daily dose
Nafcillin	150	4
Clindamycin	30	3–4
Cephazolin	100	3
Cefotaxime	150	4
Ceftriaxone	100	2
Cefuroxime	150	3
Ampicillin-Sulbactam	300	4
Gentamicin	5–7.5	3

Nursing Management

Nursing Diagnoses

- Hyperthermia related to infections
- Fluid volume deficiency risk with regard to excessive fluid loss
- Change in comfort depending on the infection, swelling and hyperthermia process in the bone

- Pain and discomfort, physical restriction of movement associated with musculoskeletal disorders
- Less nutrition than the body requirements related to loss of appetite
- Risk of deterioration in skin integrity in relation to physical immobilization
- Change in health condition, anxiety in relation to hospitalization
- Ache in relation to inflammation/infection
- Risk of injury in relation to immobilization because of spread of infections
- Limited physical activity, social isolation in relation to therapeutic isolation
- Risk of colonic constipation due to immobility.

Nursing Interventions

- Focus care on controlling infection, protecting the bone from injury and providing support.
- Encourage the patient to verbalize his concerns about his disorder.
- Encourage the patient to perform as much self-care as his conditions allows.
- Help the patient to identify care techniques and activities that promote rest and relaxation and encourage him to perform them.
- Use strict aseptic technique when changing dressings and irrigating wounds.
- Provide a well-balanced diet to promote healing.
- Support the affected limb with firm pillows.
- Provide thorough skin care.
- Provide complete cast care.
- Administer prescribed analgesics for pain.
- Assess vital signs, observe wound appearance and note any new pain which may indicate secondary infection.
- Watch for signs of pressure ulcer formation.
- Look for sudden malpositioning of the affected limb, which may indicate fracture.
- Explain all the test and treatment procedures.

Prognosis

The treatment results of children with acute hematogenous osteomyelitis who do not have complications are fine. Together with this, the prognosis is in relation with different factors. These factors include the active organism, the duration of the symptoms before the treatment, age and the duration of the antibiotics treatment.

KYPHOSIS, LORDOSIS AND SCOLIOSIS (OR) SPINE CURVATURE DISORDERS

Introduction

The spine, or backbone, is made up of small bones (vertebrae) stacked along with discs one on top of another. It provides stability to the upper part of our body. It helps to hold the body upright. It consists of series of irregularly shaped bones appearing in a straight line. The spine has two gentle curves, when looked from the side and appears to be straight when viewed from the front. When these curves are exaggerated, pronounced problems can occur such as back pain, breathing difficulties and fatigue. When abnormalities of the spine occur, the natural curvatures of the spine are misaligned or exaggerated in certain areas, as occurs with lordosis, kyphosis, and scoliosis.

Types of Spine Curvature Disorders

There are three main types of spine curvature disorders, including:

1. *Kyphosis:* Kyphosis is characterized by an abnormally rounded upper back (more than 50 degrees of curvature. It is excessive curvature of the spine in the sagittal (A-P) plane. The normal back has 20° to 45° of curvature in the upper back and anything in excess of 45° is called kyphosis.
2. *Lordosis:* Lordosis is a condition characterized by abnormal excessive curvature of the spine, sometimes called swayback. The spine of a child with lordosis curves significantly inward at the lower back.
3. *Scoliosis:* A child with scoliosis has a sideways curve to their spine. The curve is often S-shaped or C-shaped. This abnormal curvature of the spine in the coronal (lateral) plane. Scoliosis of between 10° and 20° is called mild. Less than 10° is postural variation.

KYPHOSIS

Definition

Kyphosis (ki-FO-sis) gets its name from a Greek word for bending forward. Kyphosis is an abnormal rounding of the spine that occurs in the upper and middle part of the back. Only the most serious cases will result in a hunchback or cause discomfort or breathing problems.

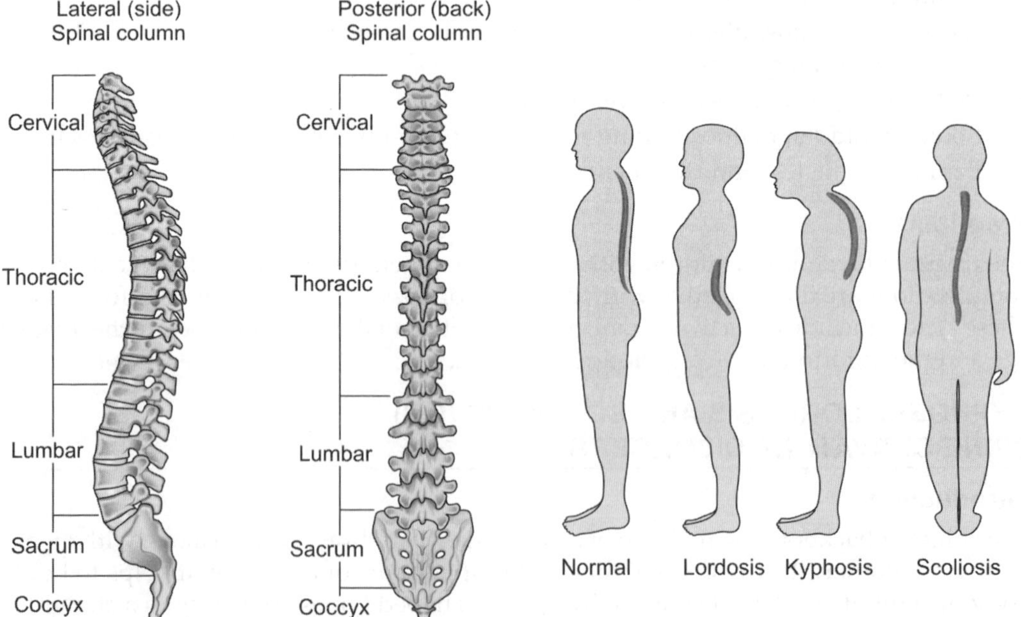

Fig. 7.111: Anatomy of spinal column

Fig. 7.112: Types of spine disorders

The origin of the condition can be idiopathic (of unknown origin) congenital (present at birth) or neuromuscular (related to the nerves and muscles). In most cases vertebral bodies appear healthy on X-ray. Abnormal development of the spinal column in the womb characterizes congenital kyphosis. The vertebrae may be formed abnormally or may be fused together.

Types of Kyphosis

- Postural kyphosis is the most common type of kyphosis and it is rarely a problem. It is more common among girls than boys and it happens when bones and muscles develop in an abnormal way as they grow, possibly because of slouching or poor posture. Child may start to notice this kind of kyphosis as they get closer to being teenagers.
- *Scheuermann's kyphosis* also usually shows up as you get closer to your teen years. It causes vertebrae to look like wedges instead of rectangles when they are viewed from the side on X-rays. Scheuermann's kyphosis is slightly more common among boys than girls and can run in families.
- *Congenital kyphosis* happens when the spine develops abnormally while a baby is still in its mother's womb. Several vertebrae can be fused together, or the bones can form improperly.

Causes of Kyphosis

- Abnormal vertebrae development in utero (congenital kyphosis)
- Poor posture or slouching (postural kyphosis)
- Scheuermann's disease, a condition that causes vertebrae to be misshaped (Scheuermann's kyphosis)

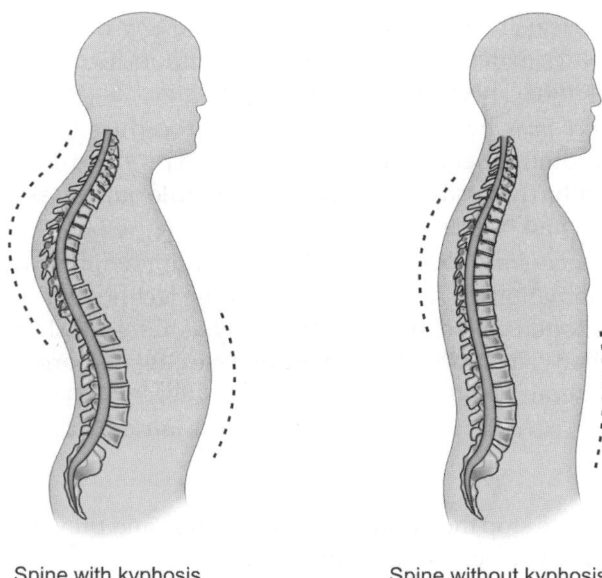

Fig. 7.113: Difference between normal and kyphosis spine

- Arthritis
- Osteoporosis
- Spina bifida, a birth defect in which the spinal column of the fetus does not close completely during development inside the womb
- Spine infections
- Spine tumors.

Signs and Symptoms

- Difference in shoulder height
- The head bends forward compared to the rest of the body
- Difference in shoulder blade height or position
- When bending forward, the height of the upper back appears higher than normal
- Tight hamstrings (back thigh) muscles.

Diagnostic Evaluation

In the most severe cases of kyphosis, there can be a visible rounding of the upper back or a hump that is easy to see. In many cases, though, kyphosis would not exhibit any obvious symptoms and can be hard to diagnose.

Diagnostic procedures may include the following:

- *X-rays:* A diagnostic test which uses invisible electromagnetic energy beams to produce images of internal tissues, bones and organs onto film. This test is used to measure and evaluate the curve. With the use of a full-spine X-ray, the doctor or radiologist measures the angle of the spinal curve. A determination for treatment can often be made based on this measurement.
- *Bone scans:* A nuclear imaging method to evaluate any degenerative and/or arthritic changes in the joints; to detect bone diseases and tumors; to determine the cause of bone pain or inflammation. This test is to rule out any infection or fractures.
- *Magnetic resonance imaging (MRI):* A diagnostic procedure that uses a combination of large magnets, radiofrequencies and a computer to produce detailed images of organs and structures within the body. This test is done to rule out any associated abnormalities of the spinal cord and nerves.
- *Computed tomography scan (also called a CT or CAT scan):* A diagnostic imaging procedure that uses a combination of X-rays and computer technology to produce horizontal, or axial, images (often called slices) of the body. A CT scan shows detailed images of any part of the body, including the bones, muscles, fat and organs. CT scans are more detailed than general X-rays.
- Blood tests

Management

The goal of treatment is to stop the progression of the curve and prevent deformity. According to the Scoliosis Research Society, treatment may include:

- *Observation and repeated examinations:* The child will need observation and repeated examinations. Progression of the curve depends on the amount of skeletal growth, or how skeletally mature the child is. Curve progression slows down or stops after the child reaches puberty.

- *Surgery:* In rare instances, surgery is recommended when the curve measures 75 degrees or more on X-ray and bracing is not successful in slowing down the progression of the curve.

Bracing

- Bracing helps positioning and function.
- Bracing can help control or correct curves.
- The brace hold child's spine in a straighter position while she is growing in order to partly correct the curve or prevent it from increasing.
- A bracing will be helpful to avoid surgery.

LORDOSIS

Definition

Lordosis is defined as the natural curve of the lower back (lumbar) area of the spine. With an extreme curve, the lower spine will have a deep curve, causing the abdomen (stomach area) to stick out and causing the pelvis (hip areas) to curve back and up. These extreme curves can be brought on from bad posture, family genetics (passed from father or mother), injury, illnesses of the spine, or surgery to the spine.

Types of Lordosis

There are 5 primary types of lordosis:

Postural Lordosis

This often comes from being overweight and lack of muscle conditioning in the stomach and back muscles. When a person carries too much weight in the front (stomach area) it pulls the back forward. When the stomach and back muscles are weak, they cannot support the spine and the pull from the weight causes the spine to curve forward.

Congenital/Traumatic Lordosis

A trauma or injury to the connecting links of the spine (pars) can cause them to break (fracture) causing pain in the low spine. In children these often occur from sports injuries. This can also be seen in children hit by a car or with falls from high areas. There can also be a defect in the way these links develop with growth, causing them to be misshaped and weak. With repetitive activities stressing this weak links, they can develop a spondylolysis (break in bone connection).

Post-surgical Laminectomy Hyperlordosis

A laminectomy is a surgical procedure where parts of the vertebrae (spinal bones) are removed to give access to the spinal cord or nerve roots. When this is done over several levels in the spine, it can cause the spine to be unstable and increase the normal curve to a hyperlordotic (overly curved) position. This is not a common problem in adults and more routinely is seen occurring in children with spinal cord tumors following surgery to remove the tumor.

Neuromuscular Lordosis

This group includes a large variety of conditions/disorders that can lead to many different types of spinal curvature problems. For each different disorder there are different treatment options.

Lordosis Secondary to Hip Flexion Contracture

This is a unique group of patients who develop a contracture of the hip joints causing the spine to be pulled out of alignment. This contracture can come from a variety of reasons including infection, injury, or muscle imbalance issues from a several different disorders.

Cause of Lordosis

- *Achondroplasia:* A disorder in which bones do not grow normally, resulting in the short stature associated with dwarfism.
- *Spondylolisthesis:* A condition in which a vertebrae, usually in the lower back, slips forward
- *Osteoporosis:* A condition in which vertebrae become fragile and can be easily broken (compression fractures)
- *Obesity:* Or being extremely overweight
- *Kyphosis:* A condition marked by an abnormally rounded upper back
- *Discitis:* Inflammation of the disc space between the bones of the spine most often caused by infection.
- Benign (harmless) juvenile lordosis.

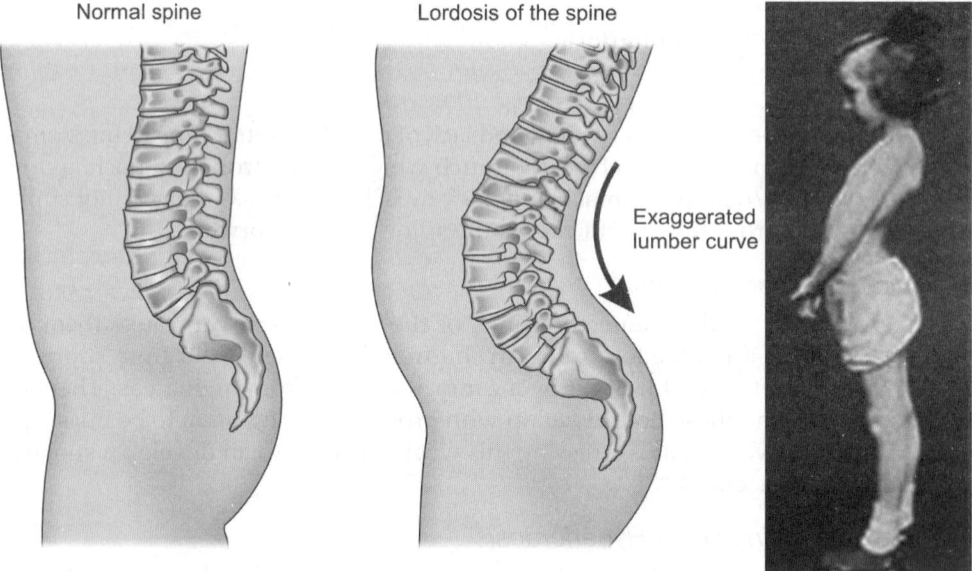

Fig. 7.114: Difference between normal and lordosis spine

Signs and Symptoms

- The major clinical feature of lordosis is a prominence of the buttocks. Symptoms will vary depending if lordosis occurs with other defects, such as:

- Muscular dystrophy
- Developmental dysplasia of the hip, or neuromuscular disorders
- Back pain, pain down the legs and changes in bowel and bladder habits are not commonly associated with lordosis
- A child experiencing these types of symptoms requires immediate medical evaluation by a physician

- The symptoms of lordosis may resemble other spinal conditions or deformities, or may be a result of an injury or infection.

Diagnostic Evaluation

- Lumbosacral spine X-ray
- Spine X-ray
- Other tests to rule out disorders that could be causing the condition
- MRI of the spine
- Laboratory tests.

Management

Treatment of lordosis includes:

- Painkiller medications to relieve the discomfort and back pain
- Wearing a back brace
- Weight loss
- Vitamin D supplementation
- Surgery
- Lordosis exercises.

Lordosis Exercises

There are many postural and muscle related factors that contribute to lordosis. These are weak core muscles, tight hip flexors, poor exercise techniques and weak gluteal muscles. Some of these problems may be corrected with lordosis exercises. These include:

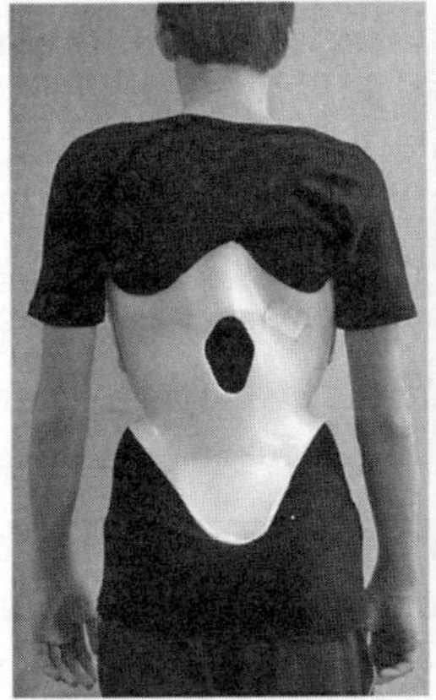

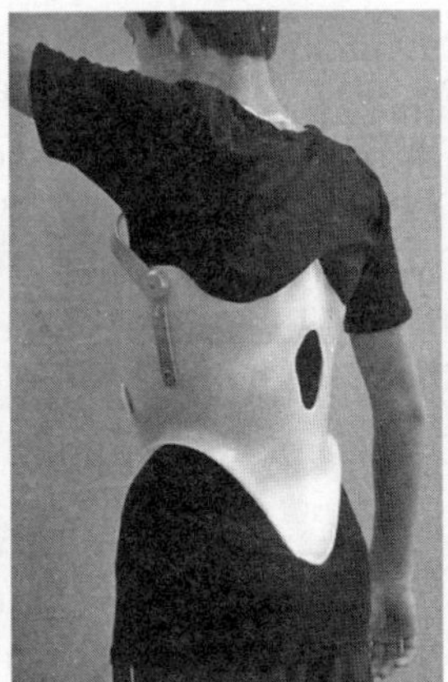

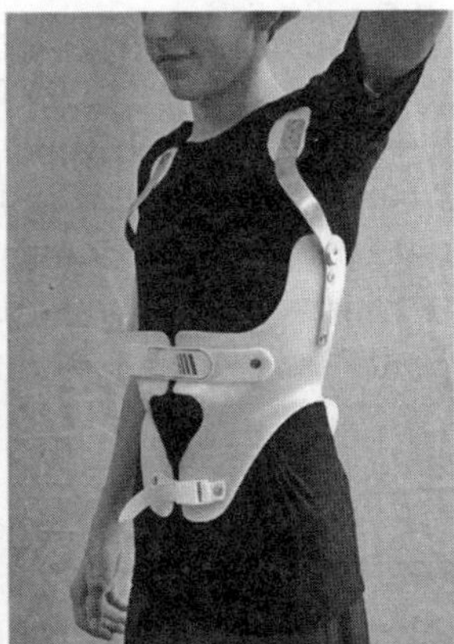

Fig. 7.115: Back brace for child with lordosis

- *Pelvic tilt*: Pelvic tilt position is the position exactly opposite of the 'arched back position'. It can help to correct lordotic posture if applied daily. The child must lie on his/her back with his/her knees bent and feet flat on the floor. Then he/she should inhale properly. After that, he/she should exhale and tilt the lower part of pelvis simultaneously. Twenty repetitions of this exercise must be performed daily.

SCOLIOSIS

Definition

Scoliosis is defined as the spinal column becomes abnormally curved from side to side into a 'C' or an 'S' shape. No one knows what the underlying cause is in the most cases of scoliosis. If the curve gets severe, it can be visible and cause discomfort. If the curve gets very severe, it can cause pain and lead to other health problems, possibly affecting the lungs, heart and joints.

Types of Scoliosis

Idiopathic Scoliosis

- Idiopathic scoliosis is the most common form, with no definite cause, mainly affecting adolescent girls, but existing in three age groups:
- Adolescent idiopathic scoliosis
- Idiopathic scoliosis
- Infantile (early-onset) idiopathic scoliosis.

Neuromuscular Scoliosis

In this type of scoliosis, there is a problem when the bones of the spine are formed. Either the bones of the spine fail to form completely or they fail to separate from each other during fetal development. Neuromuscular scoliosis is associated with a neuromuscular condition such as cerebral palsy, myopathy or spina bifida.

Congenital Scoliosis

Congenital scoliosis – exact etiology unknown; represented as malformation of one or more vertebral bodies those results in asymmetric growth.

- Type I: Failure of vertebral body formation, e.g. isolated hemivertebrae, wedged vertebra, multiple wedged vertebrae and multiple hemivertebrae.
- Type II: Failure of segmentation, e.g. unilateral unsegmented bar, bilateral block vertebra.
- Commonly associated with other congenital anomalies.

Degenerative Scoliosis

It is caused by changes in the spine due to arthritis known as spondylosis. Weakening of the normal ligaments and other soft tissues of the spine combined with abnormal bone spurs can lead to an abnormal curvature of the spine. The spine can also be affected by osteoporosis, vertebral compression fractures and disc degeneration.

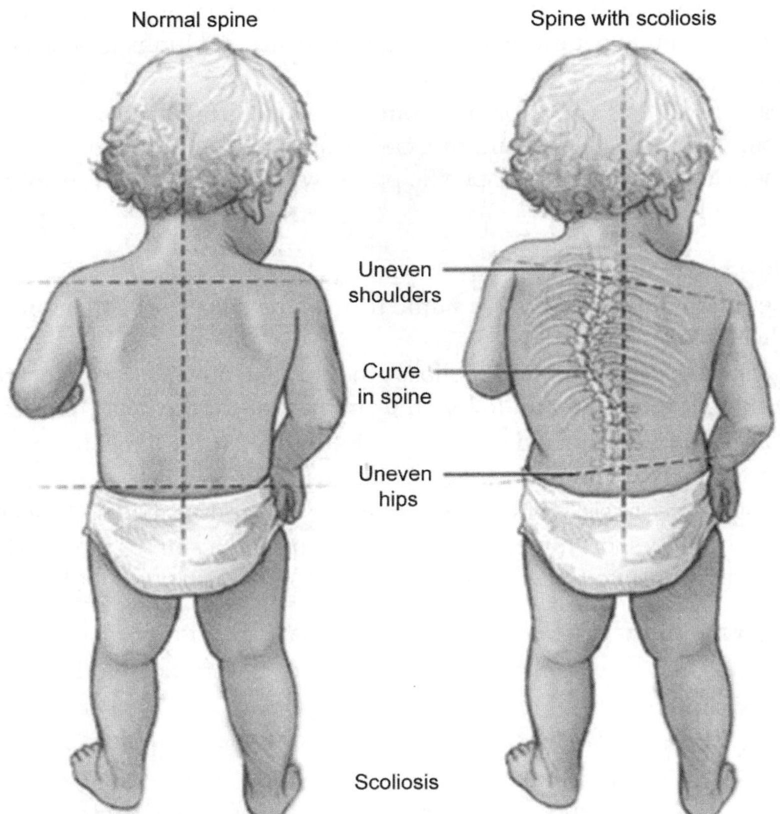

Fig. 7.116: Difference between normal and scoliosis spine

Causes of Scoliosis

In around eight out of every 10 cases a cause for scoliosis is not found. This is known as idiopathic scoliosis.

A small number of cases are caused by other medical conditions, including:

- *Cerebral palsy:* A condition associated with brain damage
- *Muscular dystrophy:* A genetic condition that causes muscle weakness
- *Marfan syndrome:* A disorder of the connective tissues.

Risk Factors

Age is a risk factor as the symptoms often begin between 9–15 years of age. Being a female increases the risk of scoliosis and females have a higher risk of worsening spine curvature than males. Although many individuals who develop the problem do not have family members with scoliosis, a family history of scoliosis increases the risk of the disease.

Signs and Symptoms

Scoliosis may cause the head to appear of center, leaning to one side or notice one hip or shoulder to be higher than the opposite side. Some of the child has a more obvious curve on one side of the rib cage on their back from twisting of the vertebrae and ribs. If the scoliosis is more severe, it can make it more difficult for the heart and lungs to work properly. This can cause shortness of breath and chest pain.

In most cases, scoliosis is not painful, but there are certain types of scoliosis that can cause back pain, rib pain, neck pain, muscle spasms, and abdominal pain. Additionally, there are other causes of these nonspecific pains, which a doctor will want to look for as well to rule out other diseases.

Complications

In most of the child with scoliosis have a mild form of the disorder; scoliosis may sometimes cause complications, including:

- *Lung and heart damage:* In severe scoliosis, the rib cage may press against the lungs and heart, making it more difficult to breathe and harder for the heart to pump.
- *Back problems:* Adults who had scoliosis as children are more likely to have chronic back pain than are people in the general population.
- *Appearance:* As scoliosis worsens, it can cause more noticeable changes—including unleveled shoulders, prominent ribs, uneven hips and a shift of the waist and trunk to the side. Individuals with scoliosis often become self-conscious about their appearance.

Diagnostic Evaluation

- History collection
- Physical examination
- Neurological examination
  - Muscle weakness
  - Numbness
  - Abnormal reflexes

Imaging study: Plain X-rays can confirm the diagnosis of scoliosis and reveal the severity of the spinal curvature and recommend additional imaging tests, such as an MRI.

Management

The majority of children with scoliosis has mild curves and no need treatment. In such cases pediatrician will recommend regular follow-ups every 4 to 6 months to monitor the curve of the spine in clinic and periodically with X-rays.

The following factors will be considered by the pediatrician:

- *Gender:* Females are more likely than males to have scoliosis that gradually gets worse.
- *Severity of the curve:* The larger the curve, the greater the risk of it worsening over time. S-shaped curves, also called 'double curves,' tend to get worse over time. C-shaped curves are less likely to worsen.
- *Curve position:* If a curve is located in the center part of the spine, it is more likely to get worse compared with curves in the lower or upper section.
- *Bone maturity:* The risk of the curve worsening is much lower if the patient's bones have stopped growing. Braces are more effective while bones are still growing.

Casting

Casting instead of bracing is sometimes used for infantile scoliosis to help the infant's spine to go back to its normal position as it grows. This can be done with a cast made of Plaster of Paris (POP). The cast is attached to the outside of the patient's body and will be worn at all times. Because the infant is growing rapidly, the cast is changed regularly.

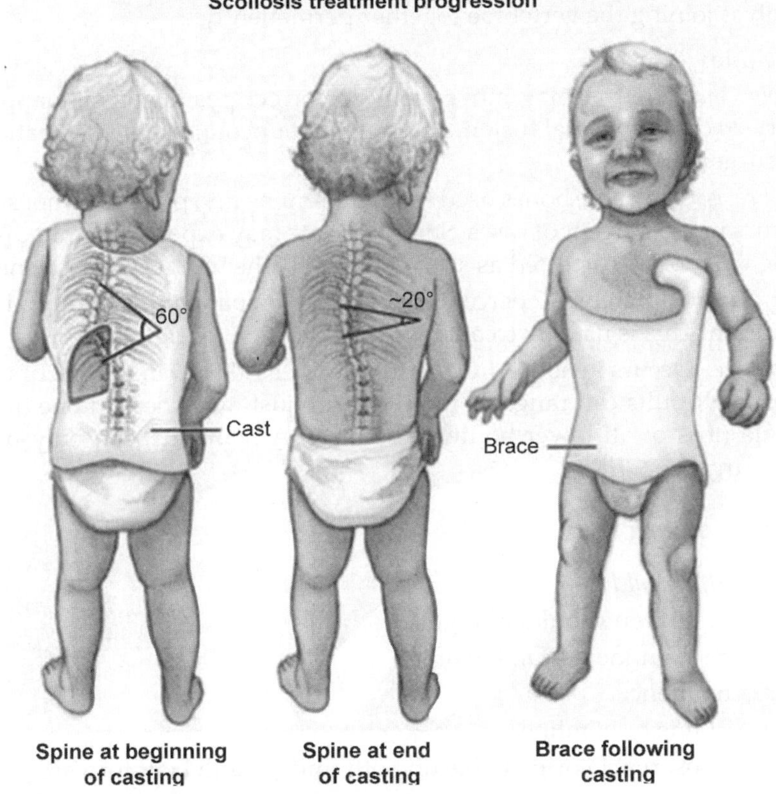

Fig. 7.117: Difference between application of cast and brace to scoliosis child

Braces

The patient has moderate scoliosis and the bones are still growing, the doctor may recommend a brace. This will prevent further curvature, but will not cure or reverse it. Braces are usually worn all the time, even at night. The more hours per day the child wears the brace, the more effective it tends to be. When the bones stop growing, braces are no longer used.

There are two types of braces:

- *Thoracolumbosacral orthosis (TLSO):* The TLSO is made of plastic and designed to fit neatly around the body's curves. It is not usually visible under clothing.
- *Milwaukee brace:* This is a full-torso brace and has a neck ring with rests for the chin and the back of the head. This type of brace is only used when the TLSO is not possible or not effective.

Surgical Management (Spinal Fusion)

The child having spine curves beyond 40 to 50 degrees are often considered for scoliosis surgery. The goal is to make sure the curve does not get worse, but surgery does not perfectly straighten the spine. During the procedure, metallic implants are utilized to correct some of the curvature and hold it in the correct position until a bone graft, placed at the time of surgery, consolidates and creates a rigid fusion in the area of the curve. Scoliosis surgery usually involves joining the vertebrae together permanently.

The risks include:

- *Rod displacement:* A rod may move from its correct position. This happens in about 1 in every 20 cases of spinal fusion. Although not uncomfortable, the patient may need further surgery.
- *Pseudarthrosis:* One of the bones used to fuse the spine into place does not stick properly. This occurs in 1–5 percent of cases. Some patients may experience mild discomfort and the spine will not be corrected as successfully. Further surgery may be needed.
- *Infection:* Approximately 1–2 percent of spinal fusion patients develop an infection after the operation. This is usually treated with medication (antibiotics).
- *Nerve damage:* Occurs in about 1 or 2 surgeries per 1,000. Damage occurs to the nerves of the spine. Results can range from mild, with just numbness in one or both legs, to paraplegia (loss of all lower bodily functions). A neurosurgeon may be present for scoliosis surgery.

Nursing Management

Assessment of the Child

- Poor posture, uneven shoulder height
- One hip more prominent than the other
- Scapular prominence
- Uneven waist line or hemline
- Spinal curve observable or palpable on both upright and bent forward
- Back pain may be present but is not a routine finding in idiopathic scoliosis
- Leg length discrepancy.

Nursing Diagnosis

- Disturbed body image related to negative feelings about spinal deformity and appearance in brace.
- Risk for impaired skin integrity related to mechanical irritation to brace.
- Risk for injury related to postoperative complications.

Nursing Interventions

- Prepare the child for casting or immobilization procedure by showing materials to be used and describing procedure in age-appropriate terms.
- Promote comfort with proper fit of brace or cast.

- Provide opportunity for the child to express fears and ask questions about deformity and brace wear.
- Assess skin integrity under and around the brace or cast frequently.
- Provide good skin care to prevent breakdown around any pressure areas.
- Instruct the patient to examine brace daily for signs of loosening or breakage.
- Instruct patient to wear cotton shirt under brace to avoid rubbing.
- Instruct about which previous activities can be continued in the brace.
- Provide a peer support person when possible so the child can associate positive outcomes and experiences from others.

FRACTURES

Introduction

The anatomy and biomechanics of pediatric bone differ from that of adult bone, leading to unique pediatric fracture patterns, healing mechanisms and management. In comparison to adult bone, pediatric bone is significantly less dense, more porous and penetrated throughout by capillary channels. Pediatric bone has a lower modulus of elasticity, lower bending strength and lower mineral content. The low bending strength induces more strain in pediatric bone than for the same stress on adult bone and the low modulus of elasticity allows for greater energy absorption before failure. The increased porosity of pediatric bone prevents propagation of fractures, thereby decreasing the incidence of comminuted fractures. The pediatric periosteum is extremely strong and thick, functioning in reduction and maintenance of fracture alignment and healing.

Anatomy of Pediatric Bone

Pediatric long bones have three main regions: Epiphysis, physis and metaphysis.

1. *Epiphysis:* Each end of a long bone with associated joint cartilage.
2. *Physis (growth plate):* Cartilage cells that create solid bone with growth.
3. *Metaphysis:* Wide area below the physis, closest to the diaphysis/shaft.

Definition

A fracture is defined as a breakdown in the bone. It can range from a thin crack to a complete break. A bone can fracture crosswise, lengthwise, in several places or into many pieces. Typically a bone can be fractured by external force or pressure.

Types

There are two types of fractures: Open and closed.

- Open fracture (also called compound fracture). The bone exits and is visible through the skin, or a deep wound that exposes the bone through the skin.
- Closed fracture (also called simple fracture). The bone is broken, but the skin is intact.

Plastic Deformation

- A force produces microscopic failure on the tensile/convex side of bone which does not propagate to the concave side. The bone is angulated beyond its elastic limit, but the energy is insufficient to produce a fracture.

- No fracture line is visible radiographically.
- Unique to children
- Most commonly seen in the ulna, occasionally in the fibula.
- Bend in the ulna of < 20° in a 4-year-old child should correct with growth.

Buckle Fracture

- Compression failure of bone that usually occurs at the junction of the metaphysis and the diaphysis
- Commonly seen in distal radius
- Inherently stable
- Heal in 3–4 weeks with simple immobilization.

Greenstick Fracture

- Bone is bent and the tensile/convex side of the bone fails.
- Fracture line does not propagate to the concave side of the bone, therefore showing evidence of plastic deformation.
- If the bone undergoes plastic deformation, it is necessary to break the bone on the concave side to restore normal alignment, as the plastic deformation recoils the bone back to the deformed position.

Complete Fracture

- Fracture completely propagates through the bone.
- Classified as spiral, transverse, or oblique, depending on the direction of the fracture line.

Spiral Fractures

- Created by a rotational force
- Low-velocity injuries
- An intact periosteal hinge enables the orthopedic surgeon to reduce the fracture by reversing the rotational injury.

Oblique Fractures

- Occur diagonally across the diaphyseal bone at 30° to the axis of the bone.
- Unstable, therefore alignment is necessary.
- Fracture reduction is attempted by immobilizing the extremity while applying traction.

Transverse Fractures

- Created by a 3-point bending force.
- Easily reduced by using the intact periosteum from the concave side of the fracture force.

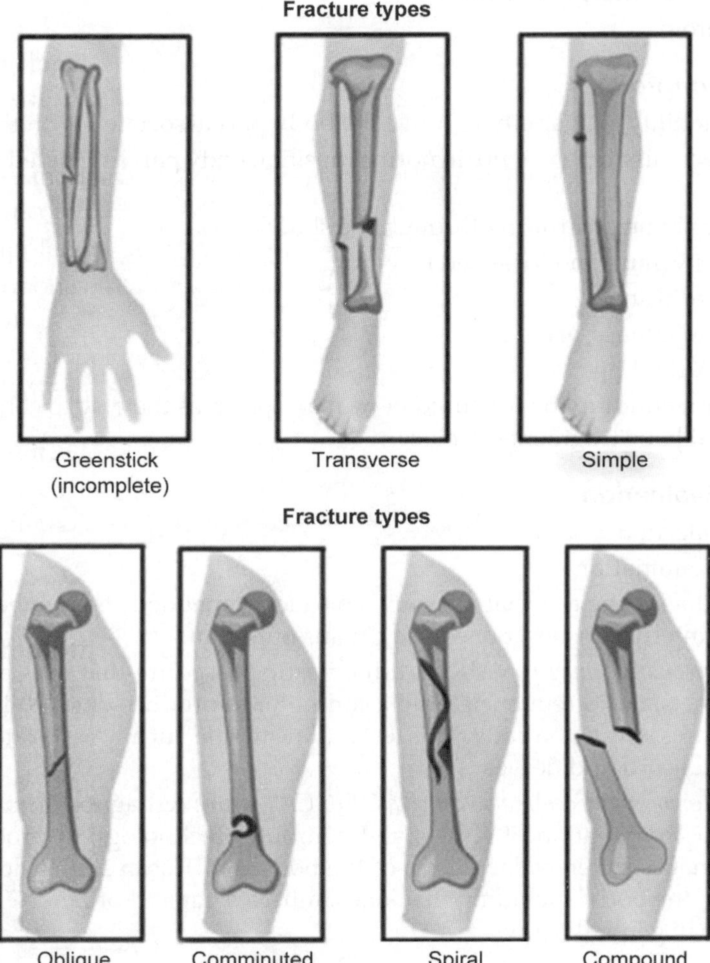

Fig. 7.118: Types of fracture

Causes

Some common causes of fractures are:

- Falls
- Direct strikes to the body
- Traumatic events such as auto accidents or gunshots
- Injuries during sports

These factors contribute to brittle bones:

- Osteoporosis
- Advanced age

- Endocrine and intestinal disorders
- Corticosteroids

Signs and Symptoms

- Limited mobility or inability to move the body part associated with the affected bone.
- A deformed, misshapen, or not in normal position body part associated with the affected bone
- An obvious bone protruding through the skin
- Localized swelling and localized bleeding
- Localized bruising
- Moderate to intense pain
- Numbness, tingling
- Muscles surrounding the fractured bone may spasm as they try to compensate to hold the affected bone fragments in place.

Diagnostic Evaluation

- History collection
- Physical examination
- *X-rays:* A diagnostic test that uses invisible electromagnetic energy beams to produce images of internal tissues, bones and organs onto film.
- *Magnetic resonance imaging (MRI):* A diagnostic procedure that uses a combination of large magnets, radiofrequencies and a computer to produce detailed images of organs and structures within the body. This test is done to rule out any associated abnormalities of the spinal cord and nerves.
- *Computed tomography scan (also called a CT or CAT scan):* A diagnostic imaging procedure that uses a combination of X-rays and computer technology to produce horizontal, or axial, images (often called slices) of the body. A CT scan shows detailed images of any part of the body, including the bones, muscles, fat and organs. CT scans are more detailed than general X-rays.

Management

- *Splint or cast:* This immobilizes the injured area to promote bone alignment and healing to protect the injured area from motion or use.
- *Medication* (for pain control)
- *Traction:* Traction is the application of a force to stretch certain parts of the body in a specific direction. Traction consists or pulleys, strings, weights and a metal frame attached over or on the bed. The purpose of traction is to stretch the muscles and tendons around the broken bone to allow the bone ends to align and heal.
- *Surgery:* This may be required to put certain types of broken bones back into place. Occasionally, internal fixation (metal rods or pins located inside the bone) or external fixation devices (metal rods or pins located outside of the body) are used to hold the bone fragments in place to allow alignment and healing.

Nursing Management

Nursing Assessment

- Assess for history of the injury, presence of factors that may cause pathologic fractures (osteoporosis, osteomyelitis, neoplastic diseases, etc.).
- Assess presence of signs of fracture (edema, pain, loss of motion, crepitus, extremity disproportion or abnormal positioning).
- Assess presence of signs and symptoms of soft tissues involvement (swelling, hemorrhage, impaired sensation in the extremity).
- Assess extremity for presence of open fracture and severe external hemorrhage.
- Assess vital signs, fluid balance and urine output.
- Assess diagnostic tests and procedures for abnormal values.
- Assess routine preoperative history.

Nursing Diagnosis

- Increased risk of hypovolemia and shock related to trauma and bleeding.
- Increased risk of bone inflammation related to open fracture.
- Increased risk of fat embolism related to fracture of the long bones.
- Increased risk of severe fluid, electrolyte and metabolic imbalances related to injury or inflammation.
- Pain and immobility, related to diagnosis of fracture.
- Increased risk of respiratory, cardiovascular, bowel and skin complications related to a long period of immobility.
- Anxiety related to the symptoms of disease and fear of the unknown.

Nursing Plan and Interventions

- Provide emergency care if requires (hemostasis, respiratory care, prevention of shock).
- Provide fracture fixation to prevent following injury of tissues.
- Observe signs of fat embolism (especially during first 48 hours after the fracture).
- Monitor fluids input and output continuously, insert IV catheter, urinary catheter.
- Monitor client's vital signs.
- Monitor client's laboratory tests results for abnormal values.
- Administer IV therapy, analgesics, antibiotics and other medications as prescribed.
- Prepare client and his family for surgical intervention if required.
- For client after surgical intervention provide routine postoperative care and teach about possible postoperative complications.
- Provide care to client with cast (observe signs of circulatory impairment – change in skin color and temperature, diminished distal pulses, pain and swelling of the extremity; protect the cast from damage).
- Provide care to client in traction (check the weights are hanging freely, observe skin for irritation and site of skeletal traction insertion for signs of infection; use aseptic technique when cleaning the site of insertion).

- In case of hip fracture and hip replacement maintain the abduction of the affected extremity.
- Provide respiratory exercises to prevent lung complications.
- Observe for signs of thrombophlebitis, report immediately.
- Provide appropriate skin care to prevent pressure sores.
- Encourage fluid intake and high-protein, high-vitamin, high-calcium diet.
- Teach the client appropriate crutch-walking techniques.
- Provide emotional support to client, explain all procedures to decrease anxiety and to obtain cooperation.
- Instruct client regarding fracture healing process, diagnostic procedures, treatment and its complications, home care, daily activities, diet, restrictions and follow-up.

PRE AND POST OPERATIVE CARE OF CHILDREN UNDERGOING SURGERY

Introduction

Preoperative care is the preparation and management of a child prior to surgery. It includes legal, physical and psychological preparation. The perioperative process can be stressful for children, their parents and the nurses who care for them. Children may experience anxiety and fear about surgery, pain, separation from parents, unfamiliar surroundings, the unknown, unpleasant sensory stimulation and loss of autonomy and control. Psychological problems can continue into the postoperative period with increased anxiety, disturbances in eating and sleeping, as well as increased pain and analgesic use.

Parents may also experience anxiety and concern about the competency of staff, possible complications and how to support their child. Unfamiliarity of surroundings and role expectations add to parental stress and this anxiety can transmit to their children.

Purpose

- The children who are physically and psychologically prepared for surgery tend to have better surgical outcomes.
- Preoperative teaching meets the child and parents need for information regarding the surgical experience, which in alleviate most of his or her fears.
- Child who are more knowledgeable about what to expect after surgery and who have an opportunity to express their goals and opinions, often cope better with postoperative pain and decreased mobility.
- Preoperative care is extremely important prior to any invasive procedure, regardless of whether the procedure is minimally invasive or a form of major surgery.
- Preoperative teaching must be individualized for each older child and parents.
- Some of the parents want as much information as possible, while others prefer only minimal information because too much knowledge may increase their anxiety.
- Children have different abilities to comprehend medical procedures; some prefer printed information, while others learn more from oral presentations.
- It is important for the parents to ask questions during preoperative teaching sessions.

Types of Preparation

A child's developmental stage can determine his level of understanding and coping mechanisms regarding the perioperative process. An appropriate developmental approach to a child is important in all phases of the surgical process, as well as all aspects of postoperative care. Developmental stages of childhood were identified by Erik Erikson and Jean Piaget. Erikson studied the impact of parents and society on a child's personality. Piaget determined that children learn about the world around them through their own actions and explorations.

It has been classified in mainly three types:

1. Legal preparation
2. Psychological preparation
3. Physical preparation

Legal Preparation (Informed Consent)

The child parents or guardians written consent for the surgery is a vital portion of preoperative care. By law, the physician who will perform the procedure must explain the risks and benefits of the surgery, along with other treatment options. However, the nurse is often the person who actually witnesses the patient's signature on the consent form. It is important that the patient understands everything he or she has been told. Sometimes, patients are asked to explain what they were told so that the health care professional can determine how much is understood.

Child who are mentally impaired, heavily sedated, or critically ill are not considered legally able to give consent. In this situation, the next of kin (spouse, adult child, adult sibling, or person with medical power of attorney) may act as a surrogate and sign the consent form. Children under age 18 must have a parent or guardian sign.

Psychological Preparation

- The children and their parents are often fearful or anxious about having surgery. It is often helpful for them to express their concerns to health care workers. This can be especially beneficial for patients who are critically ill, or who are having a high-risk procedure.
- The family needs to be included in psychological preoperative care. Pastoral care is usually offered in the hospital. If the patient has a fear of dying during surgery, this concern should be expressed and the surgeon notified. In some cases, the procedure may be postponed until the patient feels more secure.
- Children may be especially fearful. They should be allowed to have a parent with them as much as possible, as long as the parent is not demonstrably fearful and contributing to the child's apprehension. Children should be encouraged to bring a favorite toy or blanket to the hospital on the day of surgery.
- Children and families who are prepared psychologically tend to cope better with the patient's postoperative course. Preparation leads to superior outcomes since the goals of recovery are known ahead of time and the patient is able to manage postoperative pain more effectively.

Physical Preparation

- Physical preparation may consist of a complete medical history and physical exam, including the child surgical and anesthesia background. The parent should inform the physician and hospital staff if their child had an adverse reaction to anesthesia (such as anaphylactic shock), or if there is a family history of malignant hyperthermia.

- Laboratory tests may include complete blood count, electrolytes, prothrombin time, activated partial thromboplastin time, and urinalysis.
- The patient will most likely have an electrocardiogram (EKG) if he or she has a history of cardiac disease, or is over 50 years of age.
- A chest X-ray is done if the patient has a history of respiratory disease. Part of the preparation includes assessment for risk factors that might impair healing, such as nutritional deficiencies.
- Steroid use, radiation or chemotherapy, drug or alcohol abuse, or metabolic diseases such as diabetes.
- The patient should also provide a list of all medications, vitamins and herbal or food supplements that he or she uses. Supplements are often overlooked, but may cause adverse effects when used with general anesthetics (e.g. St. John's wort, valerian root). Some supplements can prolong bleeding time (e.g. garlic, gingko biloba).
- Latex allergy has become a public health concern. Latex is found in most sterile surgical gloves and is a common component in other medical supplies including general anesthesia masks, tubing and multi-dose medication vials. Children with disabilities are particularly susceptible.
- This includes children with spina bifida, congenital urological abnormalities, cerebral palsy and Dandy-Walker syndrome. At least 50% of children with spina bifida are latex-sensitive as a result of early, frequent surgical exposure.
- There is currently no cure available for latex allergy and research has found that the allergy accounts for up to 19% of all anaphylactic reactions during surgery. The best treatment is prevention, but immediate symptomatic treatment is required if the allergic response occurs. Every patient should be assessed for a potential latex reaction. Patients with latex sensitivity should have their chart flagged with a caution label. Latex-free gloves and supplies must be used for anyone with a documented latex allergy.
- Bowel clearance may be ordered if the patient is having surgery of the lower gastro-intestinal tract. The patient should start the bowel preparation early the evening before surgery to prevent interrupted sleep during the night. Some patients may benefit from a sleeping pill the night before surgery.
- The night before surgery, skin preparation is often ordered, which can take the form of scrubbing with a special soap (i.e. Hibiclens), or possibly hair removal from the surgical area. Shaving hair is no longer recommended because studies show that this practice may increase the chance of infection. Instead, adhesive barrier drapes can contain hair growth on the skin around the incision.

Preoperative Teaching

- Preoperative teaching includes instruction about the preoperative period about surgery and the postoperative period.
- Instruction about the preoperative period deals primarily with the arrival time, where the patient should go on the day of surgery and how to prepare for surgery. For example, patients should be told how long they should be NPO (nothing by mouth), which

medications to take prior to surgery and the medications that should be brought with them (such as inhalers for patients with asthma).

- Instruction about the surgery itself includes informing the patient about what will be done during the surgery and how long the procedure is expected to take. The patient should be told where the incision will be. Children having surgery should be allowed to 'practice' on a doll or stuffed animal. It may be helpful to demonstrate procedures on the doll prior to performing them on the child. It is also important for family members (or other concerned parties) to know where to wait during surgery, when they can expect progress information and how long it will be before they can see the patient.
- Knowledge about what to expect during the postoperative period is one of the best ways to improve the patient's outcome. Instruction about expected activities can also increase compliance and help prevent complications. This includes the opportunity for the patient to practice coughing and deep breathing exercises, use an incentive spirometer and practice splinting the incision. Additionally, the patient should be informed about early ambulation (getting out of bed). The patient should also be taught that the respiratory interventions decrease the occurrence of pneumonia and that early leg exercises and ambulation decrease the risk of blood clots.
- Patients hospitalized postoperatively should be informed about the tubes and equipment that they will have. These may include multiple intravenous lines, drainage tubes, dressings and monitoring devices. In addition, they may have sequential compression stockings on their legs to prevent blood clots until they start ambulating.
- Pain management is the primary concern for many patients having surgery. Preoperative instruction should include information about the pain management method that they will utilize postoperatively. Patients should be encouraged to ask for or take pain medication before the pain becomes unbearable and should be taught how to rate their discomfort on a pain scale. This instruction allows the patients and others who may be assessing them, to evaluate the pain consistently. If they will be using a patient-controlled analgesia pump, instruction should take place during the preoperative period. Use of alternative methods of pain control (distraction, imagery, positioning, mindfulness meditation, music therapy) may also be presented.

Nursing Care of Pre and Post Operative Child

The perioperative nurse in preparing children and families for the surgical process.

Infants

- Infants (birth to 1 year) develop relationships based on trust and depend on parents and caregivers to meet their needs. Separation from parents can cause distress, which is primarily expressed through crying.
- Encourage parents to remain with the infant through as much of the process as possible, as they derive comfort from familiar faces and voices. Encourage parents to bring a security object such as a blanket or stuffed animal to help soothe the infant when separated from his parents.
- Reunite the infant with his parents as soon as possible after the procedure to minimize distress. Limit the number of caregivers, if possible, as strangers also cause fear.

- Other comfort measures such as soft music, a pacifier, cuddling, gentle stroking, or rocking can help calm infants. Infants also enjoy nursery rhymes and simple rhythmic play.
- Preparation at this stage focuses on the parent due to the limited cognitive abilities of the child. Inform the parents about the procedure and provide support; their infant is likely to be less anxious if the parents are calm.

Toddlers

Toddlers (1 to 3 years) differ from infants as they are just beginning to gain autonomy by attempting to do things for themselves. This is an active period with short attention spans. Although verbal skills are limited, they understand more than they are able to say. Provide simple, concrete explanations about what the toddler will hear, feel, smell and taste. It is not necessary to cover all details of the surgery.

- In general, preparation should be done a day or two before surgery at a level the child will understand.
- Toddlers possess a limited concept of time, so use explanations the child is familiar with. For example, tell the child, 'The surgery will be before lunch.' Unfamiliar faces, routines and scary equipment may cause stress.
- Encourage family members to bring his favorite activities or toys to distract the child from boredom, fears and the new routine. Toddlers fear abandonment; as a result, separation from family can be extremely stressful.
- Minimizing separation from a parent can further a toddler's ability to cope in a stressful situation. A favorite toy, stuffed animal, or photograph that the child can hold while going to surgery can offer comfort.
- Toddlers may sometimes temporarily lose newly acquired skills such as walking or toilet training. Provide reassurance that this is okay and encourage family members to be accepting and supportive.
- It is important to answer questions about pain and separation truthfully. Also, provide simple choices whenever possible to heighten a toddler's sense of independence and control. For example, allow the toddler to choose his favorite of two character adhesive bandages for use after the IV is removed.

Preschoolers

- Preschoolers (3 to 5 years) develop their own identities, are very inquisitive and have active imaginations. Fantasies and misconceptions related to surgery are common.
- Offer simple explanations and descriptions, allowing the child to see and handle some of the medical equipment that will be used. Although their vocabulary is developing rapidly, they do not have the full ability to reason.
- Therefore, explanations about a procedure should be kept simple and matter-of-fact, focusing on what the child will hear, feel, smell, taste and see, as well as what the child is expected to do. Demonstrate with props, models and pictures whenever possible.
- As a preschooler's concept of time is limited, the nurse must review and reinforce the sequence and duration of all events. Use time concepts the child is familiar with: 'The operation will take less time than it takes to watch a cartoon.' Preparation for surgery for this developmental stage is recommended a day or two in advance.

- Preschool children fantasize and may feel that their operation is punishment for bad behavior. Reassure the child that he is not to blame and that the surgery is to fix something specific. Be honest, especially about separation and potential pain.
- Playing during the preoperative phase can help distract children who are distressed. As with all children, this age group will benefit from having a familiar toy, stuffed animal, or photograph. Offer choices whenever possible to promote a sense of control. One example might be the choice of flavored lip preparations used on the anesthesia mask to provide a more pleasing scent for the child. Another choice might be the type of transport to surgery the child would prefer such as walking, riding in a wagon, or being carried by the nurse.

School-age Children

- School-age children (5 to 12 years) devote most of their energy to school and peers. Mastery of skills, experiences and self-esteem are increasingly important issues for this age group. Although still engaged in some imaginary thinking, they are capable of concrete, logical reasoning and are gaining an increased understanding of cause and effect.
- They are better able to cooperate with treatment because they can think before they act.
- School-age children have an increased awareness of internal body parts and body function.
- They are also able to understand a series of actions and can therefore benefit from hearing about all steps involved in the surgical process.
- Preparation should begin a week in advance of the surgery. Allow the school-age child to participate in care when possible. For example, to provide a sense of control and encourage acceptance of treatment, ask the child to help hold the anesthesia mask.
- School-age children may fear other body parts will be hurt during the operation. Offer a simple explanation of what part of the body the operation will affect. Body outlines, pictures, or dolls may be helpful. For example, a child's understanding of a surgical site can be quickly assessed by asking him to mark the site on the doll. Any misconceptions revealed can then be corrected.
- Fear of death is common; the child's previous experience with illness and death will determine the explanation needed for reassurance. Be sure to express confidence in the surgeon and staff.

Adolescents

During adolescence (12 to 18 years), abstract thinking begins and adolescents can understand how the body functions, the nature of the problem and the reason for surgery. Provide honest, detailed explanations about the diagnosis and need for surgery, including what the adolescent will hear, feel, smell, taste and see. Adolescents often want to know the results of surgery and what will happen next. Involve them in decisions about their health as much as possible.

Common fears include waking during the procedure, pain and the possibility of death. They may need reassurance in their anesthesia provider's ability and an explanation that they would not wake up during the procedure but will wake up afterward.

The location and extent of surgical scars are often a major concern as adolescents may worry about how surgery will affect their appearance. If the adolescent wants to, allow him to see any changes after the procedure using mirrors as necessary. Provide reassurance that changes are temporary if that is true, but if not, be honest. Encourage parents to be available to talk after the procedure if the adolescent is willing.

Adolescents may become uncooperative or withdraw, so allow them as much independence as possible and let them know what is expected of them. Providing opportunities to make realistic choices when possible can help increase their sense of independence. For example, when ready to drink postoperatively, ask what beverage they would prefer.

Nurses should respect an adolescent's need for privacy. Always knock on the door or announce your presence before opening a curtain to avoid embarrassing them if they are undressing. This kind of courtesy can lead to increased cooperation.

During preoperative contact, encourage the family to pack the adolescent's familiar toiletries, clothing and slippers to convey a return to normalcy during the postoperative phase. Encourage the family to bring the adolescent's favorite book, magazines, word search, music with a headset, or a handheld video game to help reduce anxiety. Plan helpful coping behaviors ahead of time such as listening to music or imagining a favorite place and suggest that the family plan a favorite activity for their adolescent to look forward to after the operation.

Preparing Parents

- Preoperative preparation processes have been affected by changes in health care delivery systems and economic constraints.
- Preoperative hospital visits are now often replaced with information shared via telephone or web sites. Parents are becoming increasingly responsible for preparing their child for surgery.
- Therefore, parents should be partners in the preparation process, receiving not only information about the procedure and sequence of events, but also the guidance and tools to provide support and prepare the child for the experience. In one study, parents who received both written and verbal information expressed a preference for print materials, requiring guidance from the nurse to appropriate written resources.
- It is important to encourage parents to foster the child's normal development despite limitations that may be imposed by illness or injury.

MODEL QUESTIONS

Multiple Choice Questions

1. **Acute diarrhea is an attack of loose motion with sudden onset which usually last for ....**
   (a) 3 to 7 days (b) 25 to 30 days
   (c) 1 to 2 months (d) Up to 4 months
2. **Diarrhea with watery stools and visible blood in the stool is called ....**
   (a) Infection (b) Chronic diarrhea
   (c) Both a and b (d) Dysentery

3. Which of the following virus responsible for diarrhea?
(a) *E. coli* (b) Rotavirus
(c) Cholera vibrio (d) Candida albicans

4. The calculation of % of burn is done by ....
(a) Rule of nine (b) Rule of ten
(c) Fluid volume (d) None of there

5. Except this all are comes under the management of burns.
(a) Fluid replacements (b) Dressing
(c) Scratching of blisters (d) Nutritional supports

6. For burn patient which diet is preferred ....
(a) High protein and high calorie diet
(b) Low protein and low calorie diet
(c) Low protein and high vitamin diet
(d) All of these

7. Hydrotherapy is beneficial for .... patient
(a) Burn (b) TB
(c) Accidental (d) Allergy

8. Which one is the complication of burn?
(a) Hypovolemic shock (b) Respiratory failure
(c) Sepsis (d) All of these

9. Ectopia vesicae is also known as ....
(a) Empty bladder (b) Kidney disease
(c) Bladder exstrophy (d) None of them

10. The urethral opening present on the ventral aspect of penis is called ....
(a) Hypospadias (b) Epispadias
(c) Malformation (d) Stricture of urethra

11. Wilms tumor is the tumors of ....
(a) Eye (b) Kidney
(c) Stomach (d) Urethra

12. Wilms tumor is .... tumors
(a) Malignant (b) Benign
(c) Both a or b (d) None of them

13. The irreversible damage of kidney called
(a) Acute Glomerulonephritis (b) UTI
(c) Chronic glomerulonephritis (d) None of them

14. Nephritic syndrome is most common in
(a) Children (b) Old age
(c) Adult (d) All of these

15. Distention and rupture of the alveoli due to the loss of elasticity of the lung tissue called ..
(a) Pleural effusion (b) Atelectasis
(c) Emphysema (d) TB

16. Chronic and permanent dilation of the bronchi and bronchioles called ....

(a) Pleural effusion (b) Bronchiectasis
(c) Bronchitis (d) All of these

17. The thick pus collection in the pleural cavity called ....

(a) Empyema (b) Bronchiectasis
(c) Emphysema (d) All of these

18. The collection of air or gas in pleural space ....

(a) Pneumothorax (b) Pleural effusion
(c) Empyema (d) TB

19. Chronic inflammation bowel disease also called ....

(a) Ulcerative colitis (b) Bowel syndrome
(c) Inflammation (d) Peptic ulcer

20. Partial or total obstruction of the stomach outlet due to narrowing of the lumen is ....

(a) Pyloric stenosis (b) Stenosis
(c) Total obstruction (d) All of these

21. Tracheoesophageal fistula is fistula between ....

(a) Esophageal and trachea (b) Trachea and stomach
(c) Both a and b (d) All of these

22. Gastrostomy is done as case for ....

(a) EA with TEF (B) Liver abscess
(c) Nasal obstruction (d) Bowel inflammation disease

23. ......is the interruption in the normal flow of intestine content.

(a) Stomach obstruction (b) Gastroesophageal reflex
(c) Intestinal obstruction (d) Vomiting

24. Congenital a ganglions megacolon is also known as ....

(a) Megacolon (b) Paralytic ilius
(c) Acute liver disease (d) Large intestine

25. ...is a surgically created opening between the colon and the abdominal wall.

(a) Fistula (b) Incision
(c) Colostomy (d) All of these

26. Which of the following is the anorectal malformation...?

(a) Anal stenosis (b) Rectal atresia
(c) Rectal agenesis (d) All of these

27. The anorectal malformation corrective surgery PSARP stands for ....

(a) Peripheral sagittal anorectoplasty
(b) Post sagittal anorectoplasty
(c) Posterior sagittal anorectoplasty
(d) None of these

28. The herniation of the abdominal content through widerspread umbilicus and cover with a shiny vascular sac is. ....

(a) Exomphalos (b) Omphalocele
(c) Both a and b (d) None of these

29. The abnormal opening between the right and left ventricles called..........
(a) VSD
(b) ASD
(c) Dextroposition of aorta
(d) None of these

30. The abnormal opening between right and left atria called..........
(a) CHD
(b) VSD
(c) ASD
(d) Liver disease

31. The abnormal opening between the middle of the atrial septum is ......
(a) Ostium secondary
(b) Ostium primum
(c) Sinus venosus
(d) CHD

32. Which one is the cyanotic heart disease?
(a) VSD
(b) ASD
(c) PDA
(d) All of these

33. The most important drug used to treat CCF.
(a) Digitalis
(b) Spironolactone
(c) Amoxicillin
(d) All of these

34. According to WHO grading anemia the severe anemia happens when Hb level is ....
(a) 10 mg/dL
(b) 9 mg/dL
(c) 8 mg/dL
(d) Less than 7 mg /dL.

35. Which one is the cause of anemia?
(a) Trauma
(b) Thalassemia
(c) Dysentery
(d) All of these

36. Megaloblastic anemia is caused by the deficiency of ....
(a) Folic acid
(b) Vitamin B-12
(c) Both a and b
(d) All of these

37. Management of megaloblastic anemia is ....
(a) Folic acid and vitamin B-12
(b) Vitamin C
(c) Both a and b
(d) None of these

38. Which of the following is autosomal recessive disorder?
(a) Megaloblastic anemia
(b) Sickle cell anemia
(c) Severe anemia
(d) Thalassemia

39. Pancytopenia is ....
(a) Decrease RBC count
(b) Decrease WBC count
(c) Decrease all blood count
(d) Increase RBC count

40. Thalasemia is characterized by reduction in the synthesis of ....
(a) RBC
(b) WBC
(c) Hemoglobin
(d) All of these

41. Iron chelation therapy prevent the patient from ....
(a) Complication of repeated blood transfusion
(b) Radiation therapy
(c) Palliative therapy
(d) None of these

42. **The disease caused by deficiency of clotting factors ....**
(a) Anemia (b) Thalassemia
(c) Hemophilia (d) All of these

43. **Which one is the common type blood cancer in children?**
(a) Thalassemia (b) Leukemia
(c) Sickle cell anemia (d) All of these

44. **The inflammation of the layer covering the brain and spinal cord called...**
(a) Meningitis (b) Encephalitis
(c) Trauma (d) All of these

45. **The common antibiotics use for pyogenic bacterial meningitis is...**
(a) Corticosteroids (b) Dopamine
(c) Penicillin (d) All of these

46. **The tuberculosis meningitis caused by ....**
(a) *Mycobacterium tuberculosis* (b) *E. coli*
(c) *Streptococcus* (d) None of these

47. **The common complication of TB meningitis is ....**
(a) Infection (b) Deafness
(c) Hydrocephalus (d) Numbness

48. **The inflammation of brain tissues called ....**
(a) Meningitis (b) Encephalitis
(c) Inflammation (d) None of these

49. **The involuntary contraction or series of contraction of the voluntary muscles....**
(a) Encephalitis (b) Infection
(c) Convulsion (d) All of these

50. **Deficiency of antidiuretic hormones cause ....**
(a) Diabetes (b) Diabetes insipidus
(c) Thyroid (d) None of these

51. **Except which hormones is not secreated by anterior pituitary gland ....**
(a) Growth hormone (b) TSH
(c) Follicle stimulating hormone (d) Antidiuretic

52. **Which hormone is secreated by thyroid gland?**
(a) Thyroxine (T4) (b) Triiodothyronine
(c) Calcitonin (d) All of these

53. **The low level of thyroid hormone caused ....**
(a) Hypothyroidism (b) Hyperthyroidism
(c) Both a and b (d) None of these

54. **Goiter also known as ....**
(a) Tumor (b) Thyromegaly
(c) Swelling of throat (d) None of these

55. **Inflammation of bone called ....**
(a) Osteomyelitis (b) Ossification
(c) Arthritis (d) All of these

56. Handicapped children can be classified broadly into...

(a) Physically (b) Mentally
(c) Socially (d) All of these

57. Stammering is the ...problem

(a) Speech (b) Auditory
(c) Visual (d) All of these

Fill in the Blanks

1. The rule of nine apply for ....case.
2. The irreversible damage of the kidney known as ....renal /kidney disease.
3. Empyema is the ......collection of pleural space.
4. Malabsorption syndrome is also known as..........
5. The megaloblastic anemia caused by ....and.......deficiency.
6. Pancytopenia is the condition in which the counts of ....decrease.
7. The full form of AIDS..............
8. The cause of AIDS is............
9. Meningitis is the inflammation of ....
10. Encephalitis is the inflammation of ....

True or False

1. Kernig's sign is seen in the epilepsy patient.
2. Goiter is also known as thyromegaly.
3. Night blindness and xerophthalmia caused by deficiency of vitamin D.
4. Vitamin K is useful for the formation of the prothrombin.
5. Colitis is the inflammation of the intestine.
6. Medical management of intestinal obstruction is abdominal decompression.
7. Hirshsprung's disease is also known as congenital megacolon.
8. The thalassemia syndrome reduce the hemoglobin synthesis.
9. Hyperthyroidism also known as graves disease.
10. Hirschsprung's disease is a developmental disorder.
11. Breakage in the continuity of bone called fracture.
12. Traction used in case of fracture.

Short Answer Questions $1 \times 5 = 5$

(a) Altered state of consciousness.
(b) Write nursing management for unconscious patient.
(c) Osteomyelitis.
(d) Appendicitis.
(e) Hyperthyroidism.
(f) Pneumonia.
(g) Pleural effusion.
(h) Atelectasis.
(i) Management of child with drowning.

Long Answer Questions

1 × 15 = 15

1. (a) Define acute respiratory infection.
   (b) Classification of acute respiratory infection.
   (c) Write signs and symptoms of acute respiratory infection.
2. (a) Define asthma.
   (b) Etiological factors of asthma.
   (c) Clinical features of asthma.
   (d) Write nursing management of asthmatic patient.
3. (a) Define intestinal obstruction.
   (b) Explain the causes of intestinal obstruction.
   (c) Write the medical and surgical management of intestinal obstruction.
   (d) Write the nursing management of the child having intestinal obstruction.
4. (a) Define anemia.
   (b) Classification of anemia.
   (c) Causes of anemia.
   (d) Write medical and nursing management for anemic patient.
5. (a) Define meningitis.
   (b) Signs and symptoms of meningitis.
   (c) Write the medical and surgical management for meningitis.
   (d) Explain nursing management for meningitis patient.
6. (a) Define convulsion.
   (b) Explain the stages of convulsion.
   (c) Explain the management of convulsion
7. (a) Define burns.
   (b) Types of burns.
   (c) Write medical and nursing management of child having burns.

ANSWER KEY

Multiple Choice Questions

1. (a)	2. (d)	3. (b)	4. (a)	5. (a)	6. (a)	7. (a)
8. (d)	9. (c)	10. (a)	11. (b)	12. (a)	13. (c)	14. (a)
15. (c)	16. (b)	17. (a)	18. (a)	19. (a)	20. (a)	21. (a)
22. (a)	23. (c)	24. (a)	25. (c)	26. (d)	27. (c)	28. (c)
29. (a)	30. (c)	31. (a)	32. (d)	33. (a)	34. (d)	35. (d)
36. (c)	37. (a)	38. (c)	39. (c)	40. (c)	41. (a)	42. (c)
43. (b)	44. (a)	45. (c)	46. (a)	47. (c)	48. (b)	49. (c)
50. (b)	51. (d)	52. (d)	53. (b)	54. (c)	55. (d)	56. (a)
57. (a)						

Fill in the Blanks

1. Burns
2. Chronic
3. Pus
4. Celiac disease
5. Vitamin B-12 and folic acid
6. All blood counts
7. Acquired immune deficiency syndrome
8. HIV
9. Brain covering
10. Brain tissues

True or False

1. False	2. True	3. False	4. True
5. True	6. True	7. True	8. True
9. True	10. True	11. False	12. True

Chapter 8

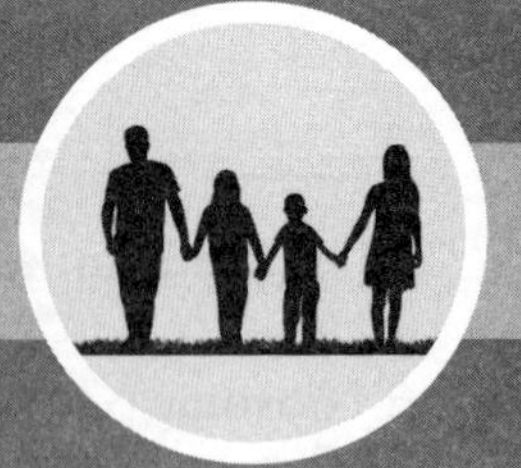

Child Welfare Services

- **Child Welfare Services and Agencies**
  - Integrated Child Development Services (ICDS)
  - Mid-day Meal Program
  - Balwadi or Anganwadi
  - Day-care Center
  - New Parent Support Program (NPSP)
- **Law Pertaining to Pediatrics**
  - National Policy on Child Labour (NPCL)
  - Child Act
  - Juvenile Justice Act
  - Internationally Accepted Rights of the Child
  - Rehabilitation of Delinquent and Destitute Children
  - Adoption Laws and Services
  - Adolescent Health Programs
  - Menstrual Hygiene
  - WIFS Program
  - Adolescent Safety Program

CHILD WELFARE SERVICES AND AGENCIES

INTRODUCTION

India has also acceded to the UN convention on the rights of the child to reiterate its commitment to the cause of children. The objective of the convention is to give every child the right to survival and development in a healthy and congenial environment. India is also party to the Millennium Development Goals and the South Asian Association for Regional Cooperation (SAARC) conventions on Child Welfare and Combating Trafficking of Women and Children is SAARC region.

Ministry of Women and Child Development has prepared a *National Plan of Action for Children* 2005 after harmonizing the goals for children set in the UN General Assembly Special

Session on Children held in 2002 and the monitorable targets set in the tenth five year plan and goals for children in related Ministries/Departments. The action plan has been prepared in consultation with concerned Ministries and Departments, States/UT Governments, nongovernmental organizations and experts. The National Plan of Action includes goals, objectives, strategies and activities for improving nutritional status of children, reducing IMR and MMR, increasing enrolment ratio and reducing dropout rates, universalization of primary education, increasing coverage for immunization, etc.

Child Welfare Programs

Several ministries and departments of the government of India are implementing various schemes and programs for the benefit of children. Some of the schemes and programs are as under:

Integrated Child Development Services (ICDS)

The integrated child development services being implemented by ministry of women and child development is the world's largest program aimed at enhancing the health, nutrition and learning opportunities of infants, young children (0–6 years) and their mothers. It is the foremost symbol of India's commitment to its children—India's response to the challenge of providing preschool education on one hand and breaking the vicious cycle of malnutrition, mortality and morbidity to the other.

The scheme provides an integrated approach for converging basic services through community based workers and helpers. The services are provided at a center called the 'Anganwadi', which literally means a courtyard play center, a childcare center located within the village itself.

The packages of services are enlisted below:

- Supplementary nutrition
- Immunization
- Health check-up
- Referral services
- Preschool nonformal education
- Nutrition and health education.

It is a centrally sponsored scheme implemented through the State Governments with 100% financial assistance from the Central Government for all inputs other than supplementary nutrition which the States were to provide from their own resources. However, from the year 2005–06, the Government of India has decided to provide Central assistance to States for supplementary nutrition also to the extent of 50% of the actual expenditure incurred by States or 50% of the cost norms, whichever is less.

Creche Scheme for the Children of Working Mothers

The Ministry of Women and Child Development has launched a new Creche scheme in January 2006. The scheme has been named as Rajiv Gandhi National Creche Scheme for the children of working mothers. These creches have been allocated to the Central Social Welfare Board, Indian Council for Child Welfare and Bhartiya Adim Jati Sevak Sangh in the ratio of 80:11:9. The priority has been given to uncovered districts/areas and tribal areas while extending the scheme to maintain balance regional coverage. Eligibility criteria under the revised scheme has also been enhanced from ₹ 1800 to ₹ 12000 per month per family.

Nutrition Program for Adolescent Girls

Nutrition component of Prime Minister Gramodya Yojana and Nutrition Programme for Adolescent Girls being implemented in 51 districts with additional central assistance provided by the Planning Commission, directly and indirectly contribute to promoting nutrition of children. A National Nutrition Mission has also been set up with a view to enable policy direction to concerned Departments of the Government for addressing the problem of malnutrition in a mission mode.

Reproductive and Child Health Programme (RCH)

Being implemented by the Ministry of Health and Family Welfare, the program provides effective maternal and child health care, micronutrient interventions for vulnerable groups, reproductive health services for adolescent, etc. Some important programs cover:

- Immunization for children for DTP, Polio and Tetanus Toxoid for women
- Vitamin-A administration
- Iron and folic acid for pregnant women.

This program integrates all family welfare and women and child health services with the explicit objective of providing beneficiaries with 'need-based, client centered, demand driven, and high quality integrated RCH services'. The strategy for the RCH program shifts the policy emphasis from achieving demographic targets to meeting the health needs of women and children.

Pulse Polio Immunization Programme

The Pulse Polio Immunization Programme being implemented by the Ministry of Health and Family Welfare covers all children blow five years. It is a massive program covers 166 million children in every round of National Immunization Day. The other immunization programs include Hepatitis B, DPT and other routine immunization.

Other notable programs for child health include, Universal immunization programme, control of deaths due to acute respiratory infections, control of diarrheal diseases, provision of essential new-born care to address the issue of the neonates, prophylactic programs for the prevention and treatment of two micronutrient deficiencies relating to vitamin A and iron, Anemia control programme, Border District Cluster Strategy and Integrated Management of Neonatal and childhood illness.

Sarva Shiksha Abhiyan

The Sarva Shiksha Abhiyan being implemented by the Department of Education provides for school infrastructure and quality improvement in education of the children. The specific objectives are:

- All children to be in school
- Universal retention by 2010
- Bridging all gender and social gaps at primary stage by 2007 and at elementary education level by 2010.

The Government of India is committed to realizing the goal of universalization of elementary education by 2010. Under Sarva Shiksha Abhiyan (SSA), the National flagship programme, the government aims to provide free and compulsory elementary education to all children in the 6–14 age groups by 2010.

National Program for Education of Girls at Elementary Level

A National Program for education of girls at elementary level is also being implemented by the Department of Education for children in difficult circumstances including drop out girls, working girls, girls from marginalized social groups, girls with low levels of achievement to gain quality elementary education and to develop self esteem of girls through a community based approach.

Kasturba Gandhi Balika Vidyalaya

The Kasturba Gandhi Balika Vidyalaya is a new scheme being implemented by the Department of Educaiton, which enables opening of 750 special residential schools for the girl child belonging to SC/ST, other backward classes and minority in educationally backward blocks having low female literacy.

Mid-day meal Scheme is also one of the important schemes of the government to aim universal enrollment and retention of children. Under the program nutrition snacks are provided to children attending schools.

Integrated Program for Street Children

The programme is being implemented by the Ministry of Social Justice and Empowerment. This programme aims at preventing destitution of children and facilitate their withdrawal from life on the streets. The programme is targeted towards children without homes and family ties, especially vulnerable to abuse and exploitation.

Integrated Program for Juvenile Justice

The program is being implemented by the Ministry of Social Justice and Empowerment with a view to providing care to children in difficult circumstances and children in conflict with the law through government institutions and through NGOs. Some special features of the scheme areas:

- Establishment of a National Advisory Board on Juvenile Justice.
- Creation of a Juvenile Justice Fund.
- Training, orientation and sensitization of judicial, administrative police and NGOs responsible for implementation of JJ Act.
- Institutions are to be used but only as a last measure by enlarging the range of suitable alternatives.
- Financial assistance to bring about a qualitative improvement in the existing infra-structure.
- Expansion of noninstitutional services such as sponsorship, foster care, probation, etc. as and an alternate to institutional care.

Child helpline: Child helpline is a toll free telephone service (1098) which anyone can call for assistance in the interest of children. Being run with the support of women and Child Welfare Ministry is working in 72 cities across the country. The *Shishu Greh Scheme* is also being implemented by the ministry to promote adoptions within the country and to ensure minimum standards in the care of abandoned/orphaned/destitute children. Grant-in-Aid upto a ceiling of Rs. 6 lakh is provided per unit of 10 children in a Shishu Greh.

The National Rural Health Mission

A scheme of health Ministry seeks to provide effective healthcare to rural population including large population of children throughout the country with special focus on 18 States, which have weak public health indicators and/or raise public spending on health from 0.9% of GDP to 2–3% of GDP. It aims to undertake architectural correction of the health system to enable it to effectively handle increased allocations as promised under the National Common Minimum Programme and promote policies that strengthen public health management and service delivery in the country.

Elimination of Child Labor

The Elimination of Child Labor is being implemented by the Ministry of Labor which sanctions projects for rehabilitation of working children and for elimination of child labor. Under the project based Action Plan of the Policy, National Child Labor Projects (NCLPs) have been set up in different areas to rehabilitate child labor. A major activity undertaken under the NCLP is the establishment of special schools to provide nonformal education, vocational training, supplementary nutrition, etc. to children withdrawn from employment. 150 Child Labor Projects have so far been sanctioned for rehabilitating children in the most endemic areas and 1.5 lakh children have already been mainstreamed in the special schools.

Prevention of Offences Against Children

After wide consultations a draft bill for offences against children has been prepared and circulated to the state governments for their comments and views. After obtaining the comments of the state governments and concerned ministries and departments, a draft has been prepared and circulated to the concerned ministries and departments for their comments and use.

Constitutional Provisions

- Article 14 provides that the state shall not deny to any person equality before the law or the equal protection of the laws within the territory of India.
- Article 15(3) provides that, 'nothing in this article shall prevent the state for making any special provision for women and children'.
- Article 21 provides that no person shall be deprived of his life or personal liberty except according to procedure established by law.
- Article 21A directs the state shall provide free and compulsory education to all children of the age of six to fourteen years in such manner as the state may by law, determine.
- Article 23 prohibits trafficking of human beings and forced labor.
- Article 24 prohibits employment of children below the age of fourteen years in factories, mines or any other hazardous occupation.
- Article 25–28 provides freedom of conscience, and free profession, practice and propagation of religion.

- Article 39(e) and (f) provide that the state shall, in particular, direct its policy towards securing to ensure that the health and strength of workers, men and women and the tender age of children are not abused and that the citizens are not forced by economic necessity to enter avocations unsuited to their age or strength and that the children are given opportunities and facilities to develop in a healthy manner and in conditions of freedom and dignity and that the childhood and youth are protected against exploitation and against moral and material abandonment.
- Article 45 envisages that the State shall endeavor to provide early childhood care and education for all children until they complete the age of six years.

Table 8.1:Child welfare programs

S. No.	Child welfare programs	Year of beginning	Objectives/Description
1	Integrated Child Development Services (ICDS)	1975	It is aimed at enhancing the health, nutrition and learning opportunities of infants, young children (0–6 years) and their mothers.
2	Creche scheme for the children of working mothers	2006	Overall development of children, childhood protection, complete immunization, awareness generation among parents on malnutrition, health and education.
3	Reproductive and Child Health Programme	1951	To provide quality Integrated and sustainable Primary Health Care services to the women in the reproductive age group and young children and special focus on family planning and Immunization.
4	Pulse Polio Immunization Programme	1995	To eradicate poliomyelitis (polio) in India by vaccinating all children under the age of five years against polio virus.
5	Sarva Shiksha Abhiyan	2001	All children in school, Education Guarantee Center, Alternate School, 'Back-to-School' camp by 2003; all children complete five years of primary schooling by 2007; all children complete eight years of elementary schooling by 2010; focus on elementary education of satisfactory quality with emphasis on education for life; bridge all gender and social category gaps at primary stage by 2007 and at elementary education level by 2010; universal retention by 2010.
6	Kasturba Gandhi Balika Vidyalaya	2004	To ensure access and quality education to the girls of disadvantaged groups of society by setting up residential schools with boarding facilities at elementary level.
7	Mid-day Meal Scheme	1995	Improving the nutritional status of children in classes I to VIII in Government, Local Body and Government aided schools, and EGS and AIE centers. Encouraging poor children, belonging to disadvantaged sections, to attend school more regularly and help them concentrate on classroom activities. Providing nutritional support to children of primary stage in drought-affected areas during summer vacation.

Contd...

Contd...

S. No.	Child welfare programs	Year of beginning	Objectives/Description
8	Integrated Program for Street Children	1993	Provisions for shelter, nutrition, health care, sanitation and hygiene, safe drinking water, education and recreational facilities and protection against abuse and exploitation to destitute and neglected street children.
9	The National Rural Health Mission	2005	Reduction in child and maternal mortality, universal access to public services for food and nutrition , sanitation and hygiene and universal access to public health care services with emphasis on services addressing women's and children's health universal immunization, etc.

INTEGRATED CHILD DEVELOPMENT SERVICES (ICDS)

Introduction

The Integrated Child Development Services was launched on 2nd October 1975 presently ICDS scheme represents one of the world's largest and most unique program for early childhood development. ICDS is the foremost symbol of India's commitment to children, India's response to the challenge of providing preschool education on one hand and breaking the vicious cycle of malnutrition, morbidity, reduced learning capacity and mortality, on the other.

Objectives

The Integrated Child Development Services (ICDS) scheme was launched in 1975 with the following objectives:

- To improve the nutritional and health status of children in the age-group 0–6 years
- To lay the foundation for proper psychological, physical and social development of the child
- To reduce the incidence of mortality, morbidity, malnutrition and school dropout
- To achieve effective coordination of policy and implementation amongst the various departments to promote child development
- To enhance the capability of the mother to look after the normal health and nutritional needs of the child through proper nutrition and health education.

Services

The above objectives are sought to be achieved through a package of services comprising:

- Supplementary nutrition
- Immunization
- Health check-up
- Referral services
- Preschool nonformal education
- Nutrition and health education.

Concept of ICDS

The concept of providing a package of services is based primarily on the consideration that the overall impact will be much larger if the different services develop in an integrated manner as the efficacy of a particular service depends upon the support, it receives from related services.

Services of ICDS

Nutrition Including Supplementary Nutrition

This includes supplementary feeding and growth monitoring; and prophylaxis against vitamin A deficiency and control of nutritional anemia. All families in the community are surveyed, to identify children below the age of six and pregnant and nursing mothers. They avail of supplementary feeding support for 300 days in a year. By providing supplementary feeding, the Anganwadi attempts to bridge the caloric gap between the national recommended and average intake of children and women in low income and disadvantaged communities.

Growth monitoring and nutrition surveillance are two important activities that are undertaken. Children below the age of three years of age are weighed once a month and children 3–6 years of age are weighed quarterly. Weight-for-age growth cards are maintained for all children below six years. This helps to detect growth faltering and helps in assessing nutritional status. Besides, severely malnourished children are given special supplementary feeding and referred to medical services.

Immunization

Immunization of pregnant women and infants protects children from six vaccine preventable diseases—poliomyelitis, diphtheria, pertussis, tetanus, tuberculosis and measles. These are major preventable causes of child mortality, disability, morbidity and related malnutrition. Immunization of pregnant women against tetanus also reduces maternal and neonatal mortality.

Health Check-ups

This includes health care of children less than six years of age, antenatal care of expectant mothers and postnatal care of nursing mothers. The various health services provided for children by anganwadi workers and Primary Health Center (PHC) staff, include regular health check-ups, recording of weight, immunization, management of malnutrition, treatment of diarrhea, de-worming and distribution of simple medicines, etc.

Referral Services

During health check-ups and growth monitoring, sick or malnourished children, in need of prompt medical attention, are referred to the Primary Health Center.

The anganwadi worker has also been oriented to detect disabilities in young children. She enlists all such cases in a special register and refers them to the medical officer of the Primary Health Center/Subcenter.

Non-formal Pre-school Education (PSE)

The Non-formal Pre-school Education (PSE) component of the ICDS may well be considered the backbone of the ICDS programme, since all its services essentially converge at the anganwadi a village courtyard. Anganwadi Center (AWC), a village courtyard – is the main platform for delivering of these services.

These AWCs have been set-up in every village in the country. In pursuance of its commitment to the cause of India's children, present government has decided to set-up an AWC in every human habitation/settlement. As a result, total number of AWC would go up to almost 1.4 million.

This is also the most joyful play-way daily activity, visibly sustained for three hours a day. It brings and keeps young children at the anganwadi center—an activity that motivates parents and communities. PSE, as envisaged in the ICDS, focuses on total development of the child, in the age up to six years, mainly from the underprivileged groups. Its program for the three-to six years old children in the anganwadi is directed towards providing and ensuring a natural, joyful and stimulating environment, with emphasis on necessary inputs for optimal growth and development.

The early learning component of the ICDS is a significant input for providing a sound foundation for cumulative lifelong learning and development. It also contributes to the universalization of primary education, by providing to the child the necessary preparation for primary schooling and offering substitute care to younger siblings, thus freeing the older ones, especially girls to attend school.

Nutrition and Health Education

Nutrition, Health and Education (NHED) is a key element of the work of the anganwadi worker. This forms part of BCC (Behavior Change Communication) strategy. This has the long-term goal of capacity-building of women – especially in the age group of 15–45 years —so that they can look after their own health, nutrition and development needs as well as that of their children and families.

Population Norms

- Community Development Block in a State should be the unit for sanction of an ICDS Project in rural/tribal areas, irrespective of number of villages/population in it.
- The existing norm of 1 lakh population for sanction of urban project may continue.

Types of Supplementary Nutrition

- *Children in the age group 0–6 months:* For Children in this age group, States/UTs may ensure continuation of current guidelines of early initiation (within one hour of birth) and exclusive breastfeeding for children for the first 6 months of life.
- *Children in the age group 6 months to 3 years:* For children in this age group, the existing pattern of Take Home Ration (THR) under the ICDS scheme will continue. However, in addition to the current mixed practice of giving either dry or raw ration (wheat and rice) which is often consumed by the entire family and not the child alone, THR should be given in the form that is palatable to the child instead of the entire family.
- *Children in the age group 3 to 6 years:* For the children in this age group, State/UTs have been requested to make arrangements to serve Hot Cooked Meal in AWCs and mini-AWCs under the ICDS Scheme. Since the child of this age group is not capable of consuming a meal of 500 calories in one sitting, States/UTs may arrange to provide a morning snack in the form of milk/banana/egg/seasonal fruits/micronutrient fortified food, etc.

Table 8.2: The concept of providing a package of services

Services	Target group	Service provided by
Supplementary Nutrition	Children below 6 years: Pregnant and Lactating Mother (P and LM)	Anganwadi Worker and Anganwadi Helper
Immunization	Children below 6 years: Pregnant and Lactating Mother (P and LM)	ANM/MO
Health Check-up	Children below 6 years: Pregnant and Lactating Mother (P and LM)	ANM/MO/AWW
Referral Services	Children below 6 years: Pregnant and Lactating Mother (P and LM)	AWW/ANM/MO
Preschool Education	Children 3–6 years	AWW
Nutrition and Health Education	Women (15–45 years)	AWW/ANM/MO

The ICDS Team Members

- Anganwadi Workers
- Anganwadi Helpers
- Supervisors
- Child Development Project Officers (CDPOs)
- District Program Officers (DPOs)

Anganwadi worker, a lady selected from the local community, is a community-based frontline honorary worker of the ICDS Programme. She is also an agent of social change, mobilizing community support for better care of young children, girls and women. Besides, the medical officers, Auxiliary Nurse Midwife (ANM) and Accredited Social Health Activist (ASHA) form a team with the ICDS functionaries to achieve convergence of different services.

International Partners of ICDS

Government of India partners with the following international agencies to supplement interventions under the ICDS:

- United Nations International Children Emergency Fund (UNICEF)
- Cooperative for Assistance and Relief Everywhere (CARE)
- World Food Programme (WFP)

Recent Initiatives

The Ministry has recently initiated a process of consultations with the states and other stakeholders to review and identify gaps in the existing training system and make suggestions to strengthen the ICDS training program including its contents/syllabi, training methodology and the existing monitoring mechanism under ICDS training program.

MID-DAY MEAL PROGRAM (OR) MID-DAY SCHOOL MEAL

Introduction

National Programme of Nutritional Support to Primary Education, popularly known as the Mid-Day Meal Scheme (MDM) was started in 1995 in an attempt to enhance enrollment, retention and attendance while simultaneously improving nutritional levels among children in school. It currently covers nearly 12 crore children. Mid-day meals program has an important role in providing balanced diet to school children. In this program, one-third of the child's daily food requirement can be fulfilled. CARE, UNICEF and many international, governmental, voluntary agencies give their contribution in this.

The main objectives of the scheme (as per the 2006 revision) are to:
- Improve the nutritional status of children in classes one through five in government schools and government aided schools
- To encourage children from disadvantaged backgrounds to attend school regularly and help them concentrate in school activities.
- As well as provide nutritional support to students in drought- ridden areas throughout summer vacation.

Aims of Mid-day School Meal

- To fulfill one-third nutrition requirement of school children
- To create interest about school and education among children
- To reduce absenteeism of children in school
- To provide relief to parents of poor children.

Concept of Program

The concept and the purpose of initiating anything is always good but when it comes to the management then we are miserable. The same thing has happened to Mid-day Meal Scheme in India. It has been found by the Human Resource Development (HRD) ministry that most of the states are receiving complaints regarding the schemes but no one is acting on these complaints that are filed against the program.

The program is being carried out by local authorities with assistance from village panchayats, village education committees, school management committees, parent teacher associations, etc. In rural areas the cooking is being done by women self-help groups. In urban areas, some NGOs have taken responsibility for cooking the food and bringing it to the primary schools. Free mid-day meals can achieve a great deal with regard to child education and health. They promote the participation of the child in school, reduce classroom hunger, facilitate the healthy growth of a child, promotes good eating habits like washing ones hands, finishing ones food, etc, and fosters social and gender equality as all children get the same food and must eat together.

Principles of Mid-day School Meal

- One-third energy and half of protein requirement of the child should be met in the daily school mid-day meal program.
- The food should be free or at a minimum cost. Cooperation from voluntary agencies should be sought for free food.
- The food should be prepared in the school itself. Hence, easily cooked and prepared food should be chosen.
- Locally available food should be used in preparing the meal. Utensils can be procured with local support but it is necessary to observe food hygiene.

- The menu should be changed to avoid boredom among children.
- The mid-day school meal program is a supplement and not substitutes of home meals. In case, there is some interruption in the mid-day school lunch program, the children can bring packed food or Tiffin from home. In any case, the children should not be deprived of mid-day lunch.

Sample Menu

Cereals	75 gm/per day per child
Pulses	30 gm/per day per child
Green leafy vegetables	30 gm/per day per child
Other vegetables	30 gm/per day per child
Oil	8 gm/per day per child

According to National Institute of Nutrition (NIN), the mid-day school meal program should be organized for at least 250 days in an educational calendar year. Teachers have an important role in school lunch program. Participation of parents is also necessary. It is also necessary to give sufficient importance to nutrition education in the curriculum of general education.

The program is being carried out by local authorities with assistance from village panchayats, village education committees, school management committees, parent teacher associations, etc. In rural areas the cooking is being done by women self-help groups. In urban areas, some NGOs have taken responsibility for cooking the food and bringing it to the primary schools. Free mid-day meals can achieve a great deal with regard to child education and health. They promote the participation of the child in school, reduce classroom hunger, facilitate the healthy growth of a child, promotes good eating habits like washing ones hands, finishing ones food, etc. and fosters social and gender equality as all children get the same food and must eat together.

Mid-day Meal Scheme

Mid-day meal scheme was launched on 15 August 1995. It is a central sponsored scheme, which was revised in 2004. Mid-day meal scheme is also called as National Programme of Nutritional Support to Primary Education. The main objective of the scheme is increasing the enrolment and reducing the absenteeism of students of primary classes.

In this scheme, central provides free supply of food grains through FCI (Food Corporation of India) to states. Along with the supply of 100 gm grain per student per day subsidy is also given for transportation of food grain. At least 300 calories and 12 gm protein is provided to all primary class students through this scheme.

BALWADI OR ANGANWADI

Introduction

The word *Anganwadi* means 'courtyard shelter' in Indian languages. They were started by the Indian government in 1975 as part of the Integrated Child Development Services program to combat child hunger and malnutrition.

A typical Anganwadi center provides basic health care in Indian villages. It is a part of the Indian public health care system. Basic health care activities include contraceptive counseling and supply, nutrition education and supplementation, as well as pre-school activities. The centers may be used as depots for oral rehydration salts, basic medicines and contraceptives.

Functions

- The basic job of Anganwadi workers is extremely important and needs to be carried out in the most efficient manner possible. They need to provide care for newborn babies and ensure that all children below the age of 6 are immunized.
- They are expected to provide antenatal care for pregnant women and ensuring that they are immunized against tetanus. In addition to this they provide post-natal care to nursing mothers.
- Since they primarily focus on poor and malnourished groups, they provide supplementary nutrition to children below the age of 6 and nursing and pregnant women.
- They ensure that regular health and medical check-ups for women 15- to 49-years-old take place and that all women and children have access to these check-ups.
- They work toward providing preschool education to children who are between 3 to 5-years-old
- The Ministry of Women and Child Development has laid down guidelines for the responsibilities of Anganwadi workers (AWW).
- These include showing community support and active participation in executing this program, to conduct regular quick surveys of all families, organize preschool activities, provide health and nutrition education to families especially pregnant women on how to breastfeed, etc. motivating families to adopt family planning, educating parents about child growth and development, assist in the implementation and execution of Kishori Shakti Yojana (KSY) to educate teenage girls and parents by organizing social awareness programs, etc. identify disabilities in children.

Advantages

India is a country suffering from overpopulation, malnourishment, poverty and high infant mortality rates. To counter the health and mortality issues there is a great need for medical and health care experts. Unfortunately India has a shortage of skilled professionals. Therefore, through the Anganwadi system, the country is trying to meet its goal of enhanced health facilities that are affordable and accessible for local populations.

In many ways an Anganwadi worker is better equipped than a physician in reaching out to the rural population. Since the worker lives with the people, she is in a better position to identify the cause of health problems and hence counter them. She has a very good insight of the health status in her region. Secondly though Anganwadi workers are not as skilled or qualified as professionals, they have better social skills thus making it easier to interact with the people. Moreover, since these workers are from the village, they are trusted which makes it easier for them to help the people. Last but not the least, Anganwadi workers are well aware of the ways of the people, are comfortable with the language, know the rural folk personally, etc. This makes it very easy for them to figure out the problems being faced by the people and ensure that they are solved.

DAY-CARE CENTER

Day-care center, also called day nursery, nursery school, or crèche (French: 'crib'), institution that provides supervision and care of infants and young children during the daytime, particularly so that their parents can hold jobs. Day-care centers were established in most European cities and industrial centers during the second half of the 19th century; the first in Great Britain, for example, was established in 1860. In the United States, the terms day nursery, day- or child-care center, and nursery schools are often used interchangeably to identify various types of day-care for children and for preschool educational programs.

It is the care of a child during the day by a person other than the child's legal guardians, typically performed by someone outside the child's immediate family. Day-care is typically an ongoing service during specific periods, such as the parents' time at work.

Services to young children and their families have a longer history in European and Asian countries than in the United States, where day-care centers are generally private and of varying quality. In many countries, day-care facilities are associated with the mother's place of work. Infant care and preschool programs are a normal provision in many developed countries, and in some countries, such as France and Italy, they are included in the regular public-school system. (For more reference see the chapter 3, page No: 109)

NEW PARENT SUPPORT PROGRAM (NPSP)

Introduction

It is a professional team of licensed social workers, counselors and registered nurses who provide educational and supportive services to military families. From the early stages of pregnancy to the development of your child up thru age 5, this program can better prepare you for parenthood. Our trained, supervised staff has extensive knowledge of the issues encountered by today's parents. Our team is sensitive to the unique challenges facing military families. We can help families cope with stress, isolation, pre and post deployment, homecoming reunions, and the everyday demands of parenting in the military. New ages and

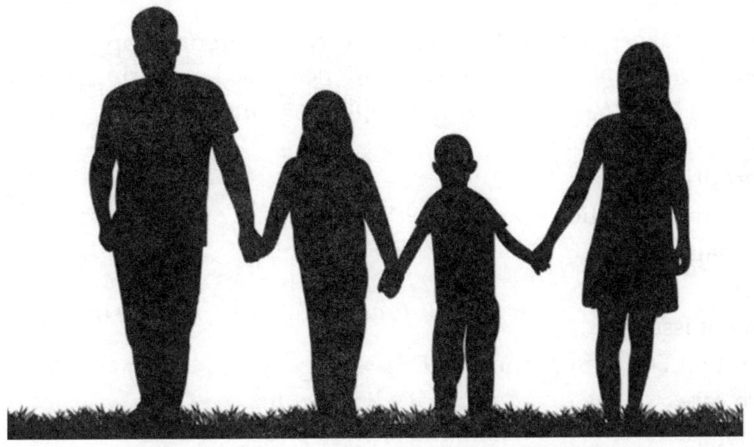

Fig. 8.1: New parent support program (NPSP)

stages in child development bring different challenges. NPSP offers you the opportunity to express your concerns and ask questions about babies, young children and family relationships.

Types of Services Provided

The needs of participating families are assessed through screening tools that help the New Parent Support Program service providers understand a family's unique needs. Most participating families use only basic services, including parenting classes, resource materials, playgroups and visits with a program staff member.

On occasion, families may be struggling with high stress, multiple challenges related to military operations, fewer parenting skills or social isolation. These families may qualify for a higher priority for service or more intensive services. What classifies as an intensive service varies from one installation to another, but it generally refers to frequent (more than three) home visits, formal referral to other support agencies or a follow-up by a provider in the Family Advocacy Program.

The New Parent Support Program is staffed by nurses, social workers, or home visitation specialists, and is supervised and monitored by the Family Advocacy Program manager, the Office of the Secretary of Defense and at the installation level the Family Advocacy Program. The program focuses on providing one-on-one support for new and expectant parents through home visits, but some installations may offer parenting classes and groups.

Services vary by service branch and by installation, but they can include:

Play Groups

Structured activities in program play groups help children improve their social and motor skills. The play groups also help new parents get to know one another and develop a support system within the military community. Play groups may also be available to families with school-aged children.

Home Visits

Home visits can take place in the home, the New Parent Support office or any other convenient and comfortable location. The evidence-based nurturing parenting curriculum is utilized during home visits. Home visit topics may include:

- Age appropriate discipline
- Age appropriate play
- Effective communication
- Stress management
- Nutrition
- Deployment issues
- Sudden Infant Death Syndrome (SIDS)
- Newborn care
- Sibling rivalry
- Toilet training.

Baby Boot Camp

This is a fun and interactive class for expectant active duty personnel and their partners. Baby Boot Camp covers everything a parent needs to know to take care of their newborn, as well as, information on resources for the whole family, including:

- The role of a parent
- Developmental stages of infants
- Basic infant care
- Child safety
- Pre and postpartum emotions

Classes are held monthly between 9 am to 4 pm. Please call for dates, registration, and class location.

Parenting Classes

A 9-week, court approved Parenting Class series for parents with children under the age of 6.

Topics

- Safety
- Communication
- Discipline
- Self-esteem
- Family structure
- All classes must be completed within one year to receive a certificate of completion. Please call New Parent Support for class dates, location and times.
- Referrals to other resources
- Sometimes you may need the assistance of additional services offered through the military health care system, your installation or the local community.
- Program professionals can help you find and take advantage of those services that suit your needs best.

LAW PERTAINING TO PEDIATRICS

NATIONAL POLICY ON CHILD LABOUR (NCLP)

Introduction

The National Policy on Child Labour (NCLP), announced in 1987, emphasizes the need for strict enforcement measures in the areas of high child labor concentration along with appropriate rehabilitative measures to curb this menace. In order to translate the policy into action, the Government of India initiated the National Child Labour Project Scheme in 1988.

The National Child Labour Policy (NCLP) stems from Government's recognition that child labor is harmful to the development of the child and has long-term adverse consequences on the cultural, economic, social and political development of a nation.

Definition

The Child Labour Policy of 1987 has envisages a plan, a legislative plan of action. It also calls for program and project-based intervention. A copy of the policy document has not been made available on the Ministry of Labor website or anywhere else according to our research. To know more about child labor in India visit either the section on National Child Labour Project or Child Labour (Prohibition and Regulation) Act, 1986.

Child Labor Policies

The policy of the government on the issue of Child Labor. The National Policy on Child Labor declared in August, 1987, contains the action plan for tackling the problem of Child Labor.

It envisages:

- *A legislative action plan:* The government has enacted the Child Labour (Prohibition and Regulation) Act, 1986 to prohibit the engagement of children in certain employments and to regulate the conditions of work of children in certain other employments.
- Focusing and convergence of general development programs for benefiting children wherever possible, A core group on convergence of various welfare schemes of the government has been constituted in the Ministry of Labour and Employment to ensure that, the families of the child labor are given priority for their upliftment.
- Project-based action plan of action for launching of projects for the welfare of working children in areas of high concentration of child labor.

Objective of the Scheme

- This is the major Central Sector Scheme for the rehabilitation of child labor.
- The scheme seeks to adopt a sequential approach with focus on rehabilitation of children working in hazardous occupations and processes in the first instance.
- Under the Scheme, survey of child labor engaged in hazardous occupations and processes has been conducted.
- The identified children are to be withdrawn from these occupations and processes and then put into special schools in order to enable them to be mainstreamed into formal schooling system.
- Project societies at the district level are fully funded for opening up of special schools/ rehabilitation centers for the rehabilitation of child labor.

The Special Schools/Rehabilitation Centers Provide

- Non-formal/bridge education
- Skilled/vocational training
- Mid day meal Stipend @ ₹ 150/- per child per month.
- Health care facilities through a doctor appointed for a group of 20 schools.

The Target Group

The project societies are required to conduct survey to identify children working in hazardous occupations and processes. These children will then form the target group for the project society. Of the children identified those in the age group 5 to 8 years will have to be mainstreamed directly to formal educational system through the SSA. Working children in the age group of 9 to 14 years will have to be rehabilitated through NCLP schools established by the project society.

Project Implementation

The entire project is required to be implemented through a registered society under the Chairmanship of administrative head of the district, namely, District Magistrate/Collector/ Dy. Commissioner of the district. Members of the society may be drawn from concerned government departments, representatives of Panchayat Raj Institutions, NGOs, Trade Unions, etc.

Funding Pattern

The projects have been taken up in the central sector, the entire funding is done by the Central Government (Ministry of Labour and Employment). Funds are released to the concerned Project Societies depending upon the progress of project activities.

CHILD ACT

Definition

Children are the important age group in all societies. Health status and health behavior of later life are laid down on this stage. National policy are made for children to improve their health status. The Children Act 1960 (amended in 1977) in India provides for the care for the maintenance, welfare, training, education and rehabilitation of the delinquent child. It covers the neglected child, destitute, socially handicapped, uncontrolled, victimized and delinquent children.

Types of Child Acts

Advisory for Eliminating of Corporal Punishment in Schools

The Right of Children to Free and Compulsory Education (RTE) Act, 2009, which has come into force with effect from 1 April 2010, prohibits, physical punishment and mental harassment, under Section 17(1) and makes it a punishable offence under Section 17(2).

These provisions read as follows:

Section 17, Prohibition of physical punishment and mental harassment to child:

- No child shall be subjected to physical punishment or mental harassment.
- Whoever contravenes the provisions of sub-section shall be liable to disciplinary action under the service rules applicable to such person.

Sections 8 and 9 of the RTE Act place a duty on the appropriate government and the local authority to 'ensure that the child belonging to weaker section and the child belonging to disadvantaged group are not discriminated against and prevented from pursuing and completing elementary education on any grounds'.

Child Labor (Prohibition and Regulation) Act, 1986

Child Labor Act Prohibition and Regulation Act, 1986. Where and how children can work and where they cannot. The act defines a child as any person who has not completed his fourteenth year of age. The act prohibits children from working in any occupation for example: Catering at railway establishments, construction work on the railway or anywhere nears the tracks, plastics factories, automobile garages, etc. The act also prohibits children from working in places for example: beedi making, tanning, soap manufacture, brick kilns and roof tiles units, etc.

Not permitted to work for more than three hour stretches and must receive an hour break after the three hours. Not permitted to work for more than six hour stretches including their break interval and cannot work between the hours of 7 p.m. and 8 a.m. No child is allowed to work overtime or work in more than one place in a given day. A child must receive a holiday from work every week. The penalty of allowing a child to work in occupations/ processes outlined in the schedule which are prohibited is a minimum of 3 months prison time and/or a minimum of ₹ 10,000 in fines. Second time offenders are subject to jail time of minimum six months.

Juvenile Justice (Care and Protection of Children) Act, 2000

This is an important statute that criminalists acts that may cause a child mental or physical suffering.

Section 23 of the JJ Act, 2000 states as follows: 'Whoever, having the actual charge of, or control over, a juvenile or the child, assaults, abandons, exposes or willfully neglects the juvenile or causes or procures him to be assaulted, abandoned, exposed or neglected in a manner likely to cause such juvenile or the child unnecessary mental or physical suffering shall be punishable with imprisonment for a term which may extend to six months, or fine, or with both.'

Section 23 covers the actions of anyone who has 'actual charge or control over' a child. While Section 23 is likely to be applied most often to personnel in childcare institutions regulated by the JJ Act, it arguably applies to cruelty by anyone in a position of authority over a child, which would include parents, guardians, teachers and employers.

Child Marriage Act

Child marriage in India, according to the Indian law, is a marriage where either the woman is below age 18 or the man is below age 21. Most child marriages involve underage women, many of whom are in poor socioeconomic conditions.

Child marriage was outlawed in 1929, under Indian law. However, in the British colonial times, the legal minimum age of marriage was set at 15 for girls and 18 for boys. Under protests from Muslim organizations in the undivided British India, a personal law Shariat Act was passed in 1937 that allowed child marriages with consent from girl's guardian.

After independence and adoption of Indian constitution in 1950, the child marriage act has undergone several revisions. The minimum legal age for marriage, since 1978, has been 18 for women and 21 for men.The child marriage prevention laws have been challenged in Indian courts with some Muslim Indian organizations seeking no minimum age and that the age matter be left to their personal law. Child marriage is an active political subject as well as a subject of continuing cases under review in the highest courts of India.

The definition of child marriage was last updated by India with its The Prohibition of Child Marriage Act of 2006, which applies only (a) to Hindus, Christians, Jains, Buddhists and those who are non-Muslims of India, and (b) outside the state of Jammu and Kashmir. For Muslims of India, child marriage definition and regulations based on Sharia and Nikah has been claimed as a personal law subject.

The Prohibition of Child Marriage Act of 2006 defines 'child marriage' means a marriage, or a marriage about to be solemnized, to which either of the contracting parties is a child; and child for purposes of marriage is defined based on gender of the person—if a male, it is 21 years of age, and if a female, 18 years of age.

Other Child Acts

- Standard Operating Procedures in safeguarding Rights of Children in contact with Railways
- The Protection of Children from Sexual Offences Act 2012
- The Right of Children to Free and Compulsory Education Act, 2009
- Bonded Labor System (Abolition) Act, 1976
- Factories Act, 1948
- Infant Milk Substitutes, Feeding Bottles and Infant Foods
- Prenatal Diagnostic Techniques Act, 1994
- Persons with Disabilities Act, 1995
- Immoral Traffic Prevention Act, 1986
- Guardians and Wards Act, 1890
- Hindu Adoption and Maintenance Act, 1956
- Right to Food Legislation and Children
- Scheduled Castes and Scheduled Tribes Act, 1989
- The India Penal Code and Child related offenses

JUVENILE JUSTICE ACT

Introduction

The first legislation on juvenile justice in India came in 1850 with the Apprentice Act which required that children between the ages of 10–18 convicted in courts to be provided vocational training as part of their rehabilitation process. This act was transplanted by the Reformatory Schools Act, 1897, the Indian Jail Committee and later the Children Act of 1960. The Juvenile Justice Bill was first introduced in the Lok Sabha on 22 August 1986. This Act was further amended in 2006 and 2011 and is now known as the Juvenile Justice (Care and Protection) Act, 2000. The State of Jammu and Kashmir has repealed its existing juvenile law of 1997 and has enacted the Jammu and Kashmir (Care and Protection of Children) Act 2013. This legislation is very similar to India's national juvenile law except that it does not contain any provision on adoption.

Section 21 of the Juvenile Justice (Care and Protection of Children) Act, 2000 (56 of 2000) as amended by the Juvenile Justice (Care and Protection of Children) Amendment Act, 2006 (33 of 2006), states that: 'Prohibition of publication of name, etc.

The Juvenile Justice Act, which allows children aged 16 to 18 years and in conflict with law to be tried as adults in cases of heinous offences, comes into force Friday. The Act, passed by the Rajya Sabha in the winter session of Parliament, received President Pranab Mukherjee's assent on December 31.

The Ministry of Woman and Child Development has passed orders stating that the Juvenile Justice (Care and Protection of Children) Act 2015 will be enforceable from January 15, 2016.

Aims of Juvenile Justice

The juvenile justice system shall emphasize the well-being of the juvenile offender must be in proportion to the circumstances of both the offender and the offence. There are two major objectives of juvenile justice. They are:

- The well-being of the juvenile
- 'The principle of proportionality', which is intended to curb' punitive sanctions expressed in just deserts in relation to the gravity of the offence', and to ensure that the response to the younger offender be based on the consideration not only of the gravity of the offence but also of the personal circumstances'.
- While the reaction must aim to ensure the welfare of the young offender, it must no go beyond necessity and, therefore infringe upon the rights of a young individual.

Some Important Points

- Juvenile Justice (Care and Protection of Children) Act, 2015 has been passed by Parliament of India. It aims to replace the existing Indian juvenile delinquency law, Juvenile Justice (Care and Protection of Children) Act, 2000, so that juveniles in conflict with Law in the age group of 16–18, involved in Heinous Offences, can be tried as adults. The Act came into force from 15 January 2016.
- The bill allows for juveniles 16 years or older to be tried as adults for heinous offences like rape and murder. Heinous offences are those which are punishable with imprisonment of seven years or more.
- The bill mandates setting up Juvenile Justice Boards and Child Welfare Committees in every district. Both must have at least one woman member each.
- Once the bill becomes law, the decision to try a juvenile 16 years or older as an adult will be taken by the Juvenile Justice Board, which will have a judicial magistrate and two social workers as members. If the board decides against it, the juvenile will be sent for rehabilitation.
- The Child Welfare Committees will look at institutional care for children in their respective districts. Each committee will have a chairperson and four other members, all specialists in matters relating to children.
- The government says it listed the bill more than a dozen times in the monsoon session and the ongoing winter session but it could not be taken up due to disruptions. The opposition, led by the Congress, had assured support to pass the bill today.
- The bill aims to 'consolidate and amend the law relating to children alleged and found to be in conflict with law and children in need of care and protection by catering to their basic needs through proper care, protection, development, treatment, social re-integration, by adopting a child-friendly approach.'
- The proposed law also aims at adjudicating and disposing cases dealing with juveniles keeping in mind 'the best interest of the children and their rehabilitation.'
- India is a signatory to the UN Convention on the Rights of the Child which mandates that all children under the age of 18 years be treated equal. The pending bill has been criticized for violation of the Convention.
- The bill also deals with adoption of children and lays down the eligibility criteria for adoptive parents. A central adoptive resource agency will frame the rules for adoption, which will be implemented by state and district level agencies.

INTERNATIONALLY ACCEPTED RIGHTS OF THE CHILD

Introduction

UNICEF considers child protection as the prevention of or responding to the incidence of abuse, exploitation, violence and neglect of children. This includes commercial sexual exploitation, trafficking, child labor and harmful traditional practices, such as female genital mutilation/cutting and child marriage. Protection also allows children to have access to their other rights of survival, development, growth and participation. UNICEF maintains that when child protection fails or is absent children have a higher risk of death, poor physical and mental health, HIV/AIDS infection, educational problems, displacement, homelessness, vagrancy and poor parenting skills later in life.

United Nations educational guides for children classify the rights outlined in the Convention on the Rights of the Child as the '3 Ps': Provision, Protection, and Participation.

- *Provision:* Children have the right to an adequate standard of living, health care, education and services, and to play and recreation. These include a balanced diet, a warm bed to sleep in, and access to schooling.
- *Protection:* Children have the right to protection from abuse, neglect, exploitation and discrimination. This includes the right to safe places for children to play; constructive child rearing behavior, and acknowledgment of the evolving capacities of children.
- *Participation:* Children have the right to participate in communities and have programs and services for themselves. This includes children's involvement in libraries and community programs, youth voice activities, and involving children as decision-makers.

Universally child rights are defined by the United Nations and United Nations Convention on the Rights of the Child (UNCRC). According to the UNCRC Child Rights are minimum entitlements and freedoms that should be afforded to all persons below the age of 18 regardless of race, color, gender, language, religion, opinions, origins, wealth, birth status or ability and therefore apply to all people everywhere. The UN finds these rights interdependent and indivisible, meaning that a right cannot be fulfilled at the expense of another right.

The purpose of the UNCRC is to outline the basic human rights that should be afforded to children. There are four broad classifications of these rights. These four categories cover all civil, political, social, economic and cultural rights of every child.

- *Right to survival:* A child's right to survival begins before a child is born. According to Government of India, a child life begins after twenty weeks of conception. Hence the right to survival is inclusive of the child rights to be born, right to minimum standards of food, shelter and clothing, and the right to live with dignity.
- *Right to protection:* A child has the right to be protected from neglect, exploitation and abuse at home, and elsewhere.
- *Right to participation:* A child has a right to participate in any decision-making that involves him/her directly or indirectly. There are varying degrees of participation as per the age and maturity of the child.
- *Right to development:* Children have the right to all forms of development: Emotional, Mental and Physical. Emotional development is fulfilled by proper care and love of a support system, mental development through education and learning and physical development through recreation, play and nutrition.

The Declaration of the Rights of the Children

- The right to equality, without distinction on account of race, religion or national origin.
- The right to special protection for the child's physical, mental and social development.
- The right to a name and a nationality.
- The right to adequate nutrition, housing and medical services.
- The right to special education and treatment when a child is physically or mentally handicapped.
- The right to understanding and love by parents and society.
- The right to recreational activities and free education.
- The right to be among the first to receive relief in all circumstances.
- The right to protection against all forms of neglect, cruelty and exploitation.
- The right to be brought up in a spirit of understanding, tolerance, friendship among people and universal brotherhood.

REHABILITATION OF DELINQUENT AND DESTITUTE CHILDREN

Definition

Delinquent Children

A delinquent child is a child of a certain age, who has violated a criminal law or engaged in a disobedient, indecent or immoral conduct. A delinquent child is usually in need of rehabilitation.

Juvenile delinquency has peak incidence around fifteen or sixteen years of age and is commonly associated with peer pressures to conform, parental neglect and lack of social opportunity to direct energy into more acceptable channels. There is often a poor school record, with truancy and resentment of authority. Most delinquents eventually learn to conform to generally acceptable patterns of behavior.

Destitute Children

According to UNICEF, children worldwide lose their parents in conflict, or due to poverty, disability, HIV/AIDS. Hence there is a large population of children that grow up without one or both of their parents. Children without parental care are at a high-risk of abuse, exploitation and neglect. Large numbers of children end up in institutional care. Inadequate individual care of institutions can socially and emotional impair children.

Children may be destitute, for the interim or permanently of parental care for many reasons including the illness, death or imprisonment of parents, separation due to migration or armed conflict, the removal by child welfare authorities and/or the courts based on the child's best interests, detention of the child, or following the child's own initiative to leave home.

In India the child parent relationship is often seen as one of obedience of a social order more so than a right of the child. Hence when a child is separated from his/her parent, it is not viewed as the duty of the state to provide that child with a family environment. None the less adoption is supervised by the state, but India does not have a long-term foster care or alternate care system outside of institutionalization.

Causes

- Broken families
- AIDS victim parents
- Extremely poor and helpless single parent or both parents
- Parent(s) died of illness other than AIDS
- Insurgency problems
- Parent(s) died either in an accident or committed suicide
- Abandoned by parents

Legal Protection Act

- The Hindu Adoption and Maintenance Act 1956
- The Guardian and Wards Act 1890
- The Juvenile Justice Act 2000

Rehabilitation

Providing them basic needs, emotional security, care and protection. This project is all about how these destitute children are taken care and rehabilitated in normal society. It also includes the perception of people towards these children and difficulties to rehabilitate them in normal society. As a social responsibility we must help or think how we can help these children in a positive and effective way.

- There are various NGO's, Government organizations taking care of these children and trying to rehabilitate them in normal society.
- As a social responsibility we must help these destitute children by financially or by physically.
- As a human-being we must help these children to rehabilitate them in normal society.

The purpose of CARA is to ensure that every orphan, destitute and surrendered child has a loving and caring family. It currently comes under the purview of the Ministry of Women and Child Development. CARA was established in 1990 under the Ministry of Welfare. Ministry of Social Justice and Empowerment conferred onto CARA the responsibility of upholding the Hague Convention on Protection of Children and Cooperation in respect of Inter-country Adoption of 1993. It became an autonomous body in 1999 by registering it under the Societies Registration Act, 1860. After the passing of the Juvenile Justice Act 2000 and its amendment in 2006, CARA was transferred to the MWCD. In India a child can be placed with a family under the Hindu Adoption and Maintenance Act 1956, Guardians and Wards Act, 1890 and Juvenile Justice Act, 2000.

Other agencies concerned with the process of adoption both in India and internationally are as follows:

- Recognized Indian Placement Agencies (RIPAs)
- Enlisted Foreign Adoption Agencies
- Adoption Coordinating Agencies (ACAs)
- Shishu Grehs
- Licensed Adoption Placement Agencies (LAPAs)
- Indian Federation of Adoptive Families Associations (IFAFA)

CARA has set out both the In-country and Inter-country guidelines and procedures for adoption.

Welfare Schemes

Scheme for welfare of orphan and destitute children is a part of Women and Child Development department. There are 85 orphanages running in the state in 28 districts with 5603 inmates. Of these 85 orphanages, 6 orphanages are managed by the Orissa State Council for Child Welfare, OSCCW, while the remaining 79 are managed by NGOs or Voluntary Organizations. From 7th August 2004, the Government has increased the maintenance grant from ₹ 300 to 500 per inmate per month. Orphan and destitute children in the age group up to 18 years for boys and up to 25 years for girls are covered.

Objectives

The objective of the program is to prevent children from turning destitute through provision of shelter, nutrition, health care, education and vocational guidance to orphaned and destitute children throughout the State. Orphans and destitute children in the age group up to 18 years for boys and up to 25 years for girls are covered. This scheme is a State Government initiative and is implemented through Voluntary Organizations or NGOs.

Funding Pattern

An amount of ₹ 1.50 crores has been provided during 2005 to 2006 under the RLTAP for KBK and ₹ 1.00 crore under state plan for this scheme. During 2006 to 2007, an amount of ₹ 78.49 lakhs has been provided in the plan budget under state plan and ₹ 266.69 lakhs under non plan for maintenance of various orphanages.

ADOPTION LAWS AND SERVICES

Definition

Adoption is defined as a social and legal process that creates a new family, giving adopted children the same rights and benefits as those born into the family. To children without a permanent family, adoption represents the hope for a better life.

The adoption procedure in India is governed by specific legislations that are applicable depending on the religion of the person who wants to adopt (called the 'adopter') a child (who is the 'adoptee'). There are two major adoptions laws that apply to adopters in India:

The Hindu Adoption and Maintenance Act, 1956 (HAMA)

This act deals with the adoption process for all Hindus in India. For legal purposes under this Act, a Hindu is defined as any person who is a Hindu, Buddhist, Jain, Brahmo, Sikh, Prarthna or Arya Samaji. An important condition of this Act is that if a couple already has a biological child, they can only adopt children belonging to the opposite sex (i.e. a girl if they already have a boy and vice versa). All cases related to adoption are handled by the city civil courts under this Act.

The Guardianship and Wards Act, 1890

This Act gives complete guardianship authority to all non-Hindus such as Christians, Muslims, Parsis and Jews who are also governed by their own religious personal laws. In this case, while the adoptive parents are conferred guardianship status, the adopted child does not automatically get inheritance rights. As per this law, guardians need to submit an investment plan and also invest a certain amount of money in the name of the ward for his/her future security. The adoption cases under this Act are handled by the High court or Family courts.

Eligibility Criteria for Prospective Adoptive Parents

- The prospective adoptive parents should be physically, mentally and emotionally stable; financially capable; motivated to adopt a child; and should not have any life-threatening medical condition
- Any prospective adoptive parent, irrespective of his marital status and whether or not he has his own biological son or daughter, can adopt a child
- Single female is eligible to adopt a child of any gender
- Single male person shall not be eligible to adopt a girl child
- In case of a couple, the consent of both spouses shall be required
- No child shall be given in adoption to a couple unless they have at least two years of stable marital relationship
- The age of prospective adoptive parents as on the date of registration shall be counted for deciding the eligibility and the eligibility of prospective adoptive parents to apply for children of different age groups shall be as under:

Age of the child	Maximum composite age of prospective adoptive parents	Maximum age of single prospective adoptive parent
Upto 4 years	90 years	45 years
Above 4 upto 8 years	100 years	50 years
Above 8 upto 18 years	110 years	55 years

  - The minimum age difference between the child and either of the prospective adoptive parents should not be less than twenty five years
  - The age for eligibility will be as on the date of registration of the prospective adoptive parents
  - Couples with more than four children shall not be considered for adoption.

Legal Procedure

- The specialized adoption agency shall file the adoption petition in the court, having jurisdiction over the place where the specialized adoption agency is located, within seven days from the date of acceptance by prospective adoptive parents for obtaining the necessary adoption orders under the Act.
- In case the child is from a children's home which is located in another district, the specialized adoption agency shall file the adoption petition in the concerned court of that district.
- The adoption petition shall contain all requisite documents as per Schedule 8.
- The court will hold the adoption proceeding in-camera and dispose of the case within a period of two months from the date of filing of the adoption petition by the specialized adoption agency.

- The specialized adoption agency shall obtain a certified copy of the adoption order from the court and will forward it to the prospective adoptive parents within ten days and it shall also post a copy of such order in the Child Adoption Resource Information and Guidance System and make necessary entries in Child Adoption Resource Information and Guidance System.
- Registration of an adoption deed shall not be necessary.
- The specialized adoption agency shall obtain the birth certificate of the child from the birth certificate issuing authority within ten days from the date of issuance of adoption order, with the name of adoptive parents, as parents, and date of birth as recorded in the adoption order.

Adoption Procedure in India

Indian citizens can adopt in India under three major legislations: the Hindu Adoption and Maintenance Act of 1956, the Guardians and Wards Act of 1890 and the Juvenile Justice (Care and Protection) Act of 2000, amended in 2006.

The Hindu Adoption and Maintenance Act, 1956 (HAMA)

This Act covers Hindus, Buddhists, Jains or Sikhs. Some relevant parts of the Act are:

- Married couples or single adults can adopt
- Legally the man adopts with the consent of his wife
- A single man or woman can adopt
- If a biological child already exists in the family, a child of the opposite sex has to be adopted
- Children adopted under this Act get the same legal rights as a biological child might
- Children under the age of 15 years can be adopted
- A single man adopting a girl should be at least 21 years older than the child
- A single woman adopting a boy should be at least 21 years older than the child
- Adoption under this act is irrevocable.

The Guardians and Wards Act, 1890 (GWA)

Before the Juvenile Justice (Care and Protection) Act of 2000, this was the only legislation that allowed non-Hindus to adopt. However, this act ended up being the first secular law that allowed for a child to be adopted in India. The salient points of this Act are:

The parent adopting is a 'guardian' and the child is a 'ward', meaning that the same rights of a biological child are not inherent

- Anyone under the age of 18 years can be a ward
- The guardianship can be revoked by the courts or by the guardian
- A will is required for any property/goods to be bequeathed to the child
- This will can be legally contested by 'blood' relatives
- Both spouses can legally be guardians (versus HAMA where the man adopts with the consent of his wife)
- Single people can adopt without any age difference restrictions.

The Juvenile Justice (Care and Protection) Act of 2000, Amended in 2006 (JJ Act)

The JJ Act is meant mainly for the care and rehabilitation of children in conflict with the law. There was the need for a law that would allow children the same rights, whether they were adopted or biological. There was also the need for a law that delinked adoption from the religion of the adoptive parent(s). The JJ Act filled this space and a tiny section was added on for adoption.

The Amendment Act of 2006 has since expanded the provisions. The main strengths of this Act are:

- Any Indian citizen can adopt a child who is legally free for adoption
- The adoptee gets the same rights that a biological child might
- The religion of the adoptive parent(s) is not relevant
- Single people can adopt
- The adoption is irrevocable
- Some time limits have been set to ensure that children are considered legally free for adoption earlier
- The thrust is on the best interest of the child.

Section 2 (aa) of the Act defines adoption as 'the process through which the adopted child is permanently separated from his biological parents and becomes the legitimate child of his adoptive parents with all rights, privileges and responsibilities that are attached to the relationship.'

While the Act covers all over India, it is only possible to adopt under this Act in areas where the JJ Boards (provided under the Act) have been constituted. This is an ongoing process, with a majority of states issuing notifications constituting these boards.

International Adoption

Indian citizens, non-resident Indians and non-Indians residing outside India can adopt a child from India. While these adoptions are also legalized under one of the three acts mentioned above, the rules related to these adoptions can be different. These differences are a function of the priority given to Indians residing in India while placing a child, the regulations of the countries in which the adoptive families reside and the relevant immigration laws.

ADOLESCENT HEALTH PROGRAMS

Definition

The term adolescence is derived from the Latin word *'adolescere'* meaning to grow, to mature. Adolescence is a journey from the world of the child to the world of the adult. It is a time of physical and emotional change as the body matures and the mind becomes more questioning and independent. This period is most crucial since these are the formative years of life of an individual when major physical, psychological and behavioral changes take place. This is also the period of preparation for undertaking greater responsibilities including healthy responsible parenthood. Future of the society depends on adolescents and they form a great human resource for the society.

Adolescents (12–18 years) constitute about one fourth of India's population and young people (12–24 years) about one third of the population. This huge section of population represents a great 'demographic dividend' and offers a dependable potential to drive and sustain economic growth that India has experienced in last few years.

In order to fulfill this potential the nation must be able to invest in their education, health and development adequately. In order to ensure that they grow healthy they require information and skills, health services and counseling as well as a safe and supportive environment.

Adolescents are generally considered healthy by themselves, their families, even health care providers and society at large. Yet they are known to suffer significant morbidity caused by risk taking behavior and inadequate access to health care. In addition, programs and services must recognize their special needs and address these in a supporting and nonjudgmental manner. This requires a better understanding of their existing status within the prevailing sociocultural settings and their vulnerabilities.

This phase of life cycle is marked by special characters:

- Rapid physical growth and development
- Physical, social and phychological maturity
- Sexual maturity and onset of sexual activity
- Beginning of menstrual cycle in girls and onset of reproduction cycle
- Development of adult mental processes and adult identity
- Transition from total socioeconomic dependence to relative independence.

The National Population Policy 2000 identified adolescents as an underserved group for which health needs and within this reproductive and sexual health interventions are to be designed. The National Youth Policy 2003 recognizes 13 to 19 years as a distinct age group which had to be covered by special programs in all sectors including health. The National Curriculum Framework 2005 for school education highlights the need for integrating adolescent reproductive and sexual health messages into school curriculum. Based on this the National Adolescence Education Programme of NACO along with the Ministry of Human Resources Development is developed.

Main Stages

- *Early adolescence (12–14):* It is characterized by a spurt of growth, and the beginnings of sexual maturation. Young people start to think abstractly.
- *In mid-adolescence (15–16):* The main physical changes are completed, while the individual develops a stronger sense of identity, and relates more strongly to his or her peer group, although families usually remain important. Thinking becomes more reflective.
- *In later adolescence (17–18):* The body fills out and takes its adult form, while the individual now has a distinct identity and more settled ideas and opinions.

Characteristics

A—Aggressive, Anemic, Abortion

D—Dynamic, Developing, Depressed

O—Overconfident, Overindulging, Obese

L—Loud but lonely and Lack information

E—Enthusiastic, Explorative and Experimenting

S—Social, Sexual and Spiritual

C—Courageous, Cheerful and Concern

E—Emotional, Eager and Emulating

N—Nervous, Never say no to peers

T—Temperamental, Teenage pregnancy.

Several important public health and social problems either peak or start during these years.

Examples include:

- Homicide
- Suicide
- Motor vehicle crashes, including those caused by drinking and driving
- Substance use and abuse
- Smoking
- Sexually transmitted infections, including human immunodeficiency virus (HIV)
- Teen and unplanned pregnancies
- Homelessness.

Strategies for Promotion of Adolescent Health

A—Adoption of healthy life style

D—Develop appropriate, i.e. strategy discourage early marriage and teenage pregnancy

O—Organize adolescent/youth friendly clinic

L—Life skill training, legal support, liaison with peers, parents

E—Educate about sexuality, safe sex, spirituality, responsible parenthood

S—Safe, secure and supportive environment to be provided

C—Counseling/curriculum in school inclusive of family life education

E—Enable and empower for responsible citizenship

N—Networking for experience sharing

T—Training for income generation, teen clubs.

Adolescent Health Programs

- Kishori Shakti Yojana: To improve the health and nutritional status of girls
- Balika Samridhi Yojana: To delay the age of marriage
- National AIDS Control Programme
- Reproductive and Child Health Programme.

Kishori Shakti Yojana

This scheme is a redesign of the already existing Adolescent Girls (AG) scheme being implemented as a component under the centrally sponsored Integrated Child Development Services (ICDS) Scheme. Kishori Shakti Yojna (KSY—a key component of ICDS scheme which aims at empowerment of adolescent girls. Kishori Shakti Yojana (KSY) seeks to empower adolescent girls, so as to enable them to take charge of their lives. The program through its interventions aims at bringing about a difference in the lives of the adolescent girls. It seeks to provide them with an opportunity to realize their full potential.

Under the scheme, the adolescent girls who are unmarried and belong to families below the poverty line and school dropouts are selected and attached to the local Anganwadi Centers for six-monthly stints of learning and training activities. This includes two sub-schemes.

- *Scheme I (Girl to Girl Approach):* The Scheme-I has been designed for adolescent girls in the age group of 12–15 years belonging to families whose income level is below ₹ 6400/- per annum.
- *Scheme II (Balika Mandal):* The Scheme-II is intended to reach to all adolescent girls in the age group of 12–18 years irrespective of income levels of the family. It may however, be mentioned that even under Scheme-II, younger girls in the age group of 12–15 years and belonging to poor families are also included.

Objective

- To improve the nutritional and health status of girls in the age group of 12–18 years
- To provide the required literacy and numeracy skills through the non-formal stream of education, to stimulate a desire for more social exposure and knowledge and to help them improve their decision making capabilities
- To train and equip the adolescent girls to improve/upgrade home-based and vocational skills
- To promote awareness of health, hygiene, nutrition and family welfare, home management and child care, and to take all measure as to facilitate their marrying only after attaining the age of 18 years and if possible, even later
- To gain a better understanding of their environment-related social issues and the impact on their lives
- To encourage adolescent girls to initiate various activities to be productive and useful members of the society.

Other Options of the Program

- IFA supplementation along with deworming
- Education for school dropouts and functional literacy among illiterate adolescent girls
- Nonformal education to adolescent girls. Emphasis on life education aspects including physical, developmental and sex education is given.
- Vocational training activities may be undertaken for adolescent girls for their economic empowerment. At Anganwadi Centers, a group of 20–25 girls may be identified by the Supervisor (Mukhya Sevika). Of these, nomination of 2 selected girls from each Anganwadi Center may be sent to the Office of District Programme Officer. District Programme Officer in consultation with CDPO, officer's in-charge of these sectors and NGOs will organize vocational training courses, nonformal education course, life education courses, health and nutrition education, legal literacy, etc. Following completion of the training, the group leaders (2 adolescent girls from each Anganwadi Center) will provide training to the remaining adolescent girls at Anganwadi Center.

Balika Samridhi Yojana

The scheme of Balika Samridhi Yojana was launched by Govt. of India in 1997 with the following objectives:

- To change negative family and community attitudes towards the girl child at birth and towards her mother.
- To improve enrollment and retention of girl children in schools
- To increase the age of marriage of girls.
- To assist the girl to undertake income generation activities.

Components of Balika Samridhi Yojana

From the start of the scheme, the mothers of newborn girl children were given a post delivery grant of ₹ 500 each in cash as a gift from the Government. There was also provision for Annual Scholarships to the girl child for attending school. (But the details/guidelines for scholarships were not received).

During 1999–2000, Govt. of India recast the scheme and the benefits and means of delivery have been redesigned to ensure that financial benefits accrue to the girl child. Now the girl children eligible under BSY are entitled to the following benefits:

- A post birth grant amount of ₹ 500
- When the girl child born on or after 15–08–1997 and covered under BSY starts attending the school, she will become entitled to annual scholarship as under for each successfully completed year of schooling:

Class	Amount of annual scholarship
I-III	₹ 300 per annum for each class
IV	₹ 500 per annum
V	₹ 600 per annum
VI-VII	₹ 700 per annum for each class
VIII	₹ 800 per annum
IX-X	₹ 1000 per annum for each class

Target Group

Under Balika Samridhi Yojana girl children belonging to families below the poverty line are given benefit, who are born on or after 15th August, 1997. The benefits are restricted to two girl children in a household irrespective of number of children in the household.

National AIDS Control Programme

Reaching youngsters at an impressionable age before they become sexually active can lay the foundation for a responsible lifestyle, including healthy relationships and safe sex habits. Under NACO Adolescent Education Programme developed which focuses primarily on prevention through awareness building.

The Adolescent Education Programme is one of the key policy initiatives of NACP II. NACO collaborated to develop this school-based program which is implemented across 144,409 secondary and senior secondary schools with the objective of reaching out to about 33 million students within two years. AEP is implemented by the Department of Education in collaboration with the State AIDS Prevention and Control Societies.

The Adolescence Education Programme (AEP)

- Co-curricular adolescence education in classes IX-XI
- Curricular adolescence education in classes IX-XI and life skills education in classes I- VIII
- Inclusion of HIV prevention education in pre-service and in-service teacher training and teacher education programs.
- Inclusion of HIV prevention education in the programs for out-of-school adolescents and young persons, and
- Incorporating measures to prevent stigma and discrimination against learners/students and educators and life skills education into education policy for HIV prevention.

Under the program, teachers and peer educators are trained who in turn conduct the program amongst the student community. The program covered 112,000 schools and trained 2,88,000 teachers. They have been provided reference material, which has been developed by NACO.

Relevant messages on safe sex, sexuality and relationships are developed and disseminated for youth via posters, booklets, panels and printed material.

Youth Unite for Victory on AIDS (YUVA)

A youth network, Yuva comprising seven youth organisations, Nehru Yuva Kendra Sangathan, National Service Scheme, Indian Red Cross Society, National Cadet Corps, Bharat Scouts and Guides, Youth Hostels Association of India and the Association of Indian Universities, working for the young people with prevention, education and life skills for promoting healthy and safe behavior and practices amongst them. The ultimate goal is to have an 'AIDS prepared Campus, AIDS prepared Community and AIDS prepared Country'.

Red Ribbon Club (RRC)

Red Ribbon Club is a voluntary on-campus intervention program for students in educational institutions. It is initiated and supported by the SACS and implemented through multi-sectoral collaboration, particularly using the services of cader officers of the State's NSS. The club is proposed to be established in every school and college to provide youth with access to information on HIV/AIDS and voluntary blood donation. The club also works towards promotion of life skills to bring about behavioral change among the youth. Already RRCs are established in more than 16,000 schools and colleges.

Reproductive and Child Health Programme

The adolescent health initiative in RCH II

Adolescent Reproductive and Sexual Health (ARSH): Services provided to all adolescent married and unmarried girls and boys.

Package of Services

- Promotive services
  - Focused care during antenatal period
  - Counseling and provision of emergency contraceptives
  - Counseling and provision of reversible contraceptives
  - Information/advice on SRH services

- Preventive services
  - Services for TT and prophylaxis against nutritional anemia
  - Nutritional counseling
  - Services for early and safe termination of pregnancy and management of post abortion complications
- Curative services
  - Treatment for common RTI/STIs
  - Treatment and counseling of menstrual disorders sexual concerns of males and female adolescents
  - Management of sexual among girls
- Referral services
  - Voluntary Counseling and Testing Center
  - Prevention of Parent to Child Transmission
- Outreach services
  - Periodic health checkups and community camps
  - Periodic health education activities
  - Co-curricular activities
- Adolescent Friendly Health Services
  - AFHS provides a broad range of preventive, promotive and curative services under one roof and which helps to ensure improved availability, accessibility and utilization of health services. It is being initiated by government, private and NGO's. The significant feature of AFHS is provision of reproductive health services, nutritional counseling, sex education and life skill education. It is kind of one-stop shopping approach which means that different needs of adolescent can be met under one roof by professional who understand their needs and are trained to address them effectively.
  - AFHS in India is first taken by Safdarjang Hospital in New Delhi that is providing a wide range of services such as clinical, mental health services, nutritional and reproductive counseling, growth monitoring and development and immunization
  - The National Institute of Research in Reproductive Health, Mumbai in collaboration with Municipal corporation of Mumbai started AHFS under the name 'Jagruti' for providing specialized sexual and reproductive services for adolescent boys and girls
  - MAMTA an NGO started AFHS in some villages.This model comprises community based Youth Information Centers (YIC's) supported by peer educators, health faclility based youth clinics at primary health centers and youth friendly centers at first referral unit.
  - In four districts of Madhya Pradesh a pilot project of AFHS launched as name 'Jigyasa' by The Family Planning Association of India (FPAI)
  - The RCH-II has a strategy to provide services for adolescent health at public health facilities and at primary health care level during routine hours and on dedicated days and times. Public health personnel such as medical officers as well as ANM's and, lady health visitors will receive training on the provision of sexual and, reproductive

health services exclusively for adolescents. Haryana is the first state in the country to launch a distinct Adolescent Reproductive and Sexual Health (ARSH) program providing AFHS at government health facilities.

Package of Health Services at AFHS

- Monitoring of growth and development
- Monitoring of behavior problems
- Offer information and counseling on developmental changes, personal care and ways of seeking help
- Reproductive health including contraceptives, STI treatment, pregnancy care and post abortion management
- Voluntary counseling and testing for HIV
- Management of sexual violence
- Mental health services including management of substance abuse.

Other Adolescent Health Programs

- *Life-skills and health and sexuality education in schools:* Well designed, well-implemented sexuality and reproductive health education can provide young people with a solid foundation of knowledge and skills to enable them to engage in safe and responsible sexual behavior.
- *Peer education:* Peer education programs are especially appropriate for young people who are not in school and for hard-to-reach, at-risk subsets of the youth population, including sex workers and street children.
- *Mass media and community mobilization:* Mass media and community mobilization efforts that engage influential adults such as parents, teachers, community and religious leaders and music and sports stars, can help normalize positive adolescent behaviors and gender roles as well as direct young people to appropriate health services.
- *Youth development programs:* Youth development programs typically address a range of key adolescent needs, including life skills, education, jobs, and psychosocial needs.
- *Clinical health services:* Although some young people seek care through the formal health system, many others do not seek health care because of attitudes of health workers, particularly when seeking care and advice on matters related to sexuality.
- *Social marketing:* This approach involves the use of public health messages to promote healthy behaviors and the use of condoms and other health products and services.
- *Workplace and private sector programs:* Programs that reach young people do so at their places of work and through private channels, such as pharmacies and for-profit medical services, where many young people prefer to seek care.

MENSTRUAL HYGIENE

Introduction

Menstruation is a natural, normal biological process experienced by all adolescent girls and women. Menstruation is still a taboo in India and it is common for people across society to feel uncomfortable about the subject. To ensure that adolescent girls and women have the necessary support and facilities, it is important that the wider society, communities and families must challenge the status quo and break the silence around menstruation.

Definitions

It is important to understand what menstruation is, and how simple management interventions along with positive attitudes can make a lasting difference to the lives of every adolescent girl and woman. The following definitions are helpful:

- *Adolescent girls:* Adolescence describes the transitional period between childhood and adulthood. Girls aged 12 to 18 are adolescents.
- *Menarche:* The first occurrence of menstruation
- *Menopause:* The time in a woman's life when her menstrual periods stop and she is no longer able to have children
- *Menstruation:* 'Monthly periods' a biological process in a woman where each month blood and other material is discharged from the lining of the uterus. Menstruation occurs from the onset of puberty until the menopause, except during pregnancy.
- *Menstrual Hygiene or Management (MHM)*
  - Articulation, awareness, information and confidence to manage menstruation with safety and dignity using safe hygienic materials together.
  - Adequate water and agents and spaces for washing and bathing with soap.
  - Disposal of used menstrual absorbents with privacy and dignity.
- *Menstrual absorbent:* A sanitary cloth, napkin, towel or pad is an absorbent item worn by an adolescent girl or woman when she is menstruating or directly after birth while she is bleeding. The material absorbs the flow of blood from her vagina.
- *Menstrual waste:* Includes a used sanitary cloth, napkin, towel or pad that contains blood.
- *Biodegradable:* Compostable, organic materials, a substance or object that is capable of being decomposed by bacteria or other living organisms and thereby avoiding pollution.

Sanitary Protection Materials and Disposal

The choice of sanitary protection is very much a personal decision based on cultural acceptability. It is often influenced by a woman's or girl's environment and access to funds, water supply and affordable options. It is critical that any program aiming to support women or girls with sanitary protection materials involves them in the planning discussions and decisions about the options to be disposable sanitary towels are the most frequently used methods of managing *menstruation*. In resource-poor settings they are often prohibitively expensive, bulky to transport and difficult to dispose of. Many women and adolescent girls from poor families cannot afford to buy these hygienic towels (APHRC 2010). Some girls may even be led to trade sex for small amounts of money in order to purchase sanitary protection materials (Kirk & Sommer 2006). But sanitary pads reduce the barriers for girls to stay in school, which are multiple: fear of soiling, fear of odor, and even if there are *WASH* facilities at school, fear of leaving visible blood in the latrine or *toilet* (WSSCC 2013).

Cloths or cloth pads may be a *sustainable* sanitary option, but it must be hygienically washed and dried in the sunlight. Sunlight is a natural sterilizer and drying the cloth pads on sunlight sterilizes them for future use. They also need to be stored in a clean dry place for *reuse*.

The menstrual cup may be an appropriate new technology for poor women and girls. It is a cup made of medical silicone rubber that is inserted into the vagina to collect menstrual blood. It needs to be removed and emptied less frequently than sanitary pads. That reduces the problems young women face in lacking privacy and facilities to change and dispose of sanitary *products* in schools and other contexts. This technology may offer a *sustainable,* practical and cost-effective alternative.

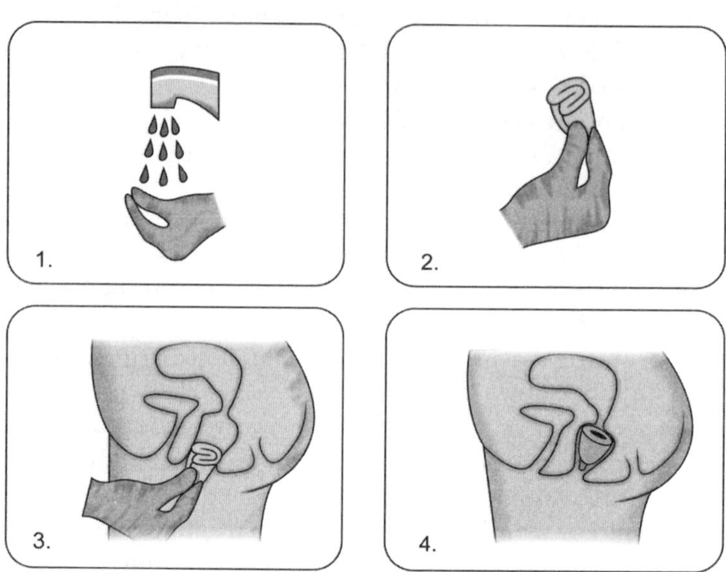

It is recommended that when using the menstrual cup one needs to maintain a high standard of hygiene especially during insertion, removal and general cleaning. Although water shortages could present challenges for its use, the amount of water required when using the menstrual cup is minimal compared to other methods (APHRC 2010). Offering menstrual cups can be a social business opportunity for the private sector, as shown by experiences from Kenya (RUBY CUP 2013).

The table below compares the advantages and disadvantages of further sanitary materials (House et al. 2012).

Sanitary protection option	Advantages	Disadvantages
Natural materials (e.g. mud, cow dung, leaves)	• Free • Locally available	• High-risk of contamination • Difficult and uncomfortable to use
Strips of clothes	• Easily available in the local market • Reusable	• If old cloths are not cleaned well they can become unhygienic • Users need somewhere private, with a water supply and soap, to *wash* and dry the cloths
Toilet paper or tissues	• Easily available in the local market	• Loses strength when wet and can fall apart • Difficult to hold in place • May be too expensive for the poorest users

Contd...

Contd...

Sanitary protection option	Advantages	Disadvantages
Reusable pads	• Available locally or on the internet • Income generation opportunity, if locally made • Cost effective as they are reusable • More environmentally-friendly than disposable pads	• Users need somewhere private, with water supply and soap to *wash* and dry the pads • If commercially produced, cost is prohibitive to many potential users
Tampons	• Convenient and comfortable to use	• Not available in many contexts • Cost is prohibitive to many potential users • Generates a lot of waste to dispose, not environmentally-friendly • May not be culturally appropriate, particularly for adolescent girls, as need to be inserted into the vagina • Hygiene and availability of water and soap for hand-washing are particularly important, as need to be inserted into the vagina
Menstrual cups	• Reusable • Only need emptying, washing and drying	• May not be culturally appropriate for use, particularly for adolescent girls, as need to be inserted into the vagina • Hygiene and availability of water and soap are particularly important, for washing hands and menstrual cup, as need to be inserted into the vagina • Expensive first investment outlay
Panties/Underwear	• Useful for keeping a sanitary *product* in place • Good for keeping the vaginal area hygienic	• Cost may be prohibitive to potential users • Cheap elastic can wear out relatively quickly

MHM Infrastructure in Schools and the Safe Disposal of Menstrual Waste

Every school is required to have basic water and sanitation infrastructure so that girls and female staff can privately manage menstruation hygienically and with dignity.

Essential facilities are:

- Separate toilets for girls and boys and ideally also for male and female teachers.
- Water supply (based on approximately 500 liters water storage capacity for 100 children),
- Soap availability for handwashing and space for washing laundering menstrual absorbent.
- Facilities for safe disposal of used menstrual absorbents.

Beyond the provision, infrastructure should be operated and maintained properly. These toilets for girls have to be so designed that they can be easily used by girls with physical disabilities. For more information on disabled friendly toilet designs, please refer to 'Handbook on Accessible Sanitation Facilities for People with Disabilities'.

Water and Soap in Every School is Essential

Both are needed for girls, boys, and staff to wash hands with soap after toilet use and before eating food. Girls and female staff must have clean, easily accessible water and soap to wash them, wash their clothing if soiled, and wash menstrual cloths or reusable napkins. Water must be inside the toilet, ideally either via a tap or a dedicated container in each cubicle. A mug should be provided to allow girls to dispense water for their own personal cleaning and to clean the toilet if required. Every person in the school community regardless of gender or caste should have access to a clean and well-maintained toilet.

Adolescent Girls and Female Teachers have Special Sanitation Requirements

- Separate toilet and sanitation blocks located in safe location to assure privacy/adequate privacy wall based on a ratio 1 toilet for every 40 girls (and or 1 urinal for every 20 girls).
- Adequate space in the cubicle for girls to change their napkins/cloth and to wash themselves.
- Toilet cubicles with a shelf, hooks or niche to keep clothing and menstrual adsorbents dry.
- A well-positioned mirror so that girls can check for stains on their clothes.
- A private bathing or changing units, including a place for drying their reusable menstrual absorbent.

Safe Disposal of Menstrual Waste

It is important to consider safe menstrual hygiene disposal options and ensure that girls and female teachers know how to use them. Common practices range from unsafe to safe, with unsafe disposal being unacceptable.

Table 8.3: Overview of common disposal practices

Unsafe	Common practices
↓	Practices throw them unwrapped into fields, rooftops, etc.
	Wrap them in paper/plastic bag and throwing them outside
	Drying, wrap in paper/plastic bag and throw in dustbins (mostly non-rural)
	Burry them for decomposting
	Throw them in latrine/toilets
	Burn it (rural areas and peri-urban areas)
	Use small scale incinerators (community or school level)
Safe	Municipal waste management/burning in health clinics (more urban)

Collection

Disposal bins are a good and affordable collection option. These must be placed within the toilet, or very close by it, ideally provided for each cubicle. Bins must be washable and must have close fitting lids to minimize seepage of odor or waste before mass disposal. Depending on the type and location of the final disposal, there might be a need for an emptying schedule of individual bins, and transport to the disposal site. It is recommended to designate a point person of the school staff to be responsible and accountable for this. To avoid transport, some incinerators have been built in with chutes directly adjacent to toilet building.

Safe Disposal

Safe disposal means ensuring that the process of destruction of used and soiled materials is done without human contact and with minimal environmental pollution. Unsafe disposal - throwing used cloth into ponds, rivers, or in the fields exposes others in the area to decaying material and should be avoided. Offsite disposal can be organized with the communal or town solid waste collection and management system. If a hospital with a safe and treatment unit for hazardous waste is nearby, this might be a best solution to explore. However, this is unfortunately not a viable option for many rural schools, and transport will be a logistical and financial challenge. Options for on-site disposal includes disposal deep burial, composting, pit burning and incineration. The right option depends on key factors such as amount and type of materials, the available budget (investment and OandM costs) and environmental considerations. The following table shows the recommendations for different types of material and disposal options.

In addition to these factors, sociocultural perceptions might play a role in choice and use of the solution. In some areas of India there is resistance to burning through incinerators, yet a burning pit may be more acceptable. There might be also the false perception that disposing of their menstrual management products in pit latrines prevents from being used in witchcraft.

WEEKLY IRON FOLIC ACID SUPPLEMENTATION (WIFS) PROGRAMME

Introduction

The Ministry of Health and Family Welfare has launched the Weekly Iron and Folic Acid Supplementation (WIFS) Programme to meet the challenge of high prevalence and incidence of anemia amongst adolescent girls and boys. WIFS is evidence-based programmatic response to the prevailing anemia situation amongst adolescent girls and boys through supervised weekly ingestion of IFA supplementation and biannual helminthic control. The long-term goal is to break the intergenerational cycle of anemia, the short-term benefits is of a nutritionally improved human capital. The program, implemented across the country both in rural and urban areas in India.

Adolescents (age 10–19 years), especially girls, are at high-risk of iron deficiency and anemia due to accelerated increase in requirements for iron, poor dietary intake of iron, malaria and worm infestation. Public health experts also attribute social and cultural factors such as early marriage, adolescent pregnancy and repeated pregnancies that make girls more vulnerable to iron deficiency and anemia.

An estimated 56 percent girl and 30 percent boys in the age group 10–19 years in India are anemic according to the third National Family Health Survey.

Considering the alarming situation, the Government of India is implementing the Weekly Iron and Folic Acid (IFA) Supplementation (WIFS) programme since January 2013, under the National Rural Health Mission (NRHM) in government/aided and municipal schools (nationwide) and Anganwadi Centers across all states in India.

The weekly iron folic acid supplementation is an evidence-based programmatic response to the prevailing anemia situation amongst adolescent's girls and boys through supervise ingestion of IFAs and bi-annual deworming. The program envisages benefiting all adolescent girls and boys enroll in all government and government aided schools including students from class 6–12, besides out of schools girls.

Objectives

- Ensure that all adolescent boys and girls in 6 to 12th standards of government/government aided/municipal schools are given a tablet of IFA once a week and Albendazole twice a year for deworming.
- To inform adolescent boys and girls of the correct dietary practices for increasing iron intake.
- To inform adolescents of the significance of preventing worm infestation and encourage adoption of correct hygiene practices, including use of footwear to prevent worm infestation.

Guidelines for the School Teacher

Distribution of IFA through the Platform of School

- Role of the Nodal Teacher School children from 6th to 12th standard, in rural and urban regions will be reached through this program. Each school will designate two teachers as the WIFS nodal teachers.
- Nodal teachers will ensure supervised ingestion of IFA tablets by adolescents enrolled in classes 6th to 12th on a fixed day preferably Monday at a fixed time after Mid-Day Meal (where applicable)/lunch.
- Teachers will also be encouraged to consume IFA. The first dose of deworming tablet i.e. 400 mg of Albendazole should ideally be administered in month of August and the second dose should be given by February (six months after the first dose).
- If the child is absent on a Monday or misses out on the consumption of the IFA tablet, subsequent follow-up during the week needs to be done to ensure that the tablet is consumed.
- The program could be initiated preferably in the month of April after beginning of new session in all schools.
- Teachers will screen adolescents for presence of moderate/severe anemia by assessing nail bed and tongue pallor and refer anemic adolescents to appropriate health facility for management of anemia.
- Three separate time should also be allotted during the school year to provide Nutrition and Health Education (NHE) to the adolescents.
- The nodal teacher should conduct monthly NHE session(s). Parents should also be oriented on WIFS and NHE during Parent Teacher Association Meetings. Before the school closes for vacations, the children can be given the requisite number of IFA tablets for consumption during the holidays under parental supervision.
- Annual supplies of IFA and Albendazole tablets should be stored in a clean, dry and dust free area away from the direct sunlight.
- The nodal teacher(s) for each school will estimate annual requirements for IFA and Albendazole tablets.

Dose

World Health Organization also recommends weekly iron-folic acid supplementation for adolescents to build iron stores in the body.

The drive to combat adolescent anemia includes–biannual (February and August) administration of Albendazole tablets to remove worm infections; weekly (Monday), supervised administration of IFA tablets (100 mg of elemental iron and 500 mg of folic acid); screening for moderate/severe anemia and referral to nearest health facility and, monthly nutrition and health education to encourage consumption of locally available iron-rich food.

Intervention

- Administration of supervised Weekly Iron-folic Acid Supplements of 100 mg elemental iron and 500 mg folic acid using a fixed day approach.
- Screening of target groups for moderate/severe anemia and referring these cases to an appropriate health facility.
- Biannual deworming (Albendazole 400 mg), six months apart, for control of helminthic infestation.
- Information and counseling for improving dietary intake and for taking actions for prevention of intestinal worm infestation.
- Convergence with key stakeholder ministries like the Ministry of Women and Child Development and Ministry of Human Resource Development is an essential part of implantation plan of the WIFS program. Key convergent areas include: joint program planning, capacity building of nodal service providers including Medical Officers, Anganwadi Worker (AWW) Staff Nurses, School teachers, monitoring and a comprehensive communication component.

District WIFS Advisory Committee

The district level WIFS Advisory Committee will be formed with participation from Health, Education and Women and Child Development Departments. The function of the committee will be to monitor the progress of the program and resolve programmatic issues. The committee would need to meet every quarter with the participation of Health, Women and Child Development and Education Block officials. Yearly meeting with nodal teachers could be organized to further streamline the implementation of program.

Committee would Monitor the Following

- Status of implementation of the program and timeliness of the submission of monthly reports.
- Facilitate convergence and ensure use of community-based platform like VHNDs for community mobilization and awareness.
- Training
- Timely and adequate supply and distribution of IFA and Albendazole tablets.
- Provision and usage of IEC materials WIFS monitoring committee.

Nutritional Advice

Nutritionists also discussed several home-based and easily available solutions to keep anemia away. These included easily available food such as spinach (palak, methi), dates (khajur), meat, fish, eggs and vitamin C rich foods (citrus fruits like Amla, Guava, Lemon). Overall, the discussions stressed on the need to focus on how the program will contribute to the physical and cognitive development of adolescents.

ADOLESCENT SAFETY PROGRAM

Introduction

Safety for adolescents is a presently focused on coping skills therapy to help people attain safety from trauma or substance abuse. The treatment is available as a book, providing both client handouts and clinician guidelines. The treatment may be conducted in group or individual format for adolescents (both females, and males) in various settings (e.g. outpatient, inpatient, residential, home care, and schools).

Goals

Safety program for adolescents are:

- Reduce trauma and/or substance abuse symptoms
- Increase safe coping in relationships
- Increase safe coping in thinking
- Increase safe coping in behavior
- Increase safe coping in emotions
- Sexual abuse

Principles

- Safety as the overarching goal (helping clients attain safety in their relationships, thinking, behavior, and emotions)
- Integrated treatment (working on both trauma and substance abuse at the same time)
- A focus on ideals to counteract the loss of ideals in both trauma and substance abuse
- Four content areas: cognitive, behavioral, interpersonal, and case management
- Attention to clinician processes (helping clinicians work on their emotional responses, self-care, and other issues).

Several Important Public Health and Social Problems Either Peak or Start During these Years

Examples include:

- Homicide
- Suicide
- Motor vehicle crashes, including those caused by drinking and driving
- Substance use and abuse
- Smoking
- Sexually transmitted infections, including human immunodeficiency virus (HIV)
- Teen and unplanned pregnancies
- Homelessness

Effective Policies and Programs that Address Adolescent Health Issues

They include:

- State graduated driver licensing programs
- Teen pregnancy prevention programs
- Violence prevention programs
- Delinquency prevention programs
- Mental health and substance abuse interventions
- HIV prevention interventions

The leading causes of illness and death among adolescents and young adults are largely preventable. Health outcomes for adolescents and young adults are grounded in their social environments and are frequently mediated by their behaviors. Behaviors of young people are influenced at the individual, peer, family, school, community, and societal levels.

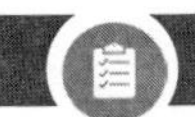

MODEL QUESTIONS

Multiple Choice Questions

1. When the international accepted right for children were approved?
(a) 14th general assembly of United Nations which approved the right?
(b) 16th general assembly of United Nations which approved the right?
(c) 18th general assembly of United Nations which approved the right?
(d) 20th century.

2. When child labor act was passed?
(a) 1988 (b) 1986
(c) 1982 (d) 1992

3. When juvenile justice act was passed?
(a) 1978 (b) 1991
(c) 1980 (d) 1986

4. When the child abuse prevention and treatment act was started?
(a) 1974 (b) 1946
(c) 1970 (d) 1949

5. In which year education for all handicapped children act was passed?
(a) 1972 (b) 1979
(c) 1975 (d) 1982

6. In which year ICDS scheme was initiated in India?
(a) 1970 (b) 1972
(c) 1975 (d) 1979

7. When the government of India adopted national nutrition policy?
(a) 1990 (b) 1984
(c) 1993 (d) 1991

8. When was national health policy approved by parliament?
(a) 1983 (b) 1991
(c) 1992 (d) 1990

9. In which year national malaria control program was launched?
(a) 1946 (b) 1950
(c) 1952 (d) 1953

10. In which year mid-day meal program started working in India?
(a) 1995 (b) 1958
(c) 1960 (d) 1962

11. When ICCW was established?
(a) 1948 (b) 1955
(c) 1950 (d) 1952

12. When India red cross society was established and how many branches it have all over India?
(a) 1920 and its have 700 branches (b) 1912 and its have 300 branches
(c) 1926 and its have 400 branches (d) 1920 and its have 400 branches

13. The FAO was stablished in
(a) 1945 (b) 1964
(c) 1946 (d) 1963

14. The Headquarters of FAO is in
(a) India (b) Geneva
(c) New York (d) Rome

15. The Headquarter of WHO is in
(a) Geneva (b) Brazil
(c) Switzerland (d) New York

Fill in the Blanks

(a) The children act was launched in ....
(b) Mid-day meal program is also known as ....
(c) It is the child's right to get special care if ....
(d) Oral polio vaccine was added to the Immunization schedule in the year ....

Short Answer Questions

1. List down the internationally accepted rights of the child.
2. Child act.
3. Juvenile justice act.
4. National child labor policy.
5. Mid-day meal program.

Long Answer Questions

1. Describe in brief about various welfare services available for challenged children in India.
2. Discuss the concept, objectives, and services provided by child guidance clinics.
3. Describe different child welfare services in detail.

ANSWER KEY

Multiple Choice Questions

1. (a)	2. (b)	3. (d)	4. (a)	5. (c)	6. (c)	7. (b)
8. (c)	9. (d)	10. (a)	11. (d)	12. (a)	13. (a)	14. (d)
15. (a)						

Fill in the Blanks

(a) 1960
(b) School lunch program
(c) Handicapped
(d) 1979.

ANNEXURES

Annexure 1

PEDIATRICS NURSING GLOSSARY

A

1. **Acne:** A chronic disorder of the hair follicles and sebaceous glands. Acne is characterized by black heads, pimple outbreaks, cysts, infected abscesses, and (sometimes) scarring.
2. **Allergen:** The substance that triggers an allergic reaction.
3. **Allergic conjunctivitis:** Red, Itchy, Watery Eyes; a result of an exposure to an allergen or an irritant.
4. **Allergy:** A physiological reaction caused when the immune system mistakenly identifies a normally harmless substance as damaging to the body.
5. **Anorexia nervosa (also called anorexia):** An eating disorder characterized by low body weight (less than 85 percent of normal weight for height and age), a distorted body image, and an intense fear of gaining weight.
6. **Antibiotic:** Chemical substances produced by living organisms or synthesized (created) in laboratories for the purpose of killing other organisms that cause disease.
7. **Asthma:** A chronic, inflammatory lung disease involving recurrent breathing problems; the most common, chronic health problem among children.
8. **Atopic dermatitis:** Red, itchy, dry skin most common in infants; a result of an exposure to an allergen or an irritant.
9. **Attention-deficit/hyperactivity disorder (ADHD):** A syndrome (a group of symptoms or signs) that is usually characterized by serious and persistent difficulties, resulting in inattentiveness or distractibility, impulsivity, and hyperactivity.
10. **Abdominal Aorta:** Section of the aorta that passes through the abdomen to supply blood to the lower part of the body.
11. **Abscess:** Swollen inflamed, tender area of infection containing pus.
12. **Accident-proneness:** Tendency of some children to have more accidents than normal. It may be due to a risk factor such as poor vision, but unconscious factors are often the cause.
13. **Acetaminophen:** Non-prescription medication used to relieve minor pain and to reduce fever. Its analgesic effects are similar to aspirin, but it does not reduce inflammation or swelling. It is less irritating to the stomach than aspirin.
14. **Achylasia:** Condition of the esophagus that disrupts normal swallowing.
15. **Acupuncture:** Method of anesthesia and treatment of pain developed by the Chinese. Needles are inserted through the skin to stimulate precise areas.
16. **Acute:** Beginning suddenly; also severe, but of short duration.
17. **Addiction:** Intense craving for substances such as alcohol, tobacco or narcotics, or a compulsive behavior such as gambling.
18. **Adenoids:** Infection-fighting tissue (part of the lymphatic system) in the upper throat, near the tonsils.

19. **Adenovirus:** Group of viruses that cause certain respiratory and eye infections.
20. **Adhesions:** Small strands of fibrous tissue that cause organs in the abdomen and pelvis to cling together abnormally, creating a risk of intestinal obstruction.
21. **Adolescence:** Time of life from the beginning of puberty until maturity.
22. **Adrenal glands:** Two glands attached to the kidneys. Each has an outer layer (cortex) that produces steroid hormones and an inner layer (medulla) that produces adrenalin.
23. **Adrenalin:** Hormone produced by the adrenal glands that increases heart rate and prepares the body for crisis. Also called epinephrine.
24. **Aging:** The normal process of gradual physical and mental decline.
25. **Airways:** Tubular passages that air passes through to the lungs; the trachea (windpipe), bronchi, and bronchioles.
26. **Albinism:** A rare, inherited disorder characterized by a lack of normal coloration of eyes, hair, skin, and sometimes shortness. The eyes are intolerant of light, move back and forth, and are affected by astigmatism. There is no treatment, except total protection from exposure to sunlight.
27. **Allergy skin tests:** A series of tests in which various substances are injected into the skin in minute amounts for the purpose of ruling in or out a person's allergy to that substance.
28. **Alveoli:** Lung cells at ends of the airways where oxygen enters the blood and waste gases leave the blood.
29. **Ambulatory medical center:** A health-care facility for patients who do not require prolonged bed rest or hospitalization.
30. **Amniocentesis:** A surgical procedure using a laparoscope (a hollow instrument with a system of lenses) that is pushed through a small incision in the abdominal wall and thence into the uterus to obtain amniotic fluid for study.
31. **Amniotic sac:** The thin, transparent membrane filled with fluid in which the fetus lives until born.
32. **Amphetamine drugs:** Habit-forming drugs that stimulate the brain and central nervous system, increase blood pressure, reduce nasal stuffiness, or suppress appetite.
33. **Amyloid deposits:** Abnormal protein material deposited in tissues, usually caused by diseases. These deposits cause impairment of certain organs.
34. **Analgesics:** Medications that relieve pain.
35. **Anemia:** Condition in which red blood cells or hemoglobin (oxygen-carrying substance in blood) is inadequate.
36. **Anesthesia, general:** Causing temporary loss of consciousness and inability to feel pain by use of inhaled gases or injected anesthetics.
37. **Aneurysm:** Abnormal swelling or ballooning of a blood vessel.
38. **Angiogram, angiography:** Study of arteries and veins by injecting material into them that X-rays can outline.
39. **Anoscopy:** Visual examination of the anus by means of a short tube called an anoscope, an optical instrument with lenses and a lighted tip.
40. **Antacid:** Medicine taken orally that reduces or neutralizes stomach acid.
41. **Antiarrhythmics:** Medications used to treat heartbeat irregularities (arrhythmias).
42. **Antibiotics:** Medications that attack germs and fight infection.
43. **Antibiotics, cephalosporin:** Class of antibiotics related to penicillin, capable of destroying more kinds of germs than penicillin.
44. **Antibiotics, erythromycin:** Class of antibiotics that destroys germs similar to those destroyed by penicillin. Often used to treat infections in patients who are allergic to penicillin.
45. **Antibodies:** Proteins created in blood and body tissue by the immune system to neutralize or destroy sources of disease.

46. **Anticancer drugs:** Medications that weaken or destroy cancerous tissues without harming healthy tissues.
47. **Anticholinergic drugs:** Medications that reduce nerve impulses in the parasympathetic nervous system. They control some activities of the gastrointestinal system, heart, bladder, and other organs.
48. **Anticoagulants:** Medications that slow or delay blood clotting.
49. **Anticonvulsants:** Medications that control seizures (convulsions), pain, or conditions in which the brain or nerves are overly sensitive.
50. **Antidepressants:** Medications that help control depression.
51. **Antiemetic drugs:** Medications that prevent or stop nausea and vomiting.
52. **Antifungal drugs:** Medications used to treat fungus diseases.
53. **Antigens:** Germs or other sources of disease that antibodies (produced by the immune system) neutralize or destroy.
54. **Antihelminthic drugs:** Medications used to treat worms in the intestines.
55. **Antihistamines:** Medications used to treat allergies.
56. **Antihyperlipidemic drugs:** Medications that reduce fat (cholesterol) in the blood. They help prevent blood-vessel disease.
57. **Antihypertensives:** Medications used to reduce blood pressure.
58. **Anti-inflammatory drugs:** Medications used to control inflammation not caused by infection.
59. **Antimalarial drugs:** Medications used to prevent or treat malaria.
60. **Antimetabolite drugs:** Medications that are used to treat some cancers and autoimmune diseases.
61. **Antimicrobial drugs:** Same as antibiotics.
62. **Antinuclear antibody:** Substance that appears in the blood, indicating presence of an autoimmune disease.
63. **Antiparkinsonism drugs:** Medications used to treat Parkinson's disease.
64. **Antiprotozoal drugs:** Medications used in treatment of single-celled parasites (protozoa).
65. **Antipruritic drugs:** Medications that reduce itching.
66. **Antispasmodic drugs:** Medications that improve digestion and relieve intestinal cramps.
67. **Anti-streptococcal titer:** Blood test that measures body's response to infection by streptococcal bacteria.
68. **Antithyroid drugs:** Medications used to counter the effects of an overactive thyroid gland.
69. **Antiviral drugs:** Medications used to treat infections caused by viruses.
70. **Anus, imperforate:** Congenital abnormality of newborn infants in which the anus cannot pass feces.
71. **Anxiety:** Uncomfortable feeling that something unpleasant or dangerous will happen.
72. **Aorta:** Body's largest blood vessel, arising from the top of the heart. It carries blood from the heart to all parts of the body.
73. **Appendage:** Body part that has a minor role (or no role at all) in normal body function. For example, the appendix is an appendage to the colon that seems to have no function.
74. **Arrhythmia:** Any variation from a normal heartbeat. Many that occur in children require no treatment. Abnormal rhythms can be caused by diseases of the heart (congenital heart disease, rheumatic heart disease) or by other diseases that may affect the heart rate (examples: Thyroid problems, blood clotting, some drugs such as digitalis). There may be no symptoms in a child or there may be a heart rate far too fast to count: 300 or over. Other symptoms include faintness, dizziness, light-headedness. Treatment depends on the cause and must be supervised by a physician.

75. **Arteriogram, arteriography:** Studying arteries by injecting material into them that x-rays can outline.
76. **Arthrograms:** X-rays of the joints taken with an arthroscope.
77. **Arthroscope:** Slender optical instrument with a lighted tip that allows direct visual examination of some joints. It can also be used to correct some defects in joints.
78. **Asphyxia:** Literally from the Greek: 'a stopping of the pulse.' Modern interpretation is the condition caused by lack of oxygen in breathed air, resulting in impending or actual cessation of life.
79. **Aspiration:** Removal of accumulated pus or fluid with a needle. Accidental inhalation of objects or fluids into the lungs.
80. **Astigmatism:** Visual impairment caused by abnormal eye shape.
81. **Asymmetrical:** Uneven in size, shape, or position.
82. **Atropine:** Medication used to treat diseases of the eye, heart, gastrointestinal system and nervous system.
83. **Autism:** A developmental disorder characterized by a lack of responsiveness to other people and by deficits in development and use of language. Cause is unknown, but may appear in conjunction with birth defects such as congenital German measles, mental retardation, or encephalitis. Treatment requires special education, training, and constant care.
84. **Autoimmune assays (ANA tests):** Blood tests to identify autoimmune disease.
85. **Autoimmune disorder:** Disease in which the immune system produces antibodies that attack the body's own tissues.
86. **Autonomic nervous system:** Part of the nervous system that controls organs that function involuntarily, such as the heart, lungs, digestive system, and blood vessels.

B

87. **Birthmark:** Abnormality of the skin that is present at birth or shortly afterward.
88. **Blister:** A raised area on the skin containing fluid. The fluid can be blood or serum, the clear liquid portion of the blood.
89. **Booster seat:** A seat to help raise a child in a vehicle so that the vehicle's seat belt fits properly.
90. **Bruise (also called contusion):** A collection of blood due to broken blood vessels underneath the skin usually caused by trauma. A bruise causes discoloration and swelling in the area.
91. **Bulimia nervosa (also known as bulimia):** A disease in which there is uncontrolled episodes of overeating that are usually followed with purging (self-induced vomiting), misuse of laxatives, enemas, or medications that cause increased production of urine, fasting, or excessive exercise to control weight.
92. **Bacteria:** One-celled microorganisms that can sometimes cause disease.
93. **Balloon angioplasty:** Treatment for obstructed arteries, especially those supplying blood to the heart and brain. A small uninflated balloon is passed up the artery to the obstruction, and then expanded to release the obstruction.
94. **Barium enema X-rays:** Examining the colon by filling it with a barium solution that is detected by X-rays.
95. **Bartholin's glands:** Small glands in the lips of the vagina that secrete a lubricating fluid, especially during sexual arousal.
96. **Belladonna:** Medication derived from a plant used to treat some diseases of the gastrointestinal system. It is similar to atropine.
97. **Beta-adrenergic blockers (beta-blockers):** Medications that reduce heart or blood-vessel overactivity to improve blood circulation. Also used to prevent migraine headaches, high blood pressure, and angina.

98. **Bilirubin:** A yellowish, red blood cell waste product in bile that the blood carries to the liver. It contributes to urine's yellowish color and can cause jaundice if it builds up in the blood.
99. **Biopsy:** Removal of a small amount of tissue or fluid for laboratory examination that aids in diagnosis.
100. **Birth control:** Two-thirds of adolescent males and one-half of adolescent females in America are sexually active. Make sure your youngster has adequate instruction in sex education and particularly birth control. Example of devices and methods include condoms, contraceptive foam, diaphragm, cervical cap, vaginal contraceptive sponge, birth control pills, intrauterine device (IUD).
101. **Birthmarks:** These are blemishes of the skin present at birth. They fit into two categories: Pigmentary and vascular. Pigmentary types include nevocellular nevi, Mongolian spots, cafe-au-lait spots, epithelial nevi, Becker's nevi, dysplastic melanocyte nevi, and white birthmarks. Vascular types include hemangiomas (also called strawberry birthmarks), port-wine stains, stork bites or salmon patches. Diagnosis requires identification by your physician. Treatment depends on the type. Most fade and disappear; others need surgical or medical treatment under a physician's guidance.
102. **Blastomycosis:** Infection caused by organisms of the genus blastomyces.
103. **Blindness and other vision problems:** The absence of vision. It may occur singly or in conjunction with other disabling handicaps. 20/200 or worse in the better eye is the legal limit of blindness.
104. **Blood chemistries:** Tests that measure chemicals in the blood.
105. **Blood vessels:** Arteries, veins, and capillaries; the tubes in which blood circulates through the body.
106. **Bone bank:** Facility where human bone is stored and made available for transplantation.
107. **Bone spurs:** Abnormal and sometimes painful protrusions of bone with sharp points near joints or tendons.
108. **Breasts:** Fat and fibrous tissue, milk-producing glands, and milk-transporting ducts. Development: most girls begin to develop breasts between 9 and 14 years of age. Average age is 10 or 11. Each girl develops at her own rate. The onset and rate of development and ultimate size are determined by heredity, level of female hormones, and nutrition. Disorders: if breasts fail to develop, if one is excessively larger than the other, if there is a lump in the breast or discharge from the nipple, consult your physician.
109. **Bronchial tubes (bronchi):** Hollow air passageways that branch from the windpipe (trachea) into the lungs. They carry oxygen into the lungs and pass waste gases (mostly carbon dioxide) out of the body.
110. **Bronchodilator drugs:** Medications used to treat diseases of the bronchi that cause shortness of breath, such as asthma. The medicines help constricted tubes to relax.
111. **Bronchogram:** Diagnosing lung diseases by placing a material in the lung that X-rays can outline.
112. **Bronchopulmonary dysplasia disease (BPD):** A chronic lung disease occurring in premature infants who have required oxygen and mechanical ventilation for a long period of time during treatment to sustain life after birth. Treatment consists of assisted breathing support, supplements of calcium and vitamin E, plus medicines to assist the heart and kidneys.
113. **Bronchoscope:** An optical instrument with a lighted tip that is passed into the windpipe, then into the bronchi.
114. **Buerger's disease:** A disease characterized by an inflammatory reaction in the arteries, veins, and nerves, which leads to a thickening of the vessel walls. It occurs mostly in young men who smoke tobacco.

C

115. **Cardiopulmonary resuscitation (CPR):** An emergency method of life-saving. Artificial respirations and chest compressions are used to restart the heart and lungs.

116. **Cephalohematoma:** An area of bleeding underneath one of the cranial bones that appears as raised lump on the baby's head.
117. **Chemical burns:** Burns due to strong acids or alkalies coming into contact with the skin and/or eyes.
118. **Chickenpox:** A highly viral infectious disease usually associated with childhood. The disease is caused by the varicella-zoster virus (VZV). Transmission occurs from person-to-person by direct contact or through the air.
119. **Circumcision:** Surgical procedure to remove the skin covering the end of the penis, called the foreskin.
120. **Colic:** A condition in an otherwise healthy baby characterized by excessive crying.
121. **Congenital**: Present at birth.
122. **Conjunctivitis:** Inflammation of the conjunctiva of the eye.
123. **Contact dermatitis:** Itchy rash; a result of an exposure to an allergen or an irritant.
124. **Cystitis:** Inflammation of the bladder, usually caused by a bacterial infection.
125. **Calcification:** A process in which calcium from the blood is deposited abnormally into tissues due to injury, infection, or aging. Often it is part of healing and not a sign of active disease.
126. **Calcium-channel blocker drugs:** Medication used to treat angina, hypertension, and heartbeat irregularities.
127. **Cancers:** Destructive tumors that can arise in almost all parts of the body. Cancer can destroy nearby healthy tissue and may spread to distant organs.
128. **Capillaries:** Microscopic vessels that supply all body cells and tissues with blood.
129. **Carbohydrates, complex:** Starches, sugars, cellulose, and gums. Complex carbohydrates are those contained in whole grains, fresh fruits, and fresh vegetables. These are considered more nutritious than simple carbohydrates.
130. **Cardiac catheter:** A slender tube that is inserted into an artery or vein and then passed into the heart. It is used to artery or vein and then passed into the heart. It is used to examine the heart and nearby blood vessels by injecting material into the heart that X-rays can detect.
131. **Caudal anesthesia:** Form of local (low-spinal) anesthesia used to reduce pain during childbirth and surgery on pelvic areas.
132. **Chemotherapy:** Treatment of cancer by injecting medications that kill cancer cells without harming healthy tissue. It is used to treat cancers that cannot be completely cured or treated with surgery or radiation.
133. **Chiggers:** Small red biting insects. Also called 'red bugs.'
134. **Children:** Person in the first 12 years of life.
135. **Chokes:** Severe breathing difficulty experienced by scuba divers and others who go from high to normal air pressure too rapidly. Bubbles of nitrogen develop in the blood stream and obstruct the blood supply to vital organs, sometimes resulting in severe injury or death.
136. **Cholangiogram, cholangiography:** X-ray procedures to diagnose diseases of the bile system (liver, gallbladder, bile ducts). Special medications are used to make the bile system visible on X-rays.
137. **Cholera:** Acute, severe, infectious disease causing extreme diarrhea and dehydration.
138. **Choroiditis:** Inflammation of the part of the eye that supports the retina and supplies blood to it.
139. **Chromosome:** Structures inside the nucleus of living cells that contain hereditary information. Defects in chromosomes cause many birth defects and inherited diseases.
140. **Chronic:** Long-term, continuing. Chronic illnesses are usually not curable, but they can often be prevented from worsening. Symptoms usually can be controlled.

141. **Cinematography:** Form of motion-picture photography used to record a fast-moving series of X-ray images.
142. **Clubfoot:** Malformation at birth of foot and ankle bones. The heel turns in under the ankle, the inner edge of the foot turns upward, and the front of the foot turns in toward the other. Treatment consisting of straightening and holding the position in casts must start within a few days of birth. New casts are applied every week until age 3 months, then at longer intervals. If casting is not successful, surgery can correct the problem.
143. **Cocaine:** Medication applied directly to mucous membranes to control pain in the nose and throat. Used illegally as a mind-altering drug, it is addicting and dangerous.
144. **Colic, colicky:** A pain that recurs in a regular pattern every few second or minutes.
145. **Collagen:** A gelatinous protein from which body tissues are formed.
146. **Colonoscopy:** Method of diagnosing diseases of the colon by visual examination of the inside of the colon through a flexible colonoscopy, a fiber-optic instrument with a lighted tip.
147. **Color-blindness:** Inability to recognize red and green, which appear to be gray. It is usually hereditary.
148. **Coma (latin: 'deep sleep'):** A state of unconsciousness from which a person cannot be aroused. Coma can be caused by any substance, disease, or injury that disrupts the brain system controlling alertness and awareness. The pulse is slower than normal and blood pressure is frequently high. Treatment includes stabilization of circulation and breathing, lowering the pressure of fluid inside the skull, and monitoring all body functions. These may require medicines, surgery, or both.
149. **Combined Immunodeficiency Disease:** Serious inherited disease in which the immune system of infants is unable to defend against disease.
150. **Complication:** Undesirable event during disease or treatment that causes further symptoms and delay in recovery.
151. **Congenital:** Abnormality of the body, present at birth, usually meaning a defect. Congenital defects may be inherited or caused by conditions occurring while the fetus grows in the uterus.
152. **Contagious:** Disease or condition that spreads from one person to another.
153. **Convalescence:** Recovery from an illness or surgery.
154. **COPD (Chronic obstructive pulmonary disease):** Several usually incurable lung diseases associated with gradually increasing breathing difficulty.
155. **Cosmetic surgery:** Surgery to improve appearance.
156. **Coxsackie viruses:** Group of viruses causing infections such as poliomyelitis, aseptic meningitis, herpangina, and myocarditis.
157. **Craniotomy:** An operation to open the cranium, the eight bones that form the vault to cradle the brain.
158. **Cryosurgery:** Destruction of abnormal tissue by applying freezing temperatures, usually with liquid nitrogen.
159. **Cryotherapy:** The use of cold (below 20 °F) temperatures in treatment.
160. **Culdocentesis:** Piercing of the space deep in the vagina under the cervix, to obtain fluid. Laboratory examination of the removed fluid aids in diagnosis of ectopic pregnancy and other disorders.
161. **Culture:** Identification of bacteria, fungi and viruses. Material (pus, blood, or urine) from an area infected is collected, placed on nutrient material, and kept warm (usually in an incubator) until the infecting agent has grown. The resulting growth is examined with a microscope.
162. **Curette:** Instrument with a sharp end used to scrape tissue from the inner lining of the uterus and to scrape away skin lesions.
163. **Cyst:** Sac or cavity filled with fluid or diseased matter.

164. **Cyst aspiration:** Removal of cyst contents for examination, or drainage for relief of symptoms.
165. **Cystoscopy:** Visual examination of the inside of the urinary bladder by means of a cystoscope, a slender optical instrument with a lighted tip.
166. **Cytotoxic drugs:** Medications used to destroy cancerous cells with minimal harm to healthy cells.

D

167. **Deciduous teeth:** Also known as 'baby' or primary teeth.
168. **Diaper rash:** An irritation of the skin in the diaper area.
169. **Diarrhea:** Increase in frequency of stools compared to normal, or looser bowel movements than usual; causes include infections of the digestive system, medications such as antibiotics, malabsorption, irritable bowel syndrome.
170. **Diphtheria:** A serious, infectious disease that produces a toxin (poison) and an inflammation in the membrane lining of the throat, nose, trachea, and other tissues.
171. **Debilitating:** Causing a general weakening or deterioration in health.
172. **Defibrillation:** Applying an electric current to the chest over the heart to interrupt fibrillation, a disturbance of heartbeat.
173. **Dehydration:** Loss of essential fluids from the tissues and blood of the body.
174. **Dependence:** Condition in which a person requires substances such as narcotics or alcohol to remain comfortable. If the substances are not used, withdrawal symptoms develop.
175. **Dermatome:** Area of the skin to which feeling (sensation) is provided by a nerve to the spinal cord.
176. **Diabetic retinopathy:** Degeneration of the retina that develops in patients with diabetes mellitus. It may cause vision impairment or blindness.
177. **Diagnosis:** Identifying disease. A complete diagnosis names the part of the body affected, the disease process (such as inflammation, cancer, or allergy) and the cause of disease.
178. **Dialysis:** Removal of natural wastes from the bloodstream. It is used to treat patients with kidney failure.
179. **Diaphragm:** Thin, broad sheet of muscle separating the chest cavity from the abdominal cavity.
180. **Diathermy:** Treatment in which mild heat is generated within the body by high-frequency radio waves.
181. **Digitalis:** A drug used to treat congestive heart failure and some other heart diseases.
182. **Dilator:** Instrument used to widen organs that have narrowed because of disease.
183. **Discolored teeth:** A yellowish-brown discoloration of the teeth frequently occurring in infants whose mothers took tetracycline while pregnant. Children may also be affected if they take tetracycline before they have their permanent teeth.
184. **Disease:** Adverse change in health; sickness or ailment. A disease can be defined by the body part involved (for example, the heart or liver), by the abnormality present (cancer, infection, allergy, degeneration, etc.) or by its cause (bacteria, poisons, injury, etc.).
185. **Diuretics:** Medications that force the kidneys to excrete more urine, sodium, and potassium than normal, which helps eliminate excessive body fluid.
186. **Diverticulum:** Small pouch or sac that develops in the wall of tubular organs such as the esophagus or colon.
187. **Dizziness:** Sensation of faintness, lightheadedness, or spinning (vertigo).
188. **Donor:** Person who gives to someone else. In transplantation surgery, the donor gives up an organ (such as a kidney) to be transplanted into the recipient.
189. **Drainage:** Passage of fluids out of the body through an opening or incision.

190. **Ductus arteriosus:** Small blood vessel connecting the aorta and the pulmonary artery, which is the main artery to the lung. The vessel is open during the time the fetus is in the uterus, but normally closes at birth.
191. **Dwarfism:** Condition of being undersized for one's age. It may be due to endocrine disorders, malnutrition, or an inherited defect.
192. **Dysproteinemia:** An abnormality of the protein content of the blood.

E

193. ***E. coli* (also called *Escherichia coli*):** Species of bacteria found in the intestines of man and healthy cattle; often the cause of urinary tract infections, diarrhea in infants, and wound infections.
194. **Electrical burns:** Burns due to contact with an electrical current.
195. **Encopresis:** Constipation and intestinal obstruction (blockage) lead to an involuntary leakage of loose stool.
196. **Enuresis:** Loss of urine, especially at night in bed.
197. **Epilepsy:** A condition in which there is a problem with the brain that causes long-term seizures in the child.
198. **Echocardiogram, echocardiography:** Studying the heart by examining sound waves created by an instrument placed on the chest. The waves reflected from the heart form an image (echocardiogram) on a monitor, aiding in diagnosis of heart diseases.
199. **Edema:** Accumulation of fluid under the skin, in the lungs, or elsewhere.
200. **EKG (electrocardiography):** Method of diagnosing heart diseases by measuring electrical activity of the heart with an electrocardiograph. The record produced is called an electrocardiogram.
201. **Electrolyte:** A chemical that is dissolved in the blood and all other body fluids. Electrolytes play an essential tole in all body functions. The major electrolytes are: sodium, potassium, chloride, calcium, phosphorus, magnesium, and carbon dioxide. Electrolytes come from food. They are regulated mostly by the kidneys and lungs.
202. **Electromyography:** Studying nerve and muscle disorders by recording electrical activity of muscles with an electromyograph. The record produced is the electromyogram.
203. **Electrosurgery:** Minor surgery performed with an electric current sent through an electric cauterizing instrument. It not only destroys tissue, but also controls bleeding.
204. **Endemic:** Disease that is constantly present in a community or group of people. Endemic disease may affect only a few people at any one time.
205. **Endocrine system:** System of organs that secrete hormones into the blood to regulate basic functions of cells and tissues. The endocrine organs are the anterior and posterior pituitary glands, thyroid and parathyroid glands, pancreas, adrenal glands, ovaries (in women), and testicles (in men).
206. **Endoscopy:** Method of diagnosing diseases in hollow organs. An endoscope (an optical instrument with a lighted tip) is inserted into the organ, which allows visual examination of the cavity. Used in the abdomen, pelvis, lumen of the bronchial tubes, or intestines.
207. **Endotracheal tube:** Tube temporarily placed in the trachea (windpipe) of patients who are unable to breathe normally because of disease or surgery.
208. **Enteric:** Relating to the small intestine. Enteric-coated medicine is coated with a hard shell that dissolves when it reaches the small intestine.
209. **Enterostomy:** Surgically created artificial opening for elimination of feces. An enterostomy nurse or enterostomy specialist is a professional who teaches patients how to care for the artificial opening.
210. **Enzymes:** Proteins manufactured by the body that regulate the rate of essential life processes (metabolism).

211. **Episcleritis:** Inflammation of tissues on the sclera (the 'white of the eye').
212. **Ergot:** Medication derived from a fungus that grows on rye plants. It is used to treat migraine headache and to increase the strength of uterine contractions during and immediately after childbirth.
213. **Esophageal varices:** Enlarged veins on the lining of the esophagus. They are subject to severe bleeding and often appear in patients with severe liver disease.
214. **Esophagoscopy:** Method of diagnosing diseases of the esophagus by means of an esophagoscope, an optical instrument with lenses and a lighted tip.
215. **Estrogen:** Female sex hormone, primarily secreted by the ovaries. It can also be produced synthetically for use in estrogen replacement therapy.
216. **Exploratory laparotomy:** Diagnosing abdominal disease by surgically opening the abdomen and examining its contents.
217. **Eyes crossed (Also called squint eyes or strabismus):** Condition in which muscles controlling the eyes are unbalanced. The eyes point in different directions.

F

218. **Fluoride:** A natural chemical that strengthens enamel—the hard outer coating on teeth—helps prevent tooth decay, and helps repair early damage to teeth.
219. **Food allergy:** A physiological reaction caused when the immune system mistakenly identifies a normally harmless food as damaging to the body.
220. **Food intolerance:** An adverse reaction of the body to a certain food(s) that does not affect the immune system, although some symptoms may be the same as in food allergy.
221. **Fractures:** A partial or complete break in the bone.
222. **Far sightedness:** Same as hypermetropia.
223. **Fascia:** Sheet or band of tough, fibrous tissue that covers muscles and other body organs.
224. **Fecal:** Relating to feces, waste products eliminated through the lower intestinal tract.
225. **Fetal monitoring:** Measuring the heart rate of the fetus during labor.
226. **Fetal-scalp electrodes:** Fine wires attached to the scalp of a fetus to measure heart rate and rhythm during labor.
227. **Fever:** A body temperature that is an elevation above normal of at least 1 degree. Critical points of fever that require treatment are as follows (all rectal temperatures): 6 months or younger-100 °F (37.8 °C) or higher; 6 months to 3 years-102 °F (38.8 °C); any age-fever accompanied by unusual drowsiness and loss of alertness, labored breathing, or otherwise appears ill. Fever is a sign of disease, not a disease itself. It may be caused by bacterial infections, viral infections, and reactions to drugs, heatstroke, dehydration, or fevers of undetermined origin. Low-grade fever can be helpful by stimulating the production of white blood cells and speeding up the body's immune system both providing useful defense mechanisms for fighting disease.
228. **Fiber:** A non-nutritious ingredient of many complex carbohydrates. Fiber increases bulk in the diet. Many nutritionists recommend including ample fiber in the diet. Experimental studies and clinical studies show that people who eat high-fiber diets are less likely to develop colon cancer, diverticulitis, atherosclerosis, and gallbladder disease.
229. **Fibrinogen:** Protein in the blood needed for blood clotting.
230. **Fibrositis:** Inflammatory conditions affecting connective tissue of muscles, joints, ligaments, and tendons.
231. **First molars:** First permanent flat teeth, used for grinding food, which appear at about age 6 to 7.
232. **Fissure:** Break in the skin or inner lining of organs.
233. **Fistula:** Abnormal passage between two organs or between the body and the outside.
234. **Flank:** Area on the side of the body below the ribs and above the hip.

235. Fleas: Tiny biting insects. Most cause minor skin irritation; some carry and transmit serious diseases such as plague and typhus.

236. Fluorescein (Dye test): Method of diagnosis using Fluorescein, a dye, to study tissues and germs. When these dyed tissues are exposed to ultraviolet light, they glow. Substances to which the dye does not cling do not glow.

237. Fluoroscopy: Method of X-ray diagnosis in which moving organs (such as the heart or intestinal tract) can be studied in action.

238. Foley catheter: Slender, flexible tube used to drain urine from the bladder of patients who are unable to urinate normally.

239. Forceps: Instrument with two blades and handles. It is used to grasp tissue, body parts, or sterile materials. Also used to deliver babies when progress of labor is slow.

240. Fracture: Break; usually used to refer to a bone or tooth.

241. Frei test: Test used to make a precise diagnosis of lymphogranuloma, a sexually transmitted disease.

242. Friedreich's ataxia: Rare, inherited nervous-system disease that causes loss of balance and coordination, awkward walking, speech difficulty, and tremors.

243. Frozen section: A study in a pathology laboratory of fresh tissue that was removed during surgery. The purpose is to determine if a suspicious area is or is not cancerous.

G

244. Galactorrhea: 1) Continued breast-milk flow after weaning. 2) Excess breast-milk flow during nursing.

245. Galactosemia: Inherited disease of infants in which milk cannot be digested. Milk should be eliminated from the infant's diet to prevent malnutrition, liver and kidney disease, and mental retardation.

246. Gallbladder: Small organ under the liver that stores bile. For digestion, the gallbladder contracts to empty bile into the intestines.

247. Gamma globulin: Protein in the blood manufactured by the immune system to help destroy or neutralize infection-causing germs. Gamma globulin derived and concentrated from blood of other humans is used to help create temporary immunity to some diseases.

248. Gamma globulinemia: Extremely low levels in the blood of gamma globulin brought about by a disease of the immune system. The deficiency causes increased susceptibility to many infections by bacteria, viruses, and fungi. Also called hypogammaglobulinemia. Gangrene—death of tissue, usually due to partial or total loss of blood supply.

249. Gastrectomy: Removal of part or all of the stomach.

250. Gastroscopy: Visual examination of the inside of the stomach by means of a gastroscope, an optical instrument with a lighted tip.

251. Gene: Basic unit of protein molecules in chromosomes of cells. Genes transmit inherited characteristics such as eye color, blood type, gender, or body shape. Defective genes cause many kinds of birth defects and inborn diseases.

252. Gene, dominant or recessive: Dominant gene, if present in either the mother's egg or father's sperm, will transmit its characteristics to the newborn child. Recessive genes must be present in both parents before its characteristics will be transmitted.

253. Genetic counseling: Counseling to help couples decide whether to have children or not when there is a risk of genetic disease being transmitted to the child.

254. Genetics: Science of determining inherited factors that result in the unique make-up of every human being; also, science that traces the appearance patterns to genetic (inherited) disease.

255. **Germs:** Organisms that cause infection such as bacteria, viruses, or fungi.
256. **Gestation:** Time spent in the mother's uterus by the fetus. Average gestation time for the human infant, from conception to delivery, is approximately 39 weeks.
257. **Gigantism:** Condition in which the body or a body part grows excessively, sometimes due to an overactive pituitary gland.
258. **Glomerulonephritis:** An inflammatory disorder of the kidney secondary to an allergic reaction to the streptococcus germ. This is one of the possible complications of a strep infection. It can usually be prevented by adequate treatment of the original strep infection with penicillin or other suitable antibiotic.
259. **Glucagon:** Hormone secreted by the pancreas that increases blood sugar. A synthetic form is sometimes used as emergency treatment for patients with diabetes who have temporarily low blood sugar.
260. **Glucose:** Major form of sugar in the blood, stored primarily in the liver. It provides energy to most tissues, organs, and systems.
261. **Glucose-tolerance test:** Method of diagnosing diabetes mellitus or functional hypoglycemia. The patient drinks a measured amount of glucose (sugar). The blood and urine are tested at measured intervals for glucose content.
262. **Gluten:** Protein found in wheat and other foods that cannot be digested by some persons because of genetic disease. A gluten-free diet allows persons with the disorder to digest food and grow normally.
263. **Gonads:** Parts of the reproductive system that produces and release female eggs (ovaries) or male sperm (testes).
264. **Growth disorders:** Conditions in children that result in underdevelopment or overdevelopment of the body. Diseases of the endocrine glands, nutritional problems, or genetic abnormalities are frequently the causes.

H

265. ***Haemophilus influenzae* (also called *H. Influenzae*):** Represents a group of bacteria that may cause different types of infections in infants and children. *H. Influenzae* most commonly causes ear, eye, or sinus infections, and pneumonia.
266. **Headache:** Pain or discomfort in the head or face area. Headaches can be single or recurrent in nature, and localized to one or more areas of the head and face.
267. **Heat exhaustion:** A form of heat-related illness that is more severe than heat cramps and results from a loss of water and salt in the body. It occurs in conditions of extreme heat and excessive sweating without adequate fluid and salt replacement. Heat exhaustion occurs when the body is unable to cool itself properly. If left untreated, heat exhaustion can progress to heat stroke.
268. **Hepatitis:** Inflammation of the liver that sometimes causes permanent damage; caused by viruses, medicines, or alcohol.
269. **H-2 blocker drugs:** Class of antihistamines that reduce the production of stomach acid for treatment of peptic ulcers.
270. **Hallucinogens:** Substances that produce hallucinations, apparent sights, sounds, or other experiences that do not actually exist.
271. **Hashimoto's Thyroiditis:** One of several kinds of inflammation of the thyroid gland.
272. **Head banging and rocking:** A common, usually harmless, habit. The child hits his head against a solid object in a rhythmical way. Head banging first appears between 6 and 12 months of age and disappears before 3 years. This habit is 3 times more common in boys than girls and occurs in 5–10% of all children. This habit is closely associated with rocking, also a harmless habit. The cause of either banging or rocking is unknown. Head banging may also be a part of the symptoms

of children with other disorders, including autism, mental retardation, blindness, and hearing loss. If rhythmical behavior begins after 18 months, consult your physician.

273. **Heart Tumors:** Rare tumors that grow in the heart wall or in the heart chambers, interfering with normal heart function.
274. **Hematocrit:** Blood test used to detect anemia and other blood disorders. It is expressed as the percentage of blood made up of red blood cells (the remainder of the blood is made up of serum or plasma). The normal hematocrit range is approximately 35% to 45%, but it varies with age and sex.
275. **Hematologist:** Doctor specially trained to diagnose and treat diseases of the blood and blood-forming organs.
276. **Hemochromatosis:** Disease in which excessive iron accumulates in the liver, pancreas, and skin, resulting in liver disease, diabetes mellitus, and a bronzed skin color.
277. **Hemoglobin:** 1) Component that carries oxygen to body tissues. 2) blood test used to detect anemia and other blood disorders, expressed in grams per 100 cubic centimeters. The normal hemoglobin range is approximately 12 to 18 grams per 100 cubic centimeters and varies according to age and sex.
278. **Hirschsprung's disease:** Congenital defect of infants in which the colon cannot eliminate feces, resulting in severe constipation.
279. **Histamine:** Chemical in body tissues that dilates the smallest blood vessels, constricts the muscle around the bronchial tubes, stimulates stomach secretions, and produces an allergic response.
280. **Holter monitor:** Instrument that detects heartbeat-rhythm abnormalities 24 hours or longer. The device is portable for patients to carry wherever they go.
281. **Hormones:** Powerful substances manufactured by the endocrine glands and carried by the blood to body tissues and organs. Hormones determine growth and structure of many organs (such as during growth and maturation) and also control many vital body functions.
282. **Host:** Person or animal with an infection that has been received from another person, animal or plant, or the environment.
283. **Hyaline-Membrane Disease (HMD):** Serious condition of premature infants in which the lungs cannot expand normally. Cause is unknown.
284. **Hydatidiform mole:** Disease occurring during early pregnancy resulting in death of the fetus and an overgrowth of tissue within the uterus.
285. **Hydramnios and polyhydramnios:** Condition in which amniotic fluid (fluid in the uterus that surrounds the fetus until birth) becomes excessive.
286. **Hyperalimentation:** Method of supplying total nutritional needs of patients unable to eat normally. The method (usually intravenous or by tube through the nose into the stomach) provides nutrients containing essential proteins, fats, carbohydrates, and vitamins.
287. **Hyperbaric chamber:** Large, sealed room in which air pressure can be raised above normal levels. It is used primarily to treat patients with either decompression sickness or severe burns (sometimes).
288. **Hypercalcemia:** Presence of excessive calcium in the blood; occasionally a sign of malignancy.
289. **Hyperlipoproteinemia:** Condition in which excessive lipoproteins (cholesterol and other fatty materials) accumulate in the blood.
290. **Hypermetropia:** Seeing distant objects clearly while nearby objects appear blurred; also called farsightedness.
291. **Hypersensitivity:** Extreme sensitivity to any agent (drugs, pollens, chemicals, etc.) that causes allergic reactions. Some reactions can be life-threatening, but most are less serious.
292. **Hypogammaglobulinemia:** An abnormally low level of all classes of gamma globulin in the blood.

293. **Hysteria:** 1) Condition in which a person becomes anxious and excitable and experiences impaired sensory and motor abilities. Sometimes, hysterical persons simulate conditions of diseases such as deafness or blindness. 2) outbreak of uncontrolled emotions, such as fits of laughing or crying.
294. **Hysterostomy:** Incision of the uterus to prepare for cesarean-section delivery of a baby.

I

295. **Immunizations (vaccines):** A set of shots given to children at different ages to help keep them from developing dangerous childhood diseases.
296. **Impetigo:** A bacterial skin infection characterized by microscopic pus-filled blisters.
297. **Influenza (also called the flu):** A viral respiratory tract infection. The influenza viruses are divided into three types: a, b, and c.
298. **Inguinal hernia:** Part of the small intestine that pushes through an opening in the abdominal muscle, causing a bulge underneath the skin in the groin area.
299. **Intravenous pyelogram:** A test that examines the urinary system using a contrast medium that can be seen on X-rays to show possible obstructions, tumors, cysts, stones, and other abnormalities.
300. **Immune, immunity:** Resistance or protection against infection by the body's natural defenses. A person may be immune to one kind of infection but not immune to another. Some infections, such as measles, chickenpox, or mumps, cause the body to become immune permanently to that infection.
301. **Immunosuppression:** Prevention of the body from forming a normal immune response. It is used to treat diseases (especially when organs must be transplanted) where certain antibodies must be inactivated.
302. **Incubation period:** The time between exposure to an infecting germ and the appearance of symptoms indicating an infection. Also describes the period of bacterial growth in laboratory cultures.
303. **Infant:** Child between the ages of 2 weeks and 1 year.
304. **Infection:** Disease caused by germs (bacteria, viruses, fungi) that enter the body and cause inflammation or other processes that have an adverse effect on health.
305. **Inflammatory process:** Process by which the body attempts to overcome illness-producing causes such as germs, injuries such as burns, or diseases such as arthritis. The process causes increased body heat (fever or local warmth), swelling, pain, and tenderness. If the inflammation is near the skin, redness results.
306. **Inhalation:** Breathing air into the lungs.
307. **Inherited:** Body characteristic that is transmitted from one generation to the next by chromosomes in the mother's egg and father's sperm. Some inherited characteristics such as brown eyes are normal; others such as Down syndrome are disorders.
308. **Inoculation:** Injection of infected material such as pus into a nutrient medium where the germs will grow, or incubate. They are then stained and analyzed through a microscope. Also describes any kind of immunization.
309. **Intermittent:** Happening only occasionally or under certain conditions.
310. **Internist:** Doctor specially trained in non-surgical diagnosis and treatment of diseases in adults.
311. **Intrauterine death:** Death of a fetus while inside the mother's uterus.
312. **Intrauterine device (IUD):** Birth-control method in which a small device placed permanently in the uterus prevents growth of fertilized eggs.
313. **Intravenous pyelogram (IVP):** See pyelogram, intravenous.
314. **IQ (intelligence quotient):** Supposedly a measure of a person's intelligence, rather than what one has learned. Recent research on intelligence raises questions about the accuracy and meaning of the IQ test.

J

315. **Jaundice:** A yellow color of the skin and eyes that is caused by too much bilirubin in the bloodstream due to liver problems.
316. **Joint replacement:** Replacement of diseased joints with mechanical joints. The wrist, hip and knee joints are among the most common joints replaced.

K

317. **Kidney and bladder ultrasound:** A diagnostic imaging technique that examines the kidney and bladder using high-frequency sound waves; to detect certain abnormalities.
318. **Ketoacidosis:** Serious complication of diabetes mellitus in which the body produces acids that cause fluid and electrolyte disorders, dehydration, and sometimes coma.
319. **Klinefelter's syndrome:** Inherited disease of young males in which secondary sex characteristics are underdeveloped. The condition does not become evident until puberty. Mental deficiency and some female characteristics are present.

L

320. **Learning disability (ID):** A disorder that affects people's ability to either interpret what they see and hear or to link information from different parts of the brain. These limitations are characterized by difficulty in reading, writing, and arithmetic.
321. **Lice:** Tiny parasites that can infest the skin; characterized by intense itching.
322. **Locking clip:** A special device used when the vehicle's lap/shoulder belts do not lock. A locking clip will help secure a child safety seat tightly into a vehicle.
323. **Laceration:** Wound with jagged edges.
324. **Lactiferous ducts:** Network of tubes in the female breast that collects milk and delivers it to the nipple.
325. **Laparoscopy:** Exploratory examination of the organs inside the abdominal cavity with a laparoscope, an optical instrument with a lighted tip. The laparoscope is inserted into the abdomen through a small incision. Visual examination can then be made of many abdominal organs.
326. **Laparotomy:** Exploratory surgery in the abdomen performed to diagnose and sometimes treat abdominal disease.
327. **Laser therapy:** Using a laser beam to treat many diseases. Sharply focused laser light creates intense heat and is valuable in cutting tissue, destroying unwanted tissue, and joining tissue together. It is most often used to treat retinal detachment, endometriosis, or atherosclerosis.
328. **Latent:** Present but inactive; something that exists in an undeveloped form.
329. **Laxatives:** Medications used to treat constipation.
330. **Lesion:** General term for injury or damage to an organ or tissue.
331. **Lethargy:** Fatigue or lack of usual physical or mental energy.
332. **Libido:** Sexual desire.
333. **Lipoproteins (high density and low density):** Components of the fluid in blood that are measured to help predict the likelihood of atherosclerosis (hardening of the arteries).
334. **Liquid nitrogen:** Nitrogen that has been cooled until it becomes a liquid. It is used most often in cryosurgery.
335. **Lumbar puncture (spinal tap):** A diagnostic procedure in which a needle is inserted between 2 bones (vertebrae) of the lower spine to collect spinal fluid for laboratory examination.
336. **Lumbar spine:** Lower part of the spine, from the lowest ribs to the bottom of the spine.
337. **Lymphatic leukemia:** Class of leukemias, involving primarily lymphatic cells, affecting children and adults.

338. **Lymphocytes:** One of several types of white blood cells that help fight infection.
339. **Lymphosarcoma:** Class of cancers of the lymphatic system.

M

340. **Measles:** A very contagious viral illness characterized by a distinct rash and a fever; spread through airborne droplets of nasal secretions.
341. **Meconium:** A sticky, greenish-black substance that forms in the intestines during fetal development and is the first bowel movement of a newborn.
342. **Meningitis:** An inflammation of the membrane that covers the brain and spinal cord.
343. **Milia:** Tiny, white, hard spots that look like pimples on a newborn's nose.
344. **Mongolian spots:** Blue or purple-colored splotches on the baby's lower back and buttocks; common in darker-skinned babies.
345. **Moro reflex:** Movement of arms and legs that occurs when a newborn is startled by a loud sound or movement.
346. **Molding:** Elongation of the shape of a baby's head due to delivery through the birth canal.
347. **Mumps:** An acute and highly contagious viral illness that usually occurs in childhood. Spread by airborne droplets from the upper respiratory tract, the disease usually takes two to three weeks to appear.
348. **Myringotomy:** A surgical opening of the eardrum to release pressure on the middle ear.
349. **Macular degeneration of the eye:** Condition of the macula (area on the retina that provides detailed vision) in which impaired blood supply causes gradual vision loss.
350. **Macula:** General term for any discolored spot or patch on the skin, such as a freckle.
351. **Malignant:** Capable of causing great harm, including death. It usually refers to cancerous growth.
352. **Mammogram, mammography:** Diagnostic method of studying the female breast by an X-ray technique that detects cancerous growths while they are still treatable. The image on X-ray film is the mammogram.
353. **Manic-depressive illness:** Mental illness in which behavior alternates between unrealistic enthusiasm and deep depression.
354. **Marrow:** Core of many bones, where most of the body's blood cells are produced.
355. **Mastoiditis:** Infection of the mastoid (bony area just behind the ear).
356. **Masturbation:** Stimulation of the genitals for pleasure. Normal behavior in infants, children, adolescents, and adults. Generally satisfying, particularly during times of separation, such as at bedtime. Stimulation of genitals will help release sexual tensions and gratify fantasies and may help control sex drives.
357. **Mediators:** Substances that: 1) help nerve impulses travel from one cell to the next; 2) participate in the allergic process.
358. **Meibomian glands:** Small glands on the inner eyelid. They secrete a fluid that helps the eyelids move easily over the surface of the eye.
359. **Membrane:** Thin tissue lining a body cavity, covering an internal organ or dividing a space.
360. **Meninges:** Three-layered membrane covering the brain.
361. **Mental retardation:** A disability in the area of thought, perception, and memory. These problems lead to slow development in language skills, learning, muscle control, poor social adaptation. Brain abnormalities from hundreds of diseases, genetic disorders, injuries, or physical deprivation.
362. **Metastases:** Cancerous cells or infectious germs that spread from their original location to other parts of the body.
363. **Metatarsal bones:** Bones in the middle of the foot.
364. **Midwife:** Nurse with special training and experience in childbirth.

365. **Mole:** Skin lesion, often dark-brown or black.
366. **Monamine oxidase (MAO) Inhibitors:** Medications used to treat some forms of depression.
367. **Motor nerve:** Nerve that transmits the stimulus that causes muscles to contract.
368. **Mucous membrane:** Thin tissue lining internal cavities (nose, mouth, vagina) and tubular systems (respiratory and gastrointestinal) that produce mucus.
369. **Mucus:** Slippery liquid produced by the lining of internal cavities and tubular systems to protect tissue.
370. **Murmur:** Sound of blood rushing through the heart and blood vessels, detected by a stethoscope. Some murmurs are innocent, meaning they are not caused by disease. Other murmurs arise from heart disease or partial obstruction in the arteries.
371. **Myelogram:** Special X-ray of the spinal canal and spinal cord, requiring a spinal tap and injection of dye that is visible on X-ray film. Myelogram frequently are used to identify the location of ruptured disks.
372. **Myopia:** Disease of the eye in which close objects are clearly visible while distant objects are blurred. Also called nearsightedness.

N

373. **Nail biting:** A frequent habit among children and adults. The majority of experts believe that nail biting results as a mechanism for discharging everyday tension, similar to thumb-sucking. Nail biting frequently accompanies fear, sadness, nervousness, or distress. Treatment: Try to provide an incentive to avoid nail biting, such as symbolic awards (stars on a calendar, etc.). Instill pride in good grooming. Do not scold or lavish attention for negative behavior.
374. **Narcotics:** Medications used to control severe pain. Narcotics should be used only when necessary because of their serious side effects: Addiction; reduced breathing; nausea and vomiting; low blood pressure; reduced cough reflex; and constipation.
375. **Nasogastric tube:** Slender tube passed through the nose into the stomach. It is used to drain away stomach secretions or to feed patients unable to eat normally.
376. **Naturopathy:** Health-care system relying on diet, sunshine, exercises, herbs, and other non-medicinal treatment.
377. **Nausea:** Unpleasant sensation of being about to vomit.
378. **Nebulizer:** Device for administering medications used to treat asthma and similar conditions. It converts medication into a fine mist that is inhaled deeply into the lungs.
379. **Needle Biopsy:** A simplified form of removing tissue for microscopic examination using a needle inserted into the tissue to be studied. Tissue is removed by suction.
380. **Nerve-Conduction Test:** Diagnostic test that measures the rate at which an electrical impulse moves along a nerve. It is used to diagnose disorders of the peripheral nerves and muscle.
381. **Neuritis:** Inflammation of a nerve.
382. **Neuroblastoma:** A solid cancerous tumor of a nerve tissue that may spread to chest, abdomen, or pelvis. Treatment combines surgery, radiation, and chemotherapy. Before age 1, 90% can be cured if treated vigorously.
383. **Neuroma:** Tumor arising from nerve tissue.
384. **Neuromuscular System:** Nerves and muscles acting together as a system to control body movements.
385. **Neurosis:** Mental illness in which anxiety is controlled by avoidance, blaming others, developing bodily complaints, or other mechanisms.
386. **Neurosurgeon:** Doctor specially trained to diagnose and treat surgically diseases of the brain, spinal cord, and nerves.

387. **Nonsteroidal anti-inflammatory drugs (NSAIDs)**: Medications that control inflammation other than that caused by infection. Usually used to treat conditions of the joints and muscles and pain such as menstrual cramps or headache. 'nonsteroidal' means they are not steroid hormones such as cortisone, prednisone, dextramethasone, and others.
388. **Nurse practitioner (NP):** Registered nurse with additional medical training who can diagnose and treat common illness. Nurse practitioners usually work closely with a doctor, although in some states the practitioner can prescribe medicine and work independently of a physician.

O

389. **Orthodontics:** Orthodontics is the dental specialty that focuses on the development, prevention, and correction of irregularities of the teeth, bite, and jaws.
390. **Otitis externa:** Inflammation of the outer part of the ear extending to the auditory canal.
391. **Otitis media:** Inflammation of the middle ear caused by infection.
392. **Otoscope:** A lighted instrument that allows the physician to see inside the ear.
393. **Outer ear:** External portion of the ear, consisting of the pinna, or auricle, and the ear canal.
394. **Overuse conditions:** Injuries due to minor trauma involving soft tissue injuries—injuries that affect the bone, muscles, ligaments, and/or tendons.
395. **Obsessions:** Unpleasant, frightening, senseless thoughts that won't go away despite reasoning.
396. **Obstetrician-gynecologist:** Doctor specially trained to treat diseases of the female reproductive system and provide health care for pregnant mothers.
397. **Obstructive pulmonary disease:** See COPD (chronic obstructive pulmonary disease).
398. **Occlusion:** Closing or obstruction. Usually used to describe blockage in blood vessels. In dentistry, it means the way the teeth come together when the mouth is closed.
399. **Oncologist:** Doctor specially trained to diagnose and treat cancer.
400. **Operative Death Rate:** Percentage of patients who die as a result of a certain surgery. It provides a general measure of the risk of a particular surgery.
401. **Ophthalmologist:** Doctor specially trained to diagnose and treat diseases of the eyes.
402. **Optic Neuritis:** Inflammation of the nerve that conducts vision impulses from the eye to the brain.
403. **Organic psychosis:** Mental illness that results from disease in the brain.
404. **Orthodontia:** Straightening teeth by applying temporary braces.
405. **Osteogenesis imperfecta:** Inherited condition in which the bones are brittle and easily broken.
406. **Otorhinolaryngologist or otolaryngologist:** See ear, nose and throat specialist.
407. **Ovary:** Female sexual gland where eggs mature and ripen for fertilization.
408. **Ovulation:** Monthly process in which an egg leaves the ovary for possible fertilization by a sperm cell.
409. **Ovum:** Egg produced by the ovary.

P

410. **Peak flow monitoring:** A measure of lung function.
411. **Pediatrics:** The branch of medicine that deals with diagnosis, treatment, and prevention of diseases in children.
412. **Personal flotation device (PFD):** Any type of item that keeps a person afloat in water. Only as coast guard-approved PFDs should be used on boats.
413. **Pertussis (also called whooping cough):** Mainly affects infants and young children; caused by a bacterium, it is characterized by paroxysms of coughing that end with the characteristic whoop as air is inhaled. Pertussis caused thousands of deaths in the 1930s and 1940s, but with the advent of a vaccine, the rate of death has declined dramatically.

414. **Pneumatic otoscope:** An instrument that blows a puff of air into the ear to test eardrum movement.
415. **Poliomyelitis:** A highly contagious infectious disease caused by various types of poliovirus. Spread though feces and airborne particles, the poliovirus usually causes no more than a mild illness. However, some of the more serious manifestations of the disease include meningitis, which can lead to extensive paralysis.
416. **Puberty:** A sequence of events by which a child becomes a young adult; characterized by secretions of hormones, development of secondary sexual characteristics, reproductive functions, and growth spurts.
417. **Pyelonephritis:** An infection of the kidney.
418. **Pain:** Unpleasant sensation arising from stimulation of sensory nerves located in almost every part of the body. Disease, injury, and strenuous activity can all cause pain.
419. **Paranoia:** Mental illness in which a person believes that he or she is being talked about or plotted against.
420. **Passive exercises:** Exercises in which a therapist moves the arms and legs of a patient while the patient relaxes. These exercises keep the joints limber until the patient is able to move without assistance.
421. **Patency:** Blood vessels or any hollow organs that clog or become blocked are said to lose their patency.
422. **Pediculicide:** Medication that cures body lice (pediculosis). Usually applied to the skin.
423. **Perfusionist:** Medical technician who controls the heart-lung machine to sustain a patient's life during open-heart and lung-transplant surgery.
424. **Peripheral neuropathy** (Also called peripheral neuritis): A group of symptoms caused by abnormalities in motor or sensory nerves. Characteristics include: Tingling, numbness, pain, usually beginning in the feet and spreading to hands and other parts of the body.
425. **Peritoneum:** Very thin, two-layered tissue. One layer lines the outer surface of all the abdominal organs. The other layer lines the abdominal wall.
426. **Peritonsillar abscess:** Abscess forming in the back of the throat near the tonsils.
427. **Pessary:** Small ring-shaped device that is inserted into the vagina to help maintain the uterus in a normal position.
428. **pH balance:** Measure of blood's acidity or alkalinity. The pH is controlled by body fluids and electrolytes. Body tissues cannot function normally if the pH varies from a limited range.
429. **Phenothiazine drugs:** Medications used to slow and regulate mental-system activity. Usually used to treat anxiety and other mental conditions; also useful in producing sleep.
430. **Phlebotomy:** Removing blood from the blood vessels. This was once believed to cure many diseases; today, it is done to remove blood for diagnostic testing.
431. **Physical therapy:** Treatment of diseases of the bone, muscular and nervous systems to help restore normal function after disease or injury.
432. **Pilocarpine:** Medication used principally in eye drops to treat glaucoma.
433. **Pituitary gland:** Small endocrine gland at the base of the brain that controls growth and regulates other endocrine glands.
434. **Plastic and reconstructive surgery:** Special surgery to repair and change body parts to improve function or appearance. The face, hands, breasts, and skin are areas most frequently treated.
435. **Pleura:** Thin tissue lining the lungs and chest cavity. Inflammation of the pleura (pleurisy) is a painful condition caused by lung diseases.
436. **Pleural effusion (pleural fluid effusion):** Fluid that collects around the lungs, usually caused by inflammation of the lungs and pleura or congestive heart failure.
437. **Polyp:** A growth, often on a stalk arising from dry mucous membranes, such as in the nose, cervix, or colon.

438. **Portal-vein system:** Veins that drain blood from the gastrointestinal system. The smaller veins empty into the portal vein, which transports blood into the liver.
439. **Postural drainage:** Exercises and body positions that promote drainage of fluid and secretions that collect in the lungs and airways.
440. **Presbyopia:** Form of nearsightedness that normally accompanies aging.
441. **Prophylaxis:** Measures taken to prevent an illness.
442. **Prophylaxis, dental:** Regular care (including cleaning) of the teeth and gums that helps prevent tooth decay and gum inflammation.
443. **Prostaglandins:** Natural substances found in semen, menstrual fluid, and many body tissues. They are involved in basic body functions such as inflammation, immune response, and activities of the lungs, heart, kidneys, uterus, and digestive system.
444. **Psychiatrist:** Doctor specially trained to diagnose and treat mental illness.
445. **Psychoanalysis:** Treatment of some mental illness that involves a detailed understanding of how past events in a person's life may have resulted in mental disturbances.
446. **Psychologist:** Health care professional specially trained to diagnose and treat some kinds of mental illness.
447. **Psychopathy:** Psychological or mental illness.
448. **Psychosomatic illness:** Illness in which thoughts and emotions play an important role.
449. **Psychotherapist:** Professional specially trained to diagnose and treat some mental illnesses.
450. **Puberty:** Period in early adolescence when hormonal changes bring about full sexual maturity and capacity to reproduce.
451. **Pulse:** Heartbeat (contraction of the heart) as felt in an artery. Heart rate is often measured by counting the pulse felt in the artery in the wrist.
452. **Pus:** Thick fluid, usually green or yellow, that forms to fight local infection. Pus often collects in an enclosed sac, an abscess, at the site of an infection.
453. **Pyelogram, retrograde:** Method of studying the kidneys, similar to an intravenous pyelogram, but in which the medication detected by X-rays is placed in the urinary system by a catheter inserted through the bladder into the ureters.

R

454. **Reye syndrome:** A potentially fatal disease that causes severe problems with the brain and other organs. Although the exact cause of the disease is not known, there has been an association with giving aspirin to children and developing the disease. It is now advised not to give aspirin to children during illnesses, unless prescribed by your child's physician.
455. **Rhinitis:** An inflammation of the mucous membrane that lines the nose; often due to allergy to pollen, dust, or other airborne substances; causes sneezing, itching, a runny nose, and nasal congestion.
456. **Rubella (also called German measles):** An acute viral infection that causes a mild illness in children and a slightly more severe illness in adults. The disease is spread person-to-person through airborne particles and takes two to three weeks to incubate.
457. **Radiation therapy or treatment:** Use of high-energy waves (generated by special X-rays machines, cobalt machines, and other devices) to treat some forms of cancer. Radiation destroys cancerous tissue but does little harm to healthy tissue.
458. **Radioisotope:** Radioactive form of chemicals normally present in the body.
459. **Radioisotope scan:** Scan of radioisotopes given orally or intravenously to a patient that become concentrated in organs such as the heart, lungs, or brain. Instruments measure the radiation given off by the radioisotopes and create a photographic image of the organ being studied.

460. **Radioisotope studies:** Radioisotopes are chemical elements that give off radiation. A radioisotope of a chemical element normally present in the body (such as carbon), if injected into the body, will mix with the non-isotopes. The body doesn't know the difference, but radiation from the isotopes can be detected with special instruments. Determining where radioisotopes go in the body allows diagnosis of diseases that cannot be detected otherwise.

461. **Radioisotope therapy:** Treatment of some cancers with radioisotopes.

462. **Radiologist:** Doctor specially trained to use X-rays and other kinds of radiation in diagnosis and treatment.

463. **Reynaud's phenomenon:** A circulatory system disorder affecting fingers and toes that is a complication of an underlying disease or emotional disturbance. Characteristics include fingers that turn pale when exposed to cold or stress. Paleness is followed by a bluish tinge and then redness.

464. **Regurgitate:** To vomit.

465. **Relapse:** Stage of illness in which the patient gets worse after having improved.

466. **Remission:** Stage of a chronic illness when the patient's condition improves.

467. **Respiratory-distress syndrome (RDS, hyaline membrane disease):** Breathing difficulty in a newborn infant. Causes: prematurity, underdeveloped lungs, deficiency of moistening and lubricating fluid in lungs and bronchial tubes. Symptoms: Trouble with breathing (rapid, shallow breathing, chest retractions, grunting, flared nostrils, bluish tint to skin).

468. **Retrolental fibroplasias:** A problem of the retina of the eyes of premature infants who required excessive amounts of oxygen to sustain life during intensive care following premature birth. If severe, retrolental fibroplasias can lead to severe visual problems or blindness.

469. **Retrovirus:** Group of viruses that cause aids (acquired immunodeficiency syndrome) and some types of lymphoma and leukemia.

470. **RH and ABO incompatibility:** When a pregnant woman during her second pregnancy has Rh negative blood and her unborn infant has Rh positive blood, incompatibility can result, causing erythroblastosis in the child at birth. Since the 1960s, preventive treatment has existed, early detection is possible, and severe erythroblastosis can be prevented. A related but much less common problem exists when a mother has type O blood and the fetus has type A or B blood. When this problem occurs, treatment requires exchange transfusion of the newborn. Rh incompatibility can be prevented by giving rhogam to an Rh negative mother within 72 hours of delivery of her first Rh positive baby.

471. **Rh negative blood:** A subtype of red blood cells. Blood subtypes are inherited. The major subtypes are types A, B, O and Rh negative.

472. **Rinne test:** Test using a tuning fork to diagnose hearing disorders.

473. **Rotator cuff:** The structure around the shoulder joint capsule composed of intermingled muscle and tendon fibers. The rotator cuff provides stability and strength to the shoulder joint.

S

474. **Sinusitis:** Inflammation of the membranes lining the facial sinuses; often caused by a bacterial or viral infection, or an allergic reaction.

475. **Stork bite or salmon patch:** Small pink or red patches often found on a baby's eyelids, between the eyes, upper lip, and back of the neck.

476. **Strawberry hemangioma:** A bright or dark red, raised or swollen, bumpy area on the skin of a baby or child.

477. **Sudden infant death syndrome (SIDS):** Unexplained, sudden death of an infant up to 1 year of age.

478. **Sunburn:** A visible reaction of the skin to overexposure to the sun's invisible ultraviolet (UV) rays.

479. **Sunscreen:** A product that protects the skin against sunburns by blocking the penetration of the sun's ultraviolet (UV) rays.
480. **Syrup of ipecac:** An emetic made from the dried root of a plant called ipecacuanha, which is grown in Brazil. An emetic is an agent that causes vomiting.
481. **Sacroiliac region:** Area of the lower back where the spine meets the pelvic bone.
482. **Saline:** Salt-containing solution similar to normal body fluid that is given intravenously to help correct fluid and electrolyte imbalances.
483. **Salivary glands:** Glands located inside the mouth around the jaw that secrete saliva into the mouth.
484. **Saphenous-femoral vein system:** Network of large veins in the legs that helps return blood from the leg to the inferior vena cava, then to the heart.
485. **Sarcoidosis:** A chronic, progressive disease involving the lungs, lymph nodes, and other tissues. There is no known treatment.
486. **Scale, scaling:** Flakes of dried skin which form as whitish skin lesions.
487. **Schizophrenia:** Mental illness characterized by a distorted sense of reality, bizarre behavior, and fragmentation of the personality.
488. **Sciatic nerve:** Large nerve that begins at the base of the spine and passes through the buttocks down the back side of the thigh and down the leg.
489. **Sciatica:** Painful condition resulting from irritation of the sciatic nerve.
490. **Scleritis:** Inflammation of the sclera (the white of the eye).
491. **Scoliosis:** Curvature of the spine.
492. **Scopolamine:** Medication used to treat hyperactive or spastic conditions of the digestive system and to prevent motion sickness.
493. **Scrotum:** Organ of the male reproductive system that contains the testicles, blood vessels, and the vas deferens.
494. **Scurvy:** Disease of bones, gums, and blood vessels caused by a deficiency of vitamin C.
495. **Second molars:** Permanent grinding teeth that appear at about age 11 to 13.
496. **Secondary infection:** Infection that results from some other problem. It may occur after surgery or develop during antibiotic treatment of another infection.
497. **Sedative:** Medication used to produce relaxation or sleep.
498. **Sensitivity studies (antibiotics):** Laboratory method of determining which antibiotic will most likely be successful in treating infections caused by bacteria.
499. **Sensory:** Ability to feel or experience sensations such as sound, light, or pain.
500. **Septic:** Infected.
501. **Serological tests**: Tests of serum (blood without cells) used to diagnose a variety of diseases, especially infections and autoimmune conditions.
502. **Serum:** Liquid portion of blood that remains after blood cells and blood clots have been removed.
503. **Serum alkaline phosphatase:** Material present in excessive amounts in the blood of patients with some bone and liver diseases.
504. **Serum electrolytes**: Same as electrolytes.
505. **Shave biopsy:** Procedure to diagnose skin disorders in which a thin layer of tissue from under a skin lesion is shaved away for laboratory examination.
506. **Shock:** Condition in which the blood pressure falls below the level needed to supply blood to the body. Signs and symptoms include weakness, paleness, rapid heartbeat, dry mouth, cold sweat, and feelings of doom.
507. **Sims-Huhner test:** Test used in diagnosis of reasons for infertility in women in which the mucus from the cervix is examined, especially for the presence of sperm after sexual intercourse.

508. Skin clips: Small u-shaped metal strips used instead of stitches to close skin that has been incised during surgery.

509. Spasmodic: Sudden intermittent symptom, or intermittent muscle spasm.

510. Spastic, spasticity: A description of muscles that are continuously contracting and in a state of excessive tension.

511. Speculum: Instrument used to examine the interior of openings such as the vagina, nose, ear, or rectum.

512. Sperm: Male reproductive cells manufactured in testicles and ejaculated in semen.

513. Spherocytosis: Abnormally shaped red blood cells caused by some anemias. These cells are sphere-shaped, in contrast to the doughnut shape of normal red blood cells.

514. Spikes, temperature: High but brief episodes of fever.

515. Spina bifida: Congenital (inherited) disorder in which the base of the spine remains open, sometimes exposing the spinal cord and nerves.

516. Spinal anesthesia: Method to provide anesthesia to the lower body by injecting an anesthetic into the fluid in the space that surrounds the lower spinal cord.

517. Spirometry: Test of lung (pulmonary) function.

518. Sputum: Secretion of the lungs, coughed up in large amounts in some lung diseases.

519. *Staphylococcus:* Bacteria that frequently cause boils, abscesses, pneumonias, bone infections, and infections in other tissues or organs.

520. *Streptococcus:* Bacteria that cause illnesses such as laryngitis, cellulitis of the skin, pneumonia, meningitis, and others. If not treated, streptococcal infections may also cause serious heart and kidney diseases as complications that appear after the original infection has cleared.

521. Symmetry, symmetrical: Refers to the arrangement of the body in pairs, such as two arms, legs, kidneys, lungs, etc.

522. Sympathomimetics: Medications similar to adrenalin in their actions.

523. Symptoms: Effects of disease that only the patient can experience, such as pain, nausea, dizziness, anxiety, depression and others.

T

524. Tetanus: An acute, sometimes fatal, disease of the central nervous system; caused by the toxin of the tetanus bacterium, which usually enters the body through an open wound. The tetanus bacterium live in soil and manure, but also can be found in the human intestine and other places.

525. Thermal burns: Burns due to external heat sources which raise the temperature of the skin and tissues and cause tissue cell death or charring. Hot metals, scalding liquids, steam, and flames, when coming in contact with the skin, cause thermal burns.

526. Tourette's syndrome: An abnormal condition characterized by tics and other movements such as eye blinks or facial twitches that cannot be controlled.

527. Tuberculosis (TB): An infectious disease that was once a major killer worldwide. The predominant TB organism is mycobacterium tuberculosis (m. Tuberculosis). Spread person-to-person in airborne droplets caused by sneezing or coughing, the bacteria usually infects the lungs. However, due to improved nutrition, housing, sanitation, medical care, and the introduction of antibiotics this century, reported TB cases in the US have declined dramatically.

528. Tympanometry: A test that allows for air and sound to be directed into the middle ear.

529. Tampons: Absorbent material to insert into the vagina during menstruation. They may be used alone, or with pads. They are safe to use as soon as menstruation begins. They should be changed about very 4 hours or more frequently. Use the smallest size possible and wear pads instead at night. Continue to take daily baths and showers. Don't use feminine sprays or douches. If the odor is really bad or a heavy discharge develops, consult your physician.

530. **Tenderness:** Condition that causes pain when pressure is applied.
531. **Thiazide diuretics:** Class of medications that promote excretion of excess fluids by the kidneys.
532. **Third molars:** Permanent grinding teeth that appear at about age 17 to 25.
533. **Thoracic duct:** The largest channel of the lymphatic system through which lymph fluid enters the vena cava.
534. **Ticks:** Small biting insects that may cause inflammation of the skin or serious infections such as rocky mountain spotted fever.
535. **Tics:** Brief, uncontrollable muscle spasms.
536. **Tissue:** Building blocks of body organs; living cells all of one type.
537. **Titer:** The quantity of a substance required to produce a reaction with a given volume of another substance.
538. **Tonsils:** Lymphatic tissues that help fight infection located at the entrance of the throat. They frequently become infected, especially in children.
539. **Topical:** Medications applied to the skin, conjunctiva, or mucous membrane of the mouth, nose, vagina, or rectum.
540. **Transplant:** Living organ (such as kidney, cornea, heart, bone marrow, or skin), removed from one person (donor), and placed in the body of another (recipient).
541. **Tricyclic antidepressant drugs (tricyclics):** Class of medications used to treat depression.
542. **Trophoblastic tumors:** See hydatidiform mole.
543. **Tube feeding:** Providing nutrients through a small tube placed in the stomach of a patient who is unable to eat. The tube may pass through the nose to the stomach or be inserted through an incision in the stomach.
544. **Tuberous sclerosis:** Rare inherited condition of the skin, nervous system, and other organs of the body.
545. **Tumor:** Literally, a swelling; usually used to refer to a benign or cancerous growth.
546. **Turner's syndrome:** A disorder in girls characterized by an abnormal chromosome pattern. They lack one of the two sex hormones. Signs and symptoms: low birth weight, skin and bone abnormalities, 'webbed' neck, swollen hands and feet, broad chest, a low hairline at the nape of the neck, congenital heart disease (frequently), absence of breast development and menstruation, or short stature. Treatment: female hormones beginning at age 13 to 15 years. Treatment is usually quite successful.

U

547. **Umbilical hernia:** A weakness in the abdominal muscles.
548. **Urethritis:** An infection limited to the urethra.
549. **Urticaria (also called hives):** A condition in which red, itchy, and swollen areas appear on the skin usually as an allergic reaction from eating certain foods or taking certain medications.
550. **Ulceration:** Wearing away of the surface or lining of an organ, exposing underlying tissue. Ulceration of the lining of the stomach exposes blood vessels, which may bleed. Ulceration may erode through the wall of an organ (perforation). Ulceration frequently affects the skin, if rubbed excessively or if diseased.
551. **Ultrasonography:** See sonography.
552. **Ultrasound treatment:** Method of treatment in which high-energy sound waves are focused on the affected area, producing mild heat that helps relieve inflammation. It is especially useful in treatment of muscular symptoms.

553. **Underlying:** Beneath, below, or more basic. Thus, losing weight may result from an underlying condition such as diabetes mellitus or cancer.
554. **Upper gastrointestinal series:** X-ray examination of the esophagus, stomach, and duodenum accomplished by having the patient swallow a barium solution that X-rays can detect.
555. **Upper respiratory system:** Upper part of the breathing system, consisting of the nose, throat, larynx, trachea, and bronchial tubes.
556. **Uremia:** A serious condition associated with kidney failure in which body wastes build up in the blood and body tissues.
557. **Uric acid:** Chemical normally produced in the body from metabolism or breakdown of protein and eliminated in the urine. If the level of uric acid rises in the body as a result of disease, gout or kidney stones may result.
558. **Urinalysis:** Laboratory test performed on a urine sample that helps diagnose diseases of the kidney and other parts of the body.
559. **Urinary studies:** Laboratory or X-ray tests of the urinary tract.
560. **Urinary tract:** Organs that produce, store, and eliminate urine. The organs are the kidneys, ureters, urinary bladder, and urethra.
561. **Uterus:** Organ of the female reproductive system on the wall of which the fertilized egg (ovum) attaches and develops to form a fetus.
562. **Uveitis:** Inflammation of the parts of the eyes that make up the iris (colored tissue encircling the clear center: The pupil).
563. **Uvula:** Soft tissue hanging down from the soft palate at the back of the throat.

V

564. **Vomiting:** The release of stomach contents through the mouth; also known as throwing-up.
565. **Vaccination:** Method of providing protection against disease (immunity) by giving a patient a small amount of the disease-causing germ that is weakened, killed, or otherwise modified so that it cannot itself cause disease. Same as immunization.
566. **Vaccine:** Medication used to provide immunity by vaccination. Vaccines are given mostly by injection or by mouth.
567. **Varicose:** Swollen and twisting, usually used to describe varicose veins.
568. **Vas deferens:** Tube that carries sperm manufactured by the testicles toward the prostate gland and seminal vesicles.
569. **Vasculitis:** Inflammation of blood vessels, the basis of any illnesses.
570. **Vasoconstrictor drugs:** Medications that cause blood vessels to contract, tighten, or become smaller.
571. **Vasodilator drugs:** Medications that cause small arteries to widen, providing more blood to an area of the body where the blood vessels are constricted by spasm, narrowed or obstructed.
572. **Vector:** 1) an imaginary line that represents both direction and quantity used to study electrocardiograms (EKGS). 2) an agent that transmits infectious germs from one organism to another.
573. **Virulent:** Extremely dangerous or harmful. Virulent bacteria are ones capable of causing diseases.
574. **Vitamins:** Chemical substances found in food that are necessary for healthy body growth, function, and tissue repair.
575. **Vitreous:** Clear fluid that fills much of the eye.
576. **Voiding cystourethrography:** An X-ray study made of the bladder and urethra after injection of a dye through a catheter inserted through the urethra into the bladder.

W

577. **Warts:** Small, often hard and rough skin growths caused by viruses that infect the skin.
578. **Wasting of body or muscles:** Severe loss of body tissues (other than surplus fat), especially muscles and vital organs, resulting in weakness, susceptibility to infection, bone fractures, and sometimes death.
579. **Weber test:** Hearing test performed with a tuning fork.
580. **Wheezes:** High-pitched sounds and whistles produced in the lungs where secretions have partially blocked air passages.
581. **Whirlpool treatment:** Method of treating minor blood-vessel and musculo-skeletal diseases by immersion in a pool where jets of warm water enter and swirl under high pressure.
582. **Wisdom teeth:** Same as third molars.
583. **Wryneck (torticollis):** A painful condition that causes a child to tip or tilt to one side. It may be present at birth (perhaps caused by injury at birth), or later in life may be caused by muscle inflammation caused by an accident, tumor, or disease. Treatment: Congenital form: A series of muscle-stretching exercises. The worst cases require surgery. Other forms: Treatment of the underlying condition.

X

584. **X-ray:** A diagnostic test which uses invisible electromagnetic energy beams to produce images of internal tissues, bones, and organs onto film.
585. **Xeroradiogram:** Method of X-ray diagnosis, usually of the female breast, which uses a process similar to that used to produce photocopies.
586. **X-rays:** High energy, invisible waves capable of penetrating the body and creating shadows on photographic film. The shadows provide images of the body tissues through which the X-rays pass.

Z

587. **Zoster:** 'Girdle,' used to describe a form of virus infection (herpes zoster, shingles) that often produces bands of inflammation across the chest or abdomen.

Annexure 2

COMMON DRUGS USED IN PEDIATRIC UNITS

Concentrations of Drugs Used in NICU

Drugs	Concentration used in NICU
Aminophylline	5 mg/ml
Caffeine base	10 mg/ml (caffeine citrate 20 mg/ml)
Dobutamine	0.05 to 3.5 mg/ml
Dopamine	0.05 to 3.5 mg/ml
Fentanyl	1.05 to 15.0 mg/ml
Heparin	0.05 to 2.0 units/ml
Indomethacin	0.05 to 1.0 mg/ml
Morphine	0.01 to 2.0 mg/ml
Prostaglandin (PGEI)	3.0 to 6.0 mg/ml
Sodium bicarbonate	6.5 mm^2/ml
Parenteral nutrition	-
Intralipid	20%

Drug Continually Used in Neonatology

Drug	Dose	Route	Frequency
Amikacin	15 mg/kg/day	IV	6 hourly
Caffeine	2 mg/kg/day	Orally	Daily
Calcium of gluconate	5 ml	IV very slow	Stat
Calcium Sandoz	1 ml	Orally	6 hourly
Cefotaxime	100 mg/kg/day	IV	6 hourly
Ceftriaxone	50 mg/kg/day	IM	Daily
Cloxacillin	100 mg/kg/day	IV	6 hourly
Dexamethasone	2 mg/kg/day	IV	6 hourly

Contd...

Contd...

Drug	Dose	Route	Frequency
Diazepam (Valium)	1 mg	Rectally Er slow ZY	Stat
Erythromycin	40 mg/kg/day	Orally or ZY	6 hourly
Ferrous Lactate (Ferro drops)	0.3 ml (term)	Orally	Daily
Folate	1 mg	Orally	Daily
Furosemide (Lasix)	1 mg/kg	Orally or IV	Stat
Gentamicin	7.5 mg/kg/day	IV	6 hourly
Indomethacin (Indocid)	0.2 mg/kg/day	IV	8 hourly × 3
Isoniazid (INH)	10 mg/kg/day	Orally	Daily
Kanamycin	15 mg/kg/day	IV	6 hourly
Lanoxin	0.01 mg/kg/day	Orally	12 hourly
Liprocil	1 ml	Orally	6 hourly
Magnesium sulfate	0.05 ml	1 M 1 sat	
Multivitamin doses	0.3 ml (term) orally	Orally	Daily
Multivitamin droops	0.6 ml (Preterm)	Orally	Daily
Naloxone (Narcan)	0.1 mg/kg (0.25 ml/kg)	IV, IM or VIO ETT	Stat
Paraldehyde	0.3 ml/kg	IMI	Stat
Penicillin – G	50,000 u/kg/day	IV	6 hourly
Penicillin Procaine	50,000 u/kg/day	Orally	12 hourly
Phenobarbitone	5 mg/kg/day	Orally	12 hourly
Phenytoin	5 mg/kg/day	Orally	12 hourly
Prostaglandins E2 (prostin)	¼ tablet	Orally	Hourly
Theophylline	4–8 mg/kg/day	Orally	6 hourly
Tobramycin	10 mg/kg/day	IV	6 hourly

Sl. No.	Drugs	Dose	Route and frequency	Action	Side effects	Nurses responsibility
1	Inj Amikacin	Inj 250 mg Inj 500 mg	Q 12 hrs Q 2 hrs	(Antibacterial) Amikacin is active against a wide range of gram-negative and gram-positive organisms including strains resistant to other antimicrobials. Amikacin exerts third generation cephalosporins	• Bone marrow suppression • Vestibular auditory toxicity	• Watch for vital signs • Check for the renal function test
2	Inj Amino-phylline	Inj 25 mg T 100 mg	IV 1 POq – 6–8 hours	(Antiasthmatics/bronchodilators) Theophylline directly relaxes bronchial smooth muscle and also pulmonary blood vessels. It increases in intracellular cyclic AMP through inhibition of phosphodiesterase	• G1 upset, arrhythmias, seizures, tachycardia	• Watch for heart rate and blood glucose level
3	Inj Albumin	10%	Q 12 hrs	(Plasma expanders) It is highly soluble. Ellipsoidal protein, accounting for 70–80% of the colloid osmotic pressure of plasma. It regulates volume of circulating blood. It is also a transport protein in circulation for naturally occurring therapeutic and toxic materials.	• Chills, fever, pulmonary edema	• Watch for the BP • Vital sign also
4	Inj Cipro-floxacin	IV 500 mg	Q 12 hr	(Antibacterial) Anti-infective. It is bactericidal against enteropathogens like Shigella, salmonella. It is active against both bacteria and protozoa.	• Constipation • Diarrhea • Joint pain	• Check the anthropometry assessment
5	Inj Dexame-thasone	4 mg	Q 6 hrs	(Corticosteroid) Glucocorticoids. Action is primarily anti-inflammatory with very little sodium retaining property. Wide spread metabolic effects and modification of immune responses can occur. Prolonged use of corticosteroids can cause suppression of the pituitary adrenal axis which may result in secondary adrenocortical insufficiency.	• Hypokalemia	• Watch for the BP
6	Tab Diazepam	Tab 5 mg Syp 2 ml	Q 15–30 min	(Anxiolytic). It has the typical activity spectrum of benzodiazepines encompassing muscular relaxation. Sleep modifying and anticonvulsant effects. Has no peripheral autonomics blocking action.	• Hyperbiliru-binemia	• Watch for respiration

Contd...

Contd...

Sl. No.	Drugs	Dose	Route and frequency	Action	Side effects	Nurses responsibility
7	Tab Digoxin	T 0.25 mg	Q 8–24 hrs in 2 doses	(Vasodilators and antiarrhythmics) Cardiac glycoside. It increases the course of myocardial contraction and slows the Heart Rate. It will increase the cardiac output.	• Bradycardia • Vomiting • Poor feeding • Hypokalemia	Check for S potassium levels
8	Inj Dobutamine	250 mg	IV	(Inotropic agents) Drugs used in CHF. It is a direct acting Inotropic agent whose primary action results from stimulation of the beta-1 receptors of the heart while producing relatively mild chronoscopic effects. It increases the stroke volume and cardiac output.		• Check for the vital signs
9	Inj Dopamine	250 mg	IV	(Inotropic agents) Antishock drug. Increase heart rate and force of contraction. At higher rates vasoconstriction in skeletal muscles and a rise in BP.	• Pulmonary hypertension antidote regitine	• Check for the BP and pulse pressure
10	Tab Enalapril	2.5 mg/5 g	Oral	(Antihypertensive) Inotropic agents.	• Hypotension • Oliguria • Hyperkalemia	• Monitor the electrolytes and heart rate and blood pressure of the child
11	Syp Erythromycin	125 g/5 ml	Q 8 hrs or Q 6 hrs as advised the doctor	(Antimicrobial). Primarily bacteriostatic against a wide range of organisms. It is used as an alternative to penciling in patients allergic to the latter group.	• Cholestasis jaundice	• Check the CBC and LFT test
12	Tab Funcornazone	50 mg	Per oral Q 72 hrs Q 48 hrs	(Antifungal). Found effective infections especially in candidiasis and cryptococcosis associated with immunosuppression as in AIDS or cancer therapy.	• Vomiting, diarrhea • Skin disorder	• Watch for the renal function and LFT

Contd...

Contd...

Sl. No.	Drugs	Dose	Route and frequency	Action	Side effects	Nurses responsibility
13	Inj Gentamicin	10 mg 20 mg	Q 12 hrs	(Antibacterial). Active against a wide range of aerobic gram-negative and some gram-positive organisms including E-coli.	• Vestibular and auditory toxicity associated with high peak levels	• Watch for the S peak levels 30 min after IV in fusion
14	Inj Heparin	0.5–10 ml of IV	IV	(Anticoagulant). It increases the incisory action of antithrombin III on factors XIIa, IXa, Xa and thrombin the major result being inhibition of the conversion of prothrombin to thrombin. It inhibits platelet function.	• Fever vomiting • Thrombocy-topenia	• PTT – 1.5–2.5 times • CT 20–30 min platelet count every time check
15	Tab Lorazepam Inj Lorazepam	T 2 mg In 2 mg/ml	Oral IM	(Sedatives). It has no appreciable effect on respiratory or cardiovascular systems. It results of facilitative effect on GABA activity.	• CNS depression • Bradycardia • Circulatory collapse • Constipation • Respiratory depression • Hypermagnesia	• Check the BP, CA, Mg, knee joint reflects
16	Inj Metronidazole Tab Metronidazole	In 500 mg T 200, 400 mg	Q 12 hrs once	(Antibacterial). Effective against wide range of organisms including Giardia. Active against gardnerella and campylobacter.	• Diarrhea • Leukemia • Thrombocy-topenia	• Check the vital signs and conscious level
17	Inj Midazolam	0.3 mg/kg dose	Intravenous Infusion IM	(Muscle relaxant) It is a short acting benzodiazepine with rapid onset of action, recovery and non painful induction and lack of venous irritation. It is a sedative and muscle relaxant.	• Respiratory distress • Apnea • Cardiac arrest • Bradycardia • Seizures reported 4–11 days after therapy	• Watch for the respiratory rate and blood pressure

Contd...

Contd...

Sl. No.	Drugs	Dose	Route and frequency	Action	Side effects	Nurses responsibility
18	Tab. Penicillin Syp. Penicillin	T 125 mg T 250 g Syp 25 mg/5 ml	Oral Oral	(Antibacterial). It constitutes one of the most important groups of antibiotics. These are bactericidal and act by interfering with the synthesis of bacterial peptidoglycans cell wall.	• Bone marrow suppression • Hemolytic anemia • Nephritis	• Watch for the blood pressure
19	Inj Phenytoin Tab Phenytoin	15–20 mg 50 mg 100 mg	IV 1 mg, 1 mg, 1 min divided in 10 mg/kg Oral	(Anticonvulsant). Acting on the motor cortex, phenytoin prevents spread of seizure activity. Reduces brain stem activity responsible for the tonic phase of convulsion.	• Hypotension • Hyperglycemia • Dermatitis • Cardiovascular collapse	• Check BUN and creatinine
20	Inj Potassium chloride	0.5 – 1 mg/1 kg	T 8 mg Syp 1.5 mg/1.5 ml Oral and IV	(Diuretic) and corticosteroid therapy	• Bradycardia • Hypotension • Peaked T waves in ECG	• Take the ECG
21	Inj Ranitidine Tab Ranitidine	2–4 mg T 150 mg	Q 8 – 12 hrs Oral or IM or IV	(H_2 Antagonist). It is stimulated gastric acid secretion through competitive blockage of H_2 receptors.	• Vomiting • Diarrhea • Pruritus • Stomatitis	• Give more fluid and educate the patient avoid chilly foods
22	Inj Taxim Tab Taximo	250 mg/1500 ml 100 mg	Oral	(Antibacterial). Highly activity against gram-negative bacteria and a variety of beta-lactamase producing organisms.	• Tachycardia • Arrhythmias • Hypertension	• Watch for the ECG monitor and check the blood pressure
23	Tab vitamin C and B_{12}	Premature 40 mg Full-term 60 mg	Per oral	(Antiasthmatics). A beta-adrenoceptor against with a selective action on beta receptors. It will reduce airways and pulmonary resistance, main effect is bronchodilator.	• Vomiting, diarrhea	• Give more fluids

Annexure 3

COMMON LABORATORY NORMAL VALUE

Common Laboratory Test

Common Laboratory Tests and Test Results

Test/Specimen	Age/gender/reference	Normal ranges			
		Conventional units		International units (SI)	
Acetaminophen serum or plasma	Therap. Conc. Toxic Conc.	10–30 μg/mL > 200 μg/mL		66–200 μmol/L > 1300 μmol/L	
Ammonia Nitrogen Plasma or serum	Newborn 0–2 wk > 1 mo Thereafter	90–150 μg/dL 79–129 μg/dL 29–70 μg/dL 0–50 μg/dL		64–107 μmol/ 56–92 μmol/L 21–50 μmol/L 0–35.7 μmol/L	
Antistreptolysin O titer (ASO) serum	2–4 yr School-age children	< 160 Todd units 170–330 Todd units			
Base excess whole blood	Newborn Infant Child Thereafter	(–10)–(–2) mEq/L (–7)–(–1) mEq/L (–4)–(+2) mEq/L (–3)–(+3) mEq/L		(–10)–(–2) mmol/L (–7)–(–1) mmol/L (–4)–(+2) mmol/L (–3)–(+3) mmol/L	
Bicarbonate (HOC$_3^-$) Serum	Arterial Venous	21–28 mEq/L 22–29 mEq/L		21–28 mmol/L 22–29 mmol/L	
Bilirubin, total Serum		Premature (mg/dL)	Full term (mg/dL)	Premature (μmol/L)	Full term (μmol/L)
	Cord	< 2.0	< 2.0	< 34	< 34
	0–1 d	< 8.0	< 6.0	< 137	< 103
	1–2 d	< 12.0	< 8.0	< 205	< 137
	2–5 d	< 16.0	< 12.0	< 274	< 205
	Thereafter	< 20.0	< 10.0	< 340	< 171
Bilirubin, direct conjugated Serum Bleeding time Blood from skin puncture	 Normal	0.0–0.2 mg/dL 2–7 min		0–3.4 μmol/L 2–7 min	

Contd...

Contd...

Test/Specimen	Age/gender/ reference	Normal ranges	
		Conventional units	International units (SI)
Simplate (G–D)	Borderline	7–11 min 2.75–8 min	7–11 min 2.75–8 min
Blood volume Whole blood	Male Female	52–83 mL/kg 50–75 mL/kg	0.052–0.083 L/kg 0.050–0.075 L/kg
C–reactive protein serum	Cord 2–12 yr	52–1330 ng/mL 67–1800 ng/mL	52–1330 μg/L 67–1800 μg/L
Calcium, ionized serum, plasma, or whole blood	Cord Newborn, 3–24 hr 24–48 hr Thereafter	5.0–6.0 mg/dL 4.3–5.1 mg/dL 4.0–4.7 mg/dL 4.8–4.92 mg/dL or 2.24–2.46 mEq/L	1.25–1.50 mmol/L 1.07–1.27 mmol/L 1.00–1.17 mmol/L 1.12–1.23 mmol/L
Calcium, total serum	Cord Newborn, 3–24 yr 24–48 hr 4–7d Child Thereafter	9.0–11.5 mg/dL 9.0–10.6 mg/dL 7.0–12.0 mg/dL 9.0–10.9 mg/dL 8.8–10.8 mg/dL 8.4–10.2 mg/dL	2.25–2.88 mmol/L 2.3–2.65 mmol/L 1.75–3.0 mmol/L 2.25–2.73 mmol/L 2.2–2.70 mmol/L 2.1–2.55 mmol/L
Carbon dioxide, partial pressure (PCO_2) whole blood, arterial	Newborn Infant Male Female	27–40 mm Hg 27–41 mm Hg 35–48 mm Hg 32–45 mm Hg	3.6–5.3 kPa 3.6–5.5 kPa 4.7–6.4 kPa 4.3–6.0 kPa
Carbon dioxide, total (tCO_2) serum or plasma	Cord Premature (1 wk) Newborn Infant, child Thereafter	14–27 mEq/L 14–22 mEq/L 13–22 mEq/L 20–28 mEq/L 23–30 mEq/L	14–22 mmol/L 14–27 mmol/L 13–22 mmol/L 20–28 mmol/L 23–30 mmol/L
Cerebrospinal fluid (CSF) Pressure Volume	 Child Adult	70–180 mm water 60–100 mL 100–160 mL	70–180 mm water 0.06–0.10 L 0.10–0.16 L
Chloride Serum or plasma Sweat	Cord Newborn Thereafter Normal (homozygote)	96–104 mEq/L 97–110 mEq/L 98–106 mEq/L < 40 mEq/L	96–104 mmol/L 97–110 mmol/L 98–106 mmol/L < 40 mmol/L

Contd...

Contd...

Test/Specimen	Age/gender/ reference	Normal ranges	
		Conventional units	International units (SI)
	Marginal (e.g., asthma, Addison disease, malnutrition)	45–60 mEq/L	45–60 mmol/L
	Cystic fibrosis	> 60 mEq/L	> 60 mmol/L
Cholesterol, total serum or plasma*	Acceptable Borderline High	< 170 mg/dL 170–199 mg/dL ≥ 200 mg/dL	< 4.4 mmol/L 4.4–5.1 mmol/L ≥ 5.2 mmol/L
Clotting time (Lee–White) White blood		5–8 min (glass tubes) 5–15 min (room temp) 30 min (silicone tube)	5–8 min 5–15 min 30 min
Creatine kinase (CK, CPK) Serum	Cord blood 5–8 hr 24–33 hr 72–100 hr Adult	70–380 U/L 214–1175 U/L 130–1200 U/L 87–725 U/L 5–130 U/L	70–380 U/L 214–1175 U/L 130–1200 U/L 87–725 U/L 5–130 U/L
Creatinine serum	Cord Newborn Infant Child Adolescent Adult: Male Female	0.6–1.2 mg/dL 0.3–1.0 mg/dL 0.2–0.4 mg/dL 0.3–0.7 mg/dL 0.5–1.0 mg/dL 0.6–1.2 mg/dL 0.5–1.1 mg/dL	53–106 μmol/L 27–88 μmol/L 18–35 μmol/L 27–62 μmol/L 44–88 μmol/L 53–106 μmol/L 44–97 μmol/L
Urine, 24 hr	Premature Full term 1.5–7 yr 7–15 yr	8.1–15,0 mg/kg/24 hr 10.4–19.7 mg/kg/24 hr 10–15 mg/kg/24 hr 5.2–41 mg/kg/24 hr	72–133 μmol/kg/24 hr 92–174 μmol/kg/24 hr 88–133 μmol/kg/24 hr 46–362 μmol/kg/24 hr
Creatinine clearance (endogenous) Serum or plasma and urine	Newborn < 40 yr: Male Female	40–65 mL/min/1.73 m^2 97–137 mL/min/1.73 m^2 88–128 mL/min/1.73 m^2	
Digoxin serum, plasma; collect at least 12 hr after dose	Therap. cone. CHF Arrhythmias	 0.8–1.5 ng/mL 1.5–2.0 ng/mL	 1.0–1.9 nmol/L 1.9–2.6 nmol/L
Serum, plasma; collect at least 12 hr after dose	Toxic conc. Child Adult	 > 2.5 ng/mL > 3.0 ng/mL	 > 3.2 nmol/L > 3.8 nmol/L

Contd...

Contd...

Test/Specimen	Age/gender/ reference	Normal ranges	
		Conventional units	International units (SI)
Eosinophil count Whole blood, capillary blood		50–250 cells/mm³ (μL)	50–250 x 10^6 cells/L
Erythrocyte (RBC) count Whole blood	Cord 1–3 d 1 wk 2 wk 1 mo 2 mo 3–6 mo 0.5–2 yr 2–6 yr 6–12 yr 12–18 yr: Male Female	3.9–5.5 million/mm³ 4.0–6.6 million/mm³ 3.9–6,3 million/mm³ 3.6–6.2 million/mm³ 3.0–5,4 million/mm³ 2.7–4.9 million/mm³ 3.1–4.5 million/mm³ 3.7–53 million/mm³ 3.9–5.3 million/mm³ 4.0–5.2 million/mm³ 4.5–5.3 million/mm³ 4.1–5.1 million/mm³	3.9–5.5 × 10^{12} cells/L 4.0–6.6 × 10^{12} cells/L 3.9–6.3 × 10^{12} cells/L 3.6–6.2 × 10^{12} cells/L. 3.0–5.4 × 10^{12} cells/L 2.7–4.9 × 10^{12} cells/L 3.1–4.5 × 10^{12} cells/L 3.7–5 3 × 10^{12} cells/L 3.9–5.3 × 10^{12} cells/L 4.0–5.2 × 10^{12} cells/L 4 5–5.3 × 10^{12} cells/L 4.1–5.1 × 10^{12} cells/L
Erythrocyte sedimentation rate (ESR) Whole blood Westergren (modified)	Child < 50 yr: Male Female	0–10 mm/hr 0–15 mm/hr 0–20 mm/hr	0–10 mm/hr 0–15 mm/hr 0–20 mm/hr
Wintrobe	Child Adult: Male Female	0–13 mm/hr 0–9 mm/hr 0–20 mm/hr	0–13 mm/hr 0–9 mm/hr 0–20 mm/hr
Fibrinogen Plasma	Newborn Thereafter	125–300 mg/dL 200–400 mg/dL	1.25–3.00 g/L 2.00–4.00 g/L
Galactose Serum	Newborn Thereafter	0–20 mg/dL < 5 mg/dL	0–1.11 mmol/L < 0.28 mmol/L
Urine	Newborn Thereafter	≤ 60 mg/dL ≤ 14 mg/24hr	≤ 3.33 mmol/L < 0.08 nmol/d
Glucose Serum	Cord Newborn, 1 d Newborn, >1 d Child Thereafter	45–96 mg/dL 40–60 mg/dL 50–90 mg/dL 60–100 mg/dL 70–105 mg/dL	2.5–5.3 mmol/L 2.2–3.3 mmol/L 2.8–5.0 mmol/L 3.3–5.5 mmol/L 3.9–5.8 mmol/L
Whole blood CSF Urine (quantitative) (qualitative) Glucose tolerance test (GTT) oral serum	Adult Adult	65–95 mg/dL 40–70 mg/dL < 0.5 g/d Negative	3.6–5.3 mmol/L 2.2–3.9 mmol/L < 2.8 mmol/d Negative

Contd...

Contd...

Test/Specimen	Age/gender/ reference	Normal ranges			
		Conventional units		International units (SI)	
Dosages Adult: 75 g Child: 1.75 g/kg of ideal Weight up to maximum of 75g		Normal	Diabetic	Normal	Diabetic
	Fasting	70–150 mg/dL	≥ 126 mg/dL	3.9–5.8 mmol/L	≥ 7.0 mmol/L
	60 min	120–170 mg/dL	≥ 200 mg/dL	6.7–9.4 mmol/L	≥ 11 mmol/L
	90 min	100–140 mg/dL	≥ 200 mg/dL	5.6–7.8 mmol/L	≥ 11 mmol/L
	120 min	70–120 mg/dL	≥ 200 mg/dL	3.9–6.7 mmol/L	≥ 11 mmol/L
Growth hormone (HGH, human growth somatotropin)	1 day 1 week 1–12 months Fasting child/ adult	5–53 ng/mL 5–27 ng/mL 2–10 ng/mL < 0.7–6.0 ng/mL		5–53 µg/L 5–27 µg/L 2–10 µg/L < 0.7–6.0 µg/L	
Hematocrit (HCT, Hct) Whole blood	1 d (cap) 2 day 3 day 2 months 6–12 years 12–18 yr: Male Female	48–69% 48–75% 44–72% 28–42% 35–45% 37–49% 36–46%		0.48–0.69 vol. fraction 0.48–0.75 vol. fraction 0.44–0.72 vol. fraction 0.28–0.42 vol. fraction 0.35–0.45 vol. fraction 0.37–0.49 vol. fraction 0.36–0.46 vol. fraction	
Hemoglobin (Hb)Whole blood	1–3 d (cap) 2 months 6–12 yr 12–18 yr: Male Female	14.5–22.5 g/dL 9.0–14.0 g/dL 11.5–15.5 g/dL 13.0–16.0 g/dL 12.0–16.0 g/dL		2.25–3.49 mmol/L 1.40–2.17 mmol/L 1.78–2.40 mmol/L 2.02–2.48 mmol/L 1.860–2.48 mmol/L	
Hemoglobin A Whole blood		> 95% of total		> 0.95 fraction of Hb	
Hemoglobin F Whole blood	1d (cap) 5 day 3 week 6–9 week 3–4 months 6 months Adult	63–92% HbF 65–88% HbF 55–85% HbF 31–75% HbF < 2–59% HbF < 2–9% HbF < 2.0% HbF		0.63–0.92 mass fraction HbF 0.65–0.88 mass fraction HbF 0.55–0.85 mass fraction HbF 0.31–0.75 mass fraction HbF < 0.02–0.59 mass fraction HbF < 0.02–0.09 mass fraction HbF < 0.02 mass fraction HbF	

Contd...

Contd...

Test/Specimen	Age/gender/ reference	Normal ranges	
		Conventional units	International units (SI)
Immuno-globulin A (IgA) Serum	Cord blood	1.4–3.6 mg/dL	14–36 mg/L
	1–3 months	1.3–53 mg/dL	13–530 mg/L
	4–6 months	4.4–84 mg/dL	44–840 mg/L
	7 months–1 yr	11–106 mg/dL	110–1060 mg/L
	2–5 years	14–159 mg/dL	140–1590 mg/L
	6–10 years	33–236 mg/dL	330–2360 mg/L
	Adult	70–312 mg/dL	700–3120 mg/L
Immuno-globulin D (IgD) Serum	Newborn	None detected	None detected
	Thereafter	0–8 mg/dL	0–80 mg/L
Immuno-globulin E (IgE) Serum	Male	0–230 lU/mL	0–230 kIU/L
	Female	0–170 lU/mL	0–170 kIU/L
Immuno-globulin G (IgG) Serum	Cord blood	636–1606 mg/dL	6.36–16.06 g/L
	1 mo	251–906 mg/dL	2.51–9.06 g/L
	2–4 mo	176–601 mg/dL	1.76–6.01 g/L
	5–12 mo	172–1069 mg/dL	1.72–10.69 g/L
	1–5 yr	345–1236 mg/dL	3.45–12.36 g/L
	6–10 yr	608–1572 mg/dL	6.08–15.72 g/L
	Adult	639–1349 mg/dL	6.39–13.49 g/L
Immuno-globulin M (IgM) Serum	Cord blood	6.3–25 mg/dL	63–250 mg/L
	1–4 mo	17–105 mg/dL	170–1050 mg/L
	5–9 mo	33–126 mg/dL	330–1260 mg/L
	10 mo–1 yr	41–173 mg/dL	410–1730 mg/L
	2–8 yr	43–207 mg/dL	430–2070 mg/L
	9–10 yr	52–242 mg/dL	520–2420 mg/L
	Adult	56–352 mg/dL	560–3520 mg/L
Iron Serum	Newborn	100–250 µg/dL	18–45 µ mol/L
	Infant	40–100 µg/dL	7–18 µmol/L
	Child	50–120 µg/dL	9–22 µmol/L
	Thereafter:		
	Male	65–170 µg/dL	12–30 µmol/L
	Female	50–170 µg/dL	9–30 µmol/L
	Intoxicated child	280–2550 µg/dL	50.12–456.5 µmol/L
	fatally poisoned child	> 1800 µg/dL	> 322.2 µmol/L

Contd...

Contd...

Test/Specimen	Age/gender/ reference	Normal ranges		
		Conventional units		International units (SI)
Iron–binding capacity, total (TIBC)	Infant Thereafter	100–400 μg/dL 250–400 μg/dL		17.90–71.60 μmol/L 44.75–71.60 μmol/L
Lead Whole blood Urine, 24 hr	Child	< 10 μg/dL < 80 μg/dL		< 0.48 μmol/L < 0.39 μmol/L
Leukocyte count (WBC count) Whole blood	Birth 24 hr 1 mo 1–3 yr 4–7 yr 8–13 yr Adult	9.0–30.0 9,4–34,0 5.0–19.5 6.0–17.5 5.5–15.5 4.5–13.5 4.5–11.0 × 1000 cells/mm^3 (μL)		9.0–30.0 9.4–34.0 5.0–19.5 6.0–17,5 5,5–15.5 4.5–13,5 4.5–11.0 × 10^6 cells/L
CSF	Premature Newborn Neonate Thereafter	0–25 mononuclear 0–10 polymorphonuclear 0–1000 RBC 0–20 mononuclear 0–10 polymorphonuclear 0–800 RBC 0–5 mononuclear 0–10 polymorphonuclear 0–50 RBC 0–5 mononuclear		0–25 0–10 0–1000 0–20 0–10 0–800 0–5 0–10 0–50 0–5
Leukocyte differential count Whole blood	Myelocytes Neutrophils ('bands')	0%	0 cells/mm^3 (μL)	Number fraction 0
	Neutrophils ('segs')	3–5%	150–400 ceils/ mm^3 (μL)	Number fraction 0.03–0.05
	Neutrophils ('segs')	54–62%	3000–5800 cells/ mm^3 (μL)	Number fraction 0.54–0.62

Contd...

Contd...

Test/Specimen	Age/gender/ reference	Normal ranges		
		Conventional units		International units (SI)
	Lymphocytes	25–33%	1500–3000 cell/mm^3 (μL)	Number fraction 0.25–0.33
	Monocytes	3–7%	285–500 cells/ mm^3 (μL)	Number fraction 0.03–0.07
	Eosinophils Basophils	1–3%	50–250 cells/ mm^3 (μL)	Number fraction 0.01–0.03
		0–0.75%	15–50 cells/ mm^3 (μL)	Number fraction 0–0.0075
Mean corpuscular hemoglobin (MCM) Whole blood	Birth 1–3 d (cap) 1 wk–1 mo 2 mo 3–6 mo 0.5–2 yr 2–6 yr 6–12 yr 12–18 yr 18–49 yr	31–37 pg/cell 31–37 pg/cell 28–40 pg/cell 26–34 pg/cell 25–35 pg/cell 23–31 pg/cell 24–30 pg/cell 25–33 pg/cell 25–35 pg/cell 26–34 pg/cell		0.48–0.57 fmol/cell 0.48–0.57 fmol/cell 0.43–0.62 fmol/cell 0.40–0.53 fmol/cell 0.39–0.54 fmol/cell 0.36–0.48 fmol/cell 0.37–0.47 fmol/cell 0.39–0.51 fmol/cell 0,39–0.54 fmol/cell 0.40–0.53 fmol/cell
Mean corpuscular hemoglobin concentration (MCHC) Whole blood	Birth	30–36% Hb/cell or g Hb/dL RBC		4.65–5.58 mmol Hb/L RBC
	1–3 d (cap)	29–37% Hb/cell or g Hb/dL RBC		4.50–5.74 mmol Hb/L RBC
	1–2 wk	28–38% Hb/cell or g Hb/dL RBC		4.34–5.89 mmol Hb/L RBC
	1–2 mo	29–37% Hb/cell or g Hb/dL RBC		4,50–5.74 mmol Hb/L RBC
	3 mo–2 yr	30–36% Hb/cell or g Hb/dL RBC		4.65–5.58 mmol Hb/L RBC
	2–18 yr	31–37% Hb/cell or g Hb/dL RBC		4:81–5.74 mmol Hb/L RBC
	> 18 yr	31–37% Hb/cell or g Hb/dL RBC		4.81–5.74 mmol Hb/L RBC
Mean corpuscular volume (MCV) Whole blood	1–3 d (cap) 0.5–2 yr 6–12 yr 12–18 yr: Male Female	95–121 μm^3 70–86 μm^3 77–95 μm^3 78–98 μm^3 78–102 μm^3		95–121 fL 70–86 fL 77–95 fL 78–98 fL 78–102 fL

Contd...

Contd...

Test/Specimen	Age/gender/ reference	Normal ranges	
		Conventional units	International units (SI)
Osmolality Serum Urine, random	Child, adult	275–295 mOsm/kg H_2O 50–1400 mOsm/kgH_2O, de pending on fluid intake; after 12–hr fluid restriction: > 850 mOsm/kg H_2O	
Urine, 24 hr Oxygen, partial pressure (PO_2) Whole blood, arterial	 Birth 5–10 min 30 min > 1 hr 1 d Thereafter (decreased with age)	≈ 300–900 mOsm/kg H_2O 8–24 mm Hg 33–75 mm Hg 31–85 mm Hg 55–80 mm Hg 54–95 mm Hg 83–108 mm Hg	 1.1–3.2 kPa 4.4–10.0 kPa 4.1–11.3 kPa 7.3–10.6 kPa 7.2–12.6 kPa 11–14.4 kPa
Oxygen saturation (SaO_2) Whole blood, arterial	Newborn Thereafter	85–90% 95–99%	Fraction saturated 0.85–9.90 Fraction saturated 0.95–0.99
Partial thromboplastin time (PTT) Whole blood (Na citrate) Nonactivated Activated		60–85 sec (platelin) 25–35 sec (differs with method)	60–85 sec 25–35 sec
PH Whole blood, arterial	 Premature Birth, full term 5–10 min 30 min > 1 hr 1 d Thereafter Must be corrected for body temperature	 7.35–7.50 7.11–7.36 7.09–7.30 7.21–7.38 7.26 7.49 7.29–7.45 7.35–7.45	H* concentration 31–44 nmol/L 43–77 nmol/L 50–81 nmol/L 41–61 nmol/L 32 54 nmol/L 35–51 nmol/L 35–44 nmol/L
Urine, random Stool	Newborn/ neonate Thereafter	5–7 4.5–8 7.0–7 5	0.1–10 µmol/L 0.01–32 µmol/L (average ≈ 1.0 µmol/L) 31–100 nmol/L

Contd...

Contd...

Test/Specimen	Age/gender/ reference	Normal ranges	
		Conventional units	International units (SI)
Phenylalanine Serum	 Premature Newborn Thereafter	 2.0–7.5 mg/dL 1.2–3.4 mg/dL 0.8–1.8 mg/dL	120–450 μmol/L 70–120 μmol/L 50–110 μmol/L 6–12 μmol/day
Urine, 24 hr	10d–2wk 3–12 yr Thereafter	12 mg/day 4–18 mg/day Trace–17 mg/day	24 110 μmol/day Trace–103 μmol/day
Plasma volume Plasma	 Male Female	 25–43 μm/kg 78–45 mL/kg	0.025–0.043 L/kg 0.028–0.045 L/kg
Platelet count (thrombocyte count) Whole blood (EDTA)	Newborn (after 1 wk, same as adult) Adult	84–478 × 103/mm³ (μL) 150–400 × 103/mm³ (μL)	84–478 × 109/L 150–400 × 109/L
Potassium Serum Plasma (heparin) Urine, 24 hr	 Newborn Thereafter	 3.0–6.0 mEq/L 3.5–5.0 mEq/L 3.4–4.5 mEq/L 2.5–125 mEq/day; varies with diet	3.0–6.0 mmol/L 3.5–5.0 mmol/L 3.4–4.5 mmol/L 2.5–125 mmol/L
Protein Serum, total	Premature Newborn 1–7 yr 8–12 yr 13–19 yr	4.3–7.6 g/dL 4.6–7.4 g/dL 6.1–7.9 g/dL 6.4–8.1 g/dL 6.6–8.2 g/dL	43–76 g/L 46–74 g/L 61–79 g/L 64–81 g/L 66–82 g/L
Total Urine, 24 hr CSF		1–14 mg/dL 50–80 mg/day (at rest) < 250 mg/day after intense exercise Lumbar: 8–32 mg/dL	10–140 mg/L 50–80 mg/day < 250 mg/day after intense exercise 80–320 mg/L
Prothrombin time (PT) One–stage (Quick)	In general	11–15 sec (varies with type of thromboplastin)	11–15 sec
Whole blood (Na citrate) Two–stage modified (ware and seegers)	Newborn	Prolonged by 2–3 sec	Prolonged by 2–3 sec

Contd...

Contd...

Test/Specimen	Age/gender/ reference	Normal ranges	
		Conventional units	International units (SI)
Whole blood (Na citrate) RBC count: see Erythrocyte count		18–22 sec	18–22 sec
Red blood cell volume Whole blood	Male Female	20–36 mL/kg 19–31 mL/kg	0.020–0.036 L/kg 0.019–0.031 L/kg
Reticulocyte count Whole blood	Adults	0.5–1.5% of erythrocytes or 25,000–75,000 mm^3 (μL)	0.005–0.015 (number fraction) or 25,000–75,000 × 10^6/L
Capillary	Id 7d 1–4wk 5–6 wk 7–8 wk 9–10 wk 11–12 wk	0.4–6.0% < 0.1–1.3% < 0.1–1.2% < 0.1–2.4% < 0.1–2.9% < 0.1–2.6% 0.1–1.3%	0.004–0.060 (number fraction) <0.001–0.013 (number fraction) <0.001–0.012 (number fraction) <0.001–0.024 (number fraction) <0.001–0.029 (number fraction) <0.001–0.026 (number fraction) 0.001–0.013 (number fraction)
Salicylates Serum, plasma	Therap. cone. Toxic cone.	15–30 mg/dL > 30 mg/dL	1.1–2.2 mmol/L > 18.5 mmol/L
Sedimentation rate: see erythrocyte sedimentation rate sodium serum or plasma	Newborn Infant Child Thereafter	134–146 mEq/L 139–146 mEq/L 138–145 mEq/L 136–146 mEq/L	134–146 mmol/L 139–146 mmol/L 138–145 mmol/L 40–220 mmol/L
Urine, 24 hr Sweat	Normal Indeterminate Cystic fibrosis	40–220 mEq/L (diet dependent) < 40 mEq/L 45–60 mEq/L > 60 mEq/L	40–220 mmol/L < 40 mmol/L 45–60 mmol/L > 60 mmol/L
Specific gravity Urine, random	Adult After 12–hr fluid restriction	1.002–1.030 > 1.025	1.002–1.030 >1.025
Theophylline Serum, plasma	Therap. cone. Bronchodilator Premature apnea Toxic cone.	10–20 μg/mL 5–10 μg/mL >20 μg/mL	56–110 μmol/L 28–56 μmol/L >110 μmol/L

Contd...

Contd...

Test/Specimen	Age/gender/ reference	Normal ranges	
		Conventional units	International units (SI)
Thrombin time whole blood (Na citrate)		Control time ± 2 sec when control is 9–13 sec	Control time ± 2 sec when control is 9–13 sec
Thyroxine, total (T,) Serum	Cord Newborn	8–13 μg/dL 11.5–24 (lower in low-birth-weight infants)	103–168 nmol/L 148–310 nmol/L
	Neonate Infant 1–5 yr 5–10 yr Thereafter Newborn screen (filter paper)	9–18 μg/dL 7–15 μg/dL 7.3–15 μg/dL 6.4–13.3 μg/dL 5–12 μg/dL 6.2–22 μg/dL	116–232 nmol/L 90–194 nmol/L 94–194 nmol/L 83–172 nmol/L 65–155 nmol/L 80–284 nmol/L
Triglycerides (TG)		Mg/dL	g/L
Serum, after ≥ 12–hr fast	 Cord blood 0–5 yr 6–11 yr 12–15 yr 16–19 yr	Male Female 10–98 10–98 30–86 32–99 31–108 35–114 36–138 41–138 40–163 40–128	Male Female 0.10–0.98 0.10–0.98 0.30–0.86 0.32–0.99 0.31–1.08 0.35–1.14 0.36–1.38 0.41–1.38 0.40–1.63 0.40–1.28
Triiodothyronine, free Serum	Cord 1–3 d 6 wk Adults (20–50 yr)	20–240 pg/dL 200–610 pg/dL 240–560 pg/dL 230–660 pg/dL	0.3–3.7 pmol/L 3.1–9.4 pmol/L 3.7–8.6 pmol/L 3.5–10.0 pmol/L
Triiodothyronine, Total (T3–RIA) Serum	Cord Newborn 1–5 yr 5–10 yr 10–15 yr Thereafter	30–70 ng/dL 72–260 ng/dL 100–260 ng/dL 90–240 ng/dL 80–210 ng/dL 115–190 ng/dL	0.46–1.08 nmol/L 1.16–4 nmol/L 1.54–4 nmol/L 1.39–3.70 nmol/L 1.23–3.23 nmol/L 1.77–2.93 nmol/L

Contd...

Contd...

Test/Specimen	Age/gender/ reference	Normal ranges	
		Conventional units	International units (SI)
Urea nitrogen			
Serum or plasma	Cord	21–40 mg/dL	7.5–14.3 mmol/L
	Premature (1 wk)	3–25 mg/dL	1.1–9 mmol/L
	Newborn	3–12 mg/dL	1.1–4.3 mmol/L
	Infant/child	5–18 mg/dL	1.8–6.4 mmol/L
	Thereafter	7–18 mg/dL	2.5–6.4 mmol/L
Urea volume			
Urine, 24 hr	Newborn	50–300 mL/d	0.050–0.3 L/day
	Infant	350–550 mL/d	0.350–0.5 L/day
	Child	500–1000 mL/d	0.500–1 L/day
	Adolescent	700–1400 mL/d	0.700–1.4 L/day
	Thereafter:	800–1800 mL/d	0.800–1.8 L/day
	Male	600–1600 mL/d (varies with	0.600–1.6 L/day
	Female	Intake and other factors)	

ABBREVIATION USED IN LABORATORY TESTS

Abbreviation	Term
Cap	capillary
CHF	congestive heart failure
Conc.	concentration
CSF	cerebrospinal fluid
d	day; diem
EDTA	ethylene diamine tetra acetate
g	gram
m	meter
hr	hour
L,l	liter
mEq	milliequivalent
min	minute
mm	millimeter
mm^3	cubic millimeter
mo	month
mol	mole

Contd...

Contd...

Abbreviation	Term
mOsmol	milliosmole
sec	second
SI	International system of units
Therap.	Therapeutic
U	International unit of enzyme activity
vol	Volume
wk	Week
yr	Year
>	Greater than
≥	Greater than or equal to
<	Less than
≤	Less than or equal to
±	Plus/minus
≈	Approximately equal to

PREFIXES DENOTING DECIMAL FACTORS

Prefix	Symbols	Amount
deci	d	one tenth (10^{-1})
centi	c	one hundredth (10^{-2})
milli	m	one thousandth (10^{-3})
micro	µ	one millionth (10^{-6})
nano	n	one billionth (10^{-9})
pico	p	one trillionth (10^{-12})
femto	f	one quadrillionth (10^{-15})

NORMAL VALUES

Normal Heart Rates for Infants and Children

	Rate (Beats/Min)		
Age	**Resting (Awake)**	**Resting (Sleeping)**	**Exercise (Fever)**
Newborn 1 week	100–180	80–160	Up to 220
3 months	100–220	80–200	Up to 220
3 months to 2 years	80–150	70–120	Up to 220

Contd...

Contd...

	Rate (Beats/Min)		
Age	**Resting (Awake)**	**Resting (Sleeping)**	**Exercise (Fever)**
2 years to 10 years	70–110	60–90	Up to 220
10 years to adult	55–90	50–90	Up to 220

From Gillette PC: Dysrhythmias. In Adams FH, Emmanouilides GC, Riemenschneider TA, editiors: Moss' heart disease in infants, children, and adolescents, ed 4, Baltimore, 1989, Williams & Wilkins.

Normal Respiratory Rates for Children

Age	Rate (Breaths/Min)
Newborn	35
1 to 11 months	30
2 years	25
4 years	23
6 years	21
8 years	20
10 years	19
12 years	19
14 years	18
16 years	17
18 years	16–18

Normal Body Temperatures for Children

Age	°F–Temperature	°C
3 months	99.4	37.5
6 months	99.5	37.5
1 years	99.7	37.7
3 years	99.0	37.2
5 years	98.6	37.0
7 years	98.3	36.8
9 years	98.1	36.7
11 years	98.0	36.7
13 years	97.8	36.6

Modified from Lowrey GH: Growth and development of children, ed 8, St Louis, 1986, Mosby.

Centigrade to Fahrenheit Temperature Conversions

°C	°F	°C	°F	°C	°F
35.0	95.0	37.0	98.6	39.0	102.2
35.2	95.4	37.2	99.0	39.2	102.6
35.4	95.7	37.4	99.3	39.4	102.9
35.6	96.1	37.6	99.7	39.6	103.3
35.8	96.4	37.8	100.0	39.8	103.6
36.0	96.8	38.0	100.4	40.0	104.0
36.2	97.2	38.2	100.8	40.2	104.4
36.4	97.5	38.4	101.1	40.4	104.7
36.6	97.96	38.6	101.5	40.6	105.1
36.8	98.2	38.8	101.8	40.8	105.4
				41.0	105.8

Conversion Formulas

°F = (°C × 9/5) + 32 or (°C × 1.8) + 32

°C = (°F – 32) × 5/9 or (°F – 32) × 0.55

Wong-Baker Faces Pain Assessment Scale

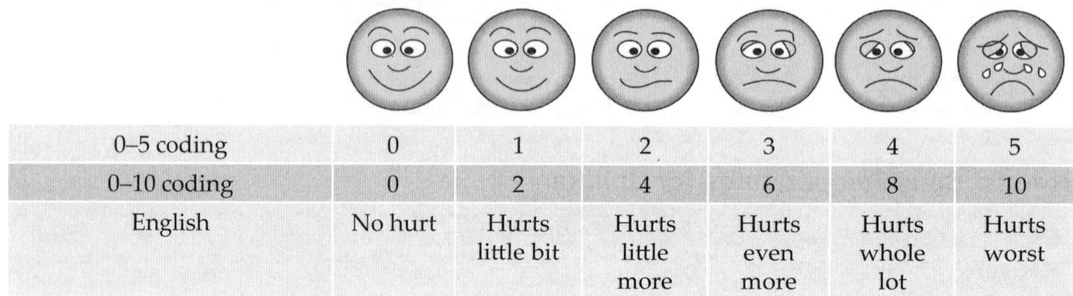

0–5 coding	0	1	2	3	4	5
0–10 coding	0	2	4	6	8	10
English	No hurt	Hurts little bit	Hurts little more	Hurts even more	Hurts whole lot	Hurts worst

Annexure 4

COMMON MEDICAL ABBREVIATIONS

AAROM	Active assistive range of motion
ABG	Arterial blood gas
ac	Before meals
A/C	Assist control
add	Adduction
ADA Diet	American diabetes association diet
ADL	Activities of daily living
AFib	Arterial fibrillation
AKA	Above knee amputation
ALS	Amyotrophic lateral sclerosis
AMA	Against medical advice
bid	Twice a day
BKA	Below knee amputation
BLBS	Bilateral breath sounds
bm	Bowel movement
BM	Bone marrow
BMR	Basal metabolism rate
BP	Blood pressure
BR	Bed rest
bs	Bowel sounds
BS	Breath sounds
B/S	Bedside
bx	Biopsy
$\bar{C}$	With (c with bar above it)
C	Celsius, centigrade
CA	Cardiac arrest
CA, ca	Carcinoma
CABG	Coronary artery bypass graft
CAD	Coronary artery disease
cal	Calorie
CBC	Complete blood count
cc	Cubic centimeter
CC	Chief complaint
CCU	Coronary care unit
CHF	Congestive heart failure, chronic heart failure
CHI	Closed head injury
cm	Centimeter
CMT	Continuing medication and treatment
CN	Cranial nerve
CNA	Certified nursing assistant
CNS	Central nervous system
c/o	Complains of
COTA	Certified occupational therapy assistant
cont	Continue (d)
COPD	Chronic obstructive pulmonary disease
CPAP	Continuous positive airway pressure
CPR	Cardiopulmonary resuscitation
CRF	Chronic renal failure
CRNP	Certified registered nurse practitioner
CSF	Cerebrospinal fluid
CT	Computerized tomography
CV	Cardiovascula
CVA	Cerebral vascular accident
CXR	Chest X-ray
d/c	Discontinue
DC	Discharge
DNK	Do not know
DNKA	Did not keep appointment
DNR	Do not resuscitate
DNT	Did not test
DOA	Dead on arrival
DOB	Date of birth
DOE	Dyspnea on exertion
d/t	Due to

Dx	Diagnosis
ECC, EKG	Electrocardiogram
ED	Emergency department
EEG	Electroencephalogram
EENT	Eye, ear, nose, throat
EMG	Electromyogram
ENT	Ear, nose, throat
ER	Emergency room
ETOH	Ethanol (alcohol)
exam	Examination
ext	External, exterior
F	Fahrenheit
FH	Family history
fib	Fibrillation
fl, fld	Fluid
FOB	Foot of bed
f/u	Follow-up
FWB	Full weight bearing
Fx	Fracture
GB	Gallbladder
GCS	Glasgow coma scale
GE	Gastroenterology
GERD	Gastroesophageal reflux disease
G/E	Gastroenteritis
gen	General
gest	Gestation
GI	Gastrointestinal
gluc	Glucose
GNA	Geriatric nursing assistant
GP	General practitioner, general paralysis
GSW	Gunshot wound
GTT	Glucose tolerance test
Gt tr	Gait training
GYN	Gynecology
H/A	Headache
HAV	Hepatitis A virus
Hb	Hemoglobin
HB	Heart block
HBP	High blood pressure
hd	At bedtime
HEENT	Head, eyes, ear, nose, throat
H_2O	Water
ho	History of
HOB	Head of bed
H&P	History and physical
HR	Heart rate
HTN	Hypertension
HVD	Hypertensive vascular disease
Hx	History
Hz	Hertz (cycles/second)
ICCU	Intensive coronary care unit
ICP	Intracranial pressure
ICU	Intensive care unit
imp	Impression
incr	Increased (ing)
inf	Infusion, inferior
inspire	Inspiration, inspiratory
int	Internal
I&O	Intake and output
IPPB	Intermittent positive pressure breathing
irreg	Irregular
IV	Intravenous(ly)
K	Potassium, kidney
L	Left, liver, liter, lower, light, lumbar
L2, L3	Second, third lumbar vertebrae
lab	Laboratory
lac	Laceration
LBW	Low birth rate
LE	Lower extremities
liq	Liquid
LOC	Loss of consciousness, level of consciousness, laxative of choice
LOS	Length of stay
LP	Lumbar puncture
LPN	Licensed practical nurse
LUE	Left upper extremity
Lx	Larynx
L&W	Living and well
max	Maximum, maxillary
MBC	Maximum breathing capacity
MBSS	Modified barium swallow study

MCA	Middle cerebral artery
MD	Muscular dystrophy
mdnt	Midnight
med	Medicine
mets	Metastasis
MG	Myasthenia gravis
MI	Myocardial infarction
min	Minute
MICU	Medical intensive care unit
mod	Moderate
MRI	Magnetic resonance imaging
MRSA	Methicillin-resistant staphylococcus aureus
mss	Massage
MVA	Motor vehicle accident
n	Nerve
Na	Sodium
NaCl	Sodium chloride
NAD	No abnormality detected
NAD	No apparent distress
neg	Negative
neur	Neurology
NG	Nasogastric
NIC	Neonatal intensive care
NICU	Neonatal intensive care unit
NKA	No known allergies
no	Number
NOS	Not otherwise specified
NPO	Nothing by mouth
NSA	No specific abnormality
NST	Non-stress test
N&V	Nausea and vomiting
NVD	Nausea, vomiting, diarrhea
N&W	Normal and well
NWB	Non-weight bearing
NYD	Not yet diagnosed
o	None, without
O	Oral
O_2	Oxygen
O_2 cap	Oxygen capacity
O_2 sat	Oxygen saturation
OA	Osteoarthritis
OB, OBG	Obstetrics
OB/GYN	Obstetrics and gynecology
Obs	Observation
OBS	Organic brain syndrome
O/E	On examination
OH	Occupational history
OHD	Organic heart disease
oint	Ointment
OM	Otitis media
OME	Otitis media with effusion
OOB, oob	Out of bed
Op	Operation
ot	Ear
Oto	Otolaryngology
OT	Occupational therapy
OR	Operating room
PA	Physician's assistant
p&a	Percussion and auscultation
PACU	Postanesthesia care unit
PAF	Paroxysmal atrial fibrillation
palp	Palpate, palpable
Path	Pathology
PA view	Posterior-anterior view on X-ray
p/c, pc	After meals
pdr	Powder
PDN	Private duty nurse
PE	Physical exam, pulmonary embolism
Ped	Pediatrics
PEEP	Positive end expiratory pressure
PEG	Percutaneous endoscopic gastrectomy
PET	Positron emission tomography
PH	Past history
pharm	Pharmacy
PHYS	Physical, physiology
PI	Present illness, pulmonary insufficiency

PICU	Pulmonary intensive care unit
PID	Pelvic inflammatory disease
plts	Platelets
PM	Afternoon, postmortem
PMH	Past medical history
PMN	Physical medicine and rehabilitation
PN	Poorly nourished, practical nurse
P&N	Psychiatry and Neurology
pneu	Pneumo, pneumonia
PNI	Peripheral nerve injury
PNX	Pneuomothorax
po	By mouth
pod	Postoperative day
pos	Positive
post	Posterior
POSTOP	Postoperative
pot	Potassium
PR	Proctology
pre-op	Preoperative
prep	Prepare for
prm	According to circumstances
prn	As often as necessary
prod	Productive
Prog	Prognosis
PROM	Passive range of motion
pron	Pronator, pronation
prosth	Prosthesis
PSH	Past surgical history
Psych	Psychiatry
pt, Pt	Patient
PT	Physical therapy
PT	Physical therapy, posterior tibial artery pulse
PTA	Prior to admission,
PUD	Peptic ulcer disease
PVD	Peripheral vascular disease
PVT	Previous trouble
PWB%	Partial weight bearing with percent
Px, PX	Physical examination
q	Every
qh	Every hour
qid	Four times a day
qt	Quart
quad	Quadriplegic
R, r	Right
R	Rub, rectal temperature
RA	Rheumatoid arthritis, right atrium
rad	Radial
ram	Rapid alternating movements
RCA	Right coronary artery
RCU	Respiratory care unit
RD	Respiratory distress
RDS	Respiratory distress syndrome
RE	Reconditioning exercise
reg	Regular
rehab	Rehabilitation
resp	Respiratory, respirations
RF	Rheumatic fever
RLA	Rancho Los Amigo Scale
R to L&A	React to light and accommodation
RLE	Right lower extremity
RN	Registered nurse
RO, R/O	Rule out
ROM	Range of motion, rupture of membranes, right otitis media
ROS	Review of symptoms
Rt	Right
RT	Radiation therapy, respiratory therapy
RUE	Right upper extremity
RV	Residual volume
Rx	Therapy, prescription
S	Without
S	Sensation, sensitive, serum

Sa	Saline
sc	Subcutaneous(ly)
SCD	Sudden cardiac death
SCI	Spinal cord injury
schiz	Schizophrenia
SCU	Special care unit
sec	Second
Sens	Sensory, sensation
sep	Separated
SGA	Small for gestational age
sgl	Without correction (without glasses)
SH	Social history
SI	Stroke index
sib	Sibling
SICU	Surgical intensive care unit
SIDS	Sudden infant death syndrome
skel	Skeletal
Sl	Slightly
SL	Under the tongue
SLP	Speech-language pathology
sm	Small
SOAP	Subjective, objective assessment plan
SOB	Shortness of breath
S/P, s/p	Status post (previous condition)
sp cd	Spinal cord
spec	Specimen
sp fl	Spinal fluid
sp&H	Speech and hearing
spin	Spine, spinal
spont	Spontaneous
s/s	Signs and symptoms
SS	Social service
ST	Speech therapy
stat, STAT	Immediately
STD	Sexually transmitted disease
subcut	Subcutaneous
subling	Sublingual
sup	Superior
supin	Supination
surg	Surgery, surgical
Sx	Symptoms
sys	System
Syst	Systolic
T	Temperature
T&A	Tonsils and adenoids,
tab	Tablet
TAH	Total abdominal
TB	Tuberculosis
TBI	Traumatic brain injury
tbsp	Tablespoon
temp	Temperature
THERAP	Therapy, therapeutic
THR	Total hip replacement
TIA	Transient ischemic attack
TKR	Total knee replacement
TNM	Tumor, nodes, and metastases
TO	Telephone order
TPN	Total parenteral nutrition
TPR	Temperature, pulse,
tr	Trace
trach	Tracheostomy
tsp	Teaspoon
Tx	Treatment, traction
U/A	Urinalysis
UCD	Usual childhood diseases
UCHD	Usual childhood diseases
UG	Upward gaze
Unilat	Unilateral
u/o	Under observation
Ur	Urine
URD	Upper respiratory disease
URI	Upper respiratory infection
Urol	Urology
u/s, US	Ultrasound
UTI	Urinary tract infection
V	Vein
VA	Visual acuity
vag	Vagina, vaginal
VC	Vital capacity (vit.cap)
VD	Venereal disease

vent	Ventilator
vert	Vertical
VF	Visual fields
Via	By way of
vit	Vitamin
VN	Visiting nurse
VO	Verbal order
VS	Vital signs
W	White
w, wk	Week
W/C, whch	Wheelchair
WBT	Weight bearing tolerance
WF	White female
WFL	Within functional limits
WM	White male
w/n	Within
WNL	Within normal limits
WP	Whirpool
wt	Weight
w/u	Workup
x	Times
yo	Years old
yrs	Years

Annexure 5

NANDA (NORTH AMERICAN NURSING DIAGNOSIS ASSOCIATION)

International-approved Nursing Diagnoses

Below is the list of the 16 new NANDA nursing diagnoses:

1. Risk for Ineffective Activity Planning
2. Risk for Adverse Reaction to Iodinated Contrast Media
3. Risk for Allergy Response
4. Insufficient Breast Milk
5. Ineffective Childbearing Process
6. Risk for Ineffective Childbearing Process
7. Risk for Dry Eye
8. Deficient Community Health
9. Ineffective Impulse Control
10. Risk for Neonatal Jaundice
11. Risk for Disturbed Personal Identity
12. Ineffective Relationship
13. Risk for Ineffective Relationship
14. Risk for Chronic Low Self-Esteem
15. Risk for Thermal Injury
16. Risk for Ineffective Peripheral Tissue Perfusion

Domain 1: Health promotion	Domain 2: Nutrition
• Deficient diversional activity	• Insufficient breast milk
• Sedentary lifestyle	• Ineffective infant feeding pattern
• Deficient community health	• Imbalanced nutrition: Less than body requirements
• Risk-prone health behavior	• Imbalanced nutrition: More than body requirements
• Ineffective health maintenance	• Risk for imbalanced nutrition: More than body requirements
• Readiness for enhanced immunization status	• Readiness for enhanced nutrition
• Ineffective protection	• Impaired swallowing
• Ineffective self-health management	• Risk for unstable blood glucose level
• Readiness for enhanced self-health management	• Neonatal jaundice
• Ineffective family therapeutic regimen management	• Risk for neonatal jaundice

Contd...

Contd...

	• Risk for impaired liver function
	• Risk for electrolyte imbalance
	• Readiness for enhanced fluid balance
	• Deficient fluid volume
	• Excess fluid volume
	• Risk for deficient fluid volume
	• Risk for imbalanced fluid volume
Domain 3: Elimination and exchange	**Domain 4: Activity/Rest**
• Functional urinary incontinence	• Insomnia
• Overflow urinary incontinence	• Sleep deprivation
• Reflex urinary incontinence	• Readiness for enhanced sleep
• Stress urinary incontinence	• Disturbed sleep pattern
• Urge urinary incontinence	– Risk for disuse syndrome
• Risk for urge urinary incontinence	– Impaired bed mobility
• Impaired urinary elimination	– Impaired physical mobility
• Readiness for enhanced urinary elimination	– Impaired wheelchair mobility
• Urinary retention	– Impaired transfer ability
• Constipation	– Impaired walking
• Perceived constipation	– Disturbed energy field
• Risk for constipation	– Fatigue
• Diarrhea	– Wandering
• Dysfunctional gastrointestinal motility	– Activity intolerance
• Risk for dysfunctional gastrointestinal motility	– Risk for activity intolerance
• Bowel incontinence	– Ineffective breathing pattern
• Impaired gas exchange	– Decreased cardiac output
	– Risk for ineffective gastrointestinal perfusion
	– Risk for ineffective renal perfusion
	– Impaired spontaneous ventilation
	– Ineffective peripheral tissue perfusion
	– Risk for decreased cardiac tissue perfusion
	– Risk for ineffective cerebral tissue perfusion
	– Risk for ineffective peripheral tissue perfusion

Contd...

Contd...

	– Dysfunctional ventilatory weaning response
	– Impaired home maintenance
	– Readiness for enhanced self-care
	– Bathing self-care deficit
	– Dressing self-care deficit
	– Feeding self-care deficit
	– Toileting self-care deficit
	– Self-neglect
Domain 5: Perception/Cognition	**Domain 6: Self-perception**
• Unilateral neglect	• Hopelessness
• Impaired environmental interpretation syndrome	• Risk for compromised human dignity
• Acute confusion	• Risk for loneliness
• Chronic confusion	• Disturbed personal identity
• Risk for acute confusion	• Risk for disturbed personal identity
• Ineffective impulse control	• Readiness for enhanced self-control
• Deficient knowledge	• Chronic low self-esteem
• Readiness for enhanced knowledge	• Risk for chronic low self-esteem
• Impaired memory	• Risk for situational low self-esteem
• Readiness for enhanced communication	• Situational low self-esteem
• Impaired verbal communication	• Disturbed body image
	• Stress overload
	• Risk for disorganized infant behavior
	• Autonomic dysreflexia
	• Risk for autonomic dysreflexia
	• Disorganized infant behavior
	• Readiness for enhanced organized infant behavior
	• Decreased intracranial adaptive capacity
Domain 7: Role-relationships	**Domain 8: Sexuality**
• Ineffective breastfeeding	• Sexual dysfunction
• Interrupted breastfeeding	• Ineffective sexuality pattern
• Readiness for enhanced breastfeeding	• Ineffective childbearing process
• Caregiver role strain	• Readiness for enhanced childbearing process
• Risk for caregiver role strain	• Risk for ineffective childbearing process

Contd...

Contd...

• Impaired parenting	• Risk for disturbed maternal-fetal dyad
• Readiness for enhanced parenting	
• Risk for impaired parenting	
• Risk for impaired attachment	
• Dysfunctional family processes	
• Interrupted family processes	
• Readiness for enhanced family processes	
• Ineffective relationship	
• Readiness for enhanced relationship	
• Risk for ineffective relationship	
• Parental role conflict	
• Ineffective role performance	
• Impaired social interaction	
Domain 9: Coping/Stress tolerance	**Domain 10: Life principles**
• Post-trauma syndrome	• Readiness for enhanced hope
• Risk for post-trauma syndrome	• Readiness for enhanced spiritual well-being
• Rape-trauma syndrome	• Readiness for enhanced decision-making
• Relocation stress syndrome	• Decisional conflict
• Risk for relocation stress syndrome	• Moral distress
• Ineffective activity planning	• Noncompliance
• Risk for ineffective activity planning	• Impaired religiosity
• Anxiety	• Readiness for enhanced religiosity
• Compromised family coping	• Risk for impaired religiosity
• Defensive coping	• Spiritual distress
• Disabled family coping	• Risk for spiritual distress
• Ineffective coping	
• Ineffective community coping	
• Readiness for enhanced coping	
• Readiness for enhanced family coping	
• Death anxiety	
• Ineffective denial	
• Adult failure to thrive	
• Fear	
• Grieving	
• Complicated grieving	
• Risk for complicated grieving	

Contd...

Contd...

• Readiness for enhanced power	
• Powerlessness	
• Risk for powerlessness	
• Impaired individual resilience	
• Readiness for enhanced resilience	
• Risk for compromised resilience	
• Chronic sorrow	
• Stress overload	
• Risk for disorganized infant behavior	
• Autonomic dysreflexia	
• Risk for autonomic dysreflexia	
• Disorganized infant behavior	
• Readiness for enhanced organized infant behavior	
• Decreased intracranial adaptive capacity	
Domain 11: Safety/Protection	**Domain 12: Comfort**
• Risk for infection	• Impaired comfort
• Ineffective airway clearance	• Readiness for enhanced comfort
• Risk for aspiration	• Nausea
• Risk for bleeding	• Acute pain
• Impaired dentition	• Chronic pain
• Risk for dry eye	• Impaired comfort
• Risk for falls	• Readiness for enhanced comfort
• Risk for injury	• Social isolation
• Impaired oral mucous membrane	
• Risk for perioperative positioning injury	
• Risk for peripheral neurovascular dysfunction	
• Risk for shock	
• Impaired skin integrity	
• Risk for impaired skin integrity	
• Risk for sudden infant death syndrome	
• Risk for suffocation	
• Delayed surgical recovery	
• Risk for thermal injury	
• Impaired tissue integrity	

Contd...

Contd...

• Risk for trauma	
• Risk for vascular trauma	
• Risk for other-directed violence	
• Risk for self-directed violence	
• Self-mutilation	
• Risk for self-mutilation	
• Risk for suicide	
• Contamination	
• Risk for contamination	
• Risk for poisoning	
• Risk for adverse reaction to iodinated contrast media	
• Risk for allergy response	
• Latex allergy response	
• Risk for latex allergy response	
• Risk for imbalanced body temperature	
• Hyperthermia	
• Hypothermia	
• Ineffective thermoregulation	

Bibliography

1. Adele Pillitteri, Maternal and child health nursing (5th ed). Philadelphia: Lippincott Publishers, 2007.
2. AN, Chowdhary, Media influenced imitative hanging: A report from West Bengal. Indian Journal of Public Health, 2008.
3. Ann J. Zwemer, Basic psychology for nurses in India (2nd ed.). Chennai: B.I. Publication, 2005.
4. Barbara Schoen Johnson. Adaptation and growth psychiatric–mental health nursing (4th ed.). Philadelphia: Lippincott publisher, 2007.
5. Basvanthappa, BT. Community health nursing, (2nd ed.). Bengaloru: Jaypee Brothers Medical Publishers, 2008.
6. Bradley S, Greenberg. Mathew Eastin, et al. Road traffic accident and emergency care for children. Indian Journal of Public Health, 2003.
7. Cheng, T L, Brenner, RA, Wright, JL, et al. Road safety education for children. Journal of Pediatrics, 2004.
8. Christakis, DA. Health education on road safety. Journal of Pediatrics, 2005.
9. Clifford, T Morgan. A brief introduction to road safety (2nd ed.). New Delhi: Tata McGraw-Hill Publisher, 2004.
10. Davison KK, Francis LA, Birch Ll. Road safety education for parents and children. Journal of Pediatrics, 2005.
11. Day RC. The accident and trauma care for children. Journal of Child health nursing, 2003.
12. Dennison BA, Russo TJ, Burdick PA et al. An intervention to reduce road safety by preschool children. Arch Pediatric Adolescent Med., 2004 158(2):170-6.
13. Dhaar GM. Foundation of community medicine (2nd ed.). New Delhi : Elsevier Publisher, 2008.
14. Durant, RH. The road safety education for teachers. Journal of Pediatrics, 2006.
15. Fosarelly, PD. Road traffic symbols and signals Journal of Developmental and Behavioral Pediatrics, 1984.
16. Francis, LA, Birch LL. First aid education for teachers, Journal of American Diet Association, 2006.
17. Ghai OP. Essential Pediatrics (7th ed.). New Delhi: CBS publishers, 2007.
18. Gupta RK, DP Saini. Impact of road safety on school children. Indian Journal of Pediatrics, 2000.
19. Gupta, VB. Externalizing behaviors and road traffic accident on children for low education parents. Journal of Clinical Pediatrics, 2001.
20. Hesketh, K, Ball, K, Crawford, D, et al. Mediators of the relationship between teacher road safety education and children's road safety education. American Journal of Preventive Medicine, 2007.
21. Hockenberry Wilson. Wongs nursing care of infants and children (8th ed.). Missouri: Mosby Publishers, 2007.
22. John, CJ. Environment factor and road traffic accident. Health Action , 2001.
23. Joseph Xavier S, Bastin Jerome V. Child and road safety problem. Health Action, 2007.
24. Judith Ann Allender. Role of Nurse in Road safety education. Child health nursing (6th ed.). Philadelphia: Lippincott Publishers, 2005.
25. Kaplan, Sadock's. Critical thinking on road safety. Health action journal (9th ed.). Philadelphia: Lippincott Publishers, 2002.

26. Kennedy Christine. Factors influencing in road traffic accident in children Journal of Pediatric Nursing, 2000.
27. Kennedy, C. Road safety measures to prevent accidents. Journal of Pediatric Nursing, 2000.
28. Kennedy, CM. Children's perception of road traffic accident and health behavior effects. Journal of Paediatric Nursing, 2003, 34(3).
29. Manganello, JA, Mckenzie, LB. Parents and child road safety. Journal of Health Education, 2008.
30. Marcia Standhope. Community and public health nursing (6th ed.). USA: Mosby Publishers, 2004.
31. Mary, C Townsend. Psychiatric mental health nursing (5th ed.). New Delhi: Jaypee Brothers Medical Publishers, 2006.
32. Normah, L Munn. Introduction to psychology (3rd ed). New Delhi: Oxford and IBH Publishers, 1999.
33. Owens, J. Sleep disturbance induced road traffic accident among school children. Journal of Pediatrics, 1992.
34. Parkar SR, Deoldhar Jayita K. Road safety measures. Pediatric Clinics of India, 1996.
35. Polit. F Hungler. Essential of nursing research, (16th ed). New York : Lippincott publishers, 1999.
36. Potter Perry. Fundamentals of nursing, (4th ed). Minssorin: Mosby publishers, 1997.
37. Ratner Adam. Road traffic accidents. Herald of Health, 2004.
38. Saibaba A. Rules and regulation of road traffic. Health Action, 2001.
39. Sundar Rao, Richard, J. An introduction to biostatistics, (3rd ed). New Delhi: Prentice Hall of India, 1999.
40. Vicky R. Bowden. Children and their families: The continuum of care (5th ed.). Philadelphia: W.B. Saunders publisher, 2007.
41. Zimmerman, F.J. Children's road traffic accident. Arch Pediatric Adolescent Med, 2005.
42. www.wikipidia.com
43. www.roadsafetyeducation.com
44. www.pediatricnursing.com
45. www.pubmed.com
46. www.questia.com
47. www.webhealthcenter.com
48. www.roadtrafficsymbols.com
49. www.healtheducation.com
50. www.googly.com
51. www.myoclinic.com

Index

Page numbers followed by *f* refer to figure and *t* refer to table, respectively.

C

D

F

I

J

K

M

Q

R

S

T

U

V

W

Y

Z